MANSON'S TROPICAL DISEASES

A classic of medical literature must, if it deals with clinical subjects, change radically over the years or risk a life spent on the library shelves disturbed only by a few scholars. 'Manson', however, perhaps because of the intellectual vigour of its past and present authors, has been no laggard in the rapidly shifting field of medicine, and it continues to be one of the most valuable textbooks on tropical medicine. In this new edition most of the text has been completely rewritten to eliminate dead wood and allow for new developments, and many new illustrations have been selected in all subjects. The contents have been rearranged to emphasize their aetiology, and special stress is laid throughout on biology, epidemiology and immunology. Carefully selected references, which will be invaluable to the research student seeking fuller information, are now included.

A growing threat of spread of the exotic diseases, brought about by the increasing mobility of populations, means that the physician's interest must extend to disorders of tropical as well as temperate climates. This standard text for the student of tropical medicine is now finding a wider readership among physicians in temperate climates whose patients have acquired a so-called 'tropical' infection.

Sir Patrick Manson
GCMG, FRS
(1844–1922)

Sir Patrick Manson,
pioneer of tropical
medicine, wrote six
editions of this book
between 1898 and
1921, distilling in to
it, in language of classical
lucidity, his immense
experience and wisdom.

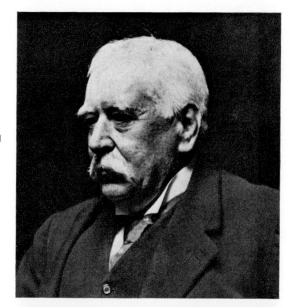

Sir Philip
Manson-Bahr
CMG, DSO
(1889–1966)

Sir Philip Manson-Bahr,
Manson's son-in-law,
prepared the next
ten editions with
sustained industry. By
constant revision, re-
writing and enlargement
he kept each one abreast
of the advances in
knowledge of its day.

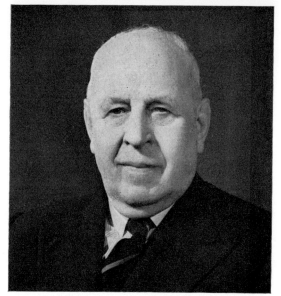

Charles Wilcocks
CMG, MD, FRCP, DTM & H

Past President and Past Honorary Secretary, Royal
Society of Tropical Medicine and Hygiene;
Formerly Medical Officer and Tuberculosis
Research Officer, Tanganyika; Formerly Director,
Bureau of Hygiene and Tropical Diseases, London

P. E. C. Manson-Bahr
MD, FRCP, DTM & H

Senior Lecturer in Clinical Tropical Medicine,
London School of Hygiene and Tropical Medicine;
Consultant Physician, The Hospital for Tropical
Diseases and Dreadnought Hospital, Greenwich,
London; Professor of Clinical Tropical Medicine,
School of Tropical Medicine and Public Health,
Tulane University, New Orleans, U.S.A.;
Formerly Senior Specialist, Colonial Medical
Service

Manson's
Tropical Diseases
Wilcocks & Manson-Bahr

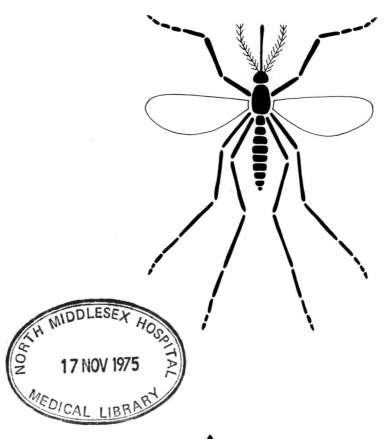

BAILLIÈRE TINDALL · LONDON

© 1972 Baillière Tindall
7 & 8 Henrietta Street, London WC2 8QE
A division of Crowell Collier and
Macmillan Publishers Ltd

First published 1898

Fifteenth edition 1960
Reprinted 1964
Sixteenth edition 1966
Reprinted 1969
Seventeenth edition 1972

ISBN 0 7020 0428 6

ELBS edition 1972 : ISBN 0 7020 0439 1

First Spanish edition (Salvat Editores, Barcelona) 1956

Published in the United States of America by
The Williams & Wilkins Company, Baltimore

Printed by The Whitefriars Press Ltd
London & Tonbridge

149

CONTENTS

COLOUR PLATES

PREFACE

In this 17th edition of *Manson's Tropical Diseases*
we have made more extensive alterations than
were possible in most earlier editions, and
consequently we have rewritten large sections
of the text, discarding or condensing much past
work, now out of date except for historical purposes,
and have added as much new material as we
felt to be consistent with our object—namely to
provide a textbook for students and a reference book
for practitioners working in the field, often isolated
from libraries.

We have rearranged the contents on the basis of
aetiology, retaining sections (again rewritten)
contributed by colleagues, and the Appendices,
which we feel have proved their value.

We have laid emphasis on diseases as they affect
both the indigenous and expatriate inhabitants of
warm climates, paying special attention to the
biology, epidemiology and immunology of tropical
infections, from both the practical and theoretical
points of view, since we regard these features as
essential for proper understanding.

We are indebted to many colleagues for help in
preparing this edition. Some who contributed whole
sections are named in those sections: Dr J. H.
Walters (Tropical Anaemias), Mr A. McKie Reid
(Ophthalmology), Dr P. H. Rees (Drugs), Dr H. A.
Reid (Clinical Notes on Snakebite), Dr D. M.
Minter (Tsetse Flies and Sandflies). Others have
read various parts of the book, criticizing the drafts
and making suggestions, which for the most part
we have accepted, and for which we are most
grateful. They include the following: Mr P. G.
Shute, Miss M. Maryon; Dr P. D. Marsden; Sir
John Boyd FRS; Dr C. A. Hoare FRS;
Professor G. S. Nelson, Dr G. Webbe, Dr D. M.
Forsyth; Dr C. E. Gordon Smith, Dr D. I. H.
Simpson; Dr W. H. Jopling, Dr D. S. Ridley, Dr
S. G. Browne; Dr L. H. Turner, Dr C. J. Hackett;
Mr M. G. R. Varma.

New illustrations have been introduced in various
sections, and we are particularly indebted to Dr
A. J. Duggan and Mr S. E. Land of the Wellcome

Museum of Medical Science for their help in this matter.

We are grateful to the Wellcome Trustees for permission to reproduce the photograph of Sir Patrick Manson which appears as the frontispiece.

As Sir Philip Manson-Bahr noted in previous editions, we have made much use of the invaluable *Tropical Diseases Bulletin* and *Abstracts on Hygiene* (formerly *Bulletin of Hygiene*), published by the Bureau of Hygiene and Tropical Diseases, and of the series of papers read at meetings of the Royal Society of Tropical Medicine and Hygiene, and published in the *Transactions* of that Society. We have also constantly referred to Faust and Russell (*Clinical Parasitology*) and Wilson and Miles (*Principles of Bacteriology and Immunity*), both standard works on their subjects, and to Martindale's *Extra Pharmacopoeia*.

We have received the greatest help from our publishers, Baillière Tindall, who have piloted the edition with care and precision.

Charles Wilcocks

May 1972   P. E. C. Manson-Bahr

SI UNITS

For this edition of *Manson's Tropical Diseases* units of measurement have been completely converted to the metric system instead of only in part, as previously. The Système International d'Unités (SI) has already been adopted by over thirty countries as their accepted system, and is recommended by the Royal Society of Medicine and the Biological Council. For full details the reader is advised to consult *Units, Symbols and Abbreviations: A Guide for Biological and Medical Editors and Authors*, published by the Royal Society of Medicine. However, for the reader's convenience some basic details are given below.

The following prefixes are used to indicate fractions or multiples of the basic units:

Fraction	Prefix	Symbol
10^{-1}	deci	d
10^{-2}	*centi	c
10^{-3}	*milli	m
10^{-6}	*micro	{†
10^{-9}	*nano	n (formerly mμ)
10^{-12}	*pico	p (formerly $\mu\mu$)
10^{-18}	atto	a

Multiple	Prefix	Symbol
10	deca	da
10^2	hecto	h
10^3	*kilo	k
10^6	mega	M
10^9	giga	G
10^{12}	tera	T

*Measurements in medicine are generally confined to these units.

†μ (micron) is no longer used.

Length

Unit = metre (m)
Conversion = 1 in = 2·54 cm
  1 ft = 0·30 m
  1 yd = 0·91 m

Weight

Unit = gramme (g)
Conversion = 1 oz = 28 g
            1 lb = 0·45 kg

Area

Unit = square metre (m²)
Conversion = 1 sq ft = 0·09 m²
            1 sq yd = 0·84 m²
            1 acre = 0·40 hectares

Volume

Unit = millilitre (ml) or cubic centimetre (cm³)
     (millilitre is preferred in most cases)
Conversion = 1 cu in = 16·38 cm³
            1 fl oz = 30 ml
            1 pt   = 0·6 litre

Temperature

Unit = degrees Celsius or Centigrade (°C)
Conversion = $°C = °F - 32 \times \frac{5}{9}$
             $°F = °C \times \frac{9}{5} + 32$

1. INTRODUCTION

PATRICK MANSON first published his *Tropical Diseases* in 1898, and all editions from 1921 onwards owe their existence to the devoted work of his son-in-law, Sir Philip Manson-Bahr, who died in 1966.

Since the first edition in 1898 there have been phenomenal advances in the knowledge and understanding of these conditions and of the complex biological processes involved. In that year the doctor did not know the causes of African sleeping sickness, Chagas's disease, leishmaniasis, bartonellosis, the rickettsial diseases, yellow fever and other arbovirus infections, the spirochaetal diseases (except relapsing fever), beriberi and pellagra. Manson did know, from his own epoch-making research on the transmission of filariasis, that mosquitoes are important intermediaries of some blood parasites, but he did not know how sleeping sickness, Chagas's disease, leishmaniasis, plague, schistosomiasis and other trematode infections, loiasis, onchocerciasis, yellow fever and the arbovirus infections or bartonellosis are spread, and even the transmission of hookworms was obscure. Pasteur had postulated viruses, but bacteriology and virology were still in their infancy.

In 1898 our forefathers had quinine, morphine, mercury, tartar emetic and a few other drugs, but the great age of chemotherapy as we understand it had not yet gone beyond the germination of ideas in the mind of Paul Ehrlich. For tuberculosis and most other bacterial diseases, and for the protozoal, rickettsial and systemic helminthic diseases, no effective drugs were known; we still lack drugs effective against the virus diseases.

Apart from smallpox vaccine and the newly discovered typhoid vaccines and diphtheria antitoxin, no immunization procedures were known in 1898. We owe the early attempts to prepare yellow fever vaccine to Edward Hindle, who is still happily with us, and the poliomyelitis and other vaccines are matters of recent history; the same is true of the toxoids.

In this edition we have not gone into the history of the great developments which have graced the present century, but in the lists of references which we have appended to the various chapters we acknowledge to some degree the careful pioneering work of our immediate predecessors and contemporaries. We have not, however, been able to do justice to the many workers who have undertaken research, often in the field and exposed to dangerous infections against which at the time they had little protection or hope of cure. They are part of a noble history, and their traditions are carried on by their younger colleagues, who still find satisfaction in the endless search for knowledge.

The diseases conventionally referred to as tropical include many which are by no means confined to the tropics. Until the era of residual insecticides, *P. vivax* malaria was endemic as far north as Holland and Moscow and in parts of the United States. Moreover, all forms of malaria are now being introduced into Britain and other temperate countries by travellers who increasingly visit endemic areas. These infections are not likely to spread in northern countries, where vectors are scarce or absent, but they provide difficult and urgent problems in diagnosis and treatment. A first attack of *P. falciparum* malaria in a European (whether child or adult) can be fatal within a few days if not diagnosed and treated, and there have been many unnecessary deaths from this cause within the last few years. In this book we stress the importance of keeping in mind the possibility of exotic diseases in patients who have travelled to endemic areas but may not report the fact, and we urge physicians to ask '*Where have you been, and when?*'

Malaria is not the only problem. African sleeping sickness has been brought to Britain, and in some cases has been misdiagnosed as encephalitis, with disastrous results. Amoebiasis has been brought in, and has progressed to liver abscess even in persons who have never been out of England; leishmaniasis is endemic in Mediterranean countries, and schistosomiasis has been acquired by holiday makers in North and East Africa, and no doubt elsewhere. Cholera has recently invaded the Near East, tropical Africa and the Mediterranean area; it reached western Europe many times in the nineteenth century, and may do so again. Typhoid, bacillary dysentery, leptospirosis, hepatitis and the worms are almost universal in countries where sanitation is poor, and travellers are at risk.

Yet though the diseases dealt with in this book are not confined to the tropics, they are most prevalent in hot countries, and there is general agreement that the category of 'tropical diseases' should be maintained, to be studied as a subject in itself; but it would be tragic if it were ignored in the training of students in temperate zones, and in the practice of doctors in those zones. The tropics are coming closer, and bringing their diseases with them.

But in this book we have paid more attention than before to diseases generally regarded as cosmopolitan, for instance tuberculosis which, though so greatly reduced in developed countries, still remains as a major killer in the tropics. Measles still devastates the children of Africa, and poliomyelitis, though becoming rare in the West, is still widely prevalent where sanitation is poor. The arbovirus diseases, though cosmopolitan, include some which are particularly rampant in hot countries, and as they are now more clearly understood than ever before, we have stressed them.

Research in tropical medicine and parasitology is moving forward strongly in many countries, and the need for it continues. In spite of the enormous advances brought by the new drugs and insecticides, there is now much evidence that the high hopes entertained some years ago have not been fulfilled, largely owing to the appearance of resistance to modern chemicals. This is now recognized. But perhaps equally serious is the growing threat to health posed by the development of industry and the consequent increase in industrial diseases, and the ailments associated with urban conditions in populations previously rural and agricultural. And in the field of agriculture the conservation of water for power, in huge dams, and the distribution of water in large permanent irrigation systems, is leading to serious extension of schistosomiasis (for which the control measures are as yet inadequate) and possibly other diseases.

This book, however, is primarily a manual for the practising physician facing the great problems of curative medicine; for the control of communicable diseases, apart from chemoprophylaxis and immunization, works on tropical public health should be consulted. We have, however, retained the Appendices, considerably rewritten, in which some control measures are mentioned in relation to the life histories of parasites and vectors.

RESIDENCE IN THE TROPICS

Tourists and expatriate workers in the tropics are living in a different environment from that to which they are normally adapted. Special protection, necessary for them if they are to remain healthy in this new environment, is considered below under the heading immunization. They should also take precautions against contracting malaria (see Chapter 4), as this is still prevalent throughout much of the tropics, and against bacterial intestinal infections (these are considered in the chapters on bacterial diseases). Acclimatization to heat is also of importance, and is considered in Chapter 36.

Immunization

All those going to the tropics or subtropics should be immunized against typhoid (TAB), tetanus, smallpox and poliomyelitis; those going to the Far East, Africa south of the Sahara, Egypt and Sudan, against cholera. Yellow fever vaccination is necessary for visits to Africa and South America. It is advisable to have BCG inoculation against tuberculosis and protection against hepatitis.

International inoculation certificates are essential for yellow fever, smallpox and cholera.

Smallpox vaccination. Unless vaccinated within the previous three years the intending traveller should be vaccinated or revaccinated against smallpox. Contra-indications are septic skin conditions, a history or presence of eczema, hypogammaglobulinaemia, leukaemia, corticosteroid or immunosuppressive therapy and pregnancy.

Pregnant women may be vaccinated under cover of antivaccinial immuno-globulin but not methisazone (Marboran), which is contra-indicated in pregnancy.

Yellow fever vaccination. Vaccination against yellow fever should be done first and at least 4 days before primary smallpox vaccination. If smallpox is done first there should be an interval of at least 21 days before yellow fever vaccination. Yellow fever vaccination should be postponed until the age of 9 months and most countries do not require a yellow fever vaccination certificate for a child aged less than 1 year.

Cholera vaccination. Vaccination against cholera is obligatory for travellers to West and East Africa, Egypt, the Sudan, the Near, Middle and Far East, Pakistan, India and Burma. These regulations may change if the present (1971) outbreaks subside.

Primary vaccination consists of two subcutaneous doses (0·5 and 1·0 ml) with an interval of 2–4 weeks in between. Only one dose is necessary to meet international requirements. Booster inoculations are given at 6-monthly intervals. Children aged 1–5 years should receive the full dose. Under 1 year of age immunization is not necessary but there is no reason why young infants should not receive the vaccine.

Validity of International Certificates of Vaccination
(Cannon 1969)

Vaccination	Valid for	Valid from
Smallpox		
Primary	3 years	8 days
Revaccination	3 years	at once
Yellow fever		
Primary	10 years	10 days
Revaccination	10 years	at once
Cholera		
Primary	6 months	6 days
Revaccination within 6 months	6 months	at once

Malaria. Prophylaxis against malaria is dealt with on page 75.

Enteric infection. All overseas travellers should be inoculated against typhoid. TAB vaccine should be given subcutaneously in 2 doses (o·5 and 1·0 ml) or intradermally (o·1 ml double strength vaccine) in 3 doses with an interval of 4–6 weeks in between. Adequate protection may be given by one dose of 1·0 ml subcutaneously or o·1 ml intradermally.

Tetanus. Primary immunization consists of three doses of tetanus toxoid with an interval of 6–12 weeks between the first and second and 6–12 months between the second and third. Tetanus toxoid is often given with TAB (TABT).

Poliomyelitis. Poliomyelitis is prevalent in many countries and travellers from non-tropical countries have little immunity against this disease. The basic course for oral immunization is 3 doses each of 3 drops with 6–8 weeks between the first and second and 6–12 months between the second and third. Those who have had previous immunization should have one dose of oral vaccine.

BCG vaccination. Young adults who are tuberculin-negative should have BCG vaccine before proceeding to the tropics. There should be an interval of 10 days between vaccination and prior or subsequent vaccination with any other live vaccine with the exception of oral polio vaccine. BCG may follow killed vaccines after a week but should not be followed by such vaccines for 10 days.

Plague and typhus vaccination are not usually required.

Hepatitis. In many countries hepatitis is prevalent and would-be residents in such areas are at some risk of developing this disease. A single intramuscular dose of human immunoglobulin (750 mg) can give protection for about 6 months (Pollock & Reid 1969).

Immunization Schedules for those going to the Tropics
(Cannon 1969)

Schedule 1

Week 1: Yellow fever vaccine
4: Smallpox vaccine
(5: Read result of smallpox vaccination)
7: TABT (1)
10: Polio vaccine (oral) (1)
13: TABT (2)
16: Polio vaccine (oral) (2)
22: Polio vaccine (oral) (3)
39: TABT (3)

Cholera vaccine in special circumstances only.

Schedule 2 (for travellers who have had little warning)

Day 1: Yellow fever and cholera (1)
Polio vaccine (oral) (1)
5: Smallpox vaccine and TABT (1)
11: Cholera (2)
(13: Read result of smallpox vaccination)
28: TABT (2)
polio vaccine (oral) (2)

TABT (3) and polio vaccine (oral) (3) will be required 6–12 months later.

Schedule 1 is preferable to schedule 2

Reinforcing injections: Yellow fever vaccine every 6 years. Smallpox vaccine every 3 years. TAB vaccine every year if at special risk, otherwise every 3 years. Tetanus toxoid every 5 years.

PATHOLOGICAL EFFECTS OF TROPICAL CLIMATE

Tropical heat produces in fair-skinned people a characteristic pallor, sometimes with a yellowish discoloration of the skin, which is to be distinguished from tropical anaemia. This appearance is due to blanching of the skin, from thickening of the surface layer and increased pigmentation.

The tropical light produces effects in the skin, which may be acute or chronic. They range from a slight sunburn to a severe erythema, accompanied by blisters and oedema, so that a reaction may set in produced by septic absorption. Sometimes this may be so severe as to produce delirium or even coma. Chronic skin irritation is shown by pigmentation and by vasomotor changes; that this is a process of natural selection is demonstrated by the skin pigmentation of most races, so that the nearer the equator, the darker the skin, while that of a European long resident in the tropics tends to darken. Chronic solar dermatitis, or sailor's skin, especially at the back of the neck or hands, is characterized by atrophy, wrinkling and pigmentation. White atrophic patches, telangiectases and warty growths (solar keratoses) develop, some of which, especially when situated on the dorsum of the hands, eventually become the seat of basal (rodent ulcer type) or squamous-cell neoplasms.

Urticaria is occasionally produced by the actinic rays. *Cheilitis actinica* is a condition of the lips caused by burning by ultra-violet light at high altitudes. Secondary carcinoma may result. For the effects of sunlight on the eyes see Chapter 44. Oedema of feet and legs in young adults is frequently noted on first entering a tropical climate. It is of peripheral vascular origin and is probably an indication of the adjustment of that system to new conditions. This oedema passes off on acclimatization.

INTESTINAL INFECTIONS

Intestinal infections causing diarrhoea are very common in the tropics and it is unusual for any period of tropical residence to be completed without some upset in bowel functions. Careful attention should be paid to the source of water for drinking and even for washing teeth. Water should be boiled, and sterilization tablets at hand for emergencies. Ice-cream and milk products should be avoided unless the source is impeccable. Salad and snacks at restaurants should be avoided in most tropical cities. Food hygiene must be strict.

INSECT BITES AND STINGS

Mosquitoes mostly bite at sundown and during the night; they may bite through a mosquito net if parts of the body of the sleeper press against the net. Women seem to be specially susceptible, and may react with extensive swellings or even blisters; severe itching is usual, and scratching may break the skin. Constant exposure, however, may eventually lead to a state of immunity.

Stings from bees, wasps and hornets may be very severe, especially if multiple, and swelling may be extensive; serious anaphylactic reactions may occur.

Treatment

Irritation and itching from mosquito bites can be relieved by applying Scrubb's ammonia, tincture of iodine or 1% menthol in 95% alcohol. An antihistamine preparation known as Thephorin (Roche), which is an ointment containing 5% of phenindamine tartrate, has been found to give almost immediate relief to patients stung or bitten by bees and other insects; it should be rubbed into the site of the sting or bite, but it can produce sensitization.

REFERENCES

CANNON, D. A. (1969) *Trans. R. Soc. trop. Med. Hyg.*, **63**, 867.
POLLOCK, T. M. & REID, D. (1969) *Lancet*, **i**, 281.

2. GENERAL DISEASES OCCURRING IN THE TROPICS

THE practice of medicine in the tropics is not only concerned with the classical tropical diseases which are a product of the tropical environment, but also with some general diseases which are or were common in temperate climates. Some of these diseases, modified by the tropical environment, and others which have become less common in temperate areas, present a considerable problem in the tropics.

PYREXIA IN THE TROPICS

Prolonged pyrexia without localizing signs presents a diagnostic problem since, in addition to the conditions found in temperate areas, there are a number of parasitic infections which are found only in the tropics. The majority of cases of prolonged pyrexia, however, are usually caused by non-tropical conditions. An essential procedure in diagnosis is a differential white cell count which will distinguish three main groups: one with a polymorphonuclear leucocytosis, another with an eosinophilia and a third with a normal white cell count or leucopenia.

Polymorphonuclear leucocytosis

This group is caused by bacterial infection or pus somewhere in the body. Pus may be localized under the diaphragm (subdiaphragmatic abscess), in the liver (liver abscess), in the lung, kidneys, pelvis or deep muscles of the abdomen. Bacterial infections which commonly cause prolonged fever and rigors are cholecystitis, cholangitis and *Escherichia coli* infections of the urinary tract.

Eosinophilic leucocytosis

Fever and eosinophilia occur in the tissue stages of many helminth infections, which are described in the appropriate sections.

Normal white cell count or leucopenia

This is the largest and most difficult group to diagnose. Non-tropical conditions are the most frequent cause, especially pulmonary and abdominal tuberculosis in the younger age-groups. Relapsing typhoid in the presence of insufficient chemotherapy, and *P. vivax* malaria, appearing many months after cessation of chemotherapy, may lead to difficulty.

The main tropical causes, such as kala-azar, brucellosis, etc., are considered in the appropriate sections. It should not be forgotten that reticulosis, hidden carcinoma, aleukaemic leukaemia and collagen disorders are not uncommon in the tropics and may be difficult to diagnose.

Diagnosis. Many other diagnostic procedures may be necessary to establish the diagnosis. Blood culture, cerebrospinal fluid examination, radiograph of the chest, sternal puncture and liver biopsy are all of great value.

FAMILIAL MEDITERRANEAN FEVER

Familial Mediterranean fever (FMF) is a genetic disorder restricted to certain ethnic groups and marked by the sporadic appearance of acute attacks of fever and the insidious development of amyloidosis (Sohar *et al.* 1967). The disease is determined by a single autosomal recessive gene which is present in Sephardic (Eastern) Jews, Iraqi Jews and Armenians, though examples have been reported in Persians, Arabs and other races. In populations at risk the gene may show a frequency of 1 : 26 and the incidence of homozygous sufferers is 1 in 2720 (Sohar *et al.* 1961). There are two types of the disease: in Phenotype I the attacks of fever appear first and in Phenotype II amyloidosis is the first manifestation.

In the first type acute attacks of fever appear during the second decade of life, each febrile period lasting 24–72 hours. The bouts recur with great regularity every 2–4 weeks. Each bout may be accompanied by abdominal pain with evidence of peritoneal irritation with ileus, pleuritic or synovial pain with effusions or an erysipelas-like rash. The rash may resemble erythema nodosum. In the second type amyloidosis is the major manifestation; the liver and spleen enlarge and there is albuminuria. The disease progresses inexorably to a nephrotic syndrome with a raised α_2 or β globulin, while the fibroginogen level of the blood is much increased. The second type may succeed the first (Blum *et al.* 1962).

The diagnosis is made from the racial and family history but cannot be confirmed in the absence of amyloid, which may be found in a rectal or renal biopsy of the patient or a sibling. Treatment is useless. No prognosis can be given when febrile attacks are the only manifestation, and life may continue for years. Some diminution of attacks has been obtained with a low-fat (20 grammes) diet. Once renal amyloidosis has developed, death is inevitable within ten years.

ALIMENTARY SYSTEM

Bilateral painless parotid glandular enlargement is not uncommon in many areas of the tropics and is associated with a low-protein, high-carbohydrate diet.

Gastric ulcer is rare in most parts of the tropics; duodenal ulcer is common in south India and in parts of Africa. Appendicitis occurs in most areas of the tropics but is commoner in urban than rural districts. It is found in Ibadan (Badoe 1967) but is uncommon in East Africa (Trowell 1960). Schistosome eggs are sometimes found in appendixes removed at operation but a causal relationship has not been established. Ulcerative colitis is generally uncommon (Trowell 1960), other than in India (Chuttani *et al.* 1967). Volvulus of the sigmoid colon accounts for a high proportion of cases of acute intestinal obstruction in many parts of Africa. The presence of a long loop of sigmoid colon with a narrow mesenteric base and distension from a high-residue diet have been suggested as causes. In Brazil volvulus of the sigmoid is associated with megacolon caused by Chagas's disease.

DIABETES MELLITUS

The incidence of diabetes mellitus in the tropics is generally considered to be low (Tulloch 1962), but there is some evidence that it is increasing, especially in the South African Bantu. A high prevalence has been recorded in Indians in Natal and East Africa. There is a lowered incidence of vascular complications, myocardial infarction, retinopathy and vascular disease excluding gangrene but a high incidence of neuropathy (Greenwood & Taylor 1968). In India a high incidence of renal changes in diabetes has been recorded.

LIVER DISEASE

Liver disease is considered to be commoner in tropical than temperate climates. The most usual type of cirrhosis seen is postnecrotic cirrhosis. Presinusoidal pipe-stem cirrhosis occurs with *Schistosoma japonicum* and *S. mansoni* infections and is considered in those sections. Biliary cirrhosis occurs with *Clonorchis sinensis* infection. Veno-occlusive disease, Indian infantile cirrhosis and African siderosis are peculiar to the tropics.

Postnecrotic cirrhosis

It is not clear whether postnecrotic cirrhosis is commoner in tropical than in temperate areas. Post-mortem figures from South Africa have not shown great differences in incidence in the Bantu, coloured and white population; however, a large proportion of cirrhotic livers in the Bantu show malignant changes.

Cirrhosis of the liver occurs in younger age-groups in the tropics and is not uncommon under the age of 20 years (Gelfand 1961).

Aetiology. Many factors are associated with the cause of tropical cirrhosis and include alcohol, malnutrition, virus and parasitic diseases and dietary toxic factors.

Alcoholism is not the same problem as in temperate areas. Crudely distilled liquors are common in urban areas but no direct causation has been shown. Malnutrition has often been considered as a cause, since dietary deficiencies have produced fatty changes in the livers of experimental animals, which has led to the belief that there is a causal relationship between protein–calorie malnutrition in childhood and cirrhosis of the liver. Follow-up studies in children suffering from kwashiorkor have not shown subsequent development of cirrhosis (Bras *et al.* 1961) and there is little justification now for this theory. Infectious hepatitis is common in the tropics but cirrhosis of the liver has rarely been found as a sequel, and there is a low incidence of cirrhosis in some regions where virus hepatitis is common, notably South America. It has been thought that viral hepatitis is more severe in malnourished people and certain patients have been shown to develop cirrhosis after hepatitis (Sherlock 1963). It is possible that different strains of virus may be responsible.

Parasitic infections include schistosomiasis, liver flukes and malaria. Schistosomiasis is associated with presinusoidal or pipe-stem cirrhosis and liver fluke with biliary cirrhosis. In areas of stable malaria stellate fibrosis of the portal tracts has been associated with the presence of malarial pigment in children gaining their immunity. However, cirrhosis is common in the South African Bantu where there is no malaria. Plant alkaloids and herbal medicines are widely used in the tropics but little is known of their effects on the liver.

Veno-occlusive disease of the liver

Veno-occlusive disease is an acute, subacute or chronic condition affecting primarily the central and sublobular hepatic veins. It has been reported mainly from the West Indies but also from North and South Africa and India.

Aetiology. It is now generally accepted that the consumption of 'bush tea' containing the alkaloids of *Crotalaria fulva* which produces a similar condition in rats is the cause in the West Indies (Hill *et al.* 1958). Alkaloids of this group of plants, *Crotalaria, Senecio* and *Heliotropium*, have produced liver injury in all animals in which they have been tested, and *Senecio* poisoning occurs naturally in animals in many parts of the world. In South Africa *C. dura* is responsible for hepatic and pulmonary lesions in horses.

Pathology. The primary pathological change involves the central and sub-lobular hepatic veins. There is subendothelial oedema followed by intimal overgrowth of connective tissue and narrowing and occlusion of the lumina. Centrizonal congestion, atrophy or necrosis of liver cells with consequent fibrosis leads to gross changes similar to those described in cardiac cirrhosis (Edington & Gilles 1969). In the West Indies cirrhosis due to veno-occlusive disease accounts for about one-third of all types of cirrhosis (Bras *et al.* 1961) The symptoms and signs are due to portal hypertension with its associated complications.

Clinical features. The condition presents as acute hepatomegaly and ascites in children. About half of those affected recover and 20% die in the acute stage. The remainder pass into a subacute and chronic stage with the develop-ment of portal hypertension (Stuart & Bras 1957).

Indian infantile cirrhosis

Infantile cirrhosis of the liver is restricted to India, where it has been reported in southern India, Calcutta and the Punjab. The disease is prevalent in Hindu children and the children of the well-to-do are attacked more freqently than those of the poor.

Aetiology. The cause is unknown. The disease tends to run in families and children of the same families succumb within a year or two of birth. It is diffi-cult to exclude dietary, toxic or deficiency factors and an undiscovered infectious agent cannot be ruled out.

Pathology. The clinicopathological findings in the acute stage are those of infectious hepatitis and in the subacute and chronic stages cirrhosis and portal hypertension. Liver biopsies have shown a severe progressive affection of the parenchymal cells which show ballooning and variation in size with enlarged pale nuclei containing nucleoli (Khanolkar 1955). Hyaline is sometimes present and in the later stages giant cell transformation and bile stasis occur. The cen-tral veins are not occluded and reticular collapse occurs in areas, and there is a proliferation of fibrous tissue in portal tracts which are infiltrated by lympho-cytes, histiocytes and occasional polymorphonuclears. The fibrosis extends periportally (Singh *et al.* 1961). There is bile duct proliferation and progressive fibrosis which eventually produces cirrhosis.

Clinical features. Clinically the condition may be fulminant, acute or subacute. It attacks children most commonly between the ages of 6 and 24 months and rarely attacks those over 3 years of age. Usually it begins during dentition or about the seventh or eighth month, running a fatal course in 3–8 months. In some cases the progress may be much more rapid and terminate in death in 2–3 weeks.

Commencing insidiously the enlargement of the liver proceeds before the disease is suspected and reaches the iliac crest in the course of 1 or 2 months. In some cases the spleen is enlarged. Nausea, anorexia and fever of a low type set in. Profound jaundice develops with bilirubinuria and clay-coloured stools. The veins become prominent on the abdominal wall and terminal ascites develops. In 5 months from the onset there is ascites, oedema of hands, feet and eyelids, and terminal gastrointestinal haemorrhage occurs. Death ensues from cholaemia. There is a terminal real lymphocytosis with counts of from 14 000 to 50 000 per mm³. Biochemically the changes of severe hepatocellular disease are present. There is a lowered serum albumin and retention of bromsulphtha-lein. The alkaline phosphatase is normal.

Treatment. There is no specific treatment. Whenever possible in a family in which several cases of this disease have occurred the latest baby should be removed from the mother and fed upon artificial baby foods.

African siderosis

Heavy iron deposits are frequently found in the tissues of South African Bantu and Ghanaians (Edington 1954). Iron deposits are not found in Africans in East Africa, Western Nigeria, Gambia or Senegal. The cause is thought to be absorption of excessive amounts of iron in the diet possibly through the use of iron cooking-pots or the fermentation of liquors in metal containers (Edington & Gilles 1969). All types of iron deposition may be found in the liver, which may closely resemble haemochromatosis. Heavy deposits of iron are also found in the duodenum, jejunum, spleen, bone marrow and upper abdominal lymph glands (Edington 1959). Where siderosis occurs, iron deficiency is relatively rare. The serum iron and iron binding capacity of the blood vary from low to normal but are occasionally high.

PANCREATIC CALCIFICATION

Fibrosis and calcification of the pancreas have been described as a common cause of diabetes mellitus in many areas of the tropics in patients under 30 years of age. It can also present as malabsorption in young children with steatorrhoea (Zuidema 1959). There is no evidence that the incidence of pancreatic calcification increases with age and neither alcoholic pancreatitis nor protein-calorie malnutrition adequately explains the incidence in some tropical countries (Shaper 1964). All patients with diabetes or steatorrhoea in the tropics should have a straight radiograph of the abdomen to exclude the possibility of pancreatic calcification.

DISEASES OF THE GALL BLADDER

Cholecystitis is rare in most tropical peoples. In Africans gall stones are usually pigment stones and are intrahepatic. They may be associated with sickle-cell disease, and cholecystitis is apt to coincide with sickling crises.

TROPICAL SPLENOMEGALY

Tropical splenomegaly is described in the section on malaria.

SPLENIC ABSCESS

Primary abscess of the spleen has been described from Rhodesia. Wallace (1922) concluded that the abscess is caused by thrombosis of the splenic vein leading to an active necrosis. A painful tumour over the spleen associated with fever and pain in the left hypochondrium in young adults is suggestive. Diagnostic aspiration reveals pus which is usually sterile and must be distinguished from that of amoebic and spirochaetal abscess. Sometimes the abscess is infected with Staphylococci.

CARDIOVASCULAR DISEASE IN THE TROPICS

With the exception of coronary artery disease and myocardial infarction the well known cardiovascular diseases occurring in temperate climates occur just as frequently in the tropics. There are two conditions which are rare in temperate climates which are quite common in some tropical areas: idiopathic cardiomegaly and endomyocardial fibrosis (EMF).

Idiopathic cardiomegaly

Idiopathic cardiomegaly is a chronic disease of unknown cause which is not atherosclerotic in origin (Goodwin 1964). It is common in West Africa and the South African Bantu. It is also found in East Africa and Rhodesia and probably occurs in most tropical areas. Viral infection, alcoholism, malnutrition, an immune mechanism and dietary deficiencies have all been considered causes, but there is no evidence for any of these.

Cases present as congestive heart failure of unknown aetiology, with generalized heart enlargement and, frequently, embolic phenomena. Electrocardiographic changes are variable and there may be ectopic ventricular beats, left bundle-branch block and left axis deviation. The main pathological changes are found in the myocardium where there are diffuse changes in the muscle cells (Schlesinger & Reiner 1955). A symptomless pericardial effusion may be found at autopsy.

Endomyocardial fibrosis (EMF)

Endomyocardial fibrosis was first described in Uganda in 1948 (Davies 1948). It has been found in Nigeria, Ghana, Kenya and Tanzania, is one of the common causes of heart failure in Uganda and also occurs in India (Williams et al. 1954). The cause is unknown but modern opinion now favours an infective immunological basis. Loa loa infection has been suggested (Ive et al. 1967), as have a plantain diet resulting in a high 5-hydroxytryptophan intake (McKinney & Crawford 1965), an unusual manifestation of the rheumatic process (Abrahams 1959) and an autoimmune process with a high frequency of circulating heart antibodies (Shaper et al. 1967).

EMF is a chronic progressive heart disease in which there is fibrosis of the inflow tract and apex of one or both ventricles, with fibrous thickening of the endothelium of the inflow tracts, the fibrous tissue extending into the myocardium. There is a considerable distortion of one or both atrioventricular valves and intracardiac thrombosis is usual in both ventricles and the atria (Fig. 1).

Clinically EMF may present in a variety of forms: the left or right heart or both may be involved. Chronic right-side heart failure with gross ascites and an enlarged liver with tricuspid incompetence and a very high venous pressure may resemble constrictive pericarditis very closely and need haemodynamic studies to make the differential diagnosis. A large pericardial effusion may be found. Left-side EMF may give rise to marked pulmonary hypertension.

Atherosclerosis and coronary artery disease

Atherosclerosis is less severe and coronary artery disease is less common in parts of the tropics. The latter has a low incidence in many parts of Africa (Walker 1963) and myocardial infarction is almost unknown in African peoples. There is also a low incidence in Japan, Thailand and China. In India the situation is variable with a high incidence in the Punjab and Madras and a low incidence in Agra. Atherosclerosis is less frequent in the Bantu than in the white population in South Africa (Anderson et al. 1959). Somalis and Masai, whose diet consists almost entirely of protein and milk, also show a low incidence. Since essential hypertension is not rare in these people the only common factor is the serum cholesterol, which is on the average low. It has been suggested that

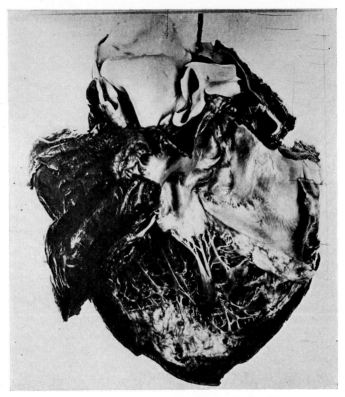

Fig. 1.—Endomyocardial fibrosis. (*Dr P. W. Hutton*)

the increased fibrinolytic activity of the African blood may be responsible (Merskey *et al.* 1960).

Rheumatic heart disease

Rheumatic heart disease is well known and an important cause of heart disease in many tropical areas. In India it is the main cardiac problem. However, acute rheumatic arthritis and chorea are relatively uncommon, although severe rheumatic endocarditis is common, and develops at an early age, with the result that well marked mitral stenosis is found in quite young children.

Anaemic heart disease

Severe iron deficiency anaemia associated with hookworm disease is common in many tropical areas, and severe anaemia is a cause of dilatation of the heart and high output failure. Removal of hookworms and iron medication procure a return to normal.

African electrocardiogram. The electrocardiogram in African people is of the 'juvenile' type and the T-waves are inverted in the right ventricular leads. This does not mean that any abnormality is present, and is a normal finding.

Tropical phlebitis

Tropical phlebitis was originally described by Fisher (1941) in Rhodesia. It occurs in healthy young males in small outbreaks which may, however, assume epidemic proportions (Manson-Bahr & Charters 1946). The long superficial veins of the lower and upper limbs are involved and the neck and intra-abdominal veins are sometimes affected. Embolism is rare. The condition may be relapsing but recovery occurs with permanent venous occlusion. There is some association between this affection and symmetrical gangrene of the feet (Gelfand 1947). No cause has been found but a virus aetiology has been considered because in the past this phlebitis has been a complication of intravenous therapy for syphilis.

MALIGNANT DISEASE IN THE TROPICS

Malignant disease is not uncommon in the tropics but in most areas the incidence of cancer is less than half that recorded in temperate areas and the pattern varies in the different regions with marked variations in neighbouring territories and in different races (Doll et al. 1966). Crude rate incidence of cancer or mortality figures cannot be used to compare the incidence of cancer in tropical and temperate zones since there is a high child mortality rate and there are few elderly people in tropical areas.

There is a relative absence of common tumours affecting the elderly in temperate zones, namely growths of the lung and large bowel. Common tumours seen in the tropics are primary liver cancer (hepatoma), bile duct carcinoma, oral, nasopharyngeal and oesophageal cancer, Burkitt's tumour, cancer of the penis, cancer of the skin and Kaposi's sarcoma (Edington & Gilles 1969).

Primary carcinoma of the liver

The highest incidence rate of liver cancer has been reported from Lourenço Marques (Prates & Torres 1965). High rates are also found in the South African Bantu, the Yoruba in Western Nigeria, in Uganda and in the Chinese living in Singapore. The relationship to cirrhosis of the liver is not clear but 50 to 80% of cirrhotic livers may become malignant, the cirrhosis usually being postnecrotic. However, cancer of the liver frequently occurs in the absence of cirrhosis. The tumour is a hepatoma and the greatest incidence is in the 20–30 age-group. The geographical distribution of hepatoma is not explained by malnutrition, infective hepatitis or parasitic infection. It has been suggested that an aflatoxin (Lancaster et al. 1961) produced by the fungus Aspergillus flavus, a contaminant of groundnuts, which causes hepatic disease in turkeys, may be responsible, acting as a carcinogen in concert with malnutrition (Linsell 1967).

Bile duct carcinoma is common in certain areas where liver flukes, especially Clonorchis sinensis, are common.

Carcinoma of the oropharynx

In most parts of India and Ceylon the incidence of cancer of the mouth and pharynx exceeds that of cancer of any other part of the body (Clifford 1970). The chewing of betel nut and tobacco is considered to be the causal factor. Histologically the tumours are squamous epitheliomas and occur on the lower lip (Khaini cancer), the mucosal lining of the cheek (betel cancer), palate (Chutta cancer) and base of tongue and tonsil.

Carcinoma of the nasopharynx

The incidence of carcinoma of the nasopharynx is high in Chinese and immigrant Chinese in Malaya, Singapore, Indonesia, Australia and America and this is the most common cancer found in Taiwan (Yeh 1966). Small foci of high incidence are seen in Kenya (Clifford 1965). The cause is unknown; snuff and smoke from woodfires have been considered. It has been noted that patients with nasopharyngeal carcinoma have a high oestrogen/androgen ratio which might alter the columnar ciliated epithelium of the nose to squamous epithelium and act in concert with carcinogens to induce malignant change (Clifford & Bulbrook 1966).

Carcinoma of the oesophagus

The incidence of cancer of the oesophagus varies widely in different areas of the tropics. It is common in China, in the Chinese in Singapore and also in the Transkei in South Africa. High frequencies have also been noted in many areas in South, Central and East Africa. The cause is not clear but deficiencies in the soil, smoking, alcohol, contamination of alcohol and the ingestion of hot foods have all been considered.

Burkitt's lymphoma

An unusual tumour was first noted by Sir Albert Cook in Uganda years ago, and Burkitt's tumour was described in 1958 (Burkitt 1958) in African children in Uganda. It occurs in a geographical belt across Africa from east to west, within which the mean average temperature does not fall below 15·6°C and the average annual rainfall is not less than 50 cm (Fig. 2). The majority of cases have occurred in Africa and New Guinea within this climatic zone, but some cases have been reported from the United States, England, Colombia, Puerto Rica, Canada, India and Vietnam.

Aetiology. The exact cause is not known. Owing to the special geographical distribution of the tumour it has been suggested that a mosquito is responsible (Burkitt 1962) and that *Anopheles* spp. are the most likely (McCrae 1968), acting as vectors of an arthropod-borne virus. Other observers consider that the disease is an atypical presentation of acute lymphocytic leukaemia.

A virus, the Epstein-Barr virus (EBV) which causes infectious mononucleosis or glandular fever, has been isolated from a number of tissue culture lines of Burkitt's lymphoma, and it is possible that malignant transformation following infection with the Epstein-Barr virus may take place against a background of chronic lymphoreticular stimulation as the result of holoendemic malaria

Epidemiology. Children of both sexes are affected and males more than females. The peak incidence is found in the 4–8-year-old group and the disease is uncommon under the age of 2 or over 16 years.

Pathology. The tumour consists of sheets of blast cells scattered among which are large histiocytes (Burkitt cells) with an eccentric nucleus and large amount of pale-staining cytoplasm containing pyknotic nuclear remnants (Edington & Gilles 1969) which give rise to a 'starry sky' appearance.

Clinical features. The commonest presentation is a tumour involving one or both jaw quadrants with gross disruption of the alveolar margins. Pain is absent until the disease is far advanced. An abdominal tumour is the second most common presentation and may originate in the retroperitoneal tissues. The tumour commonly involves ovaries, skeletal bones, thyroid, testes, suprarenals, heart and pericardium, liver and salivary glands. The central nervous system is involved in about 50% of cases and extension to the meninges causes 'Burkitt meningoencephalitis'. Paraplegia also occurs. Diffuse bone marrow involvement by tumour cells may occur and the cells may be seen in the peripheral blood.

Treatment. The tumour responds well, often dramatically, to chemotherapy. Methotrexate 5–10 mg orally or by daily intravenous drip for 5 days; nitrogen

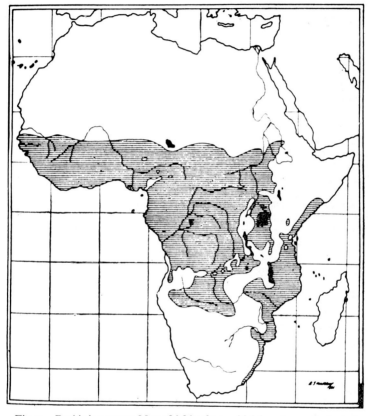

Fig. 2.—Burkitt's tumour. Map of Africa from which have been eliminated areas over 1500 m, areas where the mean temperature may fall below 15.6°C and areas where the annual rainfall is less than 50 cm. (*Burkitt 1962*)

mustard 1·0 mg/kg or Cytoxan (cyclophosphamide) 40 mg/kg intravenously as a single dose. Central nervous involvement is treated by intrathecal injection. The response to chemotherapy seems to depend upon the host immune response and a combination of specific and non-specific immunotherapy is now used in conjunction with chemotherapy (Klein *et al.* 1966). Over 70% of children with disease in one area of the body can have it eliminated for 1–3 years without maintenance therapy and some cases apparently cured for more than 3 years have been recorded.

Carcinoma of the penis

Cancer of the penis is common in many Asian countries, parts of India, South America and Africa. The incidence is high in those areas where circumcision is not practised.

Malignant disease of the skin

In Australia, New Zealand and South Africa the incidence of squamous and basal cell carcinoma is higher in white than in pigmented people. It occurs on those areas of the body which are exposed to sunlight. Kangri cancer is a squamous cell carcinoma which occurs on the abdomen and thighs in Kashmir and is associated with the habit of carrying an earthen pot containing charcoal to keep the carrier warm.

Dhoti cancer occurs in Bombay, India, and is caused by the irritation of a loin-cloth in the presence of dust, sweat and poor hygiene.

Kaposi's sarcoma

Kaposi's sarcoma is rare in most parts of the world but occurs with surprising frequency in Africa south of the Sahara with a maximum incidence along the Equator.

Kaposi's sarcoma usually presents as a circumscribed macular then nodular lesion of the skin and subcutaneous tissues of the lower limbs. It is frequently symmetrical and ulcerating and is associated with lymphoedema. The lesions may be widespread and involve mucous membranes and viscera and there is a tendency to involve the lymph glands in African children (Lothe 1963). Two types of sarcoma may be recognized: the usual type with relatively narrow spindle cells and a less differentiated type with plumper rounder cells with more mitotic figures (Lothe 1963).

Some therapeutic success has been obtained with intra-arterial nitrogen mustard.

DISEASES OF THE KIDNEY AND RENAL TRACT

Renal calculus

Vesical and renal calculi are among the most common conditions encountered in the tropics. Little is known of their causation but the explanation is thought to lie in the high concentration of urine, or an unbalanced diet with lack of vitamin A. Urinary calculi are especially common in South China.

Schistosomiasis

The effect of *Schistosoma haematobium* infection on the renal tract is considered in the section on schistosomiasis.

Nephrotic syndrome

The nephrotic syndrome is frequently seen and the connection with quartan malaria is considered in the section on malaria. Other causes encountered in the tropics are amyloidosis caused by kala-azar and a chronic infection with *Salmonella typhi*.

Escherichia coli infections

Infection of the bladder and urinary tract with *E. coli* is frequently met in both sexes in the tropics. Should the organism enter the blood stream it may give rise to a prolonged intermittent pyrexia. *E. coli* septicaemia and pyaemia may be terminal infections in debilitated persons, and are sequels of bacillary dysentery when the organisms gain entrance to the blood stream from the intestinal lesions and become arrested in the glomeruli from which they escape intermittently and appear in the urine. The attacks may be confused with malaria, and vesical and urinary symptoms are absent.

Porphyria

Two types are recognized in South Africa: (*a*) the genetically determined type confined to the white population and (*b*) a condition possibly peculiar to the Bantu (porphyria cutanea tarda). Genetically determined porphyria is due to a Mendelian dominant gene (but not sex-linked) and is common in South Africa where it is estimated there are some 8000 affected persons. The history can be traced back to a couple who married at the Cape in 1688. In men the manifestations are mainly cutaneous but in women there are usually abdominal pain and crises. Normally these people remain well but certain drugs of the barbitone group may be disastrous and in South Africa it is routine to test for porphyria before anaesthesia. In women it expresses itself from 15 to 20 years of age. Between the acute attacks the urinary and faecal excretion of porphyrins is increased. In the acute stage the urine may be reddish brown, darkening on standing, and porphyrins may be detected spectroscopically.

In the Bantu porphyria cutanea tarda is more benign and of the delayed or cutaneous type. It is recognized by blistering of the parts exposed to the sun and by a darkening of the face and hands, together with nail dystrophy. The urine is of a Burgundy red, pink, or sherry colour containing porphyrins and an abnormal amount of urobilin. There is usually hypertrichosis limited to the pre-auricular and temporal regions. More males are affected than females and in half the liver is enlarged and tests show some impairment of liver function. In some way it is connected with the drinking of illicit liquor (*skokiaan*). An epidemic of this nature has been described in Turkey where wheat which had been treated with the fungicide hexachlorbenzene was used for bread-making. The epidemic affected 5000 children who developed pigmentation of the skin, hairiness of the face and enlargement of the liver. The children were undernourished and resembled cases of porphyria cutanea tarda of the Bantu type.

AINHUM

Ainhum is a slowly progressive fibrous constriction involving usually the digital plantar fold of the fifth toe.

Aetiology

The cause is unknown but Browne (1965) considers that overproduction of fibrous tissue in response to repeated infection or injury in persons with a tendency to keloid formation is a major factor. No relationship to leprosy, scleroderma or syphilis has been noted, though a connection with yaws has been suspected.

Geographical distribution

The condition has its highest incidence in Africa, but it also occurs in those of Negro descent in South and Central America and the West Indies. A few cases have been described from India.

Pathology

The panniculus adiposus of the affected toe is much hypertrophied. The bone is infiltrated with fatty matter and the other tissues are correspondingly degenerated. Sometimes the bone is thin or altogether absorbed. At the seat of constriction a line of hypertrophy of the epithelial layers and of atrophy of the papillary layers of the skin, together with a band of fibrous tissue more or less intimately connected with the dermis, surrounds whole or in part the pedicle.

Clinical features

The disease which is most common in adult males is rare in women and children under 16. Kean and Tucker (1946), who described 45 cases from Panama, found an incidence of 1·5 per 1000 in West Indian Negro males. The disease commences as a narrow groove in the skin almost invariably on the inner and plantar side of the root of the little toe or little finger, and is usually associated

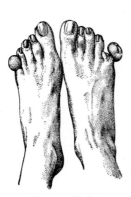

Fig. 3.—Ainhum.

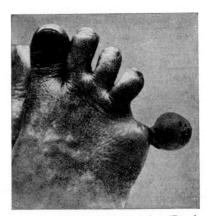

Fig. 4.—Ainhum at its height. (Dr A. B. Filho)

with plantar keratosis. It may occur in one foot only or be bilateral affecting both feet simultaneously or one foot after the other. The groove once started deepens and extends gradually round the whole circumference of the toe. As it deepens sometimes with ulceration the distal portion of the toe swells to a considerable extent as if constricted by a ligature (Figs 3, 4). The condition may be painless though Kean and Tucker (1946) found that pain may be pronounced and progressive. In the course of years the groove slowly deepens and finally the toe drops off or is amputated. The disease runs its course in from 1 to 10 years or even longer. In rare instances after the two distal phalanges have dropped off or been amputated the disease recurs in the stump and the proximal phalanx in its turn is thrown off. Radiology shows some osteoporosis and absorption of the outer layer of the cortex of the phalanx producing a tapering effect. Occasionally the terminal phalanx of the fifth digit of the hand has been affected. In a case represented in the Army Medical Museum in Washington D.C. all the toes had been thrown off and the disease was making progress in the leg.

Treatment. It has been suggested that division of the constricting fibrous band would delay the evolution of the disease. In the early stages this might be tried. When troublesome the affected toe should be amputated.

ONYALAI

Essential thrombocytopenia occurring in Africa.

Aetiology. Although onyalai is now recognized to be identical with essential thrombocytopenia, it has been asserted to be a deficiency disease or caused by various indigenous medicines, which it is not. It may be caused by sensitization to some unknown factors.

Geographical distribution. Wellman (1904) originally described the condition as a peculiar disease occurring in Africans in Angola. Since then it has been recognized in South and East Africa, Tanzania, the Congo and Zambia where it is known as 'chipola', 'kafindo' or 'akembe' (bleeding disease).

Pathology. At autopsy there is extensive haemorrhage into the tissues, with haemorrhagic vesicles found in the serous membranes, the pleura, peritoneum and diaphragm. There are usually large retroperitoneal haemorrhages. There may be haemorrhage into the brain.

Clinical features. The clinical features are the same as those of essential thrombocytopenia. The majority of cases occur in young adult males although the youngest patient was an African female child of 7 months (Stein & Miller 1943). The onset is sudden with pyrexia up to 39·4–40°C. There are widespread haemorrhages into the skin and mucous membranes. Purpura is seen most easily in the axilla but may be missed on black skins. Characteristic bullae are seen on the lips, buccal mucosa and hard palate. These are blood-filled vesicles (1·25–1·8 cm in diameter) which differ from ordinary blood-filled vesicles by the presence of numerous trabeculae and by the semicoagulation of the contents which makes the vesicle difficult to empty. There is extensive bleeding from all mucous membranes with epistaxis and subconjunctival haemorrhages. Blood may be observed in the urine and stool, and in women menstruation is profuse. The bleeding time is prolonged, usually longer than 15 minutes, and the platelets are reduced to 20 000–30 000 per mm³. The red cell count may fall to 1 000 000 per mm³. Normoblasts may be numerous in the peripheral blood. Sternal puncture may show an increase of megakaryocytes with hyalinization and failure of budding, There are both acute and chronic types, the acute type outnumbering the chronic by 7·4 : 1. In the acute type the disease is self-limiting and most cases recover. In South Africa many cases are fatal, but elsewhere recovery is the rule. In the chronic type the disease runs a remitting course with recovery and relapse.

The diagnosis has to be made from thrombocytopenia secondary to aplasia of the marrow from drugs or some other toxic factor, and from snake bite with haemorrhagic manifestations.

Treatment. Treatment with steroids has given favourable results. Other methods of treatment consist of blood transfusion of fresh blood, and the intramuscular injection into the buttocks of 18 ml of donor blood.

REFERENCES

ABRAHAMS, D. G. (1959) *Lancet,* ii, 111.
ANDERSON, M., WALKER, A. R. P., LUTZ, W. & HIGGINSON, J. (1959) *Archs Path.,* 68, 380.
BADOE, E. A. (1967) *Ghana med. J.,* 6, 69.

BLUM, A., GAFNI, J., SOHAR, E., SHIBOLETS, S. & HELLER, H. (1962) *Archs intern. Med.*, **57**, 795.
BRAS, G., BROOKES, S. E. H. & WATLER, D. C. (1961) *J. Path. Bact.*, **82**, 503.
BROWNE, S. G. (1965) *J. Bone Jt Surg.*, **47**, 52.
BURKITT, D. (1958) *Br. J. Surg.*, **46**, 315.
—— (1962) *Br. med. J.*, **ii**, 1019.
CLIFFORD, P. (1965) *E. Afr. med. J.*, **42**, 373.
—— (1970) The oropharynx. *Alimentary and Haematological Aspects of Tropical Disease* (ed. Woodruff, A. W.), pp. 5–23. London: Arnold.
—— & BULBROOK, R. D. (1966) *Lancet*, **i**, 1228.
CHUTTANI, H. K., NIGAM, S. P., SAMA, S. K., DHANDA, P. C. & GUPTA, P. S. (1967) *Br. med. J.*, **iv**, 204.
DAVIES, J. N. P. (1948) *E. Afr. med. J.*, **25**, 10.
DOLL, R., PAYNE, P. & WATERHOUSE, J. R. (1966) *Cancer Incidence in Five Continents: A Technical Report.* Berlin, Heidelberg & New York: Springer.
EDDINGTON, G. M. (1954) *Ann. trop. Med. Parasit.*, **48**, 300.
—— (1959) *Cent. Afr. J. Med.*, **5**, 186.
—— & GILLES, H. M. (1969) *Pathology in the Tropics.* London: Arnold.
FISHER, A. C. (1941) *S. Afr. med. J.*, **15**, 131.
GELFAND, M. (1947) *Br. med. J.*, **i**, 847.
—— (1961) *Acta Un. int. Cancr*, **17**, 604.
GOODWIN, J. F. (1964) *Br. med. J.*, **i**, 1527.
GREENWOOD, B. M. & TAYLOR, J. R. (1968) *Trop. geogr. Med.*, **20**, 15.
HILL, K. R., STEPHENSON, C. F. & FILSHIE, I. (1958) *Lancet*, **i**, 623.
IVE, F. A., WILLIS, A. J. P., IKEME, A. C. & BROCKINGTON, I. F. (1967) *Q. Jl Med.*, **36**, 495.
KEAN, B. M. & TUCKER, H. A. (1946) *Archs Path.*, **41**, 639.
KLEIN, G., CLIFFORD, P., KLEIN, E. & STJERNSWARD, J. (1966) *Proc. natn. Acad. Sci., U.S.A.*, **55**, 1628.
KHANOLKAR, V. R. (1955) *Indian J. med. Res.*, **43**, 723.
LANCASTER, M. C., KENKINS, F. P. & PHILIP, J. McL. (1961) *Nature, Lond.*, **192**, 1095.
LINSELL, C. A. (1967) *Lancet*, **i**, 54.
LOTHE, F. (1963) *Norwegian Monographs on Medical Science*, Oslo & London: University Books.
McCRAE, A. W. R. (1968) *E. Afr. med. J.*, **45**, 133.
McKINNEY, B. & CRAWFORD, M. A. (1965) *Lancet*, **ii**, 880.
MANSON-BAHR, P. E. C. & CHARTERS, A. D. (1946) *Lancet*, **ii**, 333.
MERSKEY, C., GORDON, H. & LACKNER, X. (1960) *Br. med. J.*, **i**, 219.
PRATES, M. D. & TORRES, F. Q. (1965) *J. natn. Cancer Inst.*, **35**, 729.
SCHLESINGER, M. J. & REINER, L. (1955) *Am. J. Path.*, **31**, 443.
SHAPER, A. G. (1964) *Br. med. J.*, **i**, 1607.
—— KAPLAN, M. H., FOSTER, W. D., MACKINTOSH, O. M. & WILKS, N. E. (1967) *Lancet*, **i**, 598.
SHERLOCK, S. (1963) *Diseases of the Liver and Biliary System*, 3rd ed. Oxford: Blackwell.
SING, A., JOLLY, S. S. & KUMAR, L. R. (1961) *Lancet*, **i**, 587.
SOHAR, E., GAFNI, J., PRAS, M. & HELLER, H. (1967) *Am. J. Med.*, **43**, 227.
—— PRAS, M., HELLER, J. & HELLER, H. (1961) *Archs intern Med.*, **107**, 529.
STEIN, H. B. & MILLER, E. (1943) *S. Afr. J. med. Sci.*, **8**, 1.
STUART, K. L. & BRAS, G. (1957) *Q. Jl Med.*, **26**, 291.
TROWELL, H. C. (1960) *Non-infective Disease in Africa.* London: Arnold.
TULLOCH, J. A. (1962) *Diabetes Mellitus in the Tropics.* Edinburgh: Livingstone.
WALKER, A. R. P. (1963) *Am. Heart J.*, **66**, 293.
WALLACE, A. F. (1922) *Med. J. S. Afr.*, **17**, 155.
WELLMAN, F. C. (1904) *J. trop. Med.*, **7**, 52.
WILLIAMS, A. W., BALL, J. D. & DAVIES, J. N. P. (1954) *Trans. R. Soc. Trop. Med. Hyg.*, **48**, 290.
YEH, S. (1966) *Int. Path.*, **7**, 24.
ZUIDEMA, P. J. (1959) *Trop. geogr. Med.*, **20**, 15.

3. THE TROPICAL ANAEMIAS

By J. H. Walters, M.D., F.R.C.P.

The following abbreviations are used in this subject:

CI $\quad$ = Colour index. $\dfrac{\text{Haemoglobin (percentage of normal)}}{\text{Red cells (percentage of normal)}} = \dfrac{100}{100} = 1$

MCV $\quad$ = Mean corpuscular volume
MCH $\quad$ = Mean corpuscular haemoglobin
MCHC = Mean corpuscular haemoglobin concentration
ESR $\quad$ = Erythrocyte sedimentation rate

Anaemia at present constitutes a major tropical disease. According to Foy and Kondi (1956) the lowest mean haemoglobin rates are found in the hot damp river valleys of the Brahmaputra and Surma (Assam) at 90–270 m. Here the mean haemoglobin for all groups was 10·9 grammes/100 ml with 16·5% of the population having levels below 8 grammes/100 ml. The lowest levels were in pregnant women; lactating women were more than 1·0 gramme higher. Mozambique is an area of similar climatic conditions, but hotter with a more extended dry season. There the mean haemoglobin level of the rural population was 10 grammes/100 ml with 32% below 8 grammes.

In high altitudes, as at Darjeeling (830–2700 m) and the Nilghiri Hills (1000–2000 m), there is an increase of the mean haemoglobin levels of the population with very few below the 8 gramme mark—this is probably attributable to altitude. In Ceylon the mean haemoglobin was higher than in India or Africa. Among pregnant women the mean was 11·0 grammes with only 11% below 8 grammes.

In addition to the examples given above, there is a wealth of evidence that anaemia of significant degree is widespread throughout the tropical world. While the iron deficiency type of anaemia predominates, many examples of macrocytic anaemia with a megaloblastic marrow reaction are to be found, and a substantial minority of patients may present with a normochromic, normocytic anaemia which results from a pure deficiency of protein in the diet (Altmann & Murray 1948; Woodruff 1955). Finally, a small minority of patients will be found whose anaemia is of a chronic haemolytic type and is due to either an inherited defect of haemoglobin production—the haemoglobinopathies and thalassaemia types—or to hypersplenism. Very many factors contribute to the aetiology of tropical anaemia and most of them are peculiar to the tropical environment. The bulk and composition of the diet is influenced by economic status and physical factors in the production of vegetables, meat and milk, and by tradition and religious prejudices. Parasites often play an important aetiological role, while, as in all underdeveloped countries with a high infant mortality and a poor economic status, frequent pregnancy throughout the ages of fertility imposes a severe stress on the blood-forming organs of the average woman. It will be appreciated that in any given patient, especially a female, multiple factors will almost certainly be operating to produce an anaemia, and this was emphasized by Trowell many years ago (1943) when he described 'dimorphic anaemia' in which the red cells showed both macrocytosis and hypochromia.

IRON DEFICIENCY ANAEMIA

A hypochromic, microcytic anaemia may result from a deficient intake of iron in the diet, from inefficient iron absorption by the small intestine or from excessive loss of iron. The normal turn-over of aged red blood cells releases in the adult about 28 mg of iron daily, of which all but about 1 mg is re-absorbed, stored and re-utilized in the synthesis of haemoglobin. The 1 mg which is lost appears in the urine, bile, skin and sweat. Though the daily supplement to be obtained from the food appears so small, it must be remembered that, under normal circumstances, only 5–10% of the total iron intake is absorbed through the gut wall. The daily requirements of iron in the diet generally recommended for people in Britain are:

Infants	6 mg daily
Children aged 1–9 years	7–10 mg daily
Children aged 9–18 years	13–15 mg daily
Adult men	10 mg daily
Adult women	10–12 mg daily
Pregnant and lactating women	15 mg daily

In women an additional loss of 1 mg/day occurs during menstruation and during pregnancy 2·7 mg a day are abstracted by the fetus, hence their greater overall requirements.

The important sources of dietary iron are animal protein, cereals, especially millets, pulses and green leafy vegetables. Many millions of people in tropical countries cannot afford to buy meat or are vegetarian for religious reasons, very little milk is available to populations in tropical Africa, and in arid areas vegetables may be difficult to obtain. Thus the total iron intake is often critically low, and any defect of absorption or increased loss will precipitate an iron deficiency anaemia.

Impaired absorption of iron tends to occur when diets contain an excess of phytic acid, due to the presence of large amounts of whole-meal cereals, which fix a proportion of the iron content in the form of insoluble phytate, and when the diet is deficient in ascorbic acid or in protein, both of which facilitate the reduction of ferric to ferrous iron. The relationship of atrophic gastritis, causing hypo- or achlorhydria, to iron absorption is a controversial subject, but the consensus of opinion is that achlorhydria causes slight impairment of absorption of the metal. In states of chronic malabsorption, as in the kwashiorkor syndrome and in tropical sprue, the absorption of iron will inevitably be impaired.

Finally, the proportionate iron absorption bears an inverse relationship to the haemoglobin concentration; in rare instances chronic pancreatic disease or a deficiency of pyridoxine may lead to an excessive absorption of iron resulting in haemosiderosis.

Increased blood loss is most commonly due to hookworm infection. Though barely 1 cm long, and as thick as a thread of sewing cotton, each worm may abstract from 0·05 to 0·5 ml of blood from the mucosa daily. Since haemoglobin resists digestion the iron contained in the blood passed through the worm's intestine is lost to the body (Foy & Kondi 1960). These workers have noted a loss of blood as high as 180 ml a day in a patient from whose faeces 834 *Ancylostoma duodenale* and 249 *Necator americanus* were recovered after thorough worming. This represented a daily loss of 33 mg of iron from this patient. It has been shown by these authors that the daily blood loss in individual patients may vary considerably, probably depending upon the numbers of worms which happen to attack over a favourable site, adjacent to an arterial capillary; *A. duodenale*, being larger than *N. americanus*, is the more voracious feeder. As the iron stores become depleted the haemoglobin concentration falls, until an equilibrium is reached between the iron absorbed and the diminishing iron content of the increasingly more anaemic blood abstracted by the hookworm. Elimination of the worms will halt this loss but prolonged oral iron therapy will be required fully to replenish the iron stores.

Other parasitic diseases predisposing to an increased iron loss are schistosomiasis, causing chronic bleeding into the urinary tract or into the bowel, and malaria, in which a proportion of the haemoglobin content of an infected erythrocyte is converted by the plasmodium into a highly insoluble pigment called haemozoin, in which the iron is fixed to a protein complex and is ultimately lost to the body.

A high rate of sweat production is another factor adding to the drain on iron resources in the population of hot, humid regions. In India, Foy and Kondi (1956) have estimated individual iron losses of 0·3–2·3 mg a day in the sweat, depending on its cellular content. Finally, intestinal blood loss from dysentery, peptic ulcer and haemorrhoids adds a further potent factor to the production of iron deficiency anaemia.

PROTEIN DEFICIENCY ANAEMIA

Protein deficiency plays a very real though unspectacular role in the aetiology of tropical anaemia. Allen and Dean (1965) have shown that on refeeding children suffering from the kwashiorkor syndrome, the haemoglobin concentration, after falling initially owing to the dilutional effect consequent on the rapid regeneration of plasma albumin, rose steadily as the activity of the impoverished bone marrow increased. Some years earlier a study on haemoglobin and plasma protein regeneration in grossly marasmic Indian ex-prisoners-of-war released from Japanese imprisonment was carried out by Walters *et al.* (1947). By making serial calculations of absolute amounts of haemoglobin and of plasma albumin they showed that, on refeeding, though there was steady regeneration of haemoglobin, the rate of regeneration of plasma was much greater so that the rapidly expanding plasma volume created a dilutional effect which caused the haemoglobin concentration actually to fall during the initial period of treatment.

MACROCYTIC ANAEMIA

Macrocytic anaemia with a megaloblastic marrow reaction is widespread in all tropical countries and is most prevalent in women of child-bearing age. Folic acid deficiency is a more common cause than an absolute dietetic deficiency of vitamin B_{12}, though the latter is often the predominating factor among strictly vegetarian communities in India. In chronic haemolytic states, such as sickle cell anaemia, the additional demand for haematinic substances, especially for folic acid, may exceed the supply in the diet, and a degree of megaloblastosis may develop. Similarly in patients suffering from severe anaemia due to ancylostomiasis, worming and oral iron therapy may cause a rise in haemoglobin concentration which fails to reach a normal level until a folic acid supplement be given: this is an example of the dimorphic anaemia of Trowell (1943). Malabsorption states, due to tropical sprue (which is not uncommon in Indian communities), to giardiasis or to chronic dysentery, may lead to a defective absorption of folic acid and occasionally of vitamin B_{12} in addition. Chronic liver disease may be associated with a macrocytic anaemia, owing to failure of storage of folic acid rather than of vitamin B_{12}, but this is seen only in advanced liver disease. A final cause of macrocytic anaemia is infection with the fish tapeworm, *Diphyllobothrium latum*, and may be seen in the Far East. This is due to the avidity for vitamin B_{12} of this, the longest tapeworm found in man, which competes successfully with its host for available supplies of the vitamin in the food.

True pernicious anaemia is rare though not unknown among tropical populations. The diagnosis is confirmed by marrow aspiration. The earliest change is the appearance of giant metamyelocytes (giant stab cells); as the condition worsens precocious haemoglobinization is seen in macronormoblasts and when the disease is fully developed megaloblasts become the predominant erythroid precursors. The marrow is hypercellular throughout. In the peripheral blood the total erythrocyte count is diminished, the red cells show anisocytosis and macrocytosis and atypical large normoblasts—later even megaloblasts—and myelocytes may appear in small numbers. The MCV exceeds 90 μm^3 and may reach 130–140 μm^3; the granulocyte count is always diminished and platelets may become scanty. Clinically the liver and spleen may be moderately enlarged, the heart may dilate and dependent oedema is often present. An extreme degree of anaemia, in which the tongue and mucous membranes appear as pale as cheese, may not infrequently be seen in India, yet the patients are still moving slowly about and even bearing sickly infants. An anaemia of so grave a degree is often accompanied by a bleeding tendency, manifested by purpura, oozing gums and retinal and subhyaloid haemorrhage.

The treatment of tropical anaemias follows conventional lines. In hookworm infections bephenium hydroxynaphthoate (Alcopar) is the drug of choice. It is completely non-toxic and can be given safely to an anaemic, marasmic child, in whom other effective drugs, such as tetrachlorethylene, would be contra-indicated owing to their hepatotoxicity. The dose is 2·5 grammes to a child up to 3 years old, 5 grammes thereafter; in heavily infected subjects a daily dose for 4 days may be necessary. The drug, which is in granular form, is administered in the early morning on an empty stomach, and no subsequent purge is given. Thereafter oral iron, as ferrous carbonate or fumarate, 200–300 mg 3 times daily, is given for several weeks, while finally a course of folic acid, 5 mg thrice daily, may be required to complete haematological recovery. The treatment of protein deficiency anaemia is described in the section on malnutrition. In megaloblastic types of anaemia oral folic acid in a dosage of 5 mg 3 or 4 times daily is required and in a minority of patients vitamin B_{12} may also be necessary; an injection of 1·0 mg weekly for 4 doses should provide an adequate supplement.

Leukaemias, polycythaemia rubra vera and erythraemic myelosis (Di Gugliemo's disease) are encountered as frequently as in Europe, but acute types of leukaemia have a higher incidence in adult life in the tropics.

Thrombocytopenia vera is not uncommon in South China and is undoubtedly to be found in many tropical peoples (see Onyalai, page 19).

DEFICIENCY OF GLUCOSE-6-PHOSPHATE DEHYDROGENASE

About 2% of all haemoglobin is oxidized daily to methaemoglobin which is useless as a respiratory pigment, and it is to limit this destructive oxidation that reduced glutathione is required in adequate amounts within the red cells

(Prankerd 1965). When the enzyme is deficient oxidation of abnormally large amounts of haemoglobin leads to the formation of Heinz inclusion bodies and erythrocytes so affected are, for reasons not yet understood, unduly susceptible to haemolysis when exposed to wide variety of oxidant substances, to the broad bean (*Vicia fava*) or its pollen, and to other plant substances. These substances are listed below:

8-Aminoquinolines	Naphthalene derivatives
Sulphonamides	Methylene blue
Sulphones	Ascorbic acid
Nitrofurans	Probenecid
Para-aminosalicylic acid	Quinidine
Acetylsalicylic acid	Trinitrotoluene
Phenacetin	Broad bean
Amidopyrine	Hibiscus flower
Antipyrine	*Verbena* spp.
Acetanilide	
Acetyl phenylhydrazine	

The enzyme within the red cells catalyses the reaction:

Glucose-6-phosphate + triphosphopyridine $\rightleftharpoons$ 6-phosphogluconic acid + triphosphopyridine hydride + hydrogen

The hydrogen thus released maintains the glutathione in its reduced state.

The defect is determined by a sex-linked gene carried on the X chromosome, which is of irregular dominance, especially in the female. Possible combinations of the gene give rise to female heterozygotes who may transmit but rarely manifest the defect, female homozygotes who show the syndrome as well as transmitting it and male homozygotes who form the bulk of the sufferers. The gene is present at a high incidence in Sephardic Jews (Jews of Mediterranean as opposed to Central European origin), in the population of the Indo-Pakistan subcontinent, especially in Parsees, in African races and in their descendants. It also occurs throughout Greece and the Levant, in Sicily and Sardinia, in Arabia, the Far East and even in remote New Guinea.

There are at least 15 qualitative variants of G-6-PD distinguishable by their differing electrophoretic mobilities, distributed in different proportions among the main racial types. This very complex problem has been studied by Porter *et al.* (1964), who noted that most Negroes have either of the main phenotypes A and B, while Caucasian races have only the main phenotype B. The deficiency of G-6-PD is less severe in Negroes whose red cells retain about 10% of normal enzymic activity, while in deficient Caucasians only about 1–3% of normal G-6-PD activity remains. Sensitivity to the broad bean, or favism, occurs only in G-6-PD deficient Caucasians, not in Negroes, and even then only a small proportion of deficient Caucasians develop favism, or suffer acute haemolysis on exposure to any of the other precipitating factors listed above. The additional factors determining such haemolytic episodes are unknown. A further effect of deficiency of G-6-PD is now recognized, for there is evidence that affected neonates may develop icterus gravis neonatorum though they show no rhesus or ABO blood group incompatibility with their mothers.

Evidence gathered in Nigeria by Gilles *et al.* (1967) that G-6-PD deficiency affords a degree of protection from malignant tertian malaria is not supported by the experience of workers in Thailand and New Guinea, and this interesting suggestion remains *sub judice*.

Various techniques are employed to demonstrate the deficiency. For field use the semi-quantitative method of Motulsky *et al.* (1959) is probably best. It depends upon the rate of reduction (decoloration) of brilliant cresyl blue by the enzymes released from haemolysed erythrocytes and added to a substratum of glucose-6-phosphate with the coenzyme nicotamide adenine dinucleotide phosphate.

Treatment aims to protect those who may carry this defect from the substances which may initiate haemolysis, and it is a good rule to insist that a patient under treatment with a drug of the 8-aminoquinoline series should spend at least the first few days of the course under observation in hospital. Acute episodes of haemolysis due to this cause require the immediate withdrawal of the precipitating substance and blood transfusion is often necessary. 100–200 mg of hydrocortisone hemisuccinate sodium may be included in the infusion, and steps should be taken to maintain an alkaline reaction of the urine, in order to avoid the precipitation of acid haematin in the renal tubules.

THE HAEMOGLOBINOPATHIES

This group of blood diseases comprises all those in which a genetically controlled variation in the structure of the globin moiety of the haemoglobin alters its physical or chemical properties. Though the thalassaemias are included in this group they arise through a somewhat different mechanism and will be described separately.

Haemoglobin consists of an iron–porphyrin complex to which are attached two chains of polypeptides, each of which is duplicated about the haem 'nucleus'. Each polypeptide chain consists of 145×2 polypeptides, arranged in a constant sequence and each named after the amino-acid from which it is derived. Each pair of polypeptide chains is under separate genetic control and is determined by a single gene carried by one germ cell.

Four distinctive polypeptide chains occur naturally in man and are designated α, β, γ and δ. They combine in the following manner to make up the types of haemoglobin normal to man:

$$\alpha_2 \beta_2 \rightarrow \text{haemoglobin A or adult haemoglobin}$$
$$\alpha_2 \gamma_2 \rightarrow \text{haemoglobin F or fetal haemoglobin}$$
$$\alpha_2 \delta_2 \rightarrow \text{haemoglobin A}_2$$

Little fetal haemoglobin persists after the third month of life, but small amounts of A_2 haemoglobin persist throughout life.

Mutation may lead to the substitution of one of the amino-acid residues (polypeptide) by another foreign to that position in each half of either the α or the β chain, and the anomalous haemoglobin which results has altered physico-chemical properties by which it can be recognized and through which, in some instances, it gives rise to a specific disease. These mutations are inherited according to Mendelian law as dominant characteristics.

The mutations which lead to significant clinical diseases involve the β polypeptide chain, giving rise to abnormal haemoglobins which have been designated S, C, E and H. Haemoglobin S (sickle) is produced when one glutamic residue is replaced by a valine residue in each half of the chain; haemoglobin C when the same amino-acid residue is replaced by that of lysine. In haemoglobin E, as in haemoglobin C, a glutamic acid residue is replaced by lysine but in a different position in the polypeptide chain. Haemoglobin H illustrates a different mechanism of variation, in which the gene governing the formation of the α chain and carried by one germ cell appears to have been lost or partially suppressed, so that an excess of β chains is produced. Those surplus β chains group themselves about haem molecules to form a haemoglobin whose formula is thus not $\alpha_2\beta_2$ but β_4. A similar mechanism gives rise to the interesting though clinically insignificant abnormal form of fetal haemoglobin, called 'haemoglobin Barts' whose composition is not $\alpha_2\gamma_2$ but γ_4.

Since alteration in the amino-acid composition of the polypeptide chains may alter the overall electric charge on the haemoglobin molecule, several of the variants can be separated and identified by their specific rate of mobility towards the anode on electrophoresis, which is usually carried out in barbiturate buffer solution at pH 8·6. The selective mobilities of a number of reported haemoglobin variants are represented in the chart (Fig. 5).

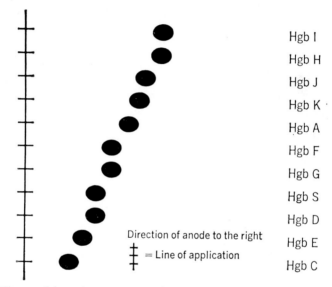

Fig. 5.—Schematic representation of the relative electrophoretic mobilities on paper of the common human haemoglobin types. (*Modern Medicine of Great Britain*)

It will be noted that haemoglobins S and D cannot be separated by this method from one another, nor can F and G. However, haemoglobin S has a specific property which determines its clinical effect and has made it notorious. In its reduced state it becomes relatively insoluble (one-hundredth as soluble as reduced haemoglobin A), and precipitates within the red cell envelope develop into filamentous liquid crystals called tactoids. These distort the red cell in characteristic fashion, so that it may be bent into a long narrow curve resembling a sickle.

Haemoglobin F has a specific property by which it can be recognized and estimated: this is its relative stability in alkaline solution, in which it differs from all other haemoglobin variants. The most convenient technique is the one minute alkaline denaturation test in which the blood suspected of containing HbF is lysed by dilution with water to a 10% solution. After estimation of the total haemoglobin content it is exposed to $N/12$ potassium hydroxide for 1 minute, after which the reaction is terminated by the addition of 50% saturated ammonium sulphate which precipitates the denatured chromogens and allows the persisting HbF to be estimated photometrically.

A simple diagram (Fig. 6) designed to show the proportionate distribution of the genes governing the formation of A (adult) or S (sickle) haemoglobin in the children resulting from the marriage of two 'sickle' heterozygotes serves to explain the principles involved.

The erythrocytes of the AS heterozygote contain both A and S haemoglobin, the former predominating; owing to the low concentration of S haemoglobin tactoid formation does not occur until a partial pressure of oxygen as low as 20 mm Hg is reached. Since so low a tension is not found under normal physiological conditions, intravascular sickling only occurs very exceptionally, though the condition has been found to be less benign than formerly thought. It has led to episodes of splenic infarction while flying in pressurized civil aircraft, in occlusion of limb vessels under conditions of stasis and cold or as a result

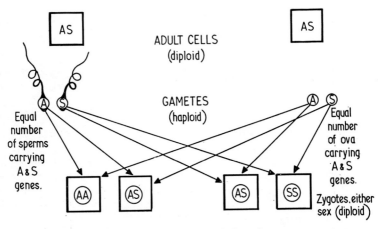

Fig. 6.—Diagram of transmission of genes.

of application of a surgical tourniquet, and it has been implicated in the production of periodic haematuria for which no other reason can be found. It is clearly an essential precaution to carry out a sickling test on any Negro patient prior to operation, and in those who are positive to ensure that the anaesthetized patient is kept warm and fully oxygenated and that no obstruction to the blood flow to a limb takes place. The homozygous condition in which the erythrocytes contain only S haemoglobin and a small, variable supplement of F (fetal) haemoglobin, results in a grave type of chronic haemolytic anaemia designated 'sickle-cell anaemia' or 'sickle-cell disease'.

In most instances, sickling begins to occur at partial pressure of oxygen between 60 and 40 mm Hg, and the percentage of sickled erythrocytes approaches 100% at 20 mm Hg. Since these oxygen tensions are within the physiological range in the capillaries of many organs, intravascular sickling can readily occur provided, as shown by Allison (1956), that the time of exposure to these low tensions exceeds 2 minutes, compared with the normal time of passage through the capillary bed of 15 seconds. Prolonged segregation of sickled cells in the spleen, possibly through loss of potassium, perpetuates the deformity in a proportion of them. Since sickled erythrocytes have an increased mechanical fragility, this moiety of irreversibly sickled cells is rapidly lysed, and a state of chronic haemolytic anaemia results. The presence of sickled cells which obstruct the smooth flow of blood cells through the capillaries leads to increased viscosity, so that a vicious circle of stasis, increasing deoxygenation and consequent increased sickling may be established in many organs and may result in multiple capillary infarction. This constitutes the most dangerous aspect of this disease. Increased coagulability of the blood, possibly due to excessive liberation of thrombokinase, has also been reported. The lives of patients suffering from sickle-cell anaemia are dominated by recurrent 'crises,' the majority of which, as pointed out by Diggs (1956), are manifestations of capillary infarction, while exacerbations of haemolysis and phases of marrow depression from intercurrent infections, may cause dangerous reduction in the red cell concentration. The majority of sickle-cell homozygotes die in crisis before puberty, but in those who do survive to adolescence the crises become infrequent and less severe. Pregnancy, carrying with it an enhanced risk of crises, is rarely survived, however, though a few males and unmarried women may attain middle life.

Geographical distribution

The gene of S haemoglobin is widely distributed throughout the Negro races, though it is very rare south of the Zambesi. It has been carried to the Caribbean Islands and to North, Central and South America. An independent focus has been found in the Thrace area of Greece by Caminopetros (1952), and may have spread thence to the whole Mediterranean littoral. It is found at a low incidence throughout Arabia; it also appears in the primitive Veddoids of Western India, and amongst races who have intermarried with them. An interesting suggestion has been made by Lehmann et al. (1956) in explanation of the wide distribution of the S gene. In neolithic times, the Arabian peninsula, which was then well watered and fertile, was inhabited by an early Veddoid race, in whom the gene arose by mutation. One section of this race later migrated down the western side of the Indian peninsula, another crossed into East Africa and a third may also have spread north into Asia Minor, each carrying the S gene with it. This S gene is not found in the negrito races of the Indian and Pacific Oceans, nor in Australian aboriginals. The incidence of the sickle-cell trait shows great variation between localities, rates as high as 40% being reported from East Africa, 20–25% from W. Africa, and 9% in U.S. Negroes. The cause of this variation, and also the persistence of high gene frequencies, despite the loss of many S genes through the premature death of S homozygotes, is not completely understood. The production of new S genes by mutation has not been observed. It seems probable that some mechanism, or mechanisms, tend to preserve selectively the heterozygous carriers of the S gene, a process termed 'balanced polymorphism'. Allison (1954) has brought forward evidence that P. falciparum malaria fulfils this role, pointing out that high S gene frequencies occur in highly malarious areas, whereas in a non-malarious area, where children who do not carry the gene have as good a chance of survival as those that do, the incidence is lower. This suggestion has been supported strongly by Gilles et al. (1967) who collected 100 children aged 6 months to 4 years who were heavily infected with P. falciparum and a similar group who were not so infected. The incidence of AS heterozygotes (4%) in the malarious group was significantly lower than in the control group (18%). This equality of survival, together with the elimination of many S genes through the early death of the sickle-cell homozygotes, would tend to dilute the S genes in the population within a few generations. This may explain the low incidence of the sickle-cell trait among the Negroes of the United States (9%), relative to that of the 20–25% among West African races, from whom they have descended. Evidence is also accumulating that deficiency of glucose-6-phosphate dehydrogenase in the red cells may similarly offer some protection against *P. falciparum* malaria, and the incidence of this anomaly too tends to follow that of sickling in areas where both occur (Gilles *et al.* 1967) but this matter is still *sub judice*.

Methods of demonstrating sickling

1. *The sealed drop method.* A drop of blood is obtained by finger-prick and is placed on a glass slide. A cover-slip is applied and is ringed with warm paraffin wax or soft paraffin. After incubation at 37°C for 24 hours, the oxygen uptake of the leucocytes will be found to have caused sickling among the erythrocytes.

2. *The bacterial reduction method.* A drop of blood is sealed beneath a cover-slip after it has been mixed with a small drop of a suspension of *Escherichia coli*. After 24 hours' incubation, sickling of the red cells is evident.

3. *The sodium metabisulphite method.* Sodium metabisulphate is a reducing agent. This is the best test for the sickling reaction. Incubate a drop of blood with a drop of freshly prepared 2% sodium metabisulphite solution, sealed under a coverslip with wax or soft paraffin, in an incubator at 38°C for 30 minutes. The intensity of the distortion produced in the erythrocytes gives an indication of their content of S haemoglobin: where this is relatively low—up to 30%—as in the heteroxygote, the characteristic pattern resembles holly leaves, whereas in the homozygous state, where the proportion of S haemoglobin is high, a bizarre set of figures with long emergent spicules is produced.

Pathology of sickle-cell anaemia

The pathological lesions comprise those of a chronic haemolytic anaemia together with the effects of multiple capillary occlusion. The red marrow is abnormally extensive; the diploëic space of the skull is widened and the outer table may be eroded over the vertex. There is marked normoblastic hyperplasia and some increase in the primitive cells of the granulocyte series. In wet, unstained marrow preparations, a mycelium-like fibrinoid network may be seen (Vandepitte & Louis 1953). Ectopic foci of haemopoiesis may be found, especially in the liver. The spleen in the early years shows grossly dilated sinusoids packed with sickled erythrocytes, while both erythropoiesis and phagocytosis of sickled cells are evident. Later, as a result of repeated infarction, it is reduced to a fibrotic vestige, containing calcium and haemosiderin crystals. The liver, which undergoes progressive enlargement with increasing age, shows, *pari passu*, increasing fibrosis. In early life the sinusoids, which are dilated, contain hypertrophied Kupffer cells, leucocytes in profusion with here and there plugs of interlocking sickled erythrocytes. A fine fibrinoid reticulum of uncertain origin usually spans the lumen. As the years pass, the stroma becomes thickened and distorted by plaques of dense fibrosis at the sites of multiple small infarctions. If adult life is attained, the liver usually shows a characteristic type of fibrosis on which nodular regeneration may be imposed. Multiple infarctions may also be found in the kidneys, brain or bones.

The bones themselves may display characteristic lesions from an early age. Ischaemic necrosis of the shaft of any long bone with marked periosteal new bone formation may be seen. Subsequently, while growth may be arrested by interference with the vascular supply in the proximal epiphyses, infarction of the diaphysis of any major long bone, such as the femur, humerus or tibia, may be found, and ischaemic necrosis of the femoral head, simulating Perthes' disease, is a well-recognized complication. Haematogenous bacterial infection (*Salmonella*) may be implanted on the infarcted area, the condition then closely resembling primary osteomyelitis. The radiological and pathological changes in the skull are indistinguishable from those of thalassaemia major, though they are to be found only in a minority (10–20%) of patients (Figs 8, 10). However, islands of sclerotic bone, a late result of infarction, may be seen in sickle-cell disease, but do not occur in thalassaemia major.

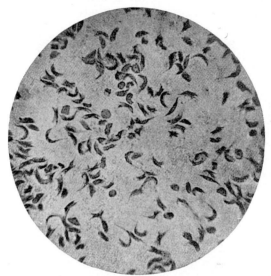

Fig. 7.—Sickle cells. (*Bulletin of the Johns Hopkins Hospital*)

Symptomatology

Owing to the inhibitory action of fetal haemoglobin on sickling, symptoms of the disease are not manifested in the early months of life during which a considerable proportion of haemoglobin F persists, but with its decline and the associated increase in the haemoglobin S concentration, which takes place from the fourth month onwards, the disease begins to declare itself. Impaired growth, anaemia with splenomegaly and slight icterus, and recurrent crises mark the progress of the disease. Stunting is commonly associated with a characteristic facial and bodily conformity, the skull being enlarged, sometimes with remarkable frontal and biparietal bossing, while an accentuated medial epicanthic fold and prominent malar bones confer a mongoloid appearance; the trunk is disproportionately short while the limbs are long and slender. Puberty is often delayed and sexually immature adults may be encountered. The spleen, which is invariably enlarged at some period during the first 5 years, as a result of multiple infarction, tends to shrink beneath the left costal margin as age increases. Hepatomegaly, which commonly appears before the age of 10 years, becomes the rule in the second decade; in surviving adults the liver may be found much enlarged, hard and irregularly nodular. The anaemia is typical of chronic haemolysis, but is subject to fluctuations due to crises of two types, that due to an exacerbation of the haemolytic process and that resulting from transient inhibition of erythropoiesis. The former may be precipitated by intercurrent infections and, in some instances, by pregnancy. The latter is commonly due to systemic infections. The anaemia with red cell counts ranging between 2 and 3·5 million is macrocytic, but the cells are fully haemoglobinized. There is a high, but variable, reticulocytosis and, usually, a considerable leucocytosis in which either polymorphs or lymphocytes may predominate. The stained film of fresh peripheral blood shows macrocytic anisocytosis, nucleated erythroblasts, whose number may equal, or even exceed, that of the leucocytes, and a few sickled erythrocytes. (The last are never found in the fresh blood of sickle-cell heterozygotes.) The platelet count tends to be increased. The serum

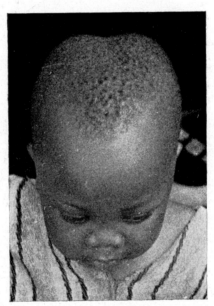

Fig. 8.—Biparietal and frontal bossing of the skull in sickle-cell anaemia. (Dr J. H. Walters)

is usually faintly icteric, and, though in early life this is due to an excess of pre-hepatic bilirubin, owing to increasing liver damage with increasing age, by the second decade a rising level of direct-acting ('post-hepatic') bilirubin is often found. An excess of fibrinogen has been noted, and also increased prothrombin activity, while coagulation time may be shortened. The marrow shows great normoblastic hyperplasia with some increase also in the myeloid series and in the megakaryocytes. In Nigeria Berry (1956) has noted evidence of the deficiency in the haemopoietic factor, namely macro-normoblastosis with precocious haemoglobinization, giant metamyelocytes and even megaloblastosis. Crises, which are usually marked by pain and fever, exhibit a variety of patterns. As pointed out by Diggs (1956) the great majority are manifestations of acute vascular occlusions, a small proportion only reflecting phases of increased haemolysis or of marrow aplasia. Joint pains, often associated with synovial effusion, occur very commonly while, as noted in East Africa by Trowell et al.

(1957), painful swelling of the metacarpals, metatarsals and phalanges is very frequent. Of equal importance is the abdominal crisis, comprising fever and tympanites, due to a degree of ileus. These attacks, provided they do not provoke surgical interference, which is harmful, usually subside on conservative treat-

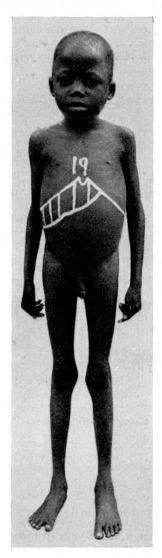

Fig. 9.—Physical characteristics of sickle-cell anaemia in a child aged 12 years: long slender limbs, short spine, frontal bossing of the skull, enlarged liver and shrunken impalpable spleen. (*Dr J. H. Walters*)

ment within 48 hours. The probable mechanism is widespread mesenteric capillary occlusion. Fatal shock may, however, terminate such an attack and in these instances acute thrombosis of the splenic vein or multiple small infarctions in liver, kidneys and suprarenals are to be found. Fever with renal pain and haematuria provides another common event. Vascular occlusion may cause focal damage to any part of the central nervous system, of which hemiplegia is a common well recognized manifestation. Retinal scars may be observed, and Edington and Sarkies (1952) have described miliary aneurysms of the retinal vessels. Painful, though transient, subcutaneous nodes may develop at any site. The heart is usually over-active and dilated; it may show signs of either right or left ventricular failure. In addition to functional haemic bruits relative incompetence of the mitral or tricuspid valve often gives rise to characteristic murmurs. A slight or moderate degree of finger clubbing is often to be seen. Chronic ulceration of the legs is very common in adults.

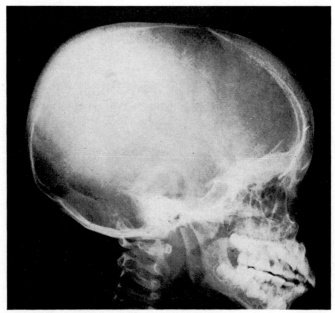

Fig. 10.—X-ray of the skull in sickle-cell disease, showing widening of the cortex and 'hair on end' appearance. (Dr J. H. Walters)

Treatment

This is unsatisfactory at the present time. Iron, except in those subjects who show evidence in the marrow of lack of essential haemopoietic substance, is of little benefit, though repeated blood transfusions may be of transient benefit during the rare haemolytic or aplastic crises. Splenectomy is not indicated, save in young children with very acute haemolysis and greatly enlarged spleens. As a vascular relaxant tolazoline hydrochloride (Priscoline) has been advocated for relief of pain in crises.

The aim of treatment is to reduce the incidence of sickling crises by preventing anoxia and febrile incidents, and to promote haemopoiesis. In malarious areas suppressive chloroquine should be given (Lewthwaite 1962); long-acting penicillin may reduce bacterial infections. A maintenance dose of folic acid, 5–10 mg daily, supports haemopoiesis. Many attempts have been made to reduce sickling, but without success. Sodium citrate, 60 ml of a 10% solution diluted in 400 ml water, may be given by mouth every 2 hours for 24 hours, and then in reduced dosage for some time. This, with codeine, reduces pain during crises, and also reduces the duration of pyrexia.

Homozygous sicklers should not travel by air.

OTHER HAEMOGLOBINOPATHIES OF CLINICAL IMPORTANCE

Haemoglobin C appears to have originated in the northern regions of Ghana, where Edington and Lehmann (1956) have found an incidence of the trait exceeding 15%, which was higher than that of the haemoglobin S trait. The gene appears to have spread laterally from this focus to a limited extent only, as far as the delta of the Niger, and has been carried to the New World, where it was first discovered in a North American Negro family. Where both C and S genes coexist, there is some tendency for the former to replace the latter since, according to Allison (1956), the haemoglobin C trait affords a selective protection comparable to that of the S trait, while there is no loss of genes due to premature death of the homozygotes as in sickle-cell anaemia. The clinical importance of this variant is its frequent association with haemoglobin S, for the heterozygous SC endowment gives rise to chronic haemolytic anaemia with splenomegaly, which, though of variable severity and always less grave than that of sickle-cell anaemia, may nevertheless cause considerable disability. Retinal micro-aneurysms are common.

In the homozygous (CC) condition the anaemia appears relatively benign and thrombotic phenomena are lacking. As in all the non-sickling haemoglobino-pathies, the presence of haemoglobin C is associated with numerous target-shaped erythrocytes in the peripheral blood. Haemoglobin D is found in the north western regions of the Indian peninsula, in Sikhs, and Punjabi Hindus, but gives rise to no symptoms. Haemoglobin E, however, is of importance in Burma, Thailand and Malaysia, where incidences exceeding 10% have been found, while a few examples have been reported from Indonesia, Sarawak and Ceylon, in which island the gene is confined to the Veddoid races. In the very occasional examples of homozygous haemoglobin E disease which have been recognized, a mild macrocytic anaemia, with numerous target cells, but without increased haemolysis, has been associated with slight hepatospleno-megaly.

Haemoglobin H has been demonstrated in populations of countries surrounding the Mediterranean, and in the Far East, but is rare in Africa. The homozygous state, in which no haemoglobin containing the α chain can be produced, is inevitably lethal in fetal life. The heterozygous state is of variable intensity, and this reflects the uncertainty which still exists as to its mode of inheritance. It has been suggested by Lehmann (1969) that the α chains are under the control of not 2 but 4 genes, and that α thalassaemia minor results from a defective function of 2 of these, whereas when the effect of 3 is suppressed, a more severe disease, called haemoglobin H disease, results.

In α thalassaemia minor, in which most of the fetal haemoglobin is of γ_4 or haemoglobin F (Bart's) type, only a minor degree of microcytosis and decreased osmotic fragility may be evident. With the disappearance of the haemoglobin F (Bart's) in early infancy, the recognition of the α thalassaemia trait may be impossible, and the carrier may show no clinical abnormality. Haemoglobin H disease, however, is a well marked clinical entity, giving rise to a chronic haemolytic state usually more severe than that seen in β thalassaemia minor. The spleen is much enlarged and there is marked anaemia. The red cells show hypochromia and polychromasia, with poikilocytes and target cells. The characteristic and diagnostic change is, however, the presence of intracellular bodies which stain with supravital stains and in the unstained cell cause stippling: these are called H bodies. Osmotic fragility is decreased and on electrophoresis a very fast-moving band outstrips HbA in its race towards the anode under standard conditions.

THALASSAEMIA, COOLEY'S OR MEDITERRANEAN ANAEMIA

This is a genetic disease in which the development of a normal adult A haemoglobin is suppressed; as a consequence fetal or F haemoglobin persists throughout life. The gene determining this anomaly is not an allelomorph of the genes governing haemoglobins A to L, though its association with any of them may give rise to an anaemia of symptomatic degree. The homozygous inheritance of the thalassaemia gene gives rise to a grave haemolytic anaemia—thalassaemia major—which usually proves lethal in the first decade, but the heterozygous condition, called thalassaemia minor, may vary in intensity from the asymptomatic thalassaemia minima to a severity approaching that of the first-named.

The defects of haemoglobin production leading to the appearance of the thalassaemic states are not yet fully understood. The concept is that the thalassaemia gene suppresses the formation of normal haemoglobin A ($\alpha_2 + \beta_2$ haemoglobin) so that fetal ($\alpha_2 + \gamma_2$) haemoglobin persists and the proportion of haemoglobin A_2 ($\alpha_2\delta_2$ haemoglobin) is raised. The defect commonly affects the β polypeptide chain, and since the thalassaemia gene is not an allelomorph of haemoglobins S, C, E, and H, the suppression of haemoglobin A may be found in association with any of these abnormalities. Thus a patient who inherits the genes of A and S haemoglobin and of thalassaemia will show only haemoglobins S and F, with perhaps some A_2.

Very rarely the thalassaemia gene appears to influence the formation of the α polypeptide chain and will then inhibit the formation of all three normal haemoglobins. The surplus β chains which result will form β_4 tetramers, that is, haemoglobin H, while surplus γ chains will form γ_4 or the abnormal type of haemoglobin F, known as 'haemoglobin Bart's'.

Throughout the world, families and individuals are occasionally found in whom, though there is no other haematological abnormality, a high level of fetal haemoglobin (12–28%) persists throughout life. This appears to be due to a failure of one gene for adult (A) haemoglobin to determine its share of β polypeptide chains, so that γ chains persist to fill their place.

The gene is now known to have a very wide distribution. Originally recognized in peoples of Mediterranean stocks, it is frequent in Burma, Thailand and Indonesia and has been recognized, though rarely, in West Africa, Arabia, Iran and India. Israëls and his associates have even discovered it in those generations of a Scottish family, in whom the possibility of an admixture of Mediterranean blood was remote (Israëls *et al.* 1955). A detailed description of the disease is beyond the scope of this book; it must suffice to describe the dominating features of thalassaemia major. The characteristic cell is the 'leptocyte', a wide, thin cell showing the 'target' or 'Mexican hat' anomaly (see page 1136) in which the concentration of haemoglobin is low, yet ample stocks of free iron can be demonstrated in the marrow and the serum iron concentration, in contrast with that seen in hypochromic anaemia due to iron deficiency, is normal or high. There is a marked resistance to lysis in hypotonic saline, yet the cell survival time is much reduced. A high sustained reticulocytosis is associated with the presence of numerous erythroblasts in the peripheral blood; a leucocytosis is common in which lymphocytes may predominate. The clinical picture comprises stunting, infantilism, marked enlargement of the spleen and liver, bossing of the skull and a mongoloid facies. There is radiological evidence of osteoporosis due to marrow hyperplasia, while the skull may show widening of the diploëic space, erosion of the outer table and the vault, the formation of new bone in vertical spicules producing a dramatic 'hair-on-end' appearance. The importance of this gene in tropical practice lies in the fact that its association with the genes of S, C and E haemoglobins results in a significant degree of anaemia. In the double heterozygote of S and thalassaemia, a severe, though non-lethal type of haemolytic anaemia termed *microdrepanocytic disease* occurs, while a very similar condition is found as haemoglobin-C-thalassaemia disease.

Treatment is difficult, but repeated blood transfusions, enough to maintain the haemoglobin at 7–10 grammes/100 ml, have been valuable. The general condition of the patient must be watched, especially the risk of siderosis from the accumulation of iron. Antibiotics are given to prevent infections, and folic acid and other vitamins are routine; the nutritional state must be maintained. Splenectomy is needed only rarely (Fessas 1967).

REFERENCES

ALLEN, D. M. & DEAN, R. F. A. (1965) *Trans. R. Soc. trop. Med. Hyg.*, **59,** 326.
ALLISON, A. C. (1954) *Br. med. J.*, i, 290.
———— (1956) *Trans. R. Soc. trop. Med. Hyg.*, **50,** 185.
ALTMANN, J. & MURRAY, A. (1948) *S. Afr. J. med. Sci.*, **13,** 91.
BERRY, C. G. (1955) *Br. med. J.*, i, 819.
CAMINOPETROS, J. (1952) *Lancet*, i, 687.
DIGGS, L. W. (1956) *Am. J. clin. Path.*, **26,** 1109.
EDINGTON, G. M. & LEHMANN, M. (1956) *Man*, **56,** 34.
———— & SARKIES, J. W. R. (1959) *Trans. R. Soc. trop. Med. Hyg.*, **46,** 59.
FESSAS, R. (1967) *Trans. R. Soc. trop. Med. Hyg.*, 61, 164.
FOY, M. & KONDI, A. (1956) *Lancet*, i, 423.
———— ———— (1960) *Trans. R. Soc. trop. Med. Hyg.*, **54,** 419.
GILLES, H. M., FLETCHER, K. A., HENDRICKSE, R. G., LINDER, R., REDDY, T. & ALLEN, N. (1967) *Lancet*, i, 138.
ISRAËLS, L. G., SUDERMAN, M. J. & HOOGSTRATEN, J. (1955) *Lancet*, ii, 1318.
LEHMANN, H. (1969) in *The Alimentary and Haematological Aspects of Tropical Diseases* (ed. Woodruff, A. W.). London: Arnold.
———— STOREY, P. & THEIM, M. (1956) *Br. med. J.*, i, 544.
LEWTHWAITE, C. J. (1962) *E. Afr. med. J.*, **39,** 196.
MOTULSKY, A. G., KRAUT, J. M., THIOME, W. J. & MUSTO, D. F. (1959) *Clin. Res.*, **7,** 89.
PRANKERD, T. A. J. (1965) *Br. med. J.*, ii, 1017.
PORTER, I. M., BOYER, S. M., WATSON-WILLIAMS, E. J., ADAMS, A., SZEINBERG, A. & SINISCALCO, M. (1964) *Lancet*, i, 895.

TROWELL, H. C. (1943) *Trans. R. Soc. trop. Med. Hyg.*, **32**, 19.
—— RAPER, A. B. & WELBOURNE, H. F. (1957) *Q. Jl Med.*, **26**, 401.
VANDEPITTE, J. M. & LOUIS, L. A. (1953) *Lancet*, **ii**, 806.
WALTERS, J. H., ROSSITER, R. J. & LEHMANN, H. (1947) *Lancet*, **i**, 244.
WOODRUFF, A. W. (1955) *Br. med. J.*, **ii**, 1415.

SECTION I

DISEASES CAUSED BY PROTOZOA

4. MALARIA

THE name malaria is derived from the Italian *mal aria*, meaning bad air. The disease is also known as paludism, from the Latin *palus*, a marsh. Both names reflect the early opinion that the disease was spread by miasma, or mist, arising in marshes.

Geographical distribution

The distribution of malaria throughout the world is shown in Fig. 11.

Aetiology

For descriptions of the various species of malaria parasites which infect man, see Appendix I.

TRANSMISSION

Transmission by mosquitoes

In nature, malaria is transmitted from man to man by *Anopheles* mosquitoes, of which there are hundreds of species, some very efficient, others not so efficient, and still others not capable of transmission. For descriptions of these mosquitoes and of the development of malaria parasites in their tissues, see Appendix I.

Transmission depends not only upon the presence of gametocytes in the blood, but also upon the infectivity of these for mosquitoes. Gametocytes are formed within red cells, but the mechanism which determines which schizonts produce them and which do not is not understood. They appear early in the infection, and they vary in infectivity for mosquitoes, following (in experiments with *Plasmodium cynomolgi*) a 48-hour cycle with peak infectivity about midnight, 84 hours after the schizogony at which they had been formed. Infectivity is high in the early days of parasitaemia, and falls abruptly when the crisis of asexual forms begins, presumably because antibodies are formed.

In the tropics children are probably the most prolific source of infective gametocytes.

Transmission other than by mosquitoes

Malaria can, however, be transmitted in other ways: by design or by accident, by the inoculation of blood from an infected person to a healthy person. In this way the asexual blood forms continue to develop in their own periodicities in the peripheral blood, producing attacks of fever in the recipients, but pre-erythrocytic and exo-erythrocytic schizonts are not formed in the liver, because these forms originate only from sporozoites inoculated by mosquitoes. Malaria transmitted by inoculation of blood is easily cured and relapses do not occur. Nevertheless, *P. falciparum* infections transmitted in this way can be fatal.

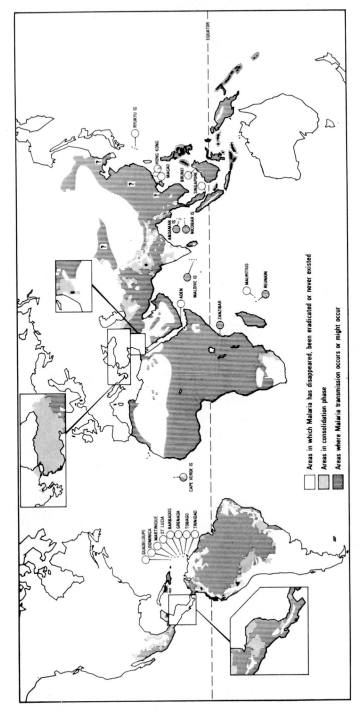

Fig. 11.—Epidemiological assessment of the malaria situation on 30 June 1968. (*WHO 1969b*)

The chief operations by which such transmission is effected are:

1. Deliberate infection in neurosyphilis for curative purposes. *P. vivax* is commonly used, but other species have also been used.

2. Unintentional infection through transfusion of blood which, unknown to the physician, contains malaria parasites. In this way *P. vivax* has been transmitted in temperate climates from donors infected 3 years before; *P. ovale* from donors infected 4 years before (Chin & Contacos 1966); *P. malariae* from donors infected as many as 17 years before, and not exposed to infection since; and *P. falciparum* present in blood from donors who were exposed 20 months to 3 years earlier (Verdrager 1964; Robinson 1966).

Refrigeration of stored blood does not eliminate malaria parasites, which can remain viable for indefinite periods at −70°C.

In non-malarious countries donors who have had malaria should not be used. In malarious countries donors should be treated with antimalaria drugs before blood is withdrawn, and non-immune recipients should also receive a course of these drugs. Dried plasma prepared from malarial blood is safe.

3. Unintentional infection is common in drug addicts who borrow syringes and needles from each other and use them without attempting to sterilize them. Many cases of *P. falciparum* infection, with many deaths, have been recorded. Such addicts also tend to suffer from hepatitis and septic phlebitis with pneumonia. *P. falciparum* has also been spread by unsterilized syringes used for injections of Salvarsan preparations.

CONGENITAL MALARIA

Evidence that congenital malaria occurs was summarized comprehensively in a critical review by Covell (1950), who concluded that intrauterine transmission from mother to child is well established, though how it occurs is not known. The placenta is normally an effective barrier, but congenital infection can occur without demonstrable damage to the placenta, and before the onset of labour. Massive infection of the placenta may break down this barrier, though concrete evidence of this is lacking, and, of course, there may be microscopic areas of damage to the placenta. All the common species of malaria parasites may be involved. Malaria in epidemic form is an important cause of abortion and stillbirth, and of deaths in newborn infants.

However, after careful studies on women in Nigeria, Madecki and Kretschmar (1966) conclude that in most cases of apparently congenital malaria there the babies are infected during parturition, and that the infection is connatal rather than congenital, and Edington (1967) states that the neonate in Nigeria does not contract malaria, and that congenital malaria does not occur. Jelliffe, E. F. P. (1966), who found one congenital case in 92 babies born to mothers with infection of the placenta, mostly due to *P. falciparum*, comments that this infection tends to result in babies of below average birth weight, and that in endemic areas chemoprophylactic drugs should be given as a routine to parturient women.

EPIDEMIOLOGY

General factors

Malaria exists where effective anopheline vectors breed in nature and where human carriers of the sexual forms of the parasites are available to these mosquitoes. In a few parts of the world anophelines have been present in the absence of malaria, but these areas are small. As a result of control and eradication procedures many former malarious areas are now clear because the anopheline population has been reduced or eliminated.

In those still great areas of the world where malaria persists, the epidemiology of the disease is the resultant of various factors, which were analysed mathematically by Macdonald (1950 a, b; 1952 a, b; 1953). They can be described as follows

Factors relating to man

1. Parasite rates in man, especially children.
2. Recovery and mortality rates from the disease.
3. State of immunity of the population.
4. Habits and living conditions of the population.

Factors relating to the parasites

1. Virulence (*P. falciparum* the most, *P. malariae* the least).
2. Persistence and tendency to relapse in man.

Factors relating to anophelines

1. Availability of water suitable for breeding, which depends largely on climate and season, governing rainfall and temperature.
2. Longevity of anophelines, and the faculty of hibernation.
3. Effectiveness as vectors; species vary in this and in their preferences for man as a source of blood meals.
4. Dose of sporozoites inoculated at a bite in man; this can vary greatly.
5. Availability of man as the donor and recipient of parasites.

These complex biological factors obviously overlap and interreact to provide various degrees of stability or instability in the prevalence of malaria. They are particularly evident in the epidemiology of *P. falciparum* malaria.

Estimation of malarial prevalence

To estimate the prevalence of malaria in a community a large number of people, especially infants and children, must be examined. The following are the methods used:

(*a*) *Spleen rate*. The spleen rate is the proportion of children (aged 2–10 years) in a community who have enlarged spleens. The spleen may be palpated with the child standing or lying, the examiner's hand being pressed gently against the abdominal wall until the spleen is felt or is found to be not palpable. An enlarged spleen, especially if only recently enlarged as a result of early attacks of malaria, is easily ruptured; care is therefore essential in palpation.

Measurement of the degree of enlargement may be made by Schüffner's method (see Fig. 12), or by estimating the number of finger-breadths below the costal margin.

The World Health Organization has proposed the following classification:

I. *Hypoendemic malaria* with spleen rate in children 2–10 years of age 0–10%.

II. *Mesoendemic malaria* with spleen rate in children 2–10 years of age 11–50%.

III. *Hyperendemic malaria* with spleen rate in children 2–10 years of age constantly over 75%. Spleen rate in adults is also high.

IV. *Holoendemic malaria* with spleen rate in children 2–10 years of age constantly over 75%. Spleen rate in adults low; it is in this type of endemicity that the strongest adult tolerance is found.

(*b*) *Parasite rate.* The parasite rate is the proportion of a population in which malaria parasites are found; some authorities use thin blood films for estimating this rate, claiming that by examining the edges of the film they can find a reasonably true rate. Other authorities rely on thick drops, arguing that fewer parasites are missed by this technique.

(*c*) *Parasite count.* The parasite count is laborious. Parasites in the blood can be counted against leucocytes, or by estimating the exact amount of blood examined and relating the count to that. Some authors have added a measured amount of fowl erythrocytes (which, being nucleated, can easily be recognized) to a measured amount of blood, and counted the parasites against these.

Serological tests (see page 64) can also be used for surveys.

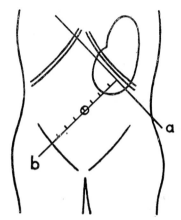

Fig. 12.—Schüffner's method of determining the degree of splenic enlargement. (a) denotes the upper limit along the left costal margin; (b) is a line drawn at right angles through the tip of the spleen and umbilicus.

Untreated malaria

In untreated or inadequately treated malaria the parasites persist in the body for months or years, and in malarious countries reinfection is the rule. After the early period of recurring fever (overt malaria) the parasites live in more or less stable equilibrium with the forces of immunity. This equilibrium is subject to fluctuations dictated by extraneous factors, chiefly connected with the characteristics of the anopheline vectors—their longevity, their prevalence (continuous or seasonal, which is related to rainfall or other factors affecting natural waters, and to the temperatures at which the mosquitoes breed), the peculiarities of their breeding places, their biting habits which may reveal preference for human blood, and their ability to act as suitable hosts for developing malaria parasites, for anophelines vary greatly in this respect.

Macdonald (1952b) analysed the epidemiology of malaria on these lines. He defined:

1. *Stable malaria,* transmitted by efficient anopheline vectors breeding

throughout the year, which bite man frequently, are moderately long-lived, and exist in climates favourable to rapid completion of the extrinsic (mosquito) life cycle of the parasite. Reduction of temperature to about 15°C would stop transmission. In stable malaria the level of immunity is high after childhood, and equilibrium is the rule.

2. *Unstable malaria*, transmitted by less efficient vectors, which bite man less frequently and may be short-lived, or which exist in climatic conditions less favourable for the development of the parasites in them. Seasonal changes in the density of mosquitoes occur. Immunity in unstable malaria is not complete, and fluctuates seasonally. Equilibrium is not attained in the population and epidemics therefore occur when mosquito breeding becomes seasonally prolific, usually in the summer months or after high rainfall though (as in Ceylon between the wars) a dry season may reduce the flow of water in rivers, leaving quiet pools favourable to the breeding of dangerous mosquitoes. The essential point of unstable malaria is lack of continuity of transmission.

Intermediate endemic forms between stable and unstable occur.

Malaria in nomads. This presents a difficult problem. Such people may not attain full immunity, and therefore require treatment; they are unlikely to take to chemoprophylaxis, and control by insecticides is difficult for people who live in temporary encampments or tents.

PATHOLOGY

The pathology of malaria is essentially the pathology of *P. falciparum* infections.

The pathogenesis of malaria has been closely studied by Maegraith (1948, 1967) and his colleagues in *P. falciparum* infections of man and the comparable *P. knowlesi* of monkeys. He does not think that these infections interfere sufficiently with haemoglobin, either by disruption of erythrocytes or by conversion to haemozoin, to affect the oxygen-carrying function of the blood, nor is the oxygenation function of the lungs sufficiently impaired. General anoxic anoxia does not occur, except possibly in extreme conditions, in which parts of an organ might be mechanically or dynamically impeded, leading eventually to relative or total anoxic anoxia.

In malaria the erythrocytes become sticky, with a coat of fibrin, and it has long been thought that this causes agglutination and obstruction in the smaller vessels (Edington & Gilles 1969) but this phenomenon occurs in peripheral areas of any form of inflammation, and is not now accepted by Maegraith as the main reason why such vessels become blocked, as they undoubtedly do. Neither clots nor emboli are involved in this process. Hypovolaemia may be a factor.

Stasis is most important. In *P. knowlesi* infections there is major constriction in the smaller branches of the portal system, which is due to the hyperactivity of the sympathetic nervous system, and which can be reversed by adrenergic drugs. It is not specific to malaria but occurs in other acute medical states. This constriction leads to stagnation and cellular damage, and a similar reaction occurs in the renal cortex, leading to renal ischaemia. In this process of stasis the endothelium of small vessels becomes permeable to the extent that heavy molecules and water pass through, and erythrocytes accumulate in the lumen, causing obstruction. In *P. knowlesi* infection, for instance, protein and water escape into the cerebrospinal fluid and tissues, a state which can be reversed by anti-inflammatory drugs such as cortisone and the antimalarials chloroquine, mepacrine and proguanil. This seems to explain the severe central nervous system signs of advanced malaria. It also explains why the erythrocytes in cerebral malaria are so heavily infected, the merozoites having easy access to new cells, in which they can develop to mature stages. Stasis, in fact, means

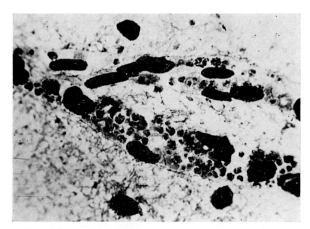

Fig. 13.—Cerebral malaria. The capillaries are packed with parasites. Field's stain. (*Dr E. C. Smith*)

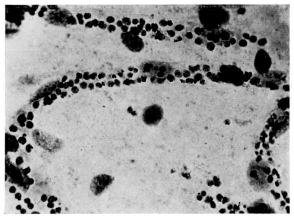

Fig. 14.—The capillaries are seen to be filled with parasites. Rosette forms are within the capillaries. (*Dr E. C. Smith*)

loss of fluid from the vessels, consequent increased viscosity of the local circulating blood and concentration of circulating erythrocytes.

Cytotoxic anoxia is generally more important than anoxic anoxia. It is probably due to some soluble factor which depresses respiration and interferes with metabolism. A malaria toxin has long been postulated, though so far never found, but Maegraith (1967) has now obtained evidence which points to two fractions in serum which may be relevant, one appearing with inorganic phosphate and one (probably acting synergically) with lactic acid. These probably interfere with mitochondrial activity, halting cellular metabolism.

Nutrition of the host is also a factor. All-milk or all-meat diets suppress malaria. Anorexia is common in malaria; the liver is depleted of glycogen and blood glucose is low, at which level competition by the parasites may be a

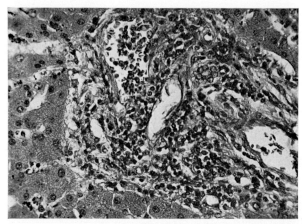

Fig. 15.—Section of the liver shows cloudy swelling, with periportal round cell infiltration. There is malaria pigment in the trabeculae and cells. (*From a specimen in the Wellcome Museum of Medical Sciences presented by Professor Gharpure, Bombay*)

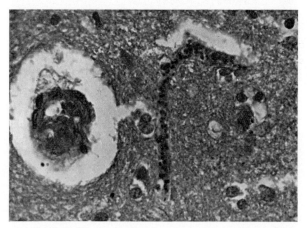

Fig. 16.—Section of the brain showing congestion in malaria. The capillaries are blocked by parasitized cells. (*From a specimen in the Wellcome Museum of Medical Sciences presented by Sir N. H. Fairley*)

factor. Absorption of xylose and an amino-acid is depressed in advanced *P. knowlesi* infection, but this can be reversed by injection of an adrenergic blocking agent (phenoxybenzamine), which presumably releases vasoconstriction.

There is obviously much room for research in this complicated subject.

Chemical changes in the blood

Plasma protein is reduced, especially albumin, though globulin is increased. The changes are not due to fever alone, but are related to upset in liver function. Hypocholesterolaemia occurs in malaria; it may rise during the rigor and falls to subnormal in the apyrexial periods. Glucose is essential for the respiration of plasmodia and rise of blood sugar occurs in both *P. falciparum* and *P. vivax* infections, possibly correlated with a change in adrenal function. Plasma potassium is raised during the fever and is at its height during segmentation and is probably due to destruction of red cells. The erythrocyte sedimentation is raised in malaria, but is restored to normal after treatment. The degree appears to be dependent upon the protein content of the plasma and activity of the surface of the cells. Acidosis is very exceptional, but as the parasites use glucose, it is probable that pyruvates and lactates may accumulate under conditions of anoxia, and such an event will result in a fall of pH and a loss of alkali reserves. Up to a point, in pathological haemoglobinaemia, the liver is capable of dealing with liberated haemoglobin, so that, when this pigment is set free in the blood, serum secretion and flow of bilirubin are correspondingly increased.

Morbid anatomy

This again is essentially the morbid anatomy of *P. falciparum* infections.

Pigment from the parasites is taken up by the reticulo-endothelial system, and is found in the liver, spleen, brain and other organs. In areas of stable malaria stellate fibrosis of the portal tracts has been associated with the presence of malarial pigment in children gaining their immunity.

Anaemia is a feature; erythrocytes are destroyed by the parasites, and parasitized red cells are taken up by phagocytes, which also engulf red cells not containing parasites. The erythropoietic centres are affected; bone marrow erythropoiesis is inhibited in acute malaria, but when parasitaemia is cleared, the marrow is hyperaemic, pigmented and active, with hyperplasia of normoblasts. In the peripheral blood there may be poikilocytosis, anisocytosis, polychromasia and basophilic stippling, resembling pernicious anaemia. Reticulocytes are much increased; *P. vivax* tends to infect reticulocytes predominantly, but *P. falciparum* infects all red cells equally.

The anaemia of malaria is not commensurate with the parasitaemia during acute infections; it is excessive and there may be a sudden dramatic fall in Hb. To explain this, one theory is that it may be the result of an autoimmune process. An antigen 'toxic' to red cells has been found, which immunizes against infection. This autoimmune process may be instrumental in clearing the blood of parasites, and this is probably the hypothesis which best explains the excessive anaemia which occurs (Cox 1966; Zuckerman 1966). Another explanation, however, is that hypersplenism causes this destruction of red cells, as has been found in *P. berghei* infections. No anti-erythrocyte antibodies could be found, and in splenectomized animals other reticulo-endothelial organs assume the sequestering function of the spleen (George *et al.* 1966).

P. knowlesi infection in rhesus monkeys causes a defibrinization syndrome which is blocked by heparin, and similar coagulation defects have been described in U.S. soldiers evacuated from Vietnam with chloroquine-resistant *P. falciparum* malaria (Dennis *et al.* 1966). In serious *P. falciparum* malaria there may be a precipitous fall in plasma fibrinogen suggesting increased consumption of fibrinogen due to intravascular coagulation, which may be of pathogenic importance (Devakul *et al.* 1966). Thrombocytopenia has been observed in

41 of 50 cases of *P. falciparum* malaria in Thailand, with a deficiency in prothrombin (Pannachet 1967).

The *liver* is commonly enlarged and congested, with parasitized red cells in sinusoids and centrilobular veins, and swollen parenchymatous and Kupffer cells. It is soft, dark chocolate red (or yellowish if fatty), or slate grey or black if there is much pigment in the Kupffer cells. The lobular structure is indistinct, and in the smaller blood vessels and sinusoids the endothelium is damaged, and there is stasis, agglutination or thrombosis. The liver cells round the central veins are sometimes atrophied and necrosed, but this is not common. The lesions resemble those of right heart failure from anoxia due to interference with flow of venous blood resulting from changes in the veins themselves, notably constriction as a result of hyperactivity of the sympathetic nervous system. Hepatic blood flow is decreased soon after sporulation, but a few hours later it is higher than normal.

As children in hyperendemic areas lose the passive immunity they inherit from their immune mothers, and begin to show clinical effects of new infection, there is a phase of hyperplasia and hypertrophy of macrophages in the liver and spleen, and large amounts of malarial pigment accumulate in the Kupffer cells throughout the whole lobule of the liver. Damage to parenchymal cells is not usual unless there is gross anaemia or malnutrition. As active immunity develops from repeated infections, stimulation of phagocytosis declines, and the production of pigment is reduced. The pigment is slowly carried away via the lymphatics, but with continuing infection some pigment remains until adult life. The hyperplasia and hypertrophy of the Kupffer cells, though reduced, does not entirely disappear, and may cause enlargement of the liver in adult life (Hutt 1971).

There may be mild jaundice with an indirect Van den Bergh reaction, and liver function tests are often abnormal. For instance, transaminases and the SGPT/SGOT ratio are increased, cephalin flocculation tests become positive, and fasting glucose and alkaline phosphatase levels are lowered. Malaria disturbs liver function even when there is no clinical evidence of hepatic insufficiency and even when parasitaemia is low. Restoration of function takes some time (Sadun *et al.* 1966).

The *kidneys* share in the anoxic process, which may lead to cortical ischaemia and epithelial changes. Acute nephritis is rare and the changes are predominantly degenerative not inflammatory. Proteinuria is common, and the renal disorganization may go on to chronic nephrosis with retention of water and sodium, and occasional azotaemia, especially in quartan malaria. Proliferative glomerulonephritis has been observed, with some tubular atrophy and increase of tubular activity. Membraneous glomerulonephritis has also been reported, but this may be due to an antigen–antibody reaction, the relationship with malaria not being proved.

Changes in the *brain* and *nervous system* are basically determined by the creation of anoxic states as a result of the vascular conditions described above. The capillaries and small vessels are dilated, grossly congested and blocked with parasitized erythrocytes. Petechial haemorrhages and so-called granulomas are found in the white matter, brain stem and cerebellum. The brain is hyperaemic and heavily pigmented, sometimes having a leaden colour. If the anaemia is intense the vessels are empty and the brain is pallid. The meninges are grossly congested and the smaller vessels are packed with parasitized red cells.

These changes reflect the clinical signs and symptoms: headache, irritability, delirium, coma, hyperpyrexia, sweating, apoplectic and epileptic attacks, convulsions, meningitis, the frontal lobe syndrome, bulbar paralysis, cerebellar disturbances, polyneuritis and tremors. In the chronic stage there may be multiple sclerosis, peripheral neuritis and amaurosis.

The *spleen* usually enlarges early in *P. vivax* and *P. falciparum* infections; later in quartan infections. The size varies with duration and the degree of exposure to superinfection, and it may be enormous, weighing up to 800 grammes in the acute stage. It is tender, and there is a considerable risk of rupture, especially during the primary attack in non-immune subjects, as in malaria induced with *P. vivax* for the treatment of neurosyphilis. Infarcts occur, and the pedicle may become twisted. The spleen is dark red to black on section, soft, congested, with haemorrhages and thromboses, and sometimes adhesions. In chronic infections it is much smaller and more fibrous, and

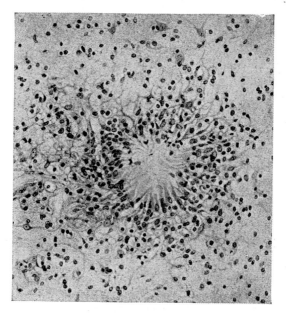

Fig. 17.—Malarial granuloma. Brain section showing plugging of capillaries of the cortex and proliferation of glial cells. (*Dürck 1925*)

contains much pigment, especially in the phagocytes. The spleen is subject to circulatory changes in the early stages, and cellular changes later. Blood flow is impeded, but the reason is not clear. Hypersplenism may be a factor in the destruction of red cells, and therefore in the aetiology of malarial anaemia. During attacks of malaria the spleen filters off and phagocytoses red cells infected with parasites.

The *suprarenals* are very important in the pathogenesis of malaria. Algid attacks sometimes take place in *P. falciparum* infections, in which the patient is in a state of collapse, with cold, clammy skin, small and fast pulse and low blood pressure; he is pale, his temperature falls rapidly and he suffers from cramps, vomiting and diarrhoea in which loss of fluid may be so great as to recall cholera (the so-called choleraic malaria). This syndrome is probably due to adrenal failure, and may be fulminating. Post mortem the adrenals are congested, with haemorrhage, or degenerated and necrotic. The condition probably results from circulatory disturbances leading to diminished supply of oxygen to the adrenals, as is the case with other organs, and this anoxia leads to a vicious circle with endocrine imbalance augmenting the condition of shock.

The *heart, lungs* and *gastro-intestinal tract* are affected by the general circulatory changes.

In the *placenta* the maternal spaces are packed with erythrocytes containing segmenting forms of the parasite, and lymphoid-macrophage cells loaded with parasites. On the fetal side of the barrier, however, the vessels are entirely free from parasites (see Congenital Malaria, page 41). In pregnancy malarial anaemia is a common cause of death, and pregnancy increases the frequency and severity of attacks, which may precipitate abortions and stillbirths. There is a relationship between low birth weight in African babies and malarial infection of the placenta.

IMMUNOLOGY

The immunology of malaria has been extensively studied in recent years, and the opinions expressed here may need modification as new work is reported. As in other infections, this immunity may be natural or acquired.

Natural immunity

This is most obvious since man is not susceptible to infection by the malaria parasites of birds or rodents, and only to some of the malaria parasites of other primates, for instance *P. inui, P. brasilianum, P. eylesi, P. cynomolgi, P. cynomolgi bastianellii, P. simium, P. shortti,* and *P. knowlesi* (Garnham 1966, 1967). It is also seen in the fact that each species of malaria parasite will develop fully only in a narrow range of invertebrate genera—the parasites of man only in *Anopheles.* The explanation of this insusceptibility of man to some animal parasites is not clear; it probably lies in differences in biochemical constitution of the various host species.

Natural immunity acts on both the asexual and the sexual erythrocytic stages of the parasite, and also on the other stages. The parasites are most susceptible when they are in contact with the body fluids of the host.

Natural, genetic immunity of man to the 'human' parasites is seen:

(*a*) In some Negro communities, for instance in North America, which are apparently relatively resistant to infection with *P. vivax,* although they have not been exposed to it for generations. The immunity may be the result of some form of natural selection; its nature is ill-defined.

(*b*) In populations long exposed to *P. falciparum,* who show some resistance to it, possibly as a result of natural selection. Resistance is most obvious in children (less so in adults) carrying the sickle-cell trait (HbS heterozygotes) or other abnormal haemoglobins (e.g. HbC); it may also be related to deficiency in glucose-6-dehydrogenase. These characters apparently do not favour the growth and development of the parasites in the red cells. But if malaria does overcome this resistance, it can be a serious precipitating cause of sickle-cell crisis, possibly in part due to dehydration and intravascular sickling.

Natural immunity can be greatly reduced by splenectomy, which can render certain animals susceptible to parasites to which normally they are resistant.

Acquired immunity

Acquired protective immunity is provoked only by the asexual erythrocytic stages of the malaria parasites, not by the liver stages or (so far as is known) by gametocytes, though gametocytes have some antigenic property, provoking antibodies which are apparently not protective. Such immunity operates only against mature schizont and free merozoite erythrocytic stages of the mammalian parasites; it does not act against gametocytes. The level of this immunity depends to a great degree on the reproductive potential of the different species of parasites, and its persistence depends on the frequency of antigenic stimulation. For instance, in *P. vivax*, *P. ovale* and *P. malariae* infection, in which some merozoites of the primary pre-erythrocytic liver phase apparently re-enter liver cells, to initiate successive exo-erythrocytic liver schizonts, and in which successive batches of merozoites from these exo-erythrocytic schizonts are released into the blood during relapses, the antigenic stimulus from these merozoites is constantly being renewed—in the case of *P. vivax* for at least 8 years, for *P. malariae* for much longer—and so, therefore, is the immune response.

In *P. falciparum* infections, however, in which no following exo-erythrocytic phases occur after the primary pre-erythrocytic liver phase, the continuing antigenic stimulus lasts only as long as recrudescences occur, and tends usually to die down after several months. The antigenic stimulus is renewed only after merozoites are released from subsequent pre-erythrocytic schizonts developed after new mosquito-borne infections.

Antigens. Acquired immunity is provoked by antigens contained in the blood stages of malaria parasites. The parasites spend most of their lives within cells of the host, first in liver cells and then in erythrocytes, from which they are set free into the plasma when the erythrocytes burst. *P. falciparum* merozoites in plasma contain soluble antigens which stimulate the production of numerous antibodies. These antigens can be found in sera of children in hyperendemic areas. Antigens are complicated, forming a mosaic with plasmodial fractions varying in solubility and enzyme composition.

These soluble antigens are present in extracts of infected erythrocytes, and in the sera of infected persons. They can be detected by double diffusion precipitation techniques. McGregor and Wilson (1971) separate them into groups:

L (labile), destroyed by heating at 56°C for 30 minutes.
R (resistant), stable at 56°C for 30 minutes.
S (stable), not destroyed at 100°C for 5 minutes.

These antigens stimulate the appropriate cells of the body to produce specific antibodies (not all protective).
The L antigens can be divided into:
La (4 antigens).
Lb (3 antigens).
Two factors are involved in acquired immunity, cellular and humoral (Leading Article, *Br. med. J.*, 1969).
The *cellular* factors are not well understood. They have been regarded as reactions mediated by actively sensitized lymphocytes such as are responsible for the rejection of grafts, but the evidence for this is inconclusive. Phagocytic activity by macrophages has long been recognized in malaria. It is probably a response to antigenic stimulus of the immunologically competent cells of the reticulo-endothelial system in the spleen and other organs, which increases the number of specifically active lymphocytes, and promotes activity by the fixed and wandering phagocytes. But phagocytosis may be stimulated by the action of malarial antibodies of IgG and IgM classes, which are known to have cytophilic properties and which can therefore promote phagocytosis of antibody-bound parasites.
Antibodies. The *humoral* factors (antibodies) are formed in response to para-

sitic antigens, and are species-specific. They are effective only against mature schizonts or free merozoites, not against intracellular forms of the parasites.

There is a close correspondence between protection against malaria and the presence of some of the antibodies, which are, in fact, regarded as the elements in the blood lethal to exposed merozoites.

Antibodies to antigen La constitute the bulk of the precipitating antibodies, and are found in the sera of almost all newborn infants in Gambia (a hyper-endemic *P. falciparum* area) where this work was done. The prevalence of these antibodies declines in later months but rises in the second year to a level of 95% at age 5–10 years, remaining high throughout life (Wilson *et al.* 1969). Antibodies to the other antigens are less common, indicating that the antigens are also less common.

It appears that antibodies to La (all in the IgG fraction of serum globulin) are probably protective. They cross the placenta from the (immune) mother's circulation, and passively protect the infant, though with diminishing effect, until the infant elaborates its own specific antibodies as a result of fresh infection with *P. falciparum*. Some antibodies may act directly on merozoites accessible to them; some may exert their known cytophilic properties to promote phago-cytosis of antibody-bound parasites. Serum antibodies appear to be the main agents in malaria immunity, but their effectiveness may depend upon a synergic action with the macrophage system (Cohen & Butcher 1971).

Immunoglobulins probably interfere with the nucleus of the parasite, pre-venting it from dividing. Although IgG seems to play the most important part, IgM probably helps, by making the parasite more acceptable to the phagocytic system of the host.

For a discussion of serological tests see diagnosis, page 64.

In *P. vivax* infection there is a rapid rise in antibody after parasites appear in the blood, but the level falls gradually when the parasites disappear, though some antibodies persist for long periods at low levels.

Antigenic variants occur, and no doubt antibody responses vary with them, but the protective antibodies to *P. falciparum* seem to be effective against different strains of the parasite. For instance, serum from immune subjects in West Africa can protect against *P. falciparum* in East Africa.

The subject is not well understood. There may be other antigens, derived from the parasites, which are either soluble but have been quickly complexed by their specific antibodies, or are relatively insoluble and therefore do not circulate for long in the body fluids.

Some soluble protein antigens, circulating in the blood, may have haemolytic properties besides their immunogenic properties, and may be responsible for the renal lesions which complicate some types of malaria.

The humoral factors (antibodies) of immunity are not dependent on comple-ment for their action. They are related to the immunoglobulins produced by the reticulo-endothelial system—IgG and IgM. The processes of immunity do not act on sporozoites, and do not, therefore, prevent superinfection. They act on the asexual blood forms and thus eventually prevent actual malarial illness. Immunity can therefore exist together with the liver stages, and even with occasional blood forms if the infection is heavy, as in the rainy season when anophelines are abundant and transmission frequent.

If the period of ill-health in childhood is successfully negotiated, a balance is achieved between infection and resistance—the stage of immune infestation or premunition. But this balance can be disturbed by intercurrent illness (especially diarrhoea and malnutrition), or long absence from the endemic area (and therefore lack of continuing antigenic stimuli), or (possibly) removal to a new endemic area and to new strains of *P. falciparum*. It can also be dramatically disturbed by splenectomy, such as for a ruptured spleen. Splenectomy abolishes acquired immunity to *P. berghei* in rats, and enables chimpanzees to be infected with *P. falciparum*, *P. vivax* and *P. ovale*, to which they are otherwise resistant. In man splenectomy may precipitate cerebral malaria in *P. falciparum* infection. The spleen is obviously a potent influence in immunity, and splenectomy can interfere with both the cellular and the humoral defence mechanisms.

Passive immunity can be induced in infants through the milk of their immune mothers, which may reflect transmission of immune substances in the milk, or may be a consequence of the deficiency in para-aminobenzoic acid (PABA) which is a known feature of milk. PABA is necessary for the full metabolism of the parasites (probably of the erythrocytic stages), and deficiency therefore inhibits them. Perhaps both factors are involved.

Autoimmune processes have been suggested as being responsible for the nephrosis observed in a minority of malaria patients.

In conditions of hyperendemicity of *P. falciparum* malaria the population has some inherited resistance, and much acquired immunity, with low blood parasite counts and low spleen rates, except in children. This leads to frequent but small sporozoite infections in the mosquitoes, because they cannot pick up enough gametocytes from the blood, except in children, to elaborate large doses. In epidemic conditions, however, the doses are much larger because the community level of parasitaemia is high, and there are many primary attacks, producing gametocytes in large numbers. Similarly, the influx into an endemic area of non-immunes, who become infected and tend to have large parasite counts, may precipitate an epidemic because the mosquitoes which bite them become heavily infected and thereafter inject large doses of sporozoites; such high doses may be enough to swamp the immunity of the local population. This swamping of immunity may explain why adult persons who live contentedly with their parasites in their own areas can react with fever if they move to other areas where sporozoite doses are heavier. Such features of the picture of immunity have been interpreted as differences in the pathogenicity or antigenic constitution of different strains of the parasites, but as McGregor *et al.* (1963) have shown, immune serum from one area (West Africa) can be effective in suppressing reactions to the parasites of another area (East Africa), and in experimental work no difference was observed between infections developed by semi-immunes when challenged with the local Liberian strain of *P. falciparum* and with strains isolated up to 250 miles away (Bray *et al.* 1962). Antigenic differences therefore may not be so great as differences in sporozoite dosages; indeed, there is a surprising degree of common antigenicity among different species of mammalian plasmodia. It should be stated, however, that in experiments with splenectomized chimpanzees and immune gamma-globulin from man taken in West Africa, Sadun *et al.* (1966) found that though the globulin protected against West African *P. falciparum* infections in the chimpanzees, it did not do so against *P. falciparum* from South-East Asia. For a discussion of this subject the reader is referred to McGregor (1965).

In experimental work on monkeys infected with *P. knowlesi* Voller and Rossan (1969) conclude that immunity to reinfection is shown by delay in the development of the infection, milder parasitaemia, or complete resistance. The immunity produced by repeated exposure to one antigenic variant is effective against challenge with heterologous variants. Populations of parasites isolated from different recrudescences of chronic *P. knowlesi* infection are antigenically distinct.

Effects of immunity

The question of immunity in malaria is not academic. The immunity gained in *P. falciparum* infections by frequent bites of infected anophelines can be partly lost if the person leaves the endemic area for a long period. Students, for instance, who come from West Africa to Europe, and stay for several years, may suffer severe attacks on return to West Africa where renewed infection takes place; it may be necessary for them to resort to chemoprophylaxis.

It is not academic in another sense because it raises the question of policy. If complete eradication of malaria is not possible, as is the case at the present time in large areas of tropical Africa, the question arises whether some degree of malaria control short of eradication should be attempted. If the numbers of infective bites are reduced to the extent that holoendemic malaria becomes mesoendemic, or if drug prophylaxis on a large scale is carried out inefficiently, or breaks down, in such an area, the resistance of adult persons is reduced, and epidemics may be expected if conditions of transmission suddenly expand, for instance as a result of excessive rainfall or other climatic change. If, on the other hand, infection is interfered with only to the extent that fever in children is treated with just enough antimalarial drugs to prevent death, and no more, and mosquito control is not attempted, their immunity is gradually built up, and epidemics do not occur. Observations in East Africa, carried out by the late D. Bagster Wilson (1936) and Margaret E. Wilson (1962) have shown that a policy of this kind is readily accepted by the population, who quickly learn to take feverish children for treatment, and the general results are reasonably favourable. It entails the setting-up of easily accessible dispensaries.

On the other hand, it has been said that if mosquito control short of eradication is attempted, by using modern insecticides, and if epidemics do occur, we have the means to deal with them. How far this is true in places where drug-resistant *P. falciparum* exists, remains to be seen.

CLINICAL FEATURES

P. falciparum MALARIA

(*Malignant Tertian, MT, Subtertian, ST*)

This is the fatal form of malaria, which can kill a non-immune person within a week or two of a primary attack unless appropriate treatment is given in time.

Pre-erythrocytic schizonts of *P. falciparum* release more merozoites than those of other species affecting man—*P. malariae* schizonts release the least. Moreover, asexual blood forms multiply to a greater extent in *P. falciparum* and in *P. vivax* than in others. *P. falciparum* therefore produces, for a given dose of sporozoites delivered by a mosquito, a far greater number of asexual blood forms than the other species, which may in part explain why it is so much the most dangerous infection. *P. malariae* is the least dangerous in this respect.

Blood volume is important. For a given dose of sporozoites the small blood volume of children means a high concentration of parasites, and children are therefore prone to heavy infection with all species. This may also be a factor in the lethality of *P. falciparum*.

P. falciparum malaria can be particularly dangerous to non-immune persons who spend short periods (even a few hours) in endemic areas, and who develop fever, with indefinite physical signs and symptoms (often diagnosed as influenza), after return to their homes in non-endemic areas, where the disease may not be suspected, and effective treatment not given. Shute and Maryon

(1969) collected records of over 2000 cases of malaria (mostly *P. falciparum*) in persons who returned to Britain after being in endemic areas; there were 58 deaths, all due to primary attacks of *P. falciparum*, mostly contracted in Africa, and all in persons who had failed to take prophylactic drugs (proguanil or pyrimethamine) for one month after arrival in Britain. There must have been others, not recognized. Death in such circumstances can be avoided by timely treatment with recognized drugs, but for this to be effective it is necessary first that the patient should inform the doctor that he or she has been in an endemic area—if the information is not given spontaneously the doctor should ask where the patient has been, and when. Secondly, the doctor should be alert to the possibility of malaria, even though the symptoms are vague, and even if the

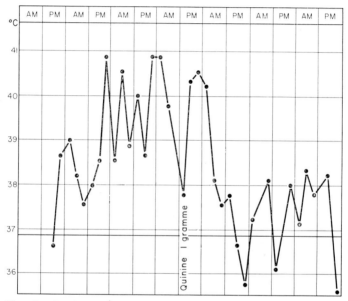

Fig. 18.—A primary aborted attack of *P. falciparum* malaria. (*Reproduced by permission of the author and Editor from Shute, P.G. (1970) Trans. R. Soc. trop. Med. Hyg., 64, 211*)

temperature does not show tertian periodicity. A doctor on his daily round may miss the rapid rise of temperature which might give a clue. The patient should also give the doctor information about the prophylactic drugs he has, or has not, taken. Blood slides taken as soon as possible can be examined at any of the hospitals for tropical diseases, or in Britain at the Malaria Reference Laboratory, Horton Hospital, Epsom, Surrey, or indeed at any hospital, but the doctor should state that he suspects malaria, because malaria has been missed in blood slides examined only for anaemia.

It is worth emphasizing also that similar reasoning applies to other tropical fevers, especially African trypanosomiasis.

These remarks on malaria are particularly relevant now that air travel is so common. It is quite usual for European schoolchildren to take their holidays with parents living in endemic areas, and schoolmasters and school doctors need to be very alert in their diagnosis of fevers in such children on return; the children may not have taken their prophylactic drugs properly. Prompt diagnosis and treatment can save life.

Primary attack. The primary attack of *P. falciparum* is the most dangerous attack. Symptoms are sometimes relatively slight in the early stages—the first

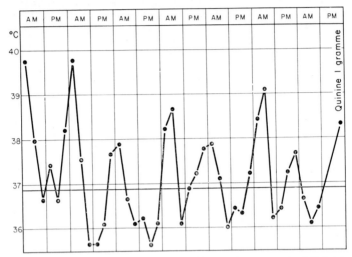

Fig. 19.—First recrudescence 10 days after a primary attack of *P. falciparum* malaria. (*Reproduced by permission of the author and Editor from Shute, P.G. (1970), Trans. R. Soc. trop. Med. Hyg.*, 64, 211)

3–4 days of such an attack are less distressing to the patient than in attacks of *P. vivax*, and the condition has often been mistaken (in non-endemic areas) for influenza. The patient may not even feel ill enough to call a doctor at first, but delay can be fatal.

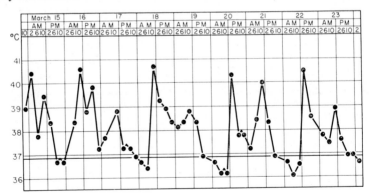

Fig. 20.—The course of the subtertian fever in *P. falciparum* malaria.

In patients from countries in which malaria is not endemic, and who therefore have no hereditary resistance, the primary attack does not at first show tertian periodicity of fever. It begins as a quotidian rise of temperature, with general malaise and a feeling of chilliness, becoming tertian a few days later.

Trophozoites are present in the blood. The pulse rate is rather slow if no treatment is given for 7 days, developing forms of the parasite, in addition to numerous trophozoites, appear in the blood, and a rigor usually occurs; the rigor, in fact, is a sign that developing forms are present, and is definitely a danger signal, indicating the need for immediate treatment. Developing forms of *P. falciparum* can be recognized by the fact that the cytoplasm never contains more than one or two pieces of pigment, whereas in the other species the forms larger than ring forms contain 20–50 individual grains (Shute 1968).

Later attacks. Later attacks of *P. falciparum* malaria are often modified by partial immunity acquired from the primary attack, but they should never be regarded lightly. Tertian periodicity of fever is more marked in later than in primary attacks, and when established, the tertian fever, like that of *P. vivax*, is accompanied by the characteristic clinical syndrome of three stages—*cold* (lasting 1–2 hours, when the patient shivers and piles on the bedclothes), *hot* (lasting 3–4 hours, when the patient's temperature is high, his skin dry, and he throws off the bedclothes) and *sweating* (lasting 2–4 hours, when the patient and his bedclothes are soaked in sweat and the temperature falls rapidly, to leave the patient relieved but exhausted). These three stages constitute the well known 'ague', which occurs on alternate days in accordance with the cycle of the parasite. The patient feels very miserable.

A double infection, with some parasites maturing on days 1, 3, 5 etc., and some on days 2, 4, 6 etc., may show daily rise of temperature (quotidian fever), but this is not common. Nevertheless, it should be remembered that malaria is not always tertian or quartan.

P. falciparum malaria is a very variable disease, mimicking many other conditions, and taking several forms which may be misleading. The parasites from various areas also vary in virulence.

Other forms of *P. falciparum* **malaria.** The forms of *P. falciparum* malaria, other than the classical form described above, are as follows:

Pernicious attacks, which usually carry high numbers of parasites in the peripheral blood, and high death rates. Parasitaemia of 100 000 parasites or more per mm³ of blood may result in death rates of about 20%. These attacks may be cerebral, with hyperpyrexia to 41·6°C (107°F) or more, and 5% or more of erythrocytes infected, some with more than a single parasite. The patient may very quickly go into low delirium or coma, with general muscular twitching, disorientation, aphasia or incontinence. Changes in behaviour, such as insolence or insubordination, may occur in the early stages, and excitement, mania and coma may follow. There may be epileptiform attacks, or signs of meningitis, or even seizures resembling apoplexy, and various forms of acute insanity may develop from damage to the brain. This syndrome has been misdiagnosed as encephalitis, with disastrous results because antimalarial treatment was not given. Differential diagnosis from heat hyperpyrexia may be difficult, and blood examination may not help in the early stages if parasites are scanty; it should be repeated daily if they are not found at first. Indeed, an attack of malaria or other fever may precipitate hyperpyrexia. Enlargement of the spleen would suggest malaria, though it is by no means always palpable in early infections. In later stages it can become enlarged and painful during the attack.

The cerebrospinal fluid is under pressure, with increase in lymphocytes and protein.

Algid malaria may result from an overwhelming infection, with collapse and peripheral vascular failure, possibly the result of acute adrenal failure. The surface of the body is cold and the temperature falls rapidly to below normal.

Blood pressure also falls alarmingly, and coma sets in, followed by death within a few hours. Developing forms of *P. falciparum* are often present in the peripheral blood.

Bilious remittent malaria, with vomiting, gastric distress and an icteric tint in the skin and conjunctivae, has been observed, and in an endemic area jaundice, indicating hepatic failure, should call for examination of the blood for malaria parasites as well as examinations for other forms of jaundice.

Other forms of *P. falciparum* malaria may lead to haemolytic anaemia, general anasarca, nephritis and haemorrhagic complications.

Mild renal failure can occur in heavy *P. falciparum* infection, and is associated with low urinary sodium, decreased clearance of para-aminohippurate and creatinine and high blood urea. There is focal vacuolization of the proximal tubules, but tubular reabsorbtion of water is maintained; the glomeruli are normal. In one series function returned to normal after treatment with intravenous and oral quinine. It is important not to overload such patients with parenteral fluids (Sitprija *et al.* 1967).

Splenic rupture, through causing severe internal haemorrhage, may produce misleading symptoms which may mimic those of rupture of the bladder by causing urinary irritability and hypogastric pain. There is often a latent period with absence of symptoms. Referred pain to the tip of the left shoulder is present in a small proportion of cases. Changes in the left lung base may serve as an aid to diagnosis. The histopathology of these friable spleens shows that a subcapsular haematoma precedes rupture and leads to capsular tear. In acute malaria small haemorrhages occur in the vicinity of the capsule or deep in the tissues. There is diffuse cellular hyperplasia, with dilated sinuses, and occasional thrombosis and infarction.

Spontaneous rupture of the chronically enlarged spleen is very rare. It may be, however, found in acute malaria in a primary attack. It is more common in therapeutic malaria, having regard to the age of the patient and the entire lack of immunity. Splenic rupture has been recorded also in portal thrombosis, torsion of the splenic pedicle, in kala-azar, acute infective hepatitis, bacterial endocarditis, splenic abscess, leukaemia, erythroblastosis fetalis, and aneurysm of the splenic artery (Covell 1955).

Recrudescence. Recrudescences occur mostly for up to 1 year and rarely up to 4 years after infection, but after the first pre-erythrocyte liver schizont there are no subsequent liver forms, and relapses characteristic of *P. vivax* and *P. malariae* are not found in infections with *P. falciparum*.

In children in hyperendemic areas the constant reinfection with *P. falciparum* tends to underlie episodes of pyrexia and diarrhoea; it is complicated by respiratory, intestinal and septic infections and malnutrition, and it leads to anaemia and therefore possibly to oedema.

MIXED INFECTIONS

Double infections with *P. vivax* and *P. falciparum* are common and may give rise to some confusion, especially when the ring (or trophozoite) stages of both parasites are present in the blood at the same time. More usually *P. vivax* is superimposed upon *P. falciparum*, so that the patient runs through the average course of the latter, and when he has apparently recovered, relapses of *P. vivax* make their appearance. This late appearance, it may be after a lapse of six months or even a year, was commonly observed in soldiers infected in war zones in both 1914–8 and in the Second World War in India and Burma (1943–5). In the endemic area of quartan malaria—for instance in S. Ceylon and Malaya—double infections with *P. vivax* and *P. malariae* are quite common, and in these cases the latter parasite survives longer.

SEQUELAE OF CHRONIC MALARIA

The term *malarial cachexia* is applied to a group of physical signs of a chronic nature the result of antecedent attacks of severe malaria where malaria is unstable and immunity is poor. The leading signs are those of anaemia, with a peculiar sallow tinting of the skin, yellow sclerotics, enlargement of the spleen and usually the liver as well. In children, the growth of the body is stunted and puberty retarded. Abortion and sterility are common effects of malarial cachexia in adult women.

Liver and gall-bladder. Chronic hepatomegaly is a not infrequent sequel of malaria, and hepatic congestion may gradually become more or less permanent. *Siderosis* is produced from chemical changes in the liver undergone by *haemosiderin.* Together with this there may be chronic engorgement of the gall-bladder, which predisposes to cholecystitis and cholelithiasis.

It has been said that stress will provoke attacks of fever in persons with latent *P. falciparum* infection, but Bruce-Chwatt (1963) failed to provoke relapses in West African volunteers by intravenous adrenaline, or by subjecting them to physical stress at high temperatures, or by giving electroconvulsive therapy to patients in a mental hospital who were suffering from chronic malaria.

P. vivax MALARIA
(*Benign Tertian, BT*)

The incubation period is usually 12–20 days, but in certain conditions (particularly with European strains) a long incubation or latent period of about 38 weeks has often been observed. The mechanism controlling this is obscure, and the several theories to explain it are unsatisfactory (Garnham 1966). Long-term relapses also occur, and are probably governed by the same conditions as the long incubation periods. Shute and Maryon (1968) think that the numbers of sporozoites injected by mosquitoes bear a relation to the incubation—if few

Table 1. Distribution of *P. vivax* Types I, II, and III, and characteristic patterns of infection

Type	Incubation period	Prolonged latency	Relapses	Names of strains	Reported distribution	Transmission
I	Short, 12–20 days	No	Frequent, at short intervals	Chesson	New Guinea Vietnam W. Malaysia	Perennial
II	Short, 12–20 days	Yes, 7–13 months	After one or more periods of prolonged latency	St Elizabeth Madagascar Nakhitchevan Volgograd	U.S.A.* U.S.S.R.* Bulgaria* Italy* Romania* Yugoslavia* Madagascar	Seasonal
III	Long, 6–9 months	Yes, 7–13 months	After delayed primary attack or subsequent prolonged latency	Kolomenski Navoflominski	Netherlands* Sweden* Finland* U.S.S.R.*	Seasonal

* With the recent recession of the range of *P. vivax*, strains of Types II and III have disappeared from all these areas (WHO 1969a).

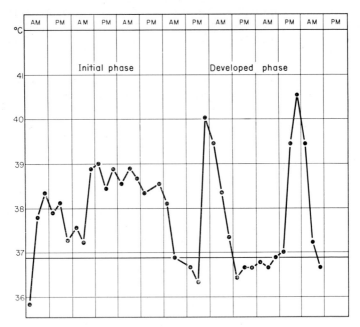

Fig. 21.—Initial phase and developed phase of *P. vivax* malaria. (*Repro-duced by permission of the author and Editor from Shute, P.G. (1970), Trans. R. Soc. trop. Med. Hyg., 64, 211*)

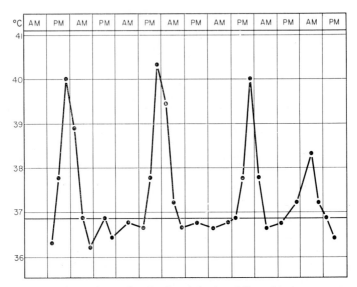

Fig. 22.—First relapse after *P. vivax* infection, followed by spontaneous recovery. (*Reproduced by permission of the author and Editor from Shute, P.G. (1970), Trans. R. Soc. trop. Med. Hyg., 64, 211*)

are injected (for instance in the autumn when the mosquitoes have almost exhausted their store of sporozoites) the period is likely to be long, and vice versa. Whatever the mechanism, the result is that an infection contracted in the autumn may not result in parasitaemia until the following spring, when the hibernating anophelines become active in time to pick up the infection and pass it on. A long latent period may also occur after insufficient chemoprophylaxis.

The various types and patterns of infection are shown in Table 1.

After the incubation period the infected person becomes ill with malaise and a temperature which may reach 40°C (104°F) or more. The malaise is often more severe than in *P. falciparum* infection. The temperature does not at first assume tertian periodicity, but this becomes marked within a week or so. Exceptionally a double infection can give persistent quotidian fever. When tertian periodicity is established the phases of cold, hot and sweating occur.

P. vivax infection can relapse for as long as 8 years, which means that the liver cycle can be repeated, with intervals in which parasitaemia cannot be detected, for that length of time. Although virulent strains of *P. vivax* have been reported by Russian workers, benign tertian malaria is not usually a killing disease.

P. ovale MALARIA
(*Ovale Tertian*)

This has been regarded as a relatively mild form of benign tertian, and this is usually so, though some of those who have contracted it have experienced quite as much distress as with *P. vivax*. Like the latter it is not a killing disease.

It is said not to relapse, and although there is evidence that second exo-erythrocytic generations do occur in the liver phase, the evidence for the occurrence of successive generations is not complete and should not be assumed (Garnham 1966). Latent periods of up to 4 years have been recorded (Chin & Contacos 1966).

P. malariae MALARIA
(*Quartan*)

The clinical feature of this infection (in the absence of multiple infections) is that the paroxysms of fever occur every fourth day. The incubation period can be as short as 15 days, corresponding with the length of the pre-erythrocytic cycle. Nothing is known about subsequent exo-erythrocytic cycles, but it is well known that blood forms can be present for many years in subjects who show no clinical signs of the infection, and that relapses can occur up to 32 (or even 53) years after infection (Garnham 1966) in people who have lived for that length of time out of the reach of reinfection. Parasitaemia can perhaps persist for life, and has been demonstrated many times in the blood of donors for transfusion who have apparently been quite well.

In general the attacks are not severe, and *P. malariae* is not a killing species. Parasites in the blood are scanty. But this infection is prone to cause nephrosis, probably owing to granular immune complexes deposited in the renal glomeruli. Kibukamusoke and Voller (1970) find that IgM levels are particularly high in patients with active nephrosis, and are associated with high malarial antibody titres.

Nephrosis has been particularly reported in Guyana, East Africa, and West Africa, where the quartan parasite is relatively common. It may not be common in some quartan areas (for instance Northern Nigeria), however, possibly because some other factor is involved (Dodge 1966). Peak incidence is at age 4–5 years, and the prognosis is poor. There is gross oedema and ascites, massive proteinuria and severe hypoproteinaemia (low plasma albumin), usually without azotaemia or hypertension. Antimalarial treatment is not helpful (Gilles & Hendrickse 1963), but treatment with a low-salt diet containing a high content of protein, and diuretics and potassium supplements if indicated, should be tried. Steroids do not help (Gilles 1968).

Quartan malaria may cause chronic ill-health, with recurrent attacks of fever, malaise, headaches, lassitude and sweating. In a series of non-African patients in Uganda the indirect fluorescent antibody test on the patients' sera, with thin

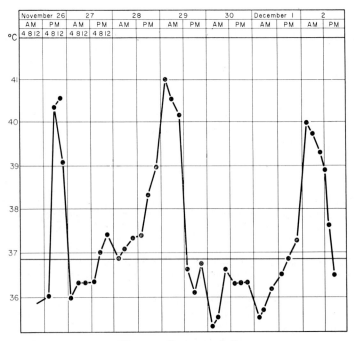

Fig. 23.—Quartan malaria.

blood films heavily infected with *P. malariae* as antigen, was strongly positive (1 : 1600 to 1 : 6400), and treatment with chloroquine and primaquine relieved the condition even though the parasites could not be demonstrated in the patient's blood. The titres of the fluorescent test also declined strongly (Wilks *et al.* 1965).

MALARIA IN CHILDREN

P. falciparum MALARIA

P. falciparum is usually very severe in children from non-endemic areas; diagnosis may be difficult, for parasites may not be found easily, and multiple blood films should be taken if the first are negative. Routine examination of thick films for 3 minutes is inadequate to detect light infections. Many gametocytes are lost from thick films; a better stain technique is needed (Dowling & Shute 1966). The incubation period is 8–15 days and there are no distinctive signs. The child is listless, restless and drowsy; he refuses food; there may be headache or nausea. Fever is usual, but variable and irregular, and tertian periodicity is uncommon. There may be diarrhoea, and an unproductive cough is common.

The spleen enlarges and is tender, but diagnosis should not depend on this. There may be infarction and perisplenitis, and rupture is possible. The liver is often large and tender, with jaundice in severe cases. Anaemia and leucopenia are variable. Herpes labialis may occur.

In the blood *P. falciparum* rings may be seen in up to 20% of red cells, though they may be difficult to find at first, and gametocytes appear after about a week, to persist for 2–3 months after cure.

P. falciparum infection is always serious, and in children this is especially true. Spontaneous clinical cure has been reported, but it is rare (except in children from endemic areas) and treatment is always urgently indicated. Recrudescence is unusual after 2 years if the child leaves the endemic area.

Complications

Anaemia is common; it is normocytic and may be severe with haemoglobin down to 5 grammes/100 ml. Haemozoin is found in polymorphs and monocytes. Transfusion of packed erythrocytes may be needed.

Cerebral malaria. In the seasonal malaria of the Dakar region, malaria in African children is a neurological illness, which kills quickly if at all (Armengaud et al. 1962). Headache, convulsions or coma are common, and there may be hepatomegaly, diarrhoea and vomiting. Bacterial and viral infection of the central nervous system must be excluded. Malnutrition is important. The mortality may reach nearly 50% (Sagnet et al. 1967). In expatriate children the disease is always most serious.

Hyperpyrexia often occurs with cerebral malaria, and it is important to reduce the temperature by methods similar to those used in heat hyperpyrexia.

Gastro-intestinal symptoms. Vomiting and diarrhoea may resemble dysentery or cholera, or the disease may mimic appendicitis. There may be jaundice indicating liver failure. Parenteral fluids may be needed, and chlorpromazine to control vomiting.

Algid malaria. There is a state of medical shock, with coma. Diastolic pressure is low, and the condition resembles acute adrenal insufficiency. Treatment is by rapid expansion of blood volume with dextran, plasma or glucose saline. Corticosteroids may be used, hydrocortisone sodium succinate 50 mg every 8 hours during the crisis, and if there is no response, noradrenaline or mephentermine may be given. Antimalarials may be given by gastric tube.

Diagnosis

This entails finding the parasites, but malaria (and trypanosomiasis) should be suspected in a sick child who has been exposed to the infection, even if supposed to have taken prophylactic drugs, in which case symptoms may not be characteristic of malaria.

P. vivax MALARIA

The incubation period is 10–15 days as a rule, but may be many months. Fever is at first remittent, going on to intermittent tertian paroxysms, with cold, hot and rarely sweating phases in children. Convulsions may occur if the fever is high, and relapses can occur after variable periods up to about 5 years. Usually about 2% of the red cells are infected.

QUARTAN MALARIA

Incubation is 10–30 days, or considerably longer. Usually less than 1% of red cells are infected. It may persist for up to 30 years.

The *nephrotic syndrome* is associated with this infection in children, though it may not be common in areas where quartan malaria occurs, possibly because some other factor—perhaps malnutrition—is involved.

For the treatment of malaria in children, see page 73.

DIAGNOSIS

Diagnosis entails recognition of the species of malaria parasites in the blood or sternal marrow. Details of staining, and the characters of the various species are given on page 948. In clinical malaria (except possibly *P. malariae* infection) examination of thin blood films is usually enough. Erythrocytes are intact and can show stippling, which helps to distinguish species, though Maurer's dots do not appear in primary *P. falciparum* infection, but only in recrudescences when the parasites may be relatively large (Shute & Maryon 1969). In *P. falciparum* infections a high proportion of red cells may contain parasites, and when 30% do so, recovery becomes unusual. In *P. vivax* infection parasites are never found in more than 2% of red cells.

For differentiation of species thin films stained with Leishman or Giemsa stain are excellent, the parasites being found most easily at the edges of the film rather than in the middle. For detecting scanty parasites, thick drops stained with Giemsa or Field stain are commonly used, but there is considerably more loss of parasites into the staining fluid from thick drops than from thin films.

Diagnosis by sternal puncture. For this a sternal puncture needle is unnecessary, and a stout truncated lumbar puncture needle can be used. It is inserted vertically at the centre of the sternum at the level of the second inter-costal space and pressed firmly through the cortex. Resistance decreases as the marrow is entered. Thick drop preparations can be made, and the fluid contains more parasites than the peripheral blood.

Serological tests. Malarial antibodies persist in blood for months or years after infection, tending to die away if no reinfection takes places. By measuring them the progression or regression of immunity can be assessed, though some of the antibodies measured appear to have no protective function; they can perhaps be regarded as pointers.

Several serological tests are useful in malaria, largely for survey or research work (Voller 1971), but also to detect infection in subjects in whom parasites are difficult to find, for instance in blood donors. They are sometimes useful in clinical diagnosis.

The oldest is *Henry's melanin flocculation test*, which detects abnormally high serum globulins; it is positive in several other conditions such as trypano-somiasis, leishmaniasis, hepatitis and others, and is therefore not specific for malaria, but it still has its uses.

The *complement fixation test* in one study in a hyperendemic area gave 98% results in children under 12 years, whether parasites were found or not. In adults with parasites the results were similar to those in children, but in adults in whom parasites were not found results were positive in only 10%. It does not measure protective capacity, and may give false positive reactions.

The *passive haemagglutination test* tends to be positive in unprotected adults, and the mean titres increase with age. In protected populations the mean titres and the positive results are lower, perhaps indicating recent but not current infections.

Infected erythrocytes are agglutinated by homologous antiserum, but *P. falciparum* is the only malaria parasite of man to produce enough infected erythrocytes for this test, and such cells tend to agglutinate spontaneously. Gametocytes, which are to some extent antigenic, do not seem to be affected, and therefore escape destruction by antibodies.

Injection of inactivated sporozoites leads to high sporozoite agglutination titres and to protection against challenge by sporozoites, and this may possibly form the basis of a vaccine.

Immunofluorescence. The function of the fluorescent dye used in this test is to unite (conjugate) in a stable association with the gamma-globulins of the serum to be tested. If the globulins contain antibodies to malaria parasites, they will adhere to the relevant malaria parasites when the conjugated serum is applied to a positive thin smear, and remain after washing, so that the parasites stand out as glistening particles under ultra-violet light, easily recognized under the fluorescence microscope. This indicates that the serum contains antibody, and is therefore positive. This is the *direct* technique.

Alternatively, by the *indirect* technique, a suspected serum (or dilution) can be flooded on to a slide having a thin positive blood smear. If the relevant antibody is present in the serum, it will adhere to the malaria parasites, and will not wash off. If then, after washing, the slide is treated with an antibody prepared (in an animal) against human serum and conjugated with the fluorescent dye, this second antibody will unite with its own antigen (the human serum containing malaria antibody) and will fluoresce with that antibody and with the malaria parasites to which it adheres, in ultra-violet light under the fluorescence microscope. This result indicates that the test serum is positive. This test, carried out on a large number of people in an area, can be taken to measure the malaria experience of the population; titres remain high for long periods, and this experience determines the development of effective immunity (Voller 1971). Serological tests measure recent and past experience of malaria, and in this have an advantage over the examination of single blood smears. It is not suggested, however, that they should replace the ordinary blood examination for clinical purposes; serological tests have a different function.

The *gel precipitation test* with an antigen from *P. falciparum* has been found positive in 86% of people in a hyperendemic area. Incidence is high at birth, to fall during the next 2 months and then increase to 89% at age 5, and 94% in adult life.

Most of these tests are adequate for the recognition of existing or latent infection, but only the fluorescent antibody test and the passive haemagglutination test with purified antigen can distinguish between the species of parasites concerned.

The techniques for these tests are complicated. Details are given by Garnham (1966), and an evaluation is given by WHO (1968b).

GENERAL TREATMENT OF MALARIA

In all forms, but especially in *P. falciparum* malaria, the usual antimalarial drugs must be given as soon as diagnosis is made. Even when *P. falciparum* is only suspected, and before the result of blood examination is received, if the patient is very ill the antimalarial drugs are indicated.

The following general treatments are also indicated.

For medical shock or dehydration, intravenous fluids may be needed. If there is gross anaemia, or if the haematocrit falls below 30%, blood transfusion may save life, but both the red cells and plasma of donor and recipient should first be cross-matched.

In cerebral malaria there may be extensive intravascular coagulation, and if the blood of a child clots abnormally quickly—within 1 minute—or if the blood cannot clot (owing to consumption of fibrinogen by intravascular coagulation), treatment with heparin should be considered, in doses of 250 units per kg, which may be added to 150–500 ml of 5% glucose or istonic saline solution, given as a continuous drip during 12 hours.

In cerebral malaria dexamethasone may be given intravenously with the idea of reducing cerebral oedema; Woodruff and Dickinson (1968) gave an initial dose of 10 mg to a comatose adult with *P. falciparum* infection (cleared by chloroquine intravenous drip), with dramatic result. They followed this with 2 injections each of 4 mg within the next 24 hours. In Vietnam dexamethasone is the standard treatment of cerebral malaria, with intravenous quinine, and dexamethasone is given (4–6 mg every 4–6 hours for up to 3 days) in other cases of *P. falciparum* malaria if no contra-indication exists, and in this way severe haemolysis, cerebral malaria, renal and pulmonary complications may be prevented or rapidly reversed (Oriscello 1968). It had been suggested that diuretics such as frusemide might reduce cerebral oedema, and that the action of dexamethasone might be due to counteracting presumable adrenal insufficiency, or even to cerebral stimulation (Hardy 1968).

For hyperpyrexia the patient may be cooled with a wet sheet and vigorous fanning, or even with ice packs, but cooling must be stopped when the rectal temperature falls to 39°C (102°F), otherwise it may fall to dangerous levels.

Cerebral malaria is an emergency, and once coma sets in, deterioration is very rapid, and the patient may die before intravenous drips can be set up. In such cases intravenous quinine, 650 mg in 10 ml distilled water should be given slowly during 10 minutes. Immediately after this 1 ml of 1 in 10 000 adrenaline should be given intramuscularly, during 5 minutes. This helps to resuscitate a collapsed patient, and has an effect on cerebral oedema (Patrick 1968).

To sum up, the dangers from *P. falciparum* malaria, especially in primary attacks, are: cerebral malaria leading to coma, impaired kidney function, and pulmonary oedema; as explained above (Pathology) there tends to be capillary stasis with damage to capillary walls, loss of fluid into the surrounding tissues, agglutination of red cells, and progressive anoxia.

To meet these conditions measures advocated by Smitskamp and Wolthuis (1971) include:

Quinine by slow intravenous injection, 1 to 2 grammes in 5% glucose solution every 24 hours.

Dexamethasone, 24 mg every 24 hours, or *prednisolone* 100 mg every 24 hours. These inhibit many inflammatory phenomena and their value in reducing cerebral oedema is established.

Low molecular weight dextran, 500 mg intravenously every 24 hours. This has an antithrombotic action and tends to prevent aggregation of erythrocytes. Dextran 40 Injection (BP) is a sterile 10% w/v solution in 5% dextrose or 0·9% sodium chloride; molecular weight about 40 000.

Heparin, 50 mg every 6 hours for at least 48 hours; this has an antithrombotic effect and may have a direct antimalarial action.

Urea, 45 grammes slowly in a single dose intravenously as a diuretic, which can be life-saving, but must not be given if kidney function is impaired.

Fluid and electrolyte balance must be rigidly maintained throughout.

Changes in this regimen must obviously be made in the light of the condition of the patient.

Maegraith (1969) considers that the life-saving effects of quinine and chloroquine are due to their pharmacological activities as anti-inflammatory compounds, and not to their antiparasitic properties. They rapidly and completely inhibit the leakage of proteins and water from the brain capillaries.

Acute renal failure may occur, more commonly than is thought, in *P. falciparum* malaria. The clinical features (confusion, restlessness, incoherence, jaundice and fever) could be mistaken for cerebral malaria, but measurements of the volume and specific gravity of the urine (below 1016) and estimation of plasma urea (progressively rising above 100 mg/100 ml) or serum urea concentration (Urastrat method) give the diagnosis. In this event lives could be saved by peritoneal dialysis (Reid *et al.* 1967). After a local anaesthetic in the lower central abdominal wall, 2 litres of fluid (for adults) or 70–100 ml/kg (for children) can be introduced through a large-bore needle, which should then be withdrawn and replaced by a catheter with cut lateral holes. The fluid contains:

Sodium lactate	0·5%
Sodium chloride	0·56%
Magnesium chloride	0·015%
Calcium chloride	0·039%
Dextrose	1·36%

and hourly exchanges of 1 litre should be made during the daytime only. Potassium chloride (250 mg) may be added to each litre if the serum potassium falls below 3·5 mEq/litre. Salt should be restricted, but a diet of normal protein and calorie value should be given. Another formula is:

Sodium acetate hydrate	0·47%
Sodium chloride	0·5%
Calcium chloride	0·032%
Magnesium chloride	0·015%
Anhydrous dextrose	1·7%

Sodium acetate seems to prevent bacterial peritonitis better than sodium lactate.

Dialysis should be continued well into the diuretic phase and until plasma urea is very considerably reduced. This treatment is possible in tropical hospitals.

Dialysis will probably be needed if the electrocardiogram records tall, narrow T-waves or other evidence of hyperkalaemia. It should also be started promptly if there are signs of overhydration such as increased breathlessness, basal crepitations and abnormal distension of the neck veins. A hypertonic dialysis fluid is highly effective in removing excess fluid.

During convalescence, anaemia may call for folic acid or iron, or for appropriate diet if the patient is malnourished.

DRUG TREATMENT OF MALARIA

Except where otherwise stated, the doses given are for non-immune adults; for children they must be scaled down. For immune or partly immune patients, in whom the disease has broken through, the first few doses are usually enough.

The treatment of acute attacks of all forms of malaria is the same in regard to the elimination of blood schizonts, but for *P. vivax*, *P. ovale* and quartan malaria the addition of an 8-aminoquinoline compound to the usual 4-amino-quinolines is advisable. The 8-aminoquinolines act on exo-erythrocytic schizonts, the 4-aminoquinolines do not. But the 8-aminoquinolines have little action on the asexual blood forms, and should not be relied upon to cure attacks if used alone.

Antimalarial drugs act on different phases of malaria parasites (Table 2).

Table 2. Action of antimalarial drugs on different phases of malaria parasites

Drug	Asexual blood parasites	Gametocytes	Tissue parasites	Sporozoites
Quinine	+ +	−†	−	−
4-Aminoquinolines (chloroquine, amodiaquine, mepacrine)	+ +	−*	−	−
8-Aminoquinolines (e.g. primaquine)	±	+	+ +	−
Dihydrofolic reductase inhibitors (proguanil, chlorproguanil, pyrimethamine, trimethoprim)	+	+	+	−
Sulphonamides and sulphones	+	+	?	−

Adapted from HMSO (1968).
* WHO (1969) Scientific Group state that the 4-aminoquinolines have action on gametocytes of *P. vivax*, *P. ovale* and *P. malariae*, but not *P. falciparum;* such action is less than that of the 8-aminoquinolines.
† See text.

Quinine dihydrochloride or bisulphate

Quinine is being called for more frequently now that strains of *P. falciparum* resistant to chloroquine and other drugs are being found. It is active against asexual blood forms, but has no action on mature gametocytes of *P. falciparum*, though it is effective against gametocytes of *P. vivax* and *P. malariae* (WHO 1967). It is particularly useful in cerebral or other dangerous forms of malaria where rapid clearance of the blood is urgently needed, though its important action, like that of chloroquine and the corticosteroids, in cerebral malaria, is anti-inflammatory, reversing the leakage of protein and water from the small vessels and restoring the circulation.

For adults the oral dose is 650 mg 3 times daily for 10–14 days. It may be combined with pyrimethamine 50–75 mg daily for the first 3 days, and this considerably reduces the proportion of recrudescences of *P. falciparum* in South-east Asia. Dapsone (25 mg daily) has been added to this régime with satisfactory results (WHO 1967).

For children the doses of quinine may be:

Under 1 year	162 mg twice daily
1–3 years	162 mg 3 times daily
4–6 years	325 mg twice daily
7–10 years	325 mg 3 times daily

Quinine dihydrochloride can be given in emergencies by slow intravenous injection of 500–650 mg (adult dose) in 15–20 ml saline or distilled water sterilized by heat. A large syringe and a fine needle should be used, and the injection should take 10 minutes. It may also be given by intravenous drip in 500 ml saline.

Quinine may also be given by deep intramuscular injection into the buttock, the dose being 500–650 mg in 10 ml of pyrogen-free sterile distilled water or saline. But intramuscular quinine tends to destroy muscle fibres, and strict sterility is necessary.

In acute attacks of *P. falciparum* malaria resistant to chloroquine, oral quinine 650 mg every 8 hours for 14 days, together with oral colchicine 0·5 mg every 2 hours for 10 doses on the first day and 0·5 mg twice on the second day, has shown considerably more activity than quinine alone (Reba & Sheehy 1967). Colchicine was chosen because of its known anti-enzyme and antimitotic activity; it is able to penetrate red cells, and has some schizontocidal activity.

4-Aminoquinolines

Chloroquine has a strong action on erythrocytic, asexual parasites of all species, and is the drug of choice for acute attacks. It becomes highly concentrated in liver cells and in parasitized erythrocytes within a few minutes of administration (Peters 1967). It has no action on mature gametocytes of *P. falciparum*, but does act against those of *P. vivax*, *P. ovale* and *P. malariae*. Chloroquine phosphate (Aralen, Avloclor, Resochin) is given by mouth in a first (immediate) dose of 600 mg of base (1000 mg salt); or chloroquine sulphate (Nivaquine) in a dose of 600 mg base (800 mg salt). This first dose is usually enough to end a mild attack of *P. falciparum* malaria in partly immune persons. In others it should be followed in 6 hours by 300 mg base, and then by 300 mg base daily for 2–4 days (occasionally more). The total dose is 1500–2400 mg base. If vomiting prevents absorption, chloroquine sulphate can be given in suppositories of 150 or 300 mg base; the rectal dose is 2 or 3 times the oral dose.

Chloroquine can also be given intravenously or intramuscularly in doses of 200–300 mg base; the injections should be made slowly (especially the intravenous injection, which should be in very dilute solution). Parenteral administration can be dangerous in children (see below).

If fever or parasitaemia persists, or if there is no clinical response after 72 hours, the diagnosis should be reviewed, or chloroquine-resistant strains of parasites should be suspected.

Weekly administration of 300–600 mg chloroquine base, orally for 4–8 weeks, may prevent recrudescence of *P. falciparum*.

Strains of *P. falciparum* resistant to chloroquine are increasingly being reported from South-east Asia and the Americas, and resistance to chloroquine is usually accompanied by resistance to other 4-aminoquinolines such as amodiaquine. For such strains other drugs, notably quinine, are being used, with the consequent risk of blackwater fever.

A schedule used in the American Army in Vietnam, for *P. falciparum* infections resistant to chloroquine, is: quinine salt 650 mg every 8 hours for 10–14 days; pyrimethamine 25 mg twice daily for 3 days. For patients with severe symptoms 650 mg quinine salt in 1 litre of 5% dextrose solution are given as an intravenous drip over 8 hours, repeated every 8 hours if necessary. Routine chemoprophylaxis (chloroquine 300 mg base, primaquine 45 mg base, once each week; dapsone 25 mg daily) was continued during treatment.

Resistance to chloroquine has not been reported in *P. vivax*, *P. ovale* or *P. malariae*.

Amodiaquine hydrochloride (Camoquin) should be given in a dose of 600 mg base (783 mg salt) immediately, followed by 400–600 mg base daily for 2 days, to a total dose of 1400–2400 mg base. If there is no response, the diagnosis should be reviewed, or resistant parasites suspected. The use of amodiaquine has not been stressed recently, reliance being placed on chloroquine.

Agranulocytosis coinciding with treatment with amodiaquine was reported in 5 cases in Papua (Booth *et al.* 1967).

Other 4-aminoquinolines being investigated include those numbered 12 278 RP, 14 153 RP, 16 126 RP. 14 153 RP given once each month appears to be rather more effective than chloroquine or 16 126 RP in suppressing *P. falciparum* parasitaemia (WHO 1967).

8-Aminoquinolines

These are used because, unlike the 4-aminoquinolines and quinine, they act on the primary tissue stages of *P. falciparum* and *P. vivax*, and the secondary exo-erythrocytic forms of *P. vivax*. They have little action on the asexual blood forms, but are used to produce radical cure after, or combined with, treatment of an attack of *P. vivax*, *P. ovale* or quartan malaria with chloroquine or other schizontocide. By virtue of their action on pre-erythrocytic schizonts of *P. falciparum* they may also help the rapid elimination of that phase. They also act on gametocytes (WHO 1967).

The earliest drug of this series was pamaquin (plasmoquine) given in doses of 10–20 mg, but this has now been superseded by primaquine phosphate, of which the dose is 13 mg (7·5 mg base) twice daily for 10–14 days. Some strains of *P. vivax* respond to shorter courses; some need higher doses. It acts chiefly on gametocytes and exo-erythrocytic schizonts.

Both pamaquin and primaquine should be used with caution. They are both potentially toxic, especially in persons with deficiency in glucose-6-phosphate dehydrogenase, in whom they may precipitate methaemoglobinaemia or acute haemolysis. This deficiency is particularly common in Africa and South-east Asia, but is also found in India and the Middle East.

To attempt radical cure while the patient remains in an endemic area where reinfection takes place seems to be pointless; it should be postponed until the patient leaves the area, and can then be useful in preventing relapses.

Acridines

The most notable acridine compound in relation to malaria is mepacrine (Atebrin, Quinacrine). It is little used at present, but was a powerful substitute for quinine in the war of 1939–45 both for treatment and prophylaxis. It is highly concentrated in liver cells and leucocytes. It has little action on strains of *P. falciparum* resistant to chloroquine (WHO 1967), and it has no action on gametocytes.

For treatment the adult dose is up to 900 mg in divided doses on the first day, 600 mg on the second day, and then 300 mg daily for 5 days. In doses of 50–200 mg it is well tolerated by children.

It is a potent prophylactic in a dose of 100 mg daily, and during the war, when it was used under discipline in this way, blackwater fever practically disappeared. It stains the skin yellow, and continued use may produce skin lesions resembling lichen planus, or cerebral excitement resembling schizophrenia.

Sulphonamides

Sulphadiazine has some antimalarial action, but is not a rapid schizontocide. In a pyrimethamine-resistant *P. falciparum* infection in an African child, 12·5 mg pyrimethamine with 1 gramme sulphadiazine, repeated after 24 hours, eliminated the parasites from the blood (McGregor *et al.* 1963), and this suggests a potentiating effect which has been studied more extensively in volunteers, and may be important.

The long-acting sulphonamide sulphormethoxine (sulphadoxine, Fanasil) can clear asexual *P. falciparum* from the blood, and is useful where chloroquine resistance is found. It gives high and early blood concentration and is excreted very slowly. In a single dose of 1 gramme in adults with pyrexia, possibly with 50 mg pyrimethamine, it may produce a radical cure, but a single dose of 1·5 grammes has been only partly effective in chloroquine-resistant *P. falciparum* infection. As little as 0·5 gramme once each week may be enough for African children with asymptomatic infections (WHO 1967).

Sulphadimethoxine (Madribon) and sulphamethoxypyridazine (Midicel) have apparently similar actions in semi-immune Bantu children (Clyde 1967).

A pyrimidine derivative (trimethoprim, a dihydrofolate reductase inhibitor), in combination with sulphalene (a long-acting sulphonamide) is useful in a single dose of 500 mg trimethoprim with 750 mg sulphalene, for chloroquine-resistant *P. falciparum* infection. There is probably a potentiating action between them.

Resistance to the sulphonamides has been reported in strains of *P. falciparum* in Africa (Bruce-Chwatt 1970).

Sulphones

Dapsone (DDS, diaphenylsulphone), the standard drug for the treatment of leprosy, has substantial schizontocidal activity against strains of *P. falciparum*, including some which are resistant to chloroquine. In a single oral dose of 200 mg it has been found useful in semi-immune subjects, but it is not a rapid schizontocide. Relatively small doses (25 or 50 mg) had a substantial effect in preventing patent infection with 2 strains of chloroquine- and pyrimethamine-resistant *P. falciparum* in volunteers; it was also effective in daily doses of 25 mg together with weekly chloroquine and primaquine (WHO 1967). Laing (1965) states that dapsone has no action on gametocytes.

It acts on asexual *P. malariae*, but not *P. vivax*. Though in general it is not reliable, it may be valuable in combination with other drugs, and in leprosy settlements it has proved effective as a suppressive of malaria. It does not act on the tissue stages of malaria parasites.

Repository preparations

Cycloguanil embonate (CI 501, Camolar, cycloguanil pamoate) exerts long-term protection against *P. falciparum* and *P. vivax*. It is given as a single intramuscular dose, in oily suspension, of 5 mg base per kg, or a standard adult dose of 350 mg. In volunteers challenge with *P. falciparum* or *P. vivax* was resisted for about 32–36 weeks; in the field in Gambia the protection lasted 2–4 months.

However, cycloguanil embonate apparently does not protect against mosquito-induced infection with chloroquine-resistant *P. falciparum*. Its use is limited by the presence of pyrimethamine- or proguanil-resistant strains (WHO 1967).

P. falciparum resistant to cycloguanil embonate has been reported from West Pakistan; the strain was also resistant to proguanil and pyrimethamine, but susceptible to mepacrine, chloroquine and quinine (Contacos *et al.* 1965).

Cycloguanil embonate (CI 501) has been mixed with 4-4′-diacetyldiamino-diphenylsulphone (acedapsone, DADDS) in a preparation with the number CI 564, for the treatment of mosquito-induced infections with multi-resistant *P. falciparum*, with clearance of parasitaemia within 3–7 days, but with radical cure in only 10 of 15 subjects. It had more preventive than curative effect. This mixture gives better results than either compound alone, and displays activity against certain strains of *P. falciparum* resistant to chloroquine and proguanil. In Tanzania this mixture as a single dose of about 12·9 mg/kg was more effective than either drug alone in children in the field, but parasites returned in 1–5 months in 11 of 24 subjects (Laing *et al.* 1966).

Table 3. Drugs recommended for non-immune persons

Drug	Base content	Adult prophylactic dose	Adult treatment dose
Chlorproguanil hydrochloride (Lapudrine, ICI)	Tab. 20 mg	20 mg once weekly	Not used
Cycloguanil embonate (Camolar, Parke, Davis)	Oily suspension 140 mg/ml	2·5 ml by deep i.m. injection once every 3–4 months	Not used
Pyrimethamine + dapsone (Maloprim, Burroughs Wellcome)	Tab. 12·5 mg + 100 mg	2 tabs 1 week before exposure, then 1 tab. once weekly	Not used
Pyrimethamine + sulphadoxine (Fansidar, Roche)	Tab. 25 mg + 500 mg	Not used	2–3 tabs as single dose
Pyrimethamine + chloroquine sulphate (Daraclor, Burroughs Wellcome)	Tab. 15 mg + 150 mg (base)	1–2 tabs once weekly	2 tabs 3 times daily on day 1; 2 tabs on day 2 and 2 on day 3

These doses are given in terms of *base*, though various brands of a preparation may contain different quantities of *salt*. Labels should specify the actual quantity of base. Chlorproguanil hydrochloride should not be used if the local strains are resistant. The paediatric dose of Maloprim is still under review.

This table is adapted from Peters (1971).

Other compounds under investigation include a pyrocatechol compound (RC 12), an acridine (CI 423), a naphthalene (377-C-54), an 8-aminoquinoline (WIN 5037), nitroguanil, and two quinoline-methanols (WHO 1967).

In addition to the drugs already mentioned, Peters (1971) recommends those shown in Table 3 for use in non-immune persons.

TESTS FOR QUININE AND CHLOROQUINE IN URINE

It is sometimes important to know if these drugs have been taken by patients who are not closely supervised. The tests are:

For quinine in urine. *Tanret-Mayer test.* Reagent 1·45 grammes mercuric chloride in 80 ml distilled water added to 5 grammes potassium iodide in 20 ml distilled water. Add a few drops to 5 ml of filtrate of boiled and filtered urine; an immediate precipitate forms if quinine is present.

This test is also positive for chloroquine in urine.

For large amounts of quinine in urine, 20 ml urine are made alkaline with ammonium hydroxide solution and extracted with an equal amount of ether or chloroform and the extract is shaken with 3 ml of 10% sulphuric acid. A blue fluorescence, more noticeable under ultra-violet light, suggests quinine or quinidine. It can be confirmed by fluorescent emission, which occurs at 450 nm when an exciting light of wavelength 250 nm is applied, if a spectrofluorimeter is available (Clarke 1969).

For chloroquine in urine. *The Wilson-Edeson test.* A few drops of Mayer's reagent (6·8 grammes $HgCl_2$, 24·9 grammes KI, 500 ml distilled water) are added to a few millilitres of urine and, if chloroquine is present, a white turbidity rapidly appears, which disappears on heating but returns on cooling. This test becomes positive 12 hours after a dose of chloroquine has been taken, and remains positive for 5–6 days after a single dose of 600 mg (Wilson & Edeson 1954).

The Haskins test (Haskins 1958)

Reagents:

10% solution of sodium hydroxide
purified ethylene dichloride
0·1% solution of methyl orange in boric acid
To 5 ml urine add 1·0 ml sodium hydroxide solution and 5 ml ethylene dichloride
Shake for 1 minute
Centrifuge if necessary to separate the layers
Draw off the ethylene dichloride layer into a clean test tube and add 0·5 ml methyl orange solution
Shake for 15–20 seconds.

The presence of a non-specific yellow colour in the ethylene dichloride layer (but not in a control urine) indicates the presence of chloroquine. It detects 2 mg/litre, and the colour is intense at 10 mg/litre.

A dose of 300 mg can produce a positive result for 10 days, negative at 12 days. It is negative with a dose of 300 mg amodiaquine, and with 25 mg pyrimethamine.

Lelijfeld and Kortmann test for amodiaquine and chloroquine (Lelijfeld & Kortmann 1968)

Reagent: 50 mg of yellowish eosin are placed in a small glass-stoppered funnel. 100 mg chloroform (reagent grade) and 1·0 ml *N* HCl are added and the mixture is shaken for a few minutes until the chloroform is light yellow as a result of solution of the eosin. The chloroform layer is allowed to separate and may be transferred to a brown, glass-stoppered bottle for storage.

The presence of chloroquine is shown if to a small test tube containing 2 ml urine, 10 drops of the reagent are added and mixed by thorough shaking for a few moments, and the colour in the chloroform layer changes from yellowish to violet-red.

SPECIFIC TREATMENT IN CHILDREN

Children tolerate oral doses of the synthetic antimalarial drugs well (Table 4), and over the age of 10 years they can usually take the full adult doses, but allowance must be made for size and weight, as well as age. If vomiting occurs within an hour of ingestion of the drug, the same dose should be repeated. Chloroquine suppositories may be used, but absorption is slow.

If follow-up treatment is impossible, single-dose oral treatment should be given as follows:

Up to 2 years	150 mg chloroquine base
3–6 years	300 mg chloroquine base
7–10 years	450 mg chloroquine base

Parenteral antimalarial treatment

Chloroquine should not be injected into infants and young children unless absolutely necessary, and even then the dose should not exceed 5 mg/kg within a 24-hour period. Sudden deaths have been attributed to parenteral administration of chloroquine in children.

Nevertheless, for cerebral malaria in children Jelliffe, D. B. (1966) advocated intramuscular chloroquine in a dose of 5 mg (base)/kg, repeated 6 hours later, or given by intragastric tube. The maximum daily dose should not exceed 10 mg (base)/ kg. He suggested that chloroquine could be given by very slow intravenous injection, or intravenous drip, in a dose of 0·5 mg (base)/kg (i.e. one-tenth of the calculated initial dose) followed by the remaining nine-tenths of the dose intramuscularly. But, as stated above, other physicians warn that chloroquine should not be given parenterally to young children.

Table 4. Oral doses of antimalarial drugs for children in uncomplicated attacks

Drug	Up to 2 years	3–6 years	7–10 years	Remarks
Chloroquine base	100 mg twice	150 mg twice	150 mg 3 times	First day
	75 mg	75 mg	150 mg	Once daily for next 4 days
Amodiaquine base	100 mg twice	150 mg twice	150 mg 3 times	First day
	100 mg	100 mg	150 mg	Once daily for next 4 days
Quinine	15 mg/kg 3 times daily	15 mg/kg 3 times daily	15 mg/kg 3 times daily	For 10 days

After Gilles (1966).

Quinine dihydrochloride, 10 mg/kg, may be given intravenously, repeated in 12 hours; the daily dose should not exceed 20 mg/kg. It may be given by intramuscular injection, but with great caution.

Intravenous infusion may also be used to correct electrolyte errors and to introduce hydrocortisone (5 mg/kg) or sedatives where these are indicated (Sagnet *et al.* 1967).

Mepacrine is contra-indicated for children under 2 years old, and some physicians never use it for any children.

Children with *P. vivax* malaria may be treated with chloroquine, amodiaquine or quinine, but for relapsing *P. vivax* malaria primaquine may be needed in daily doses. Primaquine may be toxic, producing methaemoglobinuria, haemolytic anaemia with or without haemoglobinuria (especially with glucose-6-phosphate dehydrogenase deficiency), neutropenia, colicky abdominal pain, or renal obstruction (from crystallization).

Mepacrine and primaquine should never be given simultaneously.

For children, suitable daily doses of primaquine (in coated tablets) are (modified from WHO 1967):

1–4 years	2·5 mg base
5–8 years	5·0 mg base
9–14 years	10·0 mg base
15 and over	15·0 mg base

CHEMOPROPHYLAXIS (Table 5)

For continuous administration proguanil (Paludrine, chlorguanide) is probably the drug of choice unless the local parasites are resistant to it. It has a slow action against asexual blood forms of all malaria parasites, and some action on tissue schizonts of *P. falciparum*, though less on those of *P. vivax*. The adult dose is 100–200 mg daily (according to local advice), starting the day before entry into a malarious area. As it is taken daily it is less likely to be forgotten than drugs taken only once each week.

Table 5. Summary of drug prophylaxis

Drug	Up to 2 years	3–6 years	7–10 years	Adults
Proguanil daily	25–50 mg	50–75 mg	100 mg	100–200 mg
Pyrimethamine weekly	6·25–12·5 mg	12·5–25 mg	12·5–25 mg	25 mg
Chloroquine base weekly	50–100 mg	100–200 mg	100–200 mg	300 mg or more
Amodiaquine base weekly	50–100 mg	100–200 mg	100–200 mg	400 mg or more

Pyrimethamine (Daraprim) acts mainly on gametocytes, preventing their development in mosquitoes. It acts slowly on asexual malaria parasites in the blood. For adults the usual prophylactic dose is 25–50 mg once each week. Daily doses may be toxic, giving leucopenia and irregular fever not related to parasitaemia, but toxicity may be blocked by simultaneous administration of very small doses of folic acid. Pyrimethamine has been given to African children in holoendemic areas, and they tend to remain in better health in the first few years of life than children who are not so protected, though the ultimate development of immunity as a result of continued infection is much the same in both groups. Pyrimethamine has been given at intervals of 2 or even 4 weeks in holoendemic areas, for instance to pregnant African women in Nigeria, with good results. In such cases, however, any attack of malarial fever should be treated with chloroquine or other schizontocide.

Pyrimethamine may be given in doses of 12·5 mg together with dapsone (100 mg) or with sulphormethoxine (125 or 250 mg) once each week, but these combinations may best be reserved for areas where resistance to pyrimethamine or chloroquine exists. The combination of pyrimethamine with dapsone is probably better than that with sulphormethoxine.

In children in holoendemic areas who take regular pyrimethamine, serum antibody may not be detectable by the fluorescent antibody test, though present in unprotected children.

Proguanil and pyrimethamine should be started by expatriates the day before entering a malarious area, and continued for one month after leaving.

Strains of malaria parasites resistant to chloroquine and amodiaquine are becoming more evident in some parts of the world, and they may show resistance to all other drugs except quinine, though their resistance may not be strong. It has therefore been said that the 4-aminoquinolines should not be used for chemoprophylaxis, but should be reserved for treatment. This, however, is now disputed, for instance in Africa, where chloroquine resistance has never been substantiated (Bruce-Chwatt 1970). In Tanzania resistance to proguanil and pyrimethamine is widespread, and Taylor (1968) has long since given up using them for either prophylaxis or treatment; he relies on the 4-amino-quinolines and has had no trouble. The adult dose of chloroquine for pro-phylaxis is 300 mg (base) weekly, and for amodiaquine 400 mg (base) weekly.

The adult dose of chloroquine and amodiaquine may need to be increased to 100 mg daily on 6 days each week in conditions of heavy transmission. Corre-sponding increases may be needed for children. Local advice should be taken for all these drugs.

For drug prophylaxis in West African children, a dose of 2 mg pyrimethamine with 40 mg sulphadoxine administered every 2 weeks has been used successfully (Laing 1970).

If there is resistance to proguanil, pyrimethamine and chloroquine, mepacrine may be necessary, but should be avoided if possible. The adult dose is 100 mg daily, *beginning at least 10 days before entering the malarious area*. The use of repository drugs is at present experimental.

Medicated salt. In some countries chloroquine has been added to domestic salt, for widespread supply to all the inhabitants, with the intention of suppres-sing malaria by constant dosage. In Guyana the concentration of chloroquine was 0·4%, in Iran 0·33% and in Uganda 0·38%. Parasite rates in these areas were lowered, but interruption of transmission could not be claimed with certainty, though in one experiment in Tanzania this was apparently achieved.

In this form, however, chloroquine is lost by leaching during storage, espe-cially when moisture is sealed into plastic containers, and infants and young children commonly do not receive adequate doses because they are not given salt. There is also the possibility that if strains of parasites exist which are resistant to chloroquine, they could be favoured, and spread, as a result of this pro-cedure. Moreover, Giglioli *et al.* (1967) have produced strong evidence that chloroquinized salt caused photo-allergic dermatitis in Guyana, similar to that described in rheumatoid arthritis and lupus erythematosis treated with high doses of chloroquine.

DRUG RESISTANCE

A full discussion of this subject was published by Peters (1969).

Drug resistance has been described as 'the ability of a parasite strain to survive and/or multiply despite the administration and absorption of a drug in doses equal to or higher than those usually recommended but within the limits of tolerance of the subject' (WHO 1967).

Resistance is exhibited in various grades, defined by WHO (1968a) as shown in Table 6.

Although there are variations in the responses of different strains of *P. vivax* and *P. malariae* to antimalarial drugs, for practical purposes the problem of drug resistance is confined to *P. falciparum*.

Resistance of *P. falciparum* to proguanil and cycloguanil pamoate has been reported from extensive areas of Asia and Africa, and no doubt exists elsewhere. These reports indicate that neither of these drugs should be used *alone* for *mass* chemotherapy or chemoprophylaxis, since this would almost certainly result in the appearance of resistant strains. Such strains are resistant at all stages of the life cycle, and this character is readily transmitted through the anopheline vectors.

Resistance of *P. falciparum* to pyrimethamine has been found in Asia, the Pacific, South America and Africa, where it is now widespread. It could also conceivably be spread from one species of parasite to another, as in the case of mixed (non-resistant) *P. berghei* and (resistant) *P. vinckei* in white mice (Yoeli *et al.* 1969).

Resistance of *P. falciparum* to chloroquine has been reported from South-east Asia and South America, but has not been substantiated in Africa (Bruce-Chwatt 1970). This resistance is sometimes combined with multiple resistance to other 4-aminoquinolines, and to mepacrine, proguanil and pyrimethamine,

Table 6. Grading of resistance of asexual parasites (*P. falciparum*) to schizontocidal drugs

Response	Recommended symbol	Evidence
Sensitivity	S	Clearance of asexual parasitaemia within 7 days of treatment, without recrudescence
Resistance	RI	Clearance of asexual parasitaemia within 7 days of treatment, followed by recrudescence
	RII	Marked reduction of asexual parasitaemia but no clearance
	RIII	No marked reduction of asexual parasitaemia

and some resistant strains require high doses of quinine for successful treatment. Resistance to chloroquine is usually at the RI level in South America, but in South-East Asia RII resistance is more common.

It is well known that some strains of *P. falciparum* need abnormally large doses of quinine for cure or suppression. African and Indian strains are particularly susceptible, but strains from Italy and South America have been found much more resistant. It is probably true that where primary resistance to quinine exists, there may also be a degree of resistance to chloroquine or mepacrine.

From the work of Martin and Arnold (1968) on *P. falciparum* and pyrimethamine it seems highly probable that in a large community of parasites (high parasite counts) there will be a few relatively resistant clones. The amount of drug needed to clear the blood of asexual forms is proportional to the parasite count, and any resistant forms which persist can become the dominant forms in that subject, having been selected out by the drug. But when the drug is discontinued, the proportion of resistant forms probably returns to the former state.

The growth of the incidence of resistance can therefore be attributed to the selection of existing resistant mutants through drug pressure, and as anti-malarial drugs are now widely available, the means for this pressure are now plentiful, but it is strange that chloroquine resistance has not so far appeared in

Africa. Immunity is a factor in this: the few parasites resistant to chloroquine would more easily be eliminated in African communities where immunity is high than in other areas, for instance South-east Asia, where it is less high.

A powerful plasmodicidal drug (like chloroquine) whose dose can be stepped up to 99% efficiency well within the tolerated dose is not likely to leave many resistant mutants alive at the higher dosage, whereas a less powerful plasmodistatic drug (like proguanil), which cannot be stepped up to 99% efficiency without great increase in dosage, is much more likely, in the doses commonly used, to allow many more resistant mutants to escape. In the treatment of patients with the lower degrees of chloroquine resistance, chloroquine in higher doses than usual can be successful.

Various combinations of drugs have been advocated for prophylaxis and for treatment of malaria (see those sections), but *the primary weapon against drug resistance is residual insecticide spraying to interrupt malaria transmission* (Peters 1969).

PREVENTION OF MALARIA

The anophelines which carry malaria usually bite at night, especially about dawn and dusk. Endophilic species do so inside houses, where human blood is easily available to them, but some strains of well known vectors are exophilic, biting in the open after nightfall, and resting by day in vegetation, for instance, strains of *A. gambiae* in Mauritius and elsewhere.

Many species enter houses at dusk and, after a blood meal, rest on walls or ceilings, leaving at dawn.

Protection against these vectors therefore entails:

(*a*) Siting of dwellings at distances of a kilometre or more from collections of water, or streams, where anophelines can breed. Mosquitoes can travel further than this down wind, but the distances suggested afford some protection; prevailing winds at night time should be taken into consideration. So also should elevation and exposure to wind; hill tops are usually better than valleys. Formerly, in some countries, it was found useful to interpose cattle in sheds between mosquito breeding places and human habitations, so that mosquitoes which would feed on cattle would be diverted from man. Some particularly anthropophilic species, however, cannot be diverted in this way.

(*b*) Treatment of breeding places by draining ponds or marshes, or filling them in with earth; clearing vegetation from the edges of streams, which could provide shelter for mosquito larvae.

(*c*) The use of small fish which eat mosquito larvae, especially larvae which live chiefly near the surface, such as anopheline larvae; species used include *Lebistes* and *Gambusia*.

(*d*) Removal of shade from the breeding places of anophelines which choose shaded water for breeding; or conversely, provision of shade to inhibit species which prefer direct sunlight. There is a difficulty, however, in that by altering shade, species may be attracted which prefer the altered conditions, and these may be effective vectors.

(*e*) Treatment of streams by intermittent flushing provided by special siphons constructed to hold up the flow of water until the siphon is primed and discharges the dammed-up water in a turbulent and sudden gush which washes away the mosquito larvae.

(*f*) Treatment of breeding places with larvicidal oil, or with residual insecticides in oil or water emulsions.

These methods, largely in use before the advent of the residual insecticides which are sprayed on walls and ceilings of dwellings where anophelines are known to rest, may recently have been neglected. They are, however, always important and should always be employed, particularly in places where resistance to insecticides is prevalent.

Moreover, breeding places have often been created by man, for instance when earth has been removed for the construction of railway embankments, or buildings, leaving hollows in which rain collects. This is a problem for civil engineers, but medical officers should insist on being consulted before such work is begun. The same is true for other diseases also. For instance, if a dam is built, the overflow or sluice water may create a stream ideal for the breeding of *Simulium,* or if slow-flowing irrigation canals are constructed in schistosomiasis areas, the population of vector snails may be expected to increase catastrophically. Careful attention to the manipulation of water, by engineers under the guidance of medical men, can avoid disasters of this kind. The responsibility rests primarily with the doctors.

Protection by mosquito netting is extremely important, especially for non-immune expatriates in hyperendemic areas. The windows of houses should be covered by the special metal gauze prepared for the purpose, and mosquito-proofed doors may be added to existing doors so that the latter can be kept open to allow maximum air movement inside without permitting mosquitoes to enter.

Mosquito bed nets (preferably of Terylene) are also essential, but must be scrupulously maintained to avoid tearing. The net should be suspended from metal rods connecting uprights placed at the 4 corners of the bed, and there should be no opening in the side of the net. The net should be lowered and tucked well in under the mattress before dusk, and not raised until after dawn. Mosquitoes will enter a torn or badly used net, which becomes a mosquito trap.

Mosquito boots of soft leather, reaching to just below the knee, have long been advocated. Mosquitoes tend to bite under tables and chairs, and the ankles are therefore particularly vulnerable. With or without mosquito boots, long trousers are advisable in the evenings, and long sleeves also reduce the area of skin open to mosquitoes.

Women who wear short skirts are obviously at a disadvantage in this respect, and even two pairs of stockings are not enough to prevent bites. Repellents such as dimethyl phthalate, however, can be useful when applied to the skin; they act for several hours, and proprietary preparations pleasant to use are generally available.

Spraying a room with a short-acting insecticide based on pyrethrum, from a 'Flit gun', is useful to clear it for a few hours, particular attention being paid to spaces beneath chairs and tables, and also to wardrobes, cupboards, bathrooms and lavatories, and to dark corners.

A suggestion was made (WHO 1968a) that in a holoendemic area such as Northern Nigeria, a round of drug treatment (0·6 gramme chloroquine and 45 mg pyrimethamine as an adult dose) should be given to the entire population in November 1966 and every 2 months thereafter, and that insecticide should be used in April 1967 before the onset of the rains, and repeated 4 months later. This programme could not be carried out because supplies were delayed, but the principle was accepted as a research investigation in an appropriate area.

Eradication

Complete eradication of malaria has for several years been the aim of WHO. By using residual insecticides and the newer drugs, and by antilarval methods in such places as Cyprus, eradication has been achieved in circumscribed areas, especially islands. It has almost been achieved in large areas of mainland countries, and already many millions of people have been protected. But the recent outbreak of *P. vivax* malaria in Ceylon, after that island had been dramatically cleared, or almost cleared, in the early days of residual insecticides, demonstrates how difficult it is to maintain clearance, and to ensure it.

The techniques of eradication are complex, and depend on careful organization, adequate subordinate personnel trained in the use of insecticides, and meticulous supervision. All this means finance, and the subject is beyond the scope of this book.

For a general discussion of research in relation to eradication see Bruce-Chwatt (1965).

BLACKWATER FEVER

Blackwater fever, or malarial haemoglobinuria, is a very dangerous complication of *P. falciparum* malaria, occurring most often in non-immune residents of malarious areas; it is not associated with the other malaria parasites of man. Formerly more common than it now is, it was almost invariably associated with treatment with quinine, especially when taken in full doses for an attack of fever by a person who had not been taking it regularly as a prophylactic. The two factors were *P. falciparum* and quinine, though rare cases have been reported in persons who had not taken quinine. It has also been reported, in a few cases, in indigenous inhabitants of holoendemic areas (for instance in Africa) who, perhaps, had lost some immunity, and in indigenous children in those areas.

In the war of 1939–45 blackwater fever practically disappeared from British troops stationed in Africa and other hyperendemic areas when mepacrine was substituted for quinine in prophylaxis and treatment, but it has been reported after treatment with chloroquine and pyrimethamine in a patient who had previously at some time taken quinine, which may perhaps have sensitized him in some way (Molenaar & Voors 1963).

In a sensitized person even the small doses of quinine contained in tonic water or tinned grapefruit may be enough to precipitate an attack.

The pathogenesis is still obscure though it has been greatly clarified by Maegraith (1948, 1967). There is sudden, extensive intravascular haemolysis, which may be a manifestation of some form of immunity reaction, possibly through the formation of an autoantigen, or possibly through a mechanism of sensitization, for instance to quinine. The destruction of red cells may be so great that erythrocyte counts may fall in a few hours to one million or less per mm^3. This is obviously a grave medical emergency. As a result of the haemolysis, haemoglobin is present in plasma and is passed into the urine. Methaemalbumin is also present in the plasma (and also in incompatible blood transfusion and other forms of haemoglobinuria) but is apparently unable to traverse the renal glomeruli, and therefore does not appear in the urine.

On standing, the urine settles into 2 layers—a bulky lower layer containing a brownish-grey sediment in which there are many tube casts, and perhaps some erythrocytes, and an upper, clearer, layer. If the urine is acid the haemoglobin is brown or black; if alkaline it is red. The urine contains much albumin, and may become almost solid on boiling.

Liver function is often impaired early. The liver becomes enlarged and tender, with epigastric discomfort, nausea and vomiting, followed soon by jaundice.

The dangerous feature of blackwater fever is renal failure. At one time this was thought to be due to mechanical blocking of the renal tubules by debris and the products of haemoglobin, but this mechanistic view is no longer entertained. The failure is essentially the same as that which occurs in the renal shutdown found in surgical and obstetrical shock, and crush injury. The renal changes are essentially similar to those which may occur in *P. falciparum* malaria—degenerative changes in the epithelium of the tubules, with collection of debris in them. Glomerular changes are seldom marked.

There is apparently a change in the intrarenal blood flow which leads to cortical ischaemia and anoxia, with reduction in glomerular blood flow, and therefore reduction in glomerular filtration and consequent oliguria or even anuria. A renal vasoconstrictor reflex may be involved in this process, associated with the general anoxaemia and tissue anoxia which occurs in malaria.

General circulatory changes of the nature of shock, with reduced blood volume and low blood pressure—peripheral vascular collapse—may supervene. The face is anxious and drawn, the eyes sunken, and the patient is restless; the diastolic blood pressure may fall rapidly in the final stages, and the patient dies of vascular collapse.

In the early stages the intrarenal stimulus is the important one; in the later stages of shock an extrarenal reflex, for instance from a hyperactive sympathetic system, is probably the initiating factor. In shock and similar general conditions there is evidence that the extrarenal reflex is only part of a bodily protective mechanism which involves other organs, including the adrenals and liver (Maegraith 1948).

Symptoms

Some observers have recognized a clinical condition which may be termed the *pre-blackwater state* which indicates that haemolysis is imminent and that the clinician should take precautionary measures. The patient usually gives a history of slight attacks of fever. The complexion is sallow and conjunctivae icteric. The liver is generally enlarged and tender and the spleen palpable. The urine is generally pigmented with urobilinogen. Blood examination may reveal scanty subtertian malaria rings; but, as a general rule, those with high fever and numerous parasites in the blood do not develop blackwater.

The onset is sudden. A slight or, it may be, a severe rigor is followed by irregular fever with marked bilious symptoms. Usually during the rigor the patient becomes conscious of aching pain in the loins, in the regions of liver or spleen, and when, in response to urgent desire, he passes water, he is astonished to find that his urine has become very dark in colour, possibly madeira-colour or almost black. Usually he suffers from epigastric pain, bilious vomiting to an unusual extent, and possibly bilious diarrhoea. Seldom he may be constipated. Soon he breaks into a profuse sweat and the fever gradually subsides. In milder cases the urine, which was at first scanty, now flows freely; and after passing through various paling shades, from dark brown to cherry red, becomes natural once more; coincidently the skin acquires a deep saffron-yellow tint. This icteric colour persists, or may even deepen, during the progress of the fever, and when this subsides, the patient is conscious of a feeling of great weakness. The fever, without rigor, may recur next day, or for several days. The haemoglobinuria may return with each rise of temperature or there may be only one or two outbursts. The more severe forms of blackwater are accompanied by a very great amount of bilious vomiting, intense epigastric pain and there may be severe pain in the liver and loin.

The urine may continue copious and very dark, or it may gradually get more and more scanty, acquiring a gummy consistency. Finally, urinary excretion may be completely suppressed. It is calculated that the kidneys may excrete 36% of the total haemoglobin in the blood. In severe cases, death is the rule. It may be very sudden—a matter of 7 hours, or even less. The fever may assume hyperpyrexial proportions, or sudden cerebral symptoms may supervene. Hiccough is a fatal sign. In some, the symptoms may be those consequent on sudden, profuse haemorrhage, with jactitation, sweating, sighing and syncope, or again, death may take place from sudden heart failure, or from exhaustion consequent on cyclical vomiting, or from sudden haemorrhage from stomach or bowel. Suppression of urine ends in sudden syncope, convulsions and coma.

Another aspect which is significant is that one attack of blackwater appears to predispose to a second attack; more than 2 have been noted in Nigeria in about 20% of cases, and according to Stephens, 16 is the largest number ever recorded. According to popular opinion, when a man has recovered from two attacks, the third is generally fatal. Blackwater fever is highly dangerous to pregnant women, during parturition or during the puerperium. Particular care should always be taken to guard them, in this condition, from malaria, and their blood should be frequently examined. As regards the sequelae, anaemia and debility are common but usually, under hygienic conditions, the recovery is astoundingly rapid. A curious sequel is cholelithiasis, owing to the formation of biliary calculi from inspissation of bile in the gall-bladder. Of this complication the former Editor (P. H. Manson-Bahr) had seen 2 in whom it was noted 3 weeks after cessation of blackwater and pigmented calculi were demonstrated.

Treatment

If malaria parasites are present in the blood, treatment with an antimalarial drug should be given at once; the drug of choice is chloroquine in the usual doses, but if there is evidence of resistance to chloroquine—which is increasingly being found in South-east Asia and elsewhere—for instance in a patient known to have been taking prophylactic chloroquine, some other drug must be used. In spite of the previous advice not to use quinine in *P. falciparum* malaria, in Vietnam slow intravenous infusion of quinine dihydrochloride in doses of 600 mg/24 hours has been given in such cases, sometimes changed, according to circumstances, to oral administration (650 mg every 8 hours). Blood films and electrocardiographic records should be examined frequently.

For the treatment of renal failure, which is the fatal factor, and which is of the reversible renal anoxic kind (Maegraith 1948) the artificial kidney may be life-saving, and has been used by Jackson and Woodruff (1962) in patients in whom renal biopsy or subsequent autopsy showed tubular necrosis; of 4 patients, 3 recovered. These authors make the point that patients in this state can be transported considerable distances by air to artificial kidney units, and that the concept that blackwater fever patients should not be moved must be revised.

Peritoneal dialysis can be used successfully in tropical hospitals where the artificial kidney apparatus is not available. The technique is described on page 67. In Vietnam, peritoneal dialysis in broken periods has been continued for up to 120 hours; blood urea and creatinine were high, but were cleared across the peritoneal membrane, especially when the patients improved.

Many cases of renal failure can be treated conservatively, without dialysis, by attention to fluid balance and electrolyte levels.

Corticosteroids have been used, but though favourable responses have been reported, the advantages are doubtful.

In older practice it was the custom to give large quantities of fluid by mouth, or even intravenously, in blackwater fever, but though vomiting, sweating and diarrhoea may tend to dehydrate the patient, and therefore lost fluid must be replaced (for instance by intravenous glucose saline) there is a risk that by pushing fluids, especially in oliguria and anuria, the patient may become water-logged. A balance sheet of fluid loss and intake should therefore be kept.

It was also formerly the custom to give large doses of alkalis, but careful records now indicate that this is risky. Even large doses will not render the urine alkaline, and alkalis are harmful to kidney function. They are therefore better avoided.

Transfusion of blood or of a suspension of red cells may be called for if the red cell count falls below 1 500 000. The transfusion should be given slowly, and the amount recorded in the total fluid intake. Care in cross-matching cells and serum is particularly important. If the is haemolysis is severe, red cell transfusion can be life-saving.

Cardiovascular failure is treated on general lines.

Nursing is most important in the management of blackwater. If the stomach will retain food, this should be given in the form of meat extracts, Bovril or Ovaltine, but there should be no attempt at forcible feeding. Precautions against syncope must be enforced, the patient must not be allowed to sit up, much less to get out of bed. The foot of the bed should be raised on blocks. If possible the subjects of blackwater fever should quit the endemic area and never return to it or to any malarial locality.

Some cases are so mild and transient, amounting, perhaps, to a single emission of haemoglobinous urine, that they are unattended with risk. On the other hand, the practitioner may encounter a run of severe cases, nearly all fatal. According to modern ideas, the chances of survival depend upon the number of nephrons in the kidney which have escaped destruction as the result of renal anoxia. In Southern Nigeria and in Algeria, the mortality has been as high as 50%; but as a general average, it may be assessed at about 25%. As regards prophylaxis, the answer is obvious, when it has been concluded in West Africa that, with modern advances in the prevention of malaria and the introduction of modern drugs for treatment and prophylaxis of malaria in place of quinine, the indigenous inhabitants and the Europeans have been more or less protected against blackwater fever from 1944 onwards.

TROPICAL SPLENOMEGALY
(BIG SPLEEN DISEASE)

Massive enlargement of the spleen is common in the tropics, in malaria (especially in children), kala-azar, schistosomiasis and other conditions, but in many parts of Africa and New Guinea, and probably elsewhere, it also occurs in a minority of adults in whom these causes cannot easily or fully explain it. The aetiology is not clear, but the disease is found only where malaria is endemic, and it responds to some extent to prolonged antimalarial treatment. Yet because it occurs in only a few adults in malarious areas, where the malarial splenomegaly of childhood usually regresses as immunity develops, the explanation of the adult disease does not seem to lie in malaria alone; there seems to be some other factor, probably in the individual patient, which operates in addition to malaria. The most likely explanation is that it represents an abnormal immunological response to malaria, possibly due to undefined factors in the host (which may be hereditary), or to unusual species of plasmodia, or to frequency or multiplicity of malaria infection. Certain tribes seem to be particularly liable; malnutrition may be a factor—for instance, a relatively high incidence has been observed in lactating women. For a discussion of the whole subject, see Pitney (1968) and Leading Articles (*Br. med. J.*, 1969, 1971).

Pathology

The liver is enlarged and smooth, with proliferation of lymphoid and plasma cells, and hyperplasia of the Kupffer cells containing ingested nuclear debris, lymphocytes and red cells. Some portal tracts are heavily infiltrated with cells; others not. The spleen is greatly enlarged, and may weigh 2090–4380 grammes. The sinuses are dilated, there is hyperplasia of lymphoid and plasma cells, swollen reticular cells and marked phagocytosis of red cells and leucocytes. Blood flow is increased, and may account for a systolic murmur sometimes audible over the spleen. The splenic vein is dilated and tortuous.

Anaemia, leucopenia and thrombocytopenia are common. The anaemia does not respond to anthelmintics and iron. The life-span of the red cells is reduced, but returns to normal after splenectomy. The total red cell mass is not reduced, but the plasma volume is increased. The leucopenia is probably due to sequestration of granulocytes in the enlarged spleen; it seems to be associated with ulceration of the leg.

There is an increase in the serum IgM macroglobulin concentration, which supports the view that there is an unusual immunological response to an infectious agent, probably malaria. Ziegler *et al.* (1969) found an increase in immunologically competent cells, lymphocytes and plasma cells, and of Kupffer cells and splenic histiocytes. There was no defect in immunological function, and they consider the disease to be a lymphoreticular proliferative disorder which may become neoplastic.

Other serological abnormalities occur, but are of doubtful significance.

Clinical features

These usually arise in adult life. The patient is commonly afebrile on diagnosis, and may not suffer much disability, though in severe cases this is not so. The spleen is large and firm, the liver large, the heart may be enlarged, the pulse slow and the blood pressure low. Anaemia is common. The patient in severe cases is wasted.

Treatment may not be necessary for patients who have adapted well to the condition, but for those with disabling symptoms due to anaemia or to the size and weight of the spleen, splenectomy may be advisable, but always followed by prolonged antimalaria treatment. But it should be remembered that splenectomy is likely to interfere seriously with the immune processes which protect against malaria and other dangerous infections; it should not be undertaken lightly. Chemotherapy also interferes with immunity to malaria, but often gives good results, and should be tried before splenectomy is considered. A course of 100 mg proguanil daily has been advocated, continued for long periods, possibly for life; other antimalarials may be tried. Blood transfusion may be needed for the anaemia, but with care not to overload the circulation in patients who already have increased blood volume and enlarged hearts. The response to treatment may differ in different parts of the world.

REFERENCES

ARMENGAUD, M., LOUVAIN, M. & DIOP-MAR, I. (1962) *Bull. Mém. Fac. mixte Med. Pharm. Dakar*, **10**, 171.
BOOTH, K., LARKIN, K. & MADDOCKS, I. (1967), *Br. med. J.*, **iii**, 32.
BRAY, R. S., GUNDERS, A. E., BURGESS, R. W., FREEMAN, J. B., ETZEL, E., GUTTOSO, C. & COLUSSA, B. (1962) *Riv. Malar.*, **41**, 199.
BRUCE-CHWATT, L. J. (1963) *W. Afr. med. J.*, **12**, 1.
—— (1965) *Trans. R. Soc. trop. Med. Hyg.*, **59**, 105.
—— (1970) *Trans. R. Soc. trop. Med. Hyg.*, **64**, 776.
CHIN, W. & CONTACOS, P. G. (1966) *Am. J. trop. Med. Hyg.*, **15**, 1.
CLARKE, E. G. C. (1969) *Isolation and Identification of Drugs*, p. 15. London: Pharmaceutical Press.
COHEN, S. & BUTCHER, G. A. (1971) *Trans. R. Soc. trop. Med. Hyg.*, **65**, 125.
CLYDE, D. F. (1967) *Am. J. trop. Med. Hyg.*, **16**, 7.
CONTACOS, P. G., COATNEY, G. R., LUNN, J. S. & CHIN, W. (1965) *Am. J. trop. Med. Hyg.*, **14**, 925.
COVELL, G. (1950) *Trop. Dis. Bull.*, **47**, 1147.
—— (1955) *Trop. Dis. Bull.*, **52**, 705.
COX, H. W. (1966) *Milit. Med.*, **131**, Supplement, 1195.
DENNIS, L. H., EICHELBERGER, J. W., jun., VON DOENHOFF, A. E., jun. & CONRAD, M. E. (1966) *Milit. Med.*, **131**, Supplement, 1107.
DEVAKUL, K., HARINASUTA, T. & REID, H. A. (1966) *Lancet*, **ii**, 886.
DODGE, J. S. (1966) *Br. med. J.*, **ii**, 1593.
DOWLING, M. A. C. & SHUTE, G. T. (1966) *Bull. Wld Hlth Org.*, **34**, 249.
DÜRCK, H. (1925) *Arch. Schiffs- u. Tropenhyg.*, **29**, 43.
EDINGTON, G. M. (1967) *Br. med. J.*, **i**, 715.
—— & GILLES, H. M. (1969) *Pathology in the Tropics*. London: Arnold.
GARNHAM, P. C. C. (1966) *Malaria Parasites and Other Haemosporidia*. Oxford: Blackwell.
—— (1967) *Adv. Parasit.*, **5**, 157.
GEORGE, J. N., STOKER, E. F., WICKER, D. J. & CONRAD, M. E. (1966) *Milit. Med.*, **131**, Supplement, 1217.
GIGLIOLI, G., DYRTING, A. E., RUTTEN, F. J. & GENTLE, G. H. K. (1967) *Trans. R. Soc. trop. Med. Hyg.*, **61**, 313.
GILLES, H. M. (1966) *Br. med. J.*, **ii**, 1375.
—— (1968) *Med. Today*, **2**, 6.
—— & HENDRICKSE, R. G. (1963) *Br. med. J.*, **ii**, 27.
HASKINS, W. T. (1958) *Am. J. trop. Med. Hyg.*, **7**, 199.
HARDY, A. A. (1968) *Br. med. J.*, **iii**, 680.
HMSO (1968) *Current Medical Research*, p. 13. London.
HUTT, M. S. R. (1971) *Trans. R. Soc. trop. Med. Hyg.*, **65**, 273.
JACKSON, R. C. T. & WOODRUFF, A. W. (1962) *Br. med. J.*, **ii**, 1367.
JELLIFFE, D. B. (1966) *J. Pediat.*, **69**, 483.
JELLIFFE, E. F. P. (1966) *J. trop. Pediat.*, **12**, 15.
KIBUKAMUSOKE, J. W. & VOLLER, A. (1970) *Br. med. J.*, **i**, 406.
LAING, A. B. G. (1965) *J. trop. Med. Hyg.*, **68**, 251.
—— (1970) *Bull. Wld Hlth Org.*, **43**, 513.
—— & PRINGLE, G. & LANE, F. C. T. (1966) *Am. J. trop. Med. Hyg.*, **15**, 838.
LEADING ARTICLE (1969) *Br. med. J.*, **iii**, 541; **iv**, 4.
—— (1971) *Br. med. J.*, **i**, 420, 426.
LELIJFELD, J. & KORTMANN, H. (1968) *Annual Report*, p. 23. East African Institute of Malaria and Vector-borne Diseases.
MacDONALD, G. (1950a, b) *Trop. Dis. Bull.*, **47**, 907, 915.
—— (1952a, b) *Trop. Dis. Bull.*, **49**, 569, 813.
—— (1953) *Trop. Dis. Bull.*, **50**, 817.
McGREGOR, I. A. (1965) *Trans. R. Soc. trop. Med. Hyg.*, **59**, 145.
—— WILLIAMS, K. & GOODWIN, L. G. (1963) *Br. med. J.*, **ii**, 728.

McGREGOR, I. A., WILSON, R. J. M. (1971) *Trans. R. Soc. trop. Med. Hyg.*, **65**, 136.

MADEKI, O. & KRETSCHMAR, W. (1966) *Z. Tropenmed. Parasit.*, **17**, 195.

MAEGRAITH, B. G. (1948) *Pathological Processes in Malaria and Blackwater Fever.* Oxford: Blackwell.

—— (1967) *Protozoology*, **2**, 55.

—— (1969) *Milit. Med.*, **134**, Supplement, 1130.

MARTIN, D. C. & ARNOLD, J. D. (1968) *Trans. R. Soc. trop. Med. Hyg.*, **62**, 379.

MOLENAAR, J. C. & VOORS, A. W. (1963) *Trop. geogr. Med.*, **15**, 219.

ORISCELLO, R. G. (1968) *Br. med. J.*, iii, 617.

PANNACHET, P. (1967) *Ann. trop. Med. Parasit.*, **61**, 518.

PATRICK, I. T. (1968) *Br. med. J.*, iii, 805.

PETERS, W. (1967) *Trop. Dis. Bull.*, **64**, 1145.

—— (1969) *Trans. R. Soc. trop. Med. Hyg.*, **63**, 25.

—— (1971) *Br. med. J.*, iii, 95.

PITNEY, W. R. (1968) *Trans. R. Soc. trop. Med. Hyg.*, **62**, 717.

REBA, R. C. & SHEEHY, T. W. (1967) *J. Am. med. Ass.*, **201**, 553.

REID, J. A., GOLDSMITH, H. J. & WRIGHT, F. K. (1967) *Lancet*, ii, 436.

ROBINSON, G. L. (1966) *Br. med. J.*, i, 982.

SADUN, E. H., WILLIAMS, J. S. & MARTIN, L. K. (1966) *Milit. Med.*, **131**, Supplement, 1094.

SAGNET, H., MORINAUD, J. P., REVIL, H., THOMAS, J. & MAFORT, Y. (1967) *Méd. trop.*, **27**, 606.

SHUTE, P. G. (1968) *Br. med. J.*, i, 578.

—— (1970) *Trans. R. Soc. trop. Med. Hyg.*, **64**, 210.

—— & MARYON, M. (1968) *Archs roum. Path. exp. Microbiol.*, **27**, 893.

—— —— (1969) *Br. med. J.*, ii, 781.

SITPRIJA, V., INDRAPRASIT, S., POCHANUGOOL, G., BENYAJATI, C. & PIYARATN, P. (1967) *Lancet*, i, 185.

SMITSKAMP, H. & WOLTHUIS, F. H. (1971) *Br. med. J.*, i, 714.

TAYLOR, J. (1968) *Br. med. J.*, **3**, 805.

VERDRAGER, J. (1964) *Bull. Wld Hlth Org.*, **31**, 747.

VOLLER, A. (1971) *Trans. R. Soc. trop. Med. Hyg.*, **65**, 111.

—— & ROSSAN, R. N. (1969) *Trans. R. Soc. trop. Med. Hyg.*, **63**, 507.

WILKS, N. E., TURNER, P. P., SOMERS, K. & MARKANDYA, O. P. (1965) *E. Afr. med. J.*, **42**, 580.

WILSON, D. B. (1936) *Trans. R. Soc. trop. Med. Hyg.*, **29**, 583.

—— & WILSON, M. E. (1962) *Trans. R. Soc. trop. Med. Hyg.*, **56**, 287.

WILSON, R. J. M., McGREGOR, L. A., HALL, P., WILLIAMS, K. & BARTHOLOMEW, R. (1969) *Lancet*, ii, 201.

WILSON, T. & EDESON, J. F. R. (1954) *Med. J. Malaya*, **9**, 115.

WOODRUFF, A. W. & DICKINSON, C. J. (1968) *Br. med. J.*, iii, 31.

WORLD HEALTH ORGANIZATION (1967) *Tech. Rep. Ser.*, **375**, 29.

—— (1968a) *Tech. Rep. Ser.*, **382**, 11, 19, 41.

—— (1968b) *Tech. Rep. Ser.*, **396**, 40.

—— (1969a) *Tech. Rep. Ser.*, **433**, 19.

—— (1969b) *WHO Chron.*, **23**, 514.

YOELI, M., UPMANIS, R. S. & MOST, H. (1969) *Parasitology*, **59**, 429.

ZIEGLER, J. L., COHEN, M. H. & HUTT, M. S. R. (1969) *Br. med. J.*, iv, 15.

ZUCKERMAN, A. (1966) *Milit. Med.*, **131**, Supplement, 1201.

5. AFRICAN TRYPANOSOMIASIS

Definition
Diseases produced by parasites of the genus *Trypanosoma* characterized by irregular chronic fever, skin eruptions, local oedema, adenitis, physical and mental lethargy and death. The trypanosomes are spread by tsetse flies (*Glossina*) in Africa.

Geographical distribution
The distribution of human trypanosomiasis (sleeping sickness) corresponds roughly with that of the tsetse flies *Glossina fuscipes* (*G. palpalis*), *G. tachinoides*, *G. morsitans*, *G. pallidipes* and *G. swynnertoni*.

Human sleeping sickness is found in West, Central and Eastern Africa between the 20th North and 20th South parallels as shown in the map (Fig. 24). Gambian sleeping sickness is found in West Africa, the Congo, Southern Sudan and Uganda with the main strongholds along the Congo and the Niger and their main branches. Rhodesian sleeping sickness is mainly confined to Central and Eastern Africa.

In East Africa the tsetse fly inhabits 72 million hectares out of a total of 165 million. This 'fly' country of unused, uneroded land may soon be needed when the human population rises beyond the capacity of the present settled regions to support it. For detailed information the reader is referred to Buxton (1955), Mulligan and Potts (1970) and Ford (1969).

AETIOLOGY

The three polymorphic salivarian trypanosomes *T. brucei brucei*, *T. brucei rhodesiense*, and *T. brucei gambiense* are indistinguishable morphologically.

When *T. br. brucei* and *T. br. rhodesiense* are passaged through rats and guinea-pigs a small proportion of the parasites develop nuclei located posteriorly to the kinetoplast (postero-nuclear forms) (Fig. 25, 3–6). This property was thought to be a distinguishing feature from *T. br. gambiense* but postero-nuclear trypanosomes can also be found in this form (Sicé 1937). *T. br. rhodesiense* can only be distinguished from *T. br. brucei* by its pathogenicity for man, since *T. br. brucei* is non-infective for humans. *T. br. rhodesiense* does not change into *T. br. brucei* by animal passage as was demonstrated at Tinde where for 23 years *T. br. rhodesiense* was passaged through sheep and *Glossina morsitans* without losing its pathogenicity for man, although the incubation period lengthened during this time. The main difference between *T. br. rhodesiense* and *T. br. gambiense* is a biological one. It is not yet clear whether one can change into the other with a change in the biology of the parasite. For further details and techniques for cultivation, etc., see Appendix I.

T. br. gambiense is a parasite adapted to man and transmitted by the riverine tsetse flies *Glossina fuscipes* (*G. palpalis*) and *G. tachinoides* which feed on man. *T. br. rhodesiense* is a parasite of wild game, including bushbuck, which is not so well adapted to man and is transmitted amongst animals by the game tsetse flies *G. morsitans*, *G. pallidipes* and *G. swynnertoni*.

For further details see Appendix I.

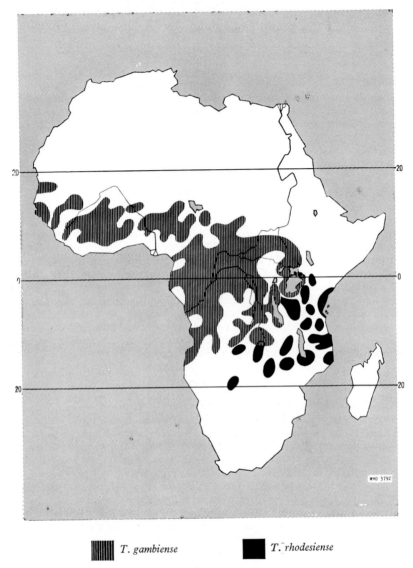

|‖‖‖| *T. gambiense*   ■ *T. rhodesiense*

Fig. 24.—Distribution of human trypanosomiasis in Africa. (*WHO 1963*)

TRANSMISSION

T. br. gambiense is not usually transmitted hereditarily in human beings although the organisms have been found in the placental blood of infected rats, as well as in the livers of their embryos, but intrauterine congenital transmission has been recorded in Germany in a European child born in Hamburg, and by Capponi (1953) in Cameroon.

In the former French Congo, Darré and his colleagues recognized congenital trypanosomiasis and demonstrated trypanosomes in the cerebrospinal fluid of a child born of an infected mother.

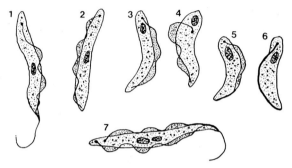

Fig. 25.—Forms of *Trypanosoma rhodesiense*. (*After Laveran*)

1, 2, Normal forms in the blood of man; 3–6, Various stages of posterior displacement of the nucleus; 7, A dividing form.

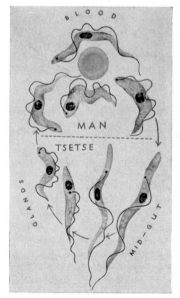

Fig. 26.—Life cycle of *Trypanosoma rhodesiense* and *T. gambiense*. (*After C. A. Hoare*)

Trypanosomes in human blood: long slender form; intermediate form; short stumpy form; stumpy form with posterior nucleus.
Stages in the tsetse fly: Trypanosome forms in the stomach and proventriculus; Crithridia and metacyclic trypanosomes in the salivary glands.
Red blood corpuscle drawn to scale.

Role of the tsetse fly as transmitting agent

There is no evidence that biting flies other than the tsetse are concerned in the spread of human trypanosomiasis, but there are apparently 2 methods by which this fly is able to transmit trypanosomes: (1) cyclical, and (2) mechanical.

(1) *Cyclical transmission.* There is no doubt that transmission ordinarily occurs through the bite of infected flies, trypanosomes passing through the salivary duct as do the sporozoites of the malaria parasite. In West Africa the major vectors, chiefly of *T. br. gambiense*, are *G. palpalis* and *G. tachinoides*.

(2) *Mechanical transmission.* Duke, in Uganda, suggested on epidemiological grounds that mechanical transmission by *Glossina* of a virulent strain of *T. br. gambiense* from man to man might be responsible for some epidemics. For further details see Appendix III.

EPIDEMIOLOGY AND EPIZOOTIOLOGY

T. br. gambiense

Gambiense trypanosomiasis is an infection of the riverine and lakeside areas of West and Central Africa. It is found wherever riverine tsetse and man are in close contact, such as river crossings, lakeside villages and waterholes frequented by man and a few infected flies. Fishermen are especially affected. Large epidemics have occurred in the past. In the Congo domestic pigs can act as occasional reservoir hosts for *T. br. gambiense*, but show no ill-effects themselves. Although eleven common species of antelope (bushbuck, reedbuck, waterbuck, etc.) can be infected artificially with *T. br. gambiense*, there is no evidence that this is a common occurrence in nature, man essentially being the reservoir.

T. br. rhodesiense

T. br. rhodesiense was first described in 1910 from a patient in the Zambesi region where the infection may have existed in an endemic form and whence it gradually spread northwards creating epidemics in various areas as far as Uganda, where it appeared in the early 1940s.

At the present time it is found sporadically in the southern part of its range, and there it is not so severe a disease as in the epidemic areas further north. It is essentially an infection of antelope (particularly the bushbuck) (Fig. 27) which has been shown by Heisch *et al.* (1958) to carry the trypanosomes in nature. In the southern area bushbuck and man are seldom in contact with each other and the strains of *T. br. rhodesiense* are not well adapted to man. In Tanzania where epidemics were severe in the 1920s and 1930s man is now infected sporadically from the animal reservoir when there is triple contact between man, the reservoir and the fly (particularly *G. pallidipes* which shows a preference for the bushbuck) which lives in a restricted area in close contact with man when he goes into the bush to collect honey or to fish. Here the strains are well adapted to man and in exceptional circumstances can be transmitted directly from man to man by *G. pallipides* in epidemic form in villages in Tanzania, Kenya and Uganda, and by *G. fuscipes* in Kenya, causing severe disease (Apted *et al.* 1963). More recently in Kenya *T. br. rhodesiense* has become adapted to the riverine tsetse, *G. fuscipes*, which has altered its habits and become peridomestic, living permanently in the rings of exotic vegetation surrounding the Luo compounds (Willett 1965), and the cattle have been found to carry *T. br. rhodesiense* (Onyango *et al.* 1966). In South-western Ethiopia *G. tachinoides* is a vector.

Feeding habits of tsetse

Weitz (1963) on evidence based upon analyses of tsetse blood meals by the precipitin test has suggested that the feeding habits of *Glossina* are genetically determined and can be grouped into 5 categories, species feeding on suids,

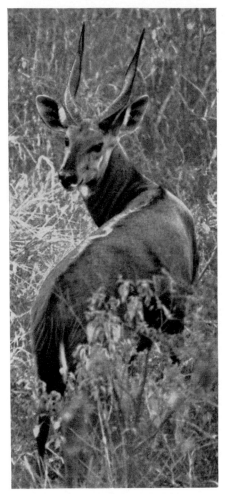

Fig. 27.—Male bushbuck (*Tragelaphus scriptus*), Kenya. (*A. W. Guggisberg, Nairobi*)

suids and bovids, bovids, mammals other than suids and bovids, and lastly most available hosts and man.

PATHOGENESIS

Most of the observations on the pathogenesis of African trypanosomiasis have been made in laboratory animals, in which as in man the growth of the parasites occurs mainly in the tissues and not in the blood (Ormerod 1970). The trypanosomes inoculated by the tsetse fly enter the tissue spaces at the site of inoculation in which they multiply, eliciting a response on the part of the host, who produces large numbers of polymorphonuclear leucocytes and other phagocytes to deal with the invader. This causes the primary chancre. The connective tissue is no barrier to the spread of the trypanosomes, which enter the lymphatics and lymph glands and spread throughout the body. The trypanosomes elicit an antibody response which is specific for each new antigenic variant produced until either the host fails to produce any more and the infection becomes overwhelming (Weitz 1962), or the infection becomes chronic, kept in check by an enhanced secondary antibody response which appears in a shorter time and is available to deal with each variant as it appears. During this process large quantities of non-specific IgM are produced and give rise to the high IgM levels which are a feature of African trypanosomiasis. The pathological effects of trypanosomiasis are produced by tissue damage and the cellular immunological response. Much of the tissue damage may be the result of kinin released by antigen–antibody reactions (Boreham 1970). There is connective tissue damage and the fibrils of voluntary muscles may also suffer (Goodwin 1970).

The immunosuppressive effect of chronic trypanosomal infection may affect the host's ability to deal with other infections resulting in an increased susceptibility to secondary infection commonly seen in advanced trypanosomiasis (Goodwin 1970).

PATHOLOGY

The chief lesions are in the lymphatic glands of the neck, submaxillary region and mesentery and in the central nervous system.

Central nervous system. Typical pathological lesions are seen only when pathogenic trypanosomes have invaded the central nervous system. No gross lesions of the nerve centres are present, but there is progressive chronic lepto-meningitis, especially in the Virchow–Robin space (where the pia sheathes the blood-vessels and the fluid acts as lymph), and also on the vertex (Dürck's nodes).

The dura may be adherent to the skull and to the arachnoid. The brain itself is congested and oedematous, the surface smooth, with convolutions flattened by increased pressure. The consistency of the brain tissue is unaltered, except for softening around any haemorrhages that may occur. The ventricles are distended with fluid. In all cases there is perivascular round-cell infiltration (perivascular cuff) throughout the brain tissue and meninges, varying in amount and in different anatomical regions (Fig. 28). The invading cells are glia cells, lymphocytes, the morula (Mott) and Marshalko cells. The 2 latter types are degenerative plasmocytes. Morula cells stain deeply, with unilateral oval nucleus and vacuolated protoplasm. Marshalko cells are large plasma cells with a blue polar zone round the nucleus, with surrounding halo and acidophilic protoplasm.

As originally demonstrated in experimental animals and in man, in advanced cases, lesions in lymphatic glands and in brain are caused by invasion of the solid tissues by trypanosomes which have migrated from the blood-stream. In the brain they have been found mainly in the frontal lobe, pons and medulla, aggregated together in masses or nests without definite relation to blood-vessels. Myelin lesions of the brain have been described by Van Bogaert (1936). The organisms also invade the cerebrospinal fluid; they enter the canal from the choroidal plexus where they congregate, as Peruzzi has shown, in active stages of division. (For eye complications, see Chapter 44.)

The spinal canal may even be blocked by cell proliferation. The cerebro-spinal fluid in early cases is under increased pressure (30–100 cm of water); the total proteins being very much increased, to 1 gramme/litre (normal 0.2 gramme).

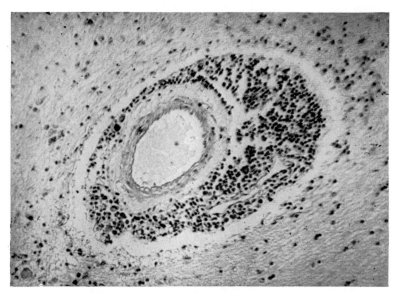

Fig. 28.—Perivascular cuffing in the cerebral cortex, due to trypano-somiasis. × 500. (*Dr A. C. Stevenson*)

The cells are increased to 15 – 500/mm³ or more (normal 2–3) and comprise lymphocytes, mononuclears, morula cells, eosinophils and trypanosomes.

Kidneys. There is glomerular nephritis, leading to fibrosis, also a generalized proliferation of the reticulo-endothelium in the capillaries.

Heart. Ecchymoses and even large haemorrhages in the epi- and endocardium have been observed. In the pathology of experimental trypanosomiasis in monkeys severe myocarditis is frequently present and is due to masses of trypanosomes within the muscle cells, and cases of myocarditis and pericardial effusion have been described in man (Hawking & Greenfield 1941; Manson-Bahr & Charters 1963).

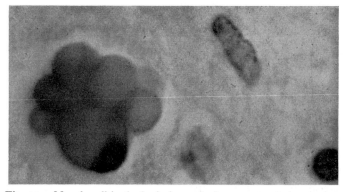

Fig. 29.—Morula cell in the brain in cerebral trypanosomiasis. × 1000.

Liver. There is spoiling of parenchyma cells, probably from toxic absorption, associated with depletion of the blood sugar. A specific central lobular necrosis has been demonstrated in experimentally infected monkeys.

Lungs. These are characterized by intravascular proliferation of the reticulo-endothelium, which may block the capillaries with fibrosis, and collapse of the alveoli.

Bone marrow. The fat is reduced and the whole tissue may be gelatinous and homogeneous.

Skin. Localized oedema, due to collections of lymphocytes, is observed in the eyelids, perineum and skin of the back.

The spleen is slightly enlarged. The Malpighian bodies are few and inconspicuous. There is a general proliferation of the reticuloendothelium, congestion at the periphery of the splenic sinuses, often focal necrosis with endothelial macrophages and ingested red blood corpuscles. Giant cells have been observed.

Lymphatic tissue shows general hyperplasia. The glands are enlarged, soft and fusiform, with great proliferation of the lymphocytes. At first there is increase of large mononuclear cells, lymphocytes and later fibroblasts. They are very vascular, with small haemorrhages containing trypanosomes (which can therefore be easily demonstrated by gland puncture).

The blood shows definite anaemia due to toxaemia and erythrophagocytosis. The haemoglobin is reduced and colour index below normal. There is usually autoagglutination of red cells with rouleaux formation (cold agglutinins). The alkali reserve is diminished and blood sugar low.

IMMUNOLOGY

Man is immune to infection with the common trypanosomes of big game, *T. congolense* and *T. vivax*. Although there is no direct evidence that man becomes immune after exposure to infection with *T. br. gambiense*, there is no doubt that when the disease has lasted any time in a district the inhabitants exhibit a degree of resistance not seen in districts more recently invaded.

Trypanosomes continually change their antigenicity and as antibodies build up new clones of trypanosomes of different antigenic structure appear against which in turn further antibodies develop. Any antibodies which develop in human trypanosomiasis are not protective. The immunoglobulins are increased and the level of IgM reaches higher than in any other protozoal infection. The sera of 85% of persons infected with *T. br. rhodesiense* agglutinate sheep red cells, while only 1 in 25 infections with *T. br. gambiense* do, a fact which can be used to detect the presence and type of trypanosomiasis in human populations (Houba & Allison 1966).

CLINICAL FEATURES

The symptoms and signs of *T. br. gambiense* and *T. br. rhodesiense* infection are similar except that in *T. br. rhodesiense* the disease runs a much more rapid course and fatal symptoms usually supervene within a year of infection. The essential clinical features are the development of a lesion at the site of the tsetse bite followed by invasion of the blood-stream and fever and at a later date invasion of the C.N.S. with encephalomyelitis and death.

Primary stage

The incubation period from natural and artificial infection is almost 2 to 3 weeks, although in some cases fever has developed as little as 5 days after the inoculation of infective trypanosomes. The bite of an infected *Glossina* is followed usually, but not invariably, by a local swelling of varying severity (in *T. br. gambiense* infections this is relatively inconspicuous), the 'trypanosomal chancre'. In *T. br. rhodesiense* transmitted by *G. morsitans* the chancre tends to be on the head and face, and on the legs in *G. pallidipes* transmission. The trypanosomal chancre is like a large boil but is relatively painless, an important point in diagnosis. The lesion subsides to be followed by invasion of the blood-stream.

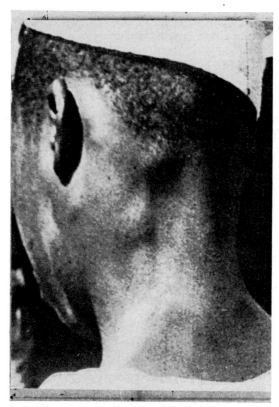

Fig. 30.—Enlargement of cervical lymph glands in trypanosomiasis (Winterbottom's sign). (*Dr F. K. Kleine*)

Blood stage

The most important symptom of invasion of the blood is fever, which is accompanied in Caucasians sometimes by a peculiar type of erythema and a certain amount of connective tissue infiltration.

Trypanosomes appear in the peripheral blood 5–21 days after the infecting bite. A form of hyperaesthesia known as 'Kerandel's sign' is usual though not invariable and is most marked over the tibiae which are tender to the touch, but the actual pain occurs after a slight delay and may cause the patient to withdraw his limbs sharply. In time the fever subsides to recur at irregular intervals of days or weeks. It is sometimes mild, sometimes severe and occasionally hyperpyrexial (41°C). It may last for weeks and the apyrexial period may be equally prolonged or it may be continuous. In time the patients become debilitated, anaemic and feeble. The spleen is usually enlarged. There is a persistent tachycardia. The cervical glands and those of other parts of the body enlarge and may become tender. Only one gland may be visibly involved or there may be polyadenitis. The implicated glands are usually most conspicuous in the posterior triangle of the neck in *T. br. gambiense* infections (Winterbottom's sign) (Fig. 30). In the early stages they are soft, later indurated. Sometimes they are painless but rarely suppurate. In *T. br. gambiense* infections this condition of irregular fever, debility, polyadenitis and slight anaemia may go on for months and even in some instances years. In *T. br. rhodesiense* infections this stage does not last more than a few months and may be as short as one month before invasion of the C.N.S. takes place.

Subclinical infection

In *T. br. gambiense* infections a proportion of cases may terminate spontaneously. Since this infection undergoes, at various stages, periods of quiescence which may be prolonged, it would be rash to call any instances of asymptomatic cases subclinical. Experiments and observations by Laveran and others in other forms of trypanosome infection as well as some cases in Caucasians justify the belief that occasionally the parasite does die out spontaneously. Observers in West Africa (Ceccaldi 1940), Katanga and Rhodesia (Blair 1939) have reported cases in which apparently healthy Africans showed trypanosomes in the peripheral blood but it is not known whether these infections were subsequently fatal or not.

Unusual manifestations

Skin rashes. In Caucasians extensive skin areas may be affected by a fugitive, patchy, frequent annular erythema (Fig. 31; Plate IV) usually most evident on the chest and back but also very often on the face, legs and elsewhere. This erythema occurs most frequently and most distinctly in the earlier stages of infection. Some of the patches may be 15 cm or even 30 cm in diameter, their margin fading off insensibly into the surrounding skin. The rash can be brought on by heat. Sometimes there is erythema nodosum.

Oedema. Oedema occurs about the site of the erythema, especially in the face. In many instances there is a general fullness of the features which is apt to convey a false impression of sound health. Transitory localized oedema may occur in the neck, abdomen, lower eyelids and sheath of the penis.

Myocarditis. Pericardial effusion and congestive heart failure have been described in *T. br. rhodesiense* infection (Manson-Bahr & Charters 1963) and mild disorders of conduction in *T. br. gambiense* infections (Bertrand *et al.* 1966).

Other features. Neuralgic pains, cramps, formication and paraesthesiae of different kinds are not uncommon; periostitis of the tibiae may occur. Toxic iridocyclitis and choroiditis are sometimes met with. There is evidence of liver dysfunction in the early stages of *T. rhodesiense* infection. Mild hepatocellular jaundice, alteration in liver function tests, decreased serum albumin and raised serum globulin can closely resemble *P. falciparum* malaria and infectious hepatitis.

Death from intercurrent disease, from rapidly developing encephalomyelitis causing convulsions, status epilepticus or coma may supervene at any stage of trypanosomiasis. Usually the case progresses into the stage known as 'sleeping sickness' which depends upon the entry of the parasite into the central nervous system.

Sleeping sickness stage (cerebral trypanosomiasis)

The terminal stage of trypanosomiasis is the result of a chronic meningo-encephalomyelitis induced by either the parasite or its toxins (Fig. 32). The characteristic symptoms are those of any chronic meningo-encephalomyelitis and consist of progressive mental deterioration proceeding to coma with in some cases localized manifestations.

In *T. br. gambiense* the interval between the start of the infection and the encephalitic stage is about 2 years, but an interval of several years, possibly 8,

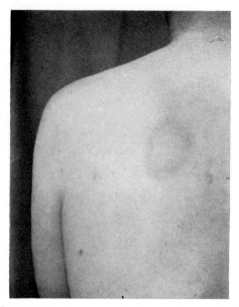

Fig. 31.—Trypanosome circinate rash. (*Cooke, Gregg and Manson-Bahr*)

may elapse. In *T. br. rhodesiense* the interval is very short, usually a few months. The average duration of this stage is from 4 to 8 months, not infrequently less, and a course of more than a year is rare.

Generally the first indications of the oncoming of sleeping sickness are an accentuation of the debility and languor usually associated with trypanosomiasis. There is disinclination to exertion, slow shuffling gait, mask-like vacant expression, puffiness and drooping of the eyelids and a tendency to lapse into sleep during the daytime, contrasting with restlessness at night. The patient will walk if forced to do so with unsteady swaying gait. There may be fibrillary twitching of the muscles, especially the tongue, tremor of the hands and more rarely of the legs. His speech is difficult to follow, becoming indistinct and staccato. By this time the patient has taken to bed and lies about in a corner of the hut indifferent to everything going on about him. He never spontaneously engages in conversation or even asks for food, but is still able to speak and take food if

T.D.—4

this is brought to him. If he is properly nursed there is no general wasting. So far the striking changes are the mental and personal changes accompanying a chronic encephalomyelitis.

As time goes on he begins to lose flesh, tremor of hands and tongue become more marked and convulsive or choreic movements may occur in the limbs or in limited muscular areas. Sometimes these convulsions are followed by local temporary paralyses. Sometimes there is meningismus with head retraction. There is generally intolerable pruritus, bed sores form, saliva dribbles from the mouth, the body wastes and finally the patient dies comatose or from slowly advancing asthenia. He may succumb to convulsions, hyperpyrexia, pneumonia, dysentery or other intercurrent infections.

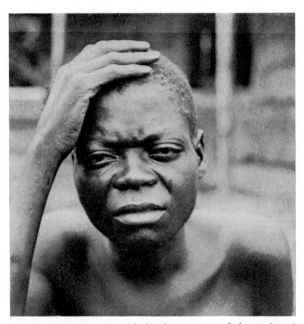

Fig. 32.—Cerebral trypanosomiasis. Appearance of the patient in the last stages of the disease. (*Dr Cuthbert Christy*)

There are considerable variations in the manifestations which may be found in any chronic meningo-encephalomyelitis. Mania is not uncommon, there may be manic-depressive episodes going on to a progressive mental deterioration and idiocy. Delusions may be present.

Localized neurological signs, such as hemiplegia, facial palsy, ophthalmoplegia and meningitic symptoms, may occur. Persistent headache is a feature (Fig. 32).

In the main 3 principal categories of trypanosomiasis may be recognized:

(*a*) Mild with few symptoms, commonest in *T. br. gambiense* infections.

(*b*) Involving the central nervous system.

(*c*) Acute, leading to death before C.N.S. symptoms develop, commonest in *T. rhodesiense* infections.

Mortality

Although spontaneous recovery may take place in the early stages of trypanosomiasis, it is believed that when the disease has arrived at the stage of sleeping sickness, in the absence of treatment, death is inevitable. Many of the African villages in Senegambia have been depopulated, and what has occurred on the Congo, in Angola and in Uganda, bears out this estimate of the gravity of the disease in epidemic form. Many islands in Lake Victoria Nyanza have been completely depopulated. The population of the implicated districts of Uganda, originally about 300 000, was reduced in 6 years to 100 000 by sleeping sickness early in this century.

DIAGNOSIS

Any fever especially if associated with enlarged cervical glands in a patient who has resided in an endemic area suggests a tentative diagnosis of trypanosomiasis, as should mental symptoms in anyone—African or Caucasian—who has been in an endemic area and who may die in an asylum of unrecognized cerebral trypanosomiasis.

Differential diagnosis

In the early stages malaria, kala-azar, tuberculosis, brucellosis, lymphoma and lymphadenoma must all be distinguished, while in the late stages, syphilitic meningomyelitis, cerebral tumour, cerebral tuberculosis and chronic virus encephalitis may all resemble each other closely.

Diagnosis may be made by finding trypanosomes in the blood, lymph gland juice or cerebrospinal fluid or by serological methods.

Examination of the blood

Parasites in the blood. In early cases of *T. br. rhodesiense* infection parasites are numerous in the blood, and may be found on direct examination of a wet drop or by concentration methods. The thick drop method should always be employed and it is estimated that it takes 20 times as long to find them in thin as in thick wet drop preparations.

Concentration method. Take into a 10 ml syringe 1 ml of 6% sodium citrate in 0·9% saline. Fill the syringe with blood from a vein. Centrifuge for 10 minutes on the low gear of the two-gear centrifuge. This brings the red cells down as a sediment, on the surface of which the leucocytes form a grey layer. Supernatant fluid is pipetted off into another tube. Examine the leucocyte layer and first sediment for trypanosomes. Re-spin supernatant fluid in the high-speed gear for 10 minutes and pipette off into a third tube. Examine the second sediment, which occasionally reveals trypanosomes (in 16%). The third sediment similarly treated often has trypanosomes in 39%. Sicé (1937) advised that the electric centrifuge should not exceed 3000 r.p.m.

Micro method. A similar method may be employed using small micro-amounts of blood in capillary tubes.

Sedimentation rate. The E.S.R. is high in patients suffering from trypanosomiasis. For this purpose the Westergren is more sensitive than the Wintrobe method. Even a delay of 5 hours after withdrawal has a negligible effect. Sedimentation readings should be made at 10-minute intervals. The median hour rate varies from 15 to 76 mm but in untreated cases may be as high as 114 mm.

The increase in E.S.R. is closely associated with red cell clumping (auto-agglutination).

Examination of lymph gland juice

Lymph gland puncture and examination of the aspirated lymph is the most certain method particularly in the early stages of the disease in gambiense infections, when the glands are soft before they have become sclerosed. The procedure is as follows:

(a) The gland is gripped between finger and thumb of the left hand and massaged.

(b) A hypodermic needle (size 14) is pushed through the skin into the substance of the gland which is then squeezed further.

(c) The needle is withdrawn and its contents gently blown out on to a slide by means of a hypodermic syringe filled with air.

(d) A coverslip is applied and the unstained preparation is *immediately* examined beneath the $\frac{1}{6}$ objective. Intensely active trypanosomes are easily recognized in a positive case. They can be subsequently fixed and stained.

Gland puncture should always be reinforced by the examination of thick blood films. The glands may be unilateral or bilateral; sometimes they reach the size of a pigeon's egg and every gradation may be shown. Although the superficial glands may be easy to palpate, deeper ones may be more difficult. Three procedures for palpation are necessary: deep palpation, superficial palpation, and palpation by passing the palmar surface of the hand over the neck. The glands should have the consistency of a ripe plum. Harding and Hawking (1944) found both gland and blood examination positive in 30–40%; gland puncture positive, blood film negative in 50–60%; and blood film positive, gland puncture negative in 10%.

Examination of the cerebrospinal fluid

Trypanosomes may be demonstrated in the centrifuged deposit of the cerebrospinal fluid but infrequently, and in cases where they cannot be found, suggestive evidence of C.N.S. involvement may be obtained by examination of the cells and estimation of the protein content. The earliest reaction from meningeal involvement is cellular, and the intensity of the reaction is shown by the number and character of the cells. The presence of leucocytes indicates recent activity, whereas plasma cells, dead cells and morula cells indicate older and more chronic lesions. The diagnosis of cerebral trypanosomiasis is not justified on a cell count below 15 or 20/mm³, the limit should be about 30 cells.

The protein is invariably raised in cerebral trypanosomiasis and the level is an indication of the duration of the infection, and the stage which the disease has reached. Prognosis and evidence of relapse are also based upon the protein level. In the field protein is best measured in a Sicard Cantaloube tube with the addition of 30% glacial acetic acid (normal 22 mg/100 ml).

The IgM level in the cerebrospinal fluid can be measured in the same way as in serum and is a useful diagnostic and prognostic tool.

Animal inoculation

Of ordinary laboratory animals the most susceptible are the guinea-pig, rat, dog and Macaca and Cercopithecus monkeys. Citrated blood, 2–10 ml, is withdrawn and inoculated intraperitoneally. The interval between the appearance of trypanosomes in the blood varies from 6 to 49 days. (*T. br. gambiense* is not pathogenic to rats.)

Cultural methods

Weinman (1963) advocates culture methods, noting that early attempts were poor because they were made with media containing blood which contained lytic substances which destroyed the trypanosomes *in vitro*. He (1960) uses a medium consisting of 2 portions: (*a*) base composed of 1·5% Difco nutrient agar (at pH 7·3) 31 grammes, plain agar 5 grammes, and distilled water 1000 ml; the ingredients are dissolved by heating, distributed in known volumes, and autoclaved; (*b*) inactivated human plasma and washed human erythrocytes at 200 ml each. Before use, blood is reconstituted by mixing equal volumes of the plasma and erythrocytes, then 3 times as much base (*a*) is cooled to 45°C and 1 part of reconstituted blood (at the same temperature) is added to 3 parts of base (*a*). The resulting medium is distributed in test tubes (5 ml each), these are slanted (2 to 3 days), and (after incubation to test sterility) stored at 4 to 8°C.

To each millilitre of blood used for cultivation is added 0·1 ml of 0·5% saline solution of anticoagulant polyvinyl sulphuric acid (PVSA) sterilized by filtration, and 2 ml of blood with PVSA are inoculated into each tube of medium, to which dihydrostreptomycin sulphate (0·5 mg in 0·1 ml saline/ml blood) has been added; the inoculum is spread over the surface of the medium by tilting the tubes, and these are incubated at 25°C in darkness. The cultures may be positive in 5 to 30 days. In one series of 34 patients 79% gave positive cultures, the remainder being contaminated, both *T. br. gambiense* and *T. br. rhodesiense* being involved. The method proved sensitive and reliable, and may reveal cases not diagnosed by other means.

Serological diagnosis. Many diagnostic techniques have been explored including agglutination, precipitation, complement fixation and neutralization. In addition auto-agglutination of red cells, adhesion of platelets or red cells to trypanosomes, agglutination inhibition of tanned red cells and agar gel precipitation have all been investigated. The most reliable methods should be complement fixation tests and the estimation of the IgM levels by means of agar gel precipitation. The indirect fluorescent antibody test also shows promise.

Complement fixation test. The test material should contain antigens common to all strains and species of trypanosomes infecting man in Africa. This should be purified to remove inhibitors and substances giving false positives. These requirements can be satisfied only in a central laboratory and the method is not suitable for field use.

Estimation of IgM. The quantitative estimation of IgM in serum is useful both for individual and mass diagnosis of trypanosomiasis in endemic areas. Cunningham *et al.* (1967) have described the test. Serum from rabbits immunized against human IgM is incorporated in agar gels. Discs of filter paper (3 mm in diameter) are soaked in the patient's blood and laid on the surface of the gel. The agar gel is thoroughly washed and dried. The zones of precipitation are then stained with Amido black and are carefully measured. Of bloods from infected people 75% gave a precipitation zone greater than 5 mm in diameter as compared with only 1 of a control group. Positive reactors should be examined further by the fluorescent antibody test.

Fluorescent antibody test. Cunningham *et al.* (1967) have described the indirect fluorescent antibody test using *T. br. rhodesiense* in rats for fluorescence on dried human blood on discs. Out of 50 known infected persons 46 gave a positive immunofluorescence whereas only 8 of 130 control persons were positive. This is a useful test for mass screening of populations.

TREATMENT

Especially in Africans, preliminary treatment directed towards eliminating superimposed infections with ancylostomes or schistosomes is advisable, on account of damage to the liver cells which renders toleration of arsenical drugs difficult.

For many years after the 1920s the most effective drugs for trypanosomiasis were suramin (Bayer 205, Antrypol, Moranyl) and tryparsamide, often given in consecutive courses. Suramin, which does not pass the blood–brain barrier, was particularly valuable in the early stages, and especially in *T. br. rhodesiense* infections; tryparsamide was most useful in the later stages.

Suramin should be given intravenously, as a freshly prepared 10% solution in distilled water, and the usual dose for an adult is 1 gramme (i.e. 10 ml of the 10% solution), repeated at intervals of 5–7 days for 5 to 6 injections. It may be wise to limit the first dose to 0·5 gramme. Suramin may injure the kidneys, and should be given only if the excretory organs are working well; the urine should be examined for albumin before each injection.

Tryparsamide is also given intravenously, in freshly prepared 20% solution in distilled water. The initial dose may be 1 gramme for an adult, followed at intervals of 5–7 days by up to 9 or 10 doses, each of 2 grammes. Tryparsamide is usually safe, but may produce optic atrophy, and careful watch must be kept on the state of visual acuity in patients treated with it. The patient may complain of a sensation of shimmering movement, as if the objects were observed through waving smoke. Soon afterwards there is a general depression of vision with diminution in central acuity. After an interval of about 2 weeks the optic discs become pale, without swelling or vascular abnormalities, and the patient may become completely blind, with inactive, partially dilated pupils. This may be followed by slow recovery of vision, partial or complete, some patients regain only a moderate degree of vision, and some remain completely blind. Ridley (1945) thought that the toxic effects may be due to impurities rather than to the tryparsamide itself.

Among the drugs used for trypanosomiasis, tryparsamide in particular has been associated with the appearance of arsenic resistance in strains of *T. br. gambiense*.

Suramin and tryparsamide have usually been given in consecutive courses, and Harding (1945), working in a *T. br. gambiense* area, advocated the following: suramin 1 gramme followed, after an interval of 3 *weeks*, by 2 further doses of suramin (1 gramme) and then 5 doses of tryparsamide (2 grammes), all at intervals of 5 *days*.

If the interval after the first dose of suramin is 2 to 3 weeks, only 1 further dose of that is given, followed by 6 doses of tryparsamide.

If the interval after the first dose of suramin is less than 2 weeks, no further suramin is given, and the course is completed with 7 doses of tryparsamide.

In more recent years, however, the introduction of pentamidine (and its dimethanesulphonate derivative lomidine) and of products with a melaminyl radicle, has strongly influenced treatment. The WHO Expert Committee on Trypanosomiasis (1962) suggested the following schedules:

T. br. gambiense infection

(1) *For treatment of patients in the stage of infection of blood and lymphatic system only.* (a) Pentamidine in doses of 3 to 4 mg of base/kg of body weight, daily for 10 days, by intramuscular injection. The solution must be freshly made. A possible hypotensive effect can be controlled by 30% hypertonic glucose solution (against hypoglycaemia), or by intravenous suramin.

(b) Suramin, if pentamidine is contra-indicated. Like suramin, pentamidine does not pass the blood–brain barrier.

(c) Mel B (Arsobal, melarsoprol). A single dose of 3·6 mg/kg can cure patients in this stage. It is not water-soluble, and must be given intravenously, in propylene glycol.

(2) *For treatment of patients in the meningo-encephalitic stage.* (a) Mel B. This should be reserved for patients in good general condition, who are free from liver or kidney trouble, and who have never presented signs of arsenical poisoning. They should be kept under medical supervision during treatment and for 12 days afterwards. Urine should be tested for albumin before each injection. Ampoules should be stored in the dark, below 25°C and the injection equipment sterilized by dry heat; the intravenous injection should be given slowly, on an empty stomach, with the patient lying down and fasting for at least 5 hours after the injection. If any signs of serious toxicity arise (encephalopathy, mental confusion, peripheral neuritis) the patient should at once be treated with BAL (dimercaptopropanol); slighter signs of intolerance (malaise, headache, vomiting, albuminuria, tendency to haemorrhage) may indicate that the drug should be stopped (Schneider 1963).

If trypanosome invasion of the nervous system is slight, 3 injections of Mel B (3·6 mg/kg to a maximum of 200 mg, i.e. 5·5 ml of a 3·6 % solution) are given intravenously, on alternate days. If the nervous system is seriously affected, 2 courses (as above) are given at an interval of 3 weeks.

An alternative schedule is to give 1 course of 3 injections of 3·6 mg/kg. when there are fewer than 20 cells/mm^3 in the cerebrospinal fluid; 2 courses when there are 20–100 cells; 3 courses when there are more than 100 cells.

It is fair to state that some physicians have found Mel B uncomfortably toxic, and advocate special care in its administration.

For patients in the later stages whose general condition is poor, pentamidine may be given on the first and third days, with 10 intravenous injections of tryparsamide on days 2, 9, 16, 23, and so on. This series may be repeated after an interval of 1 month.

An alternative is a mixture of suramin and tryparsamide (each made up fresh as 20% solution): 10 mg of suramin/kg (maximum 0·5 gramme) mixed in the syringe with 30 mg/kg of tryparsamide (maximum 1·5 grammes); this is injected intravenously every 5 days for up to 12 injections, and the course may be repeated once or twice at intervals of 1 month.

(b) Mel W (melarsonyl; 9955RP) is a water-soluble derivative of Mel B, which can be given by intramuscular injection and is less toxic than Mel B. For patients in the early stage of *T. br. gambiense* infection Schneider *et al.* (1961) gave a single injection of 4 mg/kg, intramuscularly or subcutaneously, in the form of a 5% solution. This tended to reactivate latent malaria, but had no toxic effect itself; chloroquine was therefore given at the same time. For patients in the late stages the doses were 1, 2, 3, and finally 4 mg/kg on successive days (to a maximum of 200 mg for any one injection), but for advanced late cases a second series of injections 1 to 2 weeks after the first, to a maximum single injection of 250 mg, is desirable.

Another course is a trial dose of 2 mg/kg, followed, if there is no reaction, by 4 mg/kg daily for the next 3 days. This is enough for early cases, but for more advanced cases another 4-day course of 4 mg/kg daily is given after an interval of 7–10 days (Watson 1965).

Mel W passes the blood–brain barrier, but the response may not be as dramatic as it is to treatment with Mel B, and indications of late relapse have been recorded (Watson 1962). Nevertheless, Mel W has as much effect as the older drugs, with the advantage that it can be administered easily and is less toxic; it is therefore suitable for mass treatment.

(c) Furacin (the nitrofurazone of nitro-2-furaldehyde-semicarbazone) has also been used for patients who had relapsed after other treatments. Fierlafyn (1960) reported good results from a dosage (for adults) of 1500 mg by mouth daily for 10 days, followed, if the cerebrospinal fluid did not show improvement, by a second course (though the necessity for this was later doubted). For children the daily dose was 30 mg/kg. The results were regarded as good, though some patients developed polyneuritis (reduced by treatment with thiamine), but Robertson (1961) has observed a haemolytic effect of a nitrofurazone compound, which possibly could prove serious in populations with a high incidence of G6PD deficiency. Adriaenssens (1962) has found a laevo-isomer of furaltadone effective, and less toxic, in a few cases of Rhodesian trypanosomiasis.

Diminazine aceturate (Berenil), used for animal trypanosomiasis, has been given in T. br. gambiense infection by Hutchinson and Watson (1962), in doses of 2 mg/kg of a 2% solution in 5% glucose daily for 7 days; it was given by deep intramuscular injection. The results were promising.

T. br. rhodesiense **infection**

For early cases, suramin in doses (for adults) of 1 gramme intravenously (in freshly prepared 10% solution) on days 1, 3, 7, 14, and 21, are advocated by WHO.

For cases with involvement of the nervous system (over 3 cells/mm³, or over 25 mg protein/100 ml in the cerebrospinal fluid) Mel B is regarded as the only effective drug. Mel W has not been so successful, and the effect of nitrofurazone is still not certain, though it may be tried in cases which do not respond to other drugs.

Criteria of cure

In patients treated in the haemolymph stage of the disease there should be no clinical sign of the disease, or abnormality of blood or cerebrospinal fluid, after several examinations during 2 years.

In patients treated in the meningo-encephalitic stage there should be no clinical signs (except perhaps of irreversible damage to the nervous system done before treatment); the cell count of the cerebrospinal fluid should fall steadily to below 5/mm³, and the protein content to below 0·3 mg/ml.

Prognosis

The state of the C.S.F. is most important. Increase of total protein is of more significance than cell increases. If the C.S.F. is abnormal after treatment the cell count is the more delicate indicating cure or failure. The Sicard Cantaloube method of estimating total protein (normal 22 mg/100 ml) should be used. The blood sedimentation rate is also useful.

Prophylaxis

Prophylactic measures are based principally on the habits of *Glossina palpalis*, *G. tachinoides* and other species which may transmit *T. br. gambiense*. The measures employed are so similar to those in use against *T. br. rhodesiense* and so interwoven that they must be considered together in the section on the bionomics of *Glossina* (see Appendix III).

Repellents. Little information is obtainable on this subject, but an anti-mosquito cream (containing pyrethrum) has a repellent action chiefly against *G. palpalis* for 6 hours, when applied to the skin, but this action is apt to be destroyed by heavy sweating with exposure to strong sunlight (Holden & Findlay 1944). The most popular at present is Di-Meepol which contains dimethyl phthalate and ethylhexanediol in a non-greasy base and can be dissolved in a small amount of liquid paraffin for use in fly country.

Chemoprophylaxis. The first favourable results in attempts to prevent infection by using drugs were obtained with suramin, and a dose of 25 mg/kg (1·25 grammes for a person weighing 50 kg) was reported on favourably in West Africa, though McLetchie (1948) could only put the period of protection at 12 to 16 weeks. This was in a *T. br. gambiense* area, but reports from *T. br. rhodesiense* areas were more favourable.

More recently, however, the drug most used for protection against *T. br. gambiense* has been pentamidine (especially lomidine), which is reported to give protection for about 6 months; it is given as a single dose of 4 mg of base/kg, to a maximum of 300 mg for any one person, however heavy. Its efficacy against *T. br. rhodesiense* is accepted by some authors but disputed by others. Lomidine prophylaxis has been the principal weapon used in the former French and Belgian African countries for the control of trypanosomiasis, and has un-doubtedly reduced the great epidemics to manageable proportions. It is not claimed, however, that chemoprophylaxis alone is likely to eradicate the disease.

Both suramin and pentamidine become fixed in the body tissues, and are released relatively slowly, which accounts for their prophylactic action. It has been argued that there may come a point, some months after injection, at which the drug is no longer in sufficient concentration to prevent infection, but is able to conceal it, and that this may lead to delay in diagnosis and therefore render treatment more difficult.

Control

The object of any control effort in trypanosomiasis is to break the man–tsetse fly contact. This can be done by an attack on the tsetse fly by the destruction of its habitat, removal of the food supply, or by killing with insecticides. Or it can be done by removing man from the environment by concentration of the population in certain areas or by altering the environment on a large scale.

In the event of any of the above measures being impractical a certain amount of control can be achieved by mass chemoprophylaxis in areas where only Gambian sleeping sickness occurs.

Discriminative bush clearing along rivers and in the savannah will provide an unfavourable environment for the fly in some cases. Denial of food supply to the tsetse by destruction of the big game is not practicable because alternate sources of food are usually available. Direct insecticidal attack on the fly by spraying from the air or from the ground has been useful in some special circumstances, but is expensive. By far the most useful measure of control is the creation of a new environment for the population as has been done in the Anchau experiment in Nigeria. This provided a model example of the method of clearing an area of tsetse flies as well as of benefiting the population generally and of raising their level of culture. Anchau became a tsetse-free corridor, linking two of the railway lines that diverge from Zaria, and is some 100 km long, over 155 000 hectares in extent and with a population of 50 000. The combination of partial and barrier clearings has proved effective. The work on this scheme entailed preparation of maps, surveys, construction of roads, clearing 175 km of stream, sinking of wells, study of local soils and vegetation, agricultural experiments and monthly fly surveys. The land allowance is 17·2 hectares per person. Areas are reserved for plantation of wood and grazing.

Removal of infected populations. Trypanosomiasis has interfered with the development of one-quarter of the African continent. In part of Uganda by 1900 it was estimated to have exterminated two-thirds of the local population. To preserve the hitherto uninfected from trypanosome infection, the Government transported the entire population of the Sesse Islands and neighbouring shore of Victoria Nyanza to fly-free areas in the interior. It was hoped that, the human source of trypanosome supply being thus denied them, the tsetse flies would cease to be infective. In an emergency the infected population can be removed *en masse* from a trypanosomiasis area and settled in tsetse-free villages. This was successful in Tanganyika between the two wars, but requires large areas of unoccupied land for a successful outcome, and is open to great political difficulties (Apted *et al.* 1963).

For a detailed description of tsetse flies (Figs 433–436) and preventive measures now in use, see Appendix III.

REFERENCES

ADRIENSSENS, K. (1962) *Ann. Soc. belge Méd. trop.*, **42,** 31.
APTED, F. I. C., ORMEROD, W. E., SMYLY, D. P., STRONACH, B. W. & SZLAMO, E. L. (1963) *J. trop. Med. Hyg.*, **66,** 1.
BERTRAND, E., SENTILHES, L., DUCASSE, B., VACHER, P., & BAUDIN, L. (1966) *Méd. trop.*, **25,** 603.
BLAIR, D. M. (1939) *Trans. R. Soc. trop. Med. Hyg.*, **33,** 729.
BOREHAM, P. (1970) *Trans. R. Soc. trop. Med. Hyg.*, **64,** 394.
BUXTON, P. A. (1955) *Natural History of Tsetse Flies.* London: Lewis.
CAPPONI, M. (1953) *Bull. Soc. Path. éxot.*, **46,** 667.
CECCALDI, J. (1940) *Ann. Inst. Pasteur*, 67.
CUNNINGHAM, M. D., BAILEY, N. M., & KIMBER, C. D. (1967) *Trans. R. Soc. trop. Med. Hyg.*, **61,** 696.
FIERLAFYN, E. (1960) *Ann. Soc. belge Méd. trop.*, **40,** 469.
FORD, J. (1969) *WHO Bull.*, **40,** 879.
GOODWIN, L. G. (1970) *Trans. R. Soc. trop. Med. Hyg.*, **64,** 797.
HARDING, R. D. (1945) *Trans. R. Soc. trop. Med. Hyg.*, **39,** 99.
——— & HAWKING, F. (1944) *Lancet*, **ii,** 835.
HAWKING, F. & GREENFIELD, J. C. (1941) *Trans. R. Soc. trop. Med. Hyg.*, **35,** 155.
HEISCH, R. B., McMAHON, J. P., & MANSON-BAHR, P. E. C. (1958) *Br. med. J.*, **ii,** 1203.
HOLDEN, J. R. & FINDLAY, G. M. (1944) *Trans. R. Soc. trop. Med. Hyg.*, **38,** 199.
HOUBA, V. & ALLISON, A. C. (1966) *Lancet*, **i,** 848.
HUTCHINSON, M. P. & WATSON, H. J. C. (1962) *Trans. R. Soc. trop. Med. Hyg.*, **56,** 227.
McLETCHIE, J. L. (1948) *Trans. R. Soc. trop. Med. Hyg.*, **41,** 445.
MANSON-BAHR, P. E. C. & CHARTERS, A. D. (1963) *Trans. R. Soc. trop. Med. Hyg.*, **57,** 119.
MULLIGAN, H. W. & POTTS, W. H. (1970) *The African Trypanosomiases.* London: Allen & Unwin.

ONYANGO, R. J., VAN HOEVE, K. & DE RAADT, P. (1966) *Trans. R. Soc. trop. Med. Hyg.*, **60,** 175.

ORMEROD, W. E. (1970) in *The African Trypanosomiases* (ed. Mulligan, H. W., & Potts, W.), p. 587. London: Allen and Unwin.

RIDLEY, H. (1945) *Ann. trop. Med. Parasit.*, **39,** 66.

ROBERTSON, D. H. H. (1961) *Ann. trop. Med. Parasit.*, **55,** 49.

SCHNEIDER, J. (1963) *WHO Bull.*, **28,** 763.

—— LEVEUF, J. J. & TANAGARA, S. (1961) *Bull. Soc. Path. exot.*, **54,** 345.

SICÉ, A. (1937) *La Trypanosomiase Humaine en l'Afrique Intertropical.*

VAN BOGAERT, L. (1936) *C. r. Séanc. Soc. Biol.*, **121,** 1387.

WATSON, H. J. C. (1962) *Trans. R. Soc. trop. Med. Hyg.*, **56,** 231.

WEINMAN, D. (1960) *Trans. R. Soc. trop. Med. Hyg.*, **54,** 180.

—— (1963) *WHO Bull.*, **28,** 731.

WEITZ, B. (1962) *Drugs, Parasites and Hosts* (ed. Goodwin, L. G., & Nimmo-Smith, R. H.) p. 180. London: Churchill.

—— (1963) *WHO Bull.*, **28,** 711.

WILLETT, K. C. (1965) *Trans. R. Soc. trop. Med. Hyg.*, **59,** 374.

WORLD HEALTH ORGANIZATION (1962) *Wld Hlth Org. tech. Rep. Ser.*, 247.

—— (1963) *WHO Chronicle*, **17,** 444.

6. AMERICAN TRYPANOSOMIASIS (CHAGAS'S DISEASE)

Geographical distribution

Human infection with *T. cruzi* is widespread (Fig. 33) and is found in every country in South and Central America. *T. cruzi* infection has been recorded in two patients who had never left Texas (Kagan *et al.* 1966). *T. cruzi* is also found in armadillos, racoons and opossums far outside the distribution of human trypanosomiasis and infected bugs have been found as far north as Virginia as well as in Trinidad, Curaçao and Aruba in the Caribbean (Downs 1963). Primates infected with trypanosomes resembling *T. cruzi* have been found in Indonesia (Weinman & Wiratmadja 1969), and similar trypanosomes, which were described as *T. lewisi*, were found in a sick child in Malaya (Johnson 1933), although these were probably *T. conorhini*.

AETIOLOGY

T. cruzi infection of man is the cause of South American trypanosomiasis. It is found in the blood in acute cases, but is rare in chronic cases in which infection can only be demonstrated by cultural or immunological methods. For a description of *T. cruzi* see Appendix I.

T. rangeli and *T. ariarii* (see page 963) may also be found in man, but are thought to be non-pathogenic. They can be distinguished both morphologically and by their behaviour in the bug, in which they undergo anterior development in contrast to *T. cruzi*, which always develops in the hindgut and undergoes posterior development.

TRANSMISSION

The adult trypanosomes are ingested by the invertebrate host, blood-sucking reduviid bugs either in the larval nymphal or adult stage (see page 1121). After they have passed through many stages in the intestinal canal in a period of 8–10 days fully formed trypanosomes known as 'metacyclic forms' appear in the hindgut and are passed out in the faeces of the insect. Infection takes place when the faeces are rubbed into the wound caused by the bite.

In Argentina and Chile the common vector is the 'Vinchuca' bug, *Triatoma infestans*, in Brazil *T. infestans* and *Panstrongylus megistus*, and in Venezuela *Rhodnius prolixus*. Many other species of the genera *Panstrongylus*, *Rhodnius* and *Eratyrus* can transmit the infection and bed bugs can transmit laboratory infections which may occur accidentally through ingestion of the bugs (see Appendix III).

Transmission may also take place congenitally, accidentally in a laboratory or by blood transfusion.

Congenital transmission of *T. cruzi* is probably quite common. Parasites have been found in the blood of a 15-day infant in Argentina and infection has been found in macerated fetuses and premature and stillborn infants. Several cases of accidental transmission in the laboratory have been recorded when working with cultures or infected animals. The trypanosomes may enter accidentally

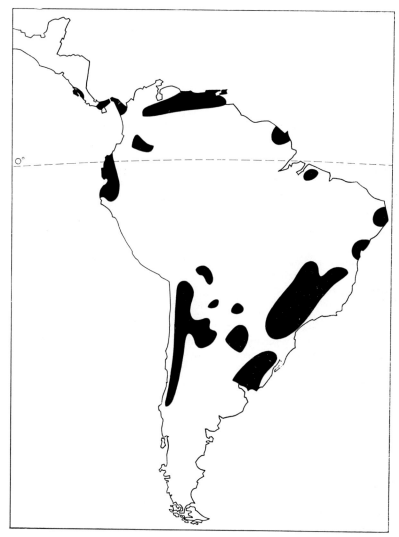

Fig. 33.—South America, showing the distribution of South American trypanosomiasis (Chagas's disease).

via the conjunctiva or abrasions in the skin. A number of observers in Brazil have reported on transmission of infection by blood transfusion and this is an obvious danger in organizing blood banks in endemic areas.

EPIDEMIOLOGY

Chagas's disease is a serious public health problem in South America. The World Health Organization estimates that 7 million people are infected and 30 million exposed to the risk of infection (WHO 1960).

Reservoir hosts

T. cruzi has been found in many wild mammalian hosts (see page 962), mainly armadillos and opossums, and in domestic animals, dogs, cats and pigs. The infection is maintained in wild mammals by various species of reduviid bugs (page 958) which are capable of transmitting *T. cruzi* but which are zoophilic and do not bite man.

Human infection

When environmental conditions permit, the reduviid bugs, which feed on man and his domestic animals, maintain the infection as a peridomestic infection. Maintenance hosts, which provide a food supply but are not infected, such as chickens, play an important part in maintaining the population of bugs. The environmental conditions which produce endemic Chagas's disease are poor adobe thatched huts in which the bugs live in close contact with man and which are present in the tropical areas of South and Central America.

PATHOLOGY

The parasites multiply rapidly at the site of inoculation where they produce a focus of infiltration with leucocytes and round cells with interstitial oedema and focal lymphangitis (chagoma). The parasites are found in the trypanosomal form in the blood during the early stage of dissemination, but they soon enter cells of mesenchymal origin (cardiac and skeletal muscle, reticulo-endothelial cells and neuroglia). In the infected cells the parasites assume the leishmanial form and multiply by binary fission until the cytoplasm is filled with large numbers of leishmaniae, producing a leishmanial pseudocyst. Since the trypanosomes do not multiply in the blood, the leishmaniae that are released by rupture of the pseudocyst must enter a new host cell promptly or die. This explains the difficulty in treatment of this disease since the parasite does not have to survive in the blood but rests safely in pseudocysts in various organs.

As the pseudocysts multiply the lymphocytes, plasma cells and histiocytes of the host appear round every focus of parasite multiplication. Granulomas, sometimes containing giant cells, form with eventual fibrosis. As the cellular and humoral immune response of the host develops, parasite multiplication is suppressed and trypanosomes become very scanty in the peripheral blood. Later even the leishmania forms become difficult to find in the tissues. The main targets are the muscle fibres of the heart, the smooth muscle of the digestive tract and the autonomic nerve ganglia. Koberle (1958) has shown that there is a great diminution in the ganglion cells of the right auricle and the enteric plexus of patients with chronic Chagas's disease and has postulated that a toxin is liberated when the pseudocysts rupture which damages the nerve cells. No toxin has been demonstrated generally, but Seneca (1969) described one, chagastoxin, which he has obtained from extracts of *T. cruzi* which has a toxic effect on cells and which causes hepatitis, myocarditis and nephropathy in mice. Chagastoxin is a lipopolysaccharide and is antigenic, giving rise to antibodies which may have toxin neutralizing properties.

Damage to the parasympathetic ganglia in the right atrium may lead to impaired sympathetic control with increased cardiac work and dilatation and hypertrophy. The myocardium may also be damaged directly by parasites with resultant inflammatory response and fibrosis. The chronic dilatation of the gut is also considered to be due to ganglion cell destruction and defective innervation. The release of cellular substances from disintegrated infected cells causing an autoimmune phenomenon has also been suggested as a cause of the pathological changes (Okamura & Corrêa Netto 1963).

As a result of these changes the classical features of chronic Chagas's disease are produced—cardiomyopathy and mega disease.

Chagas's cardiomyopathy

The characteristic macroscopic pathological features of chronic Chagas's cardiomyopathy are a greatly dilated heart, ventricular apical aneurysms, protrusion of the pulmonary conus, duplication of the heart apex and mural thrombi. Microscopic examination shows a diffuse inflammatory myocarditis with the presence of leishmanial pseudocysts. There is destruction of the muscle fibres of the myocardium, and involvement of the conduction system of the heart may occur by parasitization or secondary to adjacent fibrosis in the heart. There is a difference in opinion between observers in Brazil and Venezuela concerning the degree of neural involvement. In Brazil all cases of Chagas's cardiomyopathy show a marked decrease in the number of ganglion cells in the heart and this denervation is considered to be the essential lesion.

In Venezuela this striking reduction in ganglion cells has not been observed and the heart lesion is considered to be due to inflammatory response and to the destruction of the muscle fibres.

Numerous nodules of hyperplastic reticulo-endothelial cells and histiocyte granulomas are found in the spleen, liver and lymph nodes.

Meningo-encephalitis

Meningo-encephalitis is a severe complication of acute Chagas's disease, especially in young children. The inflammatory reaction is characterized by the invasion of neuroglia cells and the presence of glial nodules in the white and grey matter, and in the basal ganglia and cerebellum. Chronic neurological syndromes with spastic paralysis, mental deficiency and cerebellar symptoms have been ascribed to chronic Chagas's disease (Okamura & Corrêa Netto 1963).

Mega diseases

As a result, it is thought, of toxins and parasitic invasion and rupture of the pseudocysts and granulomatous inflammation, the cells of Auerbach's plexus are greatly reduced in number, resulting in discoordination of the peristaltic movement and achalasia of the cardiac sphincter, with megacolon, mega-oesophagus, megaduodenum, megajejunum, megappendix, megaureter and megabladder. Hollow organs become enormously distended.

IMMUNOLOGY

Chagas's disease is often a very chronic infection. Trypanosomes are very scanty in the blood after the early stages and the parasite maintains itself in the leishmanoid form tucked away in the reticulo-endothelial cells and protected from any possible serum antibodies. Complement fixing antibodies appear in the serum 30 days after infection, and persist for the duration but disappear with cure. Delayed hypersensitivity develops and is shown by the intradermal test of Mayer and Pifano using an extract 'cruzin' prepared from culture of *T. cruzi*. Fluorescent antibodies also develop. Much work has been done on immunization of animals against *T. cruzi*, but none has as yet proved applicable to man.

CLINICAL FEATURES

Clinically Chagas's disease may manifest itself as an acute infection in children (acute Chagas's disease) with a chagoma at the site of the infection, fever and trypanosomes in the blood and, rarely, the development of encephalo-myelitis; or it may present as a fever with trypanosomes in the blood followed by myocardial involvement with disorders of conduction and sometimes sudden death. The majority of infections are subclinical and can only be discovered by xenodiagnosis or serological tests, and some subjects with positive results show cardiomyopathy on further investigation. In some areas a proportion of these individuals develop megaoesophagus and megacolon.

Chagoma

The primary lesion which develops at the site of infection is called a chagoma. This results from invasion of the skin and surrounding tissues by proliferating trypanosomes. The chagoma is a local inflammatory swelling in which leish-manial forms of the parasite multiply within the fat cells. When the chagoma is round the eye, which is the usual site, there is oedema of the eyelids and sometimes also of the malar and temporal regions together with unilateral conjunctivitis (Romaña's sign) (Fig. 269, page 888).

There are some reasons for believing that the conjunctiva may be a common portal of entry for *T. cruzi*. In an accidental laboratory infection recorded the site of entry was undoubtedly the conjunctiva and the infection was followed by dacryocystitis, swelling of the face, pyrexia and adenitis. Dacryocystitis may be uni- or bilateral and is invariably accompanied by facial oedema. The reaction is therefore allergic in the region where reduviid bugs deposit infected faeces during sleep. Enlarged lymphatic glands containing leishmanial forms of *T. cruzi* are described in association with the inoculation chagoma and in satellite lymphatics; there may be generalized lymphadenitis.

Some 14 days after the infecting bite a rash may be seen on the chest and abdomen consisting of sharply defined red spots the size of a pin's head. There is no pain or itching and the exanthem fades entirely within 7 to 10 days. Some children develop milder disease characterized by the presence of numerous subcutaneous painful nodules throughout the body (lipochagomas).

There is hepatosplenomegaly. Cardiac arrhythmias, myocardial insufficiency and collapse are also present. There is leucocytosis with a marked lympho-cytosis, a raised sedimentation rate and a raised serum gamma-globulin.

Chagas described an acute form in infants with pyrexia and general lympha-denitis. The liver and spleen are enlarged and the child develops signs of meningo-encephalitis. In the chronic form the disease may assume a myxoede-matous, cardiac or nervous complexion. The first is frequent in children up to 15 years of age and is characterized by thyroid insufficiency, scanty urine and dry skin. The cardiac type is characterized by cardiac arrhythmia and extra-systoles with bradycardia, the nervous type by intention tremor and various paralyses.

Thyroid involvement

Areas of myxoedematous swelling appear on certain parts of the body in acute Chagas's infection and have led to the suggestion that the thyroid is implicated. It has been pointed out that it is difficult to distinguish endemic goitre and cretinism, which are frequent in the geographical range of this disease, from acute and chronic Chagas's disease. In Brazil where Chagas made his observations 75% of the population normally have goitre and there is a cretin in almost every family.

Cardiomyopathy

The cardiomyopathy of acute Chagas's disease is most frequent in infants and young children. The cardiomyopathy of chronic Chagas's disease is usually seen in subjects between 15 and 50 years of age. In endemic areas of Chagas's disease this cardiomyopathy is very prevalent. In mild cases the changes may be limited to tachycardia or extra systoles, in more severe cases there are cardiac arrhythmias, atrioventricular or right bundle-branch block and in the most severe there is dilatation of the heart with progressive myocardial insufficiency and cardiac failure. In young adults the myocarditis may be rapidly progressive, with death occurring in 6 months. Sudden death from destruction of the conducting fibres is common, especially in young men, and is a major cause for concern in Brazil.

Electrocardiographic changes. The electrocardiogram shows widening and notching of the QRS complex and abnormalities in the P and T waves. The commonest changes are disorders of rhythm, especially right bundle-branch block, both partial and complete, and complete heart block with Stokes-Adams attacks (Rosenbaum & Alvarez 1955).

Mega disease (**mal de engasco, suffocating disease**) (Koberle 1958)

In São Paulo, Brazil, there is a much higher incidence of megaoesophagus and megacolon than in other areas. This increased incidence is not seen in all *T. cruzi* endemic areas. The symptoms and signs of mega disease are the same as idiopathic achalasia of the cardia and megacolon of Hirschsprung's disease.

SUBCLINICAL INFECTIONS

In endemic areas of Chagas's disease a proportion of the population show positive complement fixation tests although they are apparently healthy and xenodiagnosis reveals *T. cruzi* in 30% of these. Surveys of these people with the electrocardiogram reveal that many show minor E.C.G. changes.

In Brazil in almost one-third of 2000 subjects examined the electrocardiogram was abnormal, and about 9% of chest radiographs showed enlargement of the cardiac shadow. It is thought that subclinical infections are by far the commonest manifestation of *T. cruzi* infection. Maekelt (1966) has stated that in Venezuela serological and xenodiagnostic methods indicated that 20% of the rural population were infected, of whom 50% showed some heart condition while most of the myocardial affections in rural inhabitants up to 40 years of age were due to Chagas's disease.

DIAGNOSIS

Diagnosis may be made by isolation of *T. cruzi* from the blood, by the demonstration of leishmanial forms, by muscle biopsy or by serological methods.

Isolation of *T. cruzi* from the blood

Trypanosomes may be found on direct blood examination in early cases of acute Chagas's disease; however they rapidly become very scanty in the blood and need methods of concentration or culture to demonstrate their presence.

Concentration. *Centrifugation.* Heparinized blood is centrifuged or allowed to settle in a haematocrit tube or microcentrifuge tube and the supernatent plasma examined just above the buffy coat or centrifuged at 2000 revolutions per minute and the deposit examined.

Phytohaemagglutinin. Five to 10 ml of blood are drawn and the red cells agglutinated by phytohaemagglutinin. The supernatant fluid is drawn off, centrifuged and the deposit examined for trypanosomes.

Culture. The blood is cultured on NNN medium. If heparinized blood is kept at room temperature *T. cruzi* will multiply and this method can be used away from laboratories.

Xenodiagnosis (Brumpt 1913)

At least 6 clean uninfected laboratory-bred reduviid bugs are allowed to feed on the suspected patient or on a specimen of blood withdrawn from the patient. Two weeks later the contents of the hindgut are examined for the presence of crithidia. It is essential to use clean insects properly protected since they can become infected by coprophagy. The bug may be macerated in saline, which is then filtered. The filtrate can be examined and inoculated into mice (Maekelt 1962).

Biopsy

Examination of biopsy material from the deltoid muscle may show granulomas, occasionally containing leishmanial forms in histiocytes.

Serological methods

Complement fixation test. The complement fixation test, the Machado–Guerreiro reaction (Guerreiro & Machado 1913), has been used with great success. The antigen which is not yet standardized is made from a freeze-dried extract of cultural flagellates. Positive titres of over 1:2 dilution are significant. There may be cross-reactions with *L. donovani* infections. Alternative serological tests are an indirect fluorescent antibody test (Fife & Muschel 1959) which can be performed on filter paper blood and a haemagglutination test (Montano & Acros 1965).

DIFFERENTIAL DIAGNOSIS

On clinical grounds Chagas's disease is to be distinguished in the acute phase from other febrile conditions and encephalomyelitis, and in the chronic stage from other cardiomyopathies, especially those of alcoholism and pregnancy, hypothyroidism, cretinism, myxoedema, Hirschsprung's disease and achalasia of the cardia.

TREATMENT

The treatment of Chagas's disease is still in a very unsettled and unsatisfactory state. An antibiotic, puromycin, had some effect on *T. cruzi* in mice and has been used in human cases with indeterminate results.

8-Aminoquinoline derivatives

Primaquine and a derivative 349C 59D (Wellcome) have been used with some success in doses of 15 mg daily for long periods up to 6 months. In acute cases trypanosomes have disappeared from the peripheral blood, and the fever has settled, but the long-term results are not yet known and positive complement fixation tests have usually remained positive.

Nitrofurazone

A nitrofurazone preparation, Bayer 2502 (Lampit), has been used successfully in the laboratory. A dose of 30 mg/kg/day for 15 days, followed by 10 mg/kg/day for 3 months, has been suggested. Immediate arrest of the chagoma and negative blood cultures for 2 years with a decreasing titre in the complement fixation test have resulted from this course. In other cases, however, there have been relapses and severe toxic effects can occur (Hawking 1964).

Chlortetracyclines and steroids should be avoided since they tend to exacerbate the infection. The treatment of mega disease is surgical.

PROGNOSIS

The prognosis of Chagas's disease both acute and chronic is very difficult. Chagas's original patient described in 1910 is still alive and well at an advanced age. Acute cases may go into remission for a long period and it is not yet known what are the chances of developing the late manifestations of cardiomyopathy, megacolon, and megaoesophagus. In the chronic stage, where there is cardiomyopathy with E.C.G. changes, disorders of rhythm may occur at any time, and sudden death is not uncommon.

PROPHYLAXIS

Since Chagas's disease in man is essentially an environmental disease, control can be effected ultimately only by changing the environment to a bug-free one. This means the construction of proper houses, so that the bugs cannot infest them. Two other approaches are possible—first vector control and secondly reservoir control.

Vector control

BHC can be used as a 1% mixture at a rate of 200 ml/m² to destroy reduviids (Chapter 45). Dieldrin, 1 gramme/m² has been used in Venezuela with success. Dwellings, hen houses and dovecotes must all be treated. Treatments must be repeated at yearly intervals according to the results on the bug population.

Reservoir control

Since armadillos are an important reservoir of infection human habitations should be placed as far away from the burrows as possible.

Personal prophylaxis

Individuals may avoid infection by refusing to sleep in adobe and thatched huts. In the endemic areas the proper use of bed nets can prevent infection since the bugs are nocturnal feeders.

Transfusion transmission of *T. cruzi* can be avoided by performing routine complement fixation tests on donors in endemic areas and eliminating positive reactors as potential donors. 25 ml of a 1:4000 solution of gentian violet should be added to each 500 ml of blood for 24 hours before transfusion. An alternative substance is a 1:5000 solution of crystal violet. All laboratory workers dealing with *T. cruzi* should have their blood examined for trypanosomes and a complement fixation test performed periodically.

REFERENCES

BRUMPT, E. (1913) *Bull. Soc. Path. éxot.*, **6,** 167.

DOWNS, W. G. (1963) *J. Parasit.*, **49,** 50.

FIFE, E. H. & MUSCHEL, L. H. (1959) *Proc. Soc. exp. Biol. Med.*, **101,** 540.

GUERREIRO, C. & MACHADO, A. (1913) *Braz.- med.*, **23,** 225.

HAWKING, F. (1964) *J. trop. Med. Hyg.*, **67,** 211.

JOHNSON, P. D. (1933) *Trans. R. Soc. trop. Med. Hyg.*, **26,** 467.

KAGAN, I. G., NORMAN, L. & ALLAIN, D. (1966) *Revta Biol. trop.*, **14,** 55.

KOBERLE, F. (1958) *Gastroenterology*, **34,** 460.

MAEKELT, G. A. (1962) *Arches venez. Med. trop.*, **4,** 277.

——— (1966) *Revta venez. Sanid. Asist. soc.*, **31,** 163.

MONTANO, G. & ACROS, H. (1965) *Boln chil. Parasit.*, **20,** 63.

OKAMURA, M. & CORRÊA NETTO, A. (1963) *Revta Hosp. Clin. Fac. Med. Univ. S Paulo*, **18,** 351.

ROSENBAUM, M. B. & ALVAREZ, A. J. (1955) *Am. Heart J.*, **50,** 492.

SENECA, H. (1969) *Trans. R. Soc. trop. Med. Hyg.*, **63,** 4.

WEINMAN, D. & WIRATMADJA, N. S. (1969) *Trans. R. Soc. trop. Med. Hyg.*, **63,** 497.

WORLD HEALTH ORGANIZATION (1960) *Wld Hlth Org. tech. Rep. Ser.*, 202.

7. LEISHMANIASIS

Definition

Leishmaniasis is caused by parasites of the genus *Leishmania*, originally parasites of rodents in which they cause a mild cutaneous disease. They are transmitted by sandflies and have become adapted to canines and man in whom they cause three main clinical types of disease.

In general there is a primary lesion of the skin to which the infection may be limited (cutaneous leishmaniasis), or which, in some areas of the world, may metastasize to the lymph glands, other areas of the skin, and mucocutaneous junctions (espundia or mucocutaneous leishmaniasis). In other areas the infection metastasizes throughout the reticulo-endothelial system of the body (kala-azar, visceral leishmaniasis). The three species of *Leishmania* which affect man cannot be distinguished morphologically, culturally or by animal inoculation but can be distinguished serologically to a certain extent.

IMMUNOLOGY

Infective *promastigotes* enter the body at the site of inoculation by the sandfly bite and cause a primary lesion which may be obvious in cutaneous leishmaniasis or small and inapparent in African kala-azar. The cellular reaction to the amastigotes which develop at the site of invasion is essentially a proliferation of histiocytes followed by the infiltration of round and plasma cells which leads to the elimination of the parasites by a process of cell-mediated immunity (CMI) mediated through sensitized lymphocytes which destroy the *Leishmania*-filled macrophages (Bray & Bryceson 1968). In diffuse cutaneous leishmaniasis this secondary invasion by lymphocytes is absent and parasites remain numerous in this form—the result of a failure of cell-mediated immunity caused by a lack of host response (Adler 1965).

In visceral leishmaniasis there is a similar proliferation of histiocytes in the reticulo-endothelial system of the affected organs and this is followed by round and plasma cell infiltration and hypergammaglobulinaemia without the elimination of parasites. The increase in immunoglobulin is in the IgG fraction and is not protective or related to the development of specific antibodies but is a product of the hypertrophied parasitized reticuloendothelial system. Specific antibodies cannot be demonstrated in *Leishmania tropica* infections, but complement fixing, haemagglutinating and fluorescent antibodies all develop in kala-azar which are specific and can be used for diagnostic purposes. The cellular reactions are accompanied by the development of delayed hypersensitivity, a positive intradermal skin reaction (leishmanin or Montenegro reaction) and the appearance of cell-mediated immunity. In *L. tropica* infections, where there are no metastases, these reactions all develop early and are associated with the elimination of the parasites. In *L. braziliensis* infection with metastasis to other areas of the skin and mucous membranes they develop later after metastasis has taken place. In *L. donovani* infection, delayed hypersensitivity and cell-mediated immunity do not appear until the visceral infection has been cured.

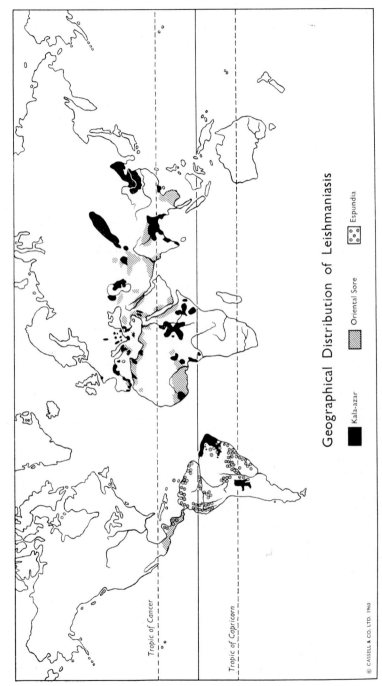

Fig. 34.—Geographical distribution of leishmaniasis.

Immunity to reinfection

Infection with all forms of leishmaniasis which is allowed to run its natural course immunizes against reinfection with the homologous strain. This immunity usually lasts for many years, possibly for life, but recent work (Guirges 1971) suggests that in both *L. donovani* and *L. tropica* infections, reinfection can occur.

Cross-immunity between the different strains is also found. *L. tropica major* protects against *L. tropica minor*, but not vice versa; it does not protect against *L. donovani*. *L. braziliensis* protects against *L. mexicana* but not vice versa. *L. donovani* does not protect against *L. tropica*.

Antigenic relationships of *Leishmania*

There is an antigenic relationship between all mammalian *Leishmania* and lizard *Leishmania* and with some mycobacteria. Adler and Adler (1955) found that *L. adleri* shared antigens with *L. donovani*, *L. braziliensis* and *L. tropica*; leishmanin can be prepared from any strain of *Leishmania* as well as flagellates such as *Strigomonas oncopelti*. Common antigens are shared with mycobacteria. The antigen for the complement fixation test in kala-azar is prepared from Kedrowsky's acid-fast bacillus or tubercle bacilli.

Leishmanin test; Montenegro reaction

This skin reaction which is a measure of delayed hypersensitivity was introduced by Montenegro (1924) in South America. Leishmanin is a suspension of washed promastigotes of *Leishmania* of any species in 0·5% phenol saline. It is used in a strength of 10^8/ml for kala-azar and New World cutaneous leishmaniasis. and 10^2/ml for Old World cutaneous leishmaniasis. The dose is 0·2 ml intradermally and the test is read after 48 or 72 hours. A positive result is an area of induration exceeding 5 mm in diameter which may be much larger and result in necrosis. A positive leishmanin reaction shows previous experience with some form of leishmanial antigen of any species, whether mammal or lizard, and indicates cell-mediated immunity to the homologous strain in the absence of any active infection.

The leishmanin reaction becomes positive early in infection with *L. tropica* and *L. mexicana* and does not denote immunity to reinfection until the leishmanial lesion has completely healed. In *L. braziliensis* the test becomes positive during the active phase of the infection. In *L. donovani* it does not become positive until 6 to 8 weeks after recovery from kala-azar.

Other serological reactions

Specific antibodies have been described only in kala-azar. Complement fixing, haemagglutinating and fluorescent antibodies all develop in kala-azar and are used for diagnosis. They are described in the section on kala-azar.

I. Kala-azar (Visceral Leishmaniasis)

Synonyms

Tropical Splenomegaly; Black Sickness; Sirkari Disease; Sahib's Disease; Burdwan Fever; Dum-dum Fever; Ponos (Greece); Mard el Bicha (Malta).

Definition

An infective disease characterized by chronicity, irregular fever, enlargement of the spleen and often of the liver, and the presence in these and other organs of *L. donovani*.

Geographical distribution

This is shown in Fig. 34.

Aetiology

Kala-azar is caused by *L. donovani* (Plate I). For details see Appendix I.

TRANSMISSION

Following the observation by Napier that there was a correlation between the distribution of *Phlebotomus argentipes* and kala-azar in India, much work was performed on the subject by Christophers, Shortt, Knowles, Napier, Barraud, Lloyd and Smith, with the result that a very rapid intensive anterior development of promastigote forms was found to occur in *P. argentipes* (see page 1078). Subsequently it was found possible to transmit the infection to hamsters by artificially infecting sandflies in the laboratory and later Swaminath *et al.* (1942) successfully transmitted kala-azar by the bites of *P. argentipes* to 7 human volunteers. This success after years of unsuccessful effort was obtained by sustaining sandflies on fruit juices during the 2 weeks of development of the parasite.

An account of the bionomics of the sandfly will be found in Appendix III. The various species transmitting kala-azar will be discussed under Epidemiology.

Other forms of transmission

Kala-azar may occasionally be a congenital infection (Lowe & Cooke 1926), and cases transmitted by blood transfusion have been reported. A case has been reported of a man with Sudanese kala-azar whose wife had never been out of England but who developed a leishmanial lesion on the vulva. It has been suggested that transmission may be direct from man to man through the faeces or via the nasal mucus, since amastigotes have been demonstrated in stools containing blood and mucus and in swabs from nasal mucosa. It is not the general opinion, however, that transmission other than through sandflies is important.

Transmission has been accomplished artificially to man by inoculating cultures of *L. donovani* intradermally into the skin. A nodule containing amastigotes developed at the site of inoculation. After a period of 4 to 6 months *Leishmania* forms were isolated on blood culture and the full-blown kala-azar syndrome developed later (Manson-Bahr 1959).

EPIDEMIOLOGY

It is best to consider the varieties of kala-azar on a biological basis. Visceral leishmaniasis with a rodent reservoir (African kala-azar), visceral leishmaniasis with a canine reservoir (Mediterranean kala-azar) and visceral leishmaniasis with a human reservoir (Indian kala-azar). Historically it is probable that *L.*

donovani was originally a parasite of rodents which became adapted to wild canines, and later, with the domestication of the dog, to the domestic dog and to man.

VISCERAL LEISHMANIASIS WITH A CANINE RESERVOIR

Kala-azar with a canine reservoir is found in many of the islands and countries of the Mediterranean basin, especially Sicily, Crete, Greece, Turkey, Portugal, Spain and southern France around Marseilles and Nice. It is also found in the Middle East, Central Asia, North China and South America.

Reservoir hosts. In the Mediterranean, Turkestan, China north of the Yangzte and Brazil kala-azar occurs in both man and dogs. In all these endemic foci the infection is far more widespread in dogs than in man. Infected dogs may be recognized by their emaciation, thickened ulcerated skin and splenomegaly; the infection rate of *Phlebotomus perniciosus* fed on dogs approached 100%, whereas when fed on human cases of kala-azar it was negligible (Adler & Theodor 1935). Human cases are of little importance as a source of infection.

In Brazil Deane and Deane (1964) have reported an infection rate of 15% in *P. longipalpis* fed on human cases as opposed to 24% fed on dogs, and on foxes (*Lycalopex vetulus*) up to 100%. In this area human cases may play a role as a source of infection although they are much less important than dogs or foxes.

In Tadjikistan in Central Asia jackals have been found infected on the outskirts of new human settlements and in Iraq kala-azar occurs on the outskirts of Baghdad where none of a number of dogs examined has been found infected (Bray & Dabbagh 1968), although an outbreak of kala-azar occurred in a pack of foxhounds in this area in 1957 and jackals have been suspected as its cause.

Mediterranean kala-azar. In the Mediterranean area kala-azar occurs sporadically especially in infants and is known as *ponos* or infantile kala-azar, although adults, especially immigrants, do not always escape. It is a seasonal disease in children and dogs on the outskirts of towns and villages and appears in April but is rare after November, and its incidence coincides with that of the sandfly season. If a child is born in October the first signs may be observed in the following August. In the Eastern Mediterranean the vector is *P. major* and in the Western Mediterranean and North Africa mainly *P. perniciosus*, *P. ariasi* and *P. longicuspis*. In Mediterranean kala-azar the disease is always endemic and sporadic, never epidemic, since canines and not man form the reservoir and maintain the infection in nature.

In Central Asia kala-azar occurs on the outskirts of towns and villages and affects mainly children. Where the jackal is a reservoir host the disease occurs in rural areas on the outskirts of settlements and adults are generally affected. In China children are affected and the vector is *P. chinensis*.

Kala-azar in the Middle East. Kala-azar occurs on the outskirts of Baghdad and sporadically in Saudi Arabia, Yemen, the Radfan area in Aden and very rarely in Iran. In none of these areas have infected dogs been found, and jackals are suspected as a source of infection.

Kala-azar in South America. Kala-azar was first discovered in South America in Paraguay in 1913. Subsequently it was found to be quite common there when the viscerotome was routinely introduced in 1936 for the diagnosis of yellow fever. The infection is found mainly in North-east Brazil, where it is epidemic, but also sporadically in Paraguay, Northern Argentina, Amazonia,

Venezuela and Colombia, and a few cases have occurred in Guatemala and Mexico.

In South America (Deane & Deane 1964) kala-azar is an infection of man, dog and the fox (*L. vetulus* and *Cerdocyon thous*), although man plays only a small part in propagating the infection. The infection is mainly sporadic but can be epidemic as in North-east Brazil. The distribution in age-groups resembles Mediterranean kala-azar although children of a somewhat higher age-group are attacked. The infection is only found where *P. longipalpis* is found in association with human habitations, feeding on man, but the distribution of this sandfly is not continuous nor are the bionomics the same in all areas.

VISCERAL LEISHMANIASIS WITH A HUMAN RESERVOIR

In India man is the ideal reservoir of infection within much of the zone of distribution of *P. argentipes*, since parasites are readily obtainable from the peripheral blood. Dogs have never been found infected though many have been examined. In Assam kala-azar occurs mainly in epidemics which have been recorded at irregular intervals since 1870, when the disease advanced slowly along the Brahmaputra valley at the rate of some 160 km in 7 years. Its introduction into a village could usually be traced to some individual from an infected locality. Generally it clung to a place for 6 years and then disappeared without any apparent change in local conditions. It is a 'house' disease, and a house which seemed to form a microfocus of infection for many months was considered dangerous to reoccupy under a year.

In India, as elsewhere, 4 males are affected to 1 female and the age-group affected is older than in the Mediterranean—most cases occur in the 10–20 age-group. *P. argentipes*, the vector, which feeds solely on man, has a distribution in India in close correspondence to that of kala-azar, is easily infected from the blood of patients suffering from kala-azar, and *P. argentipes* has transmitted the infection experimentally to human volunteers (Swaminath *et al.* 1942) in a historical experiment. *P. argentipes* is also found in Malaya but does not bite man there.

VISCERAL LEISHMANIASIS WITH A RODENT RESERVOIR (AFRICAN KALA-AZAR)

African kala-azar is found south of the Sahara from Lake Tchad eastwards to the Indian Ocean. The history of kala-azar in this area is in accord with the concept of a zoonosis with a reservoir possibly in rodents with epidemics occurring when interhuman transmission takes place. Two main types of kala-azar are found: *Sudanese kala-azar* transmitted by *P. orientalis*, and *East African kala-azar* transmitted mainly by *P. martini*; both are primarily rodent infections occurring sporadically in man when he encroaches on a 'nidus' but under certain circumstances transmitted from man to man and becoming epidemic. Severe epidemics occurred in the Sudan and in Kenya in the 1950s.

Reservoir hosts

Sudanese kala-azar. In the Sudan *Leishmania* have been isolated from wild rodents, *Arvicanthus niloticus*, *Rattus* and *Acomys* and from a serval cat and a genet (Hoogstraal & Dietlein 1964). *A. niloticus* is an excellent experimental reservoir host (Stauber *et al.* 1966) and *Leishmania* were isolated from wild

P. orientalis (Heynemann 1963). *P. orientalis* is the chief man-biting species in the Southern Sudan and strains of leishmania isolated from cases of kala-azar, rodents and *P. orientalis* were all identical serologically by Adler's test (Adler *et al.* 1966). The infection is found on the flood plain of the Nile in the southern Sudan and along other large rivers, especially the Blue Nile in the central Sudan as far as the Ethiopian border. It occurs amongst nomads and semi-nomads who occupy temporary villages near the patches of *Acacia-Balanites* woodland which has been found to harbour *P. orientalis*. Kala-azar has not been found west of Lake Tchad which is the westernmost recorded occurrence of *P. orientalis*.

East African kala-azar. East African kala-azar is found from Kapoeta in South-eastern Sudan eastwards through northern Kenya to Somalia along the Juba river and southwards in Kenya along the Tana river. Cases have occurred in the Karamoja district of northern Uganda. *Leishmania* have been isolated from rodents mainly *Tatera* (Heisch 1957), in which infection is cryptic. Strains of *Leishmania* can persist in the skin of baby mice for a long time without causing a visceral infection (Adler 1964). The relationship of animal strains to *L. donovani* is uncertain, since they caused skin nodules and not a visceral infection when inoculated into human volunteers (Manson-Bahr 1959).

In Kenya kala-azar has been found in association with eroded termite hills in microfoci (Wijers & Mwangi 1966) where *P. martini* and related species have been found to occur. *Leishmania* which caused kala-azar in man have been isolated from wild *P. martini* (Heisch *et al.* 1962; Manson-Bahr *et al.* 1963).

African kala-azar attacks males 4 times as often as females and as in India the age-group most affected is 10–20 years. Throughout its range kala-azar is sporadic, except along the Tana river in Kenya where a large epidemic started in 1953 which has continued since, and the disease has become endemic. Kala-azar has also been found to occur in Eritrea and Ethiopia in the north, but it is not known whether this is an extension of Middle Eastern kala-azar or whether this represents true African kala-azar.

PATHOLOGY

In Central Asia and Africa a *primary leishmanioma*, which may be so small as to be unapparent, forms at the site of entry. A cellular reaction of lymphocytes and plasma cells develops around the amastigote-filled histiocytes in the dermis. As the immune process develops epithelioid and giant cells appear to be followed in some cases by healing. In other cases amastigotes escape into the blood in macrophages and leucocytes and circulate and colonize the endothelial cells of the reticulo-endothelial system. Here they multiply until the cell ruptures and they are transported to fresh cells. The reticulo-endothelial cells chiefly affected are situated in the spleen, liver, bone marrow, lymphatic glands, large intestine and skin but parasites have been isolated from the ventricles of the heart, the suprarenals and the parotid gland.

The *spleen* is grossly enlarged. In the acute stage the capsule is smooth, thickened and nodular, becoming in the chronic form almost cartilaginous. The splenic pulp is increased in amount and very friable. There are usually numerous infarcts. The hypertrophy is due to the reticulo-endothelial pro-liferation and a considerable part of the spleen substance is composed of amastigote parasites. The *liver* is also enlarged, brown or mottled. The Kupffer cells are packed with amastigote parasites. There is some pressure atrophy and, finally, in the chronic stage, a fine interlobular cirrhosis.

The *bone marrow* is reddish containing abundant amastigote parasites.

The *kidneys* may contain a few amastigote parasites which are carried by the blood-stream. They may show amyloid changes in some cases.

The *lungs* show no parasites but are liable to secondary bacterial infection on account of the leucopenia which is such a constant feature of this disease. In the *gastro-intestinal* tract there is proliferation of reticulo-endothelial cells, especially in the duodenum and jejunum. The villi may become grossly hypertrophied and swollen by packed parasitized cells. Small ulcerations are not uncommon and parasites can be demonstrated in them.

The *lymphatic glands* are generally enlarged and congested, especially the mesenteric group, and the tissue is usually invaded by large numbers of *Leishmania*. There is also hypertrophy of the retropharyngeal lymphoid tissue and Leishman–Donovan bodies can be found in nasal and pharyngeal secretions.

The *skin* may contain *Leishmania*. In fatal cases of kala-azar all levels of the skin below the epidermis may contain amastigote-filled cells collected in large masses about the sweat glands and arterioles and scattered diffusely throughout the corium. Deane (1956) in Brazil and Manson-Bahr (1959) in East Africa have detected parasites in the dermis in a proportion of cases of kala-azar. There is a close resemblance between these findings and the skin rashes associated with kala-azar (page 126), and they may be of importance in the role of man in maintaining the infection in nature.

CLINICAL FEATURES

The incubation period determined experimentally lies between 4 and 10 months (Manson-Bahr *et al.* 1963), and from observations in the Sudan between 3 and 6 months (Kirk 1942). However there are considerable variations. In one case under Manson's care the time that elapsed from arrival in an endemic area and the onset of fever was under 10 days. It may be as long as 2 years (Sweeney *et al.* 1945), $2\frac{1}{2}$ and $1\frac{3}{4}$ years (Jopling 1955) or 9 years (Wright 1960). In the few cases where a primary leishmanioma has been described this develops 4 to 6 months before the onset of symptoms and may be a minute papule (Mirzoian 1941) or have the appearance of an oriental sore (Cahill 1964). The onset may be gradual or sudden. If sudden, there is high fever, which may be intermittent or remittent, often with a double rise resembling *P. falciparum* malaria (Fig. 35). It lasts from 2 to 6 weeks and occasionally longer. Waves of fever separated by apyrexial periods may often simulate undulant fever; during the apyrexial periods the spleen enlarges and may rapidly become quite large.

In cases with a gradual onset which are commonest in endemic areas there is discomfort beneath the left costal margin from an enlarging spleen and the patients often first seek medical help for an attack of pneumonia or dysentery to which they are especially liable. In these cases cough, sputum, epistaxis and diarrhoea are the presenting symptoms.

Signs

In spite of the patient's weak and emaciated condition, the pyrexia and the splenomegaly, he presents a good appetite and a clean tongue. He may be working with a temperature of (38·9°C) (102°F), quite unaware that he has fever. There may be no malaise or apathy. In this respect kala-azar differs from malaria and typhoid.

Splenomegaly. The spleen is usually enlarged from the commencement of the illness, while the liver does not become appreciably enlarged until later. The spleen usually enlarges fairly rapidly but in rare cases, especially of acute toxic kala-azar, may not be palpably enlarged.

Lymphadenopathy. Especially in the African form there is a generalized lymphadenopathy with enlargement of the inguinal and femoral glands.

Skin. In many cases, especially in Indian kala-azar, the skin acquires a strange earth grey colour. This dusky pigmentation has given rise to the name 'kala-azar' ('black fever') and is best seen on the feet, hands and abdomen in fair-skinned people, but is often missed in dark-skinned persons (Das Gupta *et al.* 1954). In African kala-azar a warty eruption may appear on the skin.

Course

Spells of fever and apyrexia occur for months, until a low form of fever, rarely over 38·9°C (102°F), becomes more or less persistent. Profuse sweats are common but rigors occur only exceptionally in the more chronic forms. When the disease is well established emaciation and anaemia become noticeable and, together with enlargement of the spleen and liver, produce a typical appearance. Oedema of the legs may be present. The hair becomes dry and brittle; haemic murmurs of the heart are heard; haemorrhages may occur from any part of the body; purpuric patches, petechiae, epistaxis and bleeding from the gums are found.

This condition of chronic fever, enlargement of the spleen, emaciation and anaemia may go on for months or even 1 or 2 years. In 96% of cases, the patient is cut off by intercurrent disease.

Goodwin (1945) and Gellhorn *et al.* (1946) have shown in hamsters that nephritic changes are common after the forty-sixth day of infection and a deposit of amyloid may take place in several organs, particularly in the kidneys. The urine frequently shows more albumin than can be accounted for by the fever and much of the oedema which is found may well be of renal origin. Death may ensue from several causes —exhaustion, dysentery (bacillary or amoebic) bronchopneumonia and coma. A mild hepatocellular jaundice is found in 10% of cases and indicates a severe infection.

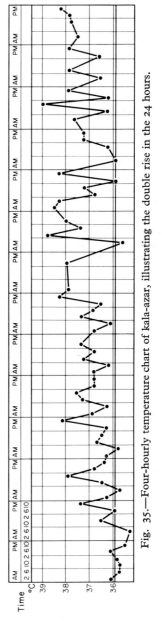

Fig. 35.—Four-hourly temperature chart of kala-azar, illustrating the double rise in the 24 hours.

Blood changes

Anaemia is invariable in advanced cases and is due to hypersplenism as demonstrated by Knight *et al.* (1967), who showed that there was a significant sequestration and haemolysis of the red cells with a half normal lifespan by an enlarged spleen, and it has been suggested that the anaemia in kala-azar is an autoimmune phenomenon. The red blood cells are often reduced to 2500 000/mm^3 with a corresponding fall in haemoglobin. The most remarkable change is *leucopenia*. The leucocytes are reduced below 3000/mm^3 in 95%, below 2000 in 75% and 1000 in 42% of cases. The proportion of leucocytes to erythrocytes, normally 1 to 750, stands at 1 to 1500 or even 1 to 2000. The differential shows a relative increase of lymphocytes, a moderate increase of large mononuclears and almost complete absence of eosinophils. The reduction in leucocytes may proceed to acute agranulocytosis.

There is usually thrombocytopenia which is responsible for the haemorrhagic tendency.

Dermal leishmanoid

A cutaneous form of leishmaniasis, in which parasites occur in nodules on the face, forearms, inner aspects of the thighs and pubic regions, was first reported by Christophers in India in 1904 and Thomson and Balfour in the

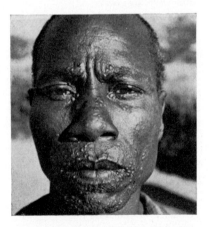

Fig. 36.—Post-kala-azar dermal leishmanoid.

Sudan in 1909. It was described by Brahmachari in India under the name of 'dermal leishmanoid' or 'post-kala-azar dermal leishmanoid'. No cases have been recorded from the Mediterranean and it is rare in China. It is certainly a sequel to generalized infection with *L. donovani*, as more than half the patients have suffered from kala-azar about one year previously and have been given antimony treatment. In Bengal up to 20% of cases develop this complication and in Africa about 2%. The longer kala-azar is endemic in an area, the more frequent does this complication become. The eruption appears in India up to 2 years after treatment and may last some years, even 20 (Sen Gupta & Mukherjee 1968). In Africa the eruption appears early during treatment and fades rapidly after cure. L-D bodies are found in smears and cultures from the nodules. This phenomenon is the result of an immune response on the part of the host and may represent a form of premunition in kala-azar since the eruption may disappear during a relapse only to reappear with recovery from the infection.

The first or depigmented stage appears as colourless patches on the face and upper extremities, gradually spreading to the remainder of the body (Fig. 36). Minute dots gradually enlarge to irregular areas 1·25 cm in diameter which occasionally break down. The second or nodular stage appears later, about 2 years after treatment in Indian and earlier in African forms. The nodules replace the depigmented patches. They may extend to the mucous membranes and ears and closely resemble leprosy (Fig. 36). In African kala-azar a punctate cutaneous eruption with leishmaniae in the larger nodules appears towards the end of antimony treatment. The epithelium is thin and the subpapillary layer oedematous with atrophy of the fibrous and elastic tissue. Subjacent to this oedematous area is a granulomatous mass of proliferating macrophages. There is also a xanthomatous form with raised orange-coloured plaques which do not ulcerate. Parasites are seen in all three types of lesion, depigmented, nodular and xanthomatous. The histopathology of leishmanoid has been described by Sen Gupta and Bhattacharjee (1953).

Parasites in the blood

Leishmania circulate in the blood-stream enclosed within large mononuclear cells and polymorphonuclear leucocytes. Direct examination of the blood is made on the buffy coat or the trailing edge of a blood film. Parasites can be demonstrated in this manner in Indian kala-azar in 90% of cases.

In African kala-azar parasites can only be recovered by blood culture in about 30% of cases. NNN tubes are inoculated with 0·25 ml of blood and allowed to stand at 28°C and examined after 7, 14 and 21 days. They should not be discarded as negative until after 28 days.

Mucocutaneous lesions

Lesions of the mucocutaneous junctions resembling those found in espundia occur occasionally in African kala-azar. There is ulceration of the nose and upper lip and destruction of the nasal bones in association with a visceral infection (Kirk 1942; Manson-Bahr 1959). Piers (1947) has described a case in Kenya who had lesions of the nose and mouth in the absence of a visceral infection. Sati and Ali (1962) have described leishmanial laryngeal granulomas after cure of kala-azar in the Sudan.

Subclinical infections

In endemic kala-azar areas in Africa, many of the inhabitants react positively to leishmanin although they have never experienced a clinical attack of kala-azar. Epidemiological studies have shown that they are relatively immune both to naturally acquired kala-azar as well as experimental infection (Southgate & Manson-Bahr 1967). It is possible that these positive leishmanin reactors have experienced a subclinical primary skin infection which has induced an immunity to both the naturally and experimentally acquired disease. Infection with non-human *Leishmania* may, however, play a part in inducing the leishmanin response.

Eye lesions

For details see Chapter 44.

Acute toxic kala-azar

During epidemics kala-azar may present as an acute haemorrhagic condition without splenomegaly. There is severe leucopenia and thrombocytopenia.

Generalized lymphadenopathy

Enlargement of the lymphatic glands is a feature of African kala-azar where the femoral group are especially involved. Rarely, however, the full-blown clinical picture may not develop and cases have been described from the Mediterranean where there was a generalized lymphatic glandular enlargement without any evidence of visceral involvement and the spleen and liver remained unaffected. The diagnosis is made by gland puncture or biopsy. The cervical group may specially be involved in these cases.

Complications

Pulmonary tuberculosis. Pulmonary tuberculosis is a common complication of untreated kala-azar. If a case of kala-azar does not respond to antimony treatment concomitant pulmonary tuberculosis should be suspected

Cancrum oris. Cancrum oris develops in late cases of kala-azar when there is severe granulopenia. It must be distinguished from mucocutaneous lesions and will not heal until the kala-azar has been treated successfully.

Cirrhosis of the liver. About 10% of cases of kala-azar show mild cirrhotic changes in the liver after treatment. One of the causes of persistent splenomegaly in spite of antimony treatment is portal hypertension caused by cirrhosis.

Geographical variation in clinical features

There are minor variations in the clinical features of the various geographical forms of kala-azar.

Mediterranean kala-azar. In Mediterranean kala-azar there is no primary lesion (except in Central Asia); *Leishmania* are not found in the skin or circulating blood. Mucocutaneous lesions have not been described and post-kala-azar dermal leishmanoid does not occur. Large doses of antimony are needed in treatment.

South American kala-azar. There is no primary leishmanioma. Parasites are found in the skin but not in the blood. Post-kala-azar dermal leishmanoid does not occur. The response to treatment is good.

Indian kala-azar. There is no primary leishmanioma. Parasites occur frequently in the blood. Mucocutaneous lesions do not occur. Post-kala-azar dermal leishmanoid is common, comes on late after treatment and lasts for a long time. The response to treatment is very good, only a few doses of antimony being required.

African kala-azar. A primary leishmanioma is present. Parasites are found in both the blood and the skin. Lymphatic gland enlargement may be marked. Mucocutaneous lesions occur. Post-kala-azar dermal leishmanoid is not uncommon, occurs during treatment and does not persist for long. Large doses of antimony are required for treatment and this is the most resistant form of kala-azar. Diamidine drugs and amphotericin B may be required. This is the only form of kala-azar in which the leishmanin test has been reported to become positive after treatment.

DIAGNOSIS

Irregular chronic fever with enlargement of the spleen and diminution in the number of leucocytes in patients from an endemic zone suggest kala-azar. Examination of the blood can at once exclude myeloid leukaemia and also malaria; the usual antimalarial drugs do not act on kala-azar (see pages 67–73). Sometimes in early infections diagnosis is very difficult when Leishman-Donovan bodies cannot be found. The formol gel test is negative and leucopenia is absent. Inoculation of material into a hamster may be necessary.

Spleen puncture is the surest method of diagnosis. Chronic myeloid leukaemia must be excluded and the prothrombin time should be normal. Contraindications are a soft spleen and a patient under the age of 5.

A dry hypodermic needle size 18 or 20 is inserted into the edge of the spleen and allowed to rest for a while. The thumb is then placed over the opening and the needle withdrawn. The object is to obtain spleen pulp and not blood. The contents of the needle are blown on to a clean slide and a smear made, or the material is cultured on NNN medium. The spleen pulp containing small sago masses will be seen in the fresh specimen. A local anaesthetic is seldom necessary.

Liver puncture is nearly as good as spleen puncture to demonstrate parasites. *Sternal puncture* is safer than spleen puncture but more painful.

Blood examination: Parasites may be seen in blood smears made from the buffy coat in Indian kala-azar and cultured from the blood on NNN in African kala-azar.

Lymphatic gland puncture is simple but is not so frequently positive as other material. The glands of the groin are usually examined, and the method is similar to that employed in trypanosomiasis (see page 100).

Hamster inoculation. Where *Leishmania* are very scanty they may be demonstrated by inoculating the material, whether spleen, liver, sternal marrow, blood or gland juice, intraperitoneally into a hamster. The hamster should be killed after 6 months if it has not died previously and the spleen, if negative, can be sub-inoculated a second time; *Leishmania* may be shown on a subsequent examination.

Immunological reactions. *Immunoglobulins.* The gamma-globulin is greatly increased in kala-azar and there is a reversal of the A/G ratio. The level of globulin may reach 4·0 grammes/100 ml with albumin 2·8 as compared with the normal 2·0 grammes/100 ml of globulin and 4·5 grammes/100 ml of albumin. The increase is in the IgG fraction (Fig. 37) (Priolesi & Giuffre 1967), which can be demonstrated by starch electrophoreisis and is responsible for the positive formol gel and aldehyde reactions. Complement fixing, haemagglutinating and fluorescent antibodies all develop in kala-azar and can be used for diagnosis.

Formol gel (aldehyde) reactions. This test has proved to be very useful in diagnosing kala-azar on a large scale. The test does not become positive until the disease is of more than 3 months' duration and reverts to negative within 6 months of cure.

About 5 ml of blood are withdrawn from a vein and allowed to stand a sufficient time for the serum to separate; 1 ml of clear serum is then placed in a test-tube (7·5 × 1·25 cm) and to this one drop of 30% formaldehyde or commercial formalin is added. The serum is well shaken and placed at room temperature. 'Jellification' with opacity like the white of a hard-boiled egg occurring within 20 minutes is a positive reaction; jellification without opacity may occur in early cases and in other conditions such as trypanosomiasis, malaria and leprosy.

Complement fixation test. Complement fixing antibodies appear in the serum within the first 3 months of symptoms and disappear in 6 months after cure. The antigen used may be prepared from Kedrowsky's acid-fast bacillus (Monsur & Khaleque 1957) or tubercle bacilli (Nussenzweig *et al.* 1957). This is the most satisfactory serological reaction in the diagnosis of kala-azar and is specific except that cross-reactions may be found with Chagas's disease, some cases of tuberculosis and lepromatous leprosy. It has been used for the mass diagnosis of kala-azar in dogs using blood smears on filter paper.

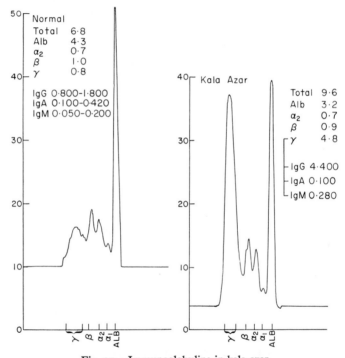

Fig. 37.—Immunoglobulins in kala-azar.

Haemagglutination test. A haemagglutination inhibition test using as antigen lyophilized promastigotes becomes positive early in the disease and reverts to negative shortly after cure.

Fluorescent antibody test. Fluorescent antibodies appear in the serum during the active phase of the disease (Duxbury & Sadun 1964) and earlier than complement fixing antibodies during the prepatent period before development of the kala-azar syndrome and persist for long after cure, as long as 10 years. Titres are higher and the test is more specific than the complement fixation test. The test can be used for the diagnosis of past infection with kala-azar. The promastigotes are used as antigen.

Leishmanin test; Montenegro reaction. In African kala-azar the leishmanin test becomes positive 6–8 weeks after cure of the infection. It is negative during the

active phase of the infection but remains positive for life after cure. In Mediterranean and Indian kala-azar the reaction remains negative.

Positive reactions can also be induced by the intradermal inoculation of
rodent strains of *L. donovani* into the skin. If the nodules which develop are
allowed to run their natural course of up to 6 months before subsiding, a
positive leishmanin reaction develops which is associated with an immunity to
inoculation with rodent or human strains of *L. donovani*. In endemic kala-azar
areas in Africa a high proportion of the people have acquired positive reactions
naturally without ever having developed clinical disease. It is not known how
they have acquired these positive reactions but they are immune to both naturally
or artificially induced kala-azar (Southgate & Manson-Bahr 1967). In these areas
leishmanin testing has been used to delineate endemic areas of leishmaniasis.

DIFFERENTIAL DIAGNOSIS

The differential diagnosis has to be made from splenic anaemia, bacterial
endocarditis, cirrhosis of the liver, febrile reticuloses such as lymphadenoma,
sarcoidosis, trypanosomiasis and Egyptian splenomegaly (caused by *Schistosoma
mansoni*), and chronic brucellosis, which may closely simulate kala-azar. In China
kala-azar may have to be differentiated from *Schistosoma japonicum* infection.
The remarkably clean tongue and good appetite serve in some measure to differentiate kala-azar from chronic malaria. Differential diagnosis has also to be made
from tropical splenomegaly or big spleen disease.

TREATMENT

Pentavalent antimony compounds

Sodium stibogluconate (sodium antimony gluconate, Pentostam, Solustibosan)
contains 30–34% of antimony and is the drug of choice in kala-azar. It is issued
in ampoules of sterile isotonic neutral solution in water so that 1 ml contains
100 mg of antimony. The adult dose is 6 ml (2 grammes sodium gluconate =
600 mg antimony) daily by intravenous or intramuscular injection. For children
aged 8–14 4 ml should be given, and 2 ml for children under 5. The total
dosage for Indian kala-azar is 6 daily injections (3·6 grammes antimony), and
for all other forms 30 daily injections (18·0 grammes antimony).

Ethyl stibamine (Neostibosan) may be used intravenously. The dose is 0·1
gramme the first day, 0·2 gramme the second and 0·3 gramme daily thereafter
for 8 injections (total 2·7 grammes).

Urea stibamine (aminostiburea, Carbostibamide, Carbantine, Stiburea) is a
compound of urea with stibamine, which is apt to undergo chemical changes if
exposed to the air. In resistant cases it may be given in conjunction with
Neostibosan. The dosage is 100 to 200 mg intravenously on alternate days for
about one month for adults. Total dosage for adults is 3·0 grammes and for
infants 0·65 gramme.

Meglumine antimionate (Glucantime) is much used in South America. The
dose is 60–100 mg/kg body weight daily by intramuscular injection, in a course
of 12–15 injections, which may be repeated after an interval of 15 days.

For toxic effects see Chapter 45.

If there is no response to pentavalent antimony drugs then diamidine drugs
must be tried. This is especially true in African kala-azar.

Diamidine drugs

Hydroxystilbamidine isethionate. The dose for adults is 250 mg daily by slow intravenous injection for 10 days followed by 7 days rest and then 2 courses each of 10 days. Total dosage 7·5 grammes. Since vasomotor symptoms constitute the main side-effects, an antihistamine preparation such as Anthisan should be given concurrently, 5–10 mg twice daily. Smaller doses suffice for Indian kala-azar which, however, seldom has to be treated with this drug. Diamidine preparations are of no use in the treatment of post-kala-azar dermal leishmanoid which should be treated with further courses of pentavalent antimony.

Pentamidine isethionate (Lomidine). This drug can be given in the same dosage used for trypanosomiasis. This drug, however, is not so successful as hydroxystilbamidine and may cause severe irreversible hypoglycaemia. For toxic effects of diamidine drugs, see Chapter 45.

Antibiotic

Amphotericin B (Fungizone). This has been used successfully in cases of kala-azar resistant to other forms of treatment. The method of administration and toxic effects are described in Chapter 45.

Splenectomy in kala-azar

Splenectomy has proved of value in cases of kala-azar resistant to all other forms of treatment (Burchenal *et al.* 1947; Manson-Bahr 1959). Further courses of antimony are necessary after the operation, the success of which may be due to the removal of a large mass of organisms from the system and the correction of the hypersplenism caused by the hypertrophied spleen. In tropical countries permanent antimalarial cover is necessary for splenectomized individuals for the rest of their lives.

PROGNOSIS AND SEQUELAE

Kala-azar is usually fatal, but responds well to treatment. Napier (1924) reported spontaneous cure in a significant proportion of Indian cases. If the temperature fails to come down and the general condition to improve with antimony treatment then an associated pulmonary tuberculosis must be suspected. If the spleen fails to diminish in size, then an associated cirrhosis of the liver, which is found in 10% of cases, should be suspected. The formol gel test should become negative and the globulin level return to normal within 6 months of successful treatment. Relapse occurs in about 2% of cases of African kala-azar up to 2 years following treatment, and can be diagnosed by an increase in the globulin and a reversal of the negative formol gel to positive.

PREVENTION AND CONTROL

Control of kala-azar may be achieved by control of the reservoir and of the vector; immunization has so far been unsuccessful.

Control of the reservoir

In Indian kala-azar, where man is the reservoir, case finding and treatment can be partially successful in control. The same has been found to be true in epidemic kala-azar in East Africa. Where there is a canine reservoir, then destruction of dogs has proved effective in Canea in the Mediterranean and in Brazil; infected dogs should be identified by mass serological testing and destroyed, since treatment is not effective in canine kala-azar.

Control of the vector

In India in the days before insecticides were developed, burning the houses which were microfoci of infection was successful to a certain extent in banishing kala-azar from Assam. With the development of DDT and residual spraying for malaria eradication, kala-azar disappeared from most of India. Spraying of kala-azar houses should be sufficient to control transmission.

In all other areas transmission does not occur in the house and residual spraying has proved ineffective in Brazil.

Immunization

Intradermal inoculation of a rodent strain of *L. donovani* was found to immunize volunteers against human strains (Manson-Bahr 1959). This rodent strain was tried as a vaccine under field conditions but failed to show any protection owing to loss of virulence on subculture.

II. Cutaneous Leishmaniasis of the Old World

Synonyms

Oriental sore; Delhi boil; Biskra button; bouton de Crête; bouton d'Alep; Aleppo evil; caneotica.

Definition

A specific ulcerating granuloma of the skin endemic in many warm countries. It is caused by *Leishmania tropica* which is a parasite of rodents (mainly gerbils) and domestic dogs and is transmitted to man by certain species of sandflies. It is characterized by an initial papule which, after scaling and crusting over, breaks down into a slowly extending and very indolent ulcer. Healing after many months, it leaves a depressed scar. The sore is inoculable and usually protective against recurrence.

AETIOLOGY

Although it is usually not possible to distinguish species of *Leishmania* morphologically or culturally, it is possible to distinguish two varieties of *L. tropica* on a biological basis (Pessôa 1961). *L. tropica major* is a parasite of the desert gerbil *Rhombomys opimus* and also to a certain extent *R. meriones*. *L. tropica minor* is a parasite of both dog and man. They can be distinguished by their different biological behaviour and cross-immunity reactions.

TRANSMISSION

Wenyon (1911) first suggested a sandfly (*Phlebotomus*) as the vector in Baghdad and found that 6% of these insects harboured promastigotes in their intestines. Later further confirmatory evidence was brought forward by Sergent *et al.* (1921) who produced oriental sores in Algiers after scarifying the skin and applying a saline suspension of crushed *P. papatasi*.

The development of *L. tropica* in the sandfly resembles that already described for *L. donovani* (Adler & Theodor 1925). *P. papatasi* can be readily infected by feeding the sandflies through a membrane or with suspensions of leishmania (Adler 1928). Adler and Ber (1941) produced 28 sores in 5 volunteers by the bites of infected sandflies.

IMMUNOLOGY

The immunology of *L. tropica* is described in the introduction. A well marked cell-mediated immunity develops, accompanied by delayed hypersensitivity. When the lesion has run its full course and subsided there is a permanent immunity to reinfection with the homologous strain. *L. tropica minor* does not protect against the *major* strain. This immunity is not accompanied by serum antibodies, but by the appearance of delayed hypersensitivity and a positive leishmanin reaction. When immunity does not develop effectively during the course of an infection, then leishmaniasis recidiva, a relapsing form of leishmaniasis results, in which there is delayed hypersensitivity without complete immunity causing a characteristic cellular reaction which is tuberculoid in nature, with epithelioid and giant cells, and closely resembles lupus vulgaris. When the immune response is absent, diffuse cutaneous leishmaniasis results (see page 143).

EPIDEMIOLOGY

Cutaneous leishmaniasis of the Old World occurs in two main forms: rural, caused by *L. tropica major*, which is an infection of the desert gerbil *Rhombomys opimus* and affects man in uninhabited areas and in villages on the edge of the desert, and urban, caused by *L. tropica minor*, which is an infection of man and dog and affects man in the big cities and towns of the Middle East.

Rural leishmaniasis (*L. tropica major*)

Rural leishmaniasis is an infection of the desert gerbil, *Rhombomys opimus*, which lives in dry desert areas of Central Asia around the Kara Kum area of the Aral Sea and in Iran. This rodent lives in burrows deep underground in colonies where it aestivates in the summer, emerging above ground only during winter and at night. In many colonies 30% of the gerbils show small sores chiefly on the ears but also on the back of the head and the base of the tail. Other rodents such as *Meriones erythrourus* and *M. meridianus* play a minor part in maintenance of the infection. Susliks, *Spermophilopsis leptodactylis,* jackals and porcupines have been found infected.

Infection in the rodents is maintained by *P. caucasicus* and *P. papatasi* and transmitted to man by *P. papatasi*. When the rodent burrows are in or near villages the rate of infection can reach 100% in the inhabitants. Groups such as soldiers and hunters can become infected after travelling in remote desert regions. In these areas the maximum incidence is aestivo-autumnal and children in exposed villages usually acquire a sore between 2 and 3 years of age; people rarely attain maturity without having had a sore.

Urban leishmaniasis (*L. tropica minor*)

Urban leishmaniasis is a natural infection of dogs and man. The organism has been demonstrated in cutaneous sores on the ears, lips, nose and inner canthus of the eye of these animals in Teheran, Tashkent and Iraq, where it is only seen in the winter months. Sinton has shown that the leishmanial sores on the noses of dogs in India are transmissible to man. The infection is maintained in dogs and man by *P. sergenti*, and can be maintained in the absence of infected dogs and vice versa. Pringle (1957) has shown that the disease spread from the Central Asia steppe to Iraq by adaptation to an anthropophilic sandfly *P. sergenti* in the Eastern and *P. papatasi* in the Western Mediterranean.

The infection is found in many of the big cities of the Middle East—Baghdad, Teheran, Aleppo, Damascus—and throughout the Mediterranean area, including Italy and North Africa. It is also found in North-west India and Pakistan. In many cities, especially Baghdad, nearly every woman bears on her face the scar of this disease. In Delhi, for example, in 1864 40–70% of the resident Europeans were affected with the local sore. Years of prevalence were succeeded by years of comparative rarity in harmony with altered sanitary conditions. In recent years there has been a great decline in the infection rate owing to the residual spraying undertaken for malaria eradication.

West African cutaneous leishmaniasis

In West Africa cutaneous leishmaniasis is found over an extensive area south of the Sahara between the 10th and 13th parallels North from near Dakar on the Atlantic coast to highland areas of Ethiopia and Kenya (Larivière 1966; Lemma *et al.* 1969). The epidemiology of the infection in this area is still not clear but *Leishmania* have been isolated from dogs and *Arvicanthus* in W. Africa and a strain of *Leishmania* isolated from both rodents and man has produced typical lesions in man. The distribution of the infection in W. Africa corresponds to that of *P. duboscqi* and in 5 other foci with *P. bergeroti*. It is likely that both rodent and canine reservoirs exist in Africa as in the Middle East. Cutaneous leishmaniasis occurs in Ethiopia (Price & Fitzherbert 1965), farther south in the Rift Valley and in South West Africa (Grove 1970). The rock hyrax has been found as a reservoir in Ethiopia where *P. longipes* is the vector (Ashford 1970) in the highlands and also probably in the Mount Elgon focus in W. Kenya.

RELATIONSHIP TO KALA-AZAR

Although oriental sore may occur in countries where kala-azar is endemic, its distribution is as a rule quite distinct. In India cutaneous leishmaniasis is confined to the west whereas kala-azar is endemic on the east coast. In Iraq and Iran, where oriental sore is common, kala-azar is very rare. In some areas, notably Central Asia and the Eastern Mediterranean, they may be found side by side in a single family. Recovery from cutaneous infection does not protect against kala-azar.

PATHOLOGY

The parasites become established in histiocytes in the dermis and there is an invasion of lymphocytes, plasma cells and large mononuclears. As immunity develops and the parasites are eliminated, epithelioid and giant cells appear. Later with healing the lesion is replaced by scar tissue. With the interplay of parasite and host reaction a histological picture develops which is variable. In the relapsing form of leishmaniasis (leishmaniasis recidiva) the histology may resemble lupus vulgaris very closely. In some cases of *L. tropica major* infection leishmania nodules may be found in the lymphatics draining a sore and *Leishmania* may be found in the local lymphatic glands. Very rarely mucous membrane lesions may occur.

CLINICAL FEATURES

Incubation period

The incubation period varies from a short period in the rural form to a longer one in the urban. It may be brief, a few days or weeks, since a sore can appear within a short time of arrival in an endemic district or after inoculation. Senekji and Beattie (1941), in studying the development of experimentally produced oriental sores in man, found that the incubation period after infection with 3 million leptomonad forms from cultures of *L. tropica* ranged from 2 to 8 weeks. Wenyon inoculated himself with oriental sore in Aleppo, but it was not until 6½ months later that a papule containing *Leishmania* developed at the site, In some cases the incubation period appears to be as much as 15 months or even as long as 3 years (Smith 1955), and depends upon the dose inoculated and the strain of infecting parasite.

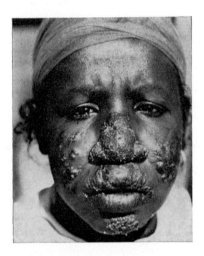

Fig. 38.—Oriental sore. (*Dr Bryceson; by courtesy of the Wellcome Museum of Medical Science*)

Symptoms

The local lesion in oriental sore commences as a minute itching papule which tends to expand somewhat as a shotty, congested infiltration of the dermis (Fig. 39). After a few days or weeks the surface of the papule becomes covered with fine, papery scales. At first these scales are dry and white; later they are moister, thicker, browner, and adherent. In this way, a crust is formed which, on falling off, or on being scratched off, uncovers a shallow ulcer. The sore now slowly extends, discharging a scanty ichorous material; this from time to time may become inspissated, and a crust forms, while the sore continues to spread underneath. The ulcer extends by the erosion of its perpendicular, sharp-cut and jagged edge, which is surrounded by an areola of congestion. The centre portion contains a horny spicule, known as the rake or 'Montpellier sign'. Subsidiary sores may arise around the parent ulcer, into which they ultimately merge. These sores, usually about 2·5 cm in diameter, may come, in some instances, to occupy an area several cm across.

After a variable period, ranging from 2 or 3 to 12 or even more months, healing sets in. Granulation is slow and frequently interrupted. Often it commences at the centre, while the ulcer may be still extending at the edge; often it is effected under a crust. Ultimately, a depressed white or pinkish cicatrix is formed. Contraction of the scar may cause considerable and unsightly deformity. Thus, on the face, scar tissue may produce retraction of the external canthus (epiphora), deformity of the naso-labial folds or eversion of the angle of the mouth.

Oriental sore may be single or multiple. Two or three sores are not uncommon; in rare instances as many as 150 have been counted on the same patient. They are mostly situated on uncovered parts—hands, feet, arms, legs, and, especially in young children, on the face; rarely on the trunk; never on the palms, soles or hairy scalp. Occasionally these ulcers may occur on the ears, tip of the nose (Fig. 39), lower lip, and even on the tongue, and 3 cases have been reported on the upper eyelids. These complications seem to be more frequent than had been supposed, and provide a link between the Old and New World leishmaniasis. A small multiple form may resemble diffuse papillomas: very rarely they occur on the buttocks or on the perineum. A former Editor (Sir Philip Manson-Bahr) recorded a case in which a diffuse indurated swelling, resembling an oriental sore, close to the anus, contained large numbers of *L. tropica.*

In a very few instances the initial papule does not proceed to ulceration, but persists as a scaling or scabbing, non-ulcerating, flattened plaque—just as sometimes happens in the primary sore of syphilis. Sometimes the ulcer is quite superficial, an erosion rather than an ulcer. Occasionally, from contamination with the organism of some other infectious acute inflammatory skin disease, the primary lesion may become complicated, and perhaps a source of serious danger. Otherwise, oriental sore is troublesome and unsightly, rather than painful or dangerous. When ulcerated, or secondarily infected, the neighbouring lymphatic glands in the area of the sore may be enlarged.

Associated subcutaneous nodules have frequently been described. Thus, Evans (1938), in a case of extensive cutaneous leishmaniasis, found, around the arm lesions, 5 separate apple-jelly-like papules. Others were seen around similar lesions on the opposite arm or leg. In size they varied from 0·25 to 1 cm in diameter; they were firm, discrete and freely movable and were not tender. On removal, they showed chronic inflammation with fibrosis, and Leishman-Donovan bodies, suggesting a chronic lymphatic infection and denoting the spread of the infection via the lymphatic route. Lymphatic nodules were described as early as 1847 by Poggioli.

In Christopherson's case (1923) there were 25 vesicular lumps of varying sizes which contained *Leishmania,* and Gonzalez *et al.* (1935) described a similar case in 1937. A sharp bout of pyrexia (temperature 39·4°–40° C, 103–104 °F) frequently precedes the appearance of the nodules.

Leishmaniasis recidiva. The relapsing tuberculoid form, most frequent in Iraq and Anatolia, involving large areas of skin, especially of the face, is an allergic manifestation and therefore analogous to cutaneous tuberculides, closely resembling lupus vulgaris (Fig. 40).

It has been termed 'metaleishmaniasis' by Marchionini. Some types resemble erysipelas with 'serviette' distribution on the face.

Relapses occur after the original lesion heals and often take the form of nodules and papules, situated at the periphery of the scar, and closely resemble 'apply-jelly' nodules. Christopherson originally described them on the cheek, and also recognized a keloid form. Leishmaniasis recidiva is resistant to all forms of treatment except the Grenz rays.

Secondary infections. Superadded staphylococcal or streptococcal infections are common. Secondary diphtheritic and streptothrical infections have been described.

DIAGNOSIS

On clinical grounds these sores have to be distinguished from the desert or veld sore (page 718), tertiary syphilis, ulcus tropicum, lupus vulgaris and blastomycosis. The distribution of the sores and the presence of the Leishman–Donovan body render the diagnosis not a difficult matter. The parasites are best demonstrated by sterilizing the skin at the edge of the ulcer, and running in a fine glass pipette through a puncture made in the skin, to get beneath the ulcer, and obtain serum and tissue cells—but not blood—if possible free from bacterial contamination. This is a better method than scraping the surface of the ulcer with a blunt needle or with a fine knife. If parasites cannot be found, cultures should always be made. The leishmanin test becomes positive within 3 months of the appearance of the lesion, and remains positive for life.

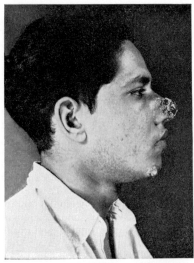

Fig. 39.—Oriental sore on the nose, showing lymphatic spread to the chin. (*By permission of the Medical Department of the Navy*)

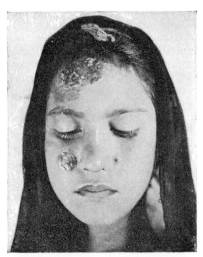

Fig. 40.—Leishmaniasis recidiva in an Egyptian girl, showing lupus-like 'apple-jelly' nodules. (*Dr H. K. Giffen, Assiut*)

Care must be taken to distinguish the Leishman–Donovan bodies from yeast cells, which are sometimes present in cutaneous ulcers and may closely simulate them.

The aldehyde test is negative and the immunoglobulins are normal.

In leishmaniasis recidiva differential diagnosis has to be made from tuberculides of the hypodermis, including Bazin's disease, and also from syphilis. Adler insists that the apple-jelly nodules so closely resemble lupus that culture on NNN medium should always be made to demonstrate parasites.

TREATMENT

The treatment of oriental sores in general, especially in a temperate climate, does not, as a rule, entail any particular difficulties, for the reaction of the tissues to the particularly indolent ulceration depends to some extent upon the general nutrition and environmental conditions. When the patient is removed from the endemic area, the disease tends to disappear spontaneously in about one year.

The main treatment is with pentavalent antimonials, which should be given as in kala-azar. More than one course may be needed. Various other drugs have been used, including Glucantime (useful), cycloguanil pamoate (fair or good), metronidazole (fair or good) and dehydroemetine resinate or dihydrochloride (good). For the administration and dosage, see Chapter 45.

Local injection of mepacrine in 15% solution or of pentavalent antimony has produced good results in some hands.

Indolent sores on the nose. These require special mention as, on account of the induration of the surrounding tissues, they are especially refractory and they do not appear to respond to the applications which are efficacious in other situations. After being cleansed, the bases should be scraped by a Volkmann's spoon and dilute nitrate of mercury ointment thoroughly rubbed in. Dry dressings and sulphonamide paste should subsequently be applied and pentavalent antimony injected intravenously.

Leishmaniasis recidiva. The recidiva form is very resistant to treatment but raising the temperature of the lesions with Grenz rays up to 40°C (104°F) has been used successfully.

PROPHYLAXIS AND CONTROL

Sandfly control

A reduction in the incidence of oriental sore will follow general sanitary measures which include removal of refuse and rubble where sandflies breed, and provision of good housing. Residual spraying for malaria control and eradication has eliminated oriental sore from many areas, but with the conclusion of many malaria eradication campaigns the sandflies and the infection have returned to the Middle East. Corradetti *et al.* (1966) noted that there were no fresh cases of cutaneous leishmaniasis in Italy for 3 years following residual spraying.

Control of the reservoir

In Central Asia colonies of gerbils have been eradicated from many villages by poisoning the burrows with picrotoxin. Burrows are treated up to 5 km from the villages. This method of control has removed the infection from large areas of country. Destruction of infected dogs can also be undertaken.

Immunization

Prophylactic inoculation with cultures of *L. tropica* has been practised successfully for many years in Russia and Palestine. A strain of *L. tropica major* is used. Sores or nodules develop at the site of inoculation after a period of 2 to 6 months and if natural development is allowed to occur an active fast immunity develops in 3 to 6 months. Katzenellenbogen (1944) undertook a successful vaccination campaign on the shores of the Dead Sea in Israel. Vaccination using live cultures is practised by the Soviet authorities.

III. Cutaneous Leishmaniasis of the New World

Synonyms

American Cutaneous Leishmaniasis; Espundia; Bubas; Uta; Pian Bois; Forest Yaws; Bosch Yaws; Bay Sore; Nasopharyngeal Leishmaniasis.

Definition

A specific ulcerating granuloma of the skin and in a proportion of cases the mucocutaneous areas, which is the result of accidental infection of man with different leishmanial parasites which are normally resident in arboreal forest rodents.

AETIOLOGY

A number of classification have been devised for American leishmaniasis. The most generally accepted one is that of Pessôa (1961):

1. *L. braziliensis braziliensis.* Metastasizes in oropharynx in 80% of cases.
2. *L. braziliensis guyanensis* (Floch & Soreau 1953). Metastasizes in nasal mucosa in 5% of cases.
3. *L. braziliensis mexicana* (Biagi 1953). Synonyms: *L. tropica mexicana; L. mexicana.* No metastases.
4. *L. braziliensis peruviana* (Velez 1913). Uta (Peru).
5. *L. braziliensis pifanoi* (Medina & Romero 1959). Diffuse cutaneous leishmaniasis.

Garnham (1962) regards *L. tropica mexicana* as a separate species (*L. mexicana*) and many workers feel that *L. braziliensis pifanoi* is not a valid subspecies. Although there is no way usually of distinguishing these varieties of *Leishmania* Lainson and Shaw (1970) have been able to distinguish two distinct strains of *L. braziliensis* in the Matto Grosso. *Strain 1* grows slowly and gives a poor growth on NNN in which it dies out after one or two transfers. The parasites grow reluctantly in hamster nose and foot skin and are scanty in the human lesions. This strain causes nasopharyngeal lesions in man. *Strain 2* is fast growing and grows luxuriantly on NNN. It grows rapidly in hamster skin in which it produces large histiocytomas. It is abundant in the skin lesions of man in whom it causes only single or diffuse cutaneous lesions.

Biological varieties

It is usual to group American leishmaniasis into the following biological varieties:

(*a*) Chicle ulcer (chiclero's ulcer) caused by *L. mexicana,* found in Mexico, Guatemala and British Honduras. Single sore; no metastases.

(*b*) Espundia. Found in South and Central America from Panama southwards. Primary sore. Metastasizes to mucocutaneous junctions in 5% of cases in Panama, and 80% of cases in Amazonia and Paraguay.

(*c*) Uta in Peru. Single sore; no metastases.

American leishmaniasis is a rural disease commonest in men who work in the forest, on the borders of forests or in rural settlements, and outbreaks occur in groups of men opening up new territories. It is obviously a zoonosis. Search for infection among animals associated with human habitations has yielded few results, a few infected dogs, a cat and a donkey and the paca have been found infected in a few cases, but the infections were visceral and probably represented 'dead end' infections.

Hertig *et al.* (1954) found natural leishmanial infections in 10% of spiny rats (*Proechimys semispinosus*) and *Hoplomys gymnurus* in Panama. These infections were cryptic and visceral and disappeared from the local rats after a time. More characteristic infections have now been found in British Honduras and Amazonia.

Reservoir hosts of American cutaneous leishmaniasis

In British Honduras leishmaniasis is a natural infection of the tree rat *Ototylomis phyllotis*. *Heteromys desmaresteanus*, a forest rat, is probably a secondary host, and *Nictomys sumichrasti*, the spiny pocket mouse, an accidental host (Williams 1970). Altogether 5 different rodents act as hosts and the incidence of infection is as high as 40% (Lainson & Strangways Dixon 1964). The *Leishmania* which cause indistinct dermal lesions on the extremities, especially the tails, cause typical cutaneous lesions in human volunteers. In the Utinga forest near Belem in Amazonia where rodents are numerous in re-grown cutover forest, leishmanial lesions have been found on the tails of *Oryzomys goeldii* and it is estimated that 70% of these rodents may experience leishmaniasis. *Leishmania* have also been found in a spiny rat (*Proechimys gyuanensis*) in lesions on the tail and have also been obtained on culture from normal ear tissue (Lainson & Shaw 1968). It is now clear that there is a patchy but intense infection in small forest rodents in these areas.

In the Matto Grosso there is evidence of the existence of two strains of the parasite. One strain grows slowly in culture and in hamsters and has a single rodent reservoir (*Orizomys concolor*). The sandfly vector is unknown. This strain causes espundia in man. The other strain grows profusely in culture and affects many rodents. The vector of the infection in these rodents is *L. flaviscutellata*. This strain causes simple and diffuse cutaneous lesions in man (Lainson & Shaw 1970).

Transmission

South American sandflies have been given specific generic status and are called *Lutzomyia*.

In South America large numbers of sandflies may be found in a single focus and it is difficult to correlate the distribution of leishmaniasis with certain species. Many sandflies show midgut and posterior infections with flagellates which usually denote non-mammalian infections. However, some midgut infections have produced sores in human volunteers.

Much work on transmission has been done in British Honduras and Panama.

In British Honduras 3 species of sandflies developed anterior infections after feeding on rodent isolates: *Lu. ylephiletrix*, *Lu. geniculatus*, and *Lu. cruciata* (Strangways Dixon & Lainson 1966; Williams 1966). However, the infection is maintained in *O. phyllotis* on or near the ground by *Lu. olmeca*, which will bite man if disturbed (Williams 1970).

In Mexico, where similar lesions have been found on rodents, a natural infection of *Lu. flaviscutellata* caused a typical lesion in a human volunteer. In Mexico and Central America *Lu. olmeca* and in South America *Lu. flaviscutellata* are two closely related species with a different distribution. In Belem in Amazonia the infection in rodents is maintained by *Lu. olmeca* which feeds on rodents and not man. Man is infected accidentally by some other species of sandfly (Lainson & Shaw 1968). In Panama natural infections of sandflies have been found in *Lu. trapidoi*, *Lu. ylephiletrix*, *Lu. gomezi*, *Lu. sanguinarius*, *Lu. panamensis* and *Lu. shannoni* (Hertig 1962); many were hindgut infections and one strain from *Lu. trapidoi* caused a typical leishmanial infection in a hamster. There is strong evidence, therefore, that South American leishmaniasis is an infection of the skin of small forest rodents which is maintained by a variety of sandflies which feed on them. The infection is transmitted occasionally to man by anthropophilic sandflies.

PATHOLOGY

The histological appearances are similar to those found in oriental sore. *Leishmania* occur in histiocytes in the dermis and are surrounded at first by plasma cells and lymphocytes. As the immune reaction develops giant and epithelioid cells appear and when healing occurs they are replaced by scar tissue When ulceration takes place there is secondary infection with polymorpho-nuclear cell infiltration.

Chicle ulcer (*L. mexicana*)

Epidemiology. Chicle ulcer occurs by itself in the Yucatan area in Mexico, the Peten area in Guatemala and in British Honduras. Elsewhere it is found in association with the metastasizing form. It is a disease of low-lying rain forest and is an occupational disease attacking gum (chicle) collecters and woodcutters. It may also affect people who live in huts in the forest. Any age may be attacked.

L. mexicana causes a benign and self-limiting disease lasting no more than 6 months. The lesion is single and does not metastasize. When it occurs on the pinna of the ear a very chronic disfiguring lesion results (Fig. 41) (Oreja de Chicleros). It occurs commonly on the face, often just beneath the lower eyelid, next on the ear and sometimes on the upper limb. A small nodule forms which ulcerates and does not spread and heals under 6 months. On the ear, the pinna becomes swollen and inflamed and the cartilage is invaded. A very chronic lesion results in which the auricle is slowly destroyed over a number of years.

Following healing there is complete immunity to reinfection with *L. mexicana*.

Espundia

Epidemiology. Espundia is usually rural in distribution, but has been seen in some towns. In Paraguay the disease has assumed epidemic character and a large proportion of the population in certain districts and 70–80% of prospecting parties and soldiers have become affected. It was a major problem to troops in the Grand Chaco war. The disease occurs at any age in either sex.

Symptoms and signs. It begins as a sore of the ordinary cutaneous type and heals in time leaving a characteristic scar. The localization of the sores has been recorded as follows: leg 30%, foot 12%, forearm 12%, head 11%, hip 4%, elbow 4%, trunk 3%, nasal mucosa 3%, knee 2%, buccal mucosa 2%, neck 2%, arm 1%, pubes 1%. The ulcers are relatively painless. In a proportion of cases metastasis to the mucocutaneous junctions occurs after a period of time which may be as long as 2 years. The proportion of cases which metastasize varies from 2% in Panama to nearly 80% in Paraguay. Metastasis to the mucocutaneous area of the nose and upper lip is commonest (Figs 42, 43) and in this area there is crusting of the anterior septum, polyp formation, ulceration and perforation of the septum with scarring and sinking of the external nose causing the typical 'tapir' nose (Fig. 42). Ulceration may destroy the whole of the nasal septum so that it is possible to look right down the larynx from the nose. Rarely the disease may involve the larynx. Sometimes the infection may metastasize into multiple cutaneous lesions (Fig. 42), sometimes of bizarre character which may resemble almost any skin disease.

Diagnosis. This is made from the typical clinical appearances and the discovery of the parasite. Espundia has to be distinguished from yaws (gangosa), lupus, syphilis, leprosy and epithelioma. Excision of a piece of granulation tissue and expression of serum on a slide affords a more ready diagnosis. The Montenegro (leishmanin) test is positive in almost all cases, becoming positive early in the infection and remaining positive after cure. No serum antibodies develop so that serodiagnosis is of no help.

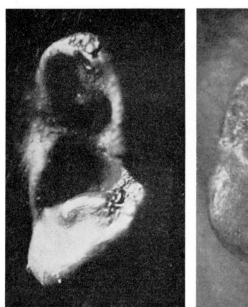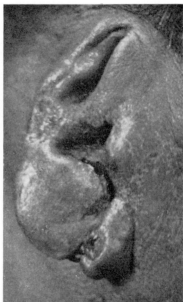

Fig. 41.—South American leishmaniasis of the pinna of the ear—oreja de chicleros. (*Dr L. A. Leon, Quito*)

Uta

Uta is found only in valleys in Peru from which it has now almost completely disappeared. The reservoir is the domestic dog and transmission between dog and man is effected by *Lu. noguchii.* It occurs in small semi-arid Andean valleys at 600 m. A single lesion like oriental sore develops which is self-limiting and heals in under one year. There are no metastases.

Diffuse cutaneous leishmaniasis (leishmaniasis diffusa, leproid or cheloid leishmaniasis)

Nodular or verrucose leishmaniasis was described from the Sudan before the First World War and was the same as the form now described as diffuse cutaneous leishmaniasis.

A similar form of cutaneous leishmaniasis has been described from Venezuela (Convit & Kerdel Vegas 1965), Ethiopia (Price & Fitzherbert 1965) and Kenya, where it is found in association with typical oriental sore. Isolated cases have been described in Tanzania and Mexico.

This form of leishmaniasis (Bryceson 1969) is very chronic and has persisted in some cases for over 20 years. It starts as a single lesion which spreads slowly until the whole body, but especially the face, limbs and buttocks, is covered with lepromatous-like nodules. There is never any ulceration, but the nose may become affected and cause obstructive symptoms. Histologically numerous *Leishmania* are found free or in macrophages in the dermis with no cellular reaction. The leishmanin test remains negative until after healing when it becomes positive. The cause of the condition is most probably a failure in the

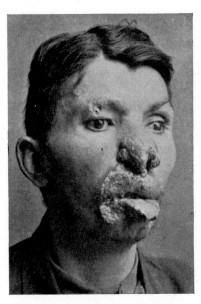

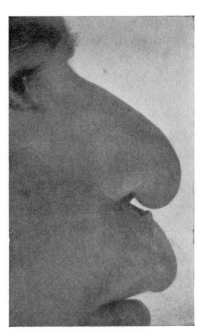

Fig. 42.—Espundia from Equador (tapir nose). (*Dr L. A. Leon, Quito*)

Fig. 43.—South American leishmaniasis (tapir nose). (*Dr L. A. Leon, Quito*)

immune response of the host and an absence of any cell-mediated immunity to eliminate the parasites. *Leishmania* have been recovered from both the blood and bone marrow. Differential diagnosis from leprosy is likely to cause trouble (Bryceson 1969).

TREATMENT

Self-limiting infections such as *L. mexicana* need no treatment unless situated on the ear. Wherever there is a chance that the lesion might metastasize because of the place where it was contracted then active treatment must be initiated.

The treatment of American leishmaniasis is the same as for oriental sore. Pentavalent antimony preparations are the drugs of choice. Glucantime and ethylstilbamine are used in the usual doses. If the condition fails to respond to antimony then pyrimethamine (Daraprim) should be given in doses of 50 mg daily for 8 days with frequent intervals of the same length.

In cases which fail to respond to any of the above treatments amphotericin B should be used.

In purely cutaneous disease cycloguanil pamoate (CI 501, Camolar) has been very effective used as one injection. Diffuse cutaneous leishmaniasis is very resistant to all forms of treatment but some success has been obtained with pentamidine isethionate in repeated courses as for trypanosomiasis. In Venezuela amphotericin B has been used with success.

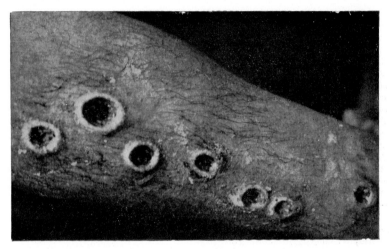

Fig. 44.—Punched-out ulcers in dermal leishmaniasis associated with espundia in Ecuador. (*Dr L. A. Leon, Quito*)

PROPHYLAXIS

Since American leishmaniasis is always a zoonosis little can be done to control the source of infection. Care should be taken in siting new settlements in the forest, leaving a cleared strip of bush a few kilometres wide around the dwellings to break contact between man and the forest. Sandfly control is not possible but repellants may be successful for a limited time when necessary work in the forest must be undertaken. Immunization using a benign strain which does not metastasize has been suggested but is not yet pract ical.

REFERENCES

ADLER, S. (1928) *Trans. R. Soc. trop. Med. Hyg.*, **22,** 177.
——— (1964) *Adv. Parasit.*, **2,** 38.
——— (1965) *Israel J. med. Sci.*, **1,** 9.
——— & ADLER, J. (1955) *Bull. Res. Coun. Israel*, **4,** 396.
——— & BER, M. (1941) *Indian J. med. Res.*, **29,** 203.
——— FONER, A. & MONTIGLIO, M. (1966) *Trans. R. Soc. trop. Med. Hyg.*, **60,** 380.
——— & THEODOR, O. (1925) *Ann. trop. Med. Parasit.*, **19,** 635.
——— ——— (1935) *Proc. R. Soc. B*, **116,** 516.
ASHFORD, R. W. (1970) *Trans. R. Soc. trop. Med. Hyg.*, **64,** 936.

BIAGI, F. F. (1953) *Medicina, Méx.*, **33,** 401.
BRAY, R. S. & BRYCESON, A. D. M. (1968) *Lancet,* **ii,** 998.
—— & DABBAGH, M. A. (1968) *J. trop. Med. Hyg.*, **71,** 46.
BRYCESON, A. D. M. (1969) *Trans. R. Soc. trop. Med. Hyg.*, **63,** 708.
BURCHENAL, J. S., BOWERS, R. F. & HAEDECKE, T. A. (1947) *Am. J. trop. Med.*, **27,** 699.
CAHILL, K. M. (1964) *Am. J. trop. Med. Hyg.*, **13,** 794.
CONVIT, J. & KERDEL VEGAS, F. T. (1965) *Archs Derm.*, **91,** 439.
CORRADETTI, A., MANTOVANI, A., ADAMS, A. J. & DELLA BRUNA, C. (1966) *Parasitologia*, **8,** 1.
DAS GUPTA, N. N., GUHA, A. & DE, N. (1954) *Exp. Cell Res.*, **6,** 353.
DEANE, L. M. (1956) *Leishmaniasis in Brazil: Study of Reservoirs in the State of Ceará.*
    Rio de Janiero: Servicio Nacional de Educacao Sanitaria.
—— & DEANE, M. P. (1964) *Archos Hig. Saúde públ.*, **29,** 89.
DUXBURY, R. E. & SADUN, E. H. (1964) *Am. J. trop. Med. Hyg.*, **13,** 525.
EVANS, R. B. (1938) *Br. J. Derm. Syph.*, **50,** 17.
FLOCH, H. & SOREAU, P. (1953) *Bull. Soc. Path. éxot.*, **46,** 297.
GARNHAM, P. C. C. (1962) *Sci. Rep. 1st sup. Sanità,* **2,** 76.
GELLHORN, A., VAN DYKE, H. B., PYLES, J. W. & TUPIKOVA, N. A. (1946) *Proc. Soc. exp. Biol. Med.*, **61,** 25.
GONZALES, G., BOGGINO, J. & RIVAROLA, J. B. (1935) *9a Réun. Soc. argent. Patol. Reg. Mendoza,* **2,** 753.
GOODWIN, L. G. (1945) *Nature, Lond.*, **156,** 476.
GROVE, S. S. (1970) *S. Afr. med. J.*, **44,** 206.
GUIRGES, S. Y. (1971) *Ann. trop. Med. Parasit.*, **65,** 197.
HEISCH, R. B. (1957) *E. Afr. med. J.*, **34,** 183.
—— WIJERS, R. B. & MINTER, D. M. (1962) *Br. med. J.*, **i,** 456.
HERTIG, M. (1962) *Rep. Gorgas meml Lab.*
—— FAIRCHILD, G. B. & JOHNSON, C. N. (1954) *Rep Gorgas meml Lab.*
HEYNEMANN, D. (1963) *Am. J. trop. Med. Hyg.*, **12,** 725.
HOOGSTRAAL, H. & DIETLEIN, D. R. (1964) *Bull. Wld Hlth Org.*, **31,** 137.
JOPLING, W. H. (1955) *Br. med. J.*, **iii,** 1013.
KATZENELLENBOGEN, I. (1944) *Archs Derm. Syph.* **50,** 239.
KIRK, R. (1942) *Trans. R. Soc. trop. Med. Hyg.*, **35,** 257.
KNIGHT, R., WOODRUFF, A. W. & PETITT, L. E. (1967) *Trans. R. Soc. trop. Med. Hyg.*, **61,** 701.
LAINSON, R. & SHAW, J. J. (1968) *Trans. R. Soc. trop. Med. Hyg.*, **62,** 385, 397.
—————— (1970) *Trans. R. Soc. trop. Med. Hyg.*, **64,** 654.
—— & STRANGWAYS DIXON, J. (1964) *Trans. R. Soc. trop. Med. Hyg.*, **58,** 136.
LARIVIERE, M. (1966) *Bull. Soc. méd. Afr. noire Lang. fr.*, **11,** 119.
LEMMA, A., FOSTER, W. A., GEMETCHU, T., PRESTON, P. M., BRYCESON, A. D. M. & MINTER, D. M. (1969) *Ann. trop. Med. Parasit.*, **63,** 455.
LOWE, G. C. & COOKE, W. E. (1926) *Lancet,* **ii,** 1209.
MANSON-BAHR, P. E. C. (1959) *Trans. R. Soc. trop. Med. Hyg.*, **53,** 123.
—— SOUTHGATE, B. A. & HARVEY, A. E. C. (1963) *Br. med. J.*, **i,** 1208.
MEDINA, R. & ROMERO, J. (1959) *Archos venez. Patol. trop. Parasit. méd.*, **1,** 298.
MIRZOIAN, I. (1941) *Medskaya Parazit.*, **10,** 101.
MONSUR, K. A. & KHALEQUE, K. A. (1957) *Trans. R. Soc. trop. Med. Hyg.*, **51,** 527.
MONTENEGRO, D. (1924) *Am. J. trop. Med.*, **4,** 331.
NAPIER, L. E. (1924) *Indian med. Gaz.*, **59,** 492.
NUSSENZWEIG, V., NUSSENZWEIG, R. S. & ALENCAR, J. E. (1957) *Hospital, Rio de J.*, **51,** 325.
PESSOA, S. B. (1961) *Archos Fac. Hig. Saúde publ. Univ. S. Paulo,* **26,** 41,
PIERS, F. (1947) *Trans. R. Soc. trop. Med. Hyg.*, **40,** 713.
PRICE, E. W. & FITZHERBERT, M. (1965) *Ethiop. med. J.*, **3,** 57.
PRINGLE, G. (1957) *Bull. endem. Dis.*, **2,** 41.
PRIOLESI, A. & GIUFFRE, L. (1967) *Pathologia Microbiol.*, **30,** 215.
SATI, M. H. & ALI, M. V. (1962) *Sudan med. J.*, **1,** 37.
SENEKJI, H. A. & BEATTIE, C. P. (1941) *Trans. R. Soc. trop. Med. Hyg.*, **23,** 523.

Sen Gupta, P. C. & Bhattacharjee, B. (1953) *J. trop. Med. Hyg.*, **56**, 110.

—— & Mukherjee, A. M. (1968) *J. Indian med. Ass.*, **50**, 1.

Sergent, Ed., Sergent, Et., Parrot, L., Donatien, A. & Beguet, M. (1921) *C. r. hebd. Séanc. Acad. Sci., Paris*, **173**, 1030.

Smith, P. A. J. (1955) *Br. med. J.*, **ii**, 1143.

Southgate, B. A. & Manson-Bahr, P. E. C. (1967) *J. trop. Med. Hyg.*, **70**, 29, 33.

Stauber, L. A., McConnell, E. & Hoogstraal, H. (1966) *Exp. Path.*, **18**, 35.

Strangways Dixon, J. & Lainson, R. (1966) *Trans. R. Soc. trop. Med. Hyg.*, **60**, 192.

Swaminath, C. S., Shortt, H. E. & Anderson, L. A. (1942) *Indian J. med. Res.*, **30**, 473.

Sweeney, J. S., Friedlander, R. D. & Queen, F. B. (1945) *J. Am. med. Ass.*, **128**, 14.

Velez, M. (1913) *Bull. Soc. Path. éxot.*, **6**, 454.

Wenyon, C. M. (1911) *J. trop. Med. Hyg.*, **14**, 103.

Wijers, D. J. B. & Mwangi, S. (1966) *Ann. trop. Med. Parasit.*, **60**, 373.

Williams, P. (1966) *Ann. trop. Med. Parasit.*, **60**, 365.

—— (1970) *Trans. R. Soc. trop. Med. Hyg.*, **64**, 317.

Wright, M. J. (1960) *Br. med. J.*, **ii**, 1218.

8. TOXOPLASMOSIS, COCCIDIOSIS, AND PNEUMOCYSTIS INFECTION

Toxoplasmosis

Definition

Infection of man and other warm-blooded animals with *Toxoplasma gondii*.

AETIOLOGY

Human toxoplasmosis is caused by *T. gondii* which belongs to the Sporozoa (Hutchinson *et al.* 1970). It is a coccidian parasite with a typical coccidial life cycle of schizogony and gametogony occurring in the intestine of cats and other warm-blooded animals. Development takes place in the mucosal cells of the small intestine and oöcysts are excreted in the faeces. The form described originally as pseudocystic, as found in man in acute cases, is probably a schizont maturing in an abnormal site and the cystic forms are oöcysts. The schizonts are intracellular and are found in acute infections. They are curved or crescent-shaped bodies. When stained by Giemsa the cytoplasm stains blue and the nucleus, which stains red or purple, is an irregular mass occupying a quarter or a fifth of the cell and eccentric in position.

The oöcysts which are found in chronic infections are usually contained in hundreds and thousands in a cyst which grows to 100 μm in diameter in the brain of warm-blooded animals; cysts can persist for years and are resistant to temperatures up to 60°C.

EPIDEMIOLOGY

Toxoplasmosis is a zoonosis and has been found in practically all warm-blooded animals but may also be found in some reptiles and fish. It has been found in dogs, guinea-pigs, gerbils, hares, mice, weasels, polecats, ferrets, macaque monkeys (*Macaca mulatta*), pigeons and several birds. In man toxoplasmosis is often associated with cats (Price 1969).

In man the infection may be congenital or acquired.

Congenital toxoplasmosis

Sabin (1942) found a high incidence of toxoplasmosis in children with mental disorders with or without hydrocephalus, microcephalus, cerebral calcification and macular choroidoretinitis. He also found neutralizing antibodies in the blood of mothers of infected children. The infection passes the placenta about the fourth month but not later in pregnancy when antibody is present, and only when infection is acquired during pregnancy can it be passed on to the fetus, 50% of which are infected (Desmonts *et al.* 1965). At birth the child's antibody titre will be the same as the mother's but in the absence of actual infection of the child it will fall to nothing after 6 months.

Acquired toxoplasmosis

The exact method by which toxoplasmosis is acquired in man is unknown. The infection can be transmitted experimentally to animals by feeding material containing the parasite, or by intranasal, intracutaneous, intraperitoneal, subcutaneous and intracerebral inoculation. *T. gondii* has been isolated from blood, saliva, urine, faeces, conjunctival exudate and mother's milk.

The main routes of infection in man are probably by ingestion or intranasal instillation by droplet spread. Weinman and Chandler (1954) showed that the disease may be contracted by eating inadequately cooked pork and that pigs may contract the infection from infected rodents. Kean *et al.* (1969) have described a small epidemic of acute toxoplasmosis in 5 medical students who ate undercooked beef hamburgers. The role of droplet spread in intranasal infection is suggested by cases presenting symptoms of meningo-encephalitis (Kunert & Schmidtke 1954).

Although arthropod vectors may have been used in earlier eras, *T. gondii* has now dispensed with this mode of transmission.

IMMUNOLOGY

Animals can be immunized against reinfection, but this immunity is not absolute and is dependent on the dose and strain of the challenge inoculum. The immunity is both cellular and humoral. In hamsters, clinical and transferable cellular immunity appears 3 weeks after infection and delayed hypersensitivity and serum antibody are present by the fifth day of infection (Frenkel 1967). Serum antibodies are both IgG and IgM and the thermolabile antitoxoplasma factor which is present is probably IgA (Strannegard 1967). IgG antibodies appear only after infection and reach their maximum after about two months. They persist for a long time and are only of significance in the diagnosis of recent acute infections if a rising or falling titre can be shown serially. IgG antibodies in the newborn are maternal in origin; if IgM antibodies are present these may be measured by immunofluorescence and denote active infection passed on from the mother. In adults a positive Sabin–Feldman test in the absence of specific IgM antibodies probably excludes active toxoplasmosis (Nicolau & Ravelo 1937; Remington *et al.* 1968).

Serum antibodies may be measured by the complement fixation test (Nicolau & Ravelo 1937), the Sabin–Feldman dye test (Sabin & Feldman 1948), a haemagglutination test (Jacobs & Lunde 1957), a fluorescent antibody test (Fulton & Voller 1964), an agar gel diffusion test, which demonstrates precipitins in the aqueous humour of the eye in cases of uveitis, and a direct agglutination test (Fulton & Turk 1959), Cross-reactions occur with *Trichomonas* infections but not with *Sarcocystis*. Delayed hypersensitivity is measured by the Frenkel test, a dermal sensitivity test using toxoplasmin (Frenkel 1948).

Complement fixation test

Fulton and Fulton (1965) have described an antigen which consists of a pure suspension of formolized *T. gondii* prepared from the peritoneal exudate of infected cotton rats which can be readily standardized by parasite counts and nitrogen estimations and which, when lyophilized in the presence of 6% salt-free dextran, remains fully potent for more than one year.

Sabin–Feldman test

The dye test is carried out by mixing peritoneal exudate from infected mice containing *Toxoplasma* with serum antibodies in the presence of a heat-labile substance called 'activator', which is of a properdin nature, and methylene blue at a pH of 11. Staining of the *Toxoplasma* cytoplasm is prevented by specific antibodies, in the absence of antibodies 90–100% of *Toxoplasma* take the stain, whereas in its presence less than 50% are stained.

A positive S–F test at titres over 1/512 is indicative of the presence of serum antibody. S–F tests are usually between 1/1000 and 1/10 000. They remain positive from several months to a year and then begin to fall, but never completely disappear.

Fluorescent antibody test

The fluorescent antibody test is reasonably specific in nature and parasites normally difficult to find in tissue smears and sections can be made visible in this way. It is economical and easy to carry out and dried blood on filter paper extracted with saline can be used.

Direct agglutination test

Using the Fulton antigen prepared for the complement fixation test Fulton (1965) used 1/10 of the original antigen and employed the micro-titration apparatus of Takatsy. The test is specific, easy to perform, repeatable and uses formolized parasites which can be kept for many months and are not infective

Frenkel skin test

About 0·1 ml of 1/500 dilution of supernatant fluid from the centrifuged peritoneal exudate of infected Swiss mice, to which Merthiolate in a dilution of 1/10 000 has been added, is injected intradermally. The test is positive when, after 48 to 72 hours, an areola and induration develops which persists and is larger than 0·5 mm. The reaction is not positive for some months after infection; it has been used to indicate the antibody status of a group but is not otherwise very informative.

PATHOLOGY

T. gondii is a parasite of the endothelial cells, mononuclear leucocytes, body fluids and tissue cells of the host. It is characteristically associated with the reticulo-endothelial system or endothelium of the circulatory system, multiplying in the cells of those tissues. The capacity of the organism to invade and develop in many types of cell is shown by the protean clinical manifestations, lymphadenopathy, typhus-like exanthemata, meningo-encephalitis and choroidoretinitis. During quiescent periods nests of toxoplasmas rest inactive inside cyst walls or tissue cells. In cysts (oöcysts) the cyst wall is derived from material secreted by the living *Toxoplasma* and may contain thousands of *Toxoplasma*. It is characteristic of strains of low virulence. Pseudocysts (schizonts) are composed of host cells which contain as many as 100 *Toxoplasma* and are characteristic of virulent strains.

The basic lesion consists of a microscopic granuloma in which organisms may be demonstrated.

In the acquired form the infection may be in the brain and cord (encephalomyelitis and meningo-encephalitis), in mononuclear cells in the bronchioles with congestion of the lungs (atypical penumonia), in the myocardium with pseudocysts lying between the muscle fibres (myocarditis) or in the lungs, myocardium, liver, spleen, bone marrow, adrenals, kidneys, lymph glands and nervous system, resembling typhus. The great majority of acquired cases are subclinical and show no signs of the infection.

In congenital infections the organisms have a predilection for the brain and retina. The mothers to whom babies affected with toxoplasmosis are born characteristically show no symptoms of infection, but maternal infection may be responsible for a significant proportion of stillbirths. Children who survive antenatal toxoplasmosis often show damage to the brain with mental retardation and epileptic seizures.

SYMPTOMS AND SIGNS

Acquired toxoplasmosis

Although the vast majority of cases of *Toxoplasma* infection are inapparent, as in mothers who give birth to infected children, there are four main types of symptomatology. The two types most commonly encountered are a febrile lymphadenitis resembling glandular fever and a non-febrile enlargement of the lymph glands without symptoms. More rarely there may be a typhus-like syndrome or a cerebrospinal form with fever, delirium and convulsions in which the cerebrospinal fluid is xanthochromic, under pressure and with a raised protein, and an increase in mononuclear cells.

Paulley *et al.* (1956) have suggested that toxoplasmosis may be responsible for Fiedler's myocarditis and other forms of cardiomegaly associated with positive serological reactions and may be responsible for endomyocardial fibrosis, although no evidence for this is forthcoming. Henry and Beverly (1969) found myocardial lesions in 71% of mice inoculated with *Toxoplasma* and a case of polymyositis as a major manifestation of *Toxoplasma* infection has been described by Chandar *et al.* (1968). *Toxoplasma* have been isolated from cases of an infectious illness resembling hepatitis.

Congenital toxoplasmosis

The disease becomes noticeable days or weeks after birth and choroido-retinitis appears in about 90%. There may be hepatosplenomegaly and ocular manifestations, nystagmus, strabismus, cataract and optic atrophy. Some children are born jaundiced with a papular or purpuric rash. In these congenital forms there is a tetrad of signs—'the syndrome of Sabin'—internal hydro-cephalus, choroidoretinitis, convulsions, and cerebral calcification, with hydrocephalus, microcephalus and psychomotor disturbances. (For ocular toxoplasmosis, see Chapter 44.)

Opportunist infection

With growth in the use of immunosuppressive agents for the treatment of malignant conditions and for transplant operations, toxoplasmosis is one of the opportunist infections that may develop when the immune responses of the body have been diminished. A case of generalized toxoplasmosis following renal transplantation has been described (Reynolds *et al.* 1966).

DIAGNOSIS

Most commonly the diagnosis of toxoplasmosis is arrived at by a combination of clinical signs and serological findings which are discussed under immunology.

Toxoplasma may rarely be found in biopsy material where they can be demonstrated by the fluorescent antibody technique. They may be isolated by inoculating biopsy or aspirated material from lymph glands or other tissues suspended in phosphate-buffered saline intraperitoneally into mice, in which *Toxoplasma*-infected peritoneal exudate will appear in 7 days.

TREATMENT

The treatment of clinical toxoplasmosis is with a combination of pyrimethamine (Daraprim) and sulphonamides. Pyrimethamine 50 mg followed by 50 mg 6 hours later and 25 mg daily for 2 to 4 weeks is given with 6·0 grammes triple sulphonamide daily (Frenkel *et al.* 1960). Megaloblastic anaemia may occur during treatment and repeated examination of the blood should be made; folic acid should be given promptly if anaemia develops.

PROGNOSIS

In older children and adults prognosis depends upon the site and degree of tissue damage. Acute toxoplasmosis in children is usually fatal. Children born to mothers with inapparent infection subsequent to the birth of an infected child will not be affected.

Coccidiosis

AETIOLOGY

Human coccidiosis is caused by two species, *Isospora belli* and *I. hominis*. The life cycle is unknown and only the oöcysts and sporocysts have been studied. However, in the closely related *I. canis* and *I. felis* sporozoites escape from oöcysts and invade the mucosa of the ileum and form trophozoites which multiply by schizogony. The parasitized cells rupture and the merozoites invade new cells.

Geographical distribution and epidemiology

Species of human *Isospora* are relatively uncommon although widely distributed in warm climates. Most infections have been found in the South-west Pacific islands, Brazil, Colombia, Natal, South Africa, Chile and the U.S.A. (Faust *et al.* 1961). Isolated infections have been reported from many other countries.

Infection is contracted from food or drink contaminated with faeces containing ripe eggs, and outbreaks have been recorded in troops and mental institutions. Dogs have been suspected to be the reservoir hosts of *I. hominis*.

PATHOLOGY

The pathology of human infections has not been studied. In dogs and cats mucosal damage results with the production of a mucous diarrhoea.

SYMPTOMS AND SIGNS

Isospora are found in healthy carriers and patients with diarrhoea and dysentery associated with other parasites. *I. belli* and *I. hominis* have sometimes been found in the absence of other parasites in association with mild diarrhoea. Oöcysts are not found in the stools until several days after the diarrhoea.

DIAGNOSIS

The oöcysts are found in the stool in unstained and iodine-stained preparations and do not persist for more than 2–4 days.

TREATMENT

No treatment is necessary as the infection is self-limiting.

Pneumocystis Infection

Synonyms

Parasitic Pneumonia; Interstitial Plasma Cell Pneumonia; Pneumocystosis.

AETIOLOGY

Pneumocystis infection is caused by *Pneumocystis carinii* probably a protozoon not uncommon in animals and pathogenic in man only as an 'opportunist' infection.

P. carinii is an intracellular parasite seen in lung smears of guinea-pigs, other animals and man, as small round 'cysts' containing 8 uninucleated bodies ('octonucleate cysts') 5–7 μm in diameter. The life history is unknown.

The method of transmission is unknown.

EPIDEMIOLOGY AND GEOGRAPHICAL DISTRIBUTION

The majority of cases have so far been reported from Yugoslavia, Germany and, more recently, from North America and Chile (Danzier *et al.* 1956; Pizzi 1956). Domestic animals, rabbits, guinea-pigs, sheep and goats form the reservoirs of infection, and the cases described from Yugoslavia were in infants and children housed in old buildings infested with rats and mice (Vanek 1951).

PATHOLOGY AND SYMPTOMATOLOGY

P. carinii infection occurs only in infants aged from 4 weeks to 4 months who suffer from immunity deficiency states, especially congenital hypogamma-globulinaemia whether sex-linked with lymphopenia, or acquired in adults secondary to cytotoxic therapy (Marshall *et al.* 1964). Cases have also occurred in immune deficiency states associated with Hodgkin's disease and other reticuloses. *Pneumocystis* infection has been found in association with cyto-megalic inclusion disease.

The *Pneumocystis* forms foam-like masses which are composed of parasites in the alveoli and bronchioles of the lung. The alveoli are filled with a cellular exudate giving a honeycomb appearance in lung sections. When stained with Giemsa, periodic acid Schiff or Gomori's methenamine silver method, the alveolar exudate is seen to be composed of masses of parasites (Baar 1955).

The symptoms and signs are those of an interstitial pneumonia and the course of the disease is acute and usually fatal unless treated. There is intense dyspnoea and cyanosis with only moderate or slight fever. The chest signs are not specific. Radiography of the chest shows characteristic ground-glass cloudiness spreading outwards from the hilum. Subsequently areas of lobular collapse produce a mottled appearance and interstitial or mediastinal emphysema may be seen (White *et al.* 1961).

DIAGNOSIS

Persistent antibiotic-resistant pneumonia with conspicuous dyspnoea and cyanosis in infants with immune deficiency states and persons receiving immunosuppressive therapy should lead to suspicion of *Pneumocystis* infection. Definitive diagnosis is by lung biopsy.

TREATMENT

Considerable success has been reported with pentamidine (Marshall *et al.* 1964). A 6-month-old infant was treated successfully with a dose of 4 mg/kg (28 mg) intravenously daily for 10 days (Rodgers & Hague 1964) with full recovery.

REFERENCES

BAAR, H. S. (1955) *J. clin. Path.*, **8,** 9.
CHANDAR, K., NAIR, H. J. & NAIR, N. S. (1968) *Br. med. J.*, **i,** 158.
DANZIER, G., WILLIS, T. & BARNETT, R. N. (1956) *Am. J. clin. Path.*, **7,** 787.
DESMONTS, G., COUVREUR, J., ALISON, E., BAUDELOT, J., GERBEAUX, J. & LELONG, M. (1965) *Rev. fr. Étude. clin. biol.*, **10,** 952.
FAUST, E. C., GIRALDO, L. E., CAICEDO, G. & BONFANTE, R. (1961) *Am. J. trop. Med. Hyg.*, **10,** 343.
FULTON, J. D. (1965) *Immunology*, **9,** 491.
────── & FULTON, F. (1965) *Nature, Lond.*, **205,** 776.
────── & TURK, J. L. (1959) *Lancet*, **ii,** 1068.
────── & VOLLER, A. (1964) *Br. med. J.*, **ii,** 1173.
FRENKEL, J. K. (1948) *Proc. Soc. exp. Biol. Med.*, **68,** 634.
────── (1967) *J. Immunol.*, **98,** 1309.
────── WEBER, R. W. & LUNDE, M. N. (1960) *J. Am. med. Ass.*, **173,** 1471.
HENRY, L. & BEVERLEY, T. K. A. (1969) *Br. J. exp. Path.*, **50,** 230.
HUTCHISON, W. M., DUNACHIE, J. F., SIIM, J. C. & WORK, K. (1970) *Br. med. J.*, **i,** 142.
JACOBS, L. & LUNDE, M. N. (1957) *J. Parasit.*, **43,** 308.
KEAN, B. H., KIMBALL, A. C. & CHRISTENSEN, W. N. (1969) *J. Am. med. Ass.*, **6,** 1002.
KUNERT, H. & SCHMIDTKE, L. (1954) *Z. Tropenmed. Parasit.*, **5,** 324.
MARSHALL, W. C., WESTON, K. J. & BODIAN, M. (1964) *Archs Dis. Childh.*, **39,** 18.
NICOLAU, S. & RAVELO, A. (1937) *Bull. Soc. Path. éxot.*, **30,** 855.
PAULLEY, J. W., JONES, R., GREEN, W. P. D. & KANE, E. P. (1956) *Br. Heart J.*, **18,** 55.
PIZZI, T. (1956) *Boln. chil. Parasit.*, **11,** 16.
PRICE, J. H. (1969) *Br. med. J.*, **iv,** 141.
REMINGTON, J. S., MILLER, M. J. & BROWNLEE, I. (1968) *Paediatrics, Springfield*, **41,** 1082.
REYNOLDS, E. S., WALLS, K. W. & PFEIFER, R. I. (1966) *Archs intern. Med.*, **4,** 401.
ROGERS, J. S. & HAGUE, H. K. (1964) *Lancet*, **i,** 1042.
SABIN, A. B. (1942) *Proc. Soc. exp. Biol. Med.*, **51,** 6.
────── & FELDMAN, H. A. (1948) *Science, N.Y.*, **108,** 660.
STRANNEGARD, O. (1967) *Acta path. microbiol. scand.*, **69,** 465.
VANEK, J. (1951) *Čas. Lék. Česk.*, **90,** 1121.
WEINMAN, D. & CHANDLER, A. H. (1954) *Proc. Soc. exp. Biol. Med.*, **87,** 211.
WHITE, W. F., SAXTON, H. M. & DAWSON, I. M. P. (1961) *Br. med. J.*, **ii,** 1327.

9. AMOEBIASIS, GIARDIASIS AND BALANTIDIASIS

Amoebiasis

THE term amoebiasis denotes the condition of harbouring *Entamoeba histolytica*, with or without clinical manifestations (WHO 1969). *E. histolytica* usually lives as a commensal organism in the bowel, feeding harmlessly on bowel contents without invading the tissues. But it can invade the bowel wall without provoking symptoms; it can produce dysentery of varying degrees of severity, and can spread from the bowel to the liver and other organs. There are many more symptomless cyst-passers than cases of amoebic dysentery or liver abscess.

Geographical distribution

In some parts of the world *E. histolytica* cysts have been found in 50–83% of the population, for instance in Egypt, South Africa, West Africa, Mexico, South America and the Far East. Rates above 30%, however, are exceptional. In such areas of widespread infection the load of *Entamoeba* in individuals is also heavy, superinfection and reinfection being the rule. Amoebiasis occurs to a greater or lesser extent throughout the tropics and subtropics, and is also found in temperate climates, for instance in Britain, northern Europe and the United States, and more especially in countries with low standards of hygiene.

AETIOLOGY

For a description of the morphology, development and cultivation of *E. histolytica*, and a discussion of its races, see Appendix III.

Despite much research, the relationship between commensal entamoebae which live harmlessly in the bowel, feeding on intestinal contents, and pathogenic entamoebae which can cause disease, remains obscure. The life history is apparently as follows (Schensnovich 1969): In healthy carriers *E. histolytica* trophozoites live in the favourable conditions of the lumen of the caecum, feeding on bacteria etc. in the fluid contents, and multiplying there.

As the contents of the bowel move on and become less fluid, the trophozoites are in a less favourable environment, and give rise to precystic and cystic forms which are discharged in the formed faeces.

If the bowel function is disturbed (for instance by diarrhoea or purgatives) the contents become more fluid, move more rapidly, and the trophozoites have no time to develop to cysts; trophozoites therefore appear in the stools.

If pathogenic trophozoites invade the bowel wall, causing ulceration, there is an exudate into the lumen which renders the contents more fluid. Stools become more frequent, and contain trophozoites which, being pathogenic, often contain ingested erythrocytes from the ulcers. The appearance of trophozoites with ingested erythrocytes, therefore, is direct evidence of invasion of the tissues and of amoebic dysentery. The presence of cysts, or of trophozoites which do not contain ingested red cells, is not proof of amoebic dysentery.

As the bowel lesions regress, remaining slight and active in the proximal colon only, and as stools become formed, patients may pass cysts, but if slight dis-

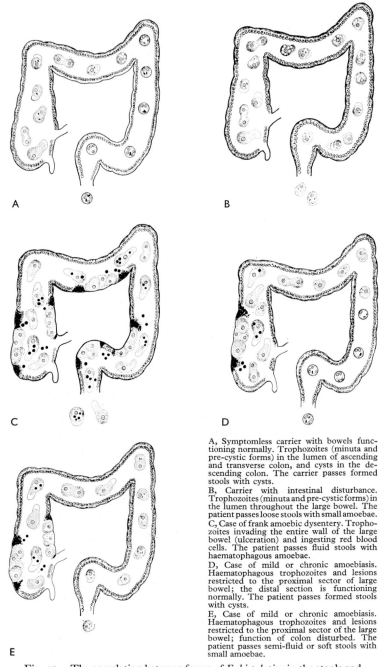

A, Symptomless carrier with bowels functioning normally. Trophozoites (minuta and pre-cystic forms) in the lumen of ascending and transverse colon, and cysts in the descending colon. The carrier passes formed stools with cysts.

B, Carrier with intestinal disturbance. Trophozoites (minuta and pre-cystic forms) in the lumen throughout the large bowel. The patient passes loose stools with small amoebae.

C, Case of frank amoebic dysentery. Trophozoites invading the entire wall of the large bowel (ulceration) and ingesting red blood cells. The patient passes fluid stools with haematophagous amoebae.

D, Case of mild or chronic amoebiasis. Haematophagous trophozoites and lesions restricted to the proximal sector of large bowel; the distal section is functioning normally. The patient passes formed stools with cysts.

E, Case of mild or chronic amoebiasis. Haematophagous trophozoites and lesions restricted to the proximal sector of the large bowel; function of colon disturbed. The patient passes semi-fluid or soft stools with small amoebae.

Fig. 45.—The correlation between forms of *E. histolytica* in the stools and clinical forms of amoebiasis. (*Reproduced from Schensnovich, V. B. (1969) Medskaya Parazit., 28, 594*)

turbance of bowel function occurs, and the stools become more fluid, the trophozoites can reappear in the faeces, along with cysts.

Cultures of pathogenic strains, when injected into the caeca of baby rats, produce characteristic lesions; cultures of non-pathogenic strains have no such action. Tested in this way, cultures of the pathogenic race breed true, retaining their virulence; non-pathogenic strains also breed true. Pathogenic strains retain pathogenicity when transferred to media containing flora which support the growth of non-pathogenic strains. Pathogenicity therefore seems to be inherent rather than induced by environmental factors.

Neal *et al.* (1968) found that patients with significant clinical symptoms harboured *E. histolytica* virulent to rats, and had positive serological tests. In

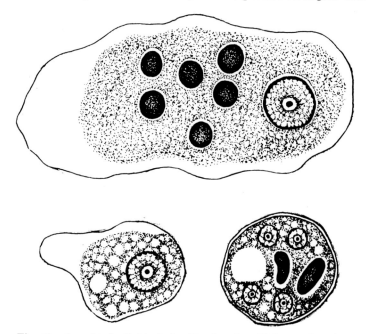

Fig. 46.—Amoebiasis. *E. histolytica*. Trophozoite with ingested erythrocytes to cysts. (*From an original drawing by B. Jobling*)

infected persons without clinical symptoms, however, the serological tests varied, but the virulence of the strains they harboured was generally low. Nevertheless, other work has shown that virulent *E. histolytica* introduced into the caeca of bacteria-free rats failed to produce lesions until bacteria were introduced, or the bowel wall was damaged by a needle. Experimental work in rats and guinea-pigs suggests that an excess of cholesterol or carbohydrate in the diet provides a suitable environment (perhaps by irritation of the bowel mucosa) for invasion by trophozoites (Neal 1968). Something of this kind may be true for man.

Virulence can apparently be increased in certain conditions; in the Durban area a gain in virulence, and hence in the frequency of invasion, is linked with rapid transmission (Powell *et al.* 1966). But factors affecting the susceptibility of the host are probably more important.

It is, however, difficult to understand why, with the return of thousands of servicemen to Britain after the two world wars, many of whom must have been excreting cysts, there were so very few instances of dysentery in them or their families, and why the incidence of cyst-passers in Britain has remained so low.

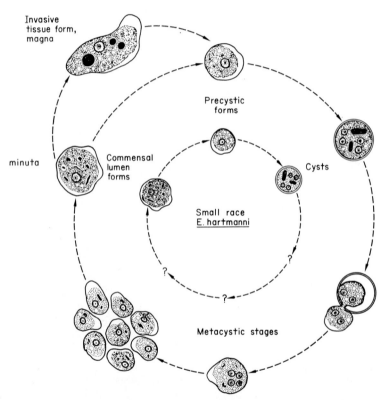

Fig. 47.—Human entamoebae with 4-nucleate cysts. Inner circle shows the life-cycle of the small race, *Entamoeba hartmanni* (interrogation marks indicate unknown metastatic stages); outer circle shows the life-cycle of the large race, *E. histolytica*, with tissue phase (invasive forms) outside the normal cycle. Arrows point to the course of development. (*Reproduced by permission of the Author and Editor from Hoare, C. A. (1957) Trans. R. Soc. trop. Med. Hyg., 51, 303*)

There may have been a change in virulence in the human host, and cyst-passers can spontaneously lose the infection; it may be that in a community in which the incidence of cyst-passers is low, and the chances of reinfection therefore also low, the threshold for continued interchange of infection is not reached.

No wholly satisfactory explanation of the relationship between pathogenic and commensal *E. histolytica* has yet been discovered. The important fact is that

in the vast majority of cases the presence of cysts in the faeces is of no pathological significance to the person who carries them.

E. hartmanni is now regarded as a species distinct from *E. histolytica* and the
minuta form. It is small, the trophozoites usually measuring under 10 μm, and
the cysts 3·8–8 μm. Certain morphological features justify its definition as a
separate species (see Appendix I). Its trophozoites never invade the tissues, and
it is therefore entirely non-pathogenic, living in the bowel contents as a commensal, and producing cysts there.

EPIDEMIOLOGY

Amoebiasis is strongly associated with slum conditions, bad sanitation,
poverty and ignorance, and probably with the general state of health and
nutrition of the people; this is true of both actual amoebic dysentery and of
symptomless infection. In the Durban area the incidence and severity of the
infection at all ages is greatest in the urban slum area, where the Africans live on
a diet largely deficient in protein. In the rural areas, on the other hand, where
conditions and diet are better, the infection in Africans is usually mild or
symptomless.

Though living in unsanitary conditions, Indians in the urban environment of
Durban are much less subject to amoebic dysentery than Africans, and Europeans least of all. It is unlikely that differences of virulence of strains are responsible, but even though sanitary conditions are probably the main factor, there
may be other influences not clearly known. Certainly diet seems to be important.

It has sometimes been suggested that amoebic dysentery is almost confined to
adults, and that it is more common in men than in women. In the Durban area,
where the general load of parasites is very heavy, however, amoebic dysentery
and its complications are often seen in children, and the same is true of Egypt,
Ghana and Nigeria, as well as elsewhere. For instance, Olatunbosun (1965)
reported 15 children who died of acute invasive amoebiasis and came to autopsy
in Lagos. One had a cerebral abscess, several had liver abscesses, several peritonitis and 2 intussusception, but the others had no extra-intestinal lesions. All
had bronchpneumonia and most were anaemic. Fulminating amoebiasis in
children is reported by Lewis and Antia (1969) in Nigeria and by Nnochiri
(1968) in Lagos, who states that 60% of all out-patients suffering from acute
amoebic dysentery at a Lagos hospital were children. Most of the mothers
were cyst-carriers. Indeed, pregnancy seems to predispose to amoebic dysentery.

E. histolytica has been found in wild rats (especially *Rattus norvegicus*),
monkeys, dogs and possibly pigs. Transmission from animals to man is rare,
from man to animals probably less so. Infected dogs and cats do not excrete
cysts and are therefore not infective to other animals.

TRANSMISSION

Man becomes infected with *E. histolytica* by swallowing the cysts (the only
infective forms). If trophozoites are swallowed they are destroyed in the
stomach, and patients in the stage of acute amoebic dysentery, passing trophozoites but not cysts, are therefore not infective to others. Cysts are formed in
response to special conditions at present ill defined; encystment appears to
require normal intestinal transit. Cysts resist cooling (as in water) for several
weeks and can remain viable in salt water for at least 12 days. They are killed
by heating (for instance in water at 50°C in 5 minutes) or deep freezing, and are

damaged by drying and putrefaction. They can pass alive through the gut of flies and cockroaches.

Cysts are presumably passed from person to person by the usual faecal–oral route, by fingers soiled with faeces, either directly into the mouth or via food which is not cooked after being handled. For instance, in West Africa, where amoebic dysentery is not unusual in young children, the mothers of such children are usually found to be excreting cysts, and the common practice of manual feeding of children affords ample opportunity for infection if the fingers are contaminated.

Amoebiasis can be a house or family infection, or can spread throughout institutions such as mental hospitals, originating from cyst-passers and producing either acute disease with diarrhoea, or quiescent infection, in other members of the community. Several instances of this have been recorded from Britain and the United States, even in families in which no member has been abroad. Association with slum conditions and bad sanitary habits is generally a feature in such cases.

The suggestion has several times been made that amoebic infection can be acquired from drinking water (for instance in Yugoslavia); this raises several points. Contaminated and untreated water obviously may contain cysts, and cysts can live in water (and faeces) for several days, though few remain alive after 2 weeks. Fully treated water is usually safe (see below, Prevention), but the possibility of infection from small supplies such as unprotected wells or water-holes cannot be excluded. For such water boiling is advised.

Amoebic dysentery does not occur in epidemics, however, as it would if water-borne (Dobell 1923; Boyd 1961). Writing from long experience, Boyd states: 'I have on no occasion encountered anything in the nature of an outbreak or epidemic of amoebic dysentery among human beings.' Yet several notorious outbreaks have been attributed to water-borne cysts, but Boyd, in a critical review of the evidence in these outbreaks, concludes that the diagnosis was sometimes at fault (as in the Chicago outbreak of intestinal infection of 1933), noting, among other things, that pathogenic amoebae were not cultivated from the suspected water. He suggests that, in other instances in which the diagnosis was correct, symptomless cyst-passers may have been precipitated into overt dysentery by bacterial infection from contaminated water, since it appears that commensal amoebae (presumably of potentially pathogenic strains) can be launched into virulence when such bacterial infection occurs, as in Westphal's experiment on himself (Westphal 1937). The high incidence of amoebic dysentery in some areas (for instance in British troops in the Burma campaigns of 1939–45) may largely be attributable to this and perhaps to the very debilitated condition of many of the patients.

PATHOLOGY

When *E. histolytica* invades the tissues of the intestine the lesions are most often found in the caecum and ascending colon or the sigmoid; the appendix may be involved and ulcers have exceptionally been found in the lower ileum. In fulminating necrotizing amoebic dysentery the whole colon may be full of ulcers, with extensive destruction in its whole length.

The early lesions are minute ulcers in the mucous membrane; they are flask-shaped in that the neck of the ulcer is much narrower than the deeper part (Fig. 48). The margins are rolled and the edges are undermined, and the ulcers are capped with dense yellow or even black sloughs. Trophozoites can be found

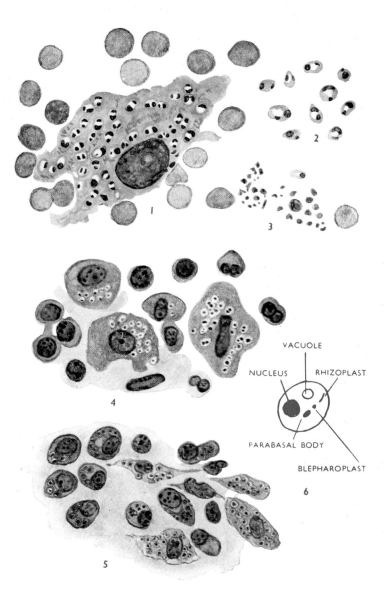

VACUOLE

NUCLEUS   RHIZOPLAST

PARABASAL BODY

BLEPHAROPLAST

6

PLATE I

Leishman–Donovan bodies in kala-azar.

1, Parasites enclosed in endothelial cells in film from spleen puncture, stained with Leishman. 2, Free forms from spleen. 3, Blood platelets in the same film for comparison. 4, Parasites enclosed within splenic pulp cells as seen in section, stained with haematoxylin. 5, Parasites in histiocytes and endothelial cells in intestinal mucosa. 6, Diagram of Leishman–Donovan body, highly magnified. × 1000.

[*To face p. 160.*]

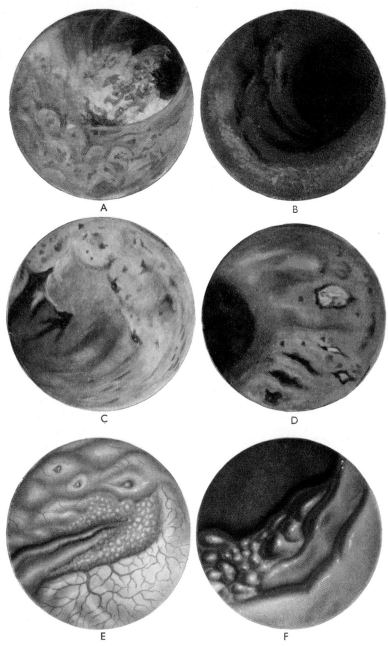

PLATE II

Sigmoidoscopic appearances of the rectum in bacilliary and amoebic
dysenteries.

A, Acute bacilliary dysentery (Shiga infection). Note the oedema of the mucosa and the
submucosal haemorrhages. (*P. Manson-Bahr*) B, Chronic bacilliary dysentery (Flexner
infection). Note the granulations on the mucous membrane. (*P. Manson-Bahr*) C, Acute
amoebic dysentery. Note the folding of the lax mucous membrane, pin-point ulcers
and surrounding submucous haemorrhages. (*P. Manson-Bahr*) D, Chronic amoebic
dysentery. Note the diamond-shaped ulcers and submucous haemorrhages. (*P. Manson-
Bahr*) E, F, Sigmoidoscopic appearance of the rectum in Eastern schistosomiasis (*S.
japonicum*). (*Originals after P'an, Huang, Chiang, Hsu and Hsu*)

in the depths of these ulcers. The mucous membrane between ulcers is usually normal and, if secondary bacterial infection does not take place, there is little evidence of inflammation. The process is essentially one of necrosis, with lysis of cells rather than inflammatory response.

The vessels at the base of the ulcer become thrombosed, but the ulcerative process may extend down to arterioles, and severe or even fatal haemorrhage may occur. Some ulcers pass through the muscular layers, perforating the bowel wall or rendering it so thin that bowel contents can seep through into the peritoneal cavity, giving rise to peritonitis or local peritoneal abscess.

In chronic cases polypoid tags may project into the lumen of the gut. When healing takes place, cicatricial pigmented scars mark the sites of former ulcers.

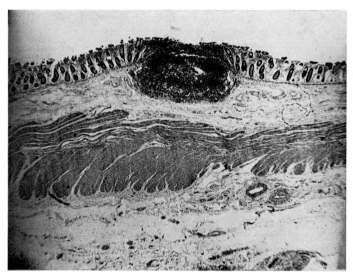

Fig. 48.—Amoebiasis. Low-power view of early amoebic ulcer in the large intestine. (*Reproduced from Ash & Spitz (1945) The Pathology of Tropical Diseases. Philadelphia: Saunders. By courtesy of the Wellcome Museum of Medical Sciences, London*)

An amoeboma, or amoebic granuloma, may result from repeated invasion of the colon by *E. histolytica*, with superadded pyogenic infection. Amoebomata are found in the rectum, rectosigmoid junction, transverse colon and caecum. There is progressive inflammation which spreads through the bowel wall to the surrounding tissues. The amoeboma may become very large, forming a hard swelling very difficult to differentiate clinically from carcinoma. Cases have been recorded in which the diagnosis of carcinoma has been contradicted by examination of tissues after death (e.g. *Br. med. J.* 1971).

Experimentally produced amoebic dysentery in kittens and dogs differs essentially from the disease in man. When introduced into the rectum of the animal, the amoebae produce a superficial excoriation within 2–3 days, and the lesions are more generalized than in man. Cysts are never found, and chronic ulceration does not occur.

IMMUNOLOGY

There is no indication that any one human race has more resistance to *E. histolytica* than any other; such differences as there are in incidence and severity are more probably due to differences in environmental conditions and diet.

There is no evidence that one attack of amoebic dysentery protects against subsequent attacks; infection does not protect against superinfection. Normal commensal *E. histolytica* does not make parenteral contact with the host, and therefore does not provoke the formation of antibodies. But invasive *E. histolytica* can provoke the formation of persisting antibodies, though these are not obviously protective. Antigenic differences between strains have, however, been demonstrated by complicated techniques.

One of these antibodies is an immunoglobulin (gamma-globulin) which can immobilize *E. histolytica* grown in culture for 24 hours, but the titre is low and the serum to be tested should be used undiluted. With this immobilization test Biagi and Buentello (1961) reported positive results in 18% of persons free from amoebiasis, but in 88% of patients with amoebic liver abscess, 90% of patients with acute amoebic dysentery and 78% of patients with chronic intestinal amoebiasis. The immobilization factor is apparently transmissible via the placenta from a positive mother to her fetus, as judged by tests on cord blood.

For serological tests involving antibodies, see Diagnosis, below.

CLASSIFICATION

The classification of the disease conditions caused by *E. histolytica* is difficult. WHO (1969) adopted the following:

1. *Asymptomatic*

2. *Symptomatic*

   a. *Intestinal amoebiasis*
   Dysentery
   Non-dysenteric colitis
   Amoeboma
   Amoebic appendicitis

   Acute dysenteric symptoms are sometimes accompanied by a tender and enlarged liver; in this condition there is thought to be no actual invasion of the liver by amoebae, and it is best referred to as non-specific hepatomegaly, which does not involve any assumption as to its exact aetiology. Complications and sequelae of intestinal amoebiasis: perforation, and peritonitis, haemorrhage, intussusception, post-dysenteric colitis, stricture.

   b. *Extra-intestinal amoebiasis*
   Hepatic
      i. Acute non-suppurative
      ii. Liver abscess
   Cutaneous

   Chronic diffuse amoebic hepatitis has been reported by some authors, but the existence of this condition has not yet been widely accepted. Complications of liver abscess: rupture or extension, bacterial infection, haematogenous spread to other organs.

      Involvement of other organs (lung, brain, spleen, etc.) without manifest liver involvement.

CLINICAL FINDINGS

An excellent account of amoebiasis was given by Wilmot (1962) who wrote from the extensive experience gained by the group of physicians in Durban, South Africa, at the large hospital there. The patients live in the surrounding area, urban and peri-urban.

Amoebiasis may coexist with other intestinal diseases, such as bacillary dysentery, typhoid, schistosomiasis, ulcerative colitis, abdominal tuberculosis and carcinoma. The finding of trophozoites in the faeces is not absolute proof that amoebiasis is the cause of the patient's illness, and the finding of cysts is a strong indication for an alternative diagnosis, since cysts are rarely found in the stools of patients with amoebic dysentery.

The *incubation period* of amoebic dysentery may be long, and is often impossible to calculate, since the patient may have had a latent infection with commensal amoebae until precipitated into dysentery by some other factor, possibly an intestinal infection with pathogenic organisms such as shigellae or schistosomes, or possibly malaria or other debilitating condition such as a low-protein diet. Persistent heavy superinfection may conceivably be a factor.

The *onset* is usually insidious, except in fulminating cases (see below), with abdominal discomfort, a mild windy looseness of the bowels, or frank diarrhoea in recurring bouts, not necessarily with blood or excessive mucus. Tenderness may develop over the caecum, simulating appendicitis, or the transverse colon, simulating peptic ulcer, or more commonly the sigmoid colon. In more severe cases there is often tenesmus.

In *mild cases* the patient is generally well nourished, sometimes even constipated, more often passing only a few dysenteric motions each day. Trophozoites are scanty on direct faecal smear, and few ulcers, or none, can be seen at proctoscopy.

In *moderately severe cases* there is some deterioration in the general condition, but not enough to force the patient to bed. Dysenteric stools number 5–15 each day, and trophozoites are numerous on direct smear. There are typical amoebic ulcers in the rectal mucosa. Africans in Durban are often incapacitated, with bloody diarrhoea, pain and tenderness, but with surprisingly little constitutional disturbance; this contrasts strongly with the condition in severe bacillary dysentery, when the patient is acutely ill, toxic and dehydrated.

Severe amoebic dysentery may occur at any age. In Nigeria children often show this form, in which the onset is relatively sudden as a result of extensive, fulminating, necrotizing amoebic colitis, and which is commonly fatal. The patient is ill and toxic, with poor general nutrition, extreme asthenia, fever, and more or less dehydration with depletion of electrolytes sometimes amounting to shock, with muscle cramps. The complexion may be subicteric or muddy. Hiccup is a bad sign. There is meteorism, vomiting, dysuria, tenesmus or even total incompetence of the anal sphincter, and the patient may pass over 15 motions in the day, though, exceptionally, there may be no diarrhoea. The rectal mucosa is severely damaged with confluent ulcers and haemorrhages. Peritonitis is a common complication, with ileus. In this condition proctoscopy is contra-indicated.

The faeces usually contain much dark and altered blood and blood-streaked mucus or even gangrenous sloughs; there are usually, but not always, abundant trophozoites containing ingested red cells.

In uncomplicated amoebic dysentery continuous pyrexia is unusual; fever may be intermittent. There is usually moderate leucocytosis of 10 000–25 000, with 70% polymorphonuclears.

In *chronic amoebic dysentery* neurasthenia is common, associated with vague bouts of abdominal discomfort. The colon may be distended with gas, and the sigmoid—and even the caecum—is sometimes palpable. Even without treatment the symptoms may subside, to reappear later, after intervals of weeks, months or years. Alternating diarrhoea and constipation are often observed, and diarrhoea may be provoked by physical exhaustion, chill or dietetic indiscretion.

Amoebic dysentery is therefore a difficult disease, to be differentiated from bacillary dysentery, duodenal ulcer, gall-bladder disease, regional ileitis, tuberculosis, diverticulitis, ulcerative colitis and carcinoma of the colon. If in a patient with trophozoites in the stools anti-amoebic treatment fails to relieve the symptoms—especially if the stools become clear—other causes of the illness should be sought.

Chronic amoebic dysentery and other forms of amoebic infection should be seriously considered in patients with ill-defined abdominal trouble, who have lived in the endemic areas; this applies particularly to enlargement of the liver, and to tumours of the colon. But it should be remembered that fatal amoebic liver abscess has been recorded in patients who have never left Britain; no doubt similar tragedies have occurred elsewhere.

An *amoeboma* can produce a tumour of the caecum, transverse colon, sigmoid or rectum, and may cause acute intussusception (especially when in the caecum). It may, rarely, lead to intestinal obstruction. Differentiation from carcinoma can be difficult, even by radiography, and cysts or trophozoites may not be found in the faeces. Clinically, an amoeboma can be mistaken for a growth of the intestine; surgical removal without anti-amoebic drugs is likely to be fatal (Stamm 1970). Medical treatment alone is effective. Amoebae can invade a tumour, and anti-amoebic treatment will reduce such a tumour, but will not cause it to disappear; this suggests carcinoma.

In invasive amoebiasis of the caecum, with local pain and tenderness, differentiation from appendicitis is difficult, but in amoebiasis the local signs in the right iliac fossa predominate over the generalized signs of toxaemia which are more usual in acute appendicitis. If signs of amoebic infection are found at operation for the removal of the appendix, specific treatment should be given at once, since operation can precipitate a fulminating exacerbation.

Sometimes, especially in elderly patients, amoebic infection in which the stools have been repeatedly negative for *E. histolytica* causes the large bowel to become greatly thickened, oedematous and friable. In such cases sigmoidoscopy may cause damage to the diseased bowel wall (Rowland 1967).

Patients who have lived in the tropics sometimes become obsessed by the idea that they are suffering from chronic amoebic infection, and tend to blame this for any irregularity of the bowel action, even for constipation. Thorough examination is needed, with reassurance if the results are negative, but the obsession is not easy to dispel.

Complications

Death may result from exhaustion, haemorrhage, perforation or liver abscess (see below). The commonest fatal complication is perforation of the bowel, leading to peritonitis. Perforation may occur during sigmoidoscopy, but apart from such trauma the bowel contents may leak or seep through the bowel wall, resulting in localized inflammatory masses, or abscesses, or generalized peritonitis. In the first two the prognosis is good, but generalized peritonitis is more common and dangerous.

General peritonitis may be of two types. In the first, which is rare, perforation occurs in the course of only moderately severe dysentery, or in patients who appear to be well controlled by treatment. The onset is abrupt, with severe abdominal pain and board-like rigidity of the abdominal muscles. In this type laparotomy is indicated, as the bowel wall can be repaired. In the second type the peritonitis is a complication of severe amoebic ulceration of the colon, though it may rarely occur in patients in whom no history, and no clinical evidence, of dysentery is found. In such patients there is usually a slow onset of abdominal distension, pain not being marked and rigidity being slight. Hiccup is a bad sign, and vomiting is even more significant. Rebound tenderness suggests peritoneal irritation but is not a certain sign of peritonitis—nor is slight distension.

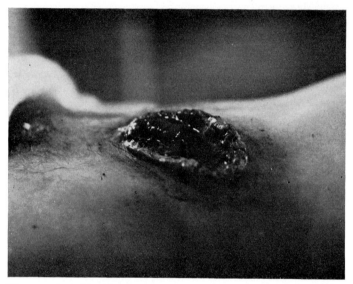

Fig. 49.—Amoebic skin ulceration surrounding a colostomy opening in a patient with an amoeboma of the colon. (*Sir Philip Manson-Bahr*)

Haemorrhage from erosion of a blood vessel by an amoebic ulcer may be serious and urgent, requiring immediate blood transfusion and energetic anti-amoebic measures. *Intussusception* is possible (usually caecocolic), and pain is then severe, with a sausage-shaped mass in the course of the colon and an empty right iliac fossa. Specific treatment should be given, but resection should not be delayed too long.

After treatment, amoebic dysentery may leave a condition of *ulcerative colitis*; it is rare and occurs only after severe dysentery. *Stricture* of the colon may develop; rectal stricture, though rare, can follow acute amoebic dysentery or even chronic infection in which dysentery is not prominent. It must be differentiated from the stricture of lymphogranuloma venereum and from malignant disease.

The *skin* around the anus, or round the stoma of a colostomy, may be extensively ulcerated (Figs 49, 50). Such distressing and unnecessary ulceration should never occur if physicians and surgeons are alive to the possibility of amoebic infection. Treatment with anti-amoebic drugs is dramatically success-ful, but the sequelae remain.

Rare complications include involvement of the prostate, and balanitis with granuloma, which may be very destructive but which responds to treatment. The vulva and vagina are sometimes infected directly from the bowel.

Abscesses have been found in the spleen, the psoas muscle, the buttocks (sometimes connected with a pararectal abscess, and secondarily infected by bacteria), and the thigh. These conditions respond well to emetine or other drugs.

Abscess of the brain sometimes occurs, especially in patients with liver abscess, and may produce pressure symptoms like those of cerebral tumour, though it is usually silent, diagnosed only at autopsy. It should be suspected in any patient showing mental deterioration, especially in association with liver abscess. For diagnosis, burr holes may be made, and abscess fluid aspirated;

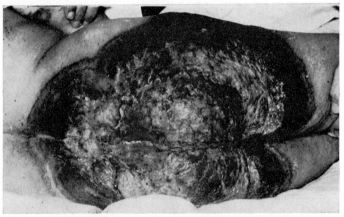

Fig. 50.—Amoebic ulceration of the skin—sacrum, coccyx and perineum.
(*Wellcome Museum of Medical Science*)

there is no meningitis. Response to emetine is very poor and it is invariably fatal.

Empyema due solely to *E. histolytica* has been reported and this may become secondarily affected with bacteria.

Amoebic infection of the urinary tract has been described, but authentic cases are rare. Trophozoites cannot live long in urine, but if they have access to the urinary passages and are passed out quickly, they may be recognizable. They may possibly gain access directly via the urethra, or via a fistula with the intes-tine, or by extension of a liver abscess into the kidney, or by blood or lymphatic spread. Care should be taken that haematophagous macrophages are not mis-taken for trophozoites. Cysts do not occur in urine.

DIAGNOSIS

History; microscopic examination

The first step in diagnosis is to have the disease in mind, and to ask patients with abdominal symptoms if they have travelled in the tropics or other endemic areas. Complaints of recurrent diarrhoea, 'haemorrhoids' or rectal bleeding should raise suspicions. Diagnosis of amoebic dysentery depends upon the history, symptoms and signs, endoscopic examination of the lower bowel, and especially upon the recognition of *E. histolytica* trophozoites in the stools or other materials, but certain other tests are useful. Trophozoites are found in the faeces of patients with amoebic dysentery, but they can usually be produced in cyst passers if a simple purgative is given (Woodruff & Bell 1967). They tend to appear in intermittent showers, and examination of 3 specimens at intervals of a week is better than examination of 3 specimens on consecutive days (Stamm 1970).

For the detection of trophozoites the faeces must be collected in a receptacle free from all traces of disinfectant, and must be examined on a warm stage while fresh. A small amount should be compressed on a slide under a coverglass so that a fairly transparent film is produced. Active trophozoites tend to be found in clumps or masses not evenly distributed throughout the stool, but best found in mucus. They may be found in one evacuation and not in the next. They can remain alive in faeces for a few hours, but become distorted in the presence of urine.

Trophozoites of *E. histolytica* have a clear, faintly greenish, transparent body several times the diameter of a red cell, and when stained by eosin they are seen to be refractile. They are actively motile, and usually elongated, producing a single blunt pseudopodium into which the endoplasm flows so rapidly that the ectoplasm may not be apparent until the amoeba slows down. But the important feature is that they contain ingested red cells, and without these, any amoeboid organism should not be diagnosed as *E. histolytica*. Large motile macrophages, such as are found in other forms of diarrhoea, and even *E. coli*, have often been mistakenly diagnosed as *E. histolytica*, with all the consequences of such a mistake.

The presence in the stool of blood, pus or mucus should be noted. Aggregations of red cells, disintegrated intestinal epithelium and Charcot–Leyden crystals may be present, but there is no characteristic exudate which is typical of amoebic dysentery (apart from an exudate which contains actively motile trophozoites containing ingested red cells). The cellular characters are no different from those of mucous colitis and other chronic lesions of the bowel. On the other hand, the exudate in acute and subacute bacillary dysentery is diagnostic (page 524). Trophozoites of *E. histolytica* may be found in a stool whose characters are typical of bacillary dysentery; in such a case the bacillary dysentery may be the cause of the patient's illness.

Cysts are more likely to be found in the faecal parts of a stool than in mucus; a small portion of faeces can be treated by zinc sulphate flotation to concentrate them. A drop of Gram's iodine added to the final preparation shows up the nuclei. Cysts of *E. histolytica* and *E. hartmanni* may be confused; both have 1–4 nuclei, but if the mean diameter of several cysts is above 10 µm they are probably *E. histolytica*, if below they are likely to be *E. hartmanni*.

If desired, thin fixed smears can be made for more careful examination, by placing the slide in Schaudinn's fixative for 30 minutes before staining with Gomori's trichrome stain or Heidenhain's iron haematoxylin.

Faeces which cannot be examined fresh may be preserved in Merthiolate-iodine-formalin (MIF) or polyvinyl alcohol (Hennessy & Elsdon-Dew 1967).

In addition to microscopic examination of material direct from the patient, *culture of entamoebae* may be called for as an aid in diagnosis. A method suitable for a clinical laboratory is described in detail by Robinson (1968); details should be sought in the original paper. He gives cultural success rates of 100% for *E. histolytica*, 70% for *Endolimax nana*, 58% for *Entamoeba coli* and 50% for

Entamoeba hartmanni (though this may be an underestimate compared with later results by improved technique). *Iodamoeba bütschlii* was never grown.

In the series of 535 cases of amoebic dysentery recorded by the former editor of this book, Sir Philip Manson-Bahr, 509 were diagnosed by microscopic examination of faeces, and the remainder by demonstration of amoebae in scrapings from amoebic ulcers. Amoebic lesions were demonstrated in 234 of 258 sigmoidoscopies.

In partly healed amoebic dysentery, lesions may be distinguished as pin-point oval or circular pits, irregularly disposed. The bowel surface may be peppered with them, and the term 'pig skin' appearances has been applied to them. They can persist even after treatment. Occasionally, solitary ulcers resembling carcinoma are seen in the rectum, even as long as 20 years after the primary infection.

Radiology is not much help in uncomplicated intestinal amoebiasis but can be valuable in detecting perforation and (by barium enema) such conditions as stricture, amoeboma and intussusception (though a barium enema in this is probably unwise if there is severe dysentery). In liver abscess a radiograph of the chest often reveals elevation of the right diaphragm.

Endoscopy by proctoscope or (better) sigmoidoscope is called for when the stools are negative, or to obtain material for examination, or to assess the results of treatment, or to differentiate from other possible diseases of the lower bowel. Amoebic ulceration occurs in the sigmoid and rectum, though it is most common in the caecum and ascending colon. No preparation of the patient is needed apart from defaecation, and the examination is best done in the knee–chest position; it is uncomfortable for the patient but need not be painful. The appearances may be normal even when lesions are present elsewhere in the bowel, so that normal endoscopic appearances do not exclude active ulcerative amoebiasis. The ulcers are usually shallow, covered with yellowish exudate, and up to 2 cm or more in diameter. The edges are raised and undermined, with some local hyperaemia though the mucous membrane between ulcers is usually normal. In large ulcers grey sloughs may be found, and in these severe cases great care is necessary in manipulating the sigmoidoscope as the bowel wall is very friable. The normal tone of the sphincter may be abolished. Material from ulcers is best removed for examination by a glass pipette, or a Volkmann spoon or a pair of bronchial biopsy forceps.

Submucous haemorrhages and blood-stained mucus are common.

Endoscopy alone cannot be relied upon to distinguish amoebic ulceration from ulcerative colitis, or bacillary or bilharzial dysentery. It is always essential to identify the parasite, and if *E. histolytica* cannot be found in material from ulcers, repeated examination of faeces is called for. The presence of *Schistosoma* eggs in the faeces or biopsy material is not proof that the ulcers or the symptoms are due to bilharzia.

Serological tests

The gel diffusion precipitin test is probably the most useful serological test. The antigen is prepared from *E. histolytica*. The antibody is, in general, a result of past or present invasion of the tissues. The test is commonly positive in acute amoebic dysentery and in post-dysenteric colitis, but may also be positive in other forms of colitis. It is therefore a help in diagnosis but is not proof of acute pathogenicity. It is almost always positive in amoebic liver abscess, and only slightly less commonly so in patients with suspected liver abscess. The test gives either positive or negative results; it does not indicate whether the infection is light or heavy. A negative result almost completely excludes amoebic invasion of the tissues.

A bedside modification of this test is used, in which equal amounts of serum and amoebic antigen are drawn into a capillary tube. A line of precipitation at the junction of serum and antigen one hour later indicates a positive reaction.

An indirect haemagglutination test (HA) is used with human Type O, Rh negative red cells preserved in citrate saline. The cells are coated with tannic acid (1 in 80 000 to 1 in 120 000) at 2°C, and sensitized with the antigen at pH 6·4 and 37°C. Titration is carried out in U-shaped wells, with 0·025 ml of sensitized cells per well, mixed with sera suitably diluted. Agglutination is usually sharply defined. In patients with amoebic liver abscess the test has been found 100% positive, in amoebic dysentery 98%; in patients without symptoms only about one-third were strongly or moderately positive, and in asymptomatic cyst-passers only 10% to two-thirds. Uninfected controls were almost all negative. In a complement fixation test with the same antigen, correlation with the HA test was complete in the liver abscess cases, but was low in cyst-passers, in whom the test often became negative within a year (Kessel et al. 1965; Neal et al. 1968).

The complement fixation test has a long history, with polyvalent antigens from various strains of E. histolytica. It is quite often positive in amoebic liver abscess or other deep-seated lesions, but is often negative in intestinal amoebiasis, and the general opinion seems to be that it cannot be relied upon in diagnosis, and it is being superseded by more modern tests. Serological tests depend upon the quality of the antigens used.

The indirect fluorescent antibody test has been used with an antigen of virulent E. histolytica on slides treated with dilutions of test sera, incubated for 30 minutes, washed in saline and then treated with fluorescein-labelled anti-human-globulin serum and incubated for 30 minutes. Results indicate that the test is useful. If the serum contains immune globulin, this is taken up by the amoebae, which in turn take up the fluorescent anti-human-globulin serum which can be detected by microscopy with near-ultra-violet light. Results have been regarded as positive at titres of 1 in 64 and over, for instance in hepatic amoebiasis. But titres of 1 in 16 or less have been found in subjects with no known evidence of amoebiasis (Jeanes 1966).

This test can be used to identify amoebae in tissue sections, which can be scanned rapidly and more effectively than by conventional staining (Parelkar et al. 1971).

An intradermal test has been used in which antigens were prepared from disintegrated E. histolytica and E. moshkovskii, extracted in 1 in 10 000 thiomersal at 37°C. 0·1 ml was injected intradermally and the result was read after 3 hours. There was some correlation with positive findings in the faeces.

Other conditions which may resemble dysentery

There are other, perhaps more familiar conditions, not necessarily of tropical origin, in which dysenteric symptoms may occur.

Of all common diseases with which mild dysentery may be confused, the first place must be given to internal haemorrhoids. A correct diagnosis may readily be made. Again, profuse offensive diarrhoeic motions with blood and mucus may be passed in tuberculous ulceration of the large bowel, which may be comparatively common in the tropics. Colitis, ulcerative, membraneous or haemorrhagic, resembles bacillary and amoebic dysenteries in clinical features and in the character of the stools, but can be differentiated by microscopic examination of the faeces, as well as by sigmoidoscopy. Idiopathic ulcerative colitis is becoming more common and has to be differentiated from the bacillary dysenteries. It is undoubtedly a disease *sui generis* and is distinguished by pyrexia, toxaemia, intense anaemia, a tendency towards spontaneous remission and great liability to relapse. Mucous colitis, or the syndrome commonly known by that name, is a frequent sequel of both bacillary and amoebic dysentery, and is frequently confused with both. Polyposis is a very distressing condition, which usually undergoes malignant degeneration. Foreign body in the rectum is another possible diagnosis. Blood and mucus are often passed in diverticulitis.

TREATMENT

The drugs used in amoebiasis are classed in several groups:

1. Direct-acting amoebicides, acting principally in the lumen of the bowel— di-iodohydroxyquinoline, arsenicals, diloxanide furoate, paromomycin.
2. Indirect-acting amoebicides, acting in the lumen and wall of the bowel, but not in the liver—tetracyclines.
3. Tissue amoebicides acting in the wall of the bowel and the liver—emetine hydrochloride, emetine and bismuth iodide, dehydroemetine.
4. Tissue amoebicides, acting principally in the liver—chloroquine.
5. Amoebicides effective at all sites—niridazole, metronidazole.

For mild to moderate cases of amoebic dysentery a combination of tetracycline, an amoebicide acting in the lumen and chloroquine is suggested. For severe cases, emetine hydrochloride or dehydroemetine, with tetracycline and an amoebicide acting in the lumen, may be used: metronidazole is safe and highly effective, and is regarded as the treatment of choice in most instances. Modern treatment is summarized in Table 7.

The original chemotherapeutic substance was *emetine*, introduced effectively in the treatment of amoebic dysentery by Sir Leonard Rogers in 1912. It had been isolated as early as 1817, and its parent substance, ipecacuanha, had been used in dysentery for more than a century. Emetine, however, was not successful when given by mouth, and it is to Rogers that we owe the knowledge of its value when given parenterally. Emetine hydrochloride is particularly effective where there is much invasion of the tissues, in metastatic lesions of the liver, lungs and skin, and in severe intestinal disease.

The hydrochloride is given by intramuscular or deep subcutaneous injection in doses of 60 mg daily for 5–10 days. It is, however, very toxic, the therapeutic and toxic doses being very close. It is a myocardial poison, and patients treated with emetine or dehydroemetine should be at rest, preferably in bed, during the course. Dehydroemetine is less toxic than emetine, but care should still be taken with it, pulse and blood pressure being recorded regularly during the course. Cardiac disease is a contra-indication, subject to the decision of the physician.

In amoebic dysentery a course of emetine is usually followed by a course of emetine bismuth iodide by mouth, in doses of 200 mg daily for 10–12 days. This tends to cause vomiting, and patients should be in bed, on a light diet, for at least the first few days. Vomiting may be controlled with tincture of opium or other sedative.

Results of treatment with emetine bismuth iodide, in patients passing trophozoites, or cysts, are very good; a 6·1% relapse rate is reported by Manson-Bahr (1941) and 3% for each category by Woodruff and Bell (1967). Dehydroemetine bismuth iodide does not produce toxic effects to the same extent as

Table 7. Summary of modern treatment of acute amoebic dysentery

Drug	Daily dose	Duration (days)	Route	Remarks
Emetine hydrochloride	60 mg single	5–10	i.m., s.c.	Toxic, patient in bed
Emetine bismuth iodide	200 mg	10–12	Oral	After the emetine
Dehydroemetine	80 mg single	10	i.m.	
Tetracycline	1000 mg	10	i.v. soln not over 0·5% w/v	Together in acute amoebic dysentery when other drugs cannot be taken
Dehydroemetine	60 mg single	3	i.m.	
Dehydroemetine resinate	1 mg/kg divided	10	Oral	After dehydroemetine
Dehydroemetine late release	60 mg divided	10	Oral	Used alone or followed by an amoebicide acting in the lumen
Dehydroemetine	60 mg single	3	i.m.	
Dehydroemetine bismuth iodide	300 mg divided	10	Oral	After dehydroemetine
Tetracycline	1000 mg divided	7–10	Oral	
Diloxanide furoate	1500 mg divided	10	Oral	Together
Chloroquine base	300 mg divided	20	Oral	
Metronidazole (Flagyl)	1200 mg divided or	6–8	Oral	Alternative regimens
	2400 mg divided or	5	Oral	Probably the drug of choice
	1600–2400 mg divided	2	Oral	
Clefamide (Mebinol)	1500–2500 mg or more divided	10–13	Oral	
Paromomycin sulphate (Humatin)	1500 mg or more divided	5	Oral	
Niridazole (Ambilhar)	1000–1500 mg divided	10	Oral	Not to be given with the emetine group. It may be too toxic in general

emetine bismuth iodide, but it should not be given until the dysenteric diarrhoea in acute amoebic dysentery has been controlled. It can be very useful in divided doses of 300 mg daily by mouth for 7–10 days after a preliminary course of dehydroemetine by injection.

Dehydroemetine resinate (RO 1–9334/19) is prepared in tablets of 10 mg. It has proved fairly successful in acute amoebic dysentery, and may with some advantage be used after a short course of parenteral dehydroemetine. Dehydro-emetine (late release tablets) has given excellent results when given alone by

Table 8. Treatment of cyst-passers

Drug	Daily dose	Duration (days)	Remarks
Dehydroemetine bismuth iodide	300 mg	7–10	
Dehydroemetine resinate	1 mg/kg	10	
Diloxanide furoate (Furamide)	1500 mg 600–1200 mg	10 7	May cause dyspepsia
Di-iodohydroxyquinoline (Diodoquin)	1000–2000 mg	15–20	
Metronidazole (Flagyl)	1200–1800 mg 1600–2400 mg	5–10 2 successive	
Clefamide (Mebinol)	1500–2500 mg	10–13	With retention enema 750 mg in 250 ml water daily for 10 days if needed
Paromomycin sulphate (Humatin)	1500 mg or more	5	Effective against other intestinal protozoa
Fumagillin	40 mg	10–14	Side-effects common
Carbarsone	500 mg	10	Or as retention enema 2000 mg in 200 ml 2% NaHCO₃ on alternate nights for 5 occasions
Milibis	1500 mg	7	
Entero-Vioform	750 mg	10	Or as retention enema

All these drugs should be administered orally in divided doses.
Cyst-passers can often be cleared of the infection by these drugs and remain clear if the opportunities for reinfection are scarce, but in endemic and hyperendemic areas the chances of reinfection are great.

mouth in acute amoebic dysentery. It should be given just before or just after meals to avoid unpleasant effects. Diloxanide furoate (Furamide) gives better results in both amoebic dysentery and in cyst-passers than diloxanide (Entamide) itself, cure rates reaching 95%. Shorter courses than 10 days are less effective.

An important new drug for amoebic dysentery (though originally introduced for the treatment of *Trichomonas vaginalis* infection) is *metronidazole* (Flagyl). This is said to be the drug of choice for acute amoebic dysentery, liver abscess and cyst-passers. It is both a contact and a tissue amoebicide, and is almost devoid of side-effects. The dosage advocated by Powell (1969) is 800 mg 3 times daily for 5 days, or even 2400 mg as a single dose daily for 3 consecutive days. Khambatta (1969) suggests 1600 mg on each of 2 successive mornings. Tetracycline can be given at the same time as metronidazole, but this addition shows little improvement on metronidazole alone (Powell 1969). Relapse appears to be rare after this treatment.

Paromomycin has also given good results; symptomatic relief is common in acute amoebic dysentery, and the cure rate in this and the chronic infection is quite high. It is also active against other intestinal protozoa, and had some effect on *Shigella sonnei* and *Sh. flexneri*. Toxic effects are rare when it is given by mouth, but if given parenterally it may affect the auditory nerve.

An older drug is carbarsone, which contains arsenic and can be used by mouth or as a retention enema. Another arsenic derivative is bismuth glycollyl-arsanilate (Milibis), often useful in clearing cyst-passers. Fumagillin is useful in cyst-passers, but ineffective in acute amoebic dysentery and liver infection. Side-effects are common, and include malaise, vertigo, nausea, vomiting, vesicular dermatitis, diarrhoea and even (after prolonged use) leucopenia.

Niridazole (Ambilhar, Ciba 32,644-Ba), originally introduced for the treatment of bilharzia (hence the trade name), is a nitrothiazole derivative. It is a direct amoebicide, giving better results than emetine preparations in amoebic dysentery, and rivalling them in amoebic liver abscess (Powell *et al.* 1966). Electrocardiographic changes are frequent but not serious, but a few patients have developed confusional states and severe headache. A later report indicates that it has proved to be too toxic (Wilmot 1968). It should not be given with emetine or dehydroemetine, and it should be reserved for use when the established forms of treatment have failed.

Di-iodohydroxyquinoline (Diodoquin) has long been used for cyst-passers. It occasionally gives rise to gastro-intestinal irritation, headache, pruritus ani and furunculosis, and may cause slight enlargement of the thyroid during treatment. For mild amoebic dysentery a combination of tetracycline, di-iodohydroxy-quinoline and chloroquine (to protect the liver) has been used, but for severe disease dehydroemetine may be necessary. For amoebic liver abscess dehydro-emetine with chloroquine and di-iodohydroxyquinoline may be used with advantage.

Clioquinol (which is present in Vioform and Entero-Vioform) has some value in cyst-passers. It is often given for traveller's diarrhoea, in which the aetiology is not known, but which is not obviously due to amoebiasis. It is said to act on various salmonellae and shigellae, though it had no effect on some salmonellae in one investigation. *Clefamide* (Mebinol) has been used with success in acute amoebic dysentery and in cyst-passers. Antibiotics of the tetracycline group are sometimes used with the true amoebicides, and may be life-saving, especially if peritonitis threatens (for instance if there is distension or vomiting) or develops. In emergency, tetracycline may be given intravenously.

Patients showing early signs of peritonitis should be given emetine hydro-chloride or dehydroemetine in full doses, together with tetracycline and fluids by mouth; intravenous fluids and intermittent or continuous gastric suction should be used if the condition deteriorates (Powell & Wilmot 1966). In a study of 75 patients with peritonitis, treated conservatively in this way, Powell and Wilmot (1966) reported death in 41%. If the onset of the peritonitis was slow, and occurred in hospital, the fatality rate was 12·5%, but if the onset was rapid death was usual.

Empyema due to *E. histolytica* demands specific treatment and continuous closed drainage, but if there is secondary infection open drainage or even decortication may be necessary.

PREVENTION

Control measures effective for enteric bacterial infections are also effective for amoebiasis. A safe and adequate water supply, and sanitary disposal of sewage and refuse, afford good protection. Ordinary chlorination of water cannot be relied upon to kill cysts, and although hyperchlorination will do so, it is expensive and gives an objectionable taste and is therefore impracticable. Filtration is necessary, but cysts can pass sand filters if the filtration rate is high. Water likely to contain cysts should therefore be treated with a coagulant and allowed to settle before sand filtration at not more than 30 litres/1000 cm²/ minute, and then chlorinated to at least 1 ppm residual chlorine. Metal micro-fabric is often used to remove particulate matter from water, but even such fabric with the smallest aperture (23 μm) will not prevent cysts from passing (Upton 1969). For personal protection where safe water is not supplied to the community, water should be boiled or treated by approved domestic measures.

Cysts can live in water (or faeces) for several days, few remaining alive after 2 weeks. Putrefaction damages them and desiccation kills them at once. A high temperature is more lethal than a low temperature, though deep freezing kills them at once, and at body temperatures they die within a few days (Dobell 1919). People who live in endemic areas should therefore be careful in the selection of foods, especially those bought from street vendors. Cooking kills the cysts, but foods commonly eaten uncooked, such as tomatoes, salads, straw-berries and others grown close to the ground and possibly fertilized with human faeces, should be avoided or thoroughly washed in safe water.

Kitchen hygiene practices which minimize the risk of exposure should be instituted, and facilities for hand-washing by cooks should be installed. All these measures should be taught to, and understood by, food handlers.

Travellers in endemic areas who stay in hotels have been advised to use water from the hot-water taps for drinking, tooth-brushing, washing dishes and cups etc., because water at 50°C kills cysts in 5 minutes. A rough test is that if the water is too hot for the hand to tolerate, it is almost certainly harmless (Neu-mann 1970). This reasoning applies also to bacterial diseases and to traveller's diarrhoea.

Cysts have been found in the vomit and faeces of flies (which also carry them on their feet) and in the droppings of cockroaches. These pests should be suppressed, and food should be protected from them.

The question of treatment of cyst-passers such as cooks, nurses etc., who might infect others, has been much discussed. In highly endemic areas reinfection is likely, and although food handlers could justifiably be given intermittent treatment, the method does not appear to have been widely used, and is not recommended by WHO except for special conditions of very high risk. As a rule nothing is required beyond the precautions normally taken to protect food and water from all types of contamination.

AMOEBIC LIVER ABSCESS

'Amoebic liver abscess continues to provide the greatest pitfall in clinical tropical medicine' (Walters 1970).

The typical liver abscess of the tropics is caused by trophozoites of *E. histo-lytica* originating in the bowel. It is commonest in patients who have, or have had, recognizable amoebic infection, but also occurs in people who give no history of amoebic dysentery. It is commonest in areas of intense infection such as Natal and parts of India, but may, very rarely, be found in persons who have never been in the tropics; Wright (1966) reports one such case and refers to others in Britain.

Liver abscess may occur after a long latent period, perhaps many years after the patient left the endemic area, and the importance of asking a patient who has an enlarged liver if he or she has been abroad cannot be overemphasized. In this as in so many other cases in which tropical diseases may be involved, it is imperative to ask the question: 'Where have you been ?' The explanation of this long latent period may be that the infection persisted without symptoms until some stimulus provoked multiplication of the entamoebae, or that the original infection induced hypersensitivity, and that reinfection provoked the reaction. Steroid therapy for some other condition may also be the stimulus.

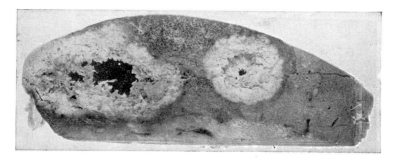

Fig. 51.—Multiple liver abscesses from a case of acute amoebic dysentery, showing the characteristic structure and zone of acute hyperaemia. One-quarter natural size.

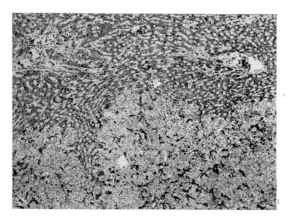

Fig. 52.—Structure of miliary amoebic hepatic abscess containing *E. histolytica*. (*P. H. Manson-Bahr, original case*)

Expatriates living in endemic areas may be more liable to liver abscess than the indigenous people, but the latter are certainly prone; McLeod *et al.* (1966) see 500–600 cases each year in Durban. Children do not escape, and many abscesses have been found before and after death in hospitals in Nigeria and Durban. Expatriate children, however, rarely get liver abscess, perhaps because they live in good sanitary conditions. Amoebic liver abscess seems to be particularly common in some ship stewards and kitchen staff, who are well nourished (Robinson 1968).

Pathology

Amoebic infection of the liver is caused by amoebae reaching the liver via the portal system. The pathological process is one of necrosis of liver cells at the centres of the lobules.

Rogers originally described a condition of 'amoebic hepatitis', as a very early stage of liver abscess. In this condition a number of small necrotic foci (or abscesses) are probably formed, which, if not treated, tend to enlarge and coalesce.

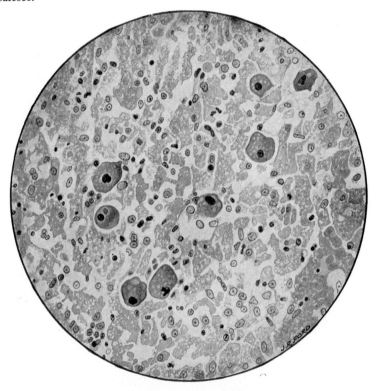

Fig. 53.—Microscopical section of a liver abscess, showing *E. histolytica* at the margin of the abscess cavity, surrounded by necrotic liver cells.

As liver abscess develops, the liver enlarges, and in the early stages contains grey, ill-defined globular necrotic patches up to 2·5 cm in diameter. These necrotic patches liquefy and coalesce, forming the characteristic ragged abscess cavities full of viscid, chocolate-brown (anchovy sauce) thick pus which contains disorganized liver tissues and clots or streaks of blood. The pus is sometimes greenish from bile. Trophozoites of *E. histolytica* can often be found in the pus after drainage of the abscess for a few days, and they are present in large numbers in the walls of the abscess cavity. Cysts are never found. The abscess can become secondarily infected with pyogenic organisms, especially if open operation is performed (which is contra-indicated); in this case trophozoites tend to disappear.

Liver abscesses may be single or multiple, and are usually (but not invariably) found in the right lobe. Multiple abscesses have been misdiagnosed as metastatic carcinoma, the correct diagnosis having been made only when histological examination revealed trophozoites in the abscess walls. A single abscess may attain great size.

An abscess in the right lobe tends to push up the right cupola of the diaphragm, and this can be seen on the radiograph, providing an important point in diagnosis. As an abscess approaches the surface of the liver, adhesions are commonly formed with the surrounding organs; they may prevent the abscess from bursting into the peritoneal cavity. Apart from the peritoneal cavity, an abscess may burst into the pleural cavity or the lung itself, though pleural

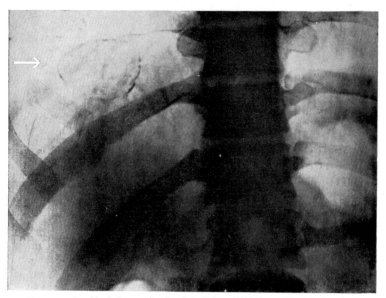

Fig. 54.—Cretified abscess in the right lobe of the liver. (*Dr M. Cordiner*)

adhesions may prevent general spread. An abscess (usually in the left lobe) may infect the pericardium, with all the serious effects of that condition.

Liver abscesses may become encysted, with thick fibrous walls, and the contents may eventually become cheesy or cretified until the cyst contracts. Calcified abscesses can sometimes be found by radiography, and must be differentiated from hydatid cysts or calcified suprarenals.

A form of subacute or chronic amoebic hepatitis has been described by Doxiades (1964) and his colleagues, in which spheroid formations having the characteristics of amoebae have been found among the liver cells, and homogenized liver tissue from such cases has been injected into the livers of animals, producing abscesses with amoebae in their walls. The condition is improved by anti-amoebic treatment. Powell (1969), however, comments that attempts to confirm these findings have been unsuccessful, in that trophozoites have not been found in the absence of necrosis.

Clinical findings

In a study of 764 cases of amoebic liver abscess in patients in hospital in Thailand, Harinasuta *et al.* (1968) give the following facts (figures given as percentages):

Presenting symptoms

Fever and pain at the right costal margin	82
Fever without pain	13
Abdominal mass	3
Others (jaundice, abdominal pain, dysentery)	2
Referred pain (right shoulder)	28

Signs

Fever	97
Hepatomegaly	91
Tenderness of the liver	95
Jaundice (usually slight)	32
X-ray, raised right diaphragm	85
Leucocytosis	87

Site of abscess

Right lobe	87
Left lobe	8
Both lobes	5
Single cavity	94

Pus

Reddish-brown	89
Creamy or yellowish green	11

Recovery of E. histolytica

From pus	11
From stool	14

Rupture of abscess	27
Pulmonary amoebiasis	3
Pleural effusion	9

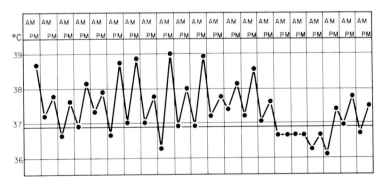

Fig. 55.—Temperature chart of a patient with amoebic abscess of the liver.

The dominant clinical condition of 'amoebic hepatitis' (the very early stage of liver abscess, see above, Pathology) is a swinging fever (Fig. 55), raised sedimentation rate, characteristic leucocytosis, and a slightly enlarged and tender liver perhaps with elevation and fixation of the right cupola of the diaphragm.

A positive complement fixation test is a help in diagnosis, for the condition is to be differentiated from typhoid, and it is important to remember that early amoebic invasion of the liver can give this swinging temperature. It is amenable to anti-amoebic treatment, and therefore aspiration or other surgical intervention can be avoided.

Symptoms. There is great variety in the symptoms of liver abscess. As a general rule, the patient is one who has long resided in the tropics and who at

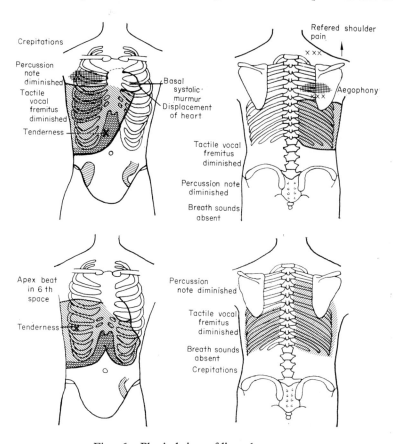

Fig. 56.—Physical signs of liver abscess.

Above: Right lobe of liver, cured by aspiration with Potain's aspirator. Leucocytes 9000. *E. histolytica* cysts in faeces.
Below: With hypertrophy of the left lobe, cured by aspiration of 1·8 litres of sterile pus. Leucocytes 12 000. *E. histolytica* cysts in faeces.

some time or other has suffered from subacute attacks of dysentery. At first he becomes conscious of a sense of weight and fullness in the right hypochondrium, and later suffers from sharp stabbing pains over the hepatic area, accentuated by coughing.

In liver abscess the onset of symptoms may be acute, or slow. Pain, usually in the right hypochondrium or chest, rarely in the left, and intercostal tenderness to finger pressure between the ribs, are prominent (Fig. 56). The pain is continuous and may be severe, made worse by movement and breathing; it may be referred to the right shoulder. There may be a pleural rub. The liver is commonly tender throughout, but usually with a spot of maximum tenderness which is often intercostal rather than subcostal; there may be oedema over the ribs in the tender area, in extreme cases showing as a very obvious swelling. If the abscess is deep in the liver, however, tenderness may not be present at first even if the liver is enlarged. There are usually signs at the base of the right lung, with cough and X-ray evidence of a raised right diaphragm. Fever is usual, with profuse sweating, the temperature often resembling that of typhoid, though it may be periodic rather than continuous, and may be mistaken for that of malaria. Leucocytosis in the range 15 000 to 35 000 is a feature; the increase is general, with polymorphs around the normal proportion of 70%. A normocytic normochromic or normocytic hypochromic anaemia is usual.

Diagnosis

Different opinions have been expressed on the subject of aspiration of amoebic liver abscess for diagnosis. Stamm (1970) states that with modern serology and non-toxic drugs, aspiration is unjustifiable for purely diagnostic purposes, and should be reserved for treatment of large abscesses liable to burst, or abscesses which fail to resolve on drug treatment.

On the other hand McLeod et al. (1966) argue that aspiration is called for if there are signs of pus in or about the liver. It is safe and the liver can confidently be explored with a long, wide-bore needle. The decision whether or not to explore is a matter of clinical judgement, but when signs of abscess are present, delay in aspiration and evacuation of the pus can lead to prolonged illness and serious complications.

For aspiration deep local analgesia usually suffices, but nervous subjects should have a general anaesthetic. If there are localizing signs, such as a tender spot, a fixed pain, localized oedema, localized pneumonic crepitus, pleuritic or peritoneal friction, these should be taken as indicating, with some probability, the seat of the abscess and the most promising spot for exploratory puncture. If no localizing sign is present, the needle should first be inserted in the anterior axillary line in the eighth or ninth interspace, but not more than 9 cm deep—the distance of the inferior vena cava from any part of the chest wall in an adult is 10 cm. This is because most liver abscesses are situated in the upper and back part of the right lobe. The needle swings when the liver is engaged and, as it does so, it should be pushed gently forward. The operator knows when he is in the abscess cavity because the needle is felt to pass into space. The syringe should then be affixed and aspiration commenced. Effusion of serum into the pleural cavity immediately near the abscess sometimes occurs.

To obtain trophozoites from hepatic pus the last part of the aspirate is collected and left until a sediment forms. Trypsin is added to digest the debris and the preparation is centrifuged. The deposit is examined for trophozoites, which may be found in 90% of abscess pus. Trophozoites may also be obtained from the wall of a liver abscess by needle biopsy at the time of aspiration.

The pus may not contain trophozoites, which are usually present in the wall of the abscess, but if they are found in the pus they are diagnostic. They are not likely to be found if anti-amoebic drugs have been given. If bacteria alone are found the abscess is probably pyogenic, though they may have been introduced during aspiration. In general, pyogenic liver abscess gives a more acute illness than the commoner type of amoebic abscess, but in acute amoebic abscess the differentiation may be impossible.

X-ray examination may confirm the upward enlargement of the liver, and bulging, 'tenting' or blurring of the outline of the right dome of the diaphragm and shadowing of the right costophrenic angle indicating effusion. Screening usually shows that it does not move on respiration (Fig. 57). Paradoxical movement (rising with inspiration) is sometimes seen. Should, however, the abscess be situated in the centre of the liver, even if of considerable size, no definite information is usually obtainable by radiography except when the abscess has become partially encysted or calcified (Fig. 54), when the outline becomes apparent by X-ray. Occasionally, however, the outline of the liver abscess may show up as a less opaque area in the liver substance, affording exact location for the exploring syringe. Air may appear in the abscess cavity and show up the fluid level. Injection of air through the aspirating syringe has been practised

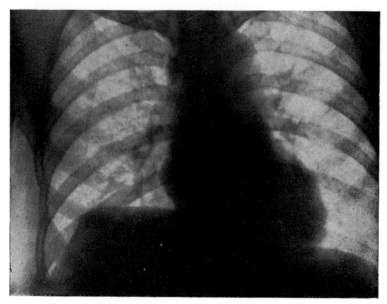

Fig. 57.—The dome of the diaphragm in liver abscess. (*Dr Carmichael Low*)

with success, and Lipiodol injection facilitates visualization (Fig. 58). The air-replacement method is useful, but examination following it should be carried out on the day after tapping. Three radiograms should be taken after screening: in the antero-posterior position, erect; in the lateral position; and in the former position with the patient on the left side. The air outlines the upper part of the abscess and by superimposing the films a correct assessment of the complete size and outline can be obtained. The outline of the diaphragm is blurred when the abscess is near the upper surface of the liver. Normally the upper margin of the hepatic shadow forms a right angle with that of the vertebral column, but when abscess is present this may become more acute.

The outline of the cavity can be shown by using a contrast medium. The pus is first drawn off by means of a long cannula, and a radio-opaque solution is injected in amounts from 5 to 60 ml, depending on the size of the cavity; air can also be added. The results can be seen on X-ray examination.

Middlemiss (1964) points out that many cases of liver abscess are still missed because they often present as pulmonary conditions. He mentions 5 radiological signs which are important:

(*a*) Elevation of the right dome of the diaphragm.
(*b*) Reduced movement of the right dome.
(*c*) Pleural effusion.
(*d*) Pulmonary collapse, often early.
(*e*) Lung abscess.

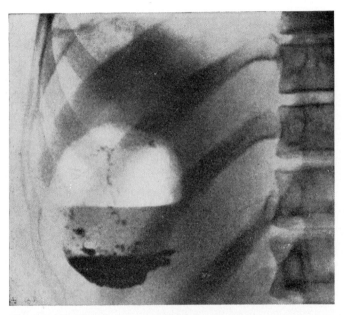

Fig. 58.—Visualization of an amoebic liver abscess by puncture and injection of Lipiodol in the erect position. (*After Snapper, Chinese Lessons to Western Medicine*)

X-ray diagnosis, to differentiate liver abscess from lower right pulmonary disease, may be facilitated by producing pneumoperitoneum by insufflating carbon dioxide (which eliminates the hazard of fatal air embolism which could occur with air or oxygen). The injection is made 2·5 cm to the left of the umbilicus and the same distance above or below it, and 250–1000 ml of carbon dioxide are injected with the patient lying on the X-ray table. Adhesions may be seen between the upper surface of the liver and the diaphragm, and distortions of the diaphragm and liver surface can be detected (Ellman *et al.* 1965).

Diagnosis can be assisted by the method of hepatoscan after intravenous injection of a suspension of 100 μCi of radioactive gold (^{198}Au). The colloidal particles are trapped by the Kupffer cells of the liver, and are detected by the isotope scanner. In the abscess areas the particles are not trapped, and these areas show as solitary or multiple non-filling or hazy areas on the hepatoscan. By serial hepatoscans after treatment Sheehy *et al.* (1968) found that most amoebic abscesses heal gradually in 2–4 months, but that occasionally the period may be as long as a year. Small abscesses do not necessarily heal more quickly than large abscesses.

Trophozoites may rarely be found in sputum if an abscess ruptures into the lung.

Diagnosis of liver abscess is not greatly helped by liver function tests.

In differential diagnosis infectious hepatitis should be considered, though jaundice is rare in liver abscess, and tenderness of the liver is more marked. Differentiation from malignant growth in the liver can be very difficult, and biopsy may be necessary; a trial of anti-amoebic drugs may be justified. Hydatid cysts are usually not as tender as abscesses, and the blood findings and a Casoni test are helpful (Wilmot 1967).

Occasionally an abscess situated near the porta hepatis may simulate empyema of the gall-bladder, with deep jaundice and exquisite local tenderness (Walters 1970).

Treatment

Most physicians recommend aspiration for evacuation of pus as soon as the pus is diagnosed, because it is thought that an amoebic abscess, once found, will not resolve on anti-amoebic drugs alone. Powell (1969) remarks that small abscesses will resolve without drainage, but that inadequate aspiration is the commonest cause for failure of treatment. An important diagnostic point is that amoebic pus is not foul-smelling.

Drug treatment is needed in addition to aspiration and is summarized in Table 9.

For amoebic liver abscess, apart from drainage, metronidazole is suggested, or a combination of either emetine hydrochloride or dehydroemetine with chloroquine and an amoebicide acting in the lumen of the bowel. If the patient also has dysentery, the dose of metronidazole should be increased, or with other regimens tetracycline should be added (WHO 1969).

Complications of amoebic liver abscess

A liver abscess may rupture into the pleural cavity, causing pleurisy, effusion or empyema. The development of this condition is often insidious but may be sudden, with marked pain and shock. The right side is more often involved than the left, and the signs are those of pleural effusion, but enlargement of the liver may suggest the diagnosis. If the effusion is aspirated the pus is usually of the anchovy paste kind and *E. histolytica* may be found in it.

An amoebic liver abscess may extend to, or rupture into, the lung, usually the right lung. The sputum often suggests amoebiasis, with small haemoptyses or quantities of reddish-brown material sometimes containing trophozoites. The diaphragm is raised and the lung is consolidated or contains an abscess. A hepatobronchial fistula may occur, and this may drain the abscess successfully.

Occasionally the pulmonary condition leads to bronchiectasis or cavitation, when surgical resection may be necessary, though not to be undertaken lightly. Treatment is conservative, with the standard drugs, and the prognosis is usually good, but adequate aspiration of the abscess is extremely important.

It is probably true that the lungs may be affected by *E. histolytica*, presumably blood-borne, in the absence of hepatic abscess, but the condition is rare. There may be single or multiple abscesses and areas of consolidation, but consolidation in the course of amoebic infection is not necessarily due to that infection. The sputum may contain amoebae, but these are likely to be *E. gingivalis*; to be labelled as *E. histolytica* a trophozoite must contain ingested red cells.

Table 9. Treatment of amoebic liver abscess

Drug	Daily dose	Duration (days)	Route	Remarks
Emetine hydrochloride	60 mg	5–10	i.m., or s.c.	Toxic, patient to be in bed
Dehydroemetine	80 mg single	10	i.m.	
Chloroquine base	600 mg at once, 300 mg 6 hours later, 300 mg daily afterwards	28	Oral	Together
Diloxanide furoate	500 mg three times daily	10	Oral	To eliminate the entamoebae from the bowel
Metranidazole (Flagyl)	1200 mg divided or 1600–2400 mg single	5 2 successive days	Oral Oral	
Niridazole (Ambilhar)	1000–1500 mg divided	10	Oral	Not to be given with the emetine group
Dehydroemetine	80 mg single	10	i.m.	
Chloroquine base	600 mg at once, 300 mg 6 hours later, 300 mg daily afterwards	28	Oral	May be used together
Di-iodohydroxyquinoline	1000–2000 mg divided	15–20	Oral	

If chloroquine is used without emetine, di-iodohydroxyquinoline may be used, but should be supplemented with tetracycline 1000 mg daily (divided) for 7 days (Wilmot 1962).

Aspiration of the abscess is important, see page 183.

An amoebic liver abscess not uncommonly ruptures into the peritoneal cavity, either suddenly or by gradual leaking. If sudden, the picture is that of acute peritonitis with shock, followed by distension and signs of free fluid. Treatment is surgical, with plasma or blood for shock. Thereafter the standard anti-amoebic treatment is indicated, together with tetracycline. In some cases there are local collections of pus, which should be drained.

Amoebic pericarditis is usually associated with abscess in the left lobe of the liver; it is rare. One type presents a pericardial rub or a clear effusion with radiographic signs of pericarditis. This indicates that the underlying liver abscess is near the pericardium; if the abscess is drained and standard treatment given the pericardial lesion resolves. Rupture of an abscess into the pericardium may be fatal in a few hours. There is pain and respiratory distress, and signs of pericardial effusion develop; it may lead to tamponade. There are also signs of the liver abscess. Diagnosis is confirmed by aspiration of characteristic pus from the pericardium; differentiation from purulent pericarditis due to bacteria is obviously important. A negative gel diffusion test excludes amoebiasis as a cause of pericarditis. Treatment is urgently needed, and is often successful. Aspiration or drainage of the pericardium and of the liver abscess is called for, together with specific treatment, and antibiotics if bacterial infection occurs. Digitalis and diuretics may be indicated. Late results may include constrictive pericarditis which may require pericardectomy. The indications for low salt diet and diuretics are the same as for other pericardial disease (Wilmot 1962).

Other rare complications of liver abscess are rupture into various hollow abdominal organs—stomach and colon—which may be followed by severe haemorrhage. The abscess may communicate with the biliary system, when the liver pus is heavily stained with bile. The liver abscess itself, usually bacteriologically sterile, may become infected by bacteria, in which case the patient tends to become toxic and the fever does not settle; the pus changes in character .

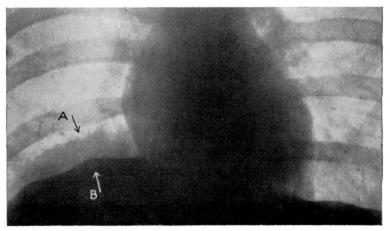

Fig. 59.—Radiograph of a liver abscess bursting through the diaphragm into the base of the right lung, where the pus is being evacuated through a branch of the right bronchus. A, Collection of pus in the pleural cavity; B, Valve-shaped opening through the diaphragm at the site of the abscess in the liver. (*Dr M. Berry*)

Treatment is with antibiotics in addition to anti-amoebic drugs, and aspiration. Surgical drainage may be needed if these measures fail.

The question of return to the tropics after recovery from liver abscess frequently crops up. If feasible, and if the patient has not to make too great a sacrifice, he ought to remain in a temperate and healthy climate. There are many instances, however, of individuals who have enjoyed permanent good health in the tropics after recovery from liver abscess. Before return the bowel should be thoroughly cleansed of amoebic infection.

PRIMARY AMOEBIC MENINGO-ENCEPHALITIS

This condition has recently been recognized in some 57 cases, from Australia, the United States, Czechoslovakia and Britain. It is caused by amoebae of the genera *Hartmannella* (*Acanthamoeba*) and *Naegleria*, free-living organisms which inhabit mud and contaminated water in slow streams, ponds and puddles, and which as cysts can resist cold and drying. The two genera are similar except that the trophozoites of *Naegleria* are smaller, and it has a flagellate phase in unfavourable conditions, for example in distilled water. The trophozoites are sluggishly motile, and show pseudopodia. They can be cultivated in artificial media. *Naegleria gruberi* has been isolated from the nose of a healthy boy after swimming in a lake in the U.S.A. (Schumaker *et al.* 1971).

Infection is apparently acquired via the nasal mucosa and the olfactory bulbs, when the patient is swimming or playing in tepid water; children are commonly affected. Most cases have occurred in summer.

Post mortem there is acute purulent meningitis with inflammation in the subarachnoid area, haemorrhages and fibrous thickening of the meninges especially over the whole base of the brain. There is superficial encephalitis from direct invasion of the cortex by the amoebae, accompanied by accumulations of inflammatory cells, thrombosis and necrosis of blood vessels, focal haemorrhages and other changes. The cerebrospinal fluid is purulent, reddish-brown, with a thick creamy deposit; it contains amoebae and red cells, but no bacteria on culture. In Australia *N. fowleri* has been isolated (Carter 1972).

In one case there was post mortem evidence of haematogenous spread, the organism being isolated from lungs, liver and spleen. There was also diffuse myocarditis, and amoebae were seen in heart blood (Duma *et al.* 1969).

The incubation period is short, and the main clinical picture is that of meningitis, which could be diagnosed as pyogenic except for the negative bacteriological tests. There may be a maculopapular rash. A feature of some cases was sore throat with purulent exudate over the tonsils.

Diagnosis depends upon recognition of the amoebae in cerebrospinal fluid soon after withdrawal, on a warm stage under phase-contrast microscopy or even dark ground illumination. In good conditions the sluggish pseudopodia can be seen in the trophozoites, which measure 6–10 μm. It is important to have this disease in mind in cases of meningitis in which the cerebrospinal fluid is bacteriologically negative.

Treatment has almost always been a failure, and the cases have almost always been fatal, though it is not known whether milder cases which have survived have been missed. The treatment perhaps most likely to have effect is to give amphotericin B together with a sulphonamide, especially sulphadiazine. Amphotericin B has been successful in experimental infections.

For reviews of this condition see Symmers (1969), Carter (1972) and Editorials in the *British Medical Journal* (1970) and the *Lancet* (1970).

Giardiasis

AETIOLOGY

Giardiasis is caused by *Giardia intestinalis* (sometimes known as *G. lamblia*) which lives in the upper part of the small intestine but may also infect the duodenum (see page 984).

TRANSMISSION AND EPIDEMIOLOGY

G. intestinalis is transmitted orally through ingesting viable cysts from contact with the excreta of an infected individual. *G. intestinalis* is most prevalent in children, especially in large families and institutions such as elementary schools and orphanages. Occasionally there is an epidemic such as has been described from Aspen, Colorado, where the cause was ascribed to a leakage of the main town sewer into part of the water supply.

PATHOLOGY

The trophozoites of *G. intestinalis* live in the small intestine and duodenum where they penetrate the epithelium; they have been observed at all levels from the epithelium to the submucosa, intestinal spaces and lamina propria (Brandborg *et al.* 1967). There is no inflammatory reaction to the parasites, which appear to be purely commensal. Mucosal changes, recorded by Hoskins *et al.* (1967), reverted to normal after treatment with mepacrine. Although there are no symptoms in the majority of infections, it is probable that when large surface areas of the upper bowel are parasitized, fat absorption is interfered with, causing steatorrhoea (Vegelhyi 1939). The gall-bladder may become infected, with obstruction of the bile passages and cholecystitis.

SYMPTOMS

The majority of cases of *Giardia* infection show no symptoms. In a minority of cases symptoms are caused which vary from a mild flatulent dyspepsia to a recurrent diarrhoea and malabsorption and steatorrhoea, which are usually associated with heavy infections. *Giardia* cysts may be found in a proportion of the normal population.

Dyspepsia

The dyspepsia associated with giardiasis resembles hepatic dysfunction with dull upper epigastric pain and flatulence. Frequently there is pain beneath the right costal margin.

Diarrhoea

The diarrhoea varies from mild with a few semi-formed stools to quite a severe watery diarrhoea which can become chronic and last for months with exacerbations and remissions.

Malabsorption and steatorrhoea

The steatorrhoea, which has been ascribed to the effect of large numbers of organisms in the small intestine and not to any pathological changes in the villi, is much less common. The stools may be typically sprue-like and associated with loss of weight and defective fat absorption, though the absorption of xylose may be reduced. The effects of malabsorption are not so apparent as in sprue and there is no anaemia. There is loss of weight but the condition resolves completely after successful treatment of the *Giardia* infection.

Unusual manifestations

Very occasionally *Giardia* invades the gall-bladder and causes cholecystitis and jaundice.

DIAGNOSIS

In cases where there is diarrhoea or malabsorption numbers of trophozoites are found in the stools. Occasionally they can be demonstrated only by duodenal intubation. *Giardia* are notoriously inconstant in their appearance and more than one stool should be examined before the infection can be excluded. Radiographic examination with barium may reveal mucosal defects in the duodenum.

TREATMENT

It is difficult to be certain of the complete extirpation of *Giardia* for they frequently reappear in numbers in the stool after an absence of several months.

Mepacrine (Atebrin): This is highly specific. 100 mg 3 times daily for 5–7 days for an adult and 100 mg twice daily for children.

Metronidazole (Flagyl): This drug has been very successful in treatment and 85% cure has been achieved (Huggins & Correia 1968) by 400 mg 3 times daily for adults and 200 mg 3 times daily for children for 5 days.

Other drugs that have been used include:

4 Aminoquinolines (Camoquin) 600 mg in a single dose for adults.

Chloroquine 300 mg daily for adults and 200 mg daily for children for 5 days.

Furazolidone (Furoxone) 100 mg 4 times a day for 5 days cured 11 of 14 cases (Chaudhuri & Chaudhuri 1965).

Relapses are common and it is often necessary to repeat the course of treatment.

Balantidiasis

Synonyms

Balantidial dysentery.

AETIOLOGY

Balantidium coli (*B. coli*) or forms morphologically indistinguishable are common parasites of many simian hosts—the rhesus monkey (*Macaca mulatta*), the orang outan, chimpanzee and New World monkeys. It also occurs in domestic pigs and rats.

It is possible that the *Balantidium* found in pigs is of a different species, *B. suis*, which is not adapted to man (Young 1950). *B. coli* is found in two forms, cysts and trophozoites (see page 984).

TRANSMISSION

B. coli cysts are relatively resistant to unfavourable environmental conditions except for direct sunlight and desiccation. The cat and monkey can be infected with human *B. coli*. Over 25% of human cases show some association with pigs but attempts to infect man with *B. coli* have been unsuccessful (Young 1950). The original infection is probably contracted from pigs and transmitted in man by oral infection with cysts from exposure to human excreta in conditions of poor environmental sanitation.

GEOGRAPHICAL DISTRIBUTION AND EPIDEMIOLOGY

Human balantidiasis is only an incidental infection in the temperate areas of the world and sporadic cases have been reported from Russia, Scandinavia, Finland, Germany, France, Austria, Holland, Italy, Spain, Siberia, China, Georgia, the Philippines, South-east Asia, the Andaman Islands, Hawaii, Mauritius, Congo, Egypt, Sudan, North America, England and Ireland. Where there are poor environmental conditions the infection may spread epidemically as in Brazil, Georgia in the U.S.S.R., and mental institutions in North America and other countries. Often there is no connection with pigs.

PATHOLOGY

In man *B. coli* is probably always a tissue invader. The cysts exist in the small intestine, and the trophozoites pass into the large intestine where they burrow into the mucosal surface and set up colonies. It is probable that lytic action helps in this process as hyaluronidase is produced by *B. coli* (Tempelis & Lysenko 1957).

Both the gross and microscopic pathology closely resemble that of amoebic infection. Ulcers are found with rounded base and wide neck and cellular infiltration round the base. Trophozoites are found in large numbers in exudates on the surface, congregated in the follicles and embedded in the tissues forming the base of the ulcers. They invade the submucosa and the muscular coat, and even enter the lumen of blood vessels and lymphatics and have been found in the mesenteric lymph glands. The early lesions appear as minute haemorrhages, then later as ulcers and abscesses. In advanced cases the colon may be a mass of ulcers throughout its length, resembling those of amoebic dysentery.

SYMPTOMS AND SIGNS

Many cases are asymptomatic; in Venezuela 80% of cases have no symptoms (Wenger 1967). Others have symptoms which are indistinguishable from those of amoebic dysentery. Diarrhoea with blood and mucus in the stool, abdominal colic and tenesmus, nausea and vomiting.

The symptoms may develop gradually or acutely. On physical examination the colon may be tender. On sigmoidoscopy the lesions resemble those of intestinal amoebiasis.

Extra-intestinal balantidiasis

Balantidia have been recorded from unusual sites. Two fatal cases of balantidial peritonitis following perforation of the colonic ulcer have been recorded (Correa Henao 1947), and balantidia have been found in the urinary tract and cases of vaginitis (Isaza Mejia 1955), and a liver abscess containing numerous trophozoites of *B. coli* was reported from Venezuela (Wenger 1967). All these cases were secondary to colonic disease.

DIAGNOSIS

Trophozoites are demonstrated in the faeces in the same way as amoebae in dysenteric stools, while cysts are found in semi-formed and formed stools.

Serodiagnosis

An immobilization test has been described to demonstrate serum antibodies in man and to identify balantidia (Zaman 1962), and a fluorescent antibody test (Zaman 1965).

TREATMENT

Most of the drugs used in the treatment of intestinal amoebiasis are effective in balantidial infection:

Metronidazole (Flagyl) 800 mg 3 times a day for 7 days.
Tetracycline 2 grammes daily for 10 days (Hoekenga 1953).
Paromomycin (Humatin) 50 to 100 mg/kg daily for 5 days (Sotolongo *et al.*
1966). Other drugs employed have been carbarsone, di-iodohydroxyquinoline (Diodoquin); they have all shown activity.

PROGNOSIS

In healthy individuals infections frequently disappear spontaneously but in
debilitated persons infection may be serious and even fatal.

PREVENTION

Preventive measures are the same as those for amoebic infection. Since
infection from pigs is common in the first case care should be taken to avoid
pigs infected with *B. coli*.

REFERENCES

BIAGI, F. F. & BUENTELLO, L. (1961) *Exp. Parasit.*, **11,** 188.
BOYD, J. S. K. (1961) *J. trop. Med. Hyg.*, **64,** 1.
BRANDBORG, L. L., TANKERSLEY, C. B., GOTTLEIB, S., BARANCIK, M. & SARTOR, V. E.
   (1967) *Gastroenterology*, **52, 143.**
Br. med. J. (1971) **iii,** 382.
CARTER, R. F. (1972) *Trans. R. Soc. trop. Med. Hyg.*, in the press.
CHAUDHURI, R. M. N. & CHAUDHURI, R. N. (1965) *Bull. Calcutta Sch. trop. Med.*, **13,**
   146.
CORREA HENAO (1947) quoted by Isaza Mejia (1955).
DOBELL, C. (1919) *The Amoebae living in Man*. London: Bale Sons and Danielsson.
——— (1923) *Official History of the War 1914–18*. London: H.M.S.O.
DOXIADES, T. (1964) *J. Am. med. Ass.*, **187,** 719.
DUMA, R. J., FERRELL, H. W., NELSON, E. C. & JONES, M. M. (1969) *New Engl. J. Med.*,
   281, 1315.
ELLMAN, B., McLEOD, I. N. & POWELL, S. J. (1965) *Br. med. J.*, **ii,** 1406.
EDITORIAL (1970) *Br. med. J.*, **ii,** 581.
——— (1970) *Lancet*, **i,** 184.
HARINASUTA, T., BUNNAG, D., JAROONVESAMA, N., CHARENLARP, K. & HARINASUTA, C.
   (1968) *Eighth International Congress on Tropical Medicine and Malaria, Teheran.*
   Abstracts and reviews 258.
HENNESSEY, E. F. & ELSDON-DEW, R. (1967) *Med. Today*, **1,** 25.
HOARE, C. A. (1957) *Trans. R. Soc. trop. Med. Hyg.*, **51,** 304.
HOEKENGA, M. T. (1953) *Am. J. trop. Med. Hyg.*, **2,** 271.
HOSKINS, L. C., WINAWER, S. J., BROITMAN, S. A., GOTTLEIB, L. S. & ZAMCHECK, N.
   (1967) *Gastroenterology*, **2,** 265.
HUGGINS, D. & CORREIA, V. (1968) *Hospital, Rio de J.*, **73,** 1833.
ISAZA MEJIA, G. (1955) *Antiquoia méd.*, **5,** 488.
JEANES, A. L. (1966) *Br. med. J.*, **ii,** 1464.
KESSEL, J. F., LEWIS, W. P., PASQUEL, C. M. & TURNER, J. A. (1965) *Am. J. trop. Med.
   Hyg.*, **14, 540.**
KHAMBATTA, R. B. (1969) *Med. Today*, **3,** 62.
LEWIS, E. A. & ANTIA, A. U. (1969) *Trans. R. Soc. trop. Med. Hyg.*, **63,** 633.
McLEOD, I. N., POWELL, S. J. & WILMOT, A. J. (1966) *Br. med. J.*, **ii,** 827.
MANSON-BAHR, P. H. (1941) *Br. med. J.*, **ii,** 255.
MIDDLEMISS, H. (1964) *Trans. R. Soc. trop. Med. Hyg.*, **58, 197.**

NEAL, R. A. (1968) *Eighth International Congress on Tropical Medicine and Malaria*, *Teheran*. Abstracts and reviews 244.
NEAL, R. A., ROBINSON, G. L., LEWIS, W. P. & KESSEL, J. F. (1968) *Trans. R. Soc. trop. Med. Hyg.*, **62,** 69.
NEUMANN, H. H. (1970) *Lancet*, **i,** 420.
NNOCHIRI, E. (1968) *Parasitic Disease and Urbanization in a Developing Country*. London: Oxford University Press.
OLATUNBOSUN, D. A. (1965) *Trans. R. Soc. trop. Med. Hyg.*, **59,** 72.
PARELKAR, S. N., STAMM, W. P. & HILL, K. R. (1971) *Br. med. J.*, **i,** 212.
POWELL, S. J. (1969) *Med. Today*, **3,** 48, 85.
—— McLEOD, I., WILMOT, A. J. & ELSDON-DEW, R. (1966) *Lancet*, **ii,** 20.
—— & WILMOT, A. J. (1966) *Trans. R. Soc. trop. Med. Hyg.*, **60,** 544.
ROBINSON, G. L. (1968) *Trans. R. Soc. trop. Med. Hyg.*, **62,** 285.
ROWLAND, H. A. K. (1967) *Med. Today*, **1,** 32.
SCHENSNOVICH, V. B. (1969) *Medskaya Parazit.*, **28,** 594.
SHEEHY, T. W., PARMLEY, L. F., JOHNSTON, G. S. & BRYCE, H. W. (1968) *Gastroenterology*, **55,** 26.
SHUMAKER, J. B., HEALY, G. R., ENGLISH, D., SCHULTZ, M. & PAGE, F. C. (1971) *Lancet*, **ii,** 602.
SOTOLONGO, F., OTERO, R. & ARGUDIN, J. (1966) *Revta cub. Med. trop.*, **18,** 103.
STAMM, W. P. (1970) *Lancet*, **ii,** 1355.
SYMMERS, W. ST. C. (1969) *Br. med. J.*, **iv,** 449.
TEMPELIS, C. H. & LYSENKO, M. G. (1957) *Exp. Parasit.*, **6,** 31.
UPTON, A. J. (1969) *Trans. R. Soc. trop. Med. Hyg.*, **63,** 542.
VEGELHYI, P. (1939) *Am. J. Dis. Children*, **57,** 894.
WALTERS, J. H. (1970) *Trans. R. Soc. trop. Med. Hyg.*, **64,** 220.
WENGER, F. (1967) *Kasmera*, **2,** 433.
WESTPHAL, A. (1937) *Arch. Schiffs- u. Tropenhyg.*, **41,** 262 (Abstract *Trop. Dis. Bull.*, **35,** 586).
WILMOT, A. J. (1962) *Clinical Amoebiasis*. Oxford: Blackwell.
—— (1967) *Med. Today*, **1,** 21.
WILMOT, A. J. (1968) *Int. Congr. trop. Med. Malar.*, 259.
WOLFENSBERGER, H. R. (1968) *Trans. R. Soc. trop. Med. Hyg.*, **62,** 831.
WOODRUFF, A. W. & BELL, S. (1967) *Trans. R. Soc. trop. Med. Hyg.*, **61,** 435.
WORLD HEALTH ORGANIZATION (1969) *Wld Hlth Org. Tech Rep. Ser.*, 421.
WRIGHT, R. (1966) *Br. med. J.*, **i,** 957.
YOUNG, M. D. (1950) *Am. J. trop. Med. Hyg.*, **30,** 71.
ZAMAN, V. (1962) *Nature, Lond.*, **194,** 404.
—— (1965) *Trans. R. Soc. trop. Med. Hyg.*, **59,** 80.

SECTION II

DISEASES CAUSED BY HELMINTHS

10. FILARIASES

Definition

A morbid condition produced by certain nematode worms (filariae). The adults of both sexes live in the lymphatics, skin, connective tissues or serous membranes, producing live embryos (microfilariae; Fig. 61) which find their way into the blood-stream, or skin, where they are capable of living, without developing further, for a period varying from less than a week in the case of *Loa loa* and *Wuchereria bancrofti* to 3 years in *Onchocerca volvulus* and *Dipetalonema perstans*.

The various filarial worms which cause filariasis in man are:

Wuchereria bancrofti (lymphatics)   *Microfilaria bancrofti* (blood, Fig. 61)
Brugia malayi (lymphatics)   *Microfilaria malayi* (blood, Fig. 61)
Onchocerca volvulus (skin)   *Microfilaria volvulus* (skin, Fig. 61)
Loa loa (connective tissues)   *Microfilaria loa* (blood, Fig. 61)
Dipetalonema perstans (serous   *Microfilaria perstans* (blood, Fig. 61)
membranes)   *Microfilaria ozzardi* (blood, Fig. 61)

I. Filariasis due to *Wuchereria bancrofti* and *Brugia malayi*

AETIOLOGY

The genus *Wuchereria* contains only one species, *W. bancrofti*, a parasite which is found only in man (Figs 62, 63). There are two biologically different forms: one periodic with nocturnal periodicity of the microfilariae, transmitted by night-biting mosquitoes, and the second subperiodic with diurnal periodicity of the microfilariae, transmitted by day-biting mosquitoes. The adult worms can survive from 10 to 18 years.

The genus *Brugia* contains 7 species: *B. malayi*, *B. pahangi*, *B. patei*, *B. beaveri*, *B. ceylonensis*, *B. guayanensis*, and *B. tupaiae*. Only *B. malayi* is known to occur as a natural infection in man, although *B. pahangi* has been transmitted experimentally to man.

TRANSMISSION

For the life cycle and development in the mosquito hosts, see Appendix II.

IMMUNITY

In a normal host there is no reaction to living worms or microfilariae. However, there is a marked immune response to both adult and larval worms

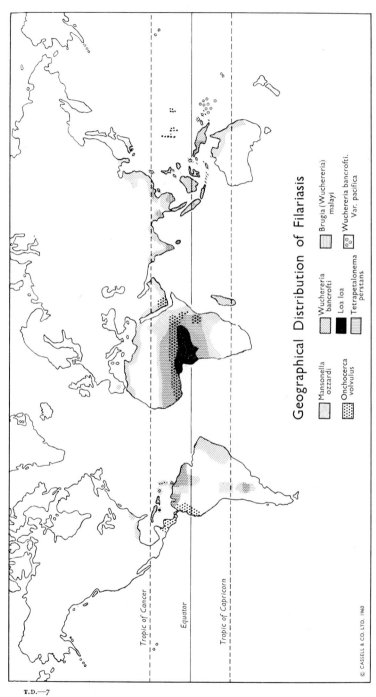

Fig. 60—Geographical distribution of filariasis.

which have been killed either naturally or by drugs. There is considerable circumstantial evidence that man develops a well marked resistance to super-infection, except in onchocerciasis. In endemic areas of *W. bancrofti*, there is an increased morbidity with age, yet many of the older people escape the serious effects of the disease.

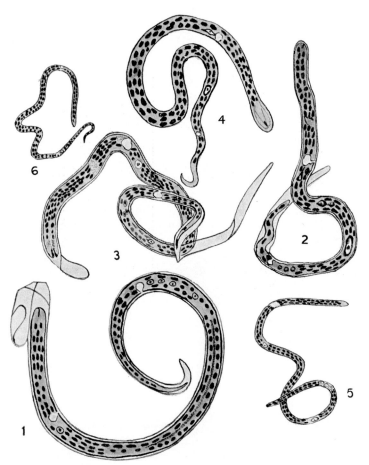

Fig. 61—Human microfilariae. 1, *Microfilaria bancrofti*, 2, *Mf. loa*. 3, *Mf. malayi*. 4, *Mf. volvulus*. 5, *Mf. perstans*. 6, *Mf. ozzardi*. (Drawn to scale)

The immune response in filariasis is both humoral and cellular, and is mainly directed against microfilariae. The humoral antibodies which are produced are complement fixing, haemagglutinating and fluorescent. In tropical eosinophilia (see page 211) there is a qualitative antibody response to microfilariae which are prevented from reaching the peripheral blood and, though there is no quantitative rise in immunoglobulins, there is invariably a high level of serum antibody. This immune response is either a genetically determined (Indian) host response to *B. malayi* or is a response to filariae of animal origin. A humoral response to dead microfilariae of immediate sensitivity type is seen in onchocerciasis following treatment with diethylcarbamazine. Humoral antibodies may result in a striking reduction of microfilariae in dogs (Wong 1964), caused by the removal of microfilariae from the blood and suppression of their formation, not by the destruction of the adult worms.

The decline in microfilaria densities in the age-group 15–20, seen in periodic *W. bancrofti* infections in man, may be due to a suppression of microfilaraemia as in dogs. A cell-mediated response of the delayed hypersensitivity type is seen in the granulomata of the lung and lymph glands in tropical eosinophilia, in

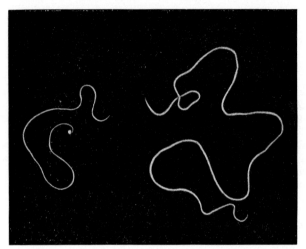

Fig. 62.—*Wuchereria bancrofti* (enlarged). Left, male; right, female.

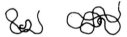

Fig. 63.—*Wuchereria bancrofti* (natural size). Left, male; right, female.

the skin in treated onchocerciasis and in the lymphatics in *W. bancrofti* infection, in which some of the reaction is directed against the dead adult worms.

Immunodiagnosis

Skin test: Intradermal reaction. This test was introduced by Fairley (1931). It is an immediate hypersensitivity reaction. The antigen is prepared from *Dirofilaria immitis* of the dog, *Dracunculus medinensis, Setaria equina* or *Setaria cervi*. WHO (1968) recommend for the skin test the antigen known as the FST Sawada, which is prepared from *D. immitis* characterized as a protein and analysed for amino acid composition. Ridley and Stott (1961) used an antigen extracted from dried *S. cervi* in saline incubated, centrifuged and sterilized by Seitz filtration in a dilution of 1/500 or 1/1000. An immediate reaction occurs, and is read after 30 minutes, when a weal of over 2 cm in diameter is regarded as positive. There is little specificity, and the skin reaction is positive in all varieties of filariasis—*W. bancrofti*, onchocerciasis and loiasis.

Cross-reactions occur with intestinal helminths and other filariae, which vitiate the use of this test both for diagnosis and in epidemiological surveys.

Complement fixation test. The complement fixation test using as antigen 1% alcoholic extract of desiccated *D. immitis* powder (Ridley 1956) and a standardized procedure, is very effective. The only form of filariasis in which positive results are obtained in a high percentage of cases (85%) is loiasis (Ridley 1956). In loiasis the test becomes positive from 1 to 3 years after infection, and remains so for 7 years, after which it reverts to negative (Kagan 1964).

Complement fixation test in filariasis (Ridley 1956)

Infection	Positive result
L. loa	85%
O. volvulus	58%
D. perstans	35%
W. bancrofti	24%

There is a considerable amount of cross-reactivity with *Ancylostoma, Schistosoma* and *Strongyloides*. In occult filariasis or tropical eosinophilia the complement fixation test is universally positive, and is a very sensitive test in the diagnosis of this condition.

Haemagglutination. The haemagglutination test for filariasis is still under development. Haemagglutinating antibodies are found in cases of filariasis when complement fixing antibodies are absent. However, 10% of patients with viral, venereal or parasitic infections gave positive results (Kagan 1964). There is cross-reactivity with trichinosis.

Fluorescent antibody test. Fluorescent antibodies develop in all forms of filariasis, but a test is not yet in general use.

EPIDEMIOLOGY

W. bancrofti

The periodic form of *W. bancrofti* with nocturnal periodicity contains two biologically different forms, one of wide tropical distribution, which is an urban strain adapted to the urban mosquitoes *Culex p. quinquefasciatus* and *C. p. atigans*. This form occurs indigenously in almost every tropical and subtropical country in a very wide but focal distribution. It has disappeared from North America and Australia and from some of the islands of the Caribbean, but is invading new areas in the growing towns of Asia and South America. The other form of *W. bancrofti* is adapted to an anopheline vector and occurs commonly in East and West Africa (*A. gambiae, A. funestus*), South East Asia, South America and New Guinea.

The diurnally subperiodic *W. bancrofti* is restricted to the South Pacific area, where it is transmitted by day-biting mosquitoes as a rural infection. In Polynesia it is transmitted by *Aedes polynesiensis, Ae. pseudoscutellaris* and *Ae. fijiensis* and in New Caledonia by *Ae. vigilax*.

B. malayi

B. malayi is predominantly an infection of rural populations, in contrast to the urban *W. bancrofti*. The periodic form has a focal distribution in Asia in rural areas of Ceylon, Thailand, Malaysia, Vietnam, China, South Korea,

Table 10. Vectors of *W. bancrofti* and *B. malayi*

	Vector	Geographical locality
Periodic *W. bancrofti*	Anophelines	
	A. bancrofti	New Guinea
	A. sinensis	Oriental
	A. whartoni	Malaya
	A. darlingi	S. America
	A. farauti	New Guinea
	A. funestus	Africa
	A. gambiae	Africa
	A. melas	West Africa
	A. koliensis	New Guinea
	A. minimus	Oriental
	Culicines	
	Mansonia uniformis	New Guinea
	Aedes kochi	New Guinea
	Ae. togoi	Oriental
	Culex annulirostris	New Guinea
	C. bitaeniorhynchus	New Guinea
	C. pipiens pallens	Oriental
	C. p. quinquefasciatus	Cosmotropical
	C. p. fatigans	Cosmotropical
Diurnally subperiodic *W. bancrofti*	Culicines	
	Aedes vigilax	New Caledonia
	Ae. fijiensis	Fiji
	Ae. polynesiensis	Polynesia
	Ae. pseudoscutellaris	Polynesia
	Culex pipiens quinquefasciatus	Polynesia
Nocturnally periodic *B. malayi*	Anophelines	
	Anopheles campestris	Malaya
	A. sinensis	China
	A. lesteri	China
	Culicines	
	Mansonia annulifera	Oriental
	M. indiana	Oriental
	M. uniformis	Oriental
Nocturnally subperiodic *B. malayi*	Culicines	
	Mansonia annulata	Malaya
	M. bonneae	Malaya
	M. dives	Malaya
	M. uniformis	Malaya

Borneo and Indonesia, and is transmitted by open swamp species of *Mansonia* (*Mansonioides*) and some anophelines. It is a parasite of man and no natural infections have been found in animals. The nocturnally subperiodic form, which is transmitted by shade swamp *Mansonia* (*Mansonioides*) and is a natural infection of a variety of animals, is a true zoonosis and is found in Malaya only along the Pahang and Perak rivers. It has, however, recently been described from Palawan Island in the Philippines (Wilson 1961).

INFECTION AND DISEASE

The infection rate, which is determined by the microfilaria rate (percentage of microfilaria carriers in the total number of people examined), and the rate of filarial disease, which is determined by the clinical signs of filariasis in the population (hydrocoele, lymphadenopathy and elephantiasis), are not identical. A high level of infection caused by a high level of endemicity is associated with a high level of clinical filariasis. *W. bancrofti* infection is prevalent in Polynesia in places where the breeding sites occur close to human habitation and there is a high output of adult mosquitoes, so that the vector density is high.

The incidence of infection is greatest in males in most countries, and it has been suggested that hormones influence the level of parasitaemia. The incidence of infection in both sexes is highest after the twentieth year and as a general rule the microfilaria rate shows a gradual but continuous rise in the 1–4 age-group and is at a peak in the 15–20 age-group. The subsequent rise is not proportionate to the increase in age. Signs of filarial disease become apparent in the 20–29 age-group. In *B. malayi* infection, owing to the shorter period of maturation of the adult worm, microfilariae have been found in a child aged $3\frac{1}{2}$ months and high microfilaria rates occur in children below the age of 5 years and a rate of 40–60% can be found in adult life.

The reasons for the variation in the incidence of filarial infection and disease around the world are not clearly understood but are dependent upon varying host–parasite relationships.

In *W. bancrofti* in East Africa there is a high proportion of hydrocoeles but elephantiasis of the legs and scrotum is less common. In West Africa elephantiasis is rare, and hydrocoele is not common, although microfilaria rates of 40–50% are recorded. In India the predominant lesion is elephantiasis of the lower limbs; hydrocoele is less common and chyluria very rare. In China the main lesions are hydrocoele, chyluria and elephantiasis of the legs and scrotum. In the Pacific chyluria is rare, but hydrocoele is not uncommon; elephantiasis is gross and enlarged lymph glands are common.

In *B. malayi* the two forms do not vary in their clinical effects but urogenital and chylous manifestations are rare. These variations in disease pattern may be due to differences in worm loads and variation in the portal of entry of the infection at the site of the infective mosquito bite.

The natural infection rates of mosquito intermediaries vary very considerably and do not form a true index of the risks of contracting filariasis in endemic areas. In Malaysia it is recognized that the majority of larval filariae in wild caught *Mansonia* (*Mansonioides*) are of avian or mammalian origin. In the Pacific high natural infection rates have been recorded: in the Cook Islands 13·5% (Iyengar 1965), in Tahiti 50%, while in Fiji the natural rate of infection in *Ae. fijiensis* is as high as 21·6%. It is quite probable that the majority of these infections are derived from avian blood for these mosquitoes feed mostly on birds. The third-stage infective larval forms can be distinguished by length, breadth, position of the anus and shape of the caudal extremity and can be used to separate *Wuchereria* and *Brugia* from almost all the animal forms that have been described. It is not possible to separate the different species of *Brugia* from one another except by injecting them into susceptible animals and waiting for their full development.

PATHOLOGY

In most cases of filarial infection the parasite does not exercise any manifest injurious influence on the host and in endemic areas of filariasis there are many people with microfilaraemia who show no clinical or pathological signs of filarial infection. In a proportion of cases there can be no doubt that damage is done mainly by the obstruction of the lymphatics by inflammation. Healthy, fully formed microfilariae are usually harmless, except in the case of occult filariasis or tropical pulmonary eosinophilia. Epidemiological surveys of different areas of human filariasis have shown that the prevalence of clinical lesions is usually correlated with the microfilaria rate and density, especially the latter.

The pathological changes produced by *W. bancrofti* and *B. malayi* are related to the three developmental stages of the parasite in the final host: developing larvae showing two moults, adult worms and, in the case of tropical eosinophilia, microfilariae.

The histological features of occult filariasis are characteristic in the lymph glands (Bras & Lie 1951), in the lung (Danaraj 1959) and in the liver (Webb *et al.* 1960). The enlarged lymph glands show a pronounced hyperplasia of the lymph follicles and reticular cells. Many yellowish grey nodules varying from 1 to 2 mm in diameter are scattered throughout the gland tissue and consist of large aggregations of eosinophils in the centre of which microfilariae or remnants may be found surrounded by hyaline material known as Meyers–Kouwenaar bodies. Epithelioid granulomas with foreign body giant cells are occasionally seen. When the spleen, lung and liver are affected they contain somewhat larger yellowish grey nodules, up to 5 mm diameter, and microfilariae are more numerous in the spleen than in the lymph glands. The nodules in the lung and liver may be few or many. Most lesions consist of epithelioid granulomas with foreign body giant cells and varying numbers of eosinophils, microfilariae and Meyer–Kouwenaar bodies.

The pathology caused by *W. bancrofti* and *B. malayi* is basically the same, although the two infections differ somewhat clinically. Developing larvae and adult worms bring about changes in the lymphatic system accompanied by acute inflammation that spreads into the adjacent tissues and causes the classical lesions of filariasis—lymphangitis, lymphadenitis, lymph varix, genital lesions, lymphoedema and ultimately elephantiasis. Lesions caused by microfilariae are less common and are not confined to the lymphatic system, but are also found in the lungs, liver and spleen. They are often associated with hypereosinophilia and lung symptoms, and this condition is known in the literature as tropical pulmonary eosinophilia, eosinophilic lung or occult or cryptic filariasis.

In classical filariasis, microfilariae are usually found in the peripheral blood whereas in occult filariasis they are absent from the blood although they are continuously being produced by the adult worms.

Classical filariasis

The early stages of filarial infection have been studied in U.S. soldiers in the Pacific (Wartman 1947) and in human volunteers infected with *B. malayi* and *B. pahangi* (Edeson *et al.* 1960), and in cats and dogs infected with third-stage larvae of *B. pahangi* (Schacher & Sahyoun 1967).

Acute inflammatory changes develop primarily in the lymphatics and lymph nodes as a result of moulting of the larvae, as a reaction to both live and dead larvae. The moulting fluid induces a severe reaction with lymphadenitis, perilymphadenitis and lymphangitis. There is an infiltration of polymorphonuclears, histiocytes and many eosinophils with a few lymphocytes. This exudative inflammatory reaction, which is soon replaced by epithelioid granulomas with foreign body giant cells surrounding the sheath of the worms, is the major cause of the rapid tissue swelling during an acute filarial attack.

Lymphatic varix

Dead adult worms are the cause of fibrous obliteration of the lymph vessels (O'Connor 1932) with the establishment of lymphatic varices of different kinds and situations. Adult worms may be found in lymphoedematous tissues especially in the breast and in the enlarged lymph glands. When the thoracic duct is obstructed the chyle poured into the vessel can reach the circulation only by a retrograde movement via the abdominal and pelvic lymphatics and the lymphatics of the groin, scrotum and abdominal wall. As a consequence these vessels

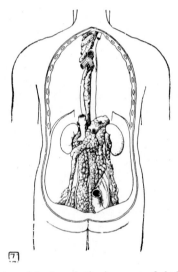

Fig. 64.—Dissection of the lymphatics in a case of chyluria, showing the dilated right and left renal lymphatics and the thoracic duct. (*Transactions of the Pathological Society of London*)

together with the thoracic duct up to the seat of obstruction become enormously dilated and when one of the vessels of the varix is pricked or ruptures the contents are found to be white or pinkish chyle (Fig. 64). When the varix involves the scrotum the result is lymph scrotum (Fig. 65), when the groin, 'varicose groin glands'. When the lymphatics of the bladder or kidneys are affected and ruptured then chyluria is the result. When those of the tunica vaginalis rupture then there is chylous dropsy of that sac, 'chylocoele'; when rupture is into the peritoneum there is chylous ascites. Occasionally varicose lymphatic glands resembling those in the groin are found in the axilla.

Filarial lymphoedema and elephantiasis

Since there are no microfilariae in most cases of lymphoedema and elephantiasis it has been suggested that there is no connection between filariasis and these conditions. However, there are strong reasons for regarding elephantiasis as a filarial disease:

(a) The geographical distributions of *W. bancrofti* and of elephantiasis correspond.

(b) Filarial lymphatic varix and elephantiasis occur in the same districts and frequently in the same individual.

(c) Lymph scrotum, unquestionably a filarial disease, terminates in elephantiasis of the scrotum.

(d) Filarial lymphatic varix and elephantiasis are both accompanied by the same type of recurring lymphangitis.

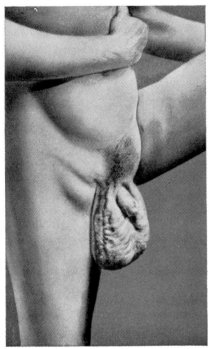

Fig. 65.—Lymph scrotum and varicose groin glands. (*Dr Rennie*)

Elephantiasis is only found in long-standing infections and takes about 20 years to develop.

The dilatation of the lymph trunks is due to failure of the valves and to blockage of the lymphatic trunks—a local reaction to the presence of adult worms (Cohen *et al.* 1961). The dilatation also destroys the valvular function, resulting in back-flow stagnation of the lymph and then lymphoedema. The size of the worm load is important and the incidence of lymphoedema increases with the increase in transmission of *W. bancrofti*. Total destruction of the lymphatics is necessary for the production of elephantiasis. The lymphatics become obstructed with dead worms undergoing disintegration, together with a reaction in the walls, blocking the lumen of the vessel (Fig. 67), and also by proliferation of the endothelium—obliterative endolymphangitis (Fig. 68)—which is due to the action of dead microfilariae which become imprisoned in the endothelial lining of the vessel. Sometimes the adult worms become calcified (Fig. 69). As a result of both stagnation of lymph and blocking of the lymphatics there is transudation into the tissues of lymph rich in protein (lymphoedema), which causes a cellular proliferation of the connective tissues and the production of elephantiasis.

Bacterial infection

Total destruction of the lymphatics may be achieved by dead worms combined with bacterial superinfection to which the lymph-soaked tissues are susceptible.

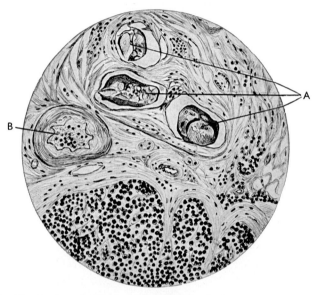

Fig. 66.—Section of a fibrosed lymphatic gland. A, Portion of a calcified *Wuchereria bancrofti* var. *pacifica*. B, Partially occluded lymphatic vessel. (*P. H. Manson-Bahr*)

This may occur in endemic areas where continuous reinfection, both bacterial and filarial, occurs. Healthy, fully formed microfilariae are harmless, but under certain conditions they may produce pathological effects (occult filariasis).

Occult filariasis (Lie Kian Joe 1962) (tropical eosinophilia; Meyers-Kouwenaar syndrome; filariasis without microfilaraemia (Beaver 1970))

Occult filariasis was first described by Meyers and Kouwenaar (1939) in Indonesia. Later Frimodt-Möller and Barton (1940) and Weingarten (1943) described tropical eosinophilia from India. The main features of this syndrome, which has now been reported from most of South-east Asia, Brazil and Africa wherever filarial infection occurs, are hypereosinophilia, lymph gland enlargement, pulmonary symptoms and the absence of microfilariae from the blood. The syndrome is the result of an unusual immune response, in which the microfilariae are destroyed in the tissues without reaching the peripheral blood.

The species of the filarial worm responsible has been the subject for discussion. The microfilariae found in South-east Asia were of the *B. malayi* type; those in India and Curaçao were similar to the *W. bancrofti* type. Other observers assume that filariae of animal origin are responsible (Danaraj *et al.* 1966).

Traditional cases of occult filariasis may show manifestations of classical filariasis, such as lymphangitis and hydrocoele (Friess *et al.* 1953). Experiments (Buckley & Wharton 1960) indicate that both human and animal parasites may induce occult filariasis, when a volunteer developed hypereosinophilia and asthma without microfilaraemia after infection with *B. pahangi* from cats, *B. malayi* from monkeys and *B. malayi* from man. The cause of occult filariasis is

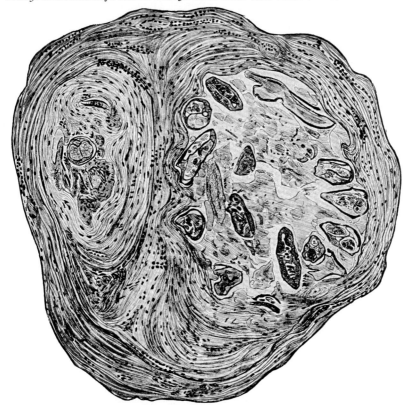

Fig. 67.—Section of a thickened brachial lymphatic, containing portions of dead filariae undergoing disintegration and blocking the lumen of the vessel. Note the large amount of fibrosis. (*P. H. Manson-Bahr*)

hypersensitivity to a specific filarial antigen no matter whether the parasite is of human or animal origin and the allergic reaction is directed towards the micro-filariae and not towards the developing larvae or dead worms. This altered immune response may have a genetic origin since the majority of cases of occult filariasis are found in persons of Indian origin (Symposium on Tropical Eosinophilia 1960).

SYMPTOMS AND SIGNS

The diseases known to be produced by association with *W. bancrofti* and *B. malayi* are abscess, lymphangitis, arthritis, synovitis, varicose groin glands,

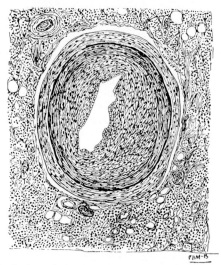

Fig. 68.—Occlusion of the lymphatic vessels by proliferation of the endothelium in filariasis (obliterative endolymphangitis).

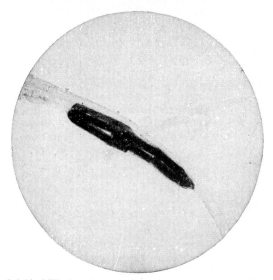

Fig. 69.—Calcified *Wuchereria bancrofti* var. *pacifica* lying in and blocking a lymphatic vessel.

varicose axillary glands, lymph scrotum, cutaneous and deep lymphatic varix, orchitis, funiculitis, hydrocoele, chyluria and elephantiasis of the leg, scrotum, vulva, arm, mamma and other parts. Chylocoele, chylous ascites, chylous diarrhoea and probably other forms of disease are caused by obstruction or varicosity of the abdominal lymphatics, and the death or injury of the parent filariae can cause a lymphatic abscess and fatal peritonitis or secondary infections by pyogenic organisms (filarial abdomen).

Abscess

Occasionally the parent filaria dies as a result of lymphangitis. The dead body is absorbed or becomes calcified. Sometimes it causes a sterile abscess in the contents of which fragments of filariae may be found. Such abscesses occurring in the limbs or scrotum will discharge in due course or may be opened. If properly treated surgically they may lead to no further trouble. Should they form in the thorax or abdomen serious consequences and even death may ensue.

Filarial fever, lymphangitis, elephantoid fever

Lymphangitis is common in all forms of filarial disease, especially in elephantiasis, varicose groin glands and lymph scrotum, and is due to secretions of the

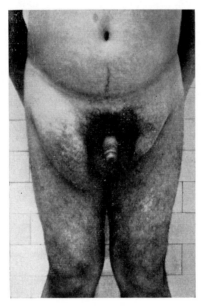

Fig. 70.—Bilateral varicose groin glands with lymph stasis and slight elephantiasis of the right leg. (*Dr F. W. O'Connor, Puerto Rico*)

worm or possible hypersensitivity (see Pathology). In the limbs it is retrograde and centrifugal, i.e., it starts near the lymph glands and spreads peripherally. There is a characteristic painful cord-like swelling of the lymphatic trunks and associated glands and the red congested streak in the superadjacent skin is usually apparent at the commencement of an attack. The limb or part of the limb affected becomes swollen during the attack, which may continue for several days and be accompanied by severe headaches, anorexia, vomiting and sometimes delirium. After a time tension of the inflamed area may relieve itself by lymphous discharge from the surface. The attack is usually accompanied by filarial fever. Lymphangitis may be confined to the groin glands, testis, spermatic cord (endemic funiculitis) or abdominal lymphatics. When it affects an extensive abdominal varix, symptoms of peritonitis rapidly develop and may prove fatal (abdominal filariasis).

Filarial fever is usually accompanied by lymphangitis, but in the Pacific Islands there is a form unassociated with obvious lymphangitis. This probably represents inflammation of deep-seated lumbar lymphatics or glands. Hetrazan treatment often provokes one of these attacks. Filarial fever occurring in association with elephantiasis is usually termed 'elephantoid fever'. In Barbados, where there is no malaria, it is called 'ague'; in Samoa it is known as 'mumu fever' and in Fiji as 'wanganga'. The fever, which tends to recur and is accompanied by rigors and sweating, may come on sometimes as late as 20 years after leaving the endemic area and recur for many years afterwards.

Varicose groin glands

Varicose groin glands (Fig. 70) are frequently associated with lymph scrotum, with chylocoele or with chyluria. Occasionally all four conditions may coexist in the same individual. As a rule the patient is not aware of the existence of varicose groin glands until they have attained considerable dimensions. Then a sense of tension or an attack of lymphangitis calls attention to the state of the groins where certain soft swelling are discovered. These swellings may be of insignificant dimensions or they may attain the size of a fist. They may involve both or only one groin. They may affect the inguinal glands or the femoral glands alone or more usually both sets.

Thickened lymphatic trunks

After the initial swelling and inflammation of lymphangitis have subsided a line of induration remains. On excising thickened tissue and carefully dissecting it minute cyst-like dilatations of the lymphatics have been found containing adult filariae alive or dead.

Filarial glandular enlargement

In the Pacific Islands great enlargement of the lymphatic glands with fibrotic changes is by far the most frequent symptom of filarial disease. The epitrochlear gland is often affected in Fiji. The groin glands are often very much enlarged, sometimes 5 or 7·5 cm in diameter, and may form permanent tumours in the groin. On section they resemble an unripe pear, the central portion being fibrotic and the peripheral glandular. The deep-seated glands—iliac, lumbar, mesenteric and mediastinal—may also be enlarged.

Lymph scrotum (Fig. 65, page 201)

In this condition the scrotum is enlarged. Though usually silky to the touch, on inspection the skin presents a few or a large number of smaller or larger lymphatic varices which, when pricked or on spontaneous rupture, discharge large quantities of milky or sanguineous-looking or straw-coloured, rapidly coagulating lymph or chyle. In some cases 225–280 ml of this substance will escape from a puncture in the course of an hour or so, in others it may go on running for many hours on end, soiling the clothes and exhausting the patient. Usually microfilariae can be discovered in the lymph so obtained or in the blood. In a large proportion of cases of lymph scrotum the inguinal and femoral glands either on one or both sides are varicose.

Chyluria and lymphuria

When a varix ruptures in the wall of the bladder or elsewhere in the urinary tract the contents of the lymphatics escape into the urine. If, as often happens, the urine contains blood the condition is known as haematochyluria. It frequently appears without warning; usually, however, pain in the back and aching sensations about the pelvis and groins, probably caused by distension of the pre-existing varix, precede it. Retention of urine from the presence of chylous or lymphous coagula is sometimes the first indication of trouble. Whether preceded by aching, by retention or by other symptoms the patient becomes suddenly aware that he is passing milky urine which may be pinkish or even red; sometimes it is white in the morning and reddish in the evening, or vice versa. Sometimes while chylous at one part of the day it is perfectly limpid at another. Chyluria is very likely to occur either for the first time or as a relapse in pregnancy or after childbirth. The presence of blood is probably caused by the rupture of small blood vessels into the dilated lymphatics; in these cases the microfilariae appear in the urine passed during the night time only.

Physical characteristics of chylous urine. Chylous urine is milky in appearance owing to suspended fat particles. If it is passed into a glass and allowed to stand it will coagulate and separate after a period of hours into 3 layers. At the top is a cream-like pellicle, at the bottom scanty reddish sediment and in the middle a mass of milky or reddish-white urine. Microscopically the deposit contains red blood cells, lymphocytes, granular fatty matter, epithelium and urinary crystals and in some cases microfilariae. If ether or xylol is shaken up with chylous urine the fatty particles dissolve and the urine becomes relatively clear. On evaporation of the ether the fat may be recovered. A considerable amount of fat is lost in the urine which may amount to 15% of the lymphatic drainage of the gut. This will have the same effect as malabsorption on the body. There is some proteinuria. In the condition known as lymphuria fatty elements are absent and the chief cellular constituent is the lymphocyte.

Chylocoele, chylous ascites, chylous diarrhoea

Chylocoele is not unusual in the tropics. A fluctuating swelling of the tunica vaginalis, which does not transmit light and which is associated with lymph scrotum or with varicose groin glands, chyluria or microfilaraemia, would suggest chylocoele. Steatorrhoea may occur owing to involvement of the mesenteric lymph glands, and may proceed to chylous diarrhoea.

Filarial orchitis, endemic funiculitis, hydrocoele

The fever attending filarial orchitis, which is usually associated with lymphangitis of the spermatic cord, has been described as 'endemic funiculitis' but is undoubtedly of filarial origin. It may be attended by inflammation of the scrotum and like filarial or elephantoid fever may closely resemble a malarial attack. The fluid aspirated from the tunica vaginalis is cloudy and contains a number of polymorphonuclear cells and occasionally red cells with microfilariae. The epididymis is enlarged and nodular. In sections dead and calcified filariae blocking the vasa efferentia cause extensive fibrotic changes and it is possible that sterility may be a direct result of this infection.

Recurrent attacks of filarial orchitis lead sooner or later to hydrocoele. This condition in some endemic areas very commonly accompanies elephantiasis of the scrotum, and is used as one of the indicators of filarial disease amongst populations. The walls of the sac are thickened and contain calcified remnants of adult filariae. The hydrocoele fluid is clear straw-coloured and may contain microfilariae, though not always, since this is not a medium particularly favourable to them. Filarial infiltrations of the cords vary in size, form and number. There may be one small single nodule or a number strung to thickened lymphatic vessels. Sometimes lymphatic obstruction affects the vessels so as to cause lymphangiectasis and lymphatic varicocoeles. It may, however, cause cystic dilatation or 'lymphocoele'. The spermatic veins are often the seat of chronic thrombophlebitis.

Filarial synovitis

Acute synovitis of the knee-joint is one of the filarial diseases, and its occurrence with filarial infection is too common to be accidental. Fibrotic ankylosis often results. In severe cases synovitis may proceed to pus formation.

Elephantiasis

In many tropical and subtropical countries elephantiasis is prevalent but especially so in the Pacific where, in Samoa and Tahiti, every second individual is affected by this disease. The relationship to filariasis is discussed on page 198 and the pathology considered on page 199.

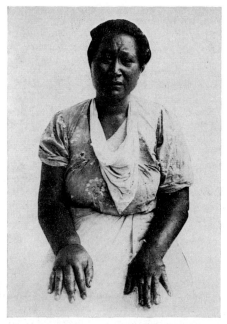

Fig. 71.—Lymphangitis of the right arm and hand of a Samoan (*Professor P.A. Buxton*)

Parts affected. In 95% of the cases the lower extremities, either one or both, alone or in combination with the scrotum or arms, are the seat of the disease. The foot and ankle only, or the foot and leg or foot, leg and thigh may each or all be involved. The arms are more rarely attacked though in the Western Pacific this is comparatively common (Fig. 71). Still more rarely involved are the mammae, vulva and circumscribed portions of the integuments of the limbs or trunk (Fig. 72).

In any of these situations the disease commences with lymphangitis, dermatitis and cellulitis accompanied by elephantoid fever. The lymphatic glands draining the affected area are generally enlarged. There is no distinct line of

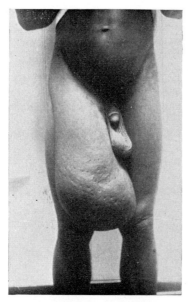

Fig. 72.—Localized elephantoid tumour of the groin in a Fijian. (*Dr R. Stuppel*)

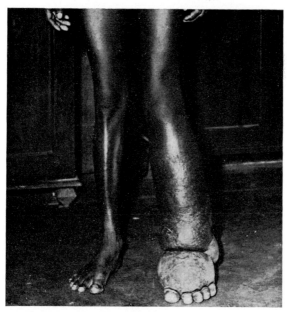

Fig. 73.—Filariasis of the leg caused by *Wuchereria bancrofti*. (*Dr C. J. Hackett*)

demarcation between healthy and diseased skin. The skin and underlying tissue is hard and dense but pits only slightly if at all and cannot be pinched up or freely glided over the deeper parts. The subjacent connective tissue is increased in bulk, having a yellowish blubbery appearance from lymphous infiltration, especially in the scrotum. A large quantity of fluid with a high protein content wells out on division of the tissues.

Elephantiasis of the legs (Fig. 73). This is usually, though by no means always, confined to below the knee. The swelling may attain enormous dimensions and involve the whole extremity, the leg attaining a circumference of several feet in aggravated cases.

Elephantiasis of the scrotum (Fig. 74). Elephantiasis of the scrotum, or scrotal tumour as it is sometimes called, may attain an enormous size; 4, 6, 8 or 9 kg are common weights for this tumour. The largest recorded weighed 102 kg.

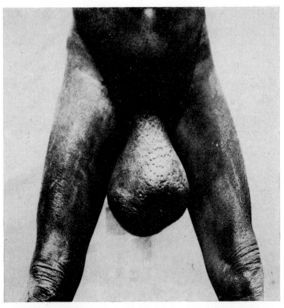

Fig. 74.—Elephantiasis of the scrotum caused by *Wuchereria bancrofti*. (*Dr J. Denfield, Nigeria*)

Anatomical characters. These tumours consist of two portions (Fig. 75): first, a dense rind of hypertrophied skin with wart-like thickenings (A, *e*), thickest towards the lower part and gradually thinning out as it merges above into the sound skin of the pubes, perineum and thighs; secondly, enclosed in this rind, a mass of lax, blubbery, dropsical, areolar tissue in which testes, cords and penis are embedded. The shape of the tumour is more or less pyriform. The upper part, or neck, on transverse section (B) is triangular, the base (B, *k*) of the triangle being in front, the apex (B, *j*) —usually somewhat bifid from dragging on the gluteal folds—towards the anus, the sides (B, *h*) towards the thighs. In the latter situation the skin, though usually more or less diseased, is, from pressure, softer and thinner than elsewhere, tempting the surgeon to utilize it for the formation of flaps—not always a wise proceeding. The penis (A, *a*; B, *f*) always lies in the upper and fore part of the neck of the mass; it is firmly attached to the pubes by the suspensory ligament. The sheath of the penis is sometimes especially hypertrophied, in some cases standing out as a projection rather like a twisted ram's horn on the anterior surface of the tumour; this, however, is unusual. Generally the sheath of the penis is incorporated in the scrotal mass, the prepuce being dragged on and inverted so as to form a long channel leading to the glans penis and opening (A, *l*) half-way down, or even lower, on the face of the tumour. The testes (A, *c*), buried in the central blubbery tissue, usually lie towards the back of the tumour, one on each side—in large tumours generally nearer the lower than the upper part. They are more or less firmly attached to the underpart of the scrotum by the hypertrophied remains of the gubernaculum testis (A, *d*)—a feature to be specially borne in mind by the surgeon. As a rule,

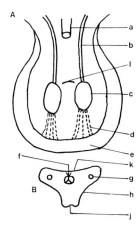

Fig. 75.—Diagram of the anatomy in elephantiasis of the scrotum. See text for details.

both testes carry large hydrocoeles with thickened tunicae vaginales. The spermatic cords also (A, *b*; B, *g*) are thickened and greatly elongated. In spite of the grave alterations in the tissues the functions of the testes remain unimpaired.

Operation. For details of operative procedures, a textbook of surgery should be consulted.

Occult filariasis, tropical esosinophilia

There is a seasonal incidence. About 90% of cases are found in people of Indian origin. Males are affected more than females and the maximum age incidence is from 20–30 years.

The symptoms are cough, lassitude, dyspnoea on exertion and asthmatic attacks especially at night occasionally with haemoptysis. There is often fever and splenomegaly. In advanced cases the condition may closely resemble chronic pulmonary tuberculosis. The most striking feature is massive eosinophilia (hypereosinophilia) which may rise as high as 60% of 60 000 white cells/mm³, which is higher than in any condition except eosinophilic leukaemia. A chest radiograph shows disseminated mottling in the lung, the average single focus being the size of a split pea. One form presents as generalized lymphadenopathy.

The differential diagnosis has to be made from spasmodic bronchial asthma, pulmonary tuberculosis, miliary tuberculosis, allergic disease of the lungs from inhaled dust, pulmonary aspergillosis, eosinophilic leukaemia and other helminthic infections, especially the tissue stages of *Ascaris, Ancylostoma, Strongyloides, Schistosoma mansoni* and *S. japonicum* infections. In all these helminthic diseases, where the parasite is in its natural host, the lung changes are of short duration and the eosinophilia does not persist for a long time. In tropical eosinophilia the eosinophilia persists for as long as the infection. Distinction has to be made from visceral larva migrans (VLM) due to toxocariasis with which it is often confused. The differentiation may be very difficult, but VLM is found mainly in children and is also sometimes associated with *Ascaris* and *Trichuris* infection. The diagnosis of tropical eosinophilia is made from the universal positive serology (see Immunodiagnosis) and the response to diethylcarbamazine therapy.

DIFFERENTIAL DIAGNOSIS

Lymphangitis and filarial fever have to be differentiated from acute bacterial lymphangitis which spreads centripetally from the periphery towards the lymph glands and from other causes of recurrent fever with rigors, septicaemia, malaria, relapsing fever, relapsing typhoid, tuberculosis, pyelonephritis, liver abscess and gall-stones.

Varicose groin glands should be distinguished from hernia, for which they are often mistaken. This can be done by observing that they are not tympanitic on percussion; that though pressure causes them to diminish they do so slowly and without the sudden dispersion accompanied by gurgling as in hernia; that they convey a relatively slight or no impulse on coughing; and that they subside slowly when the patient lies down and return slowly when the erect posture is resumed. The diagnosis is further strengthened by the coexistence of lymph scrotum, chyluria or chylous hydrocoele, or by the presence of microfilariae in the blood. They also have to be differentiated from 'hanging groins' of onchocerciasis, which are folds of atrophic skin and which are invariably associated with advanced chronic onchodermatitis elsewhere.

Filarial glandular enlargement has to be distinguished from other causes of lymphatic glandular enlargement, especially in the inguinal region: chronic infection of the feet (the inguinal glands are usually enlarged in people who wear no shoes), tuberculous adenitis, lymphogranuloma inguinale, reticuloses, lymphoma and leukaemia.

Filarial orchitis, endemic funiculitis and hydrocoele have to be distinguished from encysted hydrocoele, lipoma, spermatocoele, gonococcal epididymitis, tuberculous epididymitis, *Schistosoma haematobium* infection of the cord, strangulated hernia and suppuration of the spermatic cord. Non-filarial epidemic funiculitis has been described from Ceylon (Power 1946). It is difficult to distinguish filarial from non-filarial hydrocoele in the absence of other evidence of filarial infection, but in endemic areas of filariasis hydrocoele is accepted as an indicator of filarial disease.

Chyluria must be distinguished from other causes of lymphatic obstruction in the abdomen, especially tuberculosis.

Elephantiasis. Since microfilaraemia is usually absent in filarial lymphoedema and elephantiasis, it is difficult to prove the filarial origin of most cases of elephantiasis other than that they occur in a known area of filarial infection. Onchocerciasis and loiasis are responsible for some cases. Other causes of chronic lymphoedema and elephantiasis are familial lymphoedema or Milroy's disease, and lymphostatic verrucosis, which occurs in the higher regions of the tropics outside the endemic filarial areas. Both these conditions may be distinguished by lymphography, when absent or atrophic lymph channels may be demonstrated in contrast to the dilated channels of filariasis in which the valves are deranged and there is backflow. Other causes of elephantiasis are chronic bacterial lymphangitis (elephantiasis nostras), secondary carcinoma and surgical ablation, especially in the upper limbs.

DIAGNOSIS

Microfilariae are absent from the blood of many forms of filariasis. They are found only in the early cases of filarial disease. The absence of microfilariae in the blood does not exclude filarial disease, nor does their presence in an endemic area denote filarial disease. The presence of microfilaraemia merely denotes a microfilaria carrier.

Microfilariae in blood

In the periodic form microfilariae may be demonstrated in night blood taken at 22.00 hours; in the subperiodic forms they can be found in day blood. 30 mm^3 of blood are taken preferably from the ear lobe where the microfilariae are most numerous and prepared as a thick drop or spread as 3 parallel lines on a slide, dehaemoglobinized and stained with Giemsa or Field's stain.

Direct examination and counting of microfilariae in the blood. Microfilariae in the blood may be counted by placing multiples of 25 mm^3 of fresh capillary blood, drawn up by a capillary tube or disposable blood diluting pipette such as is used for counting white cells, in 0.5 ml of 3% acetic acid in a Sedgwick Rafter counting cell. The red cells are all destroyed and the microfilariae are fixed so that they can be seen and counted clearly under low power or the 35 magnification field of a dissecting microscope (Denham *et al.* 1971).

Diethylcarbamazine provocative test. Nocturnally periodic microfilariae may be demonstrated in the blood at any time of the day by giving 100 mg diethyl-carbamazine and taking blood 45 minutes later. Concentration methods of examining blood are very suitable for this test, which enables blood surveys to be carried out during daylight hours.

Concentration methods. Knott's method of concentrating the micro-filariae is most useful in scanty infection and for conducting filarial surveys. This consists of taking 1 ml of blood and diluting it in 9 ml of distilled water and 1 ml of 40% commercial formalin. The suspension is shaken up to haemolyse the red cells and centrifuged; the microfilariae will all be found in the deposit.

Filtration technique. Large amounts of blood may be filtered by injecting up to 10 ml of heparinized blood from a syringe through a Millipore filter Swinnex-25, containing a Nucleopore membrane filter, 5 μm in size (25 mm in diameter). The filter may be examined fresh, or stained directly in the usual way, for microfilariae.

The phytohaemagglutinin method may also be used as in trypanosomiasis (page 114).

Eosinophilia is of little use in the diagnosis of filariasis due to *W. bancrofti* and *B. malayi*, unlike most other forms of filariasis. It is present only in the early stages but is invariable and intense in that form of filariasis known as tropical eosinophilia.

Immunodiagnosis

The complement fixation test is positive in only about 94% of cases of early filariasis but is frequently negative in the later stages such as elephantiasis.

TREATMENT

The treatment of filariasis consists of chemotherapy against the adult filariae (macrofilaricidal) and microfilariae (microfilaricidal), and symptomatic treatment to contain the damage caused by the reaction of the body to the presence of adult worms.

Chemotherapy

Macrofilaricidal drugs. Since filarial disease is due mostly to the reaction of the tissues against dead, developing and adult filariae, macrofilaricidal drugs are not of much use in treatment. The death of the adult worms is shown by the disappearance of microfilariae from the blood after a period of up to 18 months. However, there is some evidence that destruction of the adult worm is accompanied by a decrease in the recurrence of lymphangitis and filarial fever.

Antimony: TWSb (Astiban) has been used in a dosage as used in schistosomiasis.

Suramin (Antrypol) may be given as 1 gramme weekly intravenously for 7 weeks.

Arsenic: Mel W has been used by Friedheim and De Jongh (1959) in doses of 100 mg intramuscularly each day for 4 days or 200 mg daily for 3 days in the form of a 5% solution (= 50 mg/ml). It has also been used in a single dose for mass chemotherapy but deaths have been recorded after its use.

Microfilaricidal drugs. Microfilaricidal drugs are used for mass chemotherapy in the control and eradication of filariasis to remove the human reservoir of infection. They are specific in the only form of filarial disease caused by microfilariae, tropical eosinophilia.

Diethylcarbamazine citrate (Hetrazan, Banocide, Notézine). This drug exerts no direct lethal action on the microfilariae, but modifies them so that they are engulfed by phagocytes of the endothelial system and thereby removed from circulation. In shut-off cavities such as hydrocoeles the microfilariae are not affected. The dose is 6 mg/kg body weight daily in 3 divided doses after meals for 2–3 weeks. Thus a patient of 70 kg should receive 450 mg daily in 3 divided doses each of 150 mg. Some workers give 600 mg daily. The microfilariae rapidly disappear from the blood but reappear after 6 months since the adult worms are not affected. Repeated courses may, however, kill some adults. *B. malayi* is more susceptible to treatment with diethylcarbamazine than *W. bancrofti*, but febrile reactions are frequent in microfilaria carriers.

Symptomatic treatment

Recurrent lymphangitis and filarial fever. Treatment should consist in removing any cause of irritation, rest, elevation of the affected part, cooling lotions, opium or morphine to relieve pain and, if tension is great, pricking or scarifying the swollen area under suitable aseptic conditions. Subsequently the parts if their position permits should be elevated and firmly bandaged.

Macrofilaricidal drugs in association with anti-inflammatory agents such as steroids have been reported to reduce the incidence of further attacks (Thooris 1956), and where filarial control measures are applied as in Tahiti, these early manifestations of filarial disease rapidly disappear from the population.

Lymph scrotum. Unless inflammation is frequent or there is frequent and debilitating lymphorrhagia, or unless the disease passes into true elephantiasis, the lymph scrotum, kept scrupulously clean, powdered with boric acid and protected, had better be left alone. Should it be deemed expedient, however, to remove the diseased tissues, this can easily be done. The scrotum should be well dragged down by an assistant while the testes are pushed up out of the way of injury. A finger knife is then passed through the scrotum and in sound tissues just clear of the testes the mass is excised by cutting backwards and forwards. No diseased tissues and hardly any flap should be left. Sufficient cover for the testes can be obtained by dragging on and if necessary dissecting up the skin of the thighs which readily yields and affords ample covering. It is a very common but a great mistake to remove too little. As a rule the wound if carefully stitched and dressed antiseptically heals rapidly.

Chyluria. Treatment should be conducted on the same lines as that of inaccessible varix elsewhere, by resting and elevating the affected part and thereby diminishing as far as possible the hydrostatic pressure in the distended vessels. The best results are obtained by putting the patient to bed on an inclined

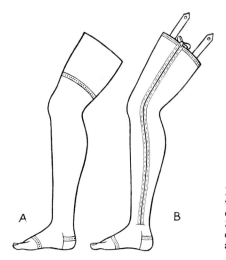

Fig. 76.—A, Plain elastic web stocking with foot piece, for slight degrees of elephantiasis of leg (James Woolley & Sons, Manchester). B, Laced form of elastic stocking with suspenders, adjustable so as to avoid pinching.

plane with feet elevated, by restricting the amount of food and fluid and by gentle purgation and absolute rest. Washing out the bladder with some bland substance such as boric acid appears to be the best form of treatment. Hetrazan may be given in the usual dosage.

Chylocoele, hydrocoele. Chylocoeles and hydrocoeles may be treated as ordinary hydrocoeles. Coagulation in the chylocoele on aspiration may be prevented by drawing off the fluid into a solution of potassium citrate. The living membranes of the sac can be obliterated by injection or open operation. Injection treatment is suitable for the small thin-walled sacs but operation is better for the others. Filarial orchitis with effusion into the tunica vaginalis is best treated by incision of the tunica vaginalis, turning out any clot that may be found in the sac and stuffing the latter with iodoform gauze.

Elephantiasis. The lymphoedema must first be reduced by prolonged firm bandaging, and then further swelling prevented by permanent support of the tissues.

Knott's method of bandaging. The patient is put to bed and firm bandaging is started from the foot upwards. Sponge rubber is used to protect the tissues from too tight bandaging. The bandages are removed every day and replaced a little tighter. Results are good even in the largest legs. Fluid is eliminated from the tissues and people who can hardly walk because of the size of their legs can become active again. After the swelling has been reduced to more manageable proportions a spiral elastic stocking on Dickson Wright's model which can be accurately fitted to the leg and which is comfortable, airy and effective is recommended (Fig. 76).

Surgical treatment

Abscesses caused by filariae must be opened and drained.

PREVENTION

The control of filariasis rests on two methods—chemotherapy and vector control (WHO 1967).

Mass chemotherapy with diethylcarbamazine

Advantages. Mass treatment produces an immediate reduction in the microfilaria level in the population. There is no known animal reservoir outside Malaya. During the last ten years it has been successful on a small scale in Tahiti (Laigret *et al.* 1966), where a quick reduction in the number of adult filariae has been obtained, and in West Africa. It is applicable to both urban and rural areas and has a beneficial effect by curing acute symptoms and thus diminishing the danger of pathological lesions. Partial control of microfilaraemia has been obtained with cooking salt medicated with diethylcarbamazine (Hawking & Marques 1967).

Disadvantages. Success depends upon obtaining good cooperation from the population, which is often difficult to achieve with large communities. The whole population must be treated, since it is not possible to determine all the microfilaria carriers at one examination.

Diethylcarbamazine is used in divided doses of 6 mg/kg once a month for 12 months (Laigret *et al.* 1965). Low doses of the drug have been incorporated in popular foods in a strength corresponding to a daily intake of 50–100 mg per person. Diethylcarbamazine is stable on boiling and autoclaving. Mel W has been used in a single dose in mass chemotherapy, but there have been some deaths, which make it unsuitable for control purposes.

Vector control

Advantages. Adult mosquito control in towns is desirable on general grounds. Larvicidal control does not depend on the cooperation of the local population.

Disadvantages. Vector control is slow to effect the prevalence of filariasis in a population. The number and longevity of the vectors must be reduced to a very low level for many years before transmission is interrupted, owing to the long life of the adult worms. Prolonged control may give rise to insecticide resistance.

Since the vectors of filariasis can be classified into 4 general groups— *Anopheles, Aedes, Mansonia* and the *Culex pipiens* complex, the diversity in the bionomics of these species calls for different control measures. Control of *Anopheles* can be undertaken as part of an antimalarial campaign, by spraying houses with DDT or dieldrin. Control of *Aedes* may be undertaken by house or aerial spraying. Villages may be protected from *Aedes* by controlling breeding places within a perimeter of 100 m, because of the short flight range of the species. Local breeding places can be controlled by village hygiene, such as was developed by Amos in Fiji. Control of the *C. pipiens* complex has failed because of insusceptibility and the development of resistance to DDT. Larval control campaigns have been of limited effectiveness.

Combined methods

A programme using both methods combined will certainly reach its goal more rapidly than a single method, but it depends upon the epidemiology of the infection in each area, the resources of the country and the personnel available.

II. Filariasis caused by *Loa loa*

History

The larval form (*Microfilaria diurna*) which closely resembles *Microfilaria bancrofti* was described by Manson in 1891. The patient from whom the specimen of blood was taken had formerly had an adult *Loa* in his eye. Later association was established between *L. loa* and the disease known as Calabar swellings and also between that disease and *Microfilaria diurna*.

Geographical distribution

Human loiasis is confined to the rain forest and swamp forest areas of West Africa and Central Africa from 8°N. to 5°S. of the equator from the Gulf of Guinea eastwards to the Great Lakes. It is especially common in the Cameroons and on the Ogowe river. Its distribution includes the coastal plain and follows the course of the Congo and its tributaries to a point about 1500 miles from the mouth (Fig. 60). It is also found in the Southern Sudan between the Bahr-el-Ghazal and the Congo between latitudes 4° and 6°N. and longitudes 27° and 31°E.

AETIOLOGY

A description of *Loa loa* is given in Appendix 11.

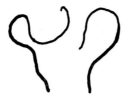

Fig. 77.—*Loa loa* (natural size).

The periodicity is the exact reverse of that of *W. bancrofti*, the embryos appear in the blood during the daytime and disappear at night (diurnal periodicity). The mechanism of this periodicity is considered in Appendix 11. The periodicity differs from that of *W. bancrofti* in that it is not so easy to invert or disturb, but changes gradually when a patient travels round the world. Human *Loa loa* is adapted to day-biting *Chrysops* of the forest canopy, *C. silacea* and *C. dimidiata*, and must be distinguished from simian *Loa loa*, a parasite of drills (*Mandrillus leucophaeus*) and to a less extent other monkeys. This simian *Loa*, which is larger, has a nocturnal periodicity and is adapted to night-biting *Chrysops, C. langi, C. longicornis* and *C. centurionis* (Duke 1961). Development takes place in the thoracic muscles and fat body of *Chrysops* (Appendix 11).

EPIDEMIOLOGY AND TRANSMISSION

Man is the only host of human *Loa loa*. Although it can be transplanted to monkeys and infect them, and even hybrids of human and simian *Loa* bred (Duke 1964), it is unlikely that natural transmission to monkeys occurs since day-biting *Chrysops* do not feed on them and night-biting *Chrysops* would not transmit the diurnal human form.

The main vectors which maintain the infection in man in nature are female *C. silacea* and *C. dimidiata*. These live in the forest canopy and are attracted mainly by dark colours and woodsmoke (Duke 1955). They need the forest canopy to rest on, and lay eggs in wet mud in swamps and river edges below the forest trees. Transmission takes place during the long wet season (April to December) by *C. silacea*, although *C. dimidiata* is absent during the heavy rains (June to October). At certain seasons the risk of transmission is great and at others negligible. In the Bahr-el-Ghazal some transmission is maintained on the edge of the forest zone into the edge of the savanna by *C. distinctipennis* and *C. longicornis* which are vectors of only secondary importance. To a less extent in the Cameroon highlands grassland area *C. zahrai* can transmit naturally (Duke 1961).

Houses built on hills at the level of the forest canopy and buildings in plantations which provide cover for flies from the forest are particularly places where human infections are acquired (Duke 1961).

PATHOLOGY

After the larva has entered the human body through the bite of a *Chrysops*, development is slow and maturity is not attained until a year or longer, although in monkeys it is about 4 months. The parasite lives and moves around in the fascial layers from which the microfilariae are liberated, travelling up the lymphatics to the blood-stream where they lodge in the lungs. In many cases the parasite does not show itself until 3 or 4 years after the patient has left the endemic area, and in one case it was extracted from the eye 13 years after the patient had left Africa. There are records of finding microfilariae in the blood for 17 years. While the active immature worm is often seen in children, the microfilariae in the blood are first found as a rule in adults as long as 7 years from the time of the original infection. This slow development accounts for the frequent failure to find microfilariae in the blood in cases from which mature parasites have been extracted. It is impossible to estimate the number of adult worms present in any given infection and whereas one particular *Loa* may show itself about the eye or elsewhere it is only one of many.

During the period of growth and development in man *L. loa* makes frequent excursions through the subdermal connective tissues. It has been noticed very often beneath the skin of the fingers, and it has been excised from under the skin of the back, from above the sternum, the left breast, the lingual fraenum, the loose skin of the penis, the eyelids, the conjunctiva, the anterior chamber of the eye and also the scalp.

The parts most frequently mentioned are the eyes and, although the worm may attract more attention in this situation, it does seem as though it has a decided predilection for the eye and its neighbourhood (Fig. 258, page 869). A patient of Manson's once stated that the average rate at which a *Loa* travelled was about 2·5 cm in 2 minutes. Both Manson and others have observed that warmth seems to attract them to the surface of the body. Chesterman in the Congo reported finding live adult worms in 10% of all cases operated on for hernia and elephantiasis, while cretified worms were frequently encountered. Calabar swellings were shown by Fülleborn to be an allergic reaction to the filarial toxins which can be reproduced by injections of extracts of the adult filariae. The recurrence of Calabar swellings on the arm or leg appears to give rise to indura- tion of the fascia and connective tissue round the tendon sheaths, causing per- manent cyst-like swellings which may cause pain on muscular movement. In one patient who had manifested these swellings over a period of 7 years all

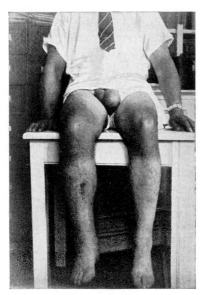

Fig. 78.—Hydrocoele and solid oedema of the right leg, caused by *Loa loa* infection from West Africa.

adult filariae appeared to die out at the same time and were discharged in a calcified state from minute chronic abscesses, which appeared on the hands, arms and legs.

Whether alive or dead this worm evokes a high eosinophilia of 30–40% and an eosinophilia is common in expatriates who have resided in endemic areas in Nigeria, the Congo and Cameroons.

Cerebral manifestations

Occasionally the adult worm may enter the central nervous system and cause cerebral symptoms.

Kivits (1952) and Toussaint and Davis (1965) have described cases of menin- go-encephalitis with choroidoretinitis and microfilariae in the cerebrospinal fluid. Browne (1954) described transient hemiparesis in a woman in the Congo who had been infected for 25 years. Schofield (1955) has described peripheral nerve involvement.

Another form of severe cerebral complication follows treatment with diethylcarbamazine of heavily infected cases of loiasis with numerous microfilariae in the blood (Downie 1966).

Lymphoedema

Solid oedema of one leg persisting for 6 weeks has been observed in a European from West Africa who had been affected for a number of years (Fig. 78), and hydrocoeles have also been reported. However, it is always difficult to exclude a double infection with *W. bancrofti*.

Other manifestations

Urticaria and dermatitis with pruritus are sometimes found in *Loa* cases. However, double infections with *Onchocerca volvulus* are difficult to exclude. Multiple intramuscular abscesses and even infections of the hip-joint have been recorded.

SYMPTOMS AND SIGNS

Expatriates of any race who come to reside in an endemic area are troubled to a much greater extent than the indigenous inhabitants, who exhibit a considerable tolerance to the presence of many worms. As a rule the migrations of the parasite give rise to no serious inconvenience but they may cause a pricking, itching, creeping sensation, neuralgia and occasionally transient oedematous swellings (Calabar swellings) in various parts of the body. When the parasite appears under the conjunctiva it may cause a considerable amount of irritation and congestion. There may be actual pain associated with swelling and inability to use the eye and perhaps tumefaction of the eyelids (Fig. 258, page 869). Should a *Loa* wander into the rima glottidis or the urethra the consequence is serious and great pain is sometimes caused. The death of a parent worm may cause a localized abscess in the groin or axilla.

Calabar swellings

The swellings are about the size of half a goose egg, painless, though somewhat hot both objectively and subjectively, not pitting on pressure and usually

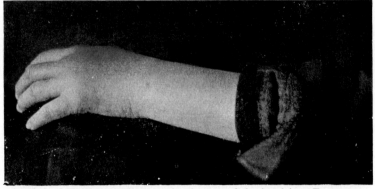

Fig. 79.—Calabar swelling on the dorsum of the hand in a European woman from the Congo.

disappearing in about 3 days. They come suddenly and disappear gradually and occur in any part of the body. They may irritate slightly but the skin maintains its normal colour. One swelling occurs at a time but recurs at irregular intervals and perhaps for years after the patient has left the endemic area. In some instances the swellings seem to be due to rubbing provoked by the irritation of a *Loa* just under the skin. In the hand or forearm they may give rise to a sense of powerlessness or soreness as if the part had received a blow. They never suppurate (Fig. 79). The effects of temperature upon these swellings is important. During the hot summer months they are frequent, but in the cold weather distinctly uncommon.

DIAGNOSIS

Microfilariae in the blood

These are found more commonly in adults than in children; they are frequently absent in early infections. They can be demonstrated in blood taken between 10.00 and 14.00 hours, either in a thick drop of 20 mm^3 or by Knott's method. In old thick drop preparations *L. loa*, and *B. malayi* have a shrunken appearance, while the other microfilariae have not. This is due to the greater permeability of the cuticle in the former, which permits faster drying and more rapid staining. *W. bancrofti* becomes shorter, and its width identifies it. Other microfilariae do not shrink in the same manner.

Eosinophilia

Eosinophilia is present to a significant degree in all cases of recent infection. A symptomless eosinophilia in an expatriate from West Africa almost always denotes loiasis or *D. perstans* infection, which are frequently associated.

Immunodiagnosis

The complement fixation test is positive in a high proportion of cases 1–3 years after infection, and remains positive for 7 years. In older infections it reverts to negative. Immunodiagnosis is considered on page 196.

TREATMENT AND PREVENTION

Diethylcarbamazine

Diethylcarbamazine rapidly immobilizes the microfilariae which are destroyed in the liver (Woodruff 1951). It also unmasks the adult parasites which are recognized as foreign and destroyed by the body's own defences. The developing worms are most susceptible, and the older ones less so.

The dose is 2–3 mg/kg body weight 3 times daily up to 600 mg daily for 21 days. The results are excellent and the microfilarial drugs used in other forms of filariasis are not necessary.

During treatment there is often fever, malaise, swelling of joints, joint pains and pruritus. If there is a heavy infection with microfilariae—1000/20 mm^3 or more—there is a great risk of encephalitis, which can be attributed to toxic material from the worms killed by treatment. Severe headache is a sign of this complication and purpura has been seen. It may be necessary to start with small doses of diethylcarbamazine as in onchocerciasis.

It has been suggested (Brumpt 1966) that exchange transfusion should be used to remove a large proportion of the microfilariae before treatment in order to avoid this reaction. Care must also be taken in treatment, as many patients are infected with *O. volvulus* and are liable to develop severe skin reactions. Steroid and antihistamine drugs are of little value in dealing with reactions during treatment of *L. loa* infections.

Chemoprophylaxis

Duke (1963) has shown that in monkeys diethylcarbamazine may act as a prophylactic by killing the young immature worms. The effective dose in man is 5 mg/kg body weight daily for 3 days each month. A course of radical curative treatment should precede that procedure.

Vector control

Control of *Chrysops* has not yet been achieved to any significant degree. The larvae can be destroyed in the mud in which they live with suspensions of dieldrin, and a whole year's crop can be destroyed at one time, since they need several months for development. However, this method of control has not proved practical at the present time.

Individuals may avoid being bitten to a great extent by wearing light-coloured clothes and avoiding wood smoke and open fires.

III. Onchocerciasis
AETIOLOGY

Human onchocerciasis is caused by *Onchocerca volvulus*, which was originally discovered by a German medical missionary in Ghana and subsequently named *Filaria volvulus* by Leuckhart in 1893. In 1899 Blanchard demonstrated that it lay in a lymphatic space in a tumour, and in 1915 Robles described it as being common in Guatemala. Brumpt classified the worms as distinct species, *O. volvulus* and *O. caecutiens*, but Strong *et al.* (1934) demonstrated that they were morphologically identical. It was suggested that the parasite had been imported into Central America by slaves from Jamaica, Sudanese servants employed by the French troops of the Emperor Maximilian or slaves imported to Venezuela to pan the rivers for gold. However, De Leon and Duke (1966) have shown that the Central American and African parasites are biologically distinct and that the American species does not develop so well in the African *Simulium*. The close adaptation of Guatemalan *O. volvulus* to *S. ochraceum* implies an association of more than 400 years. In Venezuela, on the other hand, the infection may well have been imported by slaves from Africa.

The life history of *O. volvulus* is described in Appendix 11.

GEOGRAPHICAL DISTRIBUTION

Human onchocerciasis is found in both the Old and the New Worlds. In the Americas important foci exist in Mexico, Guatemala and Venezuela (Figs 80, 81) and a small focus has recently been discovered in Colombia.

In Africa the infection occurs south of the Sahara in a wide belt stretching from west to east (Fig 82). The northern boundary of this zone coincides roughly with 15°N. and runs from Senegal to Ethiopia. South of the equator the endemic area extends down to Angola in the west and Tanzania in the east. Small foci have also been reported in the north of the Sudan republic and in the Yemen. Recent surveys have shown in Africa that onchocerciasis transmission

MEXICO AND GUATEMALA

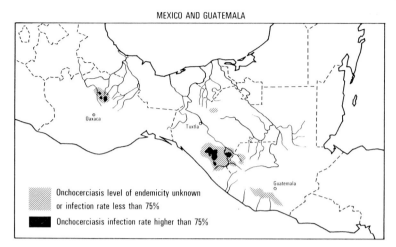

Fig. 80.—Geographical distribution of onchocerciasis in Mexico and Guatemala. (*Reproduced from WHO Chronicle (1966) 20, 379*)

VENEZUELA

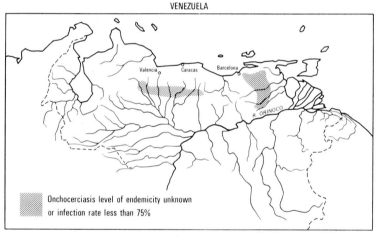

Fig. 81.—Geographical distribution of onchocerciasis in Venezuela. (*Reproduced from WHO Chronicle (1966) 20, 379*)

takes place over wider areas and extends further north in Mali and is more widespread in the forest zones of the Ivory Coast and in Cameroon. Infection rates of 6 foci are known in Tanzania, 2 in the Usambara mountains (35–40%), 1 in Mahenge (39%), 1 in Ruvuma (20%) and 2 near Morogoro (29%).

EPIDEMIOLOGY AND TRANSMISSION
(WHO 1966)

Onchocerca volvulus is transmitted by female 'black flies' of the *Simulium* genus. The development of the parasite in the arthropod host is described in Appendix 11.

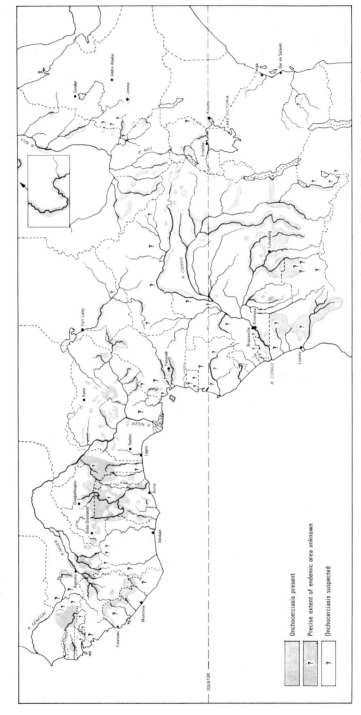

Fig. 82.—Geographical distribution of onchocerciasis in Africa. (Reproduced from *WHO Chronicle* (1966) 20, 380)

Man is the only known mammalian host, unlike *Dipetalonema streptocerca* which produces microfilariae in the human skin and is also common in the chimpanzee and gorilla in the African rain forest.

The main single factor influencing the extent of human exposure to infection is the infective density of the *Simulium* vectors. This depends upon the size of the *Simulium* population, number of infective flies, concentration of infective larvae in these flies, longevity of female *Simulium*, seasonal variation in number of flies and the distance of human dwellings from the breeding grounds. The human host factors which must be considered are occupation, seasonal migration, changes in habits of the human population, attraction of individuals of different ages, sex and racial group to *Simulium* and social and economic changes in the human population.

Ecology of the African vectors

The vectors in Africa are the *Simulium damnosum* and the *S. neavei* group (including *S. woodi*). *S. damnosum* is able to exist in large rivers and small streams provided there is an adequate velocity of the water (60–250 cm/second), adequate food supplies and suitable attachment sites existing at depths not greater than 15 cm below the water surface. *S. damnosum* has been known to fly at least 40 km for breeding purposes in savanna country during the rainy season. In the invariably dry Sudanese savanna it is only found near streams where the humidity is maintained. Female *S. damnosum* have been known to travel 85 km to establish new colonies.

There are 2 main *O. volvulus/S. damnosum* complexes, one in a Guinea forest form, in which transmission is perennial and eye lesions are rare, and the other a Sudan savanna form, in which transmission is seasonal and there is a high incidence of blindness.

The main factors governing the distribution of *S. neavei* are the existence of perennial streams containing a suitable crab host and sufficient forest cover for the adult stage. Vectors of the *S. neavei* group have a restricted flight range and are confined to forests and bush-lined rivers. *S. neavei* is not a strong flier and the maximum recorded flight is 29 km from the nearest breeding place. It is unable to migrate from one focus to another except through forest galleries.

Ecology of the American vectors

In Mexico and Guatemala the principal vector of onchocerciasis is *S. ochraceum*. *S. metallicum* and *S. callidum* are of secondary importance. *S. ochraceum* and *S. metallicum* breed in small streams at altitudes between 500 and 1500 m. *S. callidum* breeds in large rivers as well as small streams and has a greater range. All these species breed the year round but peak production takes place in the dry season. The main zone of transmission lies between altitudes of 750 and 1500 m where the coffee plantations are located. Transmission is confined to the dry season between the months of October and April. The principal vector of onchocerciasis in Venezuela is *S. metallicum*; *S. exiguum* is a vector of secondary importance.

Man-made factors

Hydroelectric schemes entailing the construction of large dams invariably inundate up-river breeding sites of Simuliidae but they create new breeding places in the spillways of the dams and in down-stream sections. Small earth dams invariably create new breeding sites.

In the human host

Infection begins in childhood as early as the first year of life. In the Red Volta district the fly infection rate is 13% and the microfilaria rate in the population is 38% under 10 years, 91% under 20 and 100% over 20. There is no decrease in the microfilaria rate with age.

General effects of onchocerciasis

Some of the most fertile valleys in tropical Africa are infested by *Simulium* and are being abandoned by the riverine population plagued by skin and eye diseases. The presence of *Simulium* flies and fear of onchocercial blindness more often than not threatens the implementation of vast irrigation and dam-building projects on which the future development of countries depends.

In many parts of West and Equatorial Africa more than 50% of the inhabitants are affected, 30% have impaired vision, and 4–10% are blind, owing chiefly to onchocerciasis. In some villages of Upper Volta and in Ghana the percentage of blindness reaches 13–35% (WHO 1966).

At Kodera in Kenya the prevalence of blindness was about 10% before control operations were undertaken in 1946, but has fallen since then to less than 1%. Mass blindness can reduce the efficiency of a primitive agricultural community below survival level. The greatest incidence of blindness is usually found in adult males who form the backbone of the labour force and as their life is not shortened they remain a burden to themselves and to the community.

PATHOLOGY (Duke 1968)

When an infective *Simulium* bites man a number of infective larvae are inoculated; each one remains a single worm which grows and matures over a period of about a year. The mature males and females collect in balls, bound together by fibrous tissue which forms the nodules typical of the infection, but mature worms can occur in the skin in the absence of nodules. Each fertilized female produces large numbers of living embryos (microfilariae) which invade the skin and remain there until they die or are ingested by a feeding *Simulium*. The time between the inoculation of infective larvae and the first appearance of microfilariae producing symptoms is commonly 15–18 months with extremes of 10–20 months. The life span of the microfilariae in the skin may be as long as 30 months and fecund female worms can live for 15 years but not more than 18 (Editorial, *Br. med. J.* 1967).

RELATIONSHIP OF INFECTION TO PATHOLOGICAL LESIONS

There is a direct relationship between the degree of infection in man and the pathological results. The heaviest infections in man are found in those who have undergone prolonged periods of exposure, and among persons thus heavily loaded with parasites for many years will be found those with the most severe lesions of the skin and eyes. It is known that dead parasites, particularly microfilariae, can cause most of the skin and eye changes as a result of tissue damage and reaction following absorption, possibly of toxins. The reaction of the host's body to the parasite and the associated immune reactions are perhaps at the root of the variable pathology of onchocerciasis.

People who first acquire a primary infection in adult life show the most intense reaction to the parasites, particularly pruritic skin rashes. Economically they are important since they are usually people on whom much economic development of the region depends. It has been suggested that the more severe and frequent ocular lesions seen in the African savanna may result from increased intensity of infection which follows intermittent transmission and the breakdown of the immune response.

The microfilariae cause pathological lesions of the skin and eyes.

Skin

Live microfilariae cause no tissue reaction (Fig. 83). Dead microfilariae cause an immediate tissue reaction which is readily seen following treatment with diethylcarbamazine; this forms the basis of the Mazzotti test (Mazzotti 1959)

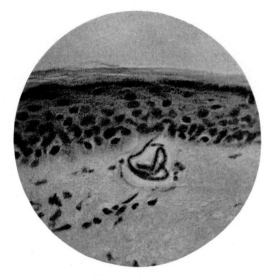

Fig. 83.—Photomicrograph of microfilaria of *Onchocerca volvulus* in subcutaneous tissue. Note the absence of any tissue reaction. (*Dr P. H. Martin*)

which is one method of diagnosing the infection. At first there is oedema and an infiltration of the dermis with eosinophil cells, which may be intense, followed by a cell-mediated response with macrophage cells, lymphocytes and sometimes giant cells forming a granuloma with subsequent fibrosis. Later, in more chronic cases, there is thickening and oedema of the subcutaneous tissues with disappearance of the elastic fibres and atrophy of the skin similar to the changes which occur in old age 'presbyderma'.

The severity of the reactions varies in individuals but is usually proportional to the weight of infection, but microfilarial densities of 50/mg of skin are sometimes seen in people with apparently normal skin. These skin reactions are responsible for onchodermatitis. In the early stages there is pruritus, a severe form of dermatitis known in Guatemala and Mexico as 'erisipela de la costa' and 'mal morado'; in the later stages there is mottled depigmentation of the skin, as well as atrophy of the skin.

These atrophic changes in the skin result in Africa in the condition known as 'hanging groin' in males and 'Hottentot apron' in females (Nelson 1958). This is a pendulous sac containing enlarged lymph glands, which predisposes to inguinal or femoral hernia (Fig. 84). Occasionally the same patients have lipomas and the looseness and atrophy of the skin of the face can produce a leonine appearance which occurs in Guatemala and Mexico.

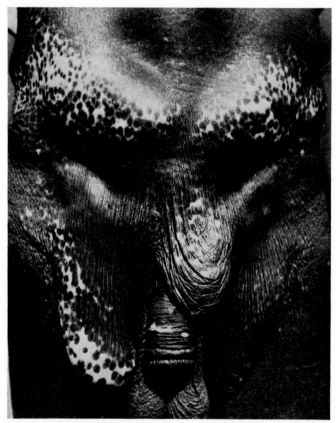

Fig. 84.—Depigmentation of the skin and 'hanging groins' in onchocerciasis. (*Dr S. G. Browne*)

Eye lesions

The most characteristic lesions are in the anterior part of the eye, and are described in the section on ophthalmology (Section XV).

In hyperendemic areas, especially in the savanna regions of Africa, onchocerciasis also causes retinopathy; there is retinitis and choroiditis which involves the optic nerve and progresses to atrophy. Microfilariae have been demonstrated in the optic nerve and retina (Rodger 1960) and there is now convincing epidemiological evidence of the aetiological association with onchocerciasis (Rodger 1957; Budden 1956). The more nodules are situated in the head and shoulders region, the greater the extent of ocular involvement. Thus in Central

America, where the nodules occur in the upper half of the body, there is a greater severity and incidence of ocular lesions.

Nodules (Fig. 85)

The adult *Onchocerca* are found in subcutaneous tumours the size of a pea to that of a pigeon's egg. One or more tumours may be present. The regions most affected are those in which the peripheral lymphatics converge, the axilla, popliteal spaces, suboccipital region, intercostal spaces and iliac crests. Nodulation frequently occurs in old scars with presumably interrupted lymph channels.

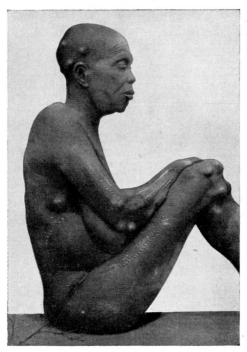

Fig. 85.—Onchocerciasis from the Congo. Note the typical nodules on the knees, elbows and scalp. (*Dr C. C. Chesterman*)

In Africa the nodules are found most commonly in the pelvic girdle area, less frequently in the shoulder girdle and least on the head. This may be connected with the fact that the vectors *S. neavei* and *S. damnosum* tend to bite on the lower parts of the body. In Central America the nodules are found mostly on the occipitofrontal and temporal regions; the vector *S. ochraceum* tends to bite about the head and neck. The situation of the nodules may be determined by the type of dress worn.

Nodules situated on the head, usually the scalp, measure 6–20 mm, rarely as much as 30 mm. They may cap and even erode the skull. Adult worms may be obtained entire by digesting the tissues with papaya juice or papain in 0·2% HCl. The tumours are never adherent to the surrounding tissues and can easily be enucleated. They are formed of a dense mass of connective tissue which envelops the parasites and encloses small cyst-like spaces filled with a greyish viscous substance consisting almost entirely of microfilariae (Fig. 86). The greater length of the coiled-up bodies of the females is embedded in the connective stroma and can only be extracted in fragments. When adult worms are encapsulated deep in the tissues they may die and cause sterile abscesses. Adult worms commonly occur free in the tissues and have been found unencapsulated during operations for hernia.

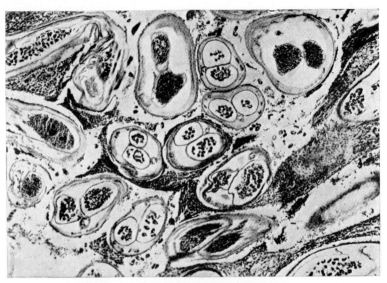

Fig. 86.—Section of an *Onchocerca volvulus* nodule, showing adult worms in the skin at various levels. × 76. (*Wanson*)

Lymphoedema

Lymphadenopathy, scrotal enlargement, hydrocoele and enlarged testes are seen in onchocerciasis, and microfilariae can be demonstrated in hydrocoele fluid as well as in lymphatic tissue.

Rodhain (1951) considered that the lymphadenopathy is due to an allergic reaction to the microfilariae in the gland. Occasionally onchocerciasis may result in some degree of elephantiasis but many of the reports of elephantiasis in onchocercal infection have failed to exclude concomitant bancroftian filariasis.

CLINICAL FEATURES

Onchocerciasis may produce no symptoms at all where transmission is light. Many onchocerciasis areas have remained undiscovered until skin snips in symptomless inhabitants have shown the presence of onchocercal infection.

Patients presenting with clinical onchocerciasis fall into two categories:

(*a*) Those with recent relatively light infections presenting with a pruritic skin rash. These are children living in endemic areas and adults, often expatriates, who come to live there without previous exposure to infection.

(*b*) Those with heavy infections of long duration who present with deteriorating vision or gross skin manifestations.

Skin symptoms and signs (onchodermatitis)

In light, recently acquired infections an adult female worm, usually impalpable, is present around the limb girdle on the affected side. Microfilariae from these worms then invade the skin of the anatomical quarter and produce the characteristic lesions. The usual picture is of a persistent itchy rash, mostly confined to one anatomical quarter of the body or on the back in a 'butterfly' distribution on the buttocks. The rash is composed of numerous small circular raised discrete papules, 1–3 mm in diameter, which are red when seen on a white skin (Fig. 87). Microfilariae are present in small numbers in these cases. In the indigenous inhabitants of areas of high endemicity the skin shows gross scarring. In Africa the skin lesions are commonest over the lower limbs but

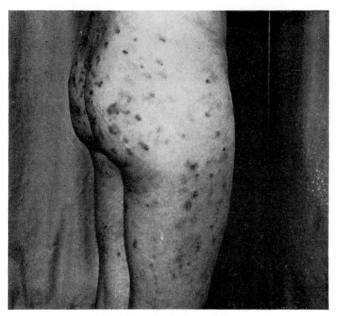

Fig. 87.—Onchodermatitis.

may cover the whole body. There is a thickening of the skin owing to subcutaneous oedema and this produces the characteristic 'peau d'orange' effect which is often associated with lymph gland enlargement, especially in the groins. Later there is a heavy lichenification and thickening of the skin (xeroderma or lizard skin) (Fig. 88), and finally there is atrophy with loss of elasticity and a premature aged appearance—presbyderma. In these cases microfilariae can readily be demonstrated in the skin, often in enormous numbers.

In Central America gross skin changes are less marked than elsewhere even when microfilariae are abundant, but some people, especially children, may show angry reddish-mauve lesions on the face ('erisipela de la costa') and adults may show a thickened smooth white face giving a leonine appearance.

Depigmentation of the skin in pretibial regions, the groins, Scarpa's triangle, over the iliac spines and rarely on the chest is distinct from onchodermatitis and may disappear if all nodules are excised. It may be due to a toxin (Browne 1960).

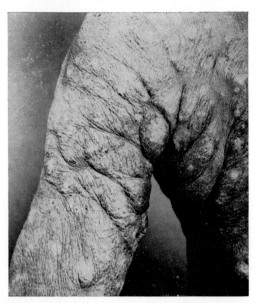

Fig. 88.—Long-standing onchodermatitis. Lichenification (*Dr P. W. Hutton*).

Eye symptoms and signs

These are considered in Section XV.

Lymphoedema

Lymphatic enlargement of the scrotum and hydrocoeles and enlarged testes have been noted in patients infected with *O. volvulus*, while the embryos can be demonstrated in hydrocoele fluid as well as in oedematous lymphatic tissue. In the Congo elephantiasis of the scrotum and legs has been described. The elephantoid scrotum is convoluted like a brain or a wrinkled walnut shell and the subcutaneous tissue is more solid and less oedematous than that in elephantiasis attributed to *W. bancrofti*, while the embryos are found in the skin.

Acute arthritis has been described in onchocerciasis (Dejou 1939) and microfilariae can be demonstrated in the synovial fluid.

Central nervous system

Onchocercal nodules on the head may erode the bone and cause epilepsy. Raper and Ladkin (1950) claim that *O. volvulus* is the aetiological agent in the Nakalanga syndrome in Uganda—the pigmy dwarfing resulting from damage to the pituitary. Microfilariae of *O. volvulus* have been found in the cerebrospinal fluid (Mazzotti 1959) and in the urine (Price 1961), probably arising from the desquamated epithelial lining of the urethra.

Laboratory findings

Eosinophilia. Except in the most advanced cases there is always a marked eosinophilia of 4000/mm³ or over. Sometimes symptomless onchocerciasis may present as an eosinophilia of which it is one of the commonest causes in people from West Africa.

Serological tests. These are discussed under immunology (page 196).

DIFFERENTIAL DIAGNOSIS

The pruritic onchodermatitis (filarial itch) must be distinguished from infection with *D. streptocerca* in which the lower limbs are rarely affected; scabies, where the typical burrows and mites can be found between the fingers; insect bites which come on early after residence in the tropics; prickly heat; contact dermatitis; and sycosis cruris, a chronic low-grade bacterial infection of the legs.

In heavy infections of long standing the skin changes must be differentiated from tertiary yaws, chronic superficial mycoses, leprosy and chronic eczema.

DIAGNOSIS

The diagnosis is made by demonstrating microfilariae of *O. volvulus* in skin snips. Skin snips (2–4) should be taken from the thighs, buttocks and iliac crests in African cases and from the scapula, buttock and face regions in American cases. After cleaning the skin with spirit and allowing to dry, a small hare-lip or entomological pin is slipped under the epidermis which is raised and sliced off with a safety razor blade, removing a small piece of skin 2–3 mm in diameter and 0·5–1·0 mm deep. The snip itself, which should be bloodless, is placed in physiological saline, torn to shreds and examined in a wet state under the microscope. The microfilariae have to be distinguished from *D. streptocerca*. The portions of skin can be weighed and the density of microfilariae per mg calculated.

Mazzotti test (Mazzotti 1959). This test consists in observing the reaction to a test dose of diethylcarbamazine given by mouth. Diethylcarbamazine, 50 or 100 mg, is given by mouth. In a positive case there will be an acute exacerbation of the rash 2–24 hours later mainly over the affected area, or a rash may appear in patients who previously had no skin symptoms. The reaction is against dead microfilariae killed by the diethylcarbamazine.

TREATMENT (Who 1966)

Three drugs are effective against *O. volvulus*: the microfilaricidal diethylcarbamazine, and the macrofilaricidal suramin and Mel W.

Diethylcarbamazine (Hetrazan, Banocide, Notézine)

Diethylcarbamazine is given in lightly infected cases to remove the microfilariae from the skin. In areas of light to moderate endemicity a great number of persons carrying *O. volvulus* have no symptoms and are in no need of treatment; in fact if they are treated the natural host–parasite relationship will be upset and subsequent reinfections may be symptomatic. If fibrosis and scarring of the skin is advanced these processes can only be arrested. To forecast reactions a small dose should be given at first: Day 1, 50 mg; Day 2, 50 mg t.d.s.; Day 3, 100 mg t.d.s.; and from Day 4 onwards 250 mg t.d.s. The accepted therapeutic course, which may be repeated 2 or 3 more times in attempts to kill the adult worms as well as the microfilariae, is 2 mg/kg body weight t.d.s. for 3 weeks.

Where the adult worms are not killed after diethylcarbamazine treatment the microfilariae will return and reach half the previous concentration within 1 year (Duke 1957). Symptoms return after a period of 3–6 months. If there is a severe reaction to treatment this may be controlled by steroids. Antihistaminics are of little use.

Suramin (Antrypol, Bayer 205)

Suramin, which acts on both the microfilariae and adult worms, is a potentially dangerous drug and great care should be taken in using it in a disease which is not fatal. Involvement of the eyes is an indication for suramin treatment.

The microfilariae should first be removed from the skin by a course of diethylcarbamazine.

After an initial dose of 100 mg, 1 gramme of suramin should be given intravenously once a week for 5–6 weeks. This can be relied upon to kill all adult worms and many nodules will disappear. In addition almost all of the microfilariae in the skin and eyes will be killed. Three to four weeks after the last dose of suramin a second course of diethylcarbamazine should be given to destroy any remaining microfilariae.

Toxic reactions to the drug are considered in Section XVI.

Reactions attributable to the death of the microfilariae are itching and swelling of the skin of the parasitized parts and a fine or coarse papular eruption and an ensuing desquamation. If the eye is involved conjunctivitis and blepharitis may occur. The reaction to the death of the adult worms is pain and tenderness in the nodules and occasionally deep intramuscular abscesses. Diarrhoea of obscure origin, sometimes fatal, has been described in patients who developed high fever, prostration arthritis, true exfoliative dermatitis and ulceration of the buccal mucosa. These symptoms should indicate the need for immediate cessation of treatment.

Mel W

Mel W has given rise to fatal arsenical encephalopathy in a quite unpredictable manner and should be used with extreme care. It has been given by intramuscular injection; 200 mg of the powder in 3 ml of pyrogen-free distilled water in courses of 200 mg/day for 4 days, being repeated after 10–14 days, or in a single dose of 7·5–10 mg/kg body weight with a ceiling of 500 mg.

Suppressive treatment

If the patient cannot tolerate suramin or if early reinfection is unavoidable weekly suppressive doses of diethylcarbamazine (50 mg) may be given. A series of reactions decreasing in severity will occur and after about 6 weeks the dosage can be increased to 200 mg which can be continued as long as desired and which will keep the skin free from microfilariae and the eyes protected from microfilarial invasion and eliminate a source of infection for *Simulium*.

Nodulectomy

Nodulectomy is a useful therapeutic measure in individual cases, particularly where the nodules occur on the head. Nodules should be removed wherever this is easy.

PREVENTION (Who 1966)

Combined control methods are those aimed at both the vector and the parasite in the human host. Campaigns directed against the parasite can be based on nodulectomy and chemotherapy.

Mass nodulectomy

This has been conducted thoroughly and efficiently in Guatemala and Mexico for the past 20 years and this has greatly reduced the incidence of severe ocular complications. However, patients from whom all palpable nodules have been removed still harbour large numbers of microfilariae which have given rise to heavy infections in *Simulium* fed on such patients.

Mass chemotherapy

Mass chemotherapy may be undertaken to reduce morbidity or to eliminate the parasite reservoir in the human host with the object of interrupting transmission.

Diethylcarbamazine is given as in suppressive treatment.

Mass treatment with drugs other than diethylcarbamazine should be confined to persons with proved infections. Great caution is called for since patients who suffer severe reactions may not report for follow-up. Suramin has been used in a similar dosage for individual treatment but has not been a success because the administration requires very careful medical supervision.

Mel W is still experimental but may hold promise since a single dose is lethal to the majority of *O. volvulus* adults but has no action on the microfilariae which can live for up to 2 years and which can maintain the individual as a source of infection until reinfection has produced new microfilariae. At some stage therefore diethylcarbamazine will have to be given to destroy the microfilaria load. It is possible that in the future populations may be treated with a single dose of Mel W, combined with diethylcarbamazine, so that the reservoir in the human population will be permanently eliminated. However, the warning on the toxicity of Mel W (see above) should not be forgotten.

Vector control measures

In order to carry out vector control it is necessary to understand the biology of the vectors in each area. In Africa larvicides have been used mainly, though adulticides have been employed also. DDT employed as a larvicide can control *S. damnosum*, but failure can be caused by lack of control of breeding sites in small tributaries. Adulticides have been applied to resting places of *S. damnosum* by dispersion from aircraft, and this has been successful in some cases where additional treatments are provided. No evidence of resistance to DDT has yet been observed.

S. naevei has been entirely eradicated from Kenya by larvicidal treatments, except for a small focus on the Uganda border. Transmission has been completely interrupted and no new cases of onchocerciasis have been reported in any of the districts since the elimination of the vector.

Control of the vector species of Simuliidae in the Americas is confined to Mexico, where larvicidal control on a yearly basis has produced a marked reduction in the density of the adult vector population.

Results. Where control has been achieved the results can be amazing. *Simulium* control along the Victoria Nile in 1952 was followed by a spectacular uncapitalized development, and previously untenable land was transformed into a major producing area of food and cash crops.

IV. Filariasis caused by *Dipetalonema perstans,* *D. streptocerca* and *Mansonella ozzardi*

AETIOLOGY

Dipetalonema is described in Appendix 11.

The microfilariae of *D. perstans* were described by Manson in 1891, and the adult form subsequently by Daniels in British Guiana.

In Africa it is also found in the chimpanzee and gorilla, and allied species occur in the New World in monkeys. The microfilariae occur in equal numbers in the blood both by day and night and can persist in the recipient for 3 years after transfusion of infected blood.

TRANSMISSION

Transmission is by midges of the species *Culicoides austeni* and to a lesser degree *C. grahami* and is described in Appendix II.

Geographical distribution

D. perstans is generally widely distributed throughout Central Africa in man and chimpanzee. In the Congo, Nigeria, Ghana, Ivory Coast, Sierra Leone, Zambia and Uganda a high proportion of the inhabitants in some areas are infected. It is also found in the New World in Venezuela, Trinidad, Guyana, Surinam, northern Argentina and Amazonia.

In Central Africa it is commonly associated with *W. bancrofti*, in West Africa with *Loa loa* and in Guyana with *Mansonella ozzardi*.

EPIDEMIOLOGY

Little is known about the epidemiology of *D. perstans*. It is found commonly in chimpanzees and gorillas in the rain forests and is a zoonosis in many areas. It is also widespread in the absence of the large apes and is a human infection in other large areas of its range.

PATHOLOGY

Adult worms occur singly in the mesentery, perirenal and retroperitoneal tissues and pericardium. They are occasionally found in subcutaneous cysts.

SYMPTOMS AND SIGNS

In the vast majority of infections, where a high proportion of the population is infected, no ill-effects can be attributed to the infection. However, some observers feel that serious clinical illness may result in some cases. Duke *et al.* (1968) have shown that the parasite is able to penetrate the central nervous system and found microfilariae in the cerebrospinal fluid of 2 cases with encephalopathy.

In other cases pains in the joints, pruritus, skin rashes and abdominal pains, especially over the hepatic area, with eosinophilia have been described (Stott 1962; Wiseman 1967). Cardiac failure and pericarditis have been described from Rhodesia (Gelfand & Wessels 1964).

Symptomless eosinophilia, which is commonly found in expatriates returning from West Africa, is commonly ascribed to *D. perstans* infection. All these symptoms which are commoner in European expatriates than Africans are considered to be allergic in nature.

TREATMENT

D. perstans is relatively unaffected by microfilaricidal or macrofilaricidal drugs, but symptoms ascribed to the parasite are reported to subside after treatment with diethylcarbamazine.

Dipetalonema streptocerca

This sheathless microfilaria was originally described in the skin of people in Ghana. It is not known if the microfilariae cause any pathology but Duke (1957) described an acute vesicular eruption on the arms and shoulders of a European in which microfilariae of *D. streptocerca* were demonstrated, and which proved susceptible to diethylcarbamazine. Development takes place in *Culicoides grahami* (Henrard & Peel 1949).

Mansonella ozzardi

Mansonella ozzardi is found in the New World in the West Indies, Peru and northern Argentina. It was originally discovered in the blood of Carib Indians and is found in rural areas, in contrast to *W. bancrofti* which is an urban infection in the New World. The vector is a midge *Culicoides furens* (Buckley 1934). Little is known of any pathology caused by this microfilaria, but Montestruc (1949; Montestruc *et al.* 1960) believes that it sometimes causes enlargement of the lymphatic glands, joint pains and an erythematous rash with eosinophilia.

V. Filariasis caused by Dirofilariae

Human dirofilariasis has been reported from the United States (Beaver & Orihel 1968; Jung & Espenan 1967; Pacheco & Schofield 1968). Unmated adult worms as well as sexually mature worms containing microfilariae have been found. Some cases have been identified as *Dirofilaria tenuis*, a parasite normally of raccoons. In most cases the adult worm does not develop fully in man and has been found in subcutaneous nodules which have appeared after death of the worm. In others involvement of the cardiopulmonary system has occurred with the production of 'coin' lesions of the lungs and infarcts which have been excised as neoplasms.

VI. Dracontiasis (Guinea-worm Infection)

GEOGRAPHICAL DISTRIBUTION

This important parasite, *Dracunculus medinensis*, is found in certain parts of Africa and India, and appears to have been imported from America. In Africa it occurs in the Valley of the Nile, Lake Chad, Bornu and West Africa; it has been observed in Uganda, but not in the Congo basin. It is also found in Iran, Turkestan, Arabia and in a very limited part of Brazil (Feira de Santa Anna). Formerly it was supposed to be endemic in Curaçao, Demerara and Surinam. *Dracunculus* is not equally diffused throughout this extensive area; it tends to special prevalence in limited districts, in some of which it is excessively common. In parts of the Deccan, for example, at certain seasons of the year nearly half the population is affected; and in places on the West Coast of Africa (Ghana) nearly every African has one or more specimens about him. In Europe, guinea-worm is seen only in natives of, or in recent visitors from, the endemic areas. In North America, according to Chitwood, it has been found in the silver fox (*Vulpes fulva*), the raccoon (*Procyon lotor*) and the mink (*Putorius vison*), but never in man. In Asia and Africa the parasite is widespread among carnivora. In some parts of Ghana this parasite has now disappeared owing to drying up of wells by drought. Indian step-wells are particularly associated with this infection.

For details of the anatomy and life history of *D. medinensis*, see Appendix II.

The evidence is now fairly complete that the life-span of the female *Dracunculus*, before she appears on the surface of the body, extends to about one year. It is not to be supposed that every species of *Cyclops* is an effective intermediary; if this were the case, guinea-worm infection would have a much wider geographical range.

Infection is largely determined by climatic conditions in that in the dry season the shallow pools are much used for drinking and washing purposes. Patients tend to bathe the affected part of the skin (usually the lower leg) in water to relieve irritation, and this causes the female worm to discharge the embryos into the water; if *Cyclops* are present they take up the embryos, and man becomes infected by swallowing the *Cyclops*. Where running water is available, or wells are properly constructed, the disease does not flourish.

PATHOLOGY AND SYMPTOMS

The gravid female worm, on attaining maturity, makes for the legs and feet; these are the parts of the human body most likely, in tropical countries, to come in contact with puddles of water, the medium in which *Cyclops*—the intermediary host—lives. The water carriers in India are very subject to guinea-worm, which, in their case, appears on the back—that is, the part of the body against which the water-skin lies when being carried. It seems that the mature guinea-worm, by instinct, seeks out that part of the body most in contact with water.

Occasionally, the guinea-worm fails to pierce the integument of her host; sometimes she dies before arriving at maturity. In either case she may give rise to abscess; or she may become cretified, and in this condition may be felt, years afterwards, as a hard convoluted cord under the skin, or be discovered on dissection.

The haunt of the female guinea-worm is the connective tissue of the limbs and trunk. When mature, she proceeds to bore her way through this tissue, travelling downwards. In 85% of cases she presents in some part of the lower extremities; occasionally in the scrotum or on the dorsum (Fig. 89) or sole of the foot; rarely in the arms; exceptionally in other parts of the body, or even in the head. In a proportion of cases the appearance of the worm at the surface of the body is preceded by slight fever and urticaria; the onset of the skin eruption is generally at night, before the blister or other localizing signs are noted. Arrived at her destination, the female worm pierces the derma. In consequence of some irritating secretion, a small blister, containing, as a rule, numerous embryos, forms and elevates the epidermis over the site of the hole in the derma. The irritation due to this act causes a burning sensation and induces the patient to immerse his foot in water. By and by the blister ruptures, disclosing a small superficial erosion 1·25–1·8 cm in diameter. At the centre of the erosion, which sometimes quickly heals spontaneously, a minute hole, large enough to admit an ordinary probe, is visible. Occasionally, when the blister ruptures, the head of the worm is seen protruding from this hole; as a rule, however, at first the worm does not show. If the neighbourhood of the ulcer is douched with a stream of cold water from a sponge, in a few seconds a droplet of fluid—at first clear, later milky—wells up through the hole and flows over the surface. Sometimes, instead of this fluid, a small, beautifully pellucid tube, the uterus, about 1 mm in diameter, is projected through the hole in response to the stimulus of the cold water. Apparently in this act the tissues of the head are exploded in order that the uterus may escape (Fig. 90).

When the tube has been extruded 2·5 cm or thereabouts, it suddenly fills

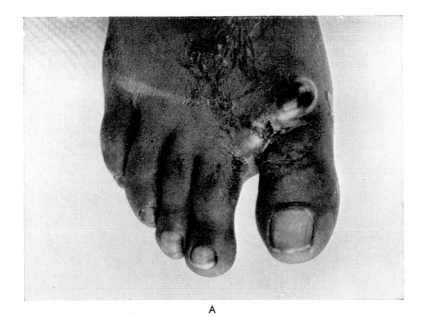

A

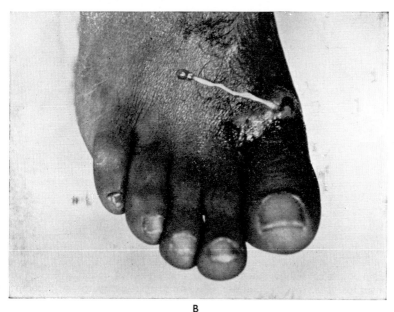

B

Fig. 89.—Guinea-worm disease. A, The primary blister produced by the head of the female prior to emergence. B, Female guinea-worm protruding from the interdigital cleft, showing the terminal expansion containing myriads of embryos. (*P. H. Manson-Bahr*)

with an opaque whitish material, ruptures, and collapses, the fluid spreading over the surface of the erosion. If a little of the fluid, either that which has welled up through the hole, or that which has escaped from the ruptured tube, is placed under the microscope, it is seen to contain myriads of *Dracunculus* embryos lying coiled up, almost motionless, with their tails projecting in a very characteristic manner (Fig. 91). If now a drop of water is instilled below the cover-glass, the embryos unroll themselves, and, in a very short time, swim about, *more suo*, with great activity. If the douching is repeated after an hour or longer, a further supply of embryos can be obtained, and this can be continued from time to time until the worm has emptied herself. Apparently the cold applied to the skin of the host stimulates the worm to contract, and thereby force out her uterus, centimetre by centimetre, until it is completely extruded. The repeated birth of a limited number of progeny each time the skin of the host comes into contact with water is therefore a wonderful provision of nature. Aberrant forms of embryos have been described (see Appendix II).

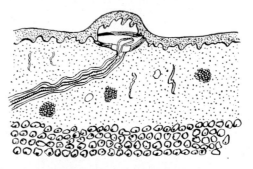

Fig. 90.—Diagram of the vesicle caused by the guinea-worm, showing prolapse of the uterus in the act of discharging embryos into the blister cavity.

The first symptoms appear usually simultaneously with the beginning of the blister formation, and consist of urticaria, nausea, vomiting, diarrhoea, asthma, giddiness and fainting and they are believed to be due to absorption of the toxin emitted by the worm to form the initial skin blister. The symptoms strongly suggest an anaphylactic reaction, and goats injected with guinea-worm extracts show similar symptoms, while injections of adrenaline bring about rapid improvement. Later symptoms result from the invasion of the ulcer by bacteria.

Should the worm become injured or lacerated while lying in the subcutaneous tissues, severe local reaction may develop. The part becomes extremely painful, inflamed and oedematous, and cellulitis may result, due to secondary downward growth of staphylococci and streptococci from the skin. Arthritis, synovitis, epididymitis, contractions of tendons and ankylosis of joints have even been known to ensue. In some patients, generalized systemic symptoms accompany the premonitory urticaria, such as pyrexia, giddiness, dyspnoea and vomiting, and gastro-intestinal symptoms have been noted during the early stages of guinea-worm infection, associated with an increase of eosinophil cells in the blood; this is due to the absorption of a specific toxin, so that alarming symptoms may be produced in laboratory animals by intravenous injections of extracts of the adult *Dracunculus*.

That the cellulitis associated with guinea-worm is due to the excretion of toxins by the mature parasite was shown by Fairley and Glen Liston, who failed to produce any local or general reaction by subcutaneous injection of the embryos themselves. Botreau-Roussel and Huard described a specific non-bacterial arthritis, especially of the knee-joint, associated with the presence of a guinea-worm in the vicinity.

Lester from Dar-es-Salaam reported the discovery of an entire guinea-worm coiled in a hernial sac; it was kept alive in the laboratory for 12 days after removal. According to Trewn, guinea-worms may present themselves after

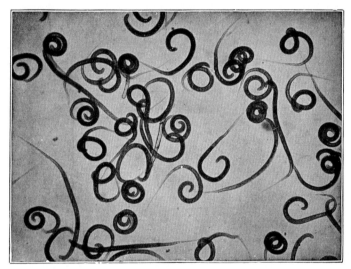

Fig. 91.—Embryos of *Dracunculus medinensis* (*Mr H. B. Bristow*)

as long an interval as 15 years from the time of infection. Massive infections are also reported, and as many as 56 adult worms have been counted in one person at the same time.

DIAGNOSIS

This is, as a rule, sufficiently obvious. In cryptic infections there is generally an eosinophilia. If the worms cannot be seen they may be felt underneath the skin. When both these methods fail, screening with X-rays has been of use; and injection of an opaque medium into the worm renders it opaque. Effete and calcified worms are easily demonstrated by skiagraphy (Fig. 92).

An *intradermal test* for diagnostic purposes was introduced by Ramsay. The antigen is obtained by adding to 100 ml of ether, 0·25 gramme of dried pow-dered guinea-worm, with frequent shakings at room temperature for 2 hours to remove the lipoids. The dried, ether-free residue is extracted with shaking for 4 hours, in 100 ml of 0·85% solution of sodium chloride at 37°C. After centrifugation, it is passed through No. 6 Seitz filter, and 0·25 ml of this is used for injection. A positive weal is 2–3 cm in diameter, with outrunners.

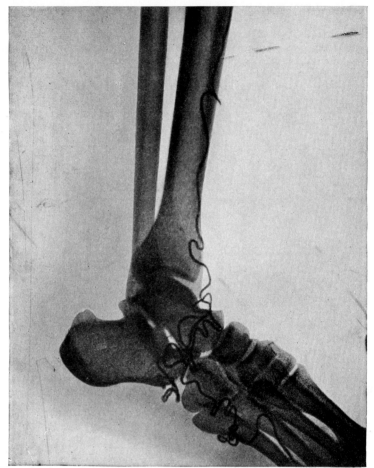

Fig. 92.—A radiograph of the leg, showing the guinea-worm injected with Lipidiol. (*Dr Botreau-Roussel*)

SEQUELAE

Subacute sterile abscesses are occasionally seen, due to premature death of the female *D. medinensis*, with the liberation of embryos into the subcutaneous tissue. The condition is diagnosed by the deeply situated fluctuating swelling, not communicating with the exterior. The track of the dead worm (if it has not been extracted completely) may become infected, with seriously disabling results. In synovitis and arthritis, the exudate may be serous or purulent. Generally, there is an associated cellulitis, the synovial membrane being involved by direct spread through the adjacent tissues. Permanent deformities and a history of prolonged illness in the recumbent position are invariably associated with sepsis. Bony ankylosis is rare. The joints mainly involved are the knee and the ankle, while the Achilles tendon and hamstrings are not infrequently contracted. O'Connor (1923) drew attention to cases diagnosed as chronic rheumatism, traumatic synovitis, periostitis or sciatica, where X-ray examination revealed calcified worms.

Dracontiasis can be an extremely disabling disease, seriously affecting the productive work of farmers at important stages of agricultural work.

TREATMENT

Formerly it was the custom, as soon as a guinea-worm showed herself, to attach the protruding part to a piece of wood and endeavour to wind her out by making a turn or two daily. Sometimes these attempts succeeded; just as often the worm snapped under the strain. The consequences of this accident were often disastrous. Myriads of young escaped from the ruptured ends into the tissues, and violent inflammation and fever, followed by abscess and sloughing, ensued; weeks, or months perhaps, elapsed before the unhappy victims of this

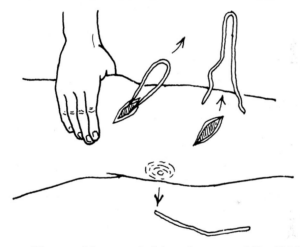

Fig. 93.—Diagram of the removal of the guinea-worm. (*After Fairley*)

rough surgery were able to get about. Too often, serious contractions and ankylosis from loss of tissue and inflammation resulted, and even death from sepsis.

If a guinea-worm is protected from injury, and the part she occupies frequently douched with water, her uterus will be gradually and naturally forced out centimetre by centimetre and emptied of embryos. Until this process is completed she resists extraction. When, in from 15 to 20 days, parturition is completed, which can easily be ascertained by the douching experiment, the worm is absorbed or tends to emerge spontaneously. A little traction then may aid extrusion. Traction, however, must not be employed so long as embryos are being emitted. When located by X-rays and an opaque medium, the worm may be dissected out.

Fairley and Glen Liston advocated aspiration of the blister fluid before extraction, followed by precautions to avoid sepsis. The surface should first be painted with tincture of iodine. After a period of 48 hours, they advised excision of the worm if lying convoluted in a limited space; failing this, intermittent traction should be combined with massage. The subcutaneous injection of 0·55–0·6 ml of 1 in 1000 adrenaline hydrochloride immediately relieves the distressing prodromal symptoms, such as urticaria and asthma, from absorption of toxins.

To complete extraction of the worm, the operative procedure is as follows. It is applicable whether a blister has formed or not, or whether a sinus is present. The skin overlying the worm at some distance from the ulcer is infiltrated with a local anaesthetic of the cocaine or procaine series containing adrenaline. An incision is made at right-angles to the line of the worm through the anaesthetized tissues. The whitish fibrous sheath of the worm being exposed, the superior surface is incised longitudinally and a small strabismus hook inserted inside its interior. By these means the female D. *medinensis* is hooked out. The loop of the worm is held tightly in the fingers while intermittent traction and massage are again employed. Should it be impossible to liberate the distal end of the parasite, a second incision is made over another palpable segment of the worm, and both ends of the central loop are cut across and the intermediary portion removed. It is most important that the proximal head portion of the worm should be removed through the sinus, not drawn through the sheath in the subcutaneous tissues in the reverse direction, or otherwise there will be pollution with organisms from the mouth of the sinus (Fig. 93).

Hetrazan

Rousset (1952) would appear to have been the first to use diethylcarbamazine in treatment and prophylaxis. The best hope for success, he thinks, is during the period of larval development in the body, a period of 9 months. Side-effects were common. Of the 31 so treated only 2 subsequently developed signs and symptoms. It was concluded that Hetrazan exerts a marked therapeutic effect. It is best given 3 months after exposure to infection. In the treatment of the adult worm, when it has penetrated the skin, Hetrazan should be given in maximal doses which result in reduction of the inflammatory oedema and render the worm more amenable to extraction.

Niridazole (Ambilhar)

Raffier (1965) has introduced Ambilhar in the treatment of guinea-worm; 20–25 mg/kg/day for 7–10 days allowed painless manual removal in 70% of the treated cases 4–17 days after starting therapy. Successful results are also reported by Reddy *et al.* (1969).

Raffier has also suggested that 25 mg/kg/day in 2 divided doses should be given to all infected persons as part of an eradication programme, combined with treatment of wells and other sources of infection.

PREVENTION

It is evident that prevention is merely a question of protecting drinking-water from pollution by guinea-worm patients. Leiper demonstrated that *Cyclops* are killed by raising by a few degrees the temperature of the water in which they live. He suggested heating by a portable steam generator the water in wells and water-holes which are known to be sources of guinea-worm infection. Alcock found that the addition of a trace of potash to the water is equally effective. In Mysore, Moorthy found that step-wells are the greatest source of infection, especially in high-caste Hindu houses. When barbel fish (*Barbus puckelli, B. ticto, Rasbora donicornicus*), which feed voraciously on *Cyclops*, are introduced, the guinea-worm disappears. Otherwise the wells may be treated every 14 days with perchloron (bleaching-powder substitute).

REFERENCES

BEAVER, P. C. (1970) *Am. J. trop. Med. Hyg.*, **19**, 181.
—— & ORIHEL, T. C. (1965) *Am. J. trop. Med. Hyg.*, **14**, 1010.
BRAS, G. & LIE KIAN JOE (1951) *Documenta neerl. indones. Morb. trop.*, **3**, 289.
BROWNE, S. G. (1954) *J. trop. Med. Hyg.*, **57**, 229.
—— (1960) *Trans. R. Soc. trop. Med. Hyg.*, **54**, 325.
BRUMPT, L. C. (1966) *Bull. Soc. méd. Hôp. Paris*, **177**, 1049.
BUCKLEY, J. J. C. (1934) *Trans. R. Soc. trop. Med. Hyg.*, **28**, 1.
—— & WHARTON, R. H. (1961) *J. Helminth. Syph.*, **17**, 4.
BUDDEN, F. H. (1956) *Trans. R. Soc. trop. Med. Hyg.*, **50**, 366.
COHEN, L. B., NELSON, G. S., WOOD, A. M., MANSON-BAHR, P. E. C. & BOWEN, R. A. (1961) *Am. J. trop. Med. Hyg.*, **10**, 834.
DANARAJ, T. J. (1959) *Archs Path.*, **67**, 515.
—— PACHECO, G., SHANMUGARATNAM, K. & BEAVER, P. C. (1966) *Am. J. trop. Med. Hyg.*, **15**, 183.
DE LEON, J. R. & DUKE, B. O. L. (1966) *Trans. R. Soc. trop. Med. Hyg.*, **60**, 735.
DENHAM, D. A., DENNIS, D. T., PONNUDURAI, T., NELSON, G. S. & GUY, F. (1971) *Trans. R. Soc. trop. Med. Hyg.*, **65**, 521.
DOWNIE, G. C. B. (1966) *Jl R. Army med. Crps*, **112**, 46.
DUKE, B. O. L. (1955) *Ann. trop. Med. Parasit.*, **49**, 260.
—— (1957) *Trans. R. Soc. trop. Med. Hyg.*, **51**, 37.
—— (1961) Patrick Buxton Memorial Prize Essay, London School of Hygiene and Tropical Medicine.
—— (1963) *Ann. trop. Med. Parasit.*, **57**, 82.
—— (1964) *Ann. trop. Med. Parasit.*, **58**, 390.
—— (1968) *Br. med. J.*, **iv**, 301.
DUKES, D. C., GELFAND, M., GADD, K. G., CLARKE, V. DE V. & GOLDSMID, J. M. (1968) *Cent. Afr. med. J.*, **14**, 21.
EDESON, D. F. B., WILSON, T., WHARTON, R. H. & LAING, A. B. G. (1960) *Trans. R. Soc. trop. Med. Hyg.*, **54**, 229.
EDITORIAL (1967) *Br. med. J.*, **i**, 3.
FAIRLEY, N. H. (1931) *Trans. R. Soc. trop. Med. Hyg.*, **24**, 635.
FRIEDHEIM, L. J. & DE JONGH, R. T. (1959) *Bull. Soc. Path. éxot.*, **53**, 43.
FREISS, J., PIERROU, M. & SEGALEN, J. (1953) *Bull. Soc. Path. éxot.*, **46**, 1037.
FRIMODT-MÖLLER, C. & BARTON, R. M. (1940) *Indian med. Gaz.*, **75**, 607.
GELFAND, M. & WESSELS, O. (1964) *Trans. R. Soc. trop. Med. Hyg.*, **58**, 552.
HAWKING, F. & MARQUES, R. J. (1967) *Bull. Wld Hlth Org.*, **37**, 405.
HENRARD, C. & PEELE, E. (1949) *Bull. Soc. Path. éxot.*, **29**, 127.
JUNG, R. C. & ESPENAN, P. H. (1967) *Am. J. trop. Med. Hyg.*, **16**, 172.
IYENGAR, M. O. T. (1965) *Epidemiology of Filariasis in the South Pacific*. Technical Paper No. 48. Noumea, New Caledonia: South Pacific Commission.
KAGAN, I. G. (1964) *J. Parasit.*, **49**, 773.
KIVITS, M. (1952) *Ann. Soc. belge Méd. trop.*, **32**, 235.
LAIGRET, J., KESSEL, J. F., BAMBRIDGE, B. & ADAMS, H. (1966) *Bull. Wld Hlth Org.*, **34**, 925.
—— MALAIDE, L. & ADAMS, H. (1965) *Bull. Soc. Path. éxot.*, **58**, 895.
LIE KIAN JOE (1962) *Am. J. trop. Med. Hyg.*, **11**, 646.
MAZZOTTI, L. (1959) *Revta Inst. Salubr. Enferm. trop., Méx.*, **19**, 1.
MEYERS, F. M. & KOUWENAAR, W. (1939) *Geneesk. Tijdschr. Ned.-Indië*, **79**, 853.
MONTESTRUC, E. (1949) *Bull. Soc. Path. éxot.*, **41**, 372.
—— COURMES, E. & FONTAN, R. (1960) *Indian J. Malar.*, **4**, 633.
NELSON, G. S. (1958) *Trans. R. Soc. trop. Med. Hyg.*, **52**, 272.
O'CONNOR, F. W. (1923) *Res. Mem. London Sch. trop. Med.*, **4**, 57.

O'CONNOR, F. W. (1932) *Trans. R. Soc. trop. Med. Hyg.*, **26**, 13.
PACHECO, G. & SCHOFIELD, H. L. (1968) *Am. J. trop. Med. Hyg.*, **17**, 180.
POWER, S. (1946) *Lancet*, **i**, 572.
PRICE, P. L. (1961) *J. Parasit.*, **47**, 572.
RAFFIER, G. (1965) *Acta trop.*, **22**, 350.
RAPER, A. B. & LADKIN, R. G. (1950) *E. Afr. med. J.*, **27**, 339.
REDDY, C. R. R. M., REDDY, M. M. & SIVA PRASAD, M. D. (1969) *Am. J. trop. Med. Hyg.*, **18**, 516.
RIDLEY, D. S. (1956) *Trans. R. Soc. trop. Med. Hyg.*, **50**, 255.
—— & STOTT, G. J. (1961) *J. trop. Med. Hyg.*, **64**, 297.
RODGER, F. C. (1957) *Br. J. Ophthal.*, **41**, 544.
—— (1960) *Am. J. Ophthal.*, **49**, 104.
RODHAIN, J. (1951) *Anais Inst. Med. trop. Lisb.*, **8**, 503.
ROUSSET, P. (1952) *Bull. med. Afr. orient. fr.*, **9**, 351.
SCHOFIELD, F. D. (1955) *Trans. R. Soc. trop. Med. Hyg.*, **49**, 588.
SCHACHER, J. F. & SAHYOUN, P. F. (1967) *Trans. R. Soc. trop. Med. Hyg.*, **61**, 234.
STOTT, G. (1962) *J. trop. Med. Hyg.*, **60**, 107.
STRONG, R. P., SANDGROUND, J. H., BEQUAERT, J. C. & MUNOZ OCHOA (1934) Contribution No. 6 from the Department of Tropical Medicine and Institute for Tropical Biology and Medicine of Harvard University. Harvard University Press.
SYMPOSIUM ON TROPICAL EOSINOPHILIA (1960) *Bull. Calcutta Sch. trop. Med.*, **3**, 82.
THOORIS, G. C. (1956) *Bull. Soc. Path. éxot.*, **49**, 306.
TOUSSAINT, D. & DAVIS, P. (1965) *Archs Ophthal.*, **74**, 470.
WARTMAN, W. B. (1947) *Medicine, Baltimore*, **26**, 333.
WEBB, J. K. G., JOB, C. K. & GAULT, E. W. (1960) *Lancet*, **i**, 835.
WEINGARTEN, R. J. (1943) *Lancet*, **i**, 103.
WISEMAN, R. A. (1967) *Trans. R. Soc. trop. Med. Hyg.*, **61**, 667.
WILSON, T. (1961) *Trans. R. Soc. trop. Med. Hyg.*, **55**, 107.
WORLD HEALTH ORGANIZATION (1966) *Wld Hlth Org. tech. Rep. Ser.*, 335.
—— (1967) *Wld Hlth Org. tech. Rep. Ser.*, 359.
—— (1968) *Second Report*. Geneva.
WONG, M. M. (1964) *Am. J. trop. Med. Hyg.*, **13**, 66.
WOODRUFF, A. W. (1951) *Trans. R. Soc. trop. Med. Hyg.*, **44**, 479.

11. OTHER NEMATODE INFECTIONS

Ascariasis

Geographical distribution

Ascaris lumbricoides is one of the commonest and most widespread human parasites. Possibly 1 in every 4 of the world's population is infected. It is found in Asia, Central and South America, Europe, Africa and North America.

Prevalence of *Ascaris* varies in different parts of the world. In China and South-east Asia it is highly prevalent. In the central Asian republics of the U.S.S.R. it is common in humid areas. In Central and South America the average rate of infection is 45% and in parts of Africa it is up to 95%. In Europe it is low in the north and light to moderate in the south. It is moderate in the southern United States.

Aetiology

For the life history of *Ascaris* see Appendix II.

EPIDEMIOLOGY

Ascaris eggs develop best in shady damp clay soil and least in sandy soil. It is mainly a family infection. The soil around the house is seeded from the droppings of small children who play on infected ground and reinfect themselves by mouth. The prevalence and intensity of infection is highest in the younger age-groups and highest in pre-school children, who are the principal agents in the spread of infection. The seed beds remain infective for a long time, and efforts to control hookworm infection have no effect on the *Ascaris* problem.

Where faeces are used as agricultural fertilizer infection is common in agricultural workers. In the overcrowded towns of non-industrialized countries prevalence may be higher in urban than in rural communities. In most damp humid areas in the tropics and subtropics transmission is perennial. In some drier areas transmission is limited to the short rainy season in the spring, and this may produce temporary outbreaks of pneumonia in the adult population.

IMMUNITY

Man acquires only a partial immunity to reinfection. The major part of the immune response is induced by the migratory stages. The antigens that elicit 'protective antibodies' are probably released at the moulting period between the second and third larval stages. The bowel phases between the fourth and fifth larval stages are also responsible for an immune response, at which time there may be a marked loss of worm burden, and this may be a regulatory mechanism in natural infections.

IMMUNODIAGNOSIS

Specific antibodies have been detected in persons infected with *A. lumbricoides* and both the complement fixation and precipitin tests have been utilized for the detection of infection. Hypersensitivity to *Ascaris* is well recognized and cutaneous tests have been used in man as diagnostic aids. There is a lack of correlation between the immunological reaction and the presence of eggs in the faeces, but in pigs the incidence of positive reactions increases with the severity of the pathology produced by the migrating parasites (Soulsby 1957). Since there is much cross-reactivity with other helminthic antigens, immunodiagnosis is of little help in *Ascaris* infections.

PATHOLOGY AND SYMPTOMS AND SIGNS

Light infections do not usually cause symptoms, though even a single worm can cause a liver abscess or block the common bile duct. The overt acute manifestations of infection are roughly proportional to the number of worms harboured. Serious disorders may be caused when the burden amounts to 100 worms or more.

The direct manifestations of ascariasis may be due to toxic symptoms caused by an allergic reaction to the adult worm or larva, the action of the adult worm on the intestinal tract and the wandering of the larvae and adults. The indirect effects are due to the carriage of micro-organisms during migration from the intestine and the possible relation of *Ascaris* to malnutrition states.

Migrating larvae

Some infected individuals manifest a peculiar sensitivity to the emanations of *Ascaris* and entry to a laboratory where the worms are being dissected is enough to cause conjunctivitis, urticaria and asthma. The skin of these people is extremely sensitive to minimal doses of *Ascaris* substance and in a few minutes after intradermal infection a red and extremely sensitive weal is produced. Urticaria and erythematous lesions may occur.

Ascaris pneumonia. During the stage of larval invasion of the lungs there may be symptoms and signs resembling tropical pulmonary eosinophilia. Loeffler's syndrome as originally described was probably caused by *Ascaris* pneumonia and a similar condition is found in pigs infected with *A. suum*. Since *A. suum* is infective for man it is a reasonable assumption that a significant proportion of respiratory illness experienced by people in contact with pigs is caused by *A. suum*.

Koino, a Japanese investigator, swallowed 2000 ripe human *Ascaris* eggs and 6 days later he was attacked by definite pneumonia with dyspnoea, cyanosis, eosinophilia and pyrexia, which lasted 7 days. The sputum was profuse from the eleventh to the sixteenth day and contained *Ascaris* larvae, of which 202 were counted. The liver was enlarged. Fifty days after infection 667 *Ascaris* worms were voided. Loeffler (1956) concluded that the majority of cases of Loeffler's syndrome were due to larval *Ascaris*. Pulmonary eosinophilia with X-ray signs of infiltration of the lungs was reported in a family of 3 who had eaten strawberries manured with infected faeces, and Beaver and Danaraj (1958) described an adult Indian who died in status asthmaticus in whom the lungs showed eosinophilic infiltration with fourth stage larvae of *A. lumbricoides* in the bronchioles. Small areas of necrosis with eosinophil cells were found in the liver. *Ascaris* pneumonia occurs after a heavy primary infection, and outbreaks of acute pneumonitis in Saudi Arabia have been due to larval ascariasis (Gelpi & Mustafa 1967). There is fever, asthma and an intense eosinophilia of short duration. Migrating larvae have been recovered from aspirated gastric juice and sputum. This condition may be distinguished from tropical pulmonary eosinophilia of filarial origin by the shorter duration of the eosinophilia and pulmonary infiltration which occurs with *Ascaris*. If the larvae reach the general circulation they may cause symptoms, depending upon their localization, which may resemble those of visceral larva migrans due to *Toxocara canis*.

Neurological disorders associated with the larvae of *Ascaris* include convulsions, meningism and epilepsy. Palpebral oedema may occur; restless sleep and tooth-grinding during the night are common. The larvae may wander into unnatural locations such as the brain or eye and cause granulomas so that larval ascariasis may simulate toxocariasis.

Adult worms

The passage of adult worms in sensitive persons may cause intolerable itching at the anus. Vomiting of worms may cause oedema of the glottis.

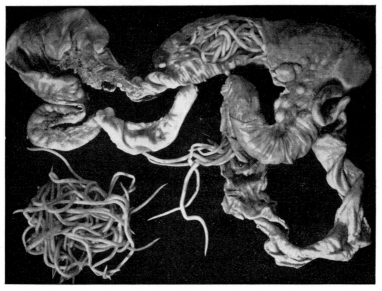

Fig. 94.—Impacted mass of ascarids in the small intestine, causing fatal intestinal obstruction. (*Atlas of Pathological Anatomy. Milan: Cioni & Palazzi*)

The effect of the adults on the intestinal tract can be severe in heavy infections. The most common complaint is intestinal colic. Aggregate masses of worms may cause volvulus or intestinal obstruction (Fig. 94) and intussusception. Wandering ascarids may reach abnormal foci and cause acute symptoms: ileus resulting from mechanical obstruction, perforation of the bowel usually in the ileocaecal region, acute appendicitis caused by a worm in the appendicular lumen, diverticulitis, gastric or duodenal trauma, blockage of the ampulla of Vater or common bile duct and obstructive jaundice, entry into the parenchyma of the liver and abscess of the liver, invasion of the genital tract, haemorrhagic pancreatitis and oesophageal perforation. In small children ascariasis is frequently complicated by larval toxocariasis (visceral larva migrans).

Ascaris liver abscess and biliary ascariasis. *Ascaris* liver abscess is caused by *Ascaris* worms migrating up the common bile duct into the liver and dying. A granulomatous reaction occurs, followed by degeneration of the worm and release of the eggs which may be demonstrated in the abscess, where they are changed by digestion of the outer coat and appear as smooth oval bodies. In some parts of the world *Ascaris* liver abscess is commoner than amoebic abscess in young children.

Biliary ascariasis has been described from the Philippines where 20% of patients treated surgically for biliary disease had live or dead *Ascaris* worms in the biliary tracts (Horrilleno *et al.* 1964). Upper abdominal colic, jaundice and a palpable gall-bladder were common. Biliary tract infections occurred and *Ascaris* worms could be demonstrated by intravenous cholangiography. At post mortem cholangitis or hepatic abscess were found. Good results followed anthelmintic therapy.

Indirect effects

There is some evidence that helminthic larvae may carry micro-organisms when they migrate from the intestines to other tissues.

Nutritional relationships

Ascariasis may contribute to protein–calorie malnutrition. From calculations in an experimental study in man (Venkatachalam & Patwardhan 1953) it has been estimated that in children infected with 13–40 worms approximately 4 grammes of protein are lost per day from a daily diet containing 35–50 grammes of protein. Kwashiorkor has been associated with *Ascaris* infection from the time when it was first recognized as a nutritional syndrome. *Ascaris* infection may contribute to vitamin A deficiency, and children suffering from night blindness have shown rapid improvement in their eye symptoms within a few days of therapeutic elimination of the worms. Infected children have also been shown to excrete a significantly lower amount of vitamin C after a test dose of ascorbic acid.

DIAGNOSIS

Established infections

Diagnosis is made by finding ova in the stools and various concentration methods may be employed (Appendix II). *Ascaris* infection is only associated with eosinophilia in the tissue stages. In established intestinal infections the eosinophil count is either normal or only slightly increased. If there is a marked eosinophilia then an associated toxocariasis or strongyloidiasis must be suspected. X-ray examination of the abdomen can be employed in diagnosis and films taken 4–6 hours after an opaque meal display the worms as cylindrical filling defects or as string-like shadows produced by the opaque substance which the worms have swallowed (Fig. 95).

Larval infections

The diagnosis of larval infections is made clinically. In *Ascaris* pneumonia the bronchial washings may show third-stage larvae. The *Ascaris* complement fixation test is of little use since it shows cross-reactivity with the filarial complement fixation test.

TREATMENT

Treatment is effective only against the adult worms. None of the anthelmintics has proved successful in killing the migrating larvae.

In any child with *Ascaris* infection who develops a febrile condition from whatever cause the *Ascaris* should be promptly treated since a rise in body temperature stimulates the migration of adult worms from the intestine to abnormal foci.

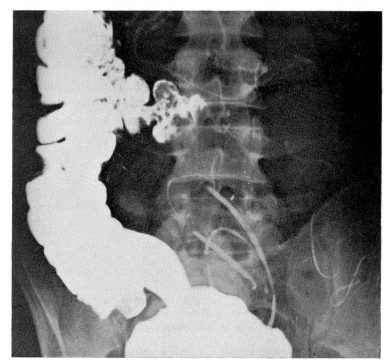

Fig. 95.—Radiographic appearances of *Ascaris lumbricoides* in the small intestine. Barium meal after evacuation. Note the worms in various stages. The barium is retained in the intestine of the worm, thus giving it a linear appearance. (*Dr T. V. Crichlow*)

Piperazines

Piperazine citrate, adipate and phosphate are equally effective *in vitro* in causing a neuroconductive block and inducing a state of narcosis in the worms. The sparingly insoluble adipate is absorbed much less than the citrate and phosphate. Piperazine compounds occasionally cause temporary attacks of ataxia and muscular hypotonia (Parsons 1971).

Piperazine citrate (Antepar). The citrate in the syrup form (Antepar) is recommended for general use. 5 ml contain the equivalent of 750 mg of the hydrate. It is given as a single dose before the evening meal and a saline purge may be given the following morning where the patient is known to be constipated. The dose of Antepar may be calculated as follows:

Body weight (kg)	Dose (ml)
5–9	5–10
10–14	15
15–19	20
over 20	30

Piperazine adipate (Entacyl). Entacyl is just as efficacious as the citrate. It is given in tablets of 300 mg. The total dose for children is 750 mg for each year of life up to 6 years, and a total dose of 4–5 grammes thereafter, given in 4 divided doses in one day.

Tetrachlorethylene

This drug is given as for ancylostomiasis (page 260) and may be used in areas where there is not enough money to buy the piperazine compounds.

Tetramisole cyclamate (R 8299)

This has been used effectively in the treatment of ascariasis in a single dose of a tablet containing 150 mg of the active substance (Huggins *et al.* 1967).

PREVENTION

Three approaches to *Ascaris* control have proved valuable:

1. The mass treatment of infected populations.
2. Measures to prevent environmental contamination with human faeces.
3. Education of the public in personal hygiene.

Mass chemotherapy

Mass chemotherapy will only produce benefits if the treatment programme is continued until the transmission rate is reduced to a level too low for widespread reinfection to occur. Japanese experience has shown that a prevalence of 63% in 1949 could be reduced to 5·3% in 1964. In this campaign as the prevalence decreased the dose frequency was reduced from twice or three times a year to once or twice yearly. Piperazine preparations, especially the citrate syrup, are the drugs of choice.

The frequency of administration will be dictated by the pattern of transmission. Where transmission is seasonal, treatment should begin 4–6 weeks after transmission starts and be given every 2 or 3 months while transmission lasts and continue for 2 months after the end of the transmission season.

Piperazine citrate syrup (Antepar) is given as a single dose up to 30 ml as previously described. If it is impractical to consider mass chemotherapy for the entire population those age-groups which exhibit the maximum intensity of infection, usually the pre-school children, should be chosen.

Environmental measures

The basic environmental measures will be concerned with the safe disposal of human excreta, the provision of adequate and safe water supplies and the prevention of food contamination by faecal material.

Health education

Health education should be based on what the people need to know, what they can do for themselves and what motivates them to participate actively.

This will need a preliminary sociological survey to determine how the programme should be developed.

Toxocariasis

Synonyms

Visceral larva migrans, granulomatous ophthalmitis, ocular toxocariasis.

Definition

Toxocariasis is the condition caused by the invasion of human tissues by the larvae of nematodes normally parasitic in lower mammals, of which the dog and cat ascarids *Toxocara canis* and *T. cati* are the commonest. Visceral larva migrans is applied to the clinical syndrome caused by visceral toxocariasis, and ocular toxocariasis or granulomatous ophthalmitis results from invasion of the eye.

HISTORY AND GEOGRAPHICAL DISTRIBUTION

Visceral larva migrans has been recognized as a clinical entity since Beaver *et al.* (1952) discovered its aetiology. Cases have been described from the southern and eastern United States, Puerto Rico, Holland, Great Britain, Mexico, Hawaii, the Philippines, Australia, South Africa and possibly Eastern Europe. Granulomatous ophthalmitis caused by *Toxocara* was first described by Wilder (1950), and was first recognized in Britain by Ashton (1960).

AETIOLOGY

Visceral larva migrans and granulomatous ophthalmitis are caused by the dog ascarid *T. canis* and occasionally the cat ascarid *T. cati*. Infective stage eggs are ingested by an unnatural host such as man. These hatch in the upper intestine, invade the intestinal wall and are carried via the mesenteric venules and lymphatics to the intestinal viscera. In the capillaries of the liver, but also to a less extent those of the lungs, brain, eye and other organs, the larvae are surrounded by a host cell reaction of a granulomatous nature which blocks their further migration.

In the unnatural host the larvae do not grow or moult but can remain alive for as long as 11 years as has been shown in a monkey. Whereas non-human strains of hookworm larvae, *Ancylostoma braziliensis* and *A. caninum,* invade the skin and cause cutaneous larva migrans, it is possible that they may enter man via the intestinal tract and form granulomas in the viscera. Intestinal auto-infection with *Strongyloides stercoralis* may produce a similar picture.

IMMUNOLOGY

The tissues of the abnormal host are sensitized to the parasite, which process is mainly responsible for the pathological changes produced. Serum antibodies, which have been used in diagnosis, are formed. In contrast to tropical eosinophilia there is a quantitative increase in the immunoglobulins. The IgM is increased, and includes an anti-γ-globulin factor which will agglutinate latex particles coated with γ-globulin. These latex factors disappear on clinical recovery (Huntley *et al.* 1966).

The serology of visceral larva migrans has been studied in haemagglutination and flocculation tests with various *Ascaris* antigens. Activity has been demonstrated, but there is no specificity between *Toxocara* and *Ascaris* (Kagan *et al.* 1959). Fluorescent antibodies are present and qualitative absorption of *Ascaris* antibodies has been successful (Bisseru & Woodruff 1968). Skin sensitivity tests have been used in diagnosis (Woodruff & Thacker 1964). Adult *Toxocara* antigens are relatively unpurified and cross-react with *Ascaris*. Antigens have been prepared from second stage larvae grown in mice and used in diagnosis.

EPIDEMIOLOGY

T. canis is a common inhabitant of adult dogs and puppies. Puppies are infected by second stage larvae in utero and are born with established intestinal infections. The puppies excrete eggs on to the ground which are ingested by small children along with *Ascaris* and *Trichuris* ova, and in urban areas in the U.S.A. lead products found in old paint. Toxocariasis is invariably associated with *Ascaris* and *Trichuris* infection and in urban areas with signs of lead poisoning. The commonest age of infection is around $2\frac{1}{2}$ years and the infection is patent from about 3 up to 5 years of age. It is uncommon at a later age unless an unusual habit of dirt-eating is present, as in mental defectives. Ocular toxocariasis is found at a later age. A statistical association between the incidence of *Toxocara* infection as shown by skin sensitivity tests and poliomyelitis and epilepsy has been shown by Woodruff *et al.* (1966). This is probably due to the introduction of the viral agents from the intestine by the migrating second stage larvae.

PATHOLOGY

The numbers of granulomatous lesions which are responsible for the clinical signs and symptoms are directly related to the numbers of second stage larvae which invade the extra-intestinal viscera. The lesions may be miliary (Dent *et al.* 1956) or they may be few. *Toxocara* granulomas are found most frequently in the liver where they can be seen as white subcapsular nodules the size of millet seed. Other sites are the lung, kidneys, heart, striated muscle, brain and eye. The microscopic picture of the granulomas is a centre of closely packed eosinophils and histiocytes surrounded by large histiocytes with pale vesicular nuclei sometimes arranged in a palisade-like manner. There is an occasional atypical multinucleate giant cell.

In recent granulomas a living second stage larva may sometimes be found, but more frequently only the remains can be seen. In the eye the granulomatous reaction forms a large subretinal mass which may closely resemble a sarcoma and later causes a patch of choroiditis. Lesions in the brain can cause epilepsy.

SYMPTOMS AND SIGNS

The clinical features of visceral larva migrans are seen most commonly in young children. There is hepatomegaly, persistent hypereosinophilia, bronchial asthma and fever. There may also be pulmonary signs, cardiac dysfunction, nephrosis or evidence of cerebral lesions. There is hyperglobulinaemia with a considerable elevation of the IgM. The eosinophil count is greatly raised to from 10 000 to 20 000/mm^3. In some urban areas there are associated signs of lead intoxication, a blue line on the gums and anaemia with stippling of the red cells.

The retinal lesion presents as a solid retinal tumour often at or near the macula. In the early stages it is raised above the level of the retina and closely mimics a retinal neoplasm. Later when the acute phase has subsided the lesion remains a clear-cut circumscribed area of retinal degeneration. Formerly these lesions were designated tuberculous, exanthematous or neoplastic. If the lesion is central the visual acuity is reduced or central vision may be lost.

Strabismus due to macular damage is often the presenting symptom. Low-grade iridocyclitis with posterior synechiae may develop and progress to general endophthalmitis and detachment of the retina. The second stage larva may rarely be seen with a slit lamp microscope in the anterior chamber of the eye. Secondary glaucoma may result.

DIAGNOSIS

The only confirmatory diagnosis is the demonstration of the larva or portion of degenerate larva in serial sections of a liver biopsy or post mortem material. The larva or its remnants are found in the centre of the granulomatous lesion. There is no reliable serological test since haemagglutination tests give cross-reactions with *Ascaris* and *Strongyloides*.

Visceral larva migrans lasts for a period of at least 2 years and must be distinguished from larval ascariasis which lasts a much shorter time and the tissue stages of *Strongyloides*. It must also be distinguished from tropical pulmonary eosinophilia, which is mainly pulmonary and occurs in adults of Indian origin.

PROGNOSIS

In some cases the outcome is fatal but usually the condition recovers completely after a period of about 2 years. In ocular toxocariasis the vision of the eye may be totally destroyed.

TREATMENT

Two drugs are used in treatment:

(a) *Diethylcarbamazine* is given in doses of 200 mg 3 times a day for 3 weeks. Courses may be repeated.

(b) *Thiabendazole* has proved of some use in this condition. Dosage is 25 mg/kg body weight twice a day for 7–28 days (Nelson *et al.* 1966). The high eosinophilia may persist for months after apparent clinical cure, which is shown by subsidence of the fever and hepatomegaly.

The above treatments have arrested ocular toxocariasis with the preservation of whatever vision which remains.

PREVENTION

It is essential to safeguard young children from exposure to dogs, especially puppies, which may convey the infection even in flats. Regular anthelmintic treatment both of adult dogs and puppies (at birth) is necessary when there are young children in the house. Dogs should be denied access to sandpits and playgrounds in the back yard.

Ancylostomiasis

Synonyms

Uncinariasis, hookworm disease, hookworm anaemia.

Definition

An infection causing, in its more pronounced forms, anaemia due to blood loss from the intestine caused by *Ancylostoma duodenale* and *Necator americanus*, nematodes which inhabit the small intestine and may be present in enormous numbers.

GEOGRAPHICAL DISTRIBUTION

The hookworm occurs in all tropical and subtropical countries (Faust & Russell 1964).

A. duodenale is essentially a parasite of southern Europe, the north coast of Africa, Northern India, North China and Japan. It was introduced by migration into Paraguay *ca* 3000 B.C. by Japanese fishermen (Manter 1967) and is the predominant hookworm in coastal Peru and Chile. It has been introduced into Western Australia and into areas where *N. americanus* is the predominant human hookworm, southern India, Burma, Malaya, the Philippines, Indonesia, Polynesia, Micronesia and Portuguese West Africa.

N. americanus is the predominant hookworm of central and southern Africa, southern Asia, Melanesia and Polynesia. It is widely distributed in the southern United States, the islands of the Caribbean, central America and northern South America where it was introduced by slaves from Africa.

AETIOLOGY

The normal habitat of both hookworms is the small intestine of man and particularly the jejunum, less so the duodenum and rarely the ileum or lower reaches of the alimentary canal. Very occasionally they are found in the stomach.

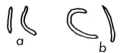

Fig. 96.—*Ancylostoma duodenale.* Natural size. *a*, Male. *b*, Female. (*Dubini*)

The male and female ancylostomes, present generally in the proportion of one male to three females, do not differ much in size. The male *A. duodenale* (Fig. 96) measures 8–11 × 0·4–0·5 mm, the female (Fig. 96) 10–13 × 0·6 mm. The worms attach themselves to the mucous membrane by means of their chitinous teeth or cutting plates, and suck the blood of the host.

N. americanus closely resembles *A. duodenale* but is shorter and more slender. The life history of these two parasites is identical (see Appendix II). The soil in the vicinity of living quarters in plantations and villages is contaminated with human faeces from which the infective larvae develop. Looss demonstrated that the larvae reach the intestinal canal by boring their way through the skin (*A. duodenale* larvae may also enter through the mouth). From the subcutaneous tissues they enter the blood vessels and lymphatics and by this channel are passively transferred to the lungs. Here they leave the capillaries, enter the air vesicles and thence along the bronchi and trachea pass into the oesophagus and so to the stomach.

IMMUNITY

Dogs develop a partial protective immunity towards *A. caninum* which in endemic areas can cause a 50% mortality from anaemia in early life. Pups that survive to adult life retain only minimal intestinal infection. After a single infection with 1000 irradiated *A. caninum* larvae a significant immunity can be demonstrated by worm counts following challenge with unirradiated larvae (Miller 1965). Primary infections in man may cause fever, eosinophilia and a moderate anaemia even when the infection is light. Such light infections do not cause symptoms of anaemia in the indigenous inhabitants of endemic areas, suggesting that a partial immunity has developed. Immediate hypersensitivity develops in hookworm infections and a skin test using an antigen prepared from *N. americanus* larvae has been used in Venezuela to indicate both prevalence and load of hookworm infection (De Hurtado & Layrisse 1968).

EPIDEMIOLOGY

The only reservoir of infection is man and the propagation of hookworm infection depends upon an adequate source of infection in the human population, the deposition of eggs in a favourable environment for extrinsic development of the parasite, appropriate conditions of the soil (moisture and warmth) to allow larvae to develop and suitable conditions for the infective larvae to penetrate the skin. In many tropical and sub-tropical countries transmission is perennial, but in cooler and drier climates transmission may take place in the warmer or wet seasons. In some temperate climates local environmental conditions may allow transmission, as in the Cornish tin-mines in the past and in the Rand in South Africa today. Cultural and agricultural practices such as the use of human faeces for fertilizer provide good opportunities for infection.

The methods which are employed to determine the amount of hookworm in a community are determination of the *prevalence* and *intensity* of infection by stool surveys and egg counts from which the worm burden can be calculated. These surveys will show whether the infection in the community is low grade, moderate or severe. Soil pollution in the area must also be studied and hookworm larvae may be recovered from the soil by the Baerman apparatus (Faust & Russell 1964). Studies of the nutritional level of the community, especially the haemoglobin level, must also be undertaken.

PATHOLOGY

Ancylostoma infection is entirely asymptomatic in the vast majority of cases, but where symptoms are produced these are at three stages of the infection:

1. Vesiculation and pustulation at the site of entry of the infective larvae (ground itch).

2. Temporary effect of the passage of larvae through the lungs—asthmatic bronchitis and eosinophilia.

3. Results of established infection in the small intestine—blood loss and vague abdominal symptoms.

The first and second of these stages are seen in individuals who receive a primary infection. These are usually Europeans or other expatriates arriving in endemic areas. The results of the third stage are seen in the inhabitants of endemic areas and lead to hookworm anaemia or hookworm disease.

Hookworm anaemia

The relationship of anaemia to hookworm infection has long been debated and the main theories which have been put forward as to the causation of anaemia are chronic blood loss and depletion of iron stores with deficiency of iron intake and toxic factors.

Hookworms have been shown to produce active suction impulses 120–200 times per minute and evidence indicates that the hookworm is indeed an habitual blood sucker or needs serum (Roche & Layrisse 1966). The blood loss has been estimated as 0·03 ml/day/worm in *N. americanus* and 0·15 ml/day/worm in *A. duodenale* infections (Roche & Layrisse 1966). There is a significant relationship between the level of haemoglobin and the worm burden, which depends upon the level of iron stores in the body (Foy & Kondi 1960). Hookworm anaemia is of the iron deficiency type and responds dramatically to iron salts by mouth, and also to removal of the hookworm burden, but after a much longer period. Light infections may cause anaemia where the iron intake is deficient and anaemia may also be caused in spite of the presence of an adequate iron intake provided that the worm burden is heavy enough.

Toxic factors. Little is known about the anaemia which develops in light primary infections. It may be related to that which develops in pups infected with *A. caninum* and be of immunological origin.

Steatorrhoea. There is a considerable amount of disagreement as to whether hookworm infection can cause malabsorption. Steatorrhoea has been reported from Ceylon in cases of *A. duodenale* infection which recovered after treatment of the hookworm infection (Rai *et al.* 1968).

In fatal cases the pathological changes are those of severe anaemia. There is plenty of fat in the usual situations. The appearance of plumpness is further increased by a greater or lesser amount of general oedema. There may be effusion in one or more of the serous cavities. The heart is dilated and flabby. The liver is fatty and the kidneys and all other organs pale.

If the post mortem examination has been made within an hour or two of death the ancylostomes in numbers ranging from a few dozen up to many hundreds will be found attached by their mouths to the mucous surfaces of the lower part of the duodenum, jejunum and perhaps the upper part of the ileum. If the examination has been delayed for some time the parasites will have loosened their hold and are then found lying in the mucus coating the bowel. Many small extravasations of blood, some fresh, others of long standing, are seen in the mucous membrane, and a minute wound in the centre of each extravasation represents the point at which a hookworm had been attached. Old extravasations are indicated by punctiform pigmentation. Occasionally streaks or large clots of blood are found in the lumen of the bowel and severe melaena may occur in children. The hookworms secrete some anticoagulant substance and may move from spot to spot, thereby increasing the damage and blood loss. The worms themselves may be seen in situ to show thin red streaks from fresh red blood in the intestinal canal; at other times they will be iron grey owing to the deposition of haemosiderin granules in the intestine.

SYMPTOMS

In the vast majority of cases of hookworm infection there are no symptoms, since these carriers have become well adapted to their infection which is not too heavy in the presence of an adequate dietary iron intake. Indeed, it has been suggested that the freedom from hookworm anaemia shown by the African population of South and Central Africa is due to the use of iron cooking-pots which is responsible for haemosiderosis. In East Africa, where other pots are used, there is no haemosiderosis but a considerable amount of hookworm anaemia.

Invasion stage

The full-blown picture of the early invasion stage may be seen in non-immune people. At the site of entry of the infective larvae there is a 'ground itch', which consists in an irritating vesicular rash limited to the exposed portion of the body, usually the soles of the feet or the hands. After 1–2 weeks pulmonary symptoms develop with a dry cough and asthmatic wheezing. Fever and a high degree of eosinophilia are found. These symptoms gradually disappear and ova of hookworm can be seen on or about the forty-second day after infection. The whole episode is self-limiting, lasting not more than 2–3 months.

Light infections

The main effects of light infections may be seen in Europeans and other expatriates who have arrived recently in an endemic area. The practitioner in the tropics should always be on the lookout for these cases, especially in children. Minor degrees of anaemia induce a tendency to fatigue and lassitude and digestive disturbances are common. Any of these symptoms in the presence of an eosinophilia should lead to the suspicion of infection. Sometimes a heavier primary infection will induce ground itch followed by fever, asthmatic bronchitis and a high eosinophilia which will be self-limiting.

Established infections in indigenous people

The essential symptoms of ancylostomiasis are connected with progressive iron deficiency anaemia associated with gastric and intestinal dyspepsia but not wasting. An early symptom is epigastric pain or discomfort which may be relieved by food and may be mistaken for duodenal ulcer. Although many people who suffer from irregular abdominal pain may show hookworm ova in the stools it does not necessarily follow that hookworm infection is the cause of the abdominal pain.

The taste may be perverted, some patients exhibiting and persistently gratifying an unnatural craving for such things as earth, mud or lime—pica or geophagy. The stools may contain blood and frank melaena may occur in children. The occult blood test is always positive in the stools in cases where symptoms are caused by hookworm.

When the iron deficiency anaemia develops then symptoms of anaemia occur. The mucous surfaces and the skin become pale. The face is puffy and the feet and ankles swollen. There are lassitude, breathlessness, palpitations, tinnitus and vertigo, mental apathy, depression and liability to syncope. There is often koilonychia. There is high output failure and haemic murmurs can be heard over the heart, seen to be enlarged on X-ray examination. Hookworm anaemia is a common cause of heart failure in the tropics and may easily be confused with rheumatic carditis. Ophthalmoscopic examination may reveal retinal haemorrhages. An irregular fever may be found in any severe anaemia.

The anaemia is typical of iron deficiency. The haemoglobin is reduced to a greater degree than the red cell count. The MCV is decreased and the MCHC may fall to as low as 22. The red cells show microcytosis and severe hypochromia. The serum iron is greatly reduced and the total iron binding capacity of the serum greatly raised, indicating that iron stores are very low. There is no marked poikilocytosis or leucocytosis, although there may be an eosinophilia of 7–14%. Because of the persistent anaemia, growth and development become stunted in children. Serum albumin is decreased.

The rate of progress varies in different cases. In some a high degree of anaemia and even death may result within a few weeks or months of the appearance of the first symptoms. More frequently the disease is chronic, ebbing and flowing or slowly progressing through a long series of years. Prolonged exposure in the European has led to the production of the 'mean white', stunted in both mental and physical capacities.

DIAGNOSIS

Provided it is suspected, ancylostomiasis is easily diagnosed. In expatriates in tropical countries, in patients coming from tropical countries and in miners who work in warm mines in cooler climates, anaemia with a concurrent eosinophilia should always suggest a microscopic examination of the faeces. In many of these patients concentration methods may be necessary such as zinc sulphate centrifugal flotation and formol ether concentration (see Appendix IV).

In established infections in indigenous people, where anaemia and other symptoms are being attributed to hookworm infection, an egg count should be undertaken and a rough estimate made of the number of adult worms.

The dyspeptic symptoms may simulate those of duodenal ulcer and it has been noted that sometimes free acidity shows a higher rise than that usually observed and that high levels may be maintained in spite of varying degrees of severe anaemia. If the eggs of *A. duodenale* or *N. americanus* are discovered and no other cause for the anaemia or digestive disturbances found, no harm is likely to result from treatment based on this supposition. The presence of occult blood and digestive disturbances has led to patients being subjected to partial gastrectomy for duodenal ulcer and the correct diagnosis only being made at a later date.

X-ray examination by barium meal is disappointing. The worms are not outlined by the opaque material, neither do they ingest the barium as does *Ascaris*. Rowland (1966a) found a close correlation between abdominal symptoms, radiological abnormality of the duodenum and haemoglobin level in hookworm patients.

TREATMENT

Treatment consists of elimination of the parasite and treatment of the anaemia. The parasite is best eliminated by tetrachlorethylene or bephenium hydroxynapthoate (WHO 1963). Tetrachlorethylene is especially effective against *N. americanus* and bephenium against *Ancylostoma*.

Elimination of parasites

Bephenium hydroxynapthoate (Alcopar). Alcopar was introduced by Goodwin *et al.* (1958) and is especially effective against *A. duodenale*. It is administered in the morning on an empty stomach in a single dose of 2·5 grammes of bephenium base (5 grammes of salt) for adults and half this amount for children under 2 years of age. It is apparently more effective if 3 grammes of the salt are combined with piperazine citrate. For children who are marasmic and anaemic the dose is 2 grammes of the salt daily for 4 days. Cases of *N. americanus* infection require 5 grammes of Alcopar daily for 3 days.

Tetrachlorethylene. Tetrachlorethylene may be given in a single dose of 2 or 3 ml for an adult in 2 portions, or 0·1–0·12 ml/kg body weight for a child, on an empty stomach without a purgative. It should not be given to persons with poor health or liver trouble.

Combined treatment with Alcopar and tetrachlorethylene is the most effective treatment for *N. americanus* (Rowland 1966b).

Thiabendazole. Thiabendazole in a dose of 25 mg/kg body weight twice daily for 2 days is effective against *A. duodenale.*

Tetramisole. Tetramisole is an effective drug for hookworm infections in a single adult dose of 2·5 mg/kg.

Anaemia

The essential basis of the treatment of the anaemia is to remove the hookworms as soon as possible and to give large doses of iron. In the vast majority of cases the anaemia responds well to ferrous sulphate 600–1200 mg daily by mouth for 3 weeks or longer. Patients whose marrow contains giant metamyelocytes also require folic acid. Where the anaemia is so severe as to threaten life, and there are signs of heart failure, transfusion of 300 ml of packed red cells should be given slowly, care being taken to avoid overloading the right side of the heart. Digitalization and diuretics may be needed.

Iron–dextran complex (Imferon) is very useful where there is difficulty in ensuring the regular administration of iron by mouth or where there has been vomiting. Treatment can be given on an out-patient basis by giving a transfusion of packed cells and the necessary amount of Imferon intravenously to raise the haemoglobin to the correct level, followed immediately by anthelmintic treatment. In those patients who had received intravenous as opposed to oral iron the haemoglobin remained high in spite of reinfection (Patel & Tulloch 1967). After this form of treatment oedema disappeared, enlarged cardiac shadows became normal, cardiac murmurs disappeared and previously palpable livers became impalpable.

PREVENTION

The basis of prophylaxis and control is the provision of proper sanitary arrangements for the disposal of faeces. This was the basis of the hookworm campaigns originally organized in the southern United States by the Rockefeller Foundation. However, the success or failure of these campaigns depended upon health education and the correct use of the latrines, and campaigns have often failed because this was not achieved.

Faecal contamination of the soil must be prevented and promiscuous deposition of faeces about huts, villages and fields must be forbidden. The Chinese plan of storing faeces for months in large cemented watertight pits is a good one since if the *Ancylostoma* larvae are kept in pure faeces they die in the absence of air and earth. After storing in this manner valuable fertilizer is secured for the agriculturist. In the tropics the larvae rarely survive longer than 6–8 weeks and do not wander outside a 10 cm radius, but can migrate to the surface from a depth of 90 cm.

After the provision of latrines, intensive mass treatment in America has been found most effective; however, mass treatment campaigns have failed in most of the tropics. The provision of cheap shoes to prevent infection has failed because they are not worn where they are most needed, that is at home.

The fortification of a staple diet with iron salts and phosphates has been suggested as a measure to build up the iron stores of the population in areas where hookworm infection is heavy and the dietary iron intake barely sufficient.

Cutaneous Larva Migrans

Synonyms

Creeping eruption, sandworm, plumber's itch, duckhunter's itch.

Definition

Creeping eruption is a cutaneous lesion resulting from exposure of the unprotected skin of man to the filariform larvae of canine, feline and occasionally
human strains of hookworm, and to human and non-human strains of *Strongyloides*. Fülleborn produced a creeping eruption in volunteers with infective
larvae of *Ancylostoma braziliensis* and Little (1965) produced a similar condition
with *Strongyloides myopotami* and *S. procyornis*.

AETIOLOGY

In nature creeping eruption is caused most commonly by the filariform larvae
of the cat and dog hookworm *A. braziliensis*, less commonly by *A. caninum* and
occasionally by the human hookworms, *N. americanus* and *A. duodenale*.
Creeping eruption of *Strongyloides* origin is caused by the human *Strongyloides*,
S. stercoralis, and by the non-human *Strongyloides* of the nutria and the racoon,
S. myopotami and *S. procyornis*.

Creeping eruptions of hookworm and *Strongyloides* origin must be distinguished from lesions caused by *Gnathostoma spinigerum* (see page 280), and
cutaneous myiasis caused by migrating fly maggots (see Appendix II). *Fasciola
hepatica* may be found under the skin and may give difficulty in diagnosis.

GEOGRAPHICAL DISTRIBUTION

Creeping eruption occurs in most warm, humid tropical and subtropical areas
and is especially common in the southern United States along the coast of the
Gulf of Mexico and Florida. It also occurs on the coasts of South, East and West
Africa and in Ceylon.

EPIDEMIOLOGY

Unprotected human skin is often exposed to soil grossly contaminated with
the faeces of cats and dogs underneath beach houses (plumber's itch), above the
high water mark on sandy beaches (sandworm) and on the mounds of nutria
and racoons in marshes (duckhunter's itch). Exposure is most common during
the summer and early fall.

PATHOLOGY

The filariform larvae of non-human hookworms are usually unable to
penetrate below the stratum germinativum of human skin. A tunnel is formed
with the corium as a floor and the stratum granulosum as a roof. Local eosinophilia and round cell infiltration occurs around the tunnels, which may persist
for months. Rarely the larvae reach the lungs where they cause transient
pulmonary symptoms and eosinophilia, and may be recovered from bronchial
washings. They do not mature in the intestine.

SYMPTOMS AND SIGNS

There is a red itchy papule at the site of entry, which becomes elevated and vesicular. The larvae move several millimetres to a few centimetres each day, and leave tunnels which become dry and crusted. The track is linear and twists and turns (Fig. 97). It causes an intense pruritus and the skin is scratched and becomes secondarily infected. The lesions may be single or multiple. The commonest sites are the hands and feet, but the abdomen is often infested in plumber's itch and the lesions may be very numerous indeed (Fig. 98).

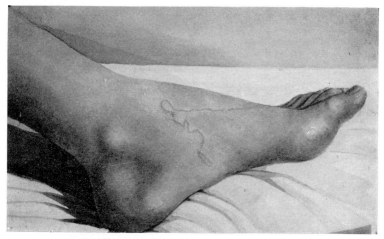

Fig. 97.—Larva migrans 4 months after probable infection at Durban. (*Philip Manson-Bahr*)

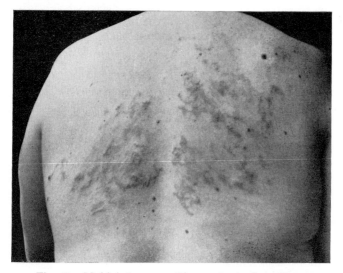

Fig. 98.—Multiple burrows of larva migrans from Ghana.

The lesions produced by non-human hookworms persist for many months, whereas those caused by *Strongyloides* last only a few weeks.

DIAGNOSIS

The diagnosis is clinical. There is usually no eosinophilia; if there is a high eosinophilia then migration of the larvae into the tissue should be suspected. There are no serological tests. It is not possible to extract and identify the larva, which is always ahead of its track.

TREATMENT

The treatment consists in the topical application of ethyl chloride or systemic therapy with thiabendazole. Local treatment consists in spraying the area with an ethyl chloride spray. Thiabendazole is given in a dose of 50 mg/kg daily in divided doses for 5 days followed by 2 days' rest and then a further 5 days' treatment may be necessary (Miller & Maynard 1967).

Itching ceases in 24 hours and the rash disappears in 10 days. *Strongyloides* responds better to this treatment than the non-human hookworms. Other dosage schedules are 50 mg/kg as a single dose, repeated each week until lesions disappear (Katz *et al.* 1965; London 1965); it may be given in divided doses for 2–4 days.

Trichinosis

AETIOLOGY

Trichinosis is caused by infection with *Trichinella spiralis* which is normally a parasite of carnivorous animals and their prey. The life history is described in Appendix II.

The adult parasite lives in the small intestine producing larvae which migrate to the muscles where they encyst, ready to be eaten by a new host which consumes the flesh of the first.

GEOGRAPHICAL DISTRIBUTION

Trichinosis is world-wide in distribution and is important as an infection of man in Europe and the United States. It is less important in the tropics and the orient but has recently been found to occur in both East and West Africa south of the Sahara.

EPIDEMIOLOGY

Man is not the normal host of *T. spiralis*, and only becomes infected when he eats raw or undercooked flesh. There are three main biological types of parasite. The usual type found in Europe and North America is an infection of the black and brown rats by which it is propagated. These rats are cannibalistic and may be eaten by domestic pigs which infect man when he eats raw or undercooked pork. This type is common wherever uncooked sausage is eaten, especially in Germany and other areas of the world to which Germans have gone, for example, North America and Chile.

Clinical illness is most likely to occur when sausage prepared from a single heavily infected pig is eaten by a family or community. Where the meat has been diluted by uninfected meat then the disease is mild or subclinical. In the U.S.A. 2 outbreaks occurred in 1956 and 1 in 1957 (Dauer & Davids 1959) and a severe epidemic occurred in England in Liverpool in 1953. Under the conditions developed by man for raising and fattening pigs, garbage which contains unsterilized pig scraps and other trimmings is the commonest source of infection in pigs in the U.S.A. at the present time. Another possible source is the ingestion of faeces of other infected animals, mice, rats, foxes and other pigs at a time when mature larvae are becoming established in the intestinal wall (Zimmerman et al. 1958). The majority of infections are symptomless and Link (1953) has estimated 350 000 new infections in the U.S.A. yearly of which only 16 000 produced symptoms. It is estimated that subclinical trichinosis can be demonstrated in 20% of the population in the U.S.A. and 1% in England by digestion of material obtained at autopsy.

The second biological type is found mainly in Alaska and the northern regions of the world (Rausch 1953). Here trichinosis is found in the white whale, walrus, hair seal, tree squirrel, black and white polar bear, dog, wolf, fox and wolverine.

The polar bear, which is at the top of the Arctic food pyramid, is usually heavily infected and is the usual source, along with the black and brown bear, of human infections. Bear meat is eaten as a luxury and as an essential food in polar regions and whole expeditions have died of trichinosis after eating polar bear meat. Maynard & Pauls (1962) have reported two epidemics in Alaska as a result of the consumption of black bear meat. In 1947 an epidemic occurred in Greenland with 300 cases and 33 deaths caused by eating walrus meat.

The third biological type is found in Africa south of the Sahara where it has recently been described from East Africa (Forrester et al. 1961) and Senegal (Onde & Carayon 1968). The infection is found in bush pigs (*Potamochoerus porcus*) and in the lion, leopard, cheetah and hyena. Man is infected when he eats the bush pig; domestic pigs are not infected. Nelson et al. (1961) think the *Trichinella* responsible is a distinct species.

IMMUNOLOGY

There is a well marked immunity to superinfection in trichinosis but it is necessary for the infective larvae to develop through to the adult stage before immunity is produced. Cell-mediated immunity is largely responsible for the immunity and Larsh (1967) has summarized the process. Immunized mice respond rapidly to a challenging infection, by an inflammatory reaction in the upper intestine with a rapid elimination of the adult worms. Cell-mediated immunity plays a prominent role in this process and can be transferred by cellular elements but is diminished by corticosteroids, adrenalectomy and whole body irradiation.

Humoral immunity

Serum antibodies develop during the infection and are important in diagnosis, but are not protective in any way.

In symptomatic cases whatever serological test is used there is a correlation between the incidence of positive reactions and the incidence of clinical disease. In asymptomatic infections when tests are used on surveys there is great difficulty in assessing the results, especially with skin tests.

A larval stage antigen is used and may vary from simple extracts in Coca's fluid to an acid soluble protein fraction, the Melcher antigen (Melcher 1943). Details of the preparation of the antigen are given by Kagan (1960).

The tests used in diagnosis are complement fixing, precipitin, flocculation, agglutination and fluorescent antibody tests. Complement fixing tests have largely been superseded by flocculation. Cross-reactions may occur with typhoid, tuberculosis collagen diseases and schistosomiasis, since schistosomal antigen can be used in the CF test.

Kline test. The Kline technique using an alkaline extract of lyophilized whole *Trichinella* (Suessenguth 1947) as antigen is satisfactory for the slide flocculation test. In a series of over 1000 human sera from diagnosed cases of trichinosis 97% were positive. False positive reactions in the general population ran at 10%, which is in accordance with the incidence of trichinosis in the general population in the U.S.A. (Norman *et al.* 1956; Kagan 1960).

Bentonite and latex flocculation test. The BFT and LFT are the tests of choice for the diagnosis of trichinosis in man. Bentonite and latex particles are added to *Trichinella* extract and glycerin saline solution.

Reagents are stable and the tests are easily and quickly performed. They detect antibodies during the acute stage of the disease (Anderson *et al.* 1963; Kagan 1960), becoming positive about day 15.

Charcoal agglutination test. The CAT is performed on plastic coated cards using cholesterol–lecithin crystals coated with a buffered saline extract of ether-treated *Trichinella* larvae to which charcoal has been added. This test is able to detect antibodies over an extended period of time.

Fluorescent antibody test (Sadun *et al.* 1962). Washed larvae from muscle tissue fixed in 10% formaldehyde in 0·5% bovine serum albumin saline absorb globulins from the test sera which are detected by fluorescent conjugated antispecies globulin sera. The antispecies serum may be replaced by a fluorescein conjugated anti-guinea-pig complement serum and the larvae exposed to the test serum in the presence of complement.

The FAT can only be performed in laboratories with trained personnel but serum extracted from dried blood specimens on filter paper can be used.

Intradermal test (Bachman test). Skin sensitivity, which is immediate, can be detected by using larval antigen 1 in 5000 to 10 000 dilution intradermally. A positive reaction appears in 15–20 minutes irrespective of the intensity of the infection. Skin sensitivity can persist for at least 10 years and as long as 20 years. When the test is used for survey purposes it is difficult to correlate positive results with the presence of infection. Cross-reactions occur with *Ascaris* and a higher incidence of positive reactions is seen in institutions than in the normal population. This test becomes positive about day 21.

PATHOLOGY

The capsule of the encysted larvae is digested in the intestine and the larvae escape at the level of the duodenum and rapidly penetrate the duodenal and jejunal mucosa where the amount of trauma and epithelial irritation is dependent on the number of invading larvae. In a period of 5–7 days the worms mature and mate and the females begin to discharge larvae into the tissues where they encyst in muscular tissues and set up an acute inflammatory reaction. When encystment is complete the local reaction subsides but generalized toxaemia becomes obvious. In the myocardium especially there is cellular infiltration, necrosis and fibrosis of the myocardial bundles in the wake of the passing larvae.

SYMPTOMS AND SIGNS

There are three stages in the development of the symptoms: (*a*) invasion (incubation), (*b*) migration of larvae, and (*c*) encystation of larvae and tissue repair.

During the incubation stage there is irritation and inflammation of the duodenal and jejunal mucosa where the encysted larvae penetrate the gut wall, with symptoms of nausea, vomiting, diarrhoea, colic and sweating resembling an attack of acute food poisoning, There may be a maculopapular eruption on the trunk and extremities. In a third of the cases respiratory symptoms occur between the second and sixth days and last about 5 days. During migration of the larvae through the tissues into the muscles there are muscular pains and some interference with muscular function, causing difficulty in breathing, mastication and swallowing. There may be some muscular paralysis especially of the extremities.

There is often a high remittent fever with typhoidal symptoms, splinter haemorrhages under the nails and there may be blood and albumin in the urine. There is characteristically a hypereosinophilia which appears by the fourteenth day and is normal by the twenty-first day. If it is absent this denotes a poor prognosis. The lymph glands may be enlarged and tender and the parotid and submental glands enlarged. Occasionally there is splenomegaly.

The 4 cardinal features at this stage are fever, orbital oedema, myalgia and eosinophilia. Severe forms have been described with haemorrhages beneath the pleura, in the stomach and intestines. Myocarditis is a most serious complication.

Larvae have been found in the cerebrospinal fluid without any cerebral or meningeal symptoms, but encephalitis, meningitis, ocular disturbances, diplegia, deafness and the syndrome of amyotrophic lateral sclerosis have been described. Larvae have been isolated from the peripheral blood by mixing blood with dilute acetic acid and centrifuging. The period of encystation is the critical third stage of the disease, with signs of severe toxaemia. There may be cachexia, oedema or extreme dehydration. The patient may collapse with a falling blood pressure. Damage to the brain may result in protean neurological signs which may clear rapidly or gradually or persist permanently. A Gram-negative septicaemia caused by the introduction of organisms with the larvae, and shock, has been reported (Punya Gupta *et al.* 1969). Spink (1935) reported a case of right-sided hemiplegia, and a case of Jacksonian epilepsy has been described as a sequel 10 years after active trichinosis.

With recovery the fever resolves but the muscular pains persist. Death may occur during the sixth or seventh week from exhaustion or complications such as lobar pneumonia, peritonitis or nephritis.

Subclinical trichinosis

The great majority of cases of *Trichinella* infections are asymptomatic and can only be detected by surveys of autopsies in the general population.

Chronic stage

When the larvae become encysted they remain alive in the tissues for many years and when calcified can be detected by radiological examination.

DIAGNOSIS

Suspected patients should be asked if they have eaten raw or undercooked pork.

The differential diagnosis is from many conditions because of the protean manifestations of the disease. Trichinosis may resemble typhoid and other fevers, nephritis, encephalitis, myositis and tetanus. The association of fever and eosinophilia may closely resemble the tissue stages of schistosomiasis (Katayama syndrome), hookworm, *Strongyloides* and other helminth infections and tropical eosinophilia. Collagen diseases may closely resemble trichinosis.

The main diagnostic features are the finding of larvae in the tissues of the muscles and diaphragm, and serology.

Trichinoscopy

The larvae can be detected in skeletal muscle by biopsy. Small samples of deltoid, biceps, gastrocnemius or, most conveniently, pectoralis major are obtained and digested in artificial gastric juice for several hours at 37°C and concentrated by centrifugation. Larvae can be seen in specimens pressed between two slides but not so easily as by concentration.

Autopsy material is obtained from the diaphragm. Light infections and the level of infection of the general population are assessed in this way.

Xenodiagnosis can be performed on diaphragmatic tissue by feeding material to uninfected albino rats and examining them one month later.

Biochemical tests

In the acute phases there are serum enzyme changes with a rise in the creatine phosphokinase, lactate dehydrogenase and myokinase levels (Hennekeuser *et al.* 1968).

TREATMENT

The aims of treatment are to counteract the toxaemia and the reaction of the body tissues to the invading larvae.

Steroids will produce a rapid amelioration in the condition of patients and may be life saving. In Kenya Forrester *et al.* (1961) used prednisone 20 mg 6-hourly for 3 days and 10 mg 5-hourly for 10 days. The only drug which has any effect on the invading larvae before encystment is thiabendazole; the dose is 50 mg/kg to a maximum of 3·0 grammes daily, given for up to 10 days and a maximum of 30 grammes (Hennekauser *et al.* 1968). This combined treatment will have a profound effect on all the signs and symptoms of acute trichinosis and should be used in all cases. In chronic trichinosis when the larvae have become encysted no treatment is necessary.

PREVENTION

The main method of prevention is thorough cooking of all meat and regular meat inspection by means of trichinoscopy of all pork. Effective treatment of pork may be instituted by means of refrigeration. Storage of pork in deep freeze units at −18°C to −15°C is effective. The cysts are destroyed by storage at −15°C for 20 days, −20°C for 10 days, −25°C for 6 and immediately by quick freezing at −37°C (Kagan 1959).

Cooking of all garbage will prevent the infection of pigs, and dressed pork may be irradiated by cobalt 60 or caesium 137 which kills the cysts. In the Arctic and sub-arctic regions bear meat should be avoided.

Strongyloidiasis

Definition

Infection of the small intestine and occasionally other tissues with *Strongyloides stercoralis*.

AETIOLOGY

Strongyloidiasis is caused by *Strongyloides stercoralis*, a nematode which has both free-living and parasitic forms. The complete life cycle (see Appendix II) (Fig. 99; Faust & Russell 1964) consists of one or more of the following phases:

1. Indirect development based on free-living growth outside the body, present primarily in the moist tropics.

2. Direct development responsible for human infection, which is the usual type present in temperate climates.

3. Auto-infection, where filariform larvae reinfect the host internally and perianally without leaving the host.

EPIDEMIOLOGY AND DISTRIBUTION

Strongyloides has a world-wide distribution in the tropics and the temperate climates. Man is the most important host, but dogs and chimpanzees have been found naturally infected with strains indistinguishable from those of man. The infective stage larvae develop in the soil and infect man via the skin. Auto-infection is responsible for infection in persons who have no direct contact with infected soil. In some areas the incidence of *Strongyloides* infection is similar to that of hookworm but this is not true in all areas. In parts of tropical Brazil, Colombia and Indochina strongyloidiasis is highly prevalent. *Strongyloides* is particularly common in institutions such as mental hospitals and prisons in warm, moist climates. It is more prevalent in adults but epidemics have occurred in homes for mentally retarded children. More recently strongyloidiasis has been a serious problem in individuals receiving immunosuppressive therapy, which reduces the natural resistance of the body to extensive tissue invasion by the adult worms.

IMMUNOLOGY

An immunity to reinfection develops in most individuals after the first primary infection, and the *Strongyloides*, adults and larvae, are confined to the intestine. Tissue hypersensitivity develops and eosinophilia and occasionally giant urticaria develop when a previously infected subject is exposed to reinfection. However, this immunity may be diminished by immunosuppressive drugs or malnutrition or overwhelmed by a massive infection which builds up with auto-infection from the bowel.

An extract of *S. ratti* has been used as an antigen for skin testing but the specificity is poor.

PATHOLOGY

The pathogenic effects begin with the entry of the infective larvae into the skin. The filariform larvae cause petechial haemorrhages at the site of invasion

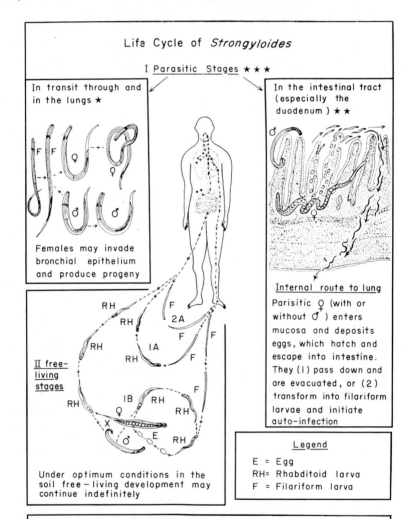

Fig. 99.—Diagrammatic representation of the potential whole life cycle of *Strongyloides*. In II, Free-living stages, X indicates fertilization of the female by the male worm. (*Reproduced from Faust & Russell (1964) Craig & Faust's Clinical Parasitology. Philadelphia: Lea & Febiger*)

accompanied by intense pruritus, congestion and oedema. The larvae migrate into cutaneous blood vessels and are carried to the lungs. In the lungs they enter the alveoli and pass up the respiratory tree where they may be delayed by the host response, become adults and invade the bronchial epithelium. Passing through the lungs the young worms may cause symptoms resembling those of bronchopneumonia with some lobular consolidation. When they have become lodged in crypts of the intestine the females mature and invade the tissues of the bowel wall but rarely penetrate the muscularis mucosae, and move in tissue channels beneath the villi, where the eggs are deposited. The eggs hatch out and the young larvae work towards the lumen of the bowel. In heavy infections sloughing of extensive patches of mucosa may occur. When the larvae reinvade the tissues autoinfection results. During their spread throughout the body they may carry micro-organisms from the bowel and an overwhelming septicaemia with *Escherichia coli* has been caused in this way. At times the filariform larvae fail to break out of the alveoli but gain access to the general circulation and may invade the brain, intestine, lymph glands, liver, lungs and, rarely, the myocardium.

SYMPTOMS

The vast majority of infections in endemic areas are symptomless. When for various reasons the number of *Strongyloides* present in the intestine increases then symptoms develop.

Diarrhoea

Watery mucous diarrhoea may develop, the degree of which depends on the intensity of the infection, its duration and the ability of the host tissues to encapsulate the worms. Frequently diarrhoea alternates with constipation. In asymptomatic or mildly symptomatic cases duodenal and jejunal biopsy has shown mononuclear and eosinophilic infiltration with positive tests for mucopolysaccharides and a collagen-like enzyme in the filariform larvae (De Paola 1961), and in heavy infections malabsorption may be found with the occurrence of a sprue-like syndrome.

Hypereosinophilia

When autoinfection takes place, hypereosinophilia and pulmonary symptoms resembling tropical pulmonary eosinophilia may occur.

Skin rashes

These are of two types. One occurring around the anus is a linear eruption which is a form of 'creeping eruption' resembling cutaneous larva migrans. The larvae move under the skin creating a pruritic reaction. The second form of skin rash is urticaria caused by allergy to the larvae penetrating the skin in an individual who has already been sensitized.

Massive strongyloidiasis

In persons debilitated by disease, malnutrition or serious illness, especially in institutions, serious illness and sometimes death may result from massive invasion of the tissues by *Strongyloides* (Bras *et al.* 1964). Treatment with immunosuppressive drugs for lymphoma and other conditions may produce the same result (Rogers & Nelson 1966). First stage larvae develop in the duodenum and jejunum, bore into the bowel wall, become adult and produce ova. In this way the number of *Strongyloides* is immensely increased and infective larvae invade the tissues and circulate, causing massive strongyloidiasis. There is a severe diarrhoea, often with malabsorption, oedema, liver enlargement and paralytic ileus. If treatment is not promptly instituted these patients will die.

DIAGNOSIS

Intestinal strongyloidiasis may be suspected where there is diarrhoea with epigastric pain and a high eosinophilia. The diagnosis is confirmed by recovery of adults or larvae from the stools or by duodenal drainage. The zinc sulphate flotation concentration method does not distort the larvae. *Strongyloides* may also be cultured from the stools (WHO 1963).

Eosinophilia

Towards the end of the early stage of infection a high leucocytosis up to 25 000/mm³ with 10 000 to 12 000 eosinophils/mm³ is characteristic. Later when the infection becomes chronic, there is neutropenia, and a moderate eosinophilia persists for years. In a chronic case a diminution of eosinophils is an indication of a poor prognosis.

Serology

The filarial complement fixation test is positive in 75% of cases of strongyloidiasis.

Course

Strongyloides may persist as an intestinal infection for many years in the absence of any reinfection from the outside. At any time the numbers of worms may increase and symptoms develop if the resistance of the host changes such as occurs during treatment with steroids. This is a real danger and any person who is on steroids should be checked for *Strongyloides* infection and treated with an anthelmintic.

TREATMENT

The drug of choice for the treatment of strongyloidiasis is thiabendazole.

Thiabendazole

The drug is given in a dose of 25 mg/kg twice a day for 2 days. This dosage cured all the patients treated (Most *et al.* 1965). Massive strongyloidiasis may respond dramatically to treatment with thiabendazole (Cahill 1967). Repeat courses are sometimes necessary.

Pyrvinium pamoate cured 87% in a single dose of 5 mg/kg (Most *et al.* 1965). Tetramisole is said to be effective in 56% of cases.

PREVENTION

The same principles as those adopted for the control of hookworm apply.

Trichuriasis

Definition

Infection of the caecum and colon with *Trichuris trichiura* (synonym *Tricocephalus dispar*), the human whipworm.

AETIOLOGY

Trichuris trichiura was first described by Linnaeus and has been found in the faeces of an Incan mummy (Faust & Russell 1964). The life history is described in Appendix II.

Pigs are commonly infected with *Trichuris suis*, and this has recently been shown to be easily capable of infecting man; a single dose of 1000 infective eggs produces a patent infection in volunteers, which can be detected 60 days later. The two species cannot be differentiated by routine parasitological methods. The implications of this finding are obvious.

EPIDEMIOLOGY

The human whipworm is cosmopolitan in distribution but is commoner in the warm moist regions of the world. In some hyperendemic areas 90% of the population are infected. In the southern part of the U.S.A. the incidence is 20–25% but the worm burden is low. The epidemiology is closely similar to that of *Ascaris*, and *Trichuris* infection is more or less coexistent with ascariasis and toxocariasis, although it is more prevalent in areas of high rainfall, high humidity and dense shade. Since infection results from the ingestion of eggs directly from the soil, the areas of high incidence and heavy worm burden are those polluted by small children who are more commonly affected than adults. Small children develop heavy infections (Jung & Beaver 1952) and the greatest prevalence is in children of primary school age who transfer fully embryonated eggs by their fingers to their mouths.

PATHOLOGY

The portal of entry into the human body is the mouth and the larva which escapes from the egg becomes attached as an adult to the intestinal mucosa in the caecum. When there are only a few worms there is little damage, but many worms cause marked irritation and inflammation of the epithelium of the caecum, appendix and ascending colon, which in some cases extends to the rectum (Fig. 100), causing dysentery and rectal prolapse (Jung & Beaver 1952). In heavily infected children in Louisiana there is a significant correlation between *Trichuris* and infection with *Entamoeba histolytica* (Jung & Beaver 1952), which may be a secondary invader of the ulcerated mucosa.

SYMPTOMS AND SIGNS

The vast majority of infections are light and cause no symptoms. In heavy infections the patient may show wasting with tenesmus and diarrhoea, blood-streaked stools and anaemia.

Hyperinfection results in rectal prolapse when the worms may actually be seen attached to the prolapsed bowel (Fig. 100). Some observers consider that epigastric pain and pain in the right iliac fossa with distension and flatulence are found in many cases (Swartzwelder 1939).

DIAGNOSIS

A heavy infection is indicated by a count of 30 000 or more eggs per gramme of faeces (Jung & Beaver 1952), which would indicate the presence of several hundred worms and the production of symptoms. Dysentery caused by *Trichuris* infection may be diagnosed by proctoscopy when numerous worms may be seen attached to a reddened and sometimes ulcerated rectal mucosa. In severe infections the clinical picture may resemble hookworm disease, acute appendicitis or amoebic dysentery. If there is a high eosinophilia then an associated *Toxocara* infection (visceral larva migrans) is most likely present.

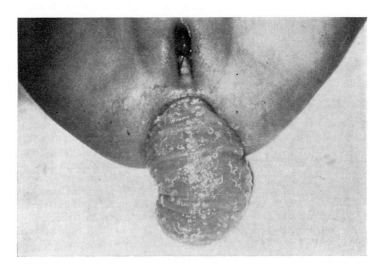

Fig. 100.—Prolapse of the rectum in a Louisiana child, due to heavy infection with *Trichuris trichiura*. (*Original photograph by Dr Paul C. Beaver and Dr Ralph V. Platou; copy by courtesy of Dr J. C. Swartzwelder. Reproduced from Faust & Russell (1964).*)

TREATMENT

The treatment of heavy infections of the rectum and colon with prolapse of the rectum is a high retention enema of hexylresorcinol: 1 gramme of hexylresorcinol crystals in 500 ml of distilled water with 50 grammes of powdered kaolin is administered and retained for 2–3 hours. The buttocks are first protected by applying a coating of petroleum jelly (Jung & Beaver 1952).

Thiabendazole 50 mg/kg is given in divided doses daily for 2 days and is sometimes effective in ordinary infections. Stilbazium iodide (Meropan) 20 mg/kg body weight twice daily for 3 days cured 80% of 40 patients (Huggins *et al.* 1969). *Trichuris* infection is, however, resistant to most anthelmintic drugs.

Capillariasis

Two species of *Capillaria* cause human capillariasis: *C. hepatica* and *C. philippinensis*.

C. hepatica

This worm is a relatively common parasite of rats and other mammals. Spurious human infections have been recorded when eggs of *C. hepatica* have appeared in the faeces. In genuine infections eggs do not appear in the stools. At least 10 cases of genuine infection have been recorded (Faust & Russell 1964).

The pathological and clinical picture is that of an acute or subacute hepatitis with eosinophilia, and there may be dissemination of the adults and eggs to the lungs and other viscera (Otto *et al.* 1954). The diagnosis is made on liver biopsy or at post mortem. There is no known treatment.

C. philippinensis

C. philippinensis was first described in 1963 and was named as a separate species by Chitwood *et al.* (1968). The eggs of the Philippine species are smaller than those of *C. hepatica* and measure 45·5 × 21 μm as compared with 52·5 × 28 μm in *C. hepatica*. They resemble the eggs of *Trichuris* but the polar plugs are flattened and much less prominent.

The method of transmission is unknown. One thousand cases with over 100 deaths have been recorded since 1963 (Dauz *et al.* 1967).

The adult *Capillaria* occur in the small intestine where they are found in the crypts without any inflammatory reaction around the parasites, which are found in enormous numbers; 40 000 adult worms were recovered from one case at autopsy. The worms cause malabsorption and there is flattening of the mucosa with extensive epithelial erosion and chronic inflammatory changes in the mucosa, which suggests serious interference with absorption and digestion.

SYMPTOMATOLOGY

In most cases there is persistent watery diarrhoea with rapid emaciation but no fever. This results in a severe protein-losing enteropathy and malabsorption of fats and sugars (Whalen *et al.* 1969).

DIAGNOSIS

The diagnosis is made by the presence of eggs in the stools; they must be distinguished from eggs of *Trichuris*. Cabrera and Silan (1968) have described an immediate skin sensitivity reaction with the intradermal injection of 0·5 ml of *Capillaria* antigen with a nitrogen content of 1 mg/ml. Of 60 cases 95% gave a positive reaction, but only 2% of 51 control subjects did.

TREATMENT

Restoration of the electrolyte imbalance and correction of the effects of malabsorption, combined with the anthelmintic therapy, is the aim of treatment. Thiabendazole 25 mg/kg/day for at least 3 weeks has proved successful (Whalen *et al.* 1969).

Enterobiasis (Oxyuriasis)

Synonyms

Threadworm, pinworm.

AETIOLOGY

Enterobius (Oxyuris) vermicularis is the cause, and the life history and morphology are described in Appendix II.

EPIDEMIOLOGY

Enterobiasis is world-wide in distribution. It is a group infection and is commoner in children than adults. It occurs especially in family groups or asylums. Transmission takes place in 4 main ways. The commonest way is by direct transmission of eggs from the anal and perianal region to the mouth by finger contamination. Schüffner (1944) considered soiled night clothes important and that this direct source of infection was common in groups of persons with similar habits. A second source of infection is exposure to viable eggs on soiled bed linen and other contaminated objects. The third source is air-borne eggs taken in by mouth; the fourth is retrofection (Schüffner 1944) in which infective stage eggs hatch on the anal mucosa and embryos migrate up the bowel.

Chimpanzees, gibbons, and marmosets can all be infected.

PATHOLOGY

The adult worm lives in the upper part of the large intestine, especially the caecum, and the lower ileum. Occasionally it is found in the female genital organs, rarely in the ear and nose. Minute ulcerations may develop at the site of attachment of the adult worms in the caecal and appendiceal mucosa. At times haemorrhages occur and secondary infection causes ulcers or submucosal abscesses. More usually symptoms are caused by gravid females which migrate out of the anus onto the perianal skin to oviposit and cause pruritus.

In the majority of infected persons there is no clinical evidence of infection.

CLINICAL FEATURES

Pruritus ani is the main symptom and varies from a mild itching to an acute pain. The pruritus provokes scratching of the perianal region and results in excoriation and secondary infection.

Appendicitis may result and adult worms are found in the lumen.

Vulvitis may be caused by worms entering the vulva causing a mucoid discharge, restlessness and insomnia.

The *general symptoms* are insomnia and restlessness and a considerable proportion of pinworm-infected children show loss of appetite, loss of weight, restlessness, irritability, emotional instability and enuresis.

Eosinophilia and *anaemia* are not pathognomonic.

De Ruiter (1962) has described local peritonitis with granulomatous lesions of the pelvic peritoneum due to *E. vermicularis* in various stages of development.

DIAGNOSIS

The diagnosis is made by finding eggs in the faeces, perianal scrapings or swabs from under the finger-nails or from finding adult worms migrating out of the bowel usually at night.

Faecal examination

Eggs are present in the faeces of no more than 5% of infected individuals. A Cellophane swab (Fig. 101) has been devised with which it is possible to obtain eggs by scraping the peri-anal area. Enclosed in a container, it may be sent through the post and examined at leisure. The Cellophane is mounted in water or *N* 10 NaOH on a slide, covered with a coverslip and examined.

The Scotch tape method, in which eggs adhere to a sticky surface, is very popular. A 5–6·25 cm strip is held sticky side out with forceps or placed over the butt end of a test-tube and rubbed over the peri-anal surface. A drop of toluene is placed on a glass slide and the tape to which the eggs adhere is spread on it and examined for eggs and adults.

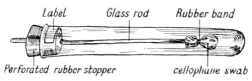

Fig. 101.—N.I.H. anal swab.

In the glass pestle method a piece of thick walled glass tubing about 1 cm in diameter with a globe at one end is used; half the surface is rough ground. The moistened globe is applied to the perianal skin with a rotary motion. The material is then dried on a slide and examined with cedarwood oil.

TREATMENT

Piperazine hydrate in the form of syrup at dose of 50–75 mg/kg daily for 7 days, repeated after an interval of 7 days if necessary, is effective. Piperazine citrate is available as Antepar elixir. Piperazine adipate (Entacyl) may be used in a similar dosage as tablets. Hexylresorcinol may be given as an enema as for *Trichuris* infection, or as hexylresorcinol crystoids in a dose of 1 gramme for adults, 600 mg for children under school age and 800 mg for those between 6 and 10 years of age.

PREVENTION

General measures must be taken. It is advisable to make the child sleep in cotton drawers and cotton gloves, to pare the finger-nails and to wash the hands frequently. Eggs are caught under the finger-nails in the act of scratching to relieve the itching round the anus and are easily transferred to the mouth. Other members of the family or school are likely to be infected.

Angiostrongyliasis

Synonyms

Eosinophilic meningitis.

Definition

A paratenic infection of man with the rodent lungworm *Angiostrongylus cantonensis.*

AETIOLOGY AND TRANSMISSION

A. cantonensis was described by Chen (1935) in the lungs of rats and the life cycle was worked out by Mackerras and Sanders (1955). The adult worms live in the pulmonary arteries of rodents where they lay eggs which hatch in the bowel and are passed out as first stage larvae. These enter the natural molluscan intermediate hosts where they develop into third stage infective larvae which are ingested with the molluscs by rats in which they migrate to the brain where they develop into adults and migrate to the pulmonary arteries.

Several species of molluscs (land snails and slugs) act as natural intermediate hosts, whereas certain species of land planarians and crustacea (crabs and freshwater prawns) are paratenic hosts in which the infection is a dead end.

In man, who is a paratenic host, the parasite does not undergo full development but dies out in the central nervous system where the eosinophilic response in the cerebrospinal fluid is a response to the metabolic products of death of the worm. Man acquires the infection by ingesting the tissues of infected molluscs, either improperly cooked intermediate hosts (snails and slugs) or paratenic or carrier hosts (crabs, prawns and land planarians).

EPIDEMIOLOGY

The rodents known at present as final hosts of *A. cantonensis* in nature are those of the genera *Rattus, Melomys* and *Bandicota* (Alicata 1969) and have been found infected in the tropical belt from 23°N. to 23° S. where there is a warm climate, moderate or heavy rainfall and abundant vegetation. Infected rodents have been reported from islands near East Africa and from South-east Asia and many islands of the Western Pacific, where the infection is associated with the presence of the giant African snail *Achatina fulica*. Alicata (1966) has produced evidence suggesting that angiostrongyliasis is a relatively new infection in the Pacific and has been introduced as a result of the spread of *Achatina fulica* to this area.

The first human cases of angiostrongyliasis were recognized on Ponape (Bailey 1948), and *A. cantonensis* was first recovered from the human brain in Hawaii (Rosen *et al.* 1962).

Eosinophilic meningitis has been found to occur in Thailand, Vietnam, Cambodia, Sumatra, Philippine islands, Taiwan, New Caledonia, Micronesia, New Hebrides, Cook Islands, Tahiti and Hawaii.

The method of infection varies in different areas of the Pacific according to the local cultural customs. In Tahiti raw freshwater prawns are consumed at feasts as special sauces from March to June which is the season of maximum incidence and small epidemics may occur (Alicata & Brown 1962). In New Caledonia the disease is acquired by eating land planaria or small molluscs on raw vegetables and the maximum incidence is during the vegetable season, June to November. Elsewhere the disease is sporadic and in Micronesia infection may have occurred as a result of eating certain species of mangrove crabs (Alicata 1969). Males and females are affected equally except under the age of 15, when twice as many males as females are affected.

IMMUNITY

There is no immunity to reinfection and second and third attacks have been described. During infection skin hypersensitivity develops and this can be measured by an intradermal test using dried adult *A. cantonensis* worm. There is, however, little specificity and cross-reactions with other helminths occur. A complement fixation test using adult worm as antigen is being developed as a diagnostic test.

PATHOLOGY

The pathological changes are associated with dead and degenerating worms. In some human cases which have come to autopsy both viable and degenerate worms have been found in the brain tissue and subarachnoid spaces. Granulomatous lesions composed of eosinophils and occasional giant cells have been described in the absence of any worms (Weinstein *et al.* 1963), and dead worms have been seen surrounded by granulomas and a diffuse eosinophilic infiltration of the meninges with many Charcot–Leyden crystals. Tracks have been found in the brain substance (Tangehai *et al.* 1967) and some tissue necrosis around dead worms (Rosen *et al.* 1967).

SIGNS AND SYMPTOMS

The disease as seen in the Pacific is of relatively short duration and terminates spontaneously without residual paralyses in the majority of cases.

At first there is headache and neck stiffness with paraesthesiae in the limbs in 50% of cases. Cranial nerve palsies, especially of the 7th nerve are common. There is a peripheral eosinophilia and the cerebrospinal fluid shows a pleocytosis with 50–75% of eosinophils in the majority of cases. Sequelae are relatively rare but may persist for several years and 3% of the patients in Tahiti showed a residual facial paralysis (Rosen *et al.* 1967).

It is not clear whether the infection is ever fatal since post mortem examinations have only been described among the inmates of mental institutions and it is not clear whether these findings are incidental to some other mental condition or have all been caused by *Angiostrongylus* infection.

DIAGNOSIS

Any patient in the Pacific exhibiting a brain syndrome with peripheral and cerebrospinal eosinophilia should be suspected of angiostrongyliasis. Other helminthic causes of a similar condition are gnathostomiasis (page 280) in South-east Asia, paragonamiasis (page 327), *Coenurus cerebralis*, hydatid disease of the brain, *Schistosoma japonicum*, ascariasis, trichinosis and disseminated strongyloidiasis. If there is an eosinophilic pleocytosis of the C.S.F. then *Angiostrongylus* or *Gnathostoma* should be seriously considered. If the intradermal test using *Angiostrongylus* antigen is negative then this infection may be ruled out (Alicata & Brown 1962).

TREATMENT

Since the pathology is caused by the death of worms there is considerable doubt as to whether any attempt should be made to kill them with drugs. Thiabendazole is active against migrating larvae in rats and might be effective in man. Marked relief of symptoms with prednisone 30 mg daily has been recorded by Cuckler *et al.* (1965).

PREVENTION AND CONTROL

Infected slugs and snails may be demonstrated by mincing them with scissors and digesting the material overnight with pepsin at 25–28°C. The larvae recovered from this material are used to inoculate white rats and the faeces are examined for first stage larvae after 40–60 days. Later the rats may be killed and the pulmonary arteries examined for adult worms.

Control methods should include public education into the manner of spread of the infection, proper cooking or freezing of crustaceans (-15°C for 12 hours), and proper washing and inspection of vegetables intended to be eaten raw (Alicata 1969).

Anisakis Infection (Herring Worm Disease)

Anisakis is an intestinal parasite of sea mammals such as the porpoise and seal. The larval stages are found in herrings and other fish which are consumed raw in some Scandinavian countries, Holland and Japan (Yokogawa & Yoshimura 1967). The larval stages may infect man in whom they cause intestinal colic, fever, eosinophilic intestinal abscesses and intestinal obstruction. Two deaths and one case of peritonitis have been described (Van Thiel *et al.* 1960).

The diagnosis is difficult, and has been studied by different immunological techniques (Suzuki 1968). Cross-reactions with *Ascaris* are common, but the indirect haemagglutination test gave higher titres with *Anisakis* than with *Ascaris* antibodies.

Gnathostomiasis

AETIOLOGY

Gnathostomiasis in man is caused by infection with the larval stage of *Gnathostoma spinigerum*, the adult stages of which are normally found in tumours in the stomach of wild and domestic cats and dogs. *G. hispidum* has been found once in a Japanese, twice as a human infection in India and once in a case of ocular gnathostomiasis in Canton.

TRANSMISSION AND EPIDEMIOLOGY

The life history of *G. spinigerum* is given in detail in Appendix II.

Eggs are extruded from the lesions in the stomach of the definitive host and are passed into water where they embryonate and hatch. The larvae are ingested by a *Cyclops* (first intermediate host) in which they develop into second stage larvae and are then eaten by a fish, frog or snake (second intermediate host) in which a third stage larva develops in the flesh. The second intermediate host is then eaten by a dog or cat and the adult stage develops in the stomach wall.

Man is infected by eating inadequately processed or cooked fish containing the third stage larva which is not fully adapted to man and in whom it migrates through the tissues causing gnathostomiasis externa.

Man cannot be infected from swallowing *Cyclops* (Miyazaki 1966). Two species of fish are mainly responsible in Japan for human infection, *Ophicephalus argus* and *O. tadianus*. In Thailand *O. striatus* is responsible.

Gnathostomiasis is commonest in Thailand but it is also found in Vietnam and some cases have been recorded from India and Malaya.

PATHOLOGY

The immature third stage larva migrates through the tissues causing relatively superficial lesions in the skin, subcutaneous tissues, muscles and more rarely the viscera and brain. Characteristically two types of lesion are found: a stationary type with abscesses and a migrating type in which deep subcutaneous channels form in which the larva migrates (larva migrans). When under the skin the larvae are found in the layer between the stratum germinativum and the corium, surrounded by eosinophils and plasma cells. Abscesses may form in any part of the body, in the breast, finger or muscles, and the tunnels may occur in the brain (cerebral gnathostomiasis).

CLINICAL FEATURES

A good account is given by Swanson (1971).

Gnathostomiasis interna

The onset of symptoms has been reported as soon as 24–48 hours after the ingestion of infected food. Symptoms start with nausea and vomiting, urticaria and eosinophilia, up to 90%. The cutaneous eruption is characteristic, with circumscribed oedema on the abdomen. Right upper quadrant pain indicates penetration of the liver and during the next few weeks attacks of pain may suggest episodes of acute cholecystitis or pulmonary lesions, with X-ray findings suggesting tuberculosis as the larva moves through the internal organs.

Within in a month the larva finds its way to a subcutaneous site, commonly on the chest, abdomen, upper extremities, head or thighs (gnathostomiasis externa). The systemic symptoms and eosinophilia subside after the subcutaneous localization of the parasite.

Gnathostomiasis externa (larva migrans)

The subsequent course is characterized by migrating intermittent subcutaneous oedema as the larva moves from one area to another, leaving a track of subsiding oedema in its wake. The episodes of swelling last 7–10 days, recurring at intervals of 2–6 weeks, which later increase. The larva may persist for as long as 10 years.

Cerebral gnathostomiasis in Thailand is a growing cause of focal cerebral lesions, often with coma resembling cerebrovascular accidents. There is marked peripheral eosinophilia, and the C.S.F. may show an eosinophilic pleocytosis.

Ocular gnathostomiasis (Chapter 44), involvement of the eye, with uveitis and retro-orbital swelling, is not uncommon.

DIAGNOSIS

Gnathostomiasis externa must be distinguished from other forms of larva migrans caused by human and non-human hookworms, cutaneous myiasis and the cutaneous lesions of paragonimiasis and sparganosis.

Cerebral gnathostomiasis must be distinguished from angiostrongyliasis and other causes of an eosinophilic meningo-encephalitis (see Angiostrongyliasis, page 277).

Intradermal test

An intradermal test using 0·05 ml of a 1/50 000 dilution of an antigen prepared from larval or adult gnathostoma gives a positive reaction in 15 minutes (Miyazaki 1960).

TREATMENT AND PREVENTION

There is no effective chemotherapeutic treatment. Worms must be removed. Infection can be prevented by the sterilization of fish, by boiling or immersion in vinegar for $5\frac{1}{2}$ hours.

REFERENCES

ALICATA, J. E. (1966) *Can. J. Zool.*, **44**, 1041.
—— (1969) *J. trop. Med. Hyg.*, **72**, 53.
—— & BROWN, R. W. (1962) *Can. J. Zool.*, **40**, 119.
ANDERSON, R. I., SADUN, E. H. & SCHOENBECHLER, M. J. (1963) *J. Parasit.*, **49**, 642.
ASHTON, N. (1960) *Br. J. Ophthal.*, **44**, 129.
BAILEY, C. A. (1948) *U.S. nav. med. Res. Inst. Proj.*, No. 005007, Report No. 7.
BEAVER, P. C. & DANARAJ, T. J. (1958) *Am. J. trop. Med. Hyg.*, **7**, 100.
—— SNYDER, C. H., CARRERA, G. M., DENT, J. H. & LAFFERTY, J. W. (1952) *Paediatrics, Springfield*, **9**, 7.
BISSERU, B. & WOODRUFF, W. W. (1968) *J. clin. Path.*, **21**, 449.
BRAS, G., RICHARDS, R. C., IRVINE, R. A., MILNER, P. F. A. & RAGBEER, M. M. S. (1964) *Lancet*, **ii**, 1257.
CABRERA, B. D. & SILAN, R. B. (1968) *Acta med. philipp.*, **4**, 157.
CAHILL, K. M. (1967) *Am. J. trop. Med. Hyg.*, **16**, 451.
CHEN, H. T. (1935) *Ann. Parasit.*, **13**, 312.
CHITWOOD, M. B., VALESQUEZ, C. & SALAZAR, N. G. (1968) *J. Parasit.*, **54**, 368.
CUCKLER, A. C., EGERTON, J. R. & ALICATA, J. E. (1965) *J. Parasit.*, **51**, 392.
DAUER, C. C. & DAVIDS, D. G. (1959) *Publ. Hlth Rep. Wash.*, **74**, 715.
DAUZ, U., CABRERA, B. D. & CANLAS, B., jun. (1967) *Acta med. philipp.*, **4**, 72.
DE HURTADO, I. & LAYRISSE, M. (1968) *Am. J. trop. Med. Hyg.*, **17**, 72.
DENT, J. H., NICHOLS, R. L., BEAVER, P. C. & CARRERA, G. M. (1956) *Am. J. Path.*, **32**, 777.
DE PAOLA, D. (1961) *Patologia da Estrongiloidiase*. Rio de Janiero: Clinica de Daencas Tropicais e Infectuosas da Faculdade de Medicina.
DE RUITER, H. (1962) *Ned. Tijdschr. Geneesk.*, **106**, 1811.
FAUST, E. C. & RUSSELL, P. F. (1964) *Craig & Faust's Clinical Parasitology*, 7th ed. Philadelphia: Lea & Febiger.
FORRESTER, A. T. T., NELSON, G. S. & SANDER, G. (1961) *Trans. R. Soc. trop. Med. Hyg.*, **33**, 503.
FOY, H. & KONDI, A. (1960) *Trans. R. Soc. trop. Med. Hyg.*, **54**, 419.
GELPI, A. P. & MUSTAFA, A. (1967) *Am. J. trop. Med. Hyg.*, **16**, 646.
GOODWIN, L. G., JAYWARDENE, L. G. & STANDEN, O. D. (1958) *Br. med. J.*, **ii**, 1572.
HENNEKEUSER, H. H., PABST, K., POEPLAU, W. & GEROK, W. (1968) *Dt. med. Wschr.*, **93**, 865.
HORRILENE, E. G., LIMBO, D. M., EUFEMIO, G. G., SILAO, J. U., jun. & GARCIA, A. H. (1964) *J. Philipp. med. Ass.*, **40**, 40.
HUGGINS, D. W., COSTA, V. D., FIGUEIRO, B., GURGEL, G. B. & ARRUDA, P. (1969) *Hospital, Rio de J.*, **75**, 511.
—— SIQUEIRA, M. W. & COSTA, V. D. (1967) *Hospital, Rio de J.*, **72**, 1577.
HUNTLEY, C. C., COSTAS, M. C., WILLIAMS, R. C., LYERLY, A. D. & WATSON, R. G. (1966) *J. Am. med. Ass.*, **197**, 552.
JUNG, R. & BEAVER, P. C. (1952) *Pediatrics, Springfield*, **8**, 548.

KAGAN, I. G. (1959) *U.S. publ. Hlth Rep.*, **74**, 159.
—— (1960) *J. infect. Dis.*, 107.
—— NORMAN, L. & ALLAIN, D. S. (1959) *J. Immunol.*, **83**, 297.
KATZ, R., ZIEGLER, J. & BLANK, H. (1965) *Archs Dermat.*, **91**, 420.
LARSH, J. E. (1967) *Am. J. trop. Med. Hyg.*, **16**, 1123.
LINK, V. B. (1953) *Pub. Hlth Rep.*, *Wash.*, **68**, 416.
LITTLE, M. D. (1965) *Am. J. trop. Med. Hyg.*, **14**, 1007.
LOEFFLER, P. (1956) *Archs int. Allergy*, **8**, 54.
LONDON, I. D. (1965) *Sth. med. J.*, *Nashville*, **58**, 1026.
MACKERRAS, M. J. & SANDERS, D. F. (1955) *Aust. J. Zool.*, **3**, 1.
MANTER, H. W. (1967) *J. Parasit.*, **53**, 3.
MAYNARD, J. E. & PAULS, F. P. (1962) *Am. J. Hyg.*, **76**, 252.
MELCHER, L. R. (1943) *J. infect. Dis.*, **73**, 31.
MILLER, M. J. & MAYNARD, G. R. (1967) *J. Can. med. Ass.*, **97**, 860.
MILLER, T. A. (1965) *J. Am. vet. med. Ass.*, **146**, 41.
MIYAZAKI, I. (1960) *Exp. Parasit.*, **9**, 338.
—— (1966) *Progress in Medical Parasitology in Japan*, Vol. III. Tokyo: Meguro Parasitological Museum.
MOST, H., YOELI, M., CAMPBELL, W. C. & CUCKLER, A. C. (1965) *Am. J. trop. Med. Hyg.*, **16**, 451.
NELSON, G. S., RICKMAN, R. & PESTER, F. R. N. (1961) *Trans. R. Soc. trop. Med. Hyg.*, **55**, 514.
NELSON, J. D., McCONNEL, T. H. & MOORE, D. V. (1966) *Am. J. trop. Med. Hyg.*, **15**, 930.
NORMAN, L., DONALDSON, A. W. & SADUN, E. H. (1956) *J. infect. Dis.*, **98**, 172.
ONDE, M. & CARAYON, A. (1968) *Bull. Soc. méd. Afr. noire Lang. fr.*, **13**, 332.
OTTO, G. F., BERTHRONG, M., APPLEBY, R. E., RAWLINS, J. C. & WILBUR, O. (1954) *Bull. Johns Hopkins Hosp.*, **94**, 319.
PARSONS, A. C. (1971) *Br. med. J.*, **iv**, 792.
PATEL, K. M. & TULLOCH, J. A. (1967) *Br. med. J.*, **i**, 605.
PUNYA, GUPTA S., COURODMITREE, C. & SIRIYADHAN, P. (1969) *J. med. Ass. Thailand*, **52**, 281.
RAI, B., SACHDEV, S. & GUPTA, S. P. (1968) *J. Ass. Physns India*, **16**, 765.
RAUSCH, R. (1953) *Publ. Hlth Rep. Wash.*, **68**, 533.
ROCHE, M. & LAYRISSE, M. (1966) *Am. J. trop. Med. Hyg.*, **15**, 1031.
ROGERS, W. A., jun. & NELSON, B. (1966) *J. Am. med. Ass.*, **195**, 685.
ROSEN, L., CHAPPELL, R., LAQUEUR, G. L., WALLACE, G. D. & WEINSTEIN, P. P. (1962) *J. Am. med. Ass.*, **179**, 620.
—— LOISON, G., LAIGRET, J. & WALLACE, G. D. (1967) *Am. J. Epidemiol.*, **85**, 17.
ROWLAND, H. A. K. (1966a) *Trans. R. Soc. trop. Med. Hyg.*, **60**, 481.
—— (1966b) *Trans. R. Soc. trop. Med. Hyg.*, **60**, 313.
SADUN, E. H., ANDERSON, R. I. & WILLIAMS, J. S. (1962) *Exp. Parasit.*, **12**, 423.
SCHÜFFNER, W. (1944) *Münch. med. Wschr.*, **31**, 411.
SOULSBY, E. J. L. (1957) *Br. vet. J.*, **113**, 439.
SPINK, W. W. (1935) *Archs int. Med.*, **56**, 238.
SUESSENGUTH, H. (1947) *Am. J. med. Techn.*, **13**, 213.
SUZUKI, T. (1968) *Jap. J. Parasit.*, **17**, 213.
SWANSON, V. L. (1971) *Pathology of Protozoal and Helminthic Diseases* (ed. Marcial-Rojas, R. A.), p. 871. Baltimore: Williams & Wilkins.
SWARTZWELDER, J. C. (1939) *Am. J. trop. Med.*, **19**, 437.
TANGEHAI, P., NYE, S. W. & BEAVER, P. C. (1967) *Am. J. trop. Med. Hyg.*, **16**, 454.
VAN THIEL, P. H., KUIPERS, F. C. & ROSKAM, T. H. (1960) *Trop. geog. Med.*, **12**, 97.
VENKATACHALAM, P. S. & PATWARDHAN, V. N. (1953) *Trans. R. Soc. trop. Med. Hyg.*, **47**, 169.
WHALEN, G. E., STRICKLAND, G. T., CROSS, J. H., ROSENBERG, E. B., GUTMAN, R. A. & WATTEN, R. H. (1969) *Lancet*, **i**, 13.
WEINSTEIN, P. P., ROSEN, L., LAQUEUR, G. & SAWYER, T. K. (1963) *Am. J. trop. Med. Hyg.*, **12**, 358.

WILDER, H. C. (1950) *Trans. Am. Acad. Ophthal.*, **55**, 99.
WOODRUFF, A. W., BISSERU, B. & BOWE, J. C. (1966) *Br. med. J.*, **i**, 1576.
WORLD HEALTH ORGANIZATION (1963) *Wld. Hlth Org. tech. Rep. Ser.*, 255.
―――― (1967) *Wld. Hlth Org. tech. Rep. Ser.*, 379.
YOKOGAWA, M. & YOSHIMURA, A. (1967) *Am. J. trop. Med. Hyg.*, **16**, 723.
ZIMMERMAN, W. J., HUBBARD, E. J. & MATTHEWS, J. (1958) *J. Parasit.*, **44**, 34.

12. TREMATODE INFECTIONS

Schistosomiasis

Definition

Schistosomiasis is the name given to a group of diseases caused by trematodes of the genus *Schistosoma*, for instance, in human infections, *S. haematobium*, *S. mansoni*, *S. japonicum*, *S. mattheei*, *S. intercalatum* and *S. bovis*. Man and other animals are definitive hosts and snails of various genera are the intermediate hosts. Certain related genera of trematodes, parasites of animals, cause skin lesions but do not mature in man.

Wilcocks (1962) discusses the history of investigations carried out in Africa on these diseases.

Table 11. Geographical distribution of *Schistosoma*

Species	Distribution
S. haematobium	Most of Africa, Madagascar, Mauritius, the Near East, Iraq, Arabia, Portugal (a small focus, now possibly extinct), India (a small focus in Bombay Province)
S. mansoni	West, Central, East and South Africa (but not Angola, though the relevant snail hosts are widely distributed there; the reason is not known), the Nile valley, Arabia, Yemen, Madagascar, South America, the Caribbean
S. japonicum	Japan, China (Yangtse valley, Fukien, Kwangtung, Yunnan), the Philippines, Celebes, Thailand, Cambodia (recently discovered)
S. intercalatum	The Congo area, Gabon, Cameroun
S. mattheei	South, Central and West Africa
S. bovis	Rare in man, in Africa

In 1965 the World Health Organization estimated that 180–200 million persons were infected throughout the world. In Egypt alone at least 37% of the 32 million population are said to be infected. Estimates of prevalence made on the basis of a single examination of urine or faeces understate the true position by at least 13–20%. The incidence is believed to be growing.

The geographical distribution of *Schistosoma* is shown in Table 11.

AETIOLOGY

For a description of these worms see Appendix II.

S. haematobium normally lives and mates in the veins of the urinary bladder of man (the only important definitive host), producing eggs with a terminal spine, which pass into the bladder wall and thence into the urine. Eggs are also often found in the mucosa of the lower bowel. *S. haematobium* has been regarded as a group of strains; it is transmitted by snails of the *Bulinus truncatus* and *B. forskali* groups (see Appendix II).

S. mansoni normally lives and mates in the veins of the mesentery of man and more rarely of some rodents and baboons, producing eggs with a lateral spine which pass into the wall of the large intestine and lower ileum, and thence into the faeces. Strains from Africa and from Puerto Rico differ in morphology, infectivity for snails and animals and pathogenicity. *S. mansoni* is transmitted by snails of the genus *Biomphalaria*.

S. japonicum normally lives and mates in the veins of the small intestine in man, cattle, water-buffalo, horses, donkeys, dogs, cats, rodents and monkeys, producing eggs with a small lateral knob-like rudimentary protrusion, which pass into the bowel wall and thence into the faeces. It produces eggs more prolifically than *S. haematobium* and *S. mansoni*.

There are several races of *S. japonicum*. The Taiwan race does not develop to maturity in man, but the Japanese, Chinese and Philippine races do, though they are not uniformly virulent. There are morphological differences between eggs of strains found in Cambodia and the classical strains. *S. japonicum* is transmitted by snails of the genus *Oncomelania*, except in Cambodia and Laos, where other snails are involved (Barbier & Brumpt 1969).

S. mattheei is essentially a parasite of sheep, goats, horses, cattle, baboons and wild game of South and East Africa. It lives in the mesenteric veins and produces eggs with a terminal spine. Human infection has been reported in 1% of persons with schistosomiasis in Rhodesia, and to the extent of 35-40% in cattle-owning people in parts of the Transvaal, always co-existing with *S. haematobium* or *S. mansoni*. Pitchford (1961) has produced evidence of possible hybridization between *S. mattheei* and *S. haematobium* in man. But Taylor *et al.* (1969) have shown that *S. mattheei* can produce eggs by parthenogenesis and suggest that in man cross-specific pairing takes place between female *S. mattheei* and male *S. haematobium* or *S. mansoni*, the males transporting the females to the bladder or bowel, and the females producing eggs characteristic of *S. mattheei*, most of which are non-viable.

S. intercalatum is a parasite of the *S. haematobium* complex, producing characteristic eggs with a terminal spine, but found exclusively in faeces. It lives in the mesenteric/portal venous system, not the vesical system.

S. bovis is a parasite of sheep and cattle, producing eggs with a terminal spine. It has occasionally been reported in man in Rhodesia, Uganda and other parts of Africa, but McMahon (1969) thinks that such infections are usually spurious, eggs appearing in the faeces of persons who have eaten the intestines of infected cattle. He has seen several subjects in whom eggs were found once but not subsequently. Nevertheless, the Uganda case was undoubtedly genuine (Raper 1951).

There are variations in the pathogenicity and infectivity of strains of schistosomes in man. The extreme example is the Taiwan strain of *S. japonicum*, which is prevalent in a wide range of animals but does not infect man or monkeys. Less pronounced variations occur in both *S. mansoni* (Saoud 1966) and *S. haematobium* (Wright & Bennett 1967). These varieties determine the infectivity to both the snails and the definitive host, and may be of considerable epidemiological significance (Nelson & Saoud 1968).

Miracidia hatched in fresh water from the eggs of schistosomes usually but not always respond to light, seeking the surface of the water, where the snail hosts mostly live. Snails inhabiting the bottom of canals have been found infected with *S. haematobium* and snails from the bottom of Lake Victoria, at a depth of about 12 m, have been found infected with *S. mansoni*. Snails frequently move up and down in water. From a single miracidium a snail may produce enormous numbers of cercariae, possibly as many as 100 000.

EPIDEMIOLOGY AND EPIZOOTIOLOGY

Schistosomiasis in all its forms is a rural disease and depends on a variety of factors:

1. Contamination of fresh water with human or animal urine or faeces containing schistosome eggs.

2. The presence in the water of snails capable of infection by miracidia hatched from those eggs, and capable of producing cercariae infective to man. Water temperature, rate of flow, acidity or alkalinity, and content of organic matter conducive to snail growth are also important.

3. Human contact with water containing living cercariae by bathing, wading or washing in it, or by drinking it. Infected children are important; they excrete large numbers of eggs and are attracted by water. The introduction of greatly increased human populations in irrigation areas adds to the chance of infection, but much transmission takes place in communities which rely on ponds or water-holes for their supplies. In South Africa there is little transmission more than 400 m from sources of polluted water, but a dense rural population adds to the incidence of the disease. In Zanzibar the incidence of *S. haematobium* infection is highly focal: in good areas wells, running streams or piped water are available and the incidence rate for *S. haematobium* is about 30% (Forsyth & Macdonald 1966); in bad areas only a few virtually stagnant streams or pools are available and infection rates reach almost 100%. In these areas the infection is not only common, it is also heavy in individual patients.

In Iraq it is a disease of fishermen and gardeners as well as agricultural workers, but is a social rather than an occupational disease, heaviest in poor people living in poor conditions.

Small dams or pools are dangerous in that they attract both bathers and snails, which may be introduced as eggs on the feet of water birds. The shores of lakes, especially near inflowing streams which are likely to be contaminated with human excreta, are also dangerous.

Irrigation is a major factor, and it is likely to increase as water conservation schemes and agricultural programmes are extended. In well maintained irrigation canals, however, snails do not thrive, but where there is silt and vegetation, unsatisfactory water management schedules, poor drainage channels with night storage dams and temporary pools, conditions suitable for the multiplication of snails exist. These factors have been responsible for the observed increase of *S. haematobium* and *S. mansoni* infections in irrigation areas.

In the Gezira plain of the Sudan, after the Sennar dam was built, over 400 000 hectares of land were opened up for irrigation and the incidence and mortality from the disease increased steadily as the population rose. The irrigation scheme has now been extended to cover another 400 000 hectares and the disease has invaded most of the new area; 25% of the people were infected by 1969.

In Egypt the old traditional basin system of irrigation was formerly the rule, in which fields alongside the Nile were divided into large basins by a system of dykes, and flood waters were kept in them long enough for valuable silt to settle. This type of irrigation depended upon the natural seasonal rise and fall of the river; it did not favour snails, and the incidence of schistosomiasis was low, about 10%. In other parts of Egypt, however, the system was introduced of perennial irrigation from reservoirs artificially created to hold the Nile water. In this system the water is released from canals as it is needed, and drainage ditches carry away the seepage water; the canals are never dried, and snails find the habitat favourable. The incidence of schistosomiasis in such areas was found to be as high as 60% of the population for both *S. haematobium* and *S. mansoni*, though in some areas where the specific snail hosts had not colonized the waters the incidence of *S. mansoni* was low. The Aswan dam has converted most of Egyptian irrigation to the perennial type and the snail hosts of both *S. haematobium* and *S. mansoni* have extended southwards, whereas with the traditional basin irrigation only the *Bulinus* snails were found in the south.

Perennial irrigation, with its ramifying canals, brings more land into cultiva- tion, and production is increased because it does not depend so much on season. There is a dilemma: better irrigation means better economics and a better standard of living, but it also usually means the spread of schistosomiasis. Restriction of irrigation is unlikely to be accepted by the economic authorities, but they must face the health hazard.

In Egypt the infection rates with *S. haematobium* and *S. mansoni* differ significantly between various areas, between different villages and even between different areas of the same village. The rates increase up to the age of 14 years, then decline somewhat to the age of 40 and remain at a level of about 30%. Infection with *S. mansoni* is acquired more slowly than with *S. haematobium*. Males are more commonly affected than females and farmers, fishermen and boatmen more than others. Of the factors affecting infection, swimming is stated to be one of the most important (Farook *et al.* 1966) and children are enthusiastic swimmers. Main drains are important sources of infection.

In parts of Africa where both *S. haematobium* and *S. mansoni* are present their prevalence is by no means equal. For instance (Forsyth 1964) the incidence in Tanzanian school-children has been recorded as follows:

	Incidence of *S. haematobium*	Incidence of *S. mansoni*
South of Lake Victoria	94%	7·9%
Tanga district	53%	30·0%

Though in Natal, South Africa and East Africa south of Lake Victoria the incidence of *S. haematobium* infection in children is very high and of *S. mansoni* low, there are parts of the eastern Congo and the southern Sudan where *S. mansoni* is very prevalent and where no *S. haematobium* has been reported (Nelson 1958). *S. mansoni* is often patchily distributed.

Infection is strongly influenced by social and religious practices in relation to contact with water. In Egypt females may have more frequent contact with water than males, in washing clothes and utensils. Males, however, tend to contaminate water more than females, except for girls under 5 years old. Summer is the period of most frequent, prolonged and extensive contact with water, and one-quarter of all exposures take place in the heat of the day, between noon and 15.00 hours, which is also the period of maximal cercarial load. Such social influences are important (Farook & Mallah 1966). Even the ablution basins built near mosques for ceremonial cleansing purposes have been incriminated in transmission.

Animal hosts

Although *S. haematobium* has (though rarely) been found in baboons, monkeys and rodents in Africa, these animals are probably not important in infecting man, who is the main reservoir. Most primates are susceptible to experimental infection.

S. *mansoni* has been found in baboons; some may have been infected from human sources, but some baboon communities can maintain the infection among themselves. Baboon faeces containing eggs and reaching a stream in Tanzania have certainly caused infection in persons bathing in the water (Fenwick 1969). The infection has also been found in other monkeys and in rodents. Calves and sheep have been infected experimentally, passing viable eggs in their faeces, a finding which may be epidemiologically important. The form described by Schwetz from rodents, which he named S. *mansoni* var. *rodentorum*, was probably S. *mansoni*.

S. *japonicum*, on the other hand, is a parasite of dogs, cats, rats, mice, cattle, water-buffalo, pigs, horses, sheep, goats and some other mammals, besides man. How much these animals pass the infection to water containing the relevant snails is not known, though in the Philippines it has been estimated that these sources account for 25% of the human infections. Rats haunting river banks are particularly involved in China. The universal use of crude human faeces for fertilizing crops greatly increases the chance of infection of snails, which are operculated, amphibious and able to survive long periods in a relatively dry state, thus conserving the infection. The Taiwan strain is pathogenic for animals but not for man.

TRANSMISSION

The snail hosts are described in Appendix II.

The snails are not vectors in the sense that mosquitoes are vectors of malaria. Snails are more or less passive intermediate hosts, playing no active part in the distribution of the disease. The distributive agent responsible for passing the disease from one snail to another is usually man (Wright 1970).

Factors relating to snails

These factors are multiple, acting together rather than individually.

1. *Composition of the water.* Snail vectors of schistosomes infecting man require fresh water, usually but not always with abundant aquatic vegetation on which to feed and on which to deposit their egg masses, though Bulinid snails also thrive in habitats almost devoid of the higher plants in most of Africa south of the Sahara. They also feed on algae and need calcium for their shells. Acidity is inimical; the alkaline and calcium-rich waters of Surinam and Venezuela are highly suitable for *Biomphalaria glabrata*, whereas the acid (pH 4·5–5·5) waters devoid of lime of British Guiana are not, and schistosomes are not found (Giglioli 1964).

2. *Temperature.* The optimum is about 22–23°C; above 39°C snails die. There is little or no transmission above an altitude of 1800 m where the water temperatures are too low.

3. *Light.* In general the snails are not found in heavily shaded or fast-flowing water, which probably explains the absence of the disease from forest areas. Most species do not survive in the dark, which is a strong argument in favour of covering the irrigation canals, or putting the water into pipes wherever possible. *Bulinus truncatus*, however, has been bred experimentally in total darkness in Iraq, but population growth was restricted. Infected *Biomphalaria* have been recovered from the bottom of Lake Victoria at a depth of about 12 m, where the light cannot possibly have been strong.

4. *Habitat.* Muddy channels favour snails, and mud absorbs molluscicides as well as encouraging vegetation, which is why concreted channels, which can be cleared, have been constructed for irrigation. Still or slow-flowing water is preferred by snails, as in ponds, dams, lakes, irrigation canals and slow streams or rivers. Swift flow is inimical. Some snails (e.g. *Biomphalaria alexandrina*) prefer permanent and stable habitats such as drains leading from canals; *Bulinus truncatus* prefers large canals. Seasonal small pools are much used for washing and bathing and watering cattle; they are the centres of intense transmission.

5. *Season.* Though there are irregular population changes independent of climate, most snail populations fall during the rainy season, to increase in the drier warmer months after the rains (for instance in East Africa). Where water temperatures are more stable some snail populations show no seasonal trends; the greatest stability is found in *Oncomelania quadrasi* in the Far East. A long hot summer leads to high death rates, though some species can aestivate and survive desiccation, for instance *Bulinus* (*Physopsis*) in Africa. *Oncomelania* (which is operculated) hibernates in cold weather in Asia. Snails can not only survive, but also carry their infection from one wet season to the next. *B.* (*P.*) *nasutus productus* infected with *S. haematobium* can survive drying for 98 days.

6. *Predators.* Ducks eat snails, and so do the large (non-vector) snails *Marisa cornuarietis* and *Tarebia granifera*, which also compete for food. They are deliberately used for snail control in the Caribbean, apparently with some success in displacing *Biomphalaria glabrata* (Webbe 1969).

7. *Snail egg masses.* These can be carried on the feet of water birds and infect other bodies of water.

Factors relating to release of cercariae and infection of man

1. *Age of snails.* Young snails are more susceptible to infection than old snails.

2. *Infection.* Snails can emit 1500–2000 cercariae daily, and continue to do so for over 200 days, but they become more susceptible than uninfected snails to adverse conditions.

3. *Season.* Active transmission in East Africa takes place for 4–5 months at the end of the main rainy season (April–August), but may occur in both wet and dry seasons; it is sometimes brief and intense, sometimes prolonged and less concentrated. In the Transvaal transmission of *S. mansoni* is seasonal, beginning in September or October at the start of the rains, but transmission of *S. haematobium* and *S. mattheei* is unpredictable. Cercariae can survive for up to 3 days in water, and even up to 6 in cold weather.

Infection rates in snails, which rise sharply in the drier months as small collections of water shrink and the density of snails increases, fall even before the snail densities decline, suggesting a high mortality in infected snails, and also suggesting that, in the absence of rain to wash excreta into the water, the snails are not being so frequently infected.

4. *Time of day.* In the laboratory most of the daily output of *S. mansoni* cercariae by *Biomphalaria* takes place between 09.00 and 14.00 hours (1–6 hours after stimulation by light), with a peak at 10.00–14.00 hours. Light is the chief stimulus causing the release of cercariae of both *S. haematobium* and *S. mansoni*. In small pools holding *B. nasutus productus* the cercariae are shed from mid-morning to late evening, and bathing at such times is therefore more hazardous than in the early morning. In the Philippines, however, where the principal hosts are nocturnal rats, the peak cercarial shedding of *S. japonicum* occurs in the evening.

5. *Velocity of water.* Experimental animals exposed to infected water at

velocities of 15–60 cm/second show high rates of infection and worm loads. The optimum rate of flow seems to be about 30 cm/second; below this few cercariae make contact, and above this the cercariae which make contact tend to be swept away. In streams most *S. mansoni* cercariae are probably swept away by mid-afternoon (Webbe 1966).

PATHOLOGY

The stages of schistosomiasis are: (*a*) invasion, (*b*) maturation, (*c*) established infection, and (*d*) late stage.

Invasion

In this stage the cercariae penetrate the skin or mucous membrane (Fig. 102), usually taking less than 15 minutes, and acting by a combination of cercarial

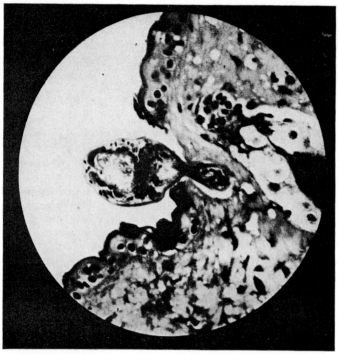

Fig. 102.—Bilharziasis. Cercarial penetration. (*Dr O. D. Standen*)

muscular action and glandular secretion. Once through the horny layer of the skin the schistosomules enter the dermis and hypodermis, where they probably remain for 4–5 days before entering the lymphatic system and thence the veins, the right heart and the lungs. After that their progress is not clearly known, but they reach the liver, where, presumably, they mature.

In unsensitized persons the reactions to the first invasion by these embryo parasites are mild, with only slight inflammatory reactions in the skin, lungs and liver (occasionally with cough, bloody sputum or even asthma), but after repeated exposures the skin shows itchy papules and local oedema. This cercarial dermatitis may be quite marked, and may indicate the date of infection. It is usually worse in infections with bird and animal schistosomes, which do not migrate. In an endemic area, however, the local people often show no local skin reaction, but in new visitors the reaction may be marked, especially after reinfection. The absence of this reaction, for instance in Africans, may be a reflection of passive immunity derived from the mother, followed by active immunity in childhood.

Maturation

This begins 2–8 weeks after infection; males and females couple and eggs are produced. The young couples of S. mansoni and S. japonicum descend the portal vein against the stream, reaching the mesenteric veins in the intestinal walls, where the main egg-laying takes place. S. haematobium probably also matures in the liver, though this has not been demonstrated, and the adult worms find their way, by some process not understood, to the veins of the genito-urinary organs.

The characteristic pathological manifestation in this stage, in moderate and heavy infections, is an acute febrile reaction, with eosinophilia up to 80%, lasting for several days or weeks. This appears to be an allergic reaction to metabolic products of the schistosomes and their eggs. There may be abdominal pain in S. mansoni infections.

Established infection

In this stage there is intense production and excretion of eggs at about 10–12 weeks after infection. Eggs are excreted via the urine or faeces according to species, and are deposited in the walls of the genito-urinary system (especially S. haematobium but also occasionally S. mansoni), or the rectum and colon (especially S. mansoni and S. japonicum, but also occasionally S. haematobium). Post mortem studies show that eggs of all species can often be found in the appendix, liver and lungs.

At this stage the eggs set up an inflammatory reaction, with the formation of granulomas, giant cells and epithelioid cells surrounded later by loose fibrous tissue. These tubercles (or granulomas) may coalesce. The eggs often become calcified. Papilloma formation and gross intestinal changes occur in mixed S. haematobium and S. mansoni infections, and in S. mansoni infections alone, especially if heavy. With S. japonicum the changes occur earlier as a result of the greater numbers of eggs involved. There is congestion and possibly micro-ulceration of the rectal mucosa, and isolated polyps may be formed, with bloody diarrhoea, abdominal pain and cramps, mainly in children. Later there is fibrosis with changes in bowel habits. Symptoms depend upon intensity of infection, from merely an irritable colon to severe trouble. This stage may last for a long time, merging into the stage of irreversible effects if not treated.

In S. haematobium infection the early inflammatory changes caused by the deposition of eggs are probably due to metabolic products of the contained miracidia, and to decomposition of dead eggs; the result is invasion by histiocytes and other cells, followed by eosinophils. As a result the epithelial cells and the adjacent muscle cells become hyperplastic. This goes on to an atrophic phase in which fibrous tissue begins to replace the granulomatous infiltration, leading to reduced blood supply. This atrophy involves epithelial, subepithelial and muscular layers, and the fibrous tissue holds eggs which later die and become calcified. Suppuration is not a feature of lesions caused by eggs, but superficial ulcers may form.

Damage to the liver is primarily due to eggs swept back by the portal circulation; lesions from adult worms can seldom be found, though dead schistosomes occasionally lead to severe thrombophlebitis, which can be found after treatment of heavily infected patients.

Late stage

This is the stage of fibrosis, and the numbers of eggs extruded are reduced. The fibrosis favours the increased formation of granulomas and the passage of eggs to the liver and lungs. Dead worms also lead to focal necrosis and granulomas, either where they have lodged or after they have been carried to other organs. In hollow organs granuloma formation may give rise to papillomas with necrosis, ulceration and secondary infection complicating the primary picture. Fibrosis and calcification may have important effects. In *S. mansoni* infections pigment from the destruction of the red cells by the worms is commonly present in Kupffer cells of the liver.

Hepatosplenic schistosomiasis results from fibrosis, which may be diffuse or localized—the periportal fibrosis of the Symmers (clay-pipe-stem) type, especially in Egypt or Brazil. When the main portal tracts are affected the resulting fibrosis prevents eggs from reaching the smaller tracts, and only the main portal tracts are involved; this is the clay-pipe-stem fibrosis which may occur in the presence of intense infection. There is no direct injury to the hepatic cells. There are many causes of cirrhosis of the liver in adults, including malnutrition, virus hepatitis and alcoholism, which can cause confusion, but in Brazil, Egypt, East Africa and Rhodesia *S. mansoni* is one definite cause of cirrhosis, even in juveniles. In the Far East *S. japonicum* is a cause.

Portal hypertension follows the fibrosis, and there may be repeated haematemesis from oesophageal varices, leading to anaemia which is worsened when haemopoiesis is disturbed owing to hypersplenism from the enlarged spleen. There may be melaena. Anaemia in the tropics, however, is caused by so many different conditions (particularly hookworm infection) that attribution is difficult. Nevertheless, Foy and Nelson (1963) conclude that blood loss and toxaemia in the early stages of schistosomiasis of all three species can cause hypochromic anaemia in children, and that in the later stages the hepatosplenic syndrome is associated with severe anaemia.

When the liver and intestine are involved, both SGOT and SGPT are raised. Liver function is usually well preserved, however, though most liver function tests show deterioration with the onset of ascites, or after haematemesis. Protein is lost from the bladder wall into the urine, apart from blood loss, in severe *S. haematobium* infection—sometimes as much as 3 grammes/litre of urine. The consequent hypoproteinaemia may be accompanied by ascites and anasarca.

Cardiopulmonary disease develops in association with hepatosplenomegaly, and eggs or parasites may be deposited in the pulmonary arteries, leading to diffuse endarteritis obliterans and cor pulmonale. Pulmonary hypertension causes overloading of the right ventricle, and heavy pooling of blood may occur in the portal circulation. Congestive heart failure may follow, but the most common cause of death is bleeding from oesophageal varices.

Cor pulmonale due to *S. mansoni* was found in 15% of patients brought to autopsy in Brazil with Symmers's fibrosis of the liver; active pulmonary arteritis was present in 90% of that group. Schistosomal cor pulmonale in the absence of Symmers's fibrosis was rare and doubtful. Severe schistosomal intestinal lesions are common in Brazil; Symmers's fibrosis was the most significant schistosomal lesion in this series (Cheever & Andrade 1967).

There is no proof that living adult worms in the veins set up any inflammatory reaction, but cor pulmonale, though due to repeated emboli of eggs in the lungs, may also be influenced by reaction to dead worms, and in pulmonary lesions dead worms may be more important than eggs, though the exact mechanisms remain obscure. There seems to be an allergic element. After treatment the adult worms may move to the lungs, causing transient changes associated with asthmatic symptoms and a great increase in eosinophil count—'verminous pneumonia'. The pathology is not known.

Nevertheless, eggs are in general the main pathogenic agents, leading to fibrosis. In *S. haematobium* infection the eggs, being already in the systemic circulation, have easy access to the lungs. In *S. mansoni* and *S. japonicum* infections the eggs enter the portal system, but can make their way to the lungs through anastomotic channels, and are therefore not filtered out by the liver.

In *S. haematobium* infection early bladder changes consist of the formation of small papules in the bladder wall, surrounded by fine capillaries, and going on to nodules which may ulcerate or become fibrosed. Calcification occurs in the bladder wall. Bleeding and dysuria are common, but tend to be overlooked by patients, although they are danger signals. The mucous membrane may later atrophy and ulcerate, or become hyperplastic with the formation of polyps. Calculi are sometimes found in the later stages.

Lesions of the bladder include the sandy patches in the posterosuperior wall near the openings of the ureters, which can be seen on cystoscopy.

Granuloma formation with oedema at the outlets of the ureters, or in the walls, can lead to dilatation or hydroureter, which can be reversed by treatment. Infection of the ureteric walls can also cause interference with their peristaltic movement and hydroureter without stenosis. Late fibrosis of the ureters, with stenosis or extensive fibrosis of the bladder itself, can also lead to hydroureter and hydronephrosis, and destruction of the ureteric sphincter leads to reflux. In advanced cases the ureters may be transformed into rigid tubes through calcification. Fibrosis and calcification of the bladder lead to contraction of that organ. The state of the ureters and bladder is important in any attempt to deal with dilatation.

The possible relationship of cancer of the bladder to urinary schistosomiasis needs elucidation. Cancer is more common in communities where schistosomiasis is prevalent and individual infection heavier than elsewhere, and has been attributed to that disease. It affects younger people in these areas, with a relatively high prevalence of the squamous type. It may be due to the combined effects of chronic inflammation due to schistosomiasis and superimposed carcinogens, possibly resulting from disordered metabolism of tryptophan as a result of treatment.

In *S. mansoni* infections gross lesions of the rectum and bowel occur in only a minority of cases; most infections are diagnosed by finding eggs in scrapings from the rectal wall. The gross lesions may consist of sandy patches in thickened mucosa containing large numbers of eggs; there may be ulceration and the formation of polyps.

Lesions of the central nervous system can occur in the brain (usually *S. japonicum*) or spinal cord (usually *S. mansoni* or *S. haematobium*). In the *S. japonicum* brain lesions there may be diffuse small lesions in the grey or white matter, either symptomless or causing epileptiform attacks. Or there may be granulomas containing large numbers of eggs; these are localized and can be removed surgically. The COP test on the cerebrospinal fluid is positive in some cases, and the fluid may be under pressure. Treatment with antimony may be useful.

In the spinal cord the lesions may take the form of transverse myelitis or granuloma formation, sometimes with severe backache, defects in bladder control, sensory changes and weakness of the legs. Eggs may be present in the lesions. A syndrome of this kind in endemic areas should suggest schistosomiasis.

IMMUNOLOGY

People of all ages are susceptible to infection; the peak incidence is between 7 and 15 years. Partial acquired immunity has been proved in experimental animals, and probably develops in man. In hyperendemic areas overwhelming infections are relatively uncommon, and the decrease in infection with age suggests an acquired immunity. Sensitization may occur, giving rise to increased skin reactions in later infections.

The schistosome egg is the primary element in provoking overt disease, stimulating first an eosinophilic reaction, followed by a granulomatous response which, as a manifestation of delayed hypersensitivity, has a basis in immunity (Warren 1968). In experimental infections, if the worms are killed before reaching maturity, or if the infections are unisexual, overt disease does not develop.

A second granulomatous reaction can be provoked by a second exposure to eggs, and this is an accelerated and augmented (anamnestic) reaction, which is specific; for instance, it does not follow previous infection with *Ascaris* eggs. It can be transferred with spleen cells or lymph node cells, but not with serum, which suggests that it is a form of delayed hypersensitivity (Warren 1968). It can be suppressed by cortisone. Superinfection can therefore occur and this, indeed, is a major feature in the epidemiology and severity of the disease; the immunity produced by a single infection is slight. One or two infections with a few (125) cercariae of *S. haematobium* confer very little immunity to challenge in hamsters (Purnell 1966). On the other hand, Smithers and Terry (1967) showed that in rhesus monkeys a single exposure to 25 normal cercariae of *S. mansoni*, which go on to maturity, produces good resistance to later challenge, but that exposure to 20 000 irradiated (and therefore inactivated) cercariae is less effective (see below). The immunizing agents are antigens from living adult worms (confirmed by experiments in which adult worms were introduced into the hepatic portal systems of the animals), and eggs are probably not important in this respect. Even the anterior halves of worms cut in half before transfer can stimulate immunity, though worms killed by freezing cannot. Injection of 500 000 live eggs into the mesenteric veins of a monkey failed to induce resistance.

Infection leads to increase in serum immunoglobulins, but their role is not understood. The various tests—COP, CHR, CF, FAT and precipitin—show no relation to protection, and passive transfer of serum has also failed to protect.

The subject is interesting and complicated. Adult schistosomes transferred surgically from infected monkeys to the portal systems of normal monkeys provide the major stimulus to immunity against challenge by cercariae, but they are not themselves affected by this immunity, and they lay their eggs normally. But if adults from mice (and other hosts) are transplanted into monkeys, the 'mouse' adult worms do not begin to produce eggs until some weeks later, presumably until they have become adapted to the new host. Moreover, if 'mouse' adult worms are transferred to monkeys which have previously been immunized against mouse body tissues, the 'mouse' worms are killed within 24–44 hours. This suggests that worms which have lived in mice have incorporated mouse antigens into their cuticular tissues, and that these antigens are attacked by the anti-mouse antibodies of the monkeys, and the worms are destroyed. The mouse antigens appear to be located on the surface of the worms, and this incorporation of host antigens to the surface of the parasites probably explains why the original 'monkey' schistosomes escape the consequences of the immunity they themselves engender (Smithers *et al.* 1968; Smithers & Terry 1969).

Heterologous immunity may be important. Nelson *et al.* (1968) studied the interaction in mice of experimental infections with *S. bovis*, *S. mattheei* and *S. rodhaini* with *S. mansoni*. Infection with *S. bovis* or *S. mattheei* reduced the expected egg load of subsequent challenge with *S. mansoni* by 74% and 85% respectively, and a similar response was observed in monkeys. This suggests that natural zooprophylaxis may be important in the human infection. In some areas man is continually exposed to infection with 'animal' schistosomes, and perhaps the severity of *S. mansoni* infections in Brazil and Egypt is in part due to the absence of concomitant transmissions of bovine schistosomes.

Unisexual infection can produce some resistance, and inoculation of irradiated cercariae can also do so. These facts suggest the possibility of protective heterologous vaccines (Amin & Nelson 1969).

The nutritional status of an animal influences the infection. In experimental *S. mansoni* infection the number of worms developing in animals on a deficient diet is usually greater than in animals on a normal diet. Rats deficient in vitamin A have less resistance to *S. mansoni* than normal rats, and a diet deficient in cystine, selenium and vitamin E has a profound effect in increasing the severity of *S. mansoni* infection in mice.

In experimental work, however, protein deficiency has a deleterious effect on *S. mansoni*, causing it to produce fewer eggs and more abnormal eggs than in animals normally fed. The abnormal eggs may be more readily absorbed in animals deficient in protein, and may more readily stimulate a granulomatous reaction; rats in this condition develop cirrhosis of the liver more readily than normal rats.

Human patients who have moderate nutritional deficiency and are infected with *S. mansoni* derive no benefit from a high-protein diet alone, but when they are treated with stibophen they respond more rapidly than usual. Treatment is less effective in vegetarians than in non-vegetarians.

CLINICAL FINDINGS

S. haematobium infection

In this form of schistosomiasis, in which the heaviest pathological burden is borne by the urinary system, the symptoms vary very greatly.

There may be irritative dermatitis in the area of penetration of the larvae soon after exposure. Thereafter the incubation period is difficult to determine, but symptoms may arise from 2 months to over 2 years after infection.

In the early stages there is often slight fever, with general weakness and prostration, but the most characteristic sign is haematuria, blood appearing especially towards the end of micturition, with or without a sense of urinary irritation. If the urine is allowed to stand, flocculi of mucus or minute blood clots settle to the bottom of the vessel, and if the sediment is examined microscopically it is seen to consist of blood cells, catarrhal products, and the characteristic terminal-spined eggs (Fig. 103). The finding of eggs is crucial for diagnosis; they occur in urine whether or not there is haematuria, and the urine should always be examined for eggs if there is any suspicion of schistosomiasis. Eggs of *S. mattheei* are sometimes found in the urine of Rhodesian European schoolboys, and eggs of *S. mansoni* in the endemic areas of that infection.

Pain is not always present, but may take the form of a dull sense of oppression in the suprapubic or perineal region, or a sense of scalding on micturition.

Frequency and urgency of micturition are early symptoms, and rectal symptoms, with passage of blood and mucus, may be present at the same time;

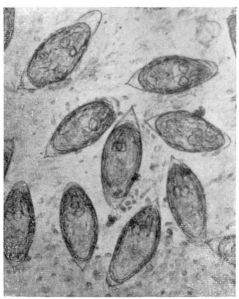

Fig. 103.—*Schistosoma haematobium* eggs in urine, showing contained miracidia. (*Dr H. K. Giffen*)

these may be due to *S. haematobium* alone, or to mixed infection with *S. mansoni*. Such symptoms and signs should lead to examination of the rectum. *S. haematobium* eggs may be present in seminal fluid (Barlow & Meleney 1949).

Haematuria is often disregarded by African children. In hyperendemic areas, in which it is almost universal, boys tend to regard it as a natural physiological phenomenon, the counterpart of menstruation in girls. It may last for months or even years, but tends to decrease if superinfection does not occur. In male Africans retention of urine with overflow and incontinence has been described.

Cystitis is likely to supervene, with all the suffering brought by that condition, and calculi may form (in 25% of cases in some reports from Egypt, but less in Zanzibar). Eggs in the bladder wall eventually become calcified, and the condition of widespread calcification can be recognized radiologically. The bladder may hypertrophy, or dilate, or even contract as a result of fibrosis, and the ureters and kidneys are often involved. Secondary infection is apparently common in Egypt, but rare in Tanzania and Rhodesia.

Excretion of leucocytes in the urine, however, is much greater in subjects with schistosomiasis of the bladder than in normal persons, in the absence of bacteriuria; quantitative examination of the cellular content of the urine is therefore not likely to be of diagnostic value in patients with renal parenchymal disease who also have urinary schistosomiasis.

Gelfand (1967) remarks: 'We all know that patients with bilharziasis, due to either *S. mansoni* or *S. haematobium*, have been diagnosed at times as having

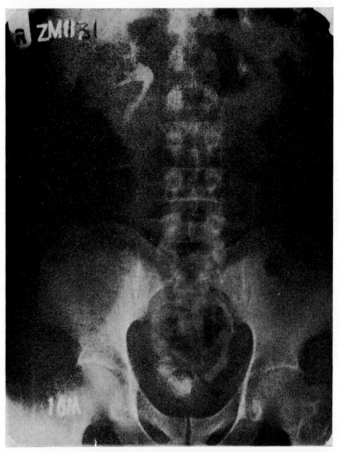

Fig. 104.—Bladder stone caused by *Schistosoma* infection. (*Dr D. M. Forsyth*)

peptic ulcer, cholecystitis, hepatitis, pancreatitis and appendicitis and that it is only when an extra specimen is taken in desperation, because the clinician is not altogether satisfied with his diagnosis, that ova are found and the patient treated correctly.' The reverse is also true, schistosomiasis being incriminated when the correct diagnosis is one of these conditions.

In patients of European extraction the allergic manifestations of the infection are prominent, and tiredness is often the chief symptom, whereas in patients of African origin there is much greater output of eggs, with severe local lesions, dysuria, haematuria and abdominal pain (Gelfand 1966). This difference may reflect the long African experience of the disease, which to the European is a relatively late comer.

In Europeans the Katayama syndrome, beginning 2–8 weeks after infection, has been reported, with fever, abdominal pain, transient generalized urticaria, cough and sometimes enlarged liver or spleen or both.

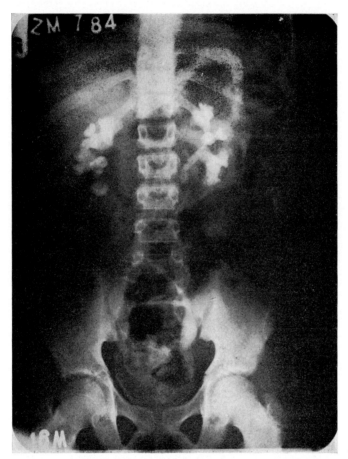

Fig. 105.—Calcified bladder in a patient aged 12, caused by *Schistosoma* infection. (*Dr D. M. Forsyth*)

There is much evidence that, though spontaneous cure often occurs in untreated infection with *S. haematobium*, it can be responsible for extensive and permanent damage to the urinary tract, with consequences which can later be fatal.

In north-west Tanzania, for instance, a hyperendemic area, the prevalence of calcification of the bladder (i.e. of the masses of calcified eggs embedded in the bladder wall), hydronephrosis and deformity of the ureters reached 8% in young children, increasing to over 30% in older children. Hydronephrosis (but not the other lesions) was much less common in girls than in boys. Growth rates may possibly be affected, and the outlook on the whole is poor, though in Zanzibar observations lasting 2½ years after treatment indicated that in schoolchildren the outlook is not quite so grave as was formerly thought; some of the treated children showed apparent resolution of the ureteric deformity and hydronephrosis, but not of the calcification (Maconald & Forsyth 1968). But it seems likely that eventually the calcified eggs may all be discharged—calcification is rarely seen in old age.

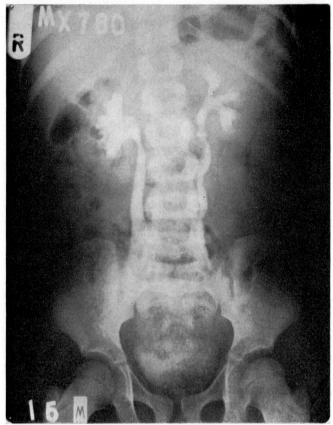

Fig. 106.—Dilated ureters, calcified bladder and hydronephrosis caused by *Schistosoma* infection. (*Dr D. M. Forsyth*)

Such abnormalities were found even in apparently healthy children, and in the same area of Tanzania hydronephrosis, ureteric lesions and non-functioning kidneys are found in over 10% of adults, and there is direct evidence that the infection causes the death of numbers of young males. In South African mine workers these lesions are substantially more common in infected than in non-infected men, urinary schistosomiasis being clearly a major cause of morbidity, and probably of mortality, in them.

In a small longitudinal study of infected children observed for up to 74 weeks in Nigeria, however, Lucas *et al.* (1966) are reasonably optimistic that nodular filling defects of the bladder, dilatation of the ureters and hydronephrosis can resolve after adequate treatment, though they do not record the same for calcification.

In Durban, South Africa, in the acute stage of urinary schistosomiasis, hydronephrosis is usually the result of ureteric obstruction by lesions which often regress; in the chronic stage it is commonly due to atonicity of the ureters, which must be distinguished from fibrous stricture, as surgical measures may have adverse effects. Although hydronephrosis was often demonstrable by excretion urography, it was not often found at autopsy; prognosis therefore seems to be reasonably favourable. Severe chronic sequelae occur in only a small proportion of patients in the Durban area (Powell *et al.* 1968).

Other effects of gross infection with *S. haematobium* include skeletal rarefaction with scoliosis and fractures of long bones. The pathological process seems to be excessive loss of phosphate, low Ca × P product and defective calcification resulting from renal tubular damage due to the infecton.

S. haematobium sometimes causes lesions in the male perineum and scrotum; stricture of the urethra is not uncommon, and fistulas may form from the floor of the urethra. The penile sheath may be infiltrated, with swelling and even obstruction to urinary flow. The cord and epididymis may be involved, but the tunica and testes are rarely affected. These lesions must be differentiated from lesions due to filariasis, tuberculosis and syphilis. The seminal vesicles are sometimes involved.

The female genitalia may be affected, particularly the cervix and tubes (with occlusion), but the vagina, vulva and ovary may also be affected. The ovaries may become fibrosed. Extension of the disease from the bladder may produce thickening and even papillomas of the urethra emerging from the external meatus; peri-urethral abscesses may form. On the vulva papillomas and ulcers may be mistaken for carcinoma, and similar excrescences round the anus and groin may be mistaken for venereal warts. Diagnosis depends on finding eggs in these tissues, but eggs can also often be found in vaginal or cervical smears.

S. haematobium can affect the spinal cord, forming a granuloma containing the characteristic eggs, which compresses the cord, giving rise to symptoms and signs of transverse myelitis or radiculitis of the cauda equina. Eggs have also been found in the brain, accounting for epileptic symptoms.

Pulmonary involvement, which is not as common as in *S. mansoni* infection, can lead to congestive heart failure and cor pulmonale. There is widespread obliteration of pulmonary arterioles and a rise in blood pressure with hypertrophy of the right ventricle. The predominating symptom is dyspnoea. On X-ray the enlargement of the right side of the heart is evident, often with diffuse and fine mottling of the lungs due to bilharzial tubercles which resemble miliary tubercles. Schistosome eggs may, rarely, be found in the deposit of sputum digested with 4% potassium hydroxide and centrifuged.

Anaemia is common and may be partly due to loss of blood in the urine, but Woodruff *et al.* (1966) have shown that the hypersplenism accompanying an enlarged spleen is probably the major factor.

A nephrotic syndrome has been reported; it is caused by an antigen–antibody complex deposited in the glomeruli (compare quartan malaria).

There is evidence to suggest that patients with typhoid or paratyphoid fever, who also have urinary schistosomiasis, remain carriers of the enteric infection much more often than patients with these infections but without schistosomiasis. Such patients may not respond to treatment with chloramphenicol until the schistosomal infection has been dealt with.

Appendicitis due to accumulation of *S. haematobium* eggs has been reported, and eggs have also been found in a tumour of the vocal cord and in a granulomatous ulcer of the lip which had been diagnosed as syphilitic.

Eggs of *S. haematobium* (and other species) have been found in the skin; for instance in the scrotum after Barlow's deliberate self infection (Barlow & Meleney 1949), in an ulcer of the lip and a chronic ulcer of the leg. They have also been found on the perineum.

For eye complications see Chapter 44.

In general, Forsyth (1969) concludes that *S. haematobium* infection in Zanzibar is not in general a chronic debilitating disease, being often compatible with good health, yet it kills some patients, probably as a result of renal failure, and is a serious public health problem.

Schistosoma intercalatum infection

This was discovered by Chesterman and studied by Fisher in the Congo region. For a description of morphology and life cycle see Appendix II. It has been found in Gabon and as far as Cameroon, and seems to be spreading with the

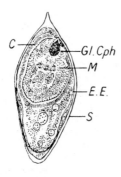

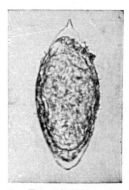

Fig. 107.—Eggs of *Schistosoma haematobium* showing the development of the miracidia.

S, Shell; *E.E.*, Embryonic envelope; *M*, Miracidium; *C*, Cilia; *Gl. Cph.*, Cephalic glands.

Fig. 108.—Eggs of *Schistosoma haematobium* showing the changes produced in the contained miracidium by antimony tartrate. (*Dr John Anderson*)

movements of workmen and nomads; its extent may be more wide than is at present known. In part of the Congo 50% of schoolchildren have been reported as infected.

The eggs, which are elongated with a terminal spine, and which closely resemble those of *S. mattheei*, are found only in faeces, and the site of infection is the bowel, which on sigmoidoscopic examination shows a 'sandpaper' appearance, with minute petechiae but no polypi or ulcers. The rectal mucosa is friable, and rectal biopsy is of great importance in diagnosis.

On the whole symptoms are said to be slight, with abdominal pain and dysenteric symptoms, or constipation and discharge of bloody mucus. Toxic manifestations, have, however, been noted, but pulmonary manifestations are practically absent. The spleen and liver may be enlarged. Abortion in the third month of pregnancy has been reported. In Gabon and Cameroon the proportion of severe cases is high, especially in young subjects and probably as a result of heavy infections. Granulomas, polypi and schistosomal tumours in the rectum and colon are common and badly tolerated, and multiple granulomas have been found in the liver, ovaries and adnexa, containing numerous eggs (Deschiens & Delas 1969).

S. mansoni infection

The prevalence of *S. mansoni* infection varies greatly, and with it the actual incidence of illness—it seems that where the infection is common, its effects are serious, probably as a result of superinfection. Symptomless infections, however, are common, and in general this infection is less severe in East Africa than in Egypt and South America.

The infection can be divided into 5 stages:

1. The stage of invasion.
2. The toxaemic and hypersensitive phase.
3. The acute intestinal disease.
4. The stage of chronic irreversible effects:
    a. Chronic intestinal form.
    b. Hepatosplenic form.
    c. Cardiopulmonary form.
5. The rare development of lesions in the nervous system, heart and skin.

1. The stage of invasion includes cercarial dermatitis (swimmer's itch), arising within 24 hours and receding within a few days. This suggests a high density of cercariae. It also includes migration and development of the schisto-somules and symptoms may start as late as 2 or 3 days after infection, with fever, pulmonary symptoms (cough), eosinophilia and moderate splenomegaly. This is rare, and probably represents a very early hypersensitive reaction seen in Europeans but not Africans.

2. The toxaemic phase develops abruptly 15–20 days after exposure, with a typhoid-like illness, hepatomegaly, splenomegaly, eosinophilia, lymphadenitis and severe enteritis with bloody stools (schistosomal dysentery, especially in Brazil). Eggs are not present in the faeces or in biopsy material, and the changes in the colon are probably due to hypersensitivity. (The stage resembles the Katayama syndrome of *S. japonicum* infection below.) Signs of encephalitis may develop in Africans.

3. The acute intestinal disease is a result of the deposition of eggs in the wall of the bowel. It may begin suddenly about 40–55 days after infection. Dysentery is prominent, with fever, weakness, anorexia, loss of weight and abdominal tenderness; it may last 6–12 months. Intestinal schistosomiasis may be present in a patient suffering from amoebic or bacillary dysentery and the diagnosis of bilharzial dysentery should not be made without excluding other more likely causes, especially in Africa where multiple infections are common. Bilharzial dysentery may be more common in South America.

4. In the stage of established disease there may be a chronic catarrhal state with swollen, granular and haemorrhagic mucous membrane, and numerous eggs in the mucosa and submucosa, especially of the rectum. Polypi and papillomas form, not only in the rectum but also in any part of the colon, or even, rarely, in the small intestine. The polypi vary in size from a few millimetres and are dusty red and blue, or rosy. They may ulcerate.

The hepatosplenic form is a late form, in which either portal hypertension or hypersplenism—or both—is present. It is fairly common in young adult patients. In the liver the clay-pipe cirrhosis of Symmers may develop in a few patients. In Rhodesia cirrhosis of the liver in adults is apparently rarely due to schistosomiasis; excessive drinking of alcohol may be a more important factor than has hitherto been realized. On the other hand, cirrhosis in juveniles is much more often due to schistosomiasis than in adults. In Brazil the bilharzial cirrhosis of Symmers is a common end result of severe infection.

In the cardiopulmonary form the lesions result from the deposition of the eggs in the pulmonary arterioles, with obstruction of new capillary formation and endarteritis with thickening of the intima.

5. Lesions are sometimes, but rarely, found in the central nervous system, the appendix (but acute appendicitis from this cause is unlikely), the female genital organs, the urinary system, the heart, the gall-bladder and the skin.

When irreversible effects occur, fewer eggs may be passed in the faeces. The main lesions result from fibrotic changes round the eggs locked in the tissues, and some lesions result from changes around dead worms.

In the early stage the most important symptom is tiredness or debility, in patients of any age, though this is more prominent in Europeans than in Africans in Rhodesia. But in that country about one-third of infected Europeans and coloured children are unaware of any infection.

Dyspepsia occurs, probably as a result of toxaemia; it is not usually severe. Patients in endemic areas who complain of this should always be examined with *S. mansoni* infection in mind. There is usually mild fever.

The Katayama syndrome is sometimes seen in *S. mansoni* infection. It starts insidiously with fever for a few weeks, resembling the fever of typhoid or brucellosis. The patient feels ill, and becomes troubled with an urticarial eruption, with weals and swelling of soft tissues about the eyes, prepuce and scrotum. Spleen and liver are slightly enlarged, and there is eosinophilia, an important diagnostic feature. Cough may be troublesome. Electrocardiographic changes with inversion of the T-waves over the left praecordial leads sometimes occur.

The Katayama syndrome is usually mild and transient, including the eosinophilia, which is an important pointer. In Africa eosinophilia should always be regarded as possibly bilharzial, and efforts should be made to find eggs, though they may not be found in the pre-patent period.

In the stage of completion of maturation the main features are lassitude, fever, headache, backache, generalized pain, anorexia, loss of weight, vomiting and diarrhoea. Eosinophilia is almost constant. The intradermal reaction does not become positive until 4–6 weeks after exposure. The intensity of symptoms depends upon the worm load.

Localizing symptoms in *S. mansoni* infection occur in rather less than half the cases, and consist of abdominal pain, sometimes diarrhoea or even dysentery, or even constipation. Other causes of dysentery should always be looked for even if eggs are found.

The question of schistosomiasis as a cause of cirrhosis of the liver is complicated by the fact that in the endemic areas there are other causes, for instance malnutrition, which no doubt operate in patients with schistosomiasis. In the Americas the association of *S. mansoni* and cirrhosis is regarded as proved—as cause and effect (Maldonado 1967). The hepatic changes usually begin insidiously, but may be acute in some cases. Eggs trapped in the finer venules cause proliferation of the vascular endothelium and the formation of granulomas, or intense endophlebitis with inflammation. With extensive involvement the fibrous tissue increases in the portal spaces, and the result is the pipe-stem cirrhosis of Symmers. The liver may be enlarged and it is usually nodular, hard but not tender, and there is no jaundice. Rarely, the abdomen and legs are oedematous. Anaemia is moderate—it is normocytic and hypochromic, with leucocytosis and a tendency to eosinophilia.

Portal congestion causes congestion of the gastric mucosa. Varices form in the stomach and oesophagus, and may bleed repeatedly and seriously. Haematemesis occurs in about one-third of such patients.

Splenomegaly is almost always present with hepatomegaly, and the spleen may be enormous (Fig. 109). Hypersplenism is sometimes a feature, leading to pooling of red cells in the spleen and destruction of those cells. Splenectomy might help such patients. Woodruff *et al.* (1966) consider that the hypersplenism which accompanies gross splenomegaly is largely responsible for the anaemia of *S. haematobium* and *S. mansoni* late infections. It is characterized by iron deficiency, shortening of the erythrocyte life span and slow plasma albumin turnover; loss of blood in urine and faeces is probably a minor factor.

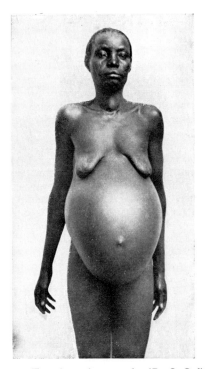

Fig. 109.—Egyptian splenomegaly. (*Dr S. C. Jones*)

In Rhodesia, however, Gelfand (1967) concludes that, though bilharzial lesions are rare in adults with cirrhosis of the liver, this is not true of Africans under the age of 20. He states that 'cirrhosis of the liver due to *S. mansoni* is probably of far more importance in tropical Africa, especially in juveniles, than any of us believed'. The same is true of cor pulmonale due to schistosomiasis. The lungs contain granulomas, and there is a strain on the right side of the heart. X-ray signs in the lungs may suggest tuberculosis; there is hilar thickening. A chief feature is cyanosis (best seen on the tongue in Africans). The jugular pressure is raised, the apex beat displaced outwards, and the ECG shows peaked P waves. X-ray shows dilatation of the pulmonary artery. The pulmonary second sound is accentuated and doubled. Heart failure may follow, with ascites. The chief symptom is dyspnoea; cyanosis may be associated with clubbing of the fingers. Hepatosplenomegaly is also usually present.

S. mansoni infection has been associated in South America with dwarfism and impairment of gonad function, and with sexual immaturity. The nephrotic syndrome due to deposit of antigen-antibody complexes in the glomeruli of the kidneys has been reported in Brazil.

In those parts of Africa where both *S. haematobium* and *S. mansoni* are prevalent, mixed infections are not rare (60% in parts of the Nile delta, 22% in European patients in Rhodesia). *S. mansoni* eggs may be found in large numbers in the faeces of patients in whom *S. haematobium* infection has gone so far as to produce calcification of the bladder, dilatation of the ureters and hydronephrosis. *S. haematobium* eggs are quite often present in faeces, but *S. mansoni* eggs are not often found in urine, though such cases do occur. For instance they have been found in 15 of 103 in-patients in St Lucia, where *S. haematobium* does not exist (Cook & Jordan 1970). Haematospermia may occur, and eggs of either *S. haematobium* or *S. mansoni* may be present in the spermatic fluid. Granulomas in the peritoneum can simulate tuberculosis.

Granulomatous masses, due to either *S. haematobium* or *S. mansoni*, can be found in association with the colon and even with the small intestine. In the colon they tend to be sausage-shaped. They can lead to obstruction or even volvulus.

S. haematobium and *S. mansoni* can both affect the central nervous system— *S. haematobium* eggs being found in the brain more often than *S. mansoni* eggs. They cause epilepsy, vertigo and other signs of cerebral damage. They may also invade the cord, leading to transverse myelitis with granuloma formation. Adult schistosomes may even enter the spinal canal. Operation to relieve pressure, together with specific treatment, may be successful in cord cases.

The general effect of schistosomiasis on the school work of children is difficult to assess, but it may well interfere with the full development of intellectual capacity. Conflicting reports have been made on this subject, which is being studied. The effect of the disease on the rate of growth, onset of menstruation, nutritional status and other features is regarded, in South Africa, as less than expected. Endocrine changes include reduction in size of the gonads and gynaecomastia, in a few patients.

S. japonicum infection

In this disease the bladder is not affected. It can be a severe disease, which, if not treated, may be fatal, but in China, the Philippines and no doubt elsewhere most people infected in childhood gradually overcome the infection. Of proved cases among American troops during the Second World War 10–40% were asymptomatic (Most *et al.* 1950).

The early (Katayama) phase occurs shortly after infection and is associated with fever, urticaria, angioneurotic oedema, abdominal pain and cramp, cough and eosinophilia (60% or more); there may be diarrhoea. A fulminating type with sudden onset has been described, in which abdominal rigidity is a feature.

The second phase is characterized by emaciation, dysentery, and enlargement of the liver (12–16%) and spleen (2–8%), with severe pain in the right hypochondrium and cough. The condition may resemble typhoid fever.

The third stage occurs some 3–5 years after the infection; liver and spleen are cirrhotic and enlarged, with ascites and oedema of the limbs, anaemia and dysentery. In chronic cases intussusception or pyloric obstruction may develop. Superficial abdominal veins are distended and varicosities occur in the oesophagus, but haemorrhage is infrequent. Signs of involvement of the central nervous system—Jacksonian epilepsy, hemiplegia or even blindness—may develop as a result of deposition of eggs in the brain. Hypopituitarism or impairment of the function of the gonads, with sexual immaturity and dwarfism may (rarely) occur. Bones may be insufficiently calcified.

In American troops, eggs of *S. japonicum* have been found in multiple pruritic papules on the chest and scrotum.

There seems to be a connection between *S. japonicum* infection and carcinoma of the colon.

Diagnosis is made by finding the eggs in the faeces, with the usual proviso that this infection may not be the true cause of the symptoms of which the

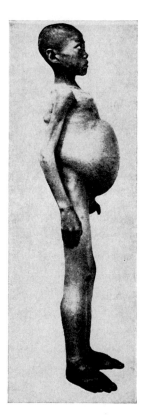

Fig. 110.—Terminal stages of Eastern schistosomiasis. (*Photograph by Dr J. A. Thomson; reproduced by courtesy of the Wellcome Bureau of Scientific Research*)

patient complains. Eggs may also be found in rectal biopsy material (very often when none can be found in the faeces), in scrape material from the wall of the rectum or in material aspirated from crypts by means of a glass pipette with a bent tip, connected to a suction pump. For a rectal snip a small portion of the membrane is obtained by curette and examined as a squash preparation between two slides, when eggs can be seen clearly under low power. This method is as accurate as examination of faeces under concentration, but each method is occasionally positive when the other is negative.

On sigmoidoscopy, in most cases, there are no visible changes, even when numerous eggs can be found on rectal snip. The earliest changes are small submucous haemorrhages, which later become small yellowish elevations of the mucosa in the rectosigmoid area; these can disappear after treatment. More rarely small ulcers and polyps may be found.

The other means of diagnosis resemble those used for *S. mansoni* infections. 'A diagnosis of *S. japonicum* infection should not be excluded unless a negative skin test, two or three negative stool examinations using concentration techniques, and a negative rectal biopsy have been obtained' (Kagan *et al.* 1962).

It need hardly be stated that in endemic areas such diagnoses as the dysenteries, typhoid, hookworm disease, tuberculosis of the intestine, carcinoma and Banti's disease should never be made without extensive examination for schistosomiasis. Multiple infections are common in the tropics, and there is no easy answer to the problems of diagnosis.

DIAGNOSIS

In *S. haematobium* infection diagnosis rests on finding eggs in the urine; they are present at all stages of micturition, and can be found especially in centrifuged specimens.

The viability of eggs in urine may be important in deciding whether treatment has succeeded in killing them. Viability can be determined by using a miracidioscope, a dull black rack for centrifuge tubes containing urinary sediment to which water has been added. Live eggs hatch quickly, and active miracidia can be seen through a hand lens against the black background. The presence of eggs in the urine does not necessarily mean that schistosomiasis is the only cause of the patient's illness; in endemic areas it may coincide with chyluria, stone, vesical tumour (benign or malignant), cystitis, pyelitis or prostatic disease which must be excluded.

Eggs may also be found in biopsy material from the bladder or rectal mucosa (which is affected quite commonly). Cystoscopic examination can be important, though rarely necessary for diagnosis. There is a danger of introducing bacterial infection, to which hydronephrotic patients are very vulnerable. It may show sparse grey or yellow discrete elevations around the ureteric orifices, or haemorrhagic papules with surrounding inflammation, which are formed by eggs passing through the mucosa. Later there are 'sandy patches' resembling ridges of sea sand, with papillomas; these are pathognomonic (Plate III). The bladder surface is generally coated with mucus, usually bloody, containing myriads of eggs; if this is detached from the surface and examined, the diagnosis is simplified.

For diagnosis of *S. mansoni* and *S. japonicum* infections, faeces should be examined microscopically for eggs, either by emulsifying a small portion in saline on a slide, to make a thin film, and covering with a coverslip, or by concentration (see Appendix IV). Biopsy material from the rectum may also be examined for eggs.

Viability of eggs can be assessed by stirring about 5 grammes of faeces in 250 ml saline, straining through a metal sieve to remove coarse particles, and allowing the fluid to stand in a conical glass or tall cylinder until the sediment has formed completely, when the supernatant is decanted. This is then repeated until the supernatant fluid is clear, when it is finally decanted. Warm tap water is then added to the sediment, and hatching of the eggs takes place. Through a hand lens the miracidia can easily be seen moving rapidly.

For the examination of faeces for worm eggs and protozoal cysts see page 1136. The method of Ridley and Hawgood (1956) is recommended (see page 1139) and other concentration techniques are described in that section. Simple sedimentation or centrifugation after shaking a small portion of faeces in saline, is also often satisfactory, but concentration gives better results.

Quantitative examination of faeces for egg content presents difficulties, which are discussed by Jordan and Webbe (1969). The favoured method seems to be that of Bell (1963), in which a sample of known weight or volume is homogenized in at least 10 volumes of water. 0·1 ml of this suspension is passed through 2 fine wire meshes (apertures of 500 and 350 μm) and then on to Whatman No. 541 filter paper in a Buchner funnel connected to a water pump. The papers are then placed on a drop of freshly made ninhydrin solution and dried. Eggs are stained blue and can easily be counted under a microscope.

Jordan and Webbe discuss other quantitative methods.

For the oögram technique of Pellegrino et al. (1962), see page 312.

Radiological examination

In *S. haematobium* infections of the bladder, calcification is relatively late. Some eggs die in the mucosa and in fibrous tissue in the bladder wall; they become necrotic, and calcify, and X-ray shows a thin line of calcification round the whole bladder, sometimes very dense around mounds of granulation tissue, and extending to the lower ureters, the seminal vesicles or even the posterior urethra. Calcification does not usually involve the muscle coat, though in rare cases it may do so.

The ureters may be narrowed, or dilated with hydroureter, hydronephrosis, or filling defects in the ureters and bladder (large filling defects are a feature of severe disease in Nigeria). It is not certain that such lesions are progressive; they may regress with treatment, but a radiologically non-functioning kidney does not regress (Forsyth 1969).

In *S. mansoni* infection, when eggs cause ulceration of the mucous membrane, healing takes place by fibrosis, and subsequent crops of eggs may become entombed, producing granulomas or polyps which can be demonstrated radiologically by barium enema, appearing as multiple small filling defects, mostly in the sigmoid. They may even produce symptoms of obstruction, and be indistinguishable radiologically from carcinoma.

Gastric varices can also be demonstrated radiologically, but oesophageal varices are more difficult.

Portal venography to demonstrate the state of the portal vein and collateral circulation, and the site of any obstruction, can be carried out by injecting 30 ml of contrast material through a wide-bore needle rapidly into the spleen, and taking serial films in rapid succession.

X-ray examination of the chest may help in the diagnosis of cor pulmonale. For instance, fluoroscopy often shows pulsation of the pulmonary artery, and enlargement of the right ventricle. Pulmonary angiography and cardiac catheterization, however, demand special techniques. The easiest way of making a presumptive diagnosis of cor pulmonale is by ECG.

The radiological changes in *S. japonicum* infection are very similar to those in *S. mansoni* infection.

Immunodiagnosis

Sadun (1967) remarks that though an intradermal test which gives results in 15–20 minutes is valuable in epidemiological studies, its value in clinical use is limited because great variations in sensitivity and specificity are common. Many antigens have been used, the most sensitive being extracts from cercariae, or from adult *S. mansoni* or *Fasciola gigantica* (some antigens being rendered lipoid-free). Cross-reactions occur where infections with *S. bovis* and other trematodes are found. The intradermal test does not become positive until 4–6 weeks after exposure.

The serological tests include complement fixation, slide flocculation, plasma card, precipitin, haemagglutination and conglutination tests, the *Cercarienhuellen* reaction, the cercarial agglutination reaction, the miracidial immobilization test, the circumoval precipitin test, the phagocytic response test and the fluorescent antibody test. Sadun quotes results obtained by various authors, which can be summarized:

Test	*Positive*
(mostly for *S. mansoni* infection)	
Complement fixation	88–94%
Slide flocculation	75–90%
Plasma card	93–98%
Fluorescent antibody (indirect)	75–99%

None of these tests is species specific, and there may be cross-reactions with other helminth infections; they may be misleading in Africa where there are many animal schistosome cercariae which may attack man.

Of the antigens used, those prepared from adult worms gave 75–99% positive results; those prepared from cercariae gave 75–98%. The complement fixation test, with either cercarial or adult worms, is highly sensitive, and will detect infection before the worms are mature. It remains positive long after active infection has ceased; it does not provide a means of assessing cure. Cross-reactions can occur, especially with *Trichuris trichiura* and non-human *Schistosoma* (e.g. swimmer's itch).

Antigens prepared from excretions and secretions of the adult worms are sensitive and specific for the slide flocculation tests. One antigen is prepared from the cercarial material adsorbed on to crystals of lecithin–cholesterol, and with this the test is sensitive. In this test the antigen is allowed to fall on a drop of inactivated serum, the slide is rotated for 2 minutes and the result is read under the microscope. In the cercarial slide flocculation test IgG and IgM are concerned.

For the plasma card test cards coated with plastic, on which a drop of plasma from a finger-puncture has been placed, are used with an antigen solution containing charcoal powder as a visualizing agent. The cards can be dried after the test and filed as records.

A conglutinative complement absorption test has proved very sensitive in patients with active *S. mansoni* infections, and negative in controls (Antunes & Pellegrino 1966). Technical details should be sought in the original paper.

A few drops of dried blood on filter paper can be used for the fluorescent antibody test, which is one of the simplest, most practical and sensitive tests, especially useful as a preliminary screen in surveys. The equipment in laboratories, however, is rather expensive, and cross-reactions occur with the various animal schistosomes. The test can also be used to detect all the stages of development of schistosomes in infected tissue. In this reaction IgM is probably involved. False negative reactions occur, especially in long-term infections. Important modifications in the technique of this test (with antigens prepared from cercariae of *S. mansoni*) are given by Cookson (1964), who also describes a fluorescent antibody test in which bentonite particles are used and a bentonite fluorescent complement fixation test.

In the *Cercarienhuellen* test a membrane is formed round cercariae immersed in immune serum, but not in control serum. The test can be valuable in the diagnosis of present and recent infections when eggs cannot be found in urine or faeces. This test becomes positive 40–70 days after successful treatment and negative 5–7 months after successful treatment; it can be used as an index of cure. IgG is involved.

The circumoval precipitin test (COP) depends upon the formation of precipitates round the schistosome eggs immersed in dilutions of sera from infected persons; these are antigen-antibody complexes formed by secretions and excretions of the living miracidia in the eggs, and specific antibodies in the sera. 0·05 ml of serum is mixed with 0·05 ml of egg suspension (which may be lyophilized) on a slide. A coverslip ringed with petroleum jelly is placed on the slide, which is then incubated at 37°C for 24 hours. Lewert and Yogore (1969) describe a simplified COP test. A similar COP may be positive in cerebral schistosomiasis due to *S. japonicum*, when eggs are incubated in the cerebrospinal fluid.

A modification of the COP, on which is superimposed the indirect FA test, is easy to perform in laboratories maintaining the parasites, eliminates non-specific reactions and simplifies the reading of results. Eggs from different species may give different results, but when several strains are available as antigens it may be possible to use the test for species-specific diagnosis. Sera are heated at 56°C for 30 minutes. Freeze-dried eggs are suspended in saline containing 1 in 10 000 Merthiolate; 0·1 ml of the suspension is added to 0·2 ml of serum, shaken and incubated for 72 hours at 37°C. 2 ml of phosphate buffer saline (*p*H 7·2) are added and the eggs are allowed to settle and are then washed twice. 0·1 ml of the sediment is placed in a tube to which is added 0·1 ml of fluorescein-labelled anti-human-globulin serum containing 20% rhodamine bovine albumin solution (this dilution is determined by titration against known positive and negative sera). The tubes are shaken at 110 rpm for 15 minutes and then incubated at 37°C for 1 hour. The eggs are washed twice in buffered saline; one drop of 90% buffered glycerin is added to each tube and the eggs are pipetted to a slide under a coverslip. Under suitably filtered ultra-violet light against a dark background the eggs are examined at a magnification of 100 (Wolstenholme 1968).

Other tests are being developed. Of particular interest are those depending on the detection of antigen rather than antibody, since they may determine whether the infection is active or not (Gold *et al.* 1969). A soluble antigen has been demonstrated in the urine in *S. haematobium* infection.

Mothers whose serum tests (*Cercarienhuellen* or FAT) are positive can transfer antibodies passively across the placenta to their fetuses, but the tests in the infants, positive at birth, are negative 6 months later. This does not prove that the antibodies so transferred are necessarily protective, though they may be so in part. It does indicate that they behave like antibodies to bacterial and viral infections (and malaria) in this respect (Lees & Jordan 1968).

An intradermal test with an antigen of an extract of an adult *S. mansoni*, standardized to contain 20–40 mg N/ml, gives a positive reaction (weal over 1·1 cm²) in infected persons. It may also be positive in persons infected with schistosomes of animals. The skin test and the fluorescent antibody tests are not reliable in areas where schistosomes of animals can infect man.

TREATMENT

The treatment of schistosomiasis cannot be regarded as satisfactory. Many drugs have shown activity, but though the excretion of eggs is usually greatly reduced or even stopped, many patients are not cured, and repetition of treatment may be needed. Patients with light infections respond better than those with heavy infections, and adults seem to respond better than children. But reports of the same drug from different authors vary, which may be a reflection of different strains of the parasite, or of methods of administration, or of the criteria of cure (Jordan 1968).

Side-effects of the commonly used drugs are not negligible; sometimes they could be serious. In debilitated children, for instance, it may be advisable to give drugs in doses considerably less than those advocated for more robust children, at the same time dealing with the other causes of debility, such as anaemia, malaria or hookworm infection.

The unfortunate fact is that, apart from exceptional circumstances, the patients return to the conditions which led to the original infection or series of infections.

The life span of the three main schistosomes of man is uncertain. It may reach 20 years or more in extreme cases, but in general is probably much less. In *S. haematobium* infection in Egypt many children under the age of 5 years apparently lose the infection spontaneously, at a rate which may be between 26 and 50% per annum; for those aged 5–6 the rate is much less, about 5%. Similarly for *S. mansoni* infection the corresponding rates are rather over 50% and about 33% respectively. These trends in losses of infection are not ascribed to the process of acquired immunity (Farook & Hairston 1966).

Most cases of *S. haematobium* infection can recover without treatment, but there is always a possibility that irreversible lesions may develop; early treatment is therefore desirable. Granulomas can resolve under drug treatment.

Various techniques are used to estimate the effectiveness of drugs in animals. One is the oögram technique (Pellegrino *et al.* 1962). Fragments of the distal parts of the small intestine of mice, after a defined course of treatment, are pressed on to slides, under coverslips, so that schistosome eggs in various stages can be counted. If mature eggs only are found, the drug has prevented the production of eggs; if immature eggs are found, the drug has been less effective. The criteria of maturity and immaturity should be sought in the original paper.

Trivalent antimony compounds

All patients under treatment with antimonial drugs should remain in bed, and blood pressure readings should be taken daily. If the systolic pressure falls by 10 mm Hg the treatment should be stopped.

These compounds inhibit the phosphofructinase enzyme system, thus depriving the worms of glycogen.

Tartar emetic (sodium or potassium antimony tartrate). This is the classical drug. It is given by not too rapid intravenous injection, on alternate days. The first (adult) dose is 30 mg in 10 ml of freshly distilled water or 5% glucose solution, and the dose is increased by 30 mg every second day to a maximum of 150 mg. This is continued to a total of 2 grammes for adult men (14 doses in all), and correspondingly reduced doses for women and children. Tartar emetic is toxic to the heart and liver if given in over-large doses, and patients should remain in bed during treatment. At one time an intensive course was used, consisting of up to 800 mg, divided into 7 or 8 doses with an interval of 16–18 hours after the first half of the course, and lasting 30 hours in all. The drug was injected very slowly and the patient was in bed. The point of this intensive course was that it could be completed at a single visit of the patient to the hospital, a consideration in places where continuity of treatment lasting for days or even weeks could not be guaranteed. But on the whole this intensive treatment has not found favour.

Antimony lithium tartrate (Anthiomaline). This is available as a 6% solution equivalent to about 10 mg antimony/ml. The dose is 0·5–5·0 ml by intramuscular injection at intervals of 2–3 days (usually 2) to a total of 40–60 ml. The average dose for adults is 1·0 ml increasing by 1·0 ml at each injection to a maximum of 4·0 ml. It is less likely than tartar emetic to cause cough or vomiting.

Stibocaptate (antimony dimercaptosuccinate) (TWSb/6, Astiban). The potassium salt is TWSb, the magnesium salt TWSb/1, and the sodium salt TWSb/6. Stibocaptate contains about 25% of trivalent antimony. It is given intramuscularly as a 10% solution (100 mg/ml) in water or 5% glucose solution (more recently in olive oil), and in doses of 10 mg (or less)/kg body weight, in the following (adult) schedules:

Daily for 3 doses (total 1500 mg)
Daily for 3–15 smaller doses (to a total of 1000–3000 mg)
Daily to a total of 15–20 ml (1500–2000 mg) during 4–5 days
Twice weekly for 5 doses (to a maximum total of 2500 mg)
Twice weekly for 5 smaller doses (total 2000 mg)
Weekly for 5 doses (total 2500 mg)
Monthly for 6 doses

Astiban may be given by very slow intravenous perfusion in glucose saline, at the rate of 1000–1300 mg over a period of 8 hours.

High cure rates are reported with Astiban, but there are side-effects (weakness, anorexia, vomiting, abdominal pain, headache and pain at the site of injection). Side-effects are less with the twice weekly schedules, which are now preferred. The drug is expensive.

Astiban and sodium antimonyl gluconate are regarded by Forsyth as the drugs of choice for *S. haematobium* infections in Tanzania. Astiban is also valuable in *S. mansoni* infections, but the results do not equal those obtained in *S. haematobium* infections.

Sodium antimonyl gluconate (Triostam). This contains 34–39% of antimony, and is given by slow intravenous injection in doses of 2·5–3·3 mg/kg body weight (usually 190 mg in 4–5 ml water for an adult of 70 kg) daily for 6 days. Solutions must be freshly made in sterile water. Higher doses (225 mg daily) have been used with success, but should not exceed 6 mg/kg daily. A total dose of 17–20 mg/kg has been given, divided over 4 days, with some success, but another report on this dosage in *S. mansoni* infection is disappointing. With a total dose of 25 mg/kg cure in *S. mansoni* infections has been reported in 96–100%. Side-effects are much less than with tartar emetic, but nausea, vomiting or urticaria may occur, usually transient and associated with the first few doses. A case of severe myocardial damage has been reported.

Stibophen (Fouadin). The dose is 100–300 mg by intramuscular injection, daily (or at longer intervals) to a total of 2400–4500 mg. Stibophen Injection (BP) contains 6·4% w/v of stibophen—about 300 mg in 5 ml.

Stibophen may cause nausea, vomiting, bradycardia or damage to the liver (if the course is prolonged); it is not advised if the liver is damaged by schistosomiasis. Haemoglobinuria and sulphaemoglobinuria have been reported, though rarely, after stibophen.

The following course has been advocated:

Day 1　　Stibophen injection (BP) 1·5 ml
Day 2　　Stibophen injection (BP) 3·5 ml
Day 3　　Stibophen injection (BP) 5·0 ml

and thereafter every second day 5·0 ml to a total of 40–75 ml.

Results are reported good for *S. haematobium* and *S. japonicum* infections, but in *S. mansoni* infections with liver damage large doses of antimony should be avoided.

Preparations not containing antimony

Lucanthone hydrochloride (*Nilodin, Miracil D*). The mode of action of lucanthone is not known, but it is fairly effective in *S. haematobium* infections, less so in *S. mansoni* infections.

It is given by mouth in doses of:

a. 0·5–1·0 gramme twice daily for 3 days (this could be repeated monthly for 3 months).
b. 200 mg once daily for 20 days together with meclizine hydrochloride 12·5 mg for each 200 mg tablet of lucanthone, to reduce side-effects.
c. 10 mg/kg daily together with tartar emetic 1·0 mg/kg daily, for 12 days. These half doses appear to act synergically.
d. 500 mg once each week for 10 weeks. This has reduced the egg loads in St Lucia (*S. mansoni*) and Tanzania by about 90%, with no side-effects (Jordan 1968). It may be that peaks of blood levels occurring weekly for several weeks are more effective than high levels for shorter periods.

Side-effects include nausea, vomiting, headache, dizziness, depression, abdominal pain and rise in blood pressure, but they seldom warrant discontinuance of the treatment. If tincture of belladonna, 0·6 ml twice daily, or mepyramine maleate 100 mg (or other similar drugs) are given with lucanthone, side-effects are considerably reduced. There may be yellow discoloration of the tongue or red-brown discoloration of the palms and soles.

A course consisting of a single dose (10 mg/kg) of TWSb followed every 2 weeks by lucanthone hydrochloride (500 mg) for 11 doses has proved satisfactory in children in Tanzania. It could be timed to coincide with the transmission season since it greatly reduces egg output, and therefore could perhaps reduce infection of snails.

Hycanthone. This is a derivative of Miracil D, and has proved successful in the treatment of *S. mansoni* infections (though still (1971) at the investigational stage). It is given by mouth in doses of 2 or 3 mg/kg daily for 5 days, producing cure rates of about 80%, mostly without serious side-effects, though vomiting may be troublesome. It has also been given by intramuscular injection in a single dose of 3·0 or 3·5 mg/kg, with similar results in both *S. haematobium* and *S. mansoni* infections. Alternatively, in *S. mansoni* infections, a course of intramuscular hycanthone, 3·0 mg/kg every 3 days for 3 doses has produced cure in over 90%. A few deaths have occurred in debilitated children after hycanthone, and it must be used with caution because of hepatotoxicity.

Amphotalide (*Schistomide, M & B 2948A, RP 6171*). This is given by mouth in doses of 250–400 mg/kg (total dose) in divided doses over 5–15 days, or of 6–29 grammes in divided doses over 7–10 days. Side-effects are minimal—some nausea and vomiting, and abdominal discomfort. Reports indicate only moderately good results in *S. haematobium* infections, and less good in *S. mansoni* infections.

Niridazole (Ambilhar, CIBA 32,644-Ba). This is given by mouth in doses of 20–30 mg/kg daily for 5–7 days. The daily dose should be divided into 2 parts, for morning and evening. Weekly doses have also been tried, but with less success; the doses were 25 mg/kg weekly for 5 weeks, but this may have been insufficient.

Single doses of 50 mg/kg, repeated every 4 weeks until eggs can no longer be found, are reported to be effective in *S. haematobium* infections. This schedule could be used in mass campaigns, but cure rates in Zanzibar were only 54% or less.

Reports of the efficacy of niridazole in *S. haematobium* infections vary. In the Durban area 94% of cures have been recorded, in Tanzania 98·5% and in Egypt 90%. In Nigeria Lucas *et al.* (1966) found that in some cases hydronephrosis and ureteric lesions showed striking improvement, or even disappeared, presumably because the obstructions were due, not to fibrosis, but to granulomas and oedema. Calcification of the bladder, however, did not change. On the other hand, nodular filling defects may be quite transitory within a short time, as seen on consecutive films during intravenous pyelography. In other cases long-term pyelograms have shown no regression of lesions in spite of apparently successful treatment.

For *S. mansoni* infections the reported results are less satisfactory, though there is great reduction in the numbers of eggs. Cure has been recorded in 89% in Brazil, in up to 50% in adults and in light infections in Africa, but lower figures are quoted for children and heavier infections. Astiban has sometimes given better results, but a higher dosage of niridazole might have been more successful.

For *S. japonicum* infections cure has been reported in about half the cases on a regimen of 20 mg/kg daily for 5 days.

Side-effects in otherwise healthy patients are infrequent, and children tolerate niridazole well. Side-effects may include headache, dizziness, insomnia, epilepsy and psychosis, tachycardia, nausea and abdominal pain; severe reactions have been reported, especially in patients with liver involvement, and niridazole should therefore be used under strict medical supervision. A young child died after 3 doses of 34 mg/kg daily; there were extensive haemorrhages in liver and kidneys. An acute confusional state was observed in 4 of over 500 patients with *S. haematobium* treated in Tanzania; in 2 of these isoniazid was also being taken, and the association of niridazole with isoniazid is to be avoided. If phenobarbital is given with niridazole this alarming complication is practically eradicated. Side-effects are most common and serious in *S. japonicum* infections; least common in *S. haematobium*.

Contra-indications to niridazole are said to be liver disease, poor general condition (especially when due to hookworm disease, anaemia and tuberculosis) and neurosis or psychosis.

Metriphonate (Trichlorphon, Dipterex, Neguvon). This is an insecticide; it has, however, been used for the treatment of helminthiasis in animals, and *S. haematobium* infections in man, in which it is apparently more successful than in *S. mansoni* infections. It is very toxic when inhaled, swallowed or spilled on to the skin in concentrated form; it is a cholinesterase inhibitor in insects and reduces cholinesterase in erythrocytes in man. Nevertheless, it has been used with success in appropriate doses by mouth, for instance 7·5 mg/kg as a single dose repeated at intervals of 2 weeks (not less), or one month, for 2–3 doses. It is supplied in capsules of 50 mg. Results in 76 lightly infected schoolboys in Tanzania were good, all ceasing to pass eggs. No toxic symptoms were noted in this series. Side-effects may be vomiting, diarrhoea, faintness, retrosternal and abdominal pain, blurring of vision, bronchial spasm, headache and tremors.

Further studies on the toxicity of this group of drugs is necessary before they can be recommended for general use.

Pararosaniline pamoate (CI-403-A). This is a complex azo dye derived from gentian violet, which acts by inhibiting the acetylcholinesterase system. It is given in hard gelatin capsules each containing 175 mg of carbonium ions and is administered before meals. In *S. japonicum* infections Pesigan *et al.* (1967) used the following schedule in the Philippines:

A. 30 mg/kg daily in 3 divided doses for 10 days
B. 35–40 mg/kg daily in 3 divided doses for 14 days
C. 35–40 mg/kg daily in 3 divided doses for 14 days, repeated after 7 days rest
D. 35–40 mg/kg daily in 3 divided doses for 14 days, followed by one full day's dose once a week for 4 weeks

Modifications of these schedules were used in later work.

The best results in this experiment on over 150 patients with *S. japonicum* were obtained with schedule C, 81% of the group being negative for eggs at 6 months; the other schedules were much less effective. Side-effects—loss of appetite, nausea vomiting, dizziness, weakness, skin eruptions—were mild except in 3 patients who had fever (schedule B). The disadvantage is that a patient of 50 kg had to swallow 3–4 capsules 3 times a day for 28 days (schedule C). But the results were encouraging. The drug is safe and the most satisfactory results are obtained when it is given for a long time or for a minimum of 28 days at a dosage of 35–40 mg/kg. It is both curative and suppressive in doses according to schedule C, followed by a full day's dose at intervals of one week for 16–24 weeks—a maximum of 52 treatment days in a total of 203 days (schedule E).

Schedule E, tested on 112 patients, in whom 72% had negative stools after 220 days, is recommended for mass treatment, especially in school-children in the Philippines. Egg counts in those still positive were reduced almost to zero.

Pararosaniline is one of the few drugs which show prophylactic action in animals.

Furapromidium (F 30066). For *S. japonicum* infection in China Chou *et al.* (1965) used furapromidium with success. It is given in capsules by mouth in daily doses of 60–100 mg/kg, divided into 4 portions, treatment lasting 1–4½ months (usually 1½–2½). The immediate result was cure in 83·8% of 136 patients; results 4–6 months after treatment showed 77% cures. Side-effects were gastro-intestinal disturbance and muscular cramps, and mild psychological changes; these all disappeared on interruption of the treatment.

Several other drugs have been tested experimentally in animals; some may eventually prove valuable but more work is needed. Certainly there is much room for improvement in the treatment of schistosomiasis. For details of the new work WHO (1966) is valuable, and experimental chemotherapy of *S. mansoni* infections is discussed at length by Pellegrino and Katz (1968).

Surgical treatment

This may be needed in the later stages of *S. haematobium* infection. Simpson (1965) uses colocystoplasty for patients whose bladder capacity is reduced to below 300 ml and who suffer from frequency, dysuria and pain. Symptoms can be relieved by this procedure. Much work has recently been done on reconstruction of the bladder, in which isolated segments of ileum and rectum are used.

A new technique, extracorporeal haemofiltration, has been used in all three types of schistosomiasis. The technique is not described in the preliminary contribution by Kean and Goldsmith (1968), but consists of filtering portal blood through an extracorporeal circulation after a dose of antimony. This is said to be a safe and practical way to remove adult schistosomes from selected patients, and could be performed whenever splenectomy or portal decompression is performed. It may have a use in acute schistosomiasis.

PREVENTION

The obvious measures of prevention are:

1. Treatment of infected persons (though this leaves the question of animal reservoirs unsolved). Large-scale treatment is reported to have reduced the overall prevalence from 54% in 1950 to 37% in 1969 in parts of Egypt.

2. Provision of latrines, especially at work places connected with irrigation channels.

3. Provision of properly constructed and controlled bathing places for children, which can be kept free from snails. Such protected swimming baths within canals have recently been suggested, to prevent indiscriminate bathing in infected water.

4. Siting of villages well away from snail-bearing irrigation canals and, if possible, other snail-bearing waters. This may not be possible if the waters are ponds forming the only water supplies for the people.

5. Provision of piped water or properly constructed wells; an easily available protected supply seems to have the greatest effect on prevalence. In this respect it should be noted that schistosome cercariae can pass in small numbers through conventional sand filters (Witenberg & Yofe 1938), and through metal microfabric Mark 1 (apertures 35 μm) though they are almost completely held back by microfabric Mark 0 (apertures 23 μm) (Webbe & James 1969).

6. Destruction of snails by molluscicides or other means, for instance by predators such as large snails (*Marisa*).

7. Education of the people.

8. Reduction of contact with snail-bearing water by covering irrigation canals, or conveying irrigation water in pipes for overhead irrigation, or by providing numerous footbridges over canals.

Macdonald (1965) has evaluated the various measures by relating them to the life cycle of the schistosomes, pointing out that in such an infection, in which sexual pairing takes place and in which there is an intermediate host, the numbers of potential pathogenic worms are enormously increased by the large numbers of eggs discharged each day by a single pair of adult worms, that they are again enormously increased if the eggs reach fresh water in which there are many snails of species susceptible to the infection, because each miracidium which develops in a snail gives rise to hundreds of cercariae.

From a mathematical analysis of factors bearing on infection he argued that reduction in the numbers of miracidia will not significantly reduce the numbers of invasive cercariae if the snails are abundant, because the miracidia can easily find the snails in which they multiply so enormously. This means that sanitary measures which reduce contamination of water by excreta to 1/15 000 of the previous level are virtually negligible in controlling spread of the infection, and that the effective measures are snail control, control of contact with water ('Safe water supplies are more important than latrines'), and treatment of infected persons.

It is only fair to say, however, that this pessimistic view of the effect of sanitary disposal of excreta does not mean that Macdonald would have restricted it in any way; improved sanitation is of the first importance in bacterial and virus diseases, and is essential to all health programmes. It must also be stated that not all authorities dealing with schistosomiasis share Macdonald's view. Wright (1970) is convinced that study of the human host and his habits, and gradual improvement in environment and behaviour, is likely to be the most effective means of long-term control. But it needs careful consideration of established customs.

This is not the place to elaborate on the techniques of snail control, but certain facts should be remembered. Snails prefer still or slowly flowing water with abundant vegetation on which they feed. They can aestivate during hot dry weather by burrowing into mud, without catastrophic reduction in their numbers, though many die. Mostly (but not invariably) they prefer water open to the sun, so that by covering a channel one can discourage them. They mostly live in shallow water, but infected *Biomphalaria* species carrying *S. mansoni* have been found at depths of 12 m in Lake Victoria. It is therefore not entirely true that bathing in deep water is safe.

Molluscicides

Details of the many molluscicides must be sought elsewhere, for instance in WHO Special Report Series (WHO 1967).

Control by molluscicides is expensive; application must be frequently repeated and needs constant supervision.

Niclosamide (Bayluscide) is very effective. It is highly toxic to snails and their eggs, and can be handled safely; it is cheap and does not upset the biological balance as much as some compounds. In some water, however, it does not diffuse effectively.

Frescon is equally effective, especially in relation to irrigation.

Sodium pentachlorophenate kills snails and their eggs and has been widely used with success, but it is irritating and potentially dangerous to the handler; its activity may be reduced by bright sunlight.

Copper sulphate (and other copper compounds) is active at low pH and is somewhat less toxic to fish than some molluscicides; it is safe to handle but is absorbed by soil and organic material and its toxicity to snails and their eggs is variable in the field. It corrodes equipment.

Other molluscicides include organo-tin and lead compounds, dinex (a dinitrophenol), carbamates, 3-trifluoromethyl-4-nitrophenol (TFM), and some plants.

Molluscicides may most profitably be used if they are related to the seasonal periodicity of snail populations. In Egypt, for instance, *Bulinus truncatus*, abundant in large canals and less abundant in drains, can double its population in 14–16 days in March, and its highest death rates are in midsummer. *Biomphalaria alexandrina*, on the other hand, is most abundant in drains and less so upstream; it reaches its maximum abundance in the presence of the water hyacinth *Eichornia crassipes*, doubling its population in 14–16 days in March, with its highest death rates in summer.

A single area-wide treatment with molluscicide in April is therefore recommended; during the rest of the year search for isolated foci of snail breeding and individual treatment of those foci will be effective in control.

In Egypt the application of Bayluscide and sodium pentachlorophenate has been shown to reduce significantly the incidence and prevalence of *S. haemato-bium* and *S. mansoni* infections. Both are highly effective, but control must be continued for many years, and in those parts of Egypt where the best results were achieved there has been failure of continuity, and reinfection has occurred.

Biological control of snails has been attempted. Ducks eat them, and have been advocated, but it seems that the snails outstrip the appetites of the ducks.

The large snail *Marisa cornuarietis* eats the egg masses of *Biomphalaria glabrata* and competes with it for food. It is used largely in Puerto Rico for control, but it is not known if it would be useful elsewhere, and though it is reputed not to affect rice, its effect on crops needs clarification. It is not, so far as is known, an intermediate host of any important parasite.

Other snails and fish, which eat snails, have been tried in control, with some success, and there have been recent developments in interspecies competition between schistosomes and other trematodes which show some promise (Lie *et al.* 1968). Embryos of some species actually devour embryos of other species (including schistosomes) within snails carrying two species.

SWIMMER'S ITCH (CLAM-DIGGER'S ITCH, CERCARIAL DERMATITIS)

This is a skin condition caused by cercariae of the human schistosomes and also by cercariae of other schistosomes which are shed from their snail inter-mediate hosts in shallow waters (usually lake shores, rice fields or even sea shores). The animal and bird cercariae can penetrate the human skin but cannot develop to maturity in man; they may possibly survive in the deeper tissues for some time.

Swimmer's itch is found in many parts of the world—the Americas, Europe, Africa and Australasia. The cercariae have been described under the names *Cercaria elvae, C. ocellata, C. herini* and others. The adult worms include *Gigantobilharzia sturniae, Trichobilharzia* spp. (from black swans and silver ducks), *Schistosomathium douthitti* (from rodents), *Austrobilharzia* spp. (from the silver gull) and *Schistosoma spindale* (from water-buffalo). Snails involved include *Lymnaea stagnalis, L. undussumae, Pyragus australis, Polypylis hemi-sphaerula* and doubtless many others.

The condition is an itching maculo-urticarial dermatitis which becomes papular or even pustular; it arises within a few days of wading or bathing in infected water. Application of 5% copper sulphate is said to relieve the itching, and 2% methylene blue to prevent bacterial infection. A protective ointment may be useful. The intradermal and complement fixation tests become positive

Fascioliasis

AETIOLOGY

Human fascioliasis is caused by infection with *Fasciola hepatica* (the sheep liver fluke) which normally inhabits the liver of sheep. In Hawaii and some other areas, Senegambia, Tashkent and Vietnam, human fascioliasis can also be caused by *F. gigantica*.

TRANSMISSION

The adult fluke lives in the biliary passages where the eggs are laid in the immature stage and are evacuated in the faeces. After maturing in water for 9–15 days the miracidia escape from the eggs and invade snails of many species of *Lymnaea* and other genera of the family Lymnaeidae. In the snail intermediate host sporocysts produce first and second generation rediae and cercariae which leave the snail and swim about in the water before encysting as metacercariae on aquatic plants. The metacercariae are ingested by mammals eating the vegetation or drinking from the bottom of contaminated pools. The metacercariae excyst in the duodenum, migrate through the intestinal wall into the peritoneal cavity, penetrate Glisson's capsule of the liver and traverse the parenchyma to the biliary passages.

The incubation period between infection and the development of the adult flukes is about 3–4 months.

Human infection

Man acquires the infection as the result of eating raw watercress on which the metacercariae have encysted from contamination of the water by sheep. In the Lebanon and Armenia the habit of eating raw sheep or goat livers causes 'halzoun' which is the result of lodgement of adult worms on the pharyngeal mucosa.

EPIDEMIOLOGY AND GEOGRAPHICAL DISTRIBUTION

Human fascioliasis is much commoner in some countries than others. Numbers of cases have been recorded from Germany, Cuba, Uruguay, Argentina, France and Russia. Isolated cases have been described from England and 6 cases were described from Ringwood in Hampshire in 1960 (Facey & Marsden 1960). In all cases infection was associated with the consumption of raw watercress.

PATHOLOGY

In the invasion stage symptoms are caused by the penetration of the intestinal wall, migration across the peritoneal cavity and entry into the liver. Small necrotic foci and micro-abscesses have been described (Belding 1965). In the stage of established infection there is hepatomegaly and eosinophilia. Most patients recover spontaneously with evacuation of the worms via the intestinal canal, or calcification (Facey & Marsden 1960). Fibrosis of the portal tracts with compression of the adjacent liver cells has been described (Biggart 1937), but the association with portal hypertension, splenomegaly and ascites is as yet unproved. The migrating larvae may be trapped in ectopic foci and flukes have been recorded from the blood vessels, lungs, subcutaneous tissues, ventricle of the brain and orbit (Neghme & Ossandon 1943).

SYMPTOMS AND SIGNS

After a short period of dyspepsia there is mild or high fever, and a dragging or cramp-like pain in the right subcostal region aggravated by coughing or movement. The liver is enlarged and tender and there is a marked peripheral eosinophilia. These signs subside and unless spontaneous recovery occurs there is mild indigestion and rarely relapse. In the stage of hepatomegaly there is a leucocytosis of 12 000 to 40 000 with 40–85% eosinophils.

Cutaneous fascioliasis has been observed in South America and France, usually in association with hepatic fascioliasis. Reddish-brown, round or oval, sub-cutaneous nodules appear on the abdomen, which migrate and are pruritic and painful. Biopsy shows eosinophilic infiltration and tunnels with necrotic walls, in which the parasite may or may not be present.

DIAGNOSIS

The association of hepatomegaly with a high eosinophilia is almost patho-gnomonic of *F. hepatica* infection. The typical eggs, which may be found in the stools, are often very scanty. Duodenal aspiration may be necessary to demon-strate the eggs.

Immunodiagnosis

A skin test using *F. hepatica* adult antigen has been described and used successfully to demonstrate exposure to infection (Pautrizel *et al.* 1962). The complement fixation test using adult *F. hepatica* antigen becomes positive shortly after infection. Cross-reactions occur with *Paragonimus* infections.

TREATMENT

Bithionol is the treatment of choice and should be given, as in *Paragonimus* infections, in a dose of 30–50 mg/kg by mouth every other day for 10–15 days.

The other treatment which has been used successfully is emetine hydro-chloride, 40 mg daily by subcutaneous injection for a week to 10 days. Chloroquine may also be useful.

HALZOUN

Temporary lodgement of adult worms on the pharyngeal mucosa causes oedematous congestion of the soft palate, pharynx, larynx, nasal fossa and Eustachian tubes, accompanied by dyspnoea, dysphagia, deafness and occa-sionally asphyxiation.

Halzoun (marrara) may also be due to nymphs of *Linguatula serrata* en-capsulated in the liver or lymph nodes of domestic herbivores, if eaten raw. They can attach themselves to the mouth, pharynx, nasal passages and other places (Schacher *et al.* 1969) (see Appendix II).

Fasciolopsiasis

Synonyms

The giant intestinal fluke.

Aetiology

Fasciolopsiasis is caused by *Fasciolopsis buski*, a parasite of the pig which constitutes the reservoir for man (see Appendix II).

TRANSMISSION

The method of transmission is similar to that of *Fasciola hepatica*. The adult fluke inhabits the small intestine and lays eggs which are excreted in the faeces into water, where ciliated miracidia hatch out after 3–7 weeks and enter fresh-water snails in which sporocysts, rediae, daughter rediae and cercariae develop—the whole cycle taking 2 months. The cercariae encyst on freshwater plants of certain species, the water calthrop (*Trapa*), water chestnut (*Eliocharis*), water bamboo (*Zigania*) and water hyacinth (*Eichornia*). The outer layers of these plants are torn off by the teeth of the definitive hosts, pigs and man, in whom the encysted metacercariae pass through the stomach and excyst in the duodenum, where the young flukes become attached to the intestinal wall and mature in 90 days.

GEOGRAPHICAL DISTRIBUTION

Human infection with *F. buski* is limited to the distribution of the water plants on which the metacercariae encyst and is associated with the cultivation of these plants in ponds manured with human and pigs' faeces (Table 12).

Table 12. Distribution of hosts of *Fasciolopsis buski*

Locality	Snails	Water plants
China Taiwan Japan	*Segmentina hemisphaerula*	*Trapa (Salvinia) natans* *Trapa bispinosa* *Eichornia crassipes*
Assam	*Segmentina trochoideus*	
China	*Hippeutis cantori*	*Eliocharis tuberosa* *Zigania aquatica*
Taiwan Japan Indochina Philippines Indonesia India	*Gyraulus convexiusculus* (*saigonensis*)	*Trapa bicornis*

F. buski is found in China, India (Assam), Malaysia, Sumatra, Borneo, Thailand and more recently in Burma. In China 5% and in Assam 50%, (Kamrup district) of the population are affected. It is estimated that there are 10 million human infections in East Asia.

PATHOLOGY

There are many asymptomatic cases.

The larvae of *F. buski* escape from the cysts in the duodenum, attach themselves to the mucosa and become adult in about 90 days. At the site of attachment, the adult flukes cause inflammatory and ulcerative lesions, and haemorrhage may result. Abscesses may develop in the intestinal wall. As many as 1000 to 2000 flukes may be found which may affect the secretion of the intestinal juices and obstruct the passage of food. Profound intoxication from and sensitization to the metabolic products of the flukes may develop.

SIGNS AND SYMPTOMS

The majority of infections in endemic areas are light and asymptomatic. In heavy infections toxic diarrhoea and hunger pains develop towards the end of the incubation period (90 days). Generalized toxic and allergic symptoms appear in the form of oedema, particularly of the face, abdominal wall and lower extremities. Ascites is common and there is generalized abdominal pain. Later signs of malabsorption appear with pale offensive stools and emaciation. Death may occur from profound intoxication. Acute ileus may result from the presence of flukes. There is a leucocytosis with eosinophilia. (For details see Daengsvang & Mangalasmaya 1941).

TREATMENT

The treatment of choice is hexylresorcinol given as crystoids 400 mg (1–7 years) and 1·0 gramme (over 13 years) in a single dose. β naphthol and tetrachlorethylene have also been used.

Opisthorchiasis

AETIOLOGY

Opisthorchiasis is caused by infection with *Opisthorchis felineus*, a normal parasite of the dog, cat, wolverine and pig, and by *O. viverrini*, a normal parasite of the civet cat, domestic dog and cat (see Appendix II).

O. felineus

Geographical distribution

Human infection with this fluke is encountered in Eastern Europe and the U.S.S.R., and it is an important human infection in north-eastern Thailand where 25% of the population are infected (Sadun 1955). A total of 2 million people are estimated to be infected.

Transmission

Transmission is essentially the same as in *Clonorchis sinensis*. Eggs are passed in the faeces of the definitive host into water. The first intermediate host is a snail, *Bithynia leachei*. The second intermediate hosts are the tench (*Tinca tinca*) and the chub (*Idus melanotus*), *Barbus barbus* and *Leuciscus rutilis*. The metacercariae encyst in the flesh of these fish and are freed in the small intestine of man whence they travel up the bile ducts in which they mature as adult flukes.

O. viverrini

Transmission is the same as in *O. felineus*. The snail hosts are unknown and metacercariae encyst in the flesh of freshwater fish, *Cyclochalicthyus* species.

Pathological and clinical features

The pathological and clinical features are the same as those of *C. sinensis*. The treatment is the same as for *C. sinensis*.

Clonorchiasis

AETIOLOGY

Clonorchiasis is caused by *Clonorchis sinensis* which is a parasite of the bile ducts of man, dogs and cats and occasionally other mammals (see Appendix II).

TRANSMISSION

The adult flukes which live in the bile ducts pass fully embryonated eggs which when excreted in water are ingested by snails (first intermediate hosts) *Parafossarulus manchouricus*, *Bithynia fuchsiana* and other related species. Miracidia hatch out after ingestion by the snail and develop into sporocysts and rediae. Cercariae escape into the water and become attached to certain fish where they discard their tails, penetrate under the skin and encyst in the flesh of fish belonging to any of 40 species of the families Cyprinidae (carp), Gobiidae, Anabantidae and Salmonidae in China, Japan, Taiwan and Korea. Cercarial glands excrete a histolytic substance which dissolves the skin of the fish allowing them to penetrate. The metacercariae secrete a viscous fluid which forms an inner true cyst which is encapsulated by a fibrous layer formed from the tissues of the host forming a complete cyst, in which the adolescercaria is protected against the gastric juice and temperatures up to 50° to 70°C for 15 minutes. In some species of fish, *Carassius auratus* and *Eleotris swinhornis*, the parasite is found under the scales; in others it is in the flesh. This may lead to the infection of domestic animals which consume offal, whereas man who consumes the flesh escapes. The cysts pass through the stomach and are digested by the succus entericus in the duodenum near the papilla of Vater. The adolescercariae escape and attach themselves to the mucosa. The young flukes at first have spines which are soon lost, attain maturity in 26 days, and ascend the bile duct by positive chemotaxis, although 95% may be digested and destroyed on the way. In the bile duct the flukes grow as large as the calibre of the ducts and can live for 12 years.

EPIDEMIOLOGY AND GEOGRAPHICAL DISTRIBUTION

The endemic areas include Japan, Korea, all of China except the north-west, Taiwan and Indochina. Autochthonous cases in Hawaii and California are infected from frozen, dried or pickled fish from endemic areas, there is but no evidence that clonorchiasis has become established outside the China Sea area. It has been estimated that 19 million people are infected in East Asia.

The important intermediate hosts are shown in Table 13. In Japan the reservoir hosts are cats and dogs. Inatomi and Kimura (1955) found 20% of dogs and 45% of cats infected.

Human infection

Man is infected by eating raw fish, which is a custom in many Eastern countries. The fish may be eaten pickled in vinegar (*sunomono*), or covered with salted soybean paste (*sashimi*).

Fish culture in ponds which contain many snails is responsible for the high incidence in Kwantung province, Canton and Chaochoufu where infection rates in some villages are 40–100% (Faust & Khaw 1927). On the east coast of

Table 13. Intermediate hosts of *Chlonorchis sinensis*

Locality	First intermediate host	Second intermediate host
China	*Parafossarulus*	*Cyprinus carpio*
Taiwan	*manchouricus*	*Carassius auratus*
Indochina		*Ctenopharygodon idellus*
Korea		*Mylopharygodon aethiops*
Japan		
South China	*Bithynia fuchsiana*	*Cultur aburnus*
China	*Alocinma longicornis*	
	Melania cancellata	
	Hua ningpoensis	

Vietnam infection rates run at 50% of the population. The incidence of infection is highest in the older age-groups and is maximum at 30–50 years. In some parts of China children under 15 have the highest incidence.

PATHOLOGY

C. sinensis inhabits the bile ducts. When the young flukes reach the bile ducts and become mature, proliferative and inflammatory changes are induced in the biliary epithelium and followed by encapsulating fibrosis of the ducts. Hsu (1939) thought that this was caused by mechanical action of the flukes. The degree of pathological change depends on the intensity and duration of the infection. There is proliferation and desquamation of the biliary epithelium with crypt formation and the appearance of new bile ducts. As the condition becomes more chronic the walls of the ducts become infiltrated with eosinophils and leucocytes. The smaller portal vessels become fibrosed with associated dilatation of the portal vein and increased portal pressure. There is fibrous formation around eggs which infiltrate the hepatic parenchyma (Faust & Khaw 1927). The bile ducts with thickened walls expand into cavities and diverticula as large as filberts in which large numbers of parasites may be found. At autopsy 21 000 flukes have been recovered (Samback & Baujean 1913). 1000 worms may be lethal but the mean intensity of infection in endemic areas is 100–200 flukes. The diverticula communicate with the bile ducts along which the eggs of the parasites, and sometimes the parasites themselves, escape into the intestine. In the cat 2400 eggs are produced daily. Yamagata and Yaegashi (1964) have described in detail changes in the pancreas, spleen, kidneys and adrenals in all of which adult flukes may be found. Changes in the pancreas may include atrophy of Langerhans cells. Ascites, the result of portal hypertension which is rare clinically, is nearly always found at autopsy, and splenomegaly was present in 22–40% of autopsies (Katsurada 1922). Secondary infection, usually due to *E. coli*, causes cholangitis, cholangiohepatitis, pyelephlebitis and abscesses. Jaundice may occur owing to bile retention and liver dysfunction. Gall-stones may form round dead worms and eggs. Worms present in the pancreatic duct may give rise to clinical symptoms of acute pancreatitis with raised enzyme levels.

Clonorchiasis and carcinoma of the liver

Adenomatous hyperplasia of the bile duct epithelium is associated with adenocarcinoma of the liver (Hou 1956) which occurs most commonly in males aged 36 and over. The carcinoma may be a polypoid adenocarcinoma or an anaplastic carcinoma arising from the bile duct epithelium, and the adenomatous tissue in the wall of the bile duct or a mixture of both types (Hou 1956). The tumours are predominantly adenocarcinomas but the anaplastic type resembles a primary liver cell carcinoma. Clonorchiasis is an important cause of primary adenocarcinoma of the liver in man (Yamagata & Yaegashi 1964).

SYMPTOMS AND SIGNS

In areas of high endemicity, where up to 50% of the population are infected with *C. sinensis*, it is not possible to assess the effects of light infections which form the majority. In endemic areas in Japan 60–80% of infections are light and are caused by no more than 100 flukes (Yamagata 1962). There is no acute stage and, although 80% were associated with vague gastro-intestinal disturbances, a control group of uninfected people showed the same symptoms (Strauss 1962).

Moderate infections are caused by 100–1000 flukes and are associated with fullness in the abdomen, an irregular appetite and oedema with hepatomegaly.

Heavy infections are caused by more than 1000 flukes. There is an acute phase which passes into a chronic phase. The onset is acute with chills and fever. The liver and spleen enlarge and become tender (Koenigstein 1949) and eggs appear in the stools in 4 weeks. The chronic stage consists of recurrent attacks of cholangitis, pancreatitis and diarrhoea with oedema.

Recurrent attacks of cholangitis with fever, chills and jaundice may lead to diffuse suppurative cholangitis usually caused by *E. coli*. Abscesses form in the liver and surgical intervention is usually necessary. Hypoglycaemia has been recorded as a complication (McFadzean & Yeung 1965). Gall-stones are common. Recurrent attacks of acute pancreatitis occur with abdominal pain and raised serum amylase. Chronic diarrhoea develops in association with the above signs and peripheral oedema is followed by cachexia and ascites which eventually proves fatal after a number of years.

Night blindness associated with vitamin A deficiency caused by the jaundice is not uncommon.

Infection with *C. sinensis* can last as long as 24 years since a case of infection 24 years after leaving an endemic area has been described by Bordes *et al.* (1963).

Eosinophilia is not a marked feature.

DIAGNOSIS

Recovery of eggs from faeces

Eggs may be found in direct smears but are scanty in infections with under 100 flukes. Concentration methods must be used. An ether sedimentation method using detergent has been described by Oshima *et al.* (1965). A solution is prepared as follows: McIlwaine buffer *p*H 4·0 and 0·5% Tween 80 with 0·01% Merthiolate as a preservative is used with the ether sedimentation method. This will increase the recovery values for eggs to 90–100% in small amounts of the sediment.

Bile aspiration

Eggs may be demonstrated in the bile when they cannot be found in the stools. A strong solution of magnesium sulphate is injected by tube into the duodenum, which paralyses the sphincter of Oddi and contracts the gall-bladder which expels bile and eggs into the duodenum.

Immunodiagnosis

Intradermal, complement fixing, precipitation and agglutination tests are all available.

Antigens. Sadun *et al.* (1959) have prepared four different antigens from adult flukes: crude fat-free (CC), lipid-free borate buffer extracted (CTP), acid soluble protein fraction (CM) and acid insoluble alkali soluble fraction (CM-ins). CC is used in the intradermal test and CM-ins and CTP in the complement fixation test.

Intradermal test. The reaction is an immediate sensitivity reaction. There is good correlation between a positive ID test and eggs in the stools. Moderate cross-reactions occur in paragonimiasis and schistosomiasis but reactions to homologous are larger than to heterologous antigen and can be distinguished by size. A positive test measures past infection and cannot be used to judge the effects of treatment.

Complement fixation test. Sadun *et al.* (1959) used CM-ins and CTP antigens for complement fixation tests. Only 2 out of 25 clonorchis sera were negative and 1 out of 20 controls positive. Cross-reactions occurred in paragonimiasis, schistosomiasis, tuberculosis and leptospirosis. The CFT becomes positive 20 days after infection and remains positive as long as there is active infection.

TREATMENT

The drug treatment of clonorchiasis is not yet entirely satisfactory. Two drugs are in use at present.

Bithionol. Yokogawa *et al.* (1965) treated dogs infected with clonorchiasis with 100 mg/kg every other day for 5 days and found no flukes at autopsy. This is the drug of choice and is given in a dose of 30–50 mg/kg by mouth on alternate days for 2–3 weeks.

Hexachlorparaxylene (Hetol). Chung *et al.* (1965) claimed 100% cure after 3 months with a dose of 50–125 mg/kg daily for 12 days. Other drugs which have been used are emetine hydrochloride by injection of 60 mg daily for 10–20 days, and trivalent and pentavalent antimony used as in schistosomiasis and leishmaniasis. Yamagata and Yaegashi (1964) claimed that the eggs disappeared from the stools in 42·8% of cases treated with antimony.

Surgical treatment

When there is diffuse suppurative cholangitis the treatment is surgical; the gall-bladder is opened and the bile ducts washed out to remove the plug of dead flukes; suitable antibiotics are administered. The bile ducts have been washed out in this way to remove the flukes with good effect in cases in which there is no suppuration (McFadzean & Yeung 1966).

Paragonimiasis

AETIOLOGY

Many species of *Paragonimus* are widespread in nature, but until recently *P. westermani* was thought to be the only species causing human infection. Recently evidence has been presented to show that *P. szechuanensis (skrjabini)*, *P. tuanshanensis (heteroterrus)* and *P. africanus* form separate species which may also infect man (Chung & Tsao 1962; Chung *et al.* 1964; Vogel & Crewe 1965).

TRANSMISSION

The most common hosts of *P. westermani* include the tiger, cat, wild cat, leopard, panther, pig and dog. Records from other animals may be from other species. In the definitive host the adult fluke lives in the lungs and other anatomical sites and the eggs reach the outside world via the sputum or are swallowed and passed into the faeces. The average life of the adults is 10 years, but more than 20 has been recorded. In other sites the eggs escape from encapsulated abscesses which rupture. After between 16 days and several weeks in water the eggs hatch and the free-swimming miracidia enter a molluscan (first intermediate) host of the genus *Melania* (synonyms *Thiaria, Semisulcospira, Brolia*). In these hosts they develop into sporocysts and rediae. They leave the molluscs as cercariae and enter crustacean (second intermediate) hosts—freshwater crabs and crayfish. In the crustacean host the metacercariae encyst in the liver, muscles and gills and are subsequently eaten by the definitive host. In this host the metacercariae enter the stomach and adolescercariae pass through the jejunum, traverse the intestinal wall, penetrate the diaphragm and pleura and enter the lungs where they encyst in the bronchioles, forming cystic cavities. For the life history see Appendix II.

EPIDEMIOLOGY AND GEOGRAPHICAL DISTRIBUTION

Flukes of the *Paragonimus* genus are found in a wide variety of mammalian hosts which feed on crabs and crayfish. *P. westermani* develops normally in man. However, human paragonimiasis is limited in its distribution to those places where food habits make infection possible. The most important endemic areas are in Korea, Japan, Formosa, Central China and the Philippines. Scattered human cases have been reported from Manchuria and Indochina. In Central Thailand there is an endemic area (Harinasuta et al. 1957) and cases have been reported from Western Nepal (Iwamura 1964). In West Africa, the Cameroons, Nigeria and the Congo human paragonimiasis has been found caused by *P. africanus* (Vogel & Crewe 1965). In China *P. szechuanensis* and *P. tuanshanensis* cause cutaneous paragonimiasis. In South America cases of human paragonimiasis have been found in the coastal regions of Ecuador and north of Lima in Peru. The eggs that have been demonstrated in the sputum of these patients belong to an unknown species of *Paragonimus* which has also been found in animals in that area (Rodriguez 1963). In Honduras eggs of an unknown species have been found in human sputum (Larach 1966).

Reservoir hosts

The reservoir hosts of *P. westermani* in all areas are wild and domestic felines. In Africa mature worms of *P. africanus* have been found in the mongoose and the dog.

Method of human infection (Yokogawa 1965)

The most important method of infection is the eating of raw or undercooked crabs. However, another possible method is the accidental transfer of the encysted metacercariae to the mouth through handling crabs when preparing them for food.

In Japan the important second intermediate host is *Eriocheir japonicus* and infection comes mostly from the preparation of crab soup.

Table 14. Intermediate hosts of *Paragonimus*

Species	Locality	First intermediate host	Second intermediate host
P. *westermani*	Japan China	*Melania libertina* (optimum host) *Melania tuberculata* *Syncera lutea*	Crabs *Eriocheir japonicus* (optimum Japan) *Eriocheir sinensis* (optimum China) *Potamon dehaani* *Potamon denticulatus* *Potamon rathbuni* Crayfish *Cambaroides similis* *Cambaroides dauricus* *Cambaroides schrenkii* *Procambarus clarkii*
	Korea	*Melania nodiperda* *Melania eberina*	*Eriocheir sinensis* *Cambaroides similis*
	Philippines	*Brolia asparata*	*Parathelphusa grapsoides* *Parathelphusa mistio*
	Taiwan	*Melania obliquegranulosa* *Melania paucicincta* *Hua amurensis*	*Potamon myazekii*
	Western Nepal	Crab and snail hosts unknown	
P. *africanus*	Africa	*Potadoma freethii*	*Sudanautes africanus* *Sudanautes pelii*

In the Philippines the juice of crabs is used to prepare a special dish, '*kinagang*', and the hands of the cooks can become contaminated from the chopping block and knife used in preparation of this dish.

In Korea *E. sinensis* is the most important source of infection since it is eaten raw. The raw juice of the crayfish *Cambaroides similis* is used as a medicine for diarrhoea.

In China the stone crab, *Potamon denticulatus*, is eaten alive, after being immersed in wine, as 'drunken crabs'. This is a dangerous method of spreading paragonimiasis.

PATHOLOGY (Diaconita & Goldis 1964)

The lesions of paragonimiasis are found in the lungs—pulmonary paragonimiasis, and outside the lungs—extrapulmonary paragonimiasis.

Pulmonary paragonimiasis

Pathological lesions are caused both by the adult flukes and the eggs. The flukes cause worm cysts (abscess cavities) and 'burrows'. The worm cysts are caused by infarction of the lung tissue and necrosis of a granulomatous or pneumonic mass with softening and distintegration of the dead worms. The granulomatous lesions are caused in the main by the eggs. These lesions show the features of a foreign body granuloma, the foreign body being the eggs with a chitinous cuticle. In the initial stage of the disease there is an eosinophilic pneumonia and bronchopneumonia with vasculitis and perivascular granulomas.

The worm cysts, which are thickly distributed over the surface of the pleura, form tumour-like swellings of a deep red colour, about the size of a grape or plum. On section these cysts are seen to be distended greyish white nodules containing irregular cavities. The lung underneath the cysts is seen to contain a number of 'burrows', which are formed of infiltrated lung tissue, containing brown material in which adult worms may lie often side by side. The septa between the tunnels may break down and a considerable cavity be produced and give the appearance of a dilated bronchus. Microscopically the walls of the cavities are composed of fibrous granulation tissue consisting of fibroblasts, mononuclear cells, plasma cells and sometimes eosinophils. Numerous *Paragonimus* eggs can be seen in and around the cavity, and granulomas due to the eggs form 'egg tubercles' consisting of epithelioid cells, lymphoid cells, plasma cells, eosinophils and peripheral fibroblasts. Giant cells both of the Langhans and foreign body type are common. The histological picture may closely resemble that of tuberculosis.

These changes are caused partly by mechanical damage produced by the adult worm as it moves around and partly as the result of immune processes and toxins.

Extrapulmonary paragonimiasis

Cerebral and spinal paragonimiasis. Cerebral paragonimiasis is probably caused by the adult worms, and cannot occur unless pulmonary foci are present. The flukes, which migrate to the brain along the soft tissues around the neck veins, may return to the lungs. Observations suggest that this occurs about 10 months after the appearance of the pulmonary disease (Lei & Yen 1957).

Cerebral or spinal paragonimiasis accounts for 30–60% of all cases of extra-pulmonary paragonimiasis. In the brain the lesion may be either solid or cystic, or may be combined. The solid foci show a central area containing eggs and giant cells, and Charcot–Leyden crystals, a middle area of connective tissue and an outer layer of plasma cells, eosinophil cells and lymphocytic infiltration.

Transverse lesions of the spinal cord may occur.

Other lesions. Paragonimus eggs may be found in the liver, peritoneum, testes, intestine, skin and muscle.

P. szechuanensis has a special predilection for the skin where it causes multiple tumours in which eggs may be found.

P. africanus causes retroauricular cysts in the Congo, as well as pulmonary disease.

SYMPTOMS AND SIGNS

Pulmonary paragonimiasis (endemic haemoptysis)

The symptoms begin insidiously. There is a chronic cough and a vague feeling of distress in the chest. The spasmodic cough produces a peculiar rusty brown pneumonic-like sputum, often in considerable quantity, which contains the eggs of *Paragonimus*. It has been estimated that the number of eggs coughed up in the 24 hours is over 13 000. There is also irregular haemoptysis which, although usually trifling, may be so profuse as to threaten life. Physical examination of the chest is essentially negative; there is usually clubbing of the fingers.

The sputum. Under the microscope the peculiar colour of the sputum is found to be due partly to red blood corpuscles and partly to a mass of dark brown thick-walled operculated eggs (Fig. 111). The eggs vary in size and shape. They are all distinctly oval and have a smooth yellow, double outlined shell and measure 80–100 × 40–60 μm. If the sputum is shaken up in water and the water renewed from time to time a ciliated miracidium forms in each egg in the course of a month to 6 weeks which can be released by pressure on a slide from a coverslip.

X-ray appearances. X-ray changes in pulmonary paragonimiasis are very similar to those of pulmonary tuberculosis. Tomography is essential for diagnosis. Abnormal shadows are found in the middle upper and lower parts of the lungs but are rarely seen in the apex, and they are commoner in the right than the left lung. There are three types of shadow which are considered typical,

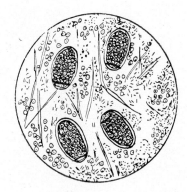

Fig. 111.—Eggs of *Paragonimus westermani* in the sputum.

nodular, ring, and infiltrative. The nodular shadow is suggestive of a tuberculoma, and has a sharply marked rounded or oval contour. The ring shadow is a cystic form with a relatively thin wall and is round, oval or irregular in shape (Fig. 112) (Diaconita & Goldis 1964).

X-ray changes at the bases strongly resemble bronchiectasis.

Cerebral paragonimiasis

The clinical symptoms of cerebral paragonimiasis are similar to those of cerebral tumour or embolism—Jacksonian epilepsy, ending in hemiplegia, aphasia, visual disturbances, homonymous hemianopia, and monoplegias of various degrees. Common eye signs are optic atrophy and papilloedema.

Radiological findings in cerebral paragonimiasis showed calcification in half the cases and pneumoencephalography showed the severity of the brain atrophy associated with the infection (Galatius-Jensen & Uhm 1965).

Other sites

Paragonimiasis should be suspected in endemic zones in cases of chronic epididymitis, enlargement of the lymph glands, liver cirrhosis and skin ulceration. In generalized paragonimiasis there is general lymphadenitis associated with the other symptoms described above, often associated with cutaneous ulcerations. These may be abdominal pain and diarrhoea and the abdominal wall is hard and may be tender. Paragonimiasis of the uterus has been described.

Clinical features of other *Paragonimus* **species**

P. szechuanensis (*skrjabini*) causes migrating subcutaneous nodules and high eosinophilia. Pulmonary symptoms are scanty and there is only a little sputum from which *Paragonimus* eggs are absent. These cases may be mistaken for

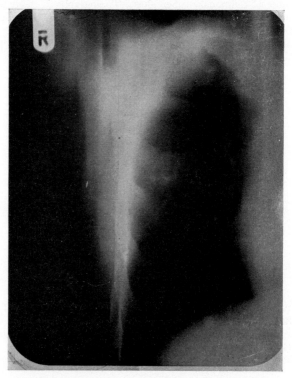

Fig. 112.—Tomogram of paragonimiasis of the lung, showing several small contiguous cavities. (*Professor W. E. Kershaw*)

schistosomiasis, since the eggs found in the skin nodules, although operculated, may be mistaken for *S. japonicum*. There is a moderate leucocytosis up to 15 000/mm³ and only a moderate eosinophilia. There was an average eosinophil count of 21% in 69 cases (Hirano 1957).

DIAGNOSIS

The stools and sputum should be examined both by direct and concentration methods. Eggs can be found in the sputum by direct smear. When there are only few eggs centrifuge sedimentation with 1–2% sodium hydroxide must be used. In light infections eggs may only be found in the stools; eggs were found only in the stools in 13·2% of cases (Komiya & Yokogawa 1953).

In the stools the eggs can be concentrated by the ether formol concentration methods. *Paragonimus* eggs can be recovered from gastric juice (Okada 1959), and on aspiration from the bronchi (Kitamoto *et al.* 1958).

Immunodiagnosis

Intradermal test. The preparation and the technique are standardized and the immediate sensitivity ID test is used widely for screening and diagnosis. A veronal buffered saline (VBS) extract of adult *P. westermani* (Yokogawa 1965), an alkaline soluble fraction standardized by the protein content and a polypeptide (PPT) antigen are all available. Of 28 individuals with eggs in the stools 23 gave positive ID tests and in another series all of 96 egg passers were positive (Yokogawa *et al.* 1960). Cross-reactions occur with *Clonorchis*. Whole populations can be screened and the positive reactors examined for infection.

Complement fixation test. The complement fixation test, using a veronal buffered saline extract of adult worms or a polypeptide antigen, has been used for diagnosis and especially to monitor the results of treatment. A positive reaction appeared in animal experiments 2–4 weeks after infection and reverted to normal following successful treatment. Cross-reactions are common with *Clonorchis* and schistosomiasis and cases of *Paragonimus* infection gave positive reactions to *Fasciola hepatica* antigen (Chung *et al.* 1965).

The intradermal test remains positive for long after recovery and only measures past infection. The complement fixation test is closely correlated with active infection. In epidemiological surveys the intradermal test should be used first and the complement fixation test should be performed on those individuals who show doubtful or positive skin reactions.

Differential diagnosis

The main difficulty in diagnosis is to differentiate paragonimiasis from pulmonary tuberculosis, and in some cases both eggs and tubercle bacilli are found in the same sputum specimen. Points of difference are the good general condition of the *Paragonimus* patients with marked X-ray signs and failure to respond to antituberculous treatment. Other conditions which resemble paragonimiasis are hydatid cyst, lung abscess, amoebic abscess, fungus infections and bronchiectasis.

Cerebral paragonimiasis has to be distinguished from cerebral schistosomiasis, cerebral gnathostomiasis and *Angiostrongylus cantonensis* infection, as well as tuberculoma of the brain, cerebral tumour and cerebrovascular disease.

Other extrapulmonary forms of paragonimiasis are apt to be mistaken for tuberculosis or schistosomiasis when the epididymis, testis or skin are involved.

TREATMENT

Bithionol is the drug of choice (Yokogawa 1961). Cure rates vary from 84% (Wang *et al.* 1964) to 100% (Kang *et al.* 1963). It is used in both pulmonary and extrapulmonary forms of the disease. A course of treatment is 30–50 mg/kg every other day by mouth for 10–15 doses. Two courses are necessary in cerebral paragonimiasis, which must be treated in the earliest stages for maximum benefit. The subcutaneous swellings associated with *P. skrjabini* disappeared with treatment but some relapsed from 4 to 9 months later and required a second course (Wang *et al.* 1964). Test of cure is disappearance of eggs from the sputum and stools, regression of the lesions and reversion of the complement fixation reaction to negative.

PREVENTION AND CONTROL

Yokogawa (1952) believes that snails are infected mainly from human sources in Japan and not from reservoir hosts.

With the development of bithionol, mass treatment for the control of para-gonimiasis is a possibility. Yokogawa (1961) treated 13 out-patients with 30 mg/kg in divided doses every other day for 10–15 doses after meals while they were leading their ordinary lives. The effects of treatment were just as good as in persons treated in hospital.

It is likely that the disease in man will gradually die out in areas where mass treatment with bithionol has been thoroughly carried out (Yokogawa 1969).

Elimination of the snail and crab hosts is not practicable. Health education in the handling and preparation of crabs for food can reduce the incidence of the disease.

REFERENCES

AMIN, M. A. & NELSON, G. S. (1969) *Bull. Wld Hlth Org.*, **41**, 225.

ANTUNES, L. J. & PELLEGRINO, J. (1966) *Bull. Wld Hlth Org.*, **35**, 721.

BARBIER, M. & BRUMPT, V. (1969) *Trans. R. Soc. trop. Med. Hyg.*, **63**, S66.

BARLOW, C. H. & MELENEY, H. E. (1949) *Am. J. trop. Med.*, **29**, 79.

BELDING, D. L. (1965) *Textbook of Clinical Parasitology*, 3rd ed. New York: Appleton Century Crofts.

BELL, D. R. (1963) *Bull. Wld. Hlth Org.*, **29**, 525.

BIGGART, J. H. (1937) *J. Path. Bact.*, **44**, 488.

BORDES, F. P., CAVALLO, A., VAILLANT, A. & MARTIN, M. (1963) *Méd. trop.*, **23**, 139.

CHEEVER, A. W. & ANDRADE, Z. A. (1967) *Trans. R. Soc. trop. Med. Hyg.*, **61**, 626.

CHOU, H. C., HUANGFU, M., CHOU, H. L. & WEI, M. H. (1965) *Chin. med. J.*, **84**, 591.

CHUNG, H. L., HO, L. Y., CHENG, L. T. & TSAO, W. C. (1964) *Chin. med. J.*, **83**, 641.

——— HSU, C. P., TSAO, W. C., K'O, H. Y., KUO, C. H., LI, P. H., CHENG, S., CHANG, H. Y., YUAN, C. T. & CHANG, Y. C. (1965) *Chin. med. J.*, **84**, 323.

——— & TSAO, W. C. (1962) *Chin. med. J.*, **81**, 354.

COOK, J. A. & JORDAN, P. (1970) *Trans. R. soc. trop. Med. Hyg.*, **64**, 793.

COOKSON, L. C. C. (1964) *Bull. Wld Hlth Org.*, **31**, 799.

DAENGSVANG, S. & MANGALASMAYA, M. (1941) *Ann. trop. Med. Parasit.*, **35**, 43.

DESCHIENS, R. & DELAS, A. E. (1969) *Trans. R. Soc. trop. Med. Hyg.*, **63**, S57.

DIACONITA, C. H. & GOLDIS, G. H. (1964) *Acta tuberc. scand.*, **44**, 51.

FACEY, R. V. & MARSDEN, P. V. (1960) *Br. med. J.*, **ii**, 619.

FAROOK, M. & HAIRSTON, N. G. (1966) *Bull. Wld Hlth Org.*, **35**, 331.

——— & MALLAH, M. B. (1966) *Bull. Wld Hlth Org.*, **35**, 377.

——— NIELSEN, J., SAMAAN, S. A., MALLAH, M. B. & ALLAM, A. S. (1966) *Bull. Wld Hlth Org.*, **35**, 293.

FAUST, E. C. & KHAW, O. K. (1927) *Am. J. Hyg.*, Monograph Series, **8**, 1.

FENWICK, A. (1969) *Trans. R. Soc. trop. Med. Hyg.*, **63**, 557.

FORSYTH, D. M. (1964) *E. Afr. med. J.*, **41**, 567.

——— (1969) *Bull. Wld Hlth Org.*, **40**, 771.

——— & MACDONALD, G. (1966) *Trans. R. Soc. trop. Med. Hyg.*, **60**, 568.

FOY, H. & NELSON, G. S. (1963) *Exp. Parasit.*, **14**, 240.

GALATIUS-JENSEN & UHM, I. (1956) *Br. J. Radiol.*, **38**, 494.

GELFAND, M. (1966) *Br. med. J.*, **ii**, 762.

——— (1967) *A Clinical Study of Intestinal Bilharziasis (Schistosoma mansoni) in Africa*. London: Arnold.

GIGLIOLI, G. (1964) *Br. med. J.*, **i**, 767.

GOLD, R., ROSEN, F. S. & WELLER, T. H. (1969) *Am. J. trop. Med. Hyg.*, **18**, 545.

HARINASUTA, T., KRUATRA CHUE, M. & TANDHANAND, S. (1957) *J. med. Ass. Thailand*, **40**, 227.

HIRANO, T. (1957) *Niigata Igakkai Zasshi*, **72**, 189.

HOU, P. C. (1956) *J. Path. Bact.*, **72**, 239.

HSU, H. F. (1939) *Chin. med. J.*, **55**, 542.

INATOMI, S. & KIMURA, M. (1955) *Okayama Igakki Zasshi*, **67**, 651.

IWAMURA, N. (1964) *Jap. J. Parasit.*, 5, 169.

JORDAN, P. (1968) *Tropical Medical Conference* 1967. London: Pitman Medical.

—— & WEBBE, G. (1969) *Human Schistosomiasis*. London: Heinemann.

KAGAN, I. G., RAIRIGH, D. W. & KAISER, R. W. (1962) *Ann. intern. Med.*, 56, 457.

KANG, S. Y., KYU, L. K., KUM, H. F. & CHYU, I. L. (1963) *Korea J. med. Ass.*, 6, 59.

KATSURADA, F. (1922) *Nisshin Igaku*, Suppl. I.

KEAN, B. H. & GOLDSMITH, E. (1968) *Eighth Int. Cong. trop. Med. Malar.*, Teheran, Abstracts and reviews 31.

KITAMOTO, O., OKADA, T., UENO, A., YOKOGAWA, M. & KIHATA, M. (1958) *Kokyuki Shinryo*, 13, 92.

KOENIGSTEIN, R. P. (1949) *Trans. R. Soc. trop. Med. Hyg.*, 42, 503.

KOMIYA, Y. & YOKOGAWA, M. (1953) *Jap. J. med. Sci. Biol.*, 6, 207.

LARACH, C. J. (1966) *Revta méd. hondur.*, 34, 111.

LEES, R. E. M. & JORDAN, P. (1968) *Trans. R. Soc. trop. Med. Hyg.*, 62, 630.

LEI, H. K. & YEN, C. K. (1957) *Chin. med. J.*, 75, 986.

LEWERT, R. M. & YOGORE, M. G. (1969) *Trans. R. Soc. trop. Med. Hyg.*, 63, 343.

LIE, K. J., BASCH, P. F., HEYNEMAN, D., BECK, W. P. & AUDY, J. R. (1968) *Trans. R. Soc. trop. Med. Hyg.*, 62, 299.

LUCAS, A. O., ADENIYI-JONES, C. C., COCKSHOTT, W. P. & GILLES, H. M. (1966) *Lancet*, i, 631.

MACDONALD, G. (1965) *Trans. R. Soc. trop. Med. Hyg.*, 59, 485, 611.

—— & FORSYTH, D. M. (1968) *Trans. R. Soc. trop. Med. Hyg.*, 62, 755.

McFAZDEAN, A. J. S. & YEUNG, R. T. T. (1965) *Trans. R. Soc. trop. med. Hyg.*, 59, 179.

—— —— (1966) *Trans. R. Soc. trop. Med. Hyg.*, 60, 466.

MALDONADO, J. F. (1967) *Schistosomiasis in America*. Barcelona: Cientifico-Medica.

McMAHON, J. E. (1969) *Trans. R. Soc. trop. Med. Hyg.*, 63, 545.

MOST, H., KANE, C. A., LAVIETAS, P. H., SCHROEDE, E. F., BEHM, A., BLUM, L., KATZIN, B. & HAYMAN, J. M., jun, (1950) *Am. J. trop. Med.*, 30, 239.

NEGHME, A. & OSSANDON, M. (1943) *Am. J. trop. Med.* 23, 545.

NELSON, G. S. (1958) *E. Afr. med. J.*, 35, 311.

—— AMIN, M. A., SAOUD, M. F. A. & TEESDALE, C. (1968) *Bull. Wld Hlth Org.*, 38, 9.

—— & SAOUD, M. F. A. (1968) *J. Helminth.*, 42, 339.

OKADA, J. (1959) *Nichon Eiseigaku Zasshi*, 13, 783.

OSHIMA, T., KAGAI, N., KIMATA, M., FUJINO, N., NOGUCHI, H. & FUJIOKA, K. (1965) *Kiseichugeka Zasshi*, 14, 195.

PAUTRIZEL, R., BAILLENGER, J., DURET, J. & TRIBONLEY, J. (1962) *Rev. Immunol.*, 26, 167.

PELLEGRINO, J. & KATZ, N. (1968) *Adv. Parasit.*, 6, 233.

—— OLIVIERA, C. A., FARIA, J. & CUNHA, A. S. (1962) *Am. J. trop. Med. Hyg.*, 11, 201.

PESIGNAN, T. P., BANZAN, T. C., SANTOS, A. T., NOSENAS, J. & ZABALA, R. G. (1967) *Bull. Wld Hlth Org.*, 36, 263.

PITCHFORD, R. J. (1961) *Trans. R. Soc. trop. Med. Hyg.*, 55, 44.

POWELL, S. J., ENGELBRECHT, H. E. & WELCHMAN, J. M. (1968) *Trans. R. Soc. trop. Med. Hyg.*, 62, 231, 238.

PURNELL, R. E. (1966) *Trans. R. Soc. trop. Med. Hyg.*, 60, 463.

RAPER, A. B. (1951) *E. Afr. med. J.*, 28, 50.

RIDLEY, D. S. & HAWGOOD, B. C. (1956) *J. clin. Path.*, 9, 74.

RODRIGUEZ, M. J. D. (1963) *Revta ecuat. Med.*, 1, 20.

SADUN, E. H. (1955) *Am. J. Hyg.*, 62, 81.

—— (1967) in *Bilharziasis* (ed. Mostofi, F.K.) Heidelberg: Springer.

—— WALTON, B. C., BUCK, A. A. & LEE, B. K. (1959) *J. Parasit.*, 45, 129.

SAMBACK, E. & BAUJEAN, R. (1913) *Bull. Soc. méd.-chir. Indochine*, 4, 425.

SAOUD, M. F. A. (1966) *Trans. R. Soc. trop. Med. Hyg.*, 60, 585.

SCHACHER, J. F., SAAB, S., GERMANOS, R. & BOUSTANY, N. (1969) *Trans. R. Soc. trop. Med. Hyg.*, 63, 854.

SIMPSON, T. R. (1965) *C. Afr. med. J.*, 11, 53.

SMITHERS, S. R. & TERRY, R. J. (1967) *Trans. R. Soc. trop. Med. Hyg.*, 61, 517.

SMITHERS, S. R. & TERRY, R. J. (1969) *Adv. Parasit.*, **7**, 41.
───── ───── & HOCKLEY, D. J. (1968) *Trans. R. Soc. trop. Med. Hyg.*, **62**, 466.
STRAUSS, W. G. (1962) *Am. J. trop. Med. Hyg.*, **11**, 625.
TAYLOR, M. G., AMIN, M. B. A. & NELSON, G. S. (1969) *J. Helminth.*, **43**, 197.
VOGEL, H. & CREWE, W. (1965) *Z. Tropenmed. Parasit.*, **16**, 109.
WANG, C., LIU, J., CHANG, T. & MIAO, H. (1964) *Chin. med. J.*, **83**, 163.
WARREN, K. S. (1968) *Eighth Int. Congr. trop. Med. Malar., Teheran,* Abstracts and reviews 12.
WEBBE, G. (1966) *Trans. R. Soc. trop. Med. Hyg.*, **60**, 280.
───── (1969) *Trans. R. Soc. trop. Med. Hyg.*, **63**, S82.
───── & JAMES, C. (1969) *Trans. R. Soc. trop. Med. Hyg.*, **63**, 541.
WILCOCKS, C. (1962) *Aspects of Medical Investigation in Africa.* London: Oxford University Press.
WITENBERG, G. & YOFE, J. (1938) *Trans. R. Soc. trop. Med. Hyg.*, **31**, 549.
WOLSTENHOLME, B. (1968) *Trans. R. Soc. trop. Med. Hyg.*, **62**, 729.
WOODRUFF, A. W., SHAFEI, A. Z., AWWAD, H. K., PETTITT, L. E. & ABAZA, H. H. (1966) *Trans. R. Soc. trop. Med. Hyg.*, **60**, 343.
WORLD HEALTH ORGANIZATION (1965) *Wld Hlth Org. tech. Rep. Ser.*, 299.
───── (1966) *Wld Hlth Org. tech. Rep. Ser.*, 317.
───── (1967) *Wld Hlth Org. tech. Rep. Ser.*, 372.
WRIGHT, C. A. (1970) in *Human Ecology in the Tropics* (ed. Garlick, J. P. & Keay, R. W. J.), p. 67. Oxford: Pergamon.
───── & BENNETT, M. S. (1967) *Trans. R. Soc. trop. Med. Hyg.*, **61**, 221, 228.
YAMAGATA, S. (1962) *S. Nakayama Shoten, Tokyo,* **1**, 134.
───── & YAEGASHI, A. (1964) *Prog. med. Parasit.*, **1**, 633.
YOKOGAWA, M. (1952) *Jap. J. med. Sci. Biol.*, **5**, 221.
───── (1961) *Kyobu Shikkan*, **5**, 965.
───── (1965) *Adv. Parasit.*, **3**, 99.
───── (1969) *Adv. Parasit.*, **7**, 375.
───── KOYAMA, H., YOSHIMURA, H. & TSAI, C. S. (1965) *Jap. J. Parasit.*, **14**, 233.
───── OKURA, K., TSUJI, M., SUZUKI, R., SHIMONO, O., HATANO, K., AMAGISHI, T., OGIDA, K. & YAMAOKO, K. (1960) *Jap. J. Parasit.*, **9**, 428.

13. CESTODE INFECTIONS

TAENIASIS (*Taenia solium*)

Synonyms

The pork tapeworm; pork tapeworm infection.

Aetiology

Taeniasis solium is caused by infection of man with *Taenia solium*, of which he is the only definitive host. Two forms of infection are found: in one the adult worm infects the small intestine and in the other (larval taeniasis) the larval stages cause cysticercosis (cysticercosis cellulosae). The intermediate stage of *T. solium* is normally found in pigs. The life history is described in Appendix II.

Geographical distribution

T. solium has a cosmopolitan distribution and is common wherever man consumes raw or insufficiently cooked pork. It is most common amongst the Slavic peoples, and in Mexico and other Latin American countries as well as North China, Manchuria and India. Larval taeniasis was formerly common in Europe, and in Africa, India and China cysticercosis is still common, as it is in Mexico, where it is a common cause of intracranial hypertension. It is also common in Brazil and Chile.

Transmission

The cysticerci are digested out of the meat in the stomach and the upper levels of the jejunum. The head evaginates from the scolex, becomes attached to the small intestine and, in 5–12 weeks, develops into a mature worm which may live up to 25 years.

Symptoms

Towards the end of the incubation period (5–12 weeks) there is a leucocytosis with a moderate eosinophilia up to 13%. In established cases of infection there is no eosinophilia. In the majority of cases there are no symptoms. The passage of segments is noticed and this may lead to psychosomatic symptoms. Occasionally there is a mild dyspepsia resembling a duodenal ulcer.

Diagnosis

Ova in the stool cannot be distinguished from *T. saginata* but examination of a gravid proglottis will show 7–13 main lateral arms of the uterus in each side (as distinguished from 15–20 for *T. saginata*). Examination of the scolex after treatment will show the armed rostellum which differentiates it from *T. saginata*.

For treatment and prevention, see page 342 and page 351.

CYSTICERCOSIS (LARVAL TAENIASIS)

Man is the only known definitive host and inadequately cooked or frozen pork is the only source of human infection with the adult worm.

Human infection with the larval stages is caused by the ingestion of eggs in contaminated food or water (hetero-infection), from soiled fingers or by internal auto-infection when the eggs are carried by reverse peristalsis back to the duodenum or stomach, where they hatch and migrate to the body tissues or viscera and cause cysticercosis. Internal auto-infection may be caused by treatment with drugs such as niclosamide, which destroy the worm and release into the small intestine the eggs, which are then regurgitated to the stomach. Such drugs are contra-indicated in *T. solium* infections. Dixon and Lipscomb (1961) found evidence of previous tapeworm infection in 26% of cases of cysticercosis.

Pathology

Whether ingested or regurgitated from the small intestine the shells of the ova disintegrate within 24–72 hours and the emergent oncospheres penetrate

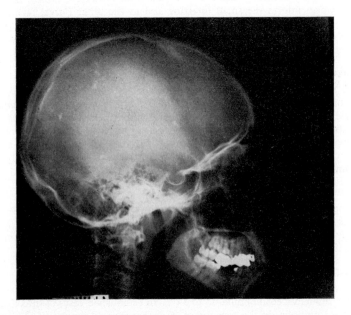

Fig. 113.—Multiple calcified lesions in the brain in cerebral cysticercosis.

through the intestinal wall, either by their hooklets or possibly by lytic secretions into the mesenteric vessels and are carried throughout the body typically filtering out between the muscles where in the course of 60–70 days they change into cysticerci (Fig. 115). Cysticerci have been found in nearly every organ and tissue of the body, most commonly in the subcutaneous tissues and muscles of the tongue neck or ribs, next in the eye and then in the brain, where they may develop in the ventricles or as cyst capsules on the surface of the brain. Less commonly they are found in the heart, liver, lungs and abdominal cavity. Except in the eye the cysticercus is surrounded by a fibrous capsule and as it grows is surrounded by a cellular reaction of neutrophils, eosinophils and, later, lymphocytes and plasma cells and sometimes giant cells.

No disturbance is caused until the cysticercus dies, when the capsule becomes necrotic and fibrosed and eventually calcified (Ch'in 1933). In the brain the cysticercus is surrounded by a wall of neuroglia which later undergoes degenerative changes and which is visible as a discoloured ring which is walled off from the normal brain by a ring of neuroglia (Fig. 114). After a variable period the parasite dies and becomes calcified, which may not affect the cyst capsule and its contents. However, the cyst wall may collapse and be flattened out by pressure of the surrounding tissues and calcify in a spindle shape. This does not happen in the brain. There is a lapse of 3 years between death of the cysticerci and calcification in the tissues but in the brain this process takes longer.

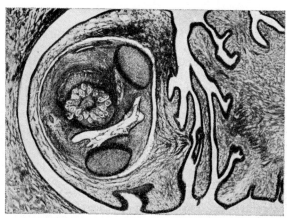

Fig. 114.—Section of cysticercus from the brain. (*Carnegie Dixon and J. D. Willis, Lancet, 1941*)

Symptoms and signs

Usually the invasion of cysticerci gives rise to no general reaction but the patient may notice the appearance of small subcutaneous nodules or intramuscular swellings. Cysts may be present in large numbers without the patient's knowledge until they are discovered accidentally on radiological examination.

Cerebral cysticercosis. *Epilepsy*. The commonest cerebral manifestation is epilepsy, and MacArthur (1933) found that 10 of 22 cases of epilepsy in British soldiers in India were due to cysticerosis. It is thought to be a common cause of epilepsy in Africans in South Africa (Powell *et al.* 1966). The fits are indistinguishable from those of idiopathic epilepsy and vary in nature from attacks of *petit mal* to Jacksonian attacks.

Other cerebral manifestations. There may be recurrent internal hydrocephalus from blocking of the aqueduct of Sylvius by a cyst, with severe headache and vomiting resembling cerebral tumour. Other cerebral manifestations are transient hemiplegia and other focal signs, psychotic states with melancholia, acute mania and disordered behaviour, and slow mental deterioration of insidious onset.

Ocular cysticercosis. The cysticerci remain alive and unencapsulated in the vitreous humour and anterior chamber of the eye, where they are constantly changing shape and may cause some discomfort from shadows cast by the larva. Other eye changes which may be caused are uveitis, retinitis, choroidal atrophy and palpebral conjunctivitis.

Other forms. Cysticerci may cause trouble in other sites, such as the bundle of His, where heart block has been recorded as the result of the presence of a cyst.

Course and prognosis

No prophecy can be made of the duration of the epileptic symptoms. Sometimes the fits cease without apparent cause, in others they persist. MacArthur (1933) recorded one cysticercus alive after 15 years. The commonest causes of death are status epilepticus and intracranial hypertension.

Diagnosis

The most helpful sign in diagnosis is the development of subcuticular nodules which provide material for biopsy and these may number from 1 to 30 or more. They may be the size of a hard pea, a hazel nut or even a pigeon's egg. Their situation varies widely. They have been found in the lips, masseter muscles, neck, chest, abdominal walls, back and groin. Unless evidence of cysticercosis is systematically sought the diagnosis may be missed, as nodules may be absent at the time of examination only to come out at a later date. Radiological evidence may not appear for some years, as calcification does not usually take place for 4 or 5 years after infection. Calcified larvae were detected in skeletal muscles in 97% of patients examined radiologically or at necropsy 5 or more years after the assumed date of infection (Dixon & Lipscomb 1961). Intracranial calcification was found in 36% within 10 years.

To demonstrate cysticerci a suitable cyst is excised under local anaesthesia and the host capsule is enucleated. The appearance of the translucent membrane with its central 'milk spot' is characteristic. If alive the parasite may evaginate the head and neck or it may be induced to do so by immersion in hot saline.

When partially calcified a good X-ray may show it as a small elongated shadow, but the completely calcified cyst gives a characteristic appearance (Fig. 115). In the muscles cysticerci are oat-shaped due to pressure, whilst in the brain they are circular. In showing up calcification, 'high penetration' is more effective than slight underexposure. The exposure should be that employed for bone detail. In the early stages the cysts are diaphanous and do not show up, so that a negative radiograph of the skull is of no significance. The size of the cysts depends mostly upon their age and situation. Eosinophilia affords no aid to diagnosis.

In cysticercosis of the brain, changes in the C.S.F. are variable. Cysticerci are rare. The pressure may be raised and there may be a pleocytosis of 5–500 cells which may be lymphocytes but sometimes eosinophils of 2 to 42% (Reinlein et al. 1951). Protein changes are non-specific. Among Africans in Durban cell changes and eosinophilia in the C.S.F. were found to be inconstant (Powell et al. 1966).

Serodiagnosis, see page 352.

Treatment

Treatment is purely symptomatic and the fits must be controlled with anti-convulsant drugs as in 'idopathic' epilepsy.

Observation on tissue stages which follow the death of intracerebral cysticerci suggest that destruction of large numbers might make matters worse. Instances of successful localization and removal of single cerebral cysts have been recorded in the literature; usually such interference is unjustifiable and in actual practice

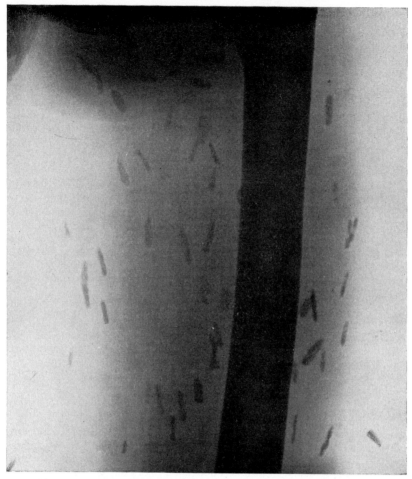

Fig. 115.—Radiograph of calcified cysticerci in the thigh. (*Major-General W. P. MacArthur*)

temporary amelioration of symptoms after removal of one or more cysts has often been followed by death.

Prevention

This can only be done by cleanliness in habits and the treatment of cases of *T. solium* infection immediately diagnosis has been made and the avoidance of drugs which cause disintegration of the worm and not expulsion of the whole worm.

TAENIASIS (*Taenia saginata*)

Synonyms

Beef tapeworm.

Geographical distribution

This is world-wide wherever beef is eaten. The worm is still found in England and is universal in Ethiopia.

Transmission

Man is the only definitive host and cattle the commonest intermediate host. Cattle become infected by grazing on ground polluted by human faeces and under suitable conditions the eggs may remain viable for 8 weeks or more Human infection is acquired from eating raw beef containing the viable cysticerci.

Pathology and symptomatology

In many cases there are no symptoms whatsoever, but because of its large size *T. saginata* is more likely than *T. solium* to cause symptoms, even acute intestinal obstruction. Towards the end of the incubation period hunger pains develop and at times nausea, post-prandial vomiting and a feeling of distension in the epigastrium may be noticed. Symptoms of peptic ulcer or gall-bladder disease may be simulated. Occasionally the proglottides, which have the habit of migrating out of the anus, may crawl down the leg and produce tickling sensations. A moderate eosinophilia occurs towards the end of the incubation period.

Diagnosis

The diagnosis is made by the presence in the stool of proglottides or eggs, which cannot be distinguished from those of *T. solium*. Gravid proglottides can, however, be distinguished by the uterine pattern. Active purgation may produce mature proglottides which will enable identification.

For treatment see page 351.

Prevention

All beef and pork consumed by man should be inspected for cysticerci. Thorough cooking of beef and ham ensures protection; the critical thermal point is 56°C. Raw hamburgers are particularly dangerous and raw ham such as is eaten in Germany. Chilled beef does not ensure protection but beef which has been frozen for 3 or more weeks is considered safe.

HYDATID DISEASE

Aetiology

Hydatid disease is caused by larvae of cestodes of the genus *Echinococcus*, the adult of which is found in carnivores which are the definitive hosts and which consume the viscera of the intermediate hosts in which the larval stages develop. These intermediate hosts are infected by swallowing eggs passed in the faeces of the definitive host. Two forms of hydatid occur in man:

1. *E. granulosus* (unilocular hydatid), which develops slowly and is adapted to large ungulates as the intermediate hosts.

2. *E. multilocularis* (multilocular or alveolar hydatid), which becomes infective in only a few months and is found in short-lived rodents as intermediate hosts (Rausch 1967).

Transmission

The adult *Echinococcus* is a parasite of carnivores whose excreta are the source of the eggs which cause infection in man, in whom the larval stage (hydatid cyst) develops. Man becomes infected by close contact with dogs, as a child or shepherd, or by handling and consuming raw vegetables and fruits contaminated by wild carnivore faeces.

E. granulosus (UNILOCULAR HYDATID)

Geographical distribution

The most extensive and endemic areas of human infection are found in the sheep-raising countries—South Australia, New Zealand, Tasmania, parts of North, South and East Africa, and the southern half of South America, particularly Argentina and southern Brazil. In addition human infection is frequently found in the south-western states of the U.S.A., southern and eastern Europe, Iraq, Syria, Lebanon, Turkey, Mongolia, Turkestan, North China, southern Japan and North Vietnam.

Epidemiology and epizootiology

E. granulosus is found in two distinct biological forms. One (*E.g. canadensis*) involves cervids (deer and moose) and wolves and is found in the high latitudes of the world, the other (*E.g. granulosus*) involves domestic ungulates (sheep and cattle) and dogs and has become part of man and his environment. In the first form (*E.g. canadensis*) in north-west Canada the natural cycle involves the wolf and the moose. Pack dogs eat the viscera of infected moose and provide the source of human infection (Miller 1953).

In the second form (*E.g. granulosus*), which is the commonest and most widespread, the dog is the optimum definitive host and in most endemic areas in the world the infection is maintained by dogs which eat the flesh of infected sheep. Sheep, cattle and pigs are the common reservoirs of the larval form of hydatid disease which is found chiefly in sheep-rearing countries. In Iceland in the past from 16 to 33% of the human population were infected with hydatid but in recent years it has disappeared. In southern Australia 40–50% of adult dogs are infected and 2% of the population in certain districts. A cycle of infection is also maintained in dingoes and wallabies.

In New Zealand hydatid disease is a major health problem with 100 new cases a year (Forbes 1962). The endemic areas where hydatid is of most concern today are the sheep- and cattle-raising areas of Argentina, Uruguay, southern Brazil and Chile (Neghme *et al.* 1949). In Chile the maximum human incidence is in the third decade and in southern Brazil in the second decade.

In addition to cattle and sheep, naturally infected animals include horses, camels, goats, monkeys, lemurs, the African elephant, argali, pronghorn antelope, moose, reindeer, caribou, elk, white-tailed deer, bison and vicuna. Other animals which have also been found infected are giraffe, gazelle, tapir, zebra, kangaroo, mongoose, wild cat, panther, jaguar, agouti, guinea-pig, rabbit, arctic fox, wolf and dingo.

Most hydatid cysts are acquired in childhood and the unilocular cyst may grow for from 5 to 20 years before it is diagnosed. There is a tendency for hydatid to be more common in members of the same family (Ferro 1946).

Pathology

The damage caused by a hydatid cyst can be both mechanical and toxic. The egg is swallowed and the onchosphere emerges; after 8 hours embryos can be found in the portal vein and liver where they are filtered out. The next filter is the lung, where a smaller number lodge. In 3 weeks the larval worm becomes vesicular and visible to the naked eye. The hydatid cyst wall (Fig. 116) is composed of an outer laminated fibrous wall formed by the host, a thick median striated layer secreted by the cyst and an inner 'germinal' layer from which the brood capsules and daughter cysts arise. There are two types of proliferation—endogenous and exogenous.

The endogenous proliferation is inwards towards the cyst cavity and a unilocular hydatid cyst is formed which is the method of development of *Echinococcus granulosus*. Exogenous proliferation is outwards and is a feature of *E. multilocularis* and a multilocular or alveolar hydatid is formed (see page 346).

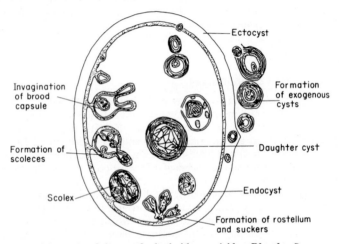

Fig. 116.—Schema of a hydatid cyst. (*After Blanchard*)

In endogenous proliferation brood capsules are formed from the germinal layer and larval scolices arise from the wall of the brood capsule, which evaginates to form a protective cup. The brood capsules become stalked and may be detached by injury or mechanical interference to form daughter cysts which with free scolices form 'hydatid sand' in the hydatid cyst cavity. Brood capsules which do not produce scolices are known as acephalocysts. Dissemination of endogenous unilocular hydatid cysts can only take place by rupture of the cyst

The contents of the cyst consist of hydatid sand and a clear watery fluid of specific gravity 1007–1015 containing albumin, and a protein allied to casein, sodium chloride (0·5%), phosphates and sulphates of sodium and calcium, succinates, traces of sugar and a toxin allied to albumin. The hydatid fluid and daughter cysts, when released into the abdominal cavity, cause anaphylactic shock.

The largest cyst ever found was in Australia and contained 50 quarts (57 litres) of fluid.

Hydatids are slow-growing and are usually sterile. In man they tend to die and calcify, but may suppurate.

The commonest site for the cysts is in the liver (57–76%), next the lung (4–14%), the omentum, mesentery and peritoneum (1·3–18·2%), pleura (0·7–0·9%), skin, subcutaneous tissues and muscles (0·7–0·9%), spleen (1·2–9·1%), brain (0·9–2%), spinal cord (0·8–0·9%), kidneys (1·6–6·1%) and bone (0·8–9·1%). In bone the result is osseous hydatid.

Symptoms

The main symptoms are caused by mechanical pressure at the site of the tumour.

Liver. A gradually increasing tumour in the right subcostal margin. Jaundice is rare.

Lung. Often found on routine examination. Other symptoms are caused by pressure on neighbouring structures, collapse of the lung and the mediastinal syndrome. In the pleural cavity a pleural effusion results.

In the kidney it resembles a hypernephroma and in the brain there will be symptoms and signs of a cerebral tumour. In bone (osseous hydatid) there may be spontaneous fracture of long bones and compression fracture of the vertebra.

The cyst may rupture with immediate pyrexia, urticaria and multiple cutaneous eruptions and in the peritoneum general peritonitis may result.

Signs

The hydatid cyst, if near the surface, appears as a smooth, round tense swelling which may give rise to a 'hydatid thrill'. If by any chance the cyst is needled a clear watery fluid is obtained which contains scolices and hooks. Otherwise the signs are those of a space-occupying lesion in the area involved.

X-ray examination. The radiological appearances of a hydatid cyst are characteristic. There is a smooth round outline and in the lung a wavy line crossing the middle of the cyst represents the 'lily' sign which looks like lilies on the surface of a pond in cross-section and is produced by the numerous daughter cysts lying inside the mother cyst (Fig. 117). Scanning of the affected organ will show a smooth round cold area. Exploratory puncture should be avoided because of the danger of spread of the daughter cysts. If it occurs then immediate operation and excision of the cyst must be undertaken.

Eosinophilia. Generalized eosinophilia is present in 20–25% of cases.

Treatment

The treatment is essentially surgical removal where possible. Cysts are removed quite easily from the liver and lung. Elsewhere removal is not so successful. The operative procedure is as follows: Expose the adventitia over the most prominent part of the tumour. Wall off the exposed surface of the wound with towels, attach a funnel to the cyst wall by a cryostat and aspirate the contents of the cyst through a large calibre needle or trochar with a closed suction apparatus. Inject 10–50 ml of 10% formalin solution into the cyst and withdraw in 5 minutes. Separate the cyst from the adventitia and remove. Swab the adventitia with 10% formalin and allow a little fluid to remain. Obliterate the cavity by sutures where possible and close the incision without drainage, anchoring the adventitia to the tissue beneath the line of incision.

Prognosis

Prognosis is fair in the unilocular form when the cyst is in an operable site and can be removed without spillage of cyst fluid into the peritoneal or pleural cavity. Recurrence of the disease from scolices spilled at the time of operation may be expected in 50% of cases.

Prevention

Infection of dogs can be prevented by controlling the disposal of raw offal. Dogs should be kept out of abattoirs and no killing of sheep or cattle should be allowed outside authorized places. Dogs may be treated with arecoline hydrobromide in a dosage of 4 mg/50 kg. Hydatid disappeared from Iceland when a change was made from the production of mutton to lamb which did not allow the hydatids time to develop and so infect the dogs on the island.

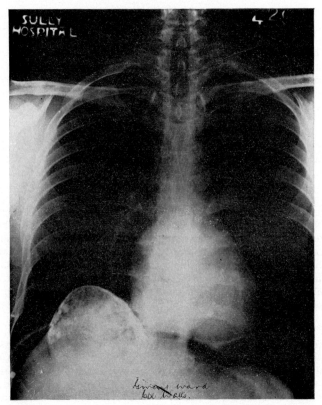

Fig. 117.—Hydatid cyst of the lung. (*Reproduced from Bennett & Thomas (1952) Br. J. Surg., 40, 161*)

E. multilocularis (MULTILOCULAR OR ALVEOLAR HYDATID CYST)

Aetiology

E. multilocularis has been recognized as a separate species (Rausch & Schiller 1951; Vogel 1955), and is the cause of multilocular or alveolar hydatid cyst. Herbivora play no part in the life history and the larval stages are found in the livers of rodents.

Geographical distribution and epidemiology

E. multilocularis has a restricted geographical distribution. In the high latitudes of North America the distribution corresponds to that of the arctic fox. There is also a focus in Central North America. It is also found in extensive areas of the U.S.S.R. from the Black Sea, with an extension into Turkey to the Far East and north to Siberia and northern Japan. Definitive records exist for France, Germany, Switzerland, Austria, Belgium and probably England and Sardinia.

In Alaska the definitive hosts are mainly the arctic fox, but also wolves and dogs, and the intermediate host in which the larval forms are found is the tundra vole (*Microtus aeconomus*) (Rausch & Schiller 1951). In St Lawrence Island in Alaska hosts of *E.m. sibericensis* are field mice (*Clethrionomys rutilis*), ground squirrels (*Citellus undulatus*) and shrews (*Sorex jacksoni*) (Thomas *et al.* 1954). In southern Germany the larval stages are found in the field mouse (*Microtus arvalis*) and the adult stages in the red fox (*Vulpes vulpes*) (Vogel 1955).

The cysts are found mainly in the liver, and in Arctic regions sledge dogs and foxes are a source of human infection. In agricultural regions man acquires the infection by eating raw fruit and vegetables contaminated by foxes and other canidae (Rausch 1956). In Europe man is infected from the contamination of strawberries, huckleberries and cranberries by foxes (Vogel 1955).

Pathology (Dew 1953)

The alveolar cyst grows by exogenous proliferation, is invasive and frequently metastasizes to other organs. It is solid and not cystic, consisting of many irregular cavities containing hyaline membrane, all enclosed in a relatively avascular fibrous adventitia. The cavities contain little or no fluid and scolices are rarely seen in them. Central necrosis and cavitation are common findings. There is a persistent cellular reaction of eosinophils in the surrounding tissues.

Symptoms and signs

Alveolar hydatid of the liver resembles a slowly developing carcinoma without fever but with hepatomegaly, splenomegaly, jaundice and ascites in the later stages (Rausch 1956).

The clinical picture is of intrahepatic portal hypertension.

Treatment

Surgical removal is not possible because there is no intact surrounding capsule. Prognosis is invariably grave.

INFECTION WITH *Coenurus cerebralis* (**BLADDER WORM**)
Aetiology

Coenurus cerebralis is the larval form of *T.* (*multiceps*) *multiceps*. The adult taenia lives in the intestine of dogs and the larval stages are normally found in the brain of sheep, in which it causes 'staggers'.

Geographical distribution

Coenurus cerebralis has been described in man from South Africa (Becker & Jacobson 1951) where it is found in sheep-raising areas, in which it may be commoner than has been realized, in Ruanda-Urundi in the Congo (Fain & Piraux 1956) and in Uganda and Kenya (Raper & Dockeray 1956). In tropical

Africa the larval stages are suspected of being the larval form of *T. brauni* which is commonly found in dogs in the Congo. There are some differences between the cases from tropical Africa and those from South Africa, which suggests a different biology.

Pathology and symptomatology

The cysts are like bladders (bladder worm), measure from a few millimetres to 2 or more centimetres in diameter and have multiple scolices dependent from the germinal wall and projecting into the bladder cavity. The cysts are normally situated in the brain where they obstruct the pathways of circulation of cerebrospinal fluid and cause raised intracranial pressure. The symptoms are those of raised intracranial pressure with headache and papilloedema. In addition there are focal signs, Jacksonian epilepsy, hemiplegia, monoplegia and cerebellar ataxia. The spinal cord may be affected with spastic paraplegia. Cysts may also occur beneath the conjunctiva and in the eyeball (Raper & Dockeray 1956).

Diagnosis

Ventriculography will show dilatation of the ventricles. Serological tests are positive as for hydatid.

Treatment

There is no treatment and the prognosis is grave. Surgical removal is usually impossible.

INFECTION WITH *Diphyllobothrium latum*

Synonyms

Broad tapeworm; fish tapeworm.

Aetiology

Diphyllobothrium infection of man is caused by the adult *D. latum* of which the first intermediate host is a freshwater crustacean, and the second intermediate host a freshwater fish (for the life history see Appendix II).

Transmission

If the eggs are passed in water a coracidium emerges and is swallowed by a freshwater crustacean—*Cyclops strenuus, C. furcifer* and *C. vicinus* in Europe; *Diaptomus oregonensis, D. sicilis* and *D. siciloides* in North America; and *Diaptomus vulgaris, D. gracilis, D. denticornis* in Norway. The coracidium develops in the crustacean into a procercoid. The crustacean is then swallowed by a freshwater fish, which is the second intermediate host: pike, perch, salmon trout and grayling in Europe; the barbel in Africa; the pike, walleye and burbot in North America; and rainbow and lake trout in Argentina and Chile. Man becomes infected by eating raw uncooked fish. Kippering does not destroy the plerocercoids, but brine saturation and freezing for 24–48 hours at −10°C does destroy them.

Geographical distribution

D. latum is a common parasite of man in northern Italy, Switzerland, parts of Germany, the Baltic countries including Poland, Lithuania, Latvia, Estonia, U.S.S.R., Finland, Sweden and Denmark. It is also common in Romania, the

Danube delta, Lake Tiberias in Israel, Siberia, Northern Manchuria and Japan. There are foci in North America in the lake region of Minnesota and Michigan. It is common in Eastern Canada and is found in Canadian and Alaskan Eskimos. It has become established in the lake district of Argentina and Chile, also in Australia, and possibly in Uganda, Botswana, Angola and Madagascar. It may occur in Papua, New Guinea.

Epidemiology

Many mammals other than man have been found infected in nature, but man is primarily responsible for the propagation of infection in most endemic areas.

Pathology and symptomatology

In man *D. latum* competes for the available supply of vitamin B_{12} in the small intestine. When this is deficient it causes a megaloblastic anaemia and, in severe cases, cord changes (Von Bonsdorff 1956). Usually there is no anaemia and 70% of the cases of anaemia have been recorded in Finland, where this tapeworm acts as a precipitating cause; elsewhere there is usually no anaemia. There is often a peripheral eosinophilia. In most persons infected with *D. latum* there is no evidence of any damage to the host. If there are a large number of worms, then mechanical obstruction of the intestine can result. The worm can live as long as 29 years.

Treatment

D. latum is treated in the same way as other tapeworms. If there is an associated megaloblastic anaemia, vitamin B_{12} injections must be given. Once the tapeworm has been removed then no further vitamin B_{12} is necessary.

SPARGANOSIS

Aetiology

Sparganosis is caused by infection of man with the plerocercoid stage of various species of *Spirometra* (*Diphyllobothrium*) worms of which the adult stage occurs in canines, the procercoid stage in *Cyclops* and the plerocercoid stage in man, frog and snakes. Various species of *Spirometra* are involved— *S. mansonioides* (the parent form of *Sparganum proliferum*) in the United States; *S. mansoni* in Japan, China, Australia and Guyana; and *S. theileri* or *S. pretoriensis* in Central Africa (Fain & Piraux 1960), where it is not uncommon among the Masai.

Transmission

Man is infected accidentally by swallowing the procercoid while drinking and thus becomes a second intermediate host, or by eating the raw flesh of frogs, snakes, or mammals, or by the Chinese custom of rubbing raw split frogs on the eye or ulcers of the skin.

Pathology

The sparganum in man measures 8–36 cm × 0·1–1·2 mm × 0·5–1·75 mm thick (Fig. 118); its body is flat and transversely wrinkled. It may be found in many parts of the body—kidneys, iliac fossae, pleural cavities, urethra, and subcutaneous tissues. Ocular sparganosis is caused by a plerocercoid in the orbit (see Chapter 44).

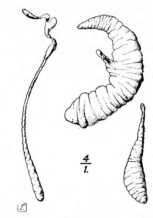

Fig. 118.—Different forms of *Sparganum proliferum*. (*After Ijima*)

Symptomatology

Swellings arise anywhere in the body, often on the chest. The invaded tissues become swollen and painful, and on incision a mass of worms can be seen in a central chylous-like area. Death of the worms may cause an intense inflammatory reaction with eosinophilic infiltration and the presence of Charcot–Leyden crystals. The lesions produced are usually incised or are excised surgically.

Hymenolepis nana INFECTION

Synonyms

Dwarf tapeworm.

Aetiology

H. nana is a small tapeworm (Appendix II) which has no intermediate host. The eggs are passed to the outside in faeces and are ingested by another host. The larva is released in the small intestine and enters a villus, forming a cercocyst. Development is rapid, and in 40–70 hours the scolex appears, in 80–90 hours the rostellum has hooks and the worm passes into the lumen of the intestine where it is attached to the villus by a short neck. After 30 days eggs appear in the faeces.

Geographical distribution and epidemiology

H. nana is found in warm countries—Egypt, Sudan, Thailand, South America, especially Cuba and Southern Europe, where it affects 10% of the children. Man is probably the only source of infection, which is commoner in children than adults and is transmitted directly from patient to patient. It is commoner in family and institutional groups than in the general population.

Pathology and symptomatology

H. nana normally causes no symptoms but may be present in large numbers, even hundreds and thousands. Occasionally there is abdominal pain and diarrhoea but of 43 patients without any other parasitoses, many complained of headache, dizziness, anorexia, pruritus ani, periodic diarrhoea and abdominal pain (Donckaster & Habibe 1958); 5% (2) had epileptiform convulsions and one-third showed an eosinophilia of over 5%.

Treatment

Atebrin treatment is usually effective. Chloroquine is also recommended. Hexylresorcinol, as used for ascariasis, Yomesan (niclosamide) and paromomycin (Humatin) are also very effective. An infected person should not sleep in the same bed as another person.

TREATMENT OF TAPEWORM INFECTIONS

General statement

Preliminary starvation appears to be necessary for one day. On this day sodium sulphate 15 grammes or castor oil 15 ml should be given to clear out the bowel; the food should be restricted to weak tea, toast and unlimited amounts of lemonade and glucose (Glucodin, Glaxo).

Filix mas treatment. Extractum filicis liquidum, dose 3–6 ml, has a disagreeable taste and is apt to cause vomiting, so the drug is best prescribed in gelatin capsules.

Capsules contain 1 ml each of the liquid extract. The dose of these is 1–6, according to the age of the patient. It is effective against *T. saginata, T. solium,* and especially against *D. latum.* The most difficult species to dislodge are *T. saginata* and *Hymenolepis nana.* On the morning of the treatment the patient should have a small cup of tea. For an adult man the full dose of filix mas is 6 ml; for a woman 4 ml. For specially resistant cases up to 8 ml may be given with safety.

> 8 a.m.: 2 capsules of extract of filix mas
> 8.30 a.m.: repeat
> 9 a.m.: repeat

The mixture in syrup is sometimes better, as follows: extract of filix mas 8 ml, acacia 8 grammes, cinnamon water 42 ml, glycerin 14 ml. Divided into 3 doses at 15-minute intervals. (This is a heavy dosage.) For children, the taste of filix mas may be disguised by blackcurrant syrup.

The patient must then lie quiet and take nothing but sips of sodium bicarbonate solution, 8 grammes dissolved in half a tumbler of hot water, with the idea of removing mucus from the small intestine. At 10.30 hours 15 grammes of sodium sulphate should be given. The bowels being opened freely by the salts, segments of the tapeworm should soon appear. All motions should be saved and strained to search for the head; should this not be seen, a soap and water enema should immediately be given.

The patient must rest in bed the whole day when undergoing treatment. A combination of filix mas with Atebrin has proved most successful. On the first day (day of preparation) the patient takes 800 mg Atebrin in 4 doses of 200 mg and on the second, the day of treatment, 200 mg directly on waking. Atebrin has an action on the head of the worm and stains the segments yellow. The filix mas course follows as above.

Treatment with filix mas must not be repeated more often than once a month, otherwise toxic symptoms, such as polyneuritis and paralysis of the iris (filicic acid poisoning), may ensue.

For the intraduodenal treatment of tapeworm 30 grammes sodium sulphate are given in the afternoon, and the patient is starved for the rest of the day. Next morning the bowels are opened by an enema, the patient swallows a catheter and is placed on his right side. The catheter enters the duodenum in 1-2 hours. The patient is then turned on his back, and a small glass funnel is attached. The standard dose of filix mas is introduced, and immediately 50 ml of warm 50% solution of sodium sulphate is poured in and the catheter extracted. Expulsion takes place in two hours.

Atebrin (mepacrine) without filix mas, has been recommended by several observers, notably Hoekenga (1951), in doses of 800 mg by the mouth followed by an aperient. Milk diet on the day before and a purge of castor oil are necessary. On the morning of treatment 600-800 mg of Atebrin are given, 200 mg every 5 minutes with water. 100 mg of phenobarbitone are given before Atebrin, to prevent vomiting. The purge is repeated 2-4 hours later and food withheld until the bowels are opened.

Seaton (1955) has improved upon this treatment by intraduodenal infiltration with Atebrin, 1 gramme, dissolved in 100 ml of warm water. Sodium amytal, 200 mg, is given as a sedative before intubation; 15-30 minutes later 60-80 ml of 30% sodium sulphate are infiltrated by the same route.

Dichlorophen (Anthiphen). This disintegrates the worms and should not be used for *T. solium* because of the risk of cysticercosis, but is said to be effective for *D. latum*. The dosage is 3-6 grammes before breakfast. No starvation or purging is necessary. It may cause some nausea or diarrhoea, and jaundice; it should not be used in patients with liver disease.

Yomesan (Bayer 2353) (niclosamide) is a new preparation which has acquired a reputation in the treatment of all forms of tapeworm infection. It is taken in tablet form, each of 500 mg. Two on the first day at an interval of one hour on a fasting stomach, and subsequently one each day for 7 days. No other measures are necessary. Another schedule is 4 tablets in 2 doses at an interval of one hour, followed usually by a saline purge. Yomesan is contraindicated in *T. solium* infections. The tablets should be chewed before being swallowed with water.

Paromomycin. Paromomycin (Humatin) has proved useful in treatment and Salem and Al Allaf (1967) treated 47 patients successfully with 50 mg/kg/day in divided doses for 5 days.

SERODIAGNOSIS OF TAPEWORM INFECTIONS

Hydatid

In general the presence of an active cyst is associated with the production of antibodies and the rupture of a cyst frequently produces a marked rise in antibody levels. Surgical removal as well as suppuration, degeneration and calcification of a cyst results in a marked reduction in antibody levels.

IgA and IgG levels are raised in active infection and the IgM is highest with active infection. IgG is responsible for the antibodies measured by the complement fixation, flocculation and fluorescent antibody tests (Kagan *et al.* 1968).

The source of antigen is usually a host species other than man and is most commonly sheep or pig.

Complement fixation test (Ghedini 1906). Unpreserved fluid from human, sheep or pig cysts is used as antigen. The CFT has proved a valuable diagnostic test especially for liver cysts. Where cerebral cysts are suspected then cerebrospinal fluid can be used for testing. The CFT can also be used as a test of cure after surgical removal of a cyst. It has a lower sensitivity than the other tests and

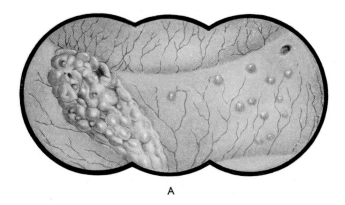

A

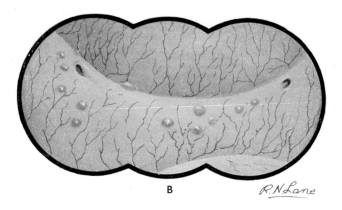

B   R.N.Lane

PLATE III

Schistosomiasis of the bladder.

Bilharzial disease of the bladder before treatment and 1 month after treatment with sodium antimony tartrate. The yellow nodules in A are the dead ova working their way through into the bladder cavity. They do not indicate active disease. (*By permission of the British Journal of Surgery, Ogier Ward and Dr J. B. Christopherson*)

[*To face p. 352.*]

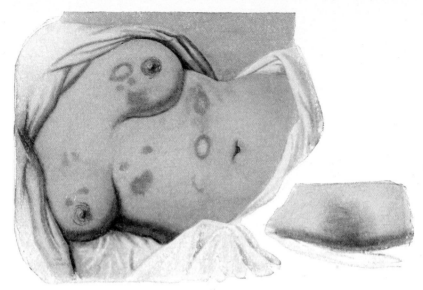

A

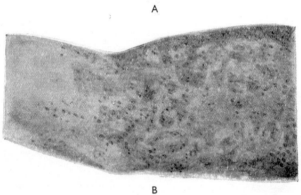

B

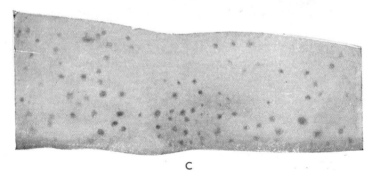

C

PLATE IV
Rashes.

A, Rash of trypanosomiasis (*Trypanosoma gambiense*). (*Dr F. Murgatroyd*)
A inset, Primary lesion of trypanosomiasis, infecting tsetse bite on the leg.
B, Dengue rash. (*After Cleland, Bradley and MacDonald*)
C, Rash of *fièvre boutoneuse* on the legs. (*After D. and J. Olmer*)

false positives may occur with patients previously immunized with vaccines such as anti-rabies vaccine.

Indirect haemagglutination test. This is a more sensitive test than the CFT. A titre of 1:400 or more in association with a positive flocculation test will distinguish true from non-specific positive reactions (Kagan 1963). No cross-reactions occur with other conditions, except that a positive reaction is found in cysticercosis (Powell *et al.* 1966). Sheep or pig preserved hydatid fluid is used and formolized red cells may be tanned, coated with antigen and lyophilized for storage.

Flocculation tests. There are two flocculation tests. The bentonite flocculation test, BFT (Norman *et al.* 1959), and the latex flocculation test, LFT (Kagan *et al.* 1966).

The LFT is equal to the BFT in specificity and sensitivity. Human cyst fluid is used as antigen with the uninactivated test serum. A fluorescent antibody test has been developed with protoscolices of fertile cysts (Sorice *et al.* 1966).

The Casoni reaction. Introduced by Casoni in 1911, this is an immediate hypersensitivity intradermal test. The sensitivity varies since there are difficulties in procuring a satisfactory antigen. Hydatid fluid, which is usually used as antigen, does not retain its antigenic properties for more than a few weeks unless Merthiolate 1:50,000 is used as a preservative. The skin antigen has been standardized to a nitrogen content of 12–15 µg/ml, which gives the highest specificity (Kagan *et al.* 1966). A few drops of the antigen are injected intradermally and a reaction appears in 10 minutes as a large wheal surrounded by erythema. It fades in an hour and a secondary reaction may appear 8 hours later. The Casoni reaction measures past as well as present infection and remains positive even after surgical removal of all cysts.

Cysticercosis

Serum antibodies do not develop in adult *T. solium* and *T. saginata* infections, but can be demonstrated in cysticercosis. The haemagglutination test has been used mainly to determine the cysticercal origin of cases of epilepsy. Of Africans known to have cysticercosis 85% gave positive reactions (Powell *et al.* 1966) and cysticercosis was found responsible for a large proportion of cases of epilepsy in Africans in Durban.

REFERENCES

BECKER, B. J. P. & JACOBSON, S. (1951) *Lancet*, **ii**, 198.
CH'IN, K. Y. (1933) *Chin. med. J.*, **49**, 429.
DEW, H. R. (1953) *Archos int. Hidatid*, **13**, 284.
DIXON, H. B. F. & LIPSCOMB, F. M. (1961) *Spec. Rep. Ser. med. Res. Coun.*, 299.
DONCKASTER, R. & HABIBE, O. (1958) *Boln chil. Parasit.*, **13**, 9.
FAIN, A. & PIRAUX, A. (1960) *Bull. Soc. Path. éxot.*, **52**, 804.
FERRO, A. (1946) *Archos int. Hidatid.*, **6**, 135.
FORBES, L. (1962) *Trans. R. Soc. trop. Med. Hyg.*, **56**, 7.
GHEDINI, G. (1906) *Gazz. Osp. Clin.*, **27**, 1616.
HOEKENGA, M. T. (1951) *Am. J. trop. Med.*, **31**, 420.
KAGAN, I. G. (1963) *Exp. Parasit.*, **13**, 57.
——— MADDISON, S. E. & NORMAN, L. (1968) *Am. J. trop. Med. Hyg.*, **17**, 79.
——— OSIMAN, J. J., VARELA, J. C. & ALLAIN, D. S. (1966) *Am. J. trop. Med. Hyg.*, **15**, 172.
MACARTHUR, W. P. (1933) *Trans. R. Soc. trop. Med. Hyg.*, **26**, 525.
MILLER, M. J. (1953) *Can. med. Ass. J.*, **68**, 423.
NORMAN, L., SADUN, E. H. & ALLAIN, D. S. (1959) *Am. J. trop. Med.*, **8**, 46.

NEGHME, R. A., FAIGENBAUM, A. J., PILOTTI, A. & SILVA CAMPOS, R. (1949) *Boln. Of. sanit. pan-am.*, **28**, 469.
POWELL, S. J., PROCTER, E. M., WILMOT, E. J. & MACLEOD, I. N. (1966) *Ann. trop. Med. Parasit.*, **60**, 152, 159.
RAPER, A. B. & DOCKERAY, G. C. (1956) *Ann. trop. Med. Parasit.*, **50**, 121.
RAUSCH, R. (1956) *Am. J. trop. Med. Hyg.*, **5**, 1086.
―――― (1967) *Annls Parasit. hum. comp.*, **42**, 19.
―――― & SCHILLER, E. L. (1951) *Science, N.Y.*, **113**, 57.
REINLEIN, J. M. ALEO, TRIGUEROS, E. ARJONA & ALCALDE, S. OBRADOR (1951) *Bull. Inst. med. Res. Madrid*, **4**, 67.
SALEM, H. H. & AL ALLAF, G. (1967) *Lancet*, **ii**, 1360.
SEATON, D. R. (1955) *Lancet*, **ii**, 644.
SORICE, R., CASTIGNARI, L. & TOLU, A. (1966) *G. Mal. infett. parassit.*, **18**, 192.
THOMAS, L. J., BABERO, B. B., GAILLICCHIO, V. & LACEY, R. J. (1954) *Science, N.Y.*, **120**, 1102.
VOGEL, H. (1955) *Dt. med. Wschr.*, **80**, 931.
VON BONSDORFF, B. (1956) *Exp. Parasit.*, **5**, 207.

SECTION III

DISEASES DUE TO VIRUSES

14. ARBOVIRUS DISEASES

THE diseases caused by arboviruses (*arthropod-borne viruses*) are zoonoses; that is they are primarily infections of vertebrates other than man, and of arthropods, and can be transmitted to man. One apparent exception is o'nyong-nyong fever, of which the only known vertebrate host is man, though others may conceivably be found later. These viruses are mostly spread by the bites of arthropods, but some of them can also be transmitted by other means (through milk, excreta or aerosols). Several definitions have been suggested. The arbovirus infections 'are maintained in nature principally, or to an important extent, through biological transmission between susceptible vertebrate hosts by haematophagous arthropods; they multiply to produce viraemia in the vertebrates, multiply in the tissues of the arthropods and are passed on to new vertebrates by the bites of arthropods after a period of extrinsic incubation' (WHO 1967). In the same publication, however, Chumakov prefers the following: 'Arboviruses are zoonotic viral agents which, when circulating in the natural foci of infection, are transmitted in a more or less regular manner by arthropods, but in certain circumstances may be transmitted in other ways than by arthropods.'

Smith (1968) suggests that the safest definition is that arboviruses are 'potential zoonotic viruses which cannot be otherwise classified.'

The matter is obviously incomplete in our present state of knowledge; much research is necessary, and is being done to clarify these points.

The names by which these viruses are known are of mixed origin. Some are dialect names for the illnesses they cause (chikungunya, o'nyong-nyong), some are place names (West Nile, Bwamba) and some derive from clinical characters (Western equine encephalitis, yellow fever).

The viruses are classified into groups (A, B, Bunyamwera and other minor groups), and this classification depends upon their antigenic characters. They may also be grouped according to their usual vectors (mosquitoes, ticks, sand-flies).

AETIOLOGY

General character of arboviruses

Most arboviruses are spherical, measuring 17–150 nm or more; a few are rod-shaped, measuring 70 × 200 nm (WHO 1967). Their morphology is very variable. Of 20 tested for nucleic acids, all were positive for RNA. Some are inactivated by ethyl ether and sodium deoxycholate. Many of the ungrouped bat viruses, and vesicular stomatitis virus, are rhabdovirus-like; African horse sickness and blue-tongue viruses are reoviruses.

Groups

The arboviruses are classified in groups. In 1967 WHO published a list of 252 arboviruses in 29 antigenic groups (plus one category of 56 marked ungrouped) but added a note that the list was not complete. Most of them are in Group A, Group B and the Bunyamwera supergroup. Many of them do not infect man. The standard reference book for details of known arboviruses is the *Catalogue of Arthropod Borne Viruses of the World* (1967). Additions are constantly being made to this list.

The arboviruses affecting man are given in Tables 15–18, but more may subsequently be found. Some cause large outbreaks, others only a few known cases; most may cause infection without clinical illness, but most can also cause symptoms and some, death.

Table 15. Arboviruses: Group A

Name of virus and abbreviation	Geographical distribution	Vector	Fever	Clinical form H	E	Rash
Chikungunya (CHIK)	South Africa East Africa Far East	Mosquito	+	+		+
Mayaro (Uruma) (MAY)	South America Trinidad, South Africa	Mosquito	+			+
Mucambo (MUC)	Brazil	Mosquito	+			
O'nyong-nyong (ONN)	Africa	Mosquito	+			+
Pixuna (PIX) (No evidence of human disease	Brazil	Mosquito ?				
Ross River (RR)	Australia	Mosquito	+			
Semliki Forest (SF)	South Africa East Africa	Mosquito	+			
Sindbis (SIN)	Africa Far East Australia	Mosquito	+			+ (Africa only)
Eastern equine encephalitis (EEE)	North America	Mosquito	+		+	
Venezuelan equine encephalitis (VEE)	North America South America British Honduras	Mosquito	+		+	
Western equine encephalitis (WEE)	North America South America	Mosquito	+		+	

H, Haemorrhagic. *E*, Encephalitis.

Group A are all transmitted by mosquitoes in nature, but in experimental work the range of mosquito species capable of transmission is larger than the known range of vectors in nature.

African strains of yellow fever possess an antigen absent from American strains, and the 17D strain, which is so successfully used as a live vaccine, has acquired an antigen absent from the original Asibi strain from which it was derived (Smith 1968).

Arboviruses of Group B are transmitted by mosquitoes or ticks; the tick-borne series includes RSSE, KFD, louping ill (LI) and Omsk haemorrhagic fever (OMSK).

Table 16. Arboviruses: Group B

Name of virus and abbreviation	Geographical distribution	Vector	Fever	Clinical forms H	Clinical forms E	Rash
Banzi (BAN)	South Africa	Mosquito	+			
Bussuquara (BSQ)	Brazil	Mosquito	?			
Dengue type 1 (DEN-1)	Africa Pacific Far East Caribbean	Mosquito	+	+		+
Dengue type 2 (DEN-2)	Far East Trinidad British Honduras	Mosquito	+	+		+
Dengue type 3 (DEN-3)	Philippines India	Mosquito	+	+		+
Dengue type 4 (DEN-4)	Philippines	Mosquito	+	+		+
Dengue type TH-36	Thailand	Mosquito	+	+		
Dengue type TH-SMAN	Thailand	Mosquito	+	+		
Ilheus (ILH)	Americas Caribbean British Honduras	Mosquito	+		+ ?	
Japanese encephalitis (JE)	Japan Far East	Mosquito	+		+	
Kumlinge (KUM)	Finland	Tick	+		+	+
Kunjin (KUN)	Australia	Mosquito	+			+
Kyasanur Forest disease (KFD)	India	Tick	+	+		
Langat (LGT)	Malaya	Tick	+		+	
Louping ill (LI)	Britain	Tick	+			+
Murray Valley encephalitis (MVE)	Australia	Mosquito	+		+	+
Negishi (NEG)	Japan	?Tick	+		+	
Omsk haemorrhagic fever (OMSK)	U.S.S.R.	Tick	+	+		+
Powassan (POW)	Canada U.S.A.	Tick	+		+	
Rio Bravo (RB)	U.S.A.	?	+ (lab.)			
Russian spring-summer encephalitis (RSSE) including Absettarov, Hanzalova and Hypr	U.S.S.R. Europe	Tick	+		+	
Spondweni (SPO)	South Africa Americas	Mosquito	+			
St Louis encephalitis (SLE)	British Honduras	Mosquito	+		+	
Wesselsbron (WSL)	South Africa	Mosquito	+			+
West Nile (WN)	Near East South Europe Africa	Mosquito	+			+
Yellow fever (YF)	Africa Americas Caribbean	Mosquito	+	+		
Zika (ZIKA)	Uganda Malaysia	?	+ (lab.)			+

H, Haemorrhagic. *E,* Encephalitis lab., Laboratory infection.

Many viruses of Group B have been isolated from the salivary glands of bats in widely separated parts of the world; they are probably transmitted from bat to bat by bite (compare rabies in Trinidad). One bat virus has caused a laboratory infection in man; others may not be concerned in human disease.

Table 17. Arboviruses: Bunyamwera supergroup

Name of virus and abbreviation	Geographical distribution	Vector	Fever	Clinical forms H	E	Rash
Bunyamwera group (BUN)						
Bunyamwera (BUN)	Africa	Mosquito	+			+
	America					
Calovo (CVO)	Czechoslovakia	Mosquito	+			.
Germiston (GER)	Africa	Mosquito	+			
Guaroa (GRO)	Brazil	Mosquito	+			
Ilesha	Americas	Mosquito	+			
	Africa					
Wyeomyia	Americas	Mosquito	+			
Bwamba group						
Bwamba (BWA)	Uganda	Mosquito	+			
Group C						
Apeu (APEU)	Brazil	Mosquito	+			
Caraparu (CAR)	Brazil	Mosquito	+			
Itaqui (ITQ)	Brazil	Mosquito	+			
Marituba (MTB)	Brazil	Mosquito	+			
Murutucu (MUR)	Brazil	Mosquito	+			
Madrid (MAD)	Panama	Mosquito	+			
Oriboca (ORI)	Brazil	Mosquito	+			
Ossa (OSSA)	Panama	Mosquito	+			
Restan (RES)	Trinidad	Mosquito	+			
	Surinam					
California group (CAL)						
California encephalitis (CE)	U.S.A.	Mosquito	+		++	
La Crosse (LAC)	U.S.A.	?	+		++	
Tahyna (Lumbo) (TAH)	Czechoslovakia	Mosquito	+			
	France					
	Africa					
Simbu group (SIM)						
Oropouche (ORO)	Trinidad	Mosquito	+			
	Brazil					
Guama group (GMA)						
Guama (GMA)	Americas	Mosquito	+			
Catu (CATU)	Americas	Mosquito	+			

H, Haemorrhagic. *E*, Encephalitis.

EPIZOOTIOLOGY AND EPIDEMIOLOGY

Vertebrate hosts

The vertebrate hosts have been differentiated as maintenance, incidental, link and amplifier hosts.

Maintenance hosts. These 'are essential for the continued existence of the virus' (Smith 1964). They usually live in symbiosis with the viruses, without actual disease, but they develop antibody.

The maintenance hosts provisionally recognized include the following, though some have only been incriminated experimentally (Simpson 1968):

Birds: Prairie chicken, red-winged blackbird, blue jay, pheasant, pigeon, cardinal, sparrow, wren, grackle, wood thrush, catbird (EEE, WEE, SLE), heron, egret (JE). Migrating birds can carry viruses over long distances (MVE, EEE, WEE, SLE).

Table 18. Arboviruses: Minor groups and ungrouped

Name of virus and abbreviation	Geographical distribution	Vector	Fever	H	E	Rash
Phlebotomus group (PHL)						
Neapolitan sandfly fever (SFN)	Mediterranean	Phlebotomus	+			
Sicilian sandfly fever (SFS)	Mediterranean	Phlebotomus	+			
Candiru (CDU)	Brazil	?	+			
Chagres (CHG)	Panama	Phlebotomus	+			
Changuinola group (CGL)						
Changuinola (CGL)	Panama	Phlebotomus	+			
Piry group (PIRY)						
Chandipura (CHP)	India	?	+			
Piry (PIRY)	Brazil	Mosquito	+			
Tacaribe group (TCR)						
Junin (JUN)*	Argentina	Mosquito	+	++		
Machupo (MAC)	Bolivia	Mosquito	+	++		
Kemerovo group (KEM)						
Kemerovo (KEM)	Siberia	Mosquito	+			
Quaranfil group (QRF)						
Quaranfil (QRF)	Egypt	Mosquito	+			
Vesicular stomatitis group (VSV)						
VSV-Indiana	U.S.A.	Mosquito	+			
Ungrouped						
Colorado tick fever (CFT)	U.S.A.	Tick	+			
Crimean haemorrhagic fever (CHF)	U.S.S.R. Bulgaria Romania	Tick	+	++		
Rift Valley fever (RVF)	Africa	Mosquito	+	+		+
Epidemic haemorrhagic fever with renal syndrome (HFRS) (Korean HF, Congo HF, haemorrhagic nephroso-nephritis)	U.S.S.R.	? Readily transmitted by animal urine	+	++		
Ganjam (GAN)	India	Tick (lab.)	+			
Nairobi sheep disease (NSD)	East Africa	Tick	+			

H, Haemorrhagic. E, Encephalitis.

* Junin virus may also be transmitted through contact with excretions of infected rodents.

New arboviruses have been described in the American Journal of Tropical Medicine and Hygiene (1970), 19, 6, suppl.

Rodents and insectivores (VEE, KFD, LGT, JUN, MAC): Vole, shrew, rat, Arvicanthus, fieldmouse, hedgehog, squirrel, lemming, chipmunk (European TBE, RSSE, LI), groundhog (POW), deermouse, porcupine (CTF), sloth, small marsupials.

Primates: Monkey (YF, ?DEN).

Leporidae: Rabbit, hare (CE, ?TAH).

Ungulates: Cattle, deer (?European TBE, LI).

Bats: (?RB, TCR).

Marsupials, reptiles and amphibia: Kangaroo, snake (?EEE, WEE), lizard, alligator, turtle (?EEE).

Incidental hosts. These become infected, but transmission from them does not occur with sufficient regularity for stable maintenance. Man is usually an incidental host, often, but not always, being a dead end in the chain. Incidental hosts may or may not show symptoms. They may be necessary for the maintenance of transmission as they are the main hosts of ticks, keeping these arthropods alive in sufficient numbers to be effective carriers.

Link hosts. These bridge a gap between maintenance hosts and man (e.g. between small mammals and man by goats (via milk) in tick-borne encephalitis, and between wild birds and man by sparrows in SLE).

Amplifier hosts. These increase the weight of infection to which man is exposed, for instance pigs, which act between wild birds (especially herons) and man in JE. Dogs may also be involved.

The mode of transmission between maintenance hosts may differ from that responsible for infection of incidental hosts, including man.

The populations and characters of the vertebrate hosts and their threshold levels of viraemia are important. Small rodents multiply rapidly and have short lives, thus providing a constant supply of susceptible individuals, especially to the tick-borne viruses. On the other hand, monkeys and pigs multiply slowly, and once they have recovered from an infection with yellow fever and JE respectively, they remain immune for life. Immunity also affects pigs in the early months of life, having been transmitted via the placenta from immune mothers, and this no doubt is a feature in other animals. African monkeys are relatively resistant to yellow fever, but Asian and American monkeys are susceptible, probably because, unlike the African monkeys, they have not been exposed continuously for centuries to the infection. It is also possible that infection with other related arboviruses may partly immunize African monkeys (and man) against yellow fever.

So far as is known, the only vertebrate host of ONN is man, and the conditions for the spread of this infection seem to depend on the human populations involved, and the multiplicity of vector mosquitoes. In urban conditions, with a concentrated human population and prolific breeding of *Aedes aegypti*, the cycle of yellow fever and dengue is also usually man–mosquito–man.

Invertebrate hosts

These include mosquitoes, sandflies and ticks, and also *Culicoides* (involved in some animal viruses).

After these vectors have imbibed virus from a vertebrate in a state of viraemia, the virus undergoes an incubation period within the arthropod, known as the extrinsic incubation period. In mosquitoes this period is short (10 days) at 30°C ambient temperature, and longer at lower temperatures, and mosquitoes remain infective for life without any apparent ill-effects. Their infectivity appears to increase with time after infection, and their effectiveness as transmitters depends upon the frequency with which they bite.

It is also possible that arthropods, whose mouthparts are contaminated by virus in the act of feeding, could transmit the virus mechanically if they feed quickly on another animal. For instance, chikungunya virus can be transmitted mechanically by *Aedes aegypti* for 8 hours after infection.

Of 181 arboviruses analysed, 131 have been recovered from mosquitoes, some from more than one species (WHO 1967):

Culex	61	Culiseta	5
Aedes	55	Trichoprosopon	4
Anopheles	23	Eretmapodites	3
Mansonia	13	Wyeomyia	3
Sabethes	10	Limatus	1
Psorophora	10	Phoniomyia	1
Haemagogus	7		

Ixodid ticks are involved in a closely interrelated subgroup of Group B arboviruses, and also in some of the other groups. Genera of ticks involved include *Haemaphysalis*, *Ixodes* and *Dermacentor*.

In general, mosquitoes are refractory to tick-borne viruses, and ticks to mosquito-borne viruses, but there may be exceptions in some conditions (WHO 1967).

Transmission by arthropods involves several processes:

1. Ingestion by the arthropods of virus in the blood (usually) or tissue fluids of the vertebrate hosts.

2. Penetration of the viruses into the tissue of the arthropods, in the gut wall, or elsewhere after passing through the gut wall ('gut barrier').

3. Multiplication of the viruses in the arthropod cells, including those of the salivary glands (WHO 1967).

Stage 2 and part of stage 3 represent the extrinsic incubation period of the disease.

The quantity of blood, and therefore the amount of virus ingested, seems to be important; each arthropod species must ingest a minimum quantity of a given virus before multiplication can take place. The same mosquito species can have two different thresholds for two different viruses, and if one species has a low threshold, other species may have high thresholds or be completely resistant. This threshold phenomenon is extremely important in determining the efficiency of a vector, and may also vitally affect the course of an epidemic.

The viruses persist in Ixodid ticks for months or years, and in mosquitoes for practically their whole lives, though there may be a gradual decrease of concentration of the virus with time. Viruses have been reported to persist in overwintering mosquitoes, and this could be important, for instance in *C. tritaeniorhynchus* infected with JE, and *C. tarsalis* infected with WEE (infective by bite up to 8 months).

Trans-stadial persistence of virus is normal in ticks, and transovarial passage has been observed in some species; both are of great epidemiological importance. There is no evidence that these phenomena can occur in mosquitoes. Arthropods do not appear to be harmed by these infections.

Factors in transmission by arthropods

Important factors in transmission by arthropods are:

1. Susceptibility of the arthropods to infection, and ability to transmit it. There is wide variation in this.

2. Breeding habits of the arthropods, and preferred habitats, whether near man and other hosts of the virus.

3. Biting habits of the arthropods; in mosquitoes whether they are anthropophilic or zoophilic, exophilic or endophilic.

4. Longevity of the arthropods, which depends to a great extent on temperature, humidity and (especially in ticks) on the availability of hosts to feed on.

Overwintering mosquitoes can carry virus from one year to the next—*C. tarsalis* can carry WEE for 8 months.

5. Abundance of the arthropods; for mosquitoes the availability of suitable breeding places (and therefore the rainfall) is a major factor. An efficient vector may have a wide range of animals on which to feed, but if the arthropod species is abundant, and even if it bites man only infrequently in the presence of other (and preferred) animals, the large numbers enable it to maintain transmission to man. For instance, *C. tritaeniorhynchus*, which mostly bites birds, Bovidae, dogs

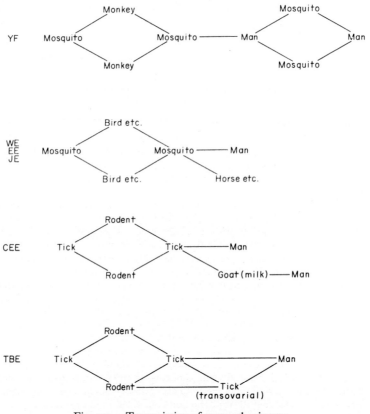

Fig. 119.—Transmission of some arboviruses.

and especially porcines, and only to a limited extent man, can maintain transmission of JE from pigs to man by sheer numbers. *C. tarsalis* feeds indiscriminately on mammals in summer, when WEE and SLE tend to occur in man and horses, but at other times it feeds on birds, which carry the virus.

6. Migratory birds can help by spreading virus which is circulating in their blood, or by carrying infected ticks.

7. Ecological systems are of primary importance in transmission, and biocenosis determines the formation of natural foci of infection. A case in point is the circulation of yellow fever virus among forest monkeys and tree-living mosquitoes, occasionally reaching mosquitoes haunting banana plantations

raided by the monkeys, and thence reaching man and perhaps spreading from man to man by peridomestic mosquitoes. Similarly, man becomes infected with KFD when he enters the domain of infected monkeys and picks up infected ticks. Other mosquito-borne and tick-borne infections are variations on the same theme.

The mosquito-borne and tick-borne infections differ in that ticks attach themselves to vertebrates for relatively long periods, and can therefore overlap a viraemic phase. In the case of KFD the populations of ticks are maintained at high levels by domestic cattle, on which they feed, and the cattle are close enough to the sources of viraemia (monkeys, and possibly birds and small rodents) to maintain enough ticks to carry on the cycle in animals. Man is an intruder, and though he becomes infected, he is not a link in the chain. The subject is discussed in more detail in the section on KFD, below.

Transmission may be represented diagrammatically, as in Fig. 119.

Other factors in transmission

Although transmission of arboviruses usually takes place through the bites of arthropods, it is important to remember that some of the viruses can, exceptionally, be transmitted in other ways. European tick-borne encephalitis can be acquired by drinking the milk of infected goats, Junin virus through contact with excreta of infected rodents, VEE (in cotton rats) apparently via urine or faeces infecting the nasopharynx, WEE possibly through aerosol from a patient and EEE (in pheasants) by one bird pecking another. Laboratory infections have been reported with Kunjin virus in Australia, and others. Korean HF can be transmitted by aerosol from infected rodents.

Many human activities encourage transmission of these animal viruses to man. Irrigation often promotes the breeding of enormous numbers of mosquitoes. For instance, the development of rice fields encourages *C. tritaeniorhynchus* in Sarawak, spreading JE, and *Mansonia uniformis* and *Anopheles gambiae* in Kenya, spreading chikungunya, ONN, possibly WN and Sindbis, and malaria. The seasonal cutting of old vegetation in Sarawak produces heavily polluted pools, which support massive populations of culicines. The keeping of cattle, driven into marginal forest areas in India, promotes the growth and transport of ticks, and the intrusion of man into forest areas lays him open to infection with yellow fever and the tick-borne diseases.

For a fuller discussion of these points the paper on epidemiology by Smith *et al.* (1970) should be consulted.

PATHOLOGY

The pathology of arbovirus diseases is described from the fatal cases of the haemorrhagic and encephalitic forms. The pathology of yellow fever is described separately in the section on that disease (page 376).

Haemorrhagic fevers

The viruses have special affinity for the endothelium of capillaries and small vessels, which are severely affected, resulting in increased permeability. This may be the result of antigen–antibody complexes formed in the blood stream and deposited in the vessel walls, where they are thought to release mediating substances, with damage to the capillaries. These lesions involve the autonomic nervous system, the internal organs and the blood.

The vascular abnormalities lead to capillary fragility (positive tourniquet test), bleeding from mucous membranes and even cerebral haemorrhages. If they are widespread there may be extravasation through capillary walls, producing hyperconcentration of the blood, hypovolaemia (placing strain on the heart), hypoxia of the tissues, acidosis and hyperkalaemia. Vomiting may induce dehydration. This combination may lead to shock, which can rapidly become irreversible unless treated very early. The syndrome is not peculiar to haemorrhagic arbovirus diseases, but is general to other forms of shock.

In haemorrhagic fevers in Thai children, post mortem findings have shown interstitial pneumonitis and scattered haemorrhages on the pleurae. There was slight enlargement of the liver with diffuse fatty degeneration of the liver cells and foci of lymphocytes. The spleen was slightly enlarged, with granulomatous lesions in the Malpighian bodies, and mesenteric lymph nodes were enlarged. Focal haemorrhages in the heart and patchy myocardial degeneration were also seen.

In fatal dengue haemorrhagic fever in the Far East the lesions found at autopsy were not pathognomonic. There were haemorrhages in various organs, evidence of reticulo-endothelial cell reaction (proliferation of lymphocytes and plasmacytoid cells and increase in phagocytosis), arrest of maturation of megakaryocytes or hypocellularity of bone marrow often followed by hyperplasia and early degenerative or infiltrative changes in the liver (focal hyaline or acidophilic necrosis of parenchymal and Kupffer cells and infiltration of portal areas of sinusoids by lymphoid cells, or paracentral necrosis of liver cells without inflammatory reaction). Capillary damage resulted in leakage of fluid, plasma and erythrocytes into interstitial spaces or into serous cavities.

Infection by a dengue virus may sensitize the tissues so that subsequent infection with a related virus may lead to a hypersensitivity reaction.

Serious renal lesions in haemorrhagic dengue are rare, but have been reported in Korea. Pituitary lesions have not been reported, but changes consistent with depletion of adrenal cortical cells are common, though adrenal haemorrhage is rare. Haemorrhage is not a common cause of death, but can be fatal if it is intracerebral or massively gastro-intestinal. Indeed, in most Thai patients no pathological abnormalities have been found which could be sufficient to account for death (WHO 1967).

Epidemic HF (Korean HF, haemorrhagic nephroso-nephritis, HF with renal syndrome) is often accompanied by shock, and is often fatal. There are marked haemorrhagic manifestations, including gross haematuria, pituitary lesions, thrombocytopenia and marked proteinuria. This disease is readily transmitted by the urine of infected animals (WHO 1967); the virus may not be a true arbovirus.

The haemorrhagic arbovirus diseases are probably expressions of acute disseminated intravascular coagulation, consequent on the vascular lesions, and treatment with heparin has tentatively been tried, apparently with some success (McKay & Margaretten 1967).

Encephalitis

In fatal cases the findings are those of meningo-myelo-encephalitis, with widespread cortical damage, degeneration of ganglion cells, focal perivascular lymphocytic infiltration, destruction of the Purkinje cells of the cerebellum and changes in the cord almost identical with those of poliomyelitis. The brain is hyperaemic and shows small haemorrhages; the general histological picture is typical of virus encephalitis in general.

IMMUNOLOGY

After a vertebrate has been infected by an arbovirus, the virus probably multiplies first in the regional lymph glands, where the earliest formation of antibodies also probably takes place. The antibodies are haemagglutination inhibiting (HI), complement fixing (CF) and neutralizing (N). In general HI antibodies appear early and may be long-lasting; CF antibodies appear later and may last 2–5 years; and N antibodies appear early and are long-lasting. But there are differences; some arboviruses do not produce high titres of antibodies in man, and some antibodies are short-lived or appear late.

Of these antibodies, HI and CF are important in diagnosis, but the only protective antibody is N, which is also the most specific antibody.

Arboviruses are grouped according to antigenic characters, but after inoculation of one virus into a fresh animal, not only the homologous antibodies, but also heterologous antibodies reacting with other viruses of the same group tend to appear. Recovery from an infection by a member of one group of arboviruses may provide some degree of resistance to a subsequent infection by another member of the same group; for instance, infection with West Nile virus may have modified the Ethiopian epidemic of yellow fever in 1962 (Pinto 1967). Again, the effect of prior infection with Zika, Uganda S and other related viruses in the forest belt of Nigeria, leading to a high incidence of related antibodies, is suggested as the explanation of the absence of epidemic yellow fever in man in that area. These related infections probably modify the disease rather than prevent infection (Macnamara *et al.* 1959).

Active immunity

A person who recovers from an attack of yellow fever possesses a solid immunity against reinfection. Neutralizing antibodies can be found as early as a few days after the beginning of the disease, and are found constantly for many years in the sera of such persons. This persistence of immunity does not depend upon exogenous reinfection, and the mechanism by which the antibodies are produced is not clear. Boyd (1961) comments that a mosquito infected with yellow fever is not harmed by it, but continues to excrete the virus throughout life. This means a continuous release of virus, probably from epithelial cells of the salivary glands. The virus enters man (or other animals) and gains the liver and other epithelium, provoking the early antibodies in the blood, which neutralize circulating viruses. But antibodies which can be detected for so many years in man must stem from a continuing stimulus, and the sensitive cells and their progeny probably have a prophage equivalent of the virus incorporated into their genetic structure, with occasional reversion to productive development which provides the stimulus for further antibody formation. The solid and fundamental immunity probably lies at the genetic level. A degree of immunity of this kind may possibly be provided when a related virus invades epithelial cells.

Epidemics of MV, JE and WN are not reported in the endemic areas of dengue, possibly because of cross-protection. There seems to be an analogy with the protective effect in schistosomiasis of infection with heterologous schistosomes.

The immunology of arbovirus infections is in line with the immunological principles of virus infections in general.

Passive immunity

Infant rhesus monkeys and human infants born of mothers immune to yellow fever have protective antibodies in their sera at birth, which persist for several months. These immune bodies are probably transmitted via the placenta rather than in the mothers' milk, because antibodies may disappear from infant sera while they are still suckling. This passive immunity is transient. Passive immunity induced by injection of homologous immune serum, however, has been used for protection against TBE in circumstances of special risk, and similar sera could be used against other infections, particularly after laboratory accidents.

CLINICAL FEATURES

After the virus enters the body it reaches the lymphatic system, where it multiplies and from which it is released into the blood (viraemic phase), and thence to the organs affected.

Basic clinical manifestations

Most arbovirus infections are inapparent (producing no symptoms), or mild (producing some fever and occasionally a rash), diagnosable retrospectively by serological methods. For instance, in an epidemic of Japanese encephalitis it was estimated that for each case of apparent disease there were 500–1000 inapparent infections. The proportions no doubt vary with circumstances.

If clinical manifestations arise after infection they do so after an intrinsic incubation period, usually lasting for a few days to a week or more. There is a general pattern of biphasic illness, with a systemic and a central nervous system phase, either of which may predominate. The first phase is associated with viraemia and ends when antibodies appear in the blood.

The onset of clinical manifestations is nearly always abrupt, generally occurring after the onset of viraemia. *Fever* is usual, and is sometimes the only sign. In many cases the clinical manifestations last only while the virus is disseminated, recovery following without sequelae, but in other cases there is *remission*, short or long. If long, the disease is biphasic. After this *fever returns* with signs indicating localization of the virus in certain organs: albuminuria, jaundice, meningeal signs, encephalitis and myelitis. If the period of viraemia has been without symptoms, and the virus becomes localized in the central nervous system, encephalitis appears late and may seem to be primary. In haemorrhagic cases there is a special risk of shock, which can rapidly become irreversible unless treated promptly.

All degrees of involvement may be observed in a single epidemic, but some arboviruses cause generally mild disease, others tend to severity.

The syndromes may be grouped as follows:

1. Systemic febrile diseases.
2. Haemorrhagic fevers (HF) including yellow fever (YF).
3. Encephalitides.

1. Systemic febrile diseases

This is the largest group, and the mild forms of all arbovirus diseases are of this kind. The course may be biphasic, and the infection may go on to the more serious haemorrhagic or encephalitic forms.

In addition to fever, which may suggest influenza, the following symptoms may occur:

1. *Anorexia*, with nausea and vomiting (phlebotomus fevers), or respiratory symptoms may predominate (Tahyna).
2. A *rash*, erythematous or itchy maculo-papular, with congestion of the face and neck (phlebotomus), inflammation of the palate, vesicles on the feet (Sindbis), or even petechiae or more extensive haemorrhages.
3. *Conjunctivitis*, with photophobia and orbital pain (phlebotomus) or even central retinitis and chorioretinitis (Rift Valley).
4. *Epidemic polyarthritis* (Ross River in Australia).
5. *Arthralgia* (o'nyong-nyong, chikungunya) or myalgia (especially in dengue), which can be responsible for excruciating pain, sometimes so severe as to render the patient incapable of movement ('break-bone fever'); lumbar pain is also common (phlebotomus).
6. *Inflammation* and enlargement of the lymphatic glands (o'nyong-nyong, chikungunya, West Nile).
7. *Leucopenia*, which is common, and thrombocytopenia (Colorado).

Sindbis (in South Africa) produces fever, rash and, in severe cases, vesicles on the feet, from the fluid of which the virus has been recovered. It is transmitted by *Culex univittatus* in South Africa.

O'nyong-nyong is transmitted by *Anopheles gambiae* and *A. funestus*. It causes fast-spreading epidemics, with sudden onset, and a benign, dengue-like disease with marked arthralgia, an itchy skin rash, low fever, inflammation of the palate, lymphadenitis and conjunctivitis.

Chikungunya (transmitted by *Aedes aegypti* or possibly *Ae. taylori* and *Ae. furcifer*) is usually also mild, producing pronounced cervical and inguinal adenitis, and an irritating maculo-papular rash after the febrile phase; but it can be severe. In an epidemic in South India, where subclinical infections were rare, an outstanding symptom was arthralgia. It has been associtaed with dengue haemorrhagic fever. In Thailand it was a febrile illness with minor haemorrhagic manifestations, without shock, and did not threaten life. Chikungunya has a forest cycle involving monkeys (vervet monkeys, baboons) and other mammals, with transmission by *Aedes luteocephalus*, and an urban cycle in man with transmission by *Ae. aegypti*. Ross River virus produces similar outbreaks in Australia.

In the diseases marked by arthralgia there may be relapses of the arthralgia without fever.

Dengue is transmitted by *Aedes aegypti*, *Ae. albopictus* and experimentally by members of the *Ae. scutellaris* group. It is endemic in South-east Asia, the Pacific area, Africa and the Americas, where there have been large and explosive outbreaks, as in Puerto Rico. It is biphasic and usually mild, but may be more severe, myalgia appearing early ('break-bone fever'). There is an early erythematous rash, and after a few days an eruption resembling that of measles or scarlet fever may appear, beginning on the extremities and accompanied by generalized lymphadenopathy. The liver is moderately enlarged. The second phase usually lasts 2–3 days, and convalescence is long and distressing. In some outbreaks dengue goes on to a severe haemorrhagic form with shock, which can be fatal (for a fuller description of dengue haemorrhagic fever see page 373).

Antibodies have been found in monkeys in South-east Asia, but their significance is doubtful.

Chandipura virus has been isolated from 2 patients in India suffering from a dengue-like illness, and antibodies have been found in horses, camels, cattle and monkeys.

West Nile (WN), present in the Near East and Africa, has now spread to man and horses (causing encephalitis) in southern France. The infection can closely resemble dengue, but inflammation of lymph nodes is often more marked, and there may be a meningeal syndrome and myocarditis. In old people encephalitis may occur and be fatal, but in children the infection may be inapparent. *Culex modestus*, *C. univittatus* and *C. antennatus* are vectors; pigeons and crows are hosts.

Tahyna (Lumbo) has been found, causing respiratory symptoms, in Czechoslovakia, and it has been isolated in southern France; antibodies have been found in Corsica.

Oropouche virus can cause epidemics, and has been isolated from patients with fever, and from one healthy person, in Brazil. Neutralizing (N) antibodies have been found in monkeys.

Bwamba virus is transmitted by *Anopheles gambiae*. Rift Valley fever shows leucocytosis at first, with leucopenia during convalescence, and sometimes central retinitis or persistent chorioretinitis.

The sandfly fevers due to the Neapolitan and Sicilian viruses, spread by *Phlebotomus* species, are clinically alike. A very characteristic feature is congestion of the face and neck, resembling sunburn, which suggests 'sunstroke'. Relapses sometimes occur.

Colorado tick fever is usually mild and often biphasic, sometimes with a maculo-papular rash or petechiae, and sometimes causing haemorrhages or even encephalitis in children, who mostly recover without sequelae.

2. Haemorrhagic fevers

There are common features in this group. The first systemic phase is dominant, severe and often fatal. The incubation period may be short (3–6 days in YF though sometimes possibly more), 7–12 (Crimean HF, Junin), 3–25 (dengue HF) or 12–23 (HFRS).

The onset may be slow, with conjunctival injection, palpebral oedema and vesicles on the palate (Junin), or more usually it is brusque, with fever, pain in the lower back and limbs, headache and prostration. Gastro-intestinal disturbances are common, and there may be respiratory symptoms (dengue HF).

Bleeding is a feature, from gums, nose, gastro-intestinal tract, uterus, lungs and kidneys (with oliguria and anuria, later going on to polyuria (HFRS)). Bleeding may occur in the spleen, with splenomegaly, the liver, with hepatomegaly (dengue HF) and the pituitary or brain (HFRS, Machupo) with loss of equilibrium (Junin). There may be insterstitial pneumonitis (Machupo).

Haemorrhagic rashes are common, petechial or purpuric (Crimean HF). Leucopenia and thrombocytopenia are also common (Omsk, HFRS), and lymphadenopathy occurs.

Serious cases can go on to shock, in which the extremities are cold and clammy, the trunk warm and the face flushed, with peripheral vascular congestion; the patient is restless, sweating and often shows a petechial or maculo-papular rash. The blood pressure is low, or cannot even be determined, and the pulse pressure is below 20 mm Hg, the pulse being rapid and weak. ECG changes indicate myocardial damage (Junin). The liver may be enlarged, and SGOT values are often high. There is sometimes pleural effusion.

A positive tourniquet test, with thrombocytopenia and prolonged bleeding time and arrest of maturation of megakaryocytes, indicates a serious disturbance of the haemostatic mechanism.

Deepening shock and coma carry a grave prognosis, with a case mortality rate which may be as high as 50–60%: in lesser degrees of shock the rate may be 1–10% (Omsk), 2–15% (Crimean HF) or 20% (Junin).

The haemorrhagic fevers caused by arboviruses are due to viruses of several of the groups, most of which can also cause mild infections. Some are associated with conspicuous kidney or liver changes.

Devastating epidemics have occurred in the Far East and in South America. Some are mosquito-borne, some tick-borne; some may be connected with rodents through mites or by direct contact with rodent excreta.

The most important of these diseases are: *Group A*, chikungunya (often associated with dengue); *Group B*, yellow fever, dengue, Omsk HF, Kyasanur Forest disease (KFD); *Tacaribe Group*, Junin (Argentinian HF), Machupo (Bolivian HF); *Ungrouped*, HFRS (Korean HF, haemorrhagic nephroso-nephritis), Crimean HF. For convenience, and because of their importance, or because much work has been done on them, dengue HF, YF, and KFD are discussed in detail separately (pages 372–9).

Omsk HF and KFD, both transmitted by ticks, have similarities with each other. Omsk HF is found in steppe forest and KFD in or near Indian forest. HFRS occurs in river valleys inhabited by small rodents, and is probably transmitted by gamesoid ticks. Four types are described: typhoido-influenzal, gastro-intestinal, uraemic and meningo-encephalitic (Zdanov 1966). The virus has been isolated from the vole *Clethrionomys glareolus*, and is neutralized by convalescent serum. It can readily be transmitted by the urine of infected animals, and may not be a true arbovirus.

Crimean HF is found in steppe areas; hares are the suspected reservoir and *Amblyomma plumbeum* the suspected vector (Zdanov 1966).

Argentinian HF (Junin virus) and Bolivian HF (Machupo virus), with case mortality rates around 20%, are often severe, resembling HFRS (Korean HF, haemorrhagic nephroso-nephritis). Junin virus has been reported to have been isolated from mites, but evidence suggests transmission by other means than an arthropod, i.e. rodent urine.

The Machupo virus has been isolated from blood and spleen, and one patient was apparently infected by her husband. Rodents (*Calomys*) may be the reservoir; they increased greatly in San Joachim (Bolivia) where an outbreak took place. In this disease eosinophil inclusions are found in the Kupffer cells; and cells of the reticulo-endothelial system in the liver, spleen and lymph nodes proliferate widely. There is marked interstitial pneumonitis.

The haemorrhagic fevers of South-East Asia are essentially diseases of the indigenous children, mostly caused by the dengue viruses (all types, but especially types 1 and 2); the chikungunya virus (a Group A virus) has occasionally also been involved. Of 10 367 patients in Thailand (694 deaths), all except 24 were under 14 years old. Foreign residents of these areas are subject to dengue fever of the classical, milder type, but not, apparently, to this dangerous haemorrhagic form.

The reason for this distribution is not clear, but though sensitization by previous infection may be a factor, it is perhaps more likely that different strains of the viruses are involved, the highly pathogenic strains (perhaps mutants or perhaps introduced) are more likely to affect local children than the usually better protected expatriates (Hammon 1966).

3. The encephalitides

Almost all arboviruses are neurotropic in mice, and are therefore presumably able to cause encephalitis, though only a few are known to do so in man after natural infection. The most important of these viruses causing epidemics of encephalitis are: *Group A*, EEE, WEE, VEE; *Group B*, JE, MVE, SLE, RSSE; and at least one member of the *California (CE) Group*. West Nile virus can cause encephalitis or meningitis in old people.

Though these viruses are associated in general with encephalitis, most of them produce mild, undifferentiated febrile illnesses, with headache but no loss of consciousness, or non-bacterial (aseptic) meningitis, far more often than encephalitis. In one epidemic of JE the findings suggest up to 1000 infections for each case of encephalitis. On the other hand, in many areas of EEE activity very few persons show serological evidence of infection without encephalitis.

The encephalitides are biphasic illnesses, the encephalitis occurring as a second phase after the preliminary fever, and after the end of viraemia, when circulating antibody can be detected.

The general picture of encephalitis and encephalo-myelitis is broadly the same. There is acute fever with progressively severe headache, nausea and vomiting, stiff neck and back, dysarthria, tight hamstring muscles, going on in severe cases to nystagmus, stupor, coma, ataxia, paralyses (flaccid or spastic), localizing neurological changes, personality changes and possibly convulsions, especially in children. There are, however, many variations. The TBE of central Europe tends to have a longer febrile course. In Far Eastern TBE flaccid paralyses involving especially the shoulder girdle are more common; in JE and WEE paralyses are likely to be more spastic. Mental as well as motor sequelae may occur after any encephalitis in arbovirus disease, especially in children and old people.

EEE has been found in the United States, Central and South America and the Caribbean, mainly in freshwater swamp areas. It is carried by *Culiseta melanura* and *Aedes sollicitans*, and its natural hosts are wild and domestic birds, though it spills over to man and horses. Though inapparent infections occur, in general this illness is severe and sometimes fatal. In 1962 there was an epidemic of 6762 cases in Venezuela, 0·6% fatal.

WEE is found on the western side of North America. It is carried by *Culex tarsalis* and its hosts are wild and domestic birds, from which it is conveyed to man and horses. One big epidemic was related to extensive floods. It is less severe than EEE, involving chiefly infants and young children; inapparent infections are common. Sore throat may be common, and respiratory infections leading to haemorrhagic patches in the lungs (as seen at post mortem). The main symptoms of central nervous system involvement include somnolence, unconsciousness or convulsions. Gastro-intestinal or renal symptoms may be prominent.

VEE is found in South America, causing mainly a mild or inapparent infection in man, though this is not always the pattern—a few years ago it produced an epidemic of over 30 000 cases, with 200 deaths (and many cases in horses, often fatal). Most patients were children under 15, and most had an influenza-like disease; encephalitis occurred in only a few. In some cases the virus was isolated from throat swabs, suggesting air spread.

SLE, reported in 14 states of the U.S.A., has been responsible for many outbreaks, often urban, probably carried by *Culex tarsalis* and the *C. pipiens* complex (especially *quinquefasciatus*), though in Florida the main vector was

C. nigripalpus, and *Aedes crucians* was infected. The hosts are passerine birds, blue jays, pigeons, geese, mocking birds and possibly bats. Like other arbovirus infections it can be inapparent, or merely a mild fever, and the incidence has been calculated as 59 inapparent infections for each overt case; in Florida 53% of the Negro rural adults have shown HI antibodies. But SLE is severe in children and old people, and in those with diabetes, high blood pressure, tuberculosis, pre-existing brain damage and alcoholism. In these groups sequelae and mortality are high. In one series of 222 cases of overt disease in Florida (1962), 22% had fever and headache only, 12% had aseptic meningitis, 62% had encephalitis without paralysis, 4% had encephalitis with paralysis and 19% died. There may be confusion and tremor. The cerebrospinal fluid contains more cells than usual, chiefly mononuclears. Abnormalities of isolated cranial nerves, nystagmus and abnormal reflexes may be found, and there may be increased cells in urinary deposits not associated with bacterial infection.

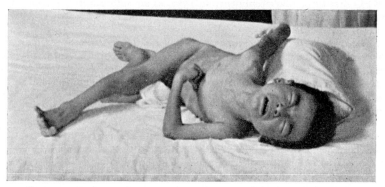

Fig. 120.—A 5-year-old male with Japanese encephalitis. Fortieth day of illness. (*W. Hammond*)

JE, which, like other virus infections, can be transmitted by blood taken for transfusion in the period of viraemia, is carried in East and South Asia by *C. tritaeniorhynchus* breeding in rice fields, and by *C. gelidus*. Like other arbovirus infections it can be inapparent, or can cause serious disease with a case mortality rate of 7%, or even, as in Taiwan in 1961, as high as 28% of the diagnosed cases. It mostly affects children under 5 (for instance in Singapore) and tends to leave many sequelae. The incubation period is 6–8 days and the onset may be acute or gradual, with high fever, rigidity and exaggerated reflexes, headache and dizziness, convulsions or even delusions and later coma. Meningeal symptoms may predominate (Fig. 120). JE is endemic in some tropical areas, but causes severe epidemics in sub-tropical and temperate regions, with peaks when the temperature is highest and humidity lowest (e.g. in July). Many vertebrates including pigs, a sparrow, herons, certain lizards and possibly bats, are infected, maintaining a continuous chain of infection.

RSSE is characterized by an incubation period of 10–14 days, and in severe cases by fever, flaccid paralysis of the peripheral type, the brachial plexus and muscles of the neck being sometimes permanently paralysed; bulbar disturbances are also seen. The mortality may reach 30% of recognized cases. The hosts are rodents and the vectors ticks (*Ixodes persulcatus*); a related virus (Langat) has been isolated from *Ixodes granulatus* from forest rats in Malaysia. In the U.S.S.R. RSSE occurs in thickly forested areas of the Far East.

European tick-borne encephalitis is less severe than RSSE, appearing as a biphasic meningo-encephalitis which, exceptionally, is fatal. The main vector is *Ixodes ricinus* but infection may follow the drinking of the milk of infected goats, which develop only unstable immunity and are liable to reinfection.

California encephalitis exists in a rodent–*Aedes* cycle, the rodents being squirrels (grey, red, fox and ground squirrels), and the mosquitoes *Aedes canadensis* and *Ae. triseriatus*. It is a disease of some considerable public health importance, as a rural forest infection of man, widely reported in North America. There are various antigenic types.

KYASANUR FOREST DISEASE (KFD)

Epizootiology and epidemiology

KFD first came into prominence in 1957, as an outbreak in man associated with a high mortality in forest monkeys, in the Sagar-Sorab area of Mysore State, India (Boshell 1969).

The vectors are ticks: *Haemaphysalis spinigera*, *H. turturis* and *H. papuana kinneari* in that order of importance; the virus has also been found in pools of certain other species of *Haemaphysalis*. It is also carried by *Ixodes petauristae* and *I. ceylonensis*, and has been recovered from *Dermacentor* nymphs. These ticks show fluctuations in numbers according to season, *Haemaphysalis* adults reaching a peak in the rainy months, and *Ixodes* having a phase fluctuation roughly alternating with that of *Haemaphysalis*.

Vertebrate hosts. Man is bitten by nymphs of *H. spinigera* and other ticks, which have been infected in the larval stage from some other animal. Man, however, is a dead end in this cycle, which is maintained in nature by other hosts, the virus probably circulating in ticks and rodents. Monkeys spend enough time at ground level in forest to collect tick larvae in numbers adequate to ensure the survival of nymphs in sufficient numbers. The larvae fall from the monkeys when they are resting on the ground, and then the larvae burrow, later emerging as nymphs. But monkeys have a high death rate from KFD, and survivors show high immunity. It seems, therefore, that the monkey population is not adequate to support the circulation of the virus.

Cattle, though showing a low degree of susceptibility to KFD, are important in that they ensure the propagation of *H. spinigera* and other ticks by harbouring the adults, and cattle are kept by man in contact with forest. They therefore constitute a man-made factor in the epizootiology of the disease.

Small mammals (rats, squirrels, mice and shrews) are relatively inefficient carriers of the virus, and do not carry the same load of ticks as monkeys and birds, but the virus has been isolated from the spleens of small mammals caught at all seasons, including the forest shrew *Suncus murinus*. In this the virus circulates in relatively high concentrations for many days, and the rate of reproduction of the shrew is high, indicating a rapid turn-over of the population.

A high proportion of birds captured in the area have antibodies to KFD, and are infested by ticks; experimentally the virus can multiply in these birds, and young chicks can be infected by tick bite. Birds have therefore been suspected of taking some part in maintaining the disease, but it is not clear.

Amplifying mechanism. The rate of tick infestation of man in contact with forest is low, and only a high rate of infection in the vectors could offset this. To raise a latent zoonosis to epizootic proportions it is necessary to increase the numbers and density of the vectors, and this is done by domestic cattle. The abundant larvae must also find an efficient source of infection, and in KFD the monkeys meet this requirement, having the virus in high titre, with a high rate of infestation by larvae, and moving about the forest freely enough to form foci of infected nymphs. The squirrels, rats, mice, shrews and birds are less effective (Boshell 1969).

Man has favoured the spread of KFD, partly by steadily expanding rice cultivation at the expense of forest, and by extending the timber industry. These changes have created thousands of miles of interface between forest and cultivated land, and both vectors and hosts are activated by such changes. In particular, this interface is colonized by lantana thicket, a dense bush some 9–15 feet high, in which many species of birds nest, and which is crossed by innumerable runways of ground birds and small mammals, and narrow trails and tunnels used by cattle, deer and even elephants. The whole subject is discussed by Boshell (1969).

Clinical findings

KFD can be a severely prostrating disease. The incubation period is 3–9 days, and the onset is sudden, with fever and headache, followed by severe pain in the back and limbs, and marked prostration. The conjunctivae are inflamed and there is often a papular or vesicular eruption on the palate. Other features are bradycardia and hypotension, diarrhoea, vomiting and bleeding from gums, mouth, nose, stomach or intestine. There is marked leucopenia, and casts are commonly found in the urine. If a second phase occurs there may be encephalitic changes.

Pyrexia lasts 5–10 days, and patients who recover remain asthenic for a long time.

In fatal cases there is focal necrosis of the liver, with parenchymatous degeneration. The kidneys show acute degeneration of the proximal and collecting tubules. The case mortality rate is about 5% with modern treatment; formerly it was considerably higher.

DENGUE HAEMORRHAGIC FEVER

Apart from yellow fever, this disease has caused more deaths in recent years than any other arbovirus disease. It is particularly associated with urban conditions and abundant *Aedes aegypti*, breeding in domestic water-containers. Foreign residents living in good conditions in Bangkok, with piped water, tend

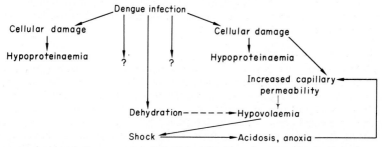

Fig. 121.—The evolution of the shock syndrome in dengue haemorrhagic fever. (*After Balankura et al. 1966*)

to escape. An outbreak started in Manila in 1953, invading Thailand (where there were 150 000–200 000 cases) and South Vietnam (1963). It has been complicated by a large number of infections with the chikungunya virus, transmitted by the same mosquito, *Ae. aegypti*. Chikungunya virus can cause a haemorrhagic fever, but without shock.

The evolution of the shock syndrome has been suggested to be that shown in Fig. 121. The mechanisms leading to cellular damage are not known, but it seems certain that dengue can initiate the cycle. When the circulating blood volume is reduced to a critical low level, shock with acidosis and cellular anoxia occurs. Acidosis and anoxia produce more cellular damage, which tends to make the shock more severe—a vicious circle. The final, irreversible step, which occurs in fatal cases, is rapidly developing, severe hyperkalaemia.

In dengue haemorrhagic fever the responses to HI and CF tests are rapid and broadly reactive within Group B, suggesting that dengue may have been superimposed on a previous infection with a Group B virus.

YELLOW FEVER

Geographical distribution

West Africa was probably the original home of yellow fever, and it may have been transported to the Americas by ships carrying infected mosquitoes. In the Americas it has been reported from as far north as Baltimore and Philadelphia in the United States, to as far south as southern Brazil and northern Argentina. In Africa it has been reported throughout the tropical area and as far south as Rhodesia. Enormous epidemics occurred in the Nuba mountains of the southern Sudan in 1940 (with about 17 000 cases and a fatality rate of some 10%) and in south-western Ethiopia along the river Omo in 1960–62, with not less than 15 000 (possibly 30 000) deaths, the apparent fatality rate as high as 85% in some areas. All age-groups were affected. The fatality rate can be calculated only on diagnosed cases, but, as with other arbovirus diseases, it is highly probable that there were also many mild or inapparent cases which were not recognized. *Aedes simpsoni* was firmly incriminated as the vector to man in Ethiopia, but *Ae. africanus* and *Ae. dentatus* were also found infected. Virus was also isolated from the monkey *Colobus abyssinicus*. An epidemic in 1965–6 in Senegal mainly affected children under 10 years old, with a case mortality rate of about 15%. Mass vaccination had been suspended since 1960.

Yellow fever has been brought by ship to Europe, but has never established itself there, because the relevant mosquitoes do not exist there. It has never been reported from Asia or Australasia, though potential vectors (especially *Ae. aegypti* in South-east Asia) abound. If it should be introduced into Asia the result could be catastrophic, and for this reason the strictest controls of immigrants and aircraft are in force.

Epizootiology and epidemiology

After the discovery that yellow fever is transmitted by *Ae. aegypti* it was thought that this was the only mosquito involved, and that the cycle was exclusively man–*Ae. aegypti*–man. In 1910, however, Manson, discussing a paper by Boyce on the history of yellow fever, suggested that the virus (he used this term in a general sense) could be inoculated into lower animals if they were bitten by the mosquito, and from them, perhaps to man in an attenuated form. This was pure speculation, but was near the truth. Then in 1914 Balfour recorded the common belief in Trinidad that yellow fever could be predicted if dead and dying red howler monkeys were found in the forests, and he suggested that in West Africa the blood of monkeys should be examined.

Since then there has been abundant evidence that yellow fever is enzootic in the forest monkeys of Central and South America and Africa, that it is transmitted among them by mosquitoes which haunt the forest canopy in which the monkeys live, and that epizootics occasionally sweep through the monkey communities, the most notable being the great wave which swept northwards from Panama, at a rate of about 13 miles a month, reaching Guatemala in October 1955, where it seems to have exterminated the forest primates. The monkeys involved in the Americas were *Cebus* (capuchin monkeys), *Ateles* (spider monkeys) and *Alouatta* (howler monkeys), *Cebus* surviving in Honduras and possibly acting as an important reservoir. Other American animals which have proved susceptible to the virus by experimental mosquito bite or injection of crushed infected mosquito tissues, or infected blood, either intracerebrally or extracerebrally, include: *Saimiri* (squirrel monkey), *Lagothrix* (woolly monkey), *Hapale* (*Callithrix*; marmoset), bats, coatis, wild cats, agoutis, armadillos and opossums.

Susceptible African animals include *Pan* (chimpanzee), *Cercopithecus* (grivet, tantalus, diana, patas, mona monkeys), *Cercocebus* (mangabey), *Colobus*, *Papio* (baboon), *Galago* (bush baby) and *Erinaceus* (hedgehog).

Asian monkeys are very susceptible: *Macaca* (rhesus, bonnet, kra monkeys) (Corson 1945).

Transmission

In nature, yellow fever is transmitted by mosquitoes of several genera.

In the Americas, apart from *Aedes aegypti* which has been responsible for many urban outbreaks, the mosquitoes chiefly involved are *Haemagogus capricorni*, *H. spegazzinii falco*, *H. mesodentatus*, *H. equinus*, *Ae. leucocelaenus* and *Sabethes chloropterus*. Virus has also been isolated from *Ae. fulvus* in Brazil.

In Africa the mosquitoes chiefly involved are *Ae. aegypti* (for instance in Senegal 1965–6), *Ae. africanus*, which maintains the monkey–mosquito–monkey cycle in the forests, and *Ae. simpsoni* which breeds closer to man (for instance in axils of plants in Ethiopia) and becomes infected when monkeys raid banana plantations, which the mosquito haunts, passing on the infection to man.

The question of the maintenance of the forest cycle is not regarded as completely settled, since in East Africa some species of bush baby (*Galago*) have been found susceptible to the virus, and have also been found to have yellow fever antibodies, as shown by the mouse protection test. This has led to the suggestion that the virus may circulate in these nocturnal animals, probably not transmitted by mosquitoes but by other ectoparasites, and may be passed on in some way not clearly understood, to other susceptible primates, and thence, sporadically, to man (Haddow & Ellice 1964).

Yellow fever not only involves forest animals and their vector mosquitoes (or other ectoparasites), but is profoundly affected by the ecological conditions which man creates for himself. In forest areas sporadic human cases may occur, and at the forest edges sporadic cases may give rise to small outbreaks, but in towns and cities, wherever the domestic *Ae. aegypti* proliferates, sporadic yellow fever can be converted into epidemic yellow fever. In survivors of such epidemics, who have had only mild attacks, the rate of residual immunity is high, and even if the virus is introduced again it is not likely to spread widely for some years until a new generation of non-immunes has grown up. Where man is constantly in contact with virus-carrying mosquitoes, for instance near forests, infection is common in childhood, and may be slight, leading nevertheless to solid immunity, and epidemics do not occur. But in populations in which contact with the virus rarely occurs, whether in urban or rural surroundings, introduction of the virus can produce violent epidemics, as in the Sudan and Ethiopia. In the tropical rain forest area of West Africa, yellow fever is rarely recognized in the indigenous people, but antibody surveys show a steady increase in immunity with age, until in adolescence most people are immune.

Pathology

The virus affects highly specialized epithelial or myocardial cells only; stroma cells are not involved. The changes are toxic, beginning with cloudy swelling and going on to degenerative fatty changes and coagulative necrosis. There is no inflammatory response.

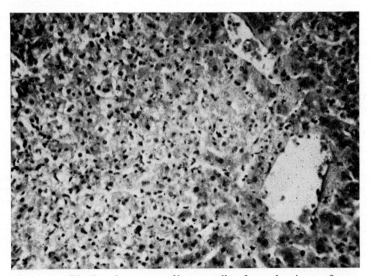

Fig. 122.—The liver from a case of human yellow fever, showing confluent mid-zonal necrosis. The degree of destruction near the centrilobular vein is characteristic of yellow fever. (*Dr G. Beanscroft*)

The liver. Typical lesions may not be found in biopsy specimens from patients who later recover, and serological evidence is necessary for diagnosis in such cases. In fatal cases, however, the liver is not shrunken; it may be reddish yellow, and feels greasy. The typical lesions form a characteristic triad: microglobular fatty degeneration of epithelial liver cells throughout the hepatic lobule; dissociation of the hepatic lobule, most marked in the mid-zone (but some normal liver cells always remain around the central zone); and coagulative necrosis of the epithelial liver cells mainly affecting the mid-zone. The nuclei of the liver cells are pyknotic and the coagulated contents of the cells stain deeply with eosin, the Councilman bodies resulting from this degeneration taking on a salmon-pink colour. Under low power a stained section looks as if red pepper has been scattered on it (Fig. 122).

Other organs. The lesions are variable—some degree of nephritis or nephrosis (with transient proteinuria in mild cases), adrenal lesions, lesions of the heart (fatty changes, even in the sino-auricular node and the bundle of His, corresponding with the clinical bradycardia), and lesions of the brain (perivascular haemorrhages). In the kidneys there are fatty changes with necrosis of tubular epithelium, and casts in both cortex and medulla. Encephalitis was not formerly thought to be part of the picture of naturally occurring yellow fever, but meningo-encephalitis was a dominant feature of the epidemic of 1959 in the Sudan and Ethiopia. Severe haemorrhages may take place in the digestive system, the internal cavities, the lungs (common), liver, spleen and kidneys. Death results from failure of the liver or kidneys or both, though cardiac damage may contribute. Patients who recover show complete replacement of lost tissue by direct regeneration and hypertrophy of surviving cells.

Clinical findings

As in many other virus infections, there are many inapparent infections, leading to immunity without a phase of overt illness.

In most overt cases the disease is of the undifferentiated fever type, without haemorrhage, jaundice, significant albuminuria or signs of involvement of the central nervous system. In populations constantly exposed from infancy to infection, for instance in those who live in the rain forest area of Africa, the infection is likely to be inapparent, or so mild that the diagnosis cannot be made except retrospectively by serological tests. The virus, however, is highly pantropic and in severe cases haemorrhagic manifestations are often more prominent than the jaundice from which it gets its name. A well known adage is that ' everything is congested at the outset, everything bleeds at the end '.

In all clinically recognizable forms the onset is sudden, with fever up to 39·4–40°C, tending to fall during the next few days. If severe, this is accompanied by an initial chill or rigor, headache (a prominent feature), nausea and vomiting and pain in the abdomen, back, loins and even limbs, which can be very distressing. The patient is likely to be dehydrated, with a dry tongue and foul breath. There may be a yellow tint in the conjunctivae, which tends to deepen on subsequent days, when the skin also shows jaundice.

At first the pulse is full and strong at 100–120/minute, and the blood pressure is normal, but as the disease progresses the pulse becomes disproportionally weaker and slower than the temperature would suggest. This is the well known Faget's sign—a falling pulse rate with a constant temperature, or a constant pulse rate with a rising temperature. The blood pressure may fall to seriously low figures. Anaemia is not a feature at first, but may develop later; leucopenia is common.

A short period of calm may follow the initial fever, and in mild cases recovery takes place. In severe cases, however, the patient's condition then rapidly deteriorates and a hepatorenal condition develops. The abdominal pain continues, and the patient vomits 'coffee-ground' or black ('black vomit') material, signifying altered blood, or even fresh blood. Some diarrhoea is common, and there may be blood in the stools. Bleeding may take place from eyes, nose, mouth, bladder, uterus and other organs. Jaundice becomes more evident, there is proteinuria with a tendency to suppression, and granular casts with spectroscopic evidence of haemoglobin can be found in the urine. Blood urea rises in the terminal stages. The state of shock is common, as in other haemorrhagic arbovirus diseases. Death may be due to haemorrhage, shock, uraemic coma or myocarditis, and in fulminating cases may take place as early as the third day.

Signs that the central nervous system is affected suggest meningitis or encephalitis, and include slurred speech, nystagmus, incoordination of movements, with tremor of the hands, and brisk tendon reflexes. There may be convulsions followed by sudden death. Overall case mortality in overt disease is usually 5–10%, but as in Ethiopia is sometimes much higher. If the patient recovers from a severe attack, convalescence tends to be long, but usually without sequelae.

Virus can be detected in the blood for up to 107 hours after the onset, possibly more.

Diagnosis

Post mortem diagnosis has been very useful in determining the extent of yellow fever in a community, and in South America was greatly helped by the use of the viscerotome, an instrument with which specimens of liver or other organs can be taken after death when full autopsy is not possible.

The severe form of leptospirosis, the true Weil's disease, can very easily be mistaken for yellow fever. Relapsing fever and acute infective hepatitis can also lead to confusion, even in histological diagnosis, as in the well known case of the missionary who died at Torit in the southern Sudan. A section from his liver was diagnosed as yellow fever, but Boyd (1965), who subsequently examined the section, concluded that the appearances were characteristic of infective hepatitis, with which he was very familiar. In the case described by Tulloch and Patel (1965) the first diagnosis was gastro-enteritis, and later infective hepatitis with liver failure; but after death, yellow fever virus was isolated from the patient's blood.

Although proteinuria is a feature of classical yellow fever, it is inconstant and transitory in mild cases, and its absence does not rule out the disease. Liver biopsy may also be unhelpful in mild cases, Councilman cells being rare. In such cases serological evidence is essential. Malaria and malnutrition can complicate the liver picture. In icteric cases the transaminase levels are high, up to 2766 SGOT and 660 SGPT units. Elevation in these indices precedes the onset of jaundice. In benign, anicteric, cases the levels are only slightly raised (SGOT 192, SGPT 117), but they support the diagnosis. These tests, however, do not differentiate between yellow fever and infectious hepatitis.

Isolation of the virus by inoculation of blood in the first few days into infant mice has already been discussed; the virus can be identified by the neutralization test.

Retrospective diagnosis is made by the mouse protection test. Equal parts of the serum to be tested, or the control serum, and a dilution of virus calculated to deliver 100 LD_{50} when combined with the serum, are mixed, incubated for a fixed period, and inoculated intracerebrally into mice of strains known to be susceptible to yellow fever virus. The intracerebral dose is 0·03 ml. Immune serum protects, whereas with non-immune control serum the mice die of yellow fever encephalitis in 4–10 days. The average survival time of mice given the virus with the serum is a more sensitive key to the detection of weakly positive sera than the survival ratio.

An intraperitoneal test in mice has been extensively used for serum surveys. An essential part of this test is the inoculation of sterile 2% starch solution into the brain to produce mild trauma which permits the virus to become localized there from the blood; this is done because, normally, intraperitoneal inoculation of the virus has little effect. This route permits the administration of a larger volume of serum and obviates the necessity for meticulous assay of the virus, which is essential in the intracerebral test (Strode 1951).

Treatment

There is no specific treatment, and patients with yellow fever should be dealt with like patients with other severe arbovirus diseases.

DIAGNOSIS OF ARBOVIRUS INFECTIONS

Virological diagnosis

Blood should be taken as soon as possible after the onset of the disease, part being reserved for isolation of the virus (only useful in the first few days), and part for serological tests. Suckling mice, hamsters, guinea-pigs and tissue-culture techniques are used for isolation of the virus.

If there are meningeal signs, the cerebrospinal fluid may be used for isolation, and is occasionally positive in tick-borne encephalitis, Colorado fever, Japanese encephalitis, WEE, SLE and yellow fever. Cells may be sedimented and examined by the fluorescent antibody technique.

After death, specimens of tissue should be taken as soon as possible, emulsified and quickly inoculated into suckling mice 1–3 days old, or adult mice, newborn hamsters, chick embryos or even guinea-pigs (Junin virus). The material to be inoculated is usually treated with antibiotics, and part is kept frozen for confirmation by re-isolation of the virus.

Serological diagnosis

After infection the virus probably first multiplies in the regional lymph glands, where the earliest antibody formation also probably starts. Serological diagnosis is based on the detection of agglutination inhibiting (HI), complement fixing (CF) and neutralizing (N) antibodies, and on the variations in titre found in paired sera at various stages. HI antibodies are cross-reactive within the arbovirus groups, and may need confirmation by tests for N antibodies. CF antibodies are separate and distinct from N antibodies. N antibodies are usually the most specific.

If the patient has been exposed to an arbovirus of the same group as the one responsible for his illness, serological diagnosis is difficult because group antibodies are at high titre—even to some extent the N antibodies.

The gel precipitin test has been used successfully with antigens produced in cell cultures, for tests on paired sera. It has also been used to differentiate various viruses, though consistently satisfactory antisera for this purpose may be difficult to obtain.

The fluorescent antibody test has been used as a reliable test for antigen in acute-phase blood clots in Colorado tick fever, and on post mortem material, for instance in JE.

Some of the reagents—antigens and immune fluids—used for tests are described in WHO (1967).

TREATMENT OF SEVERE ARBOVIRUS INFECTIONS

There is no specific treatment; nursing and general care are all-important. To avoid infecting local mosquitoes, patients with mosquito-borne infections should be nursed under a bed net during the period of viraemia. Blood should be examined for malaria and other parasites.

Restlessness may be treated with sedatives and headache with codeine sulphate. Glucose in doses of 4 grammes, or intravenously as a 5% solution (up to 300 ml), may help the liver condition. Phentolamine and cortisone have been used for shock in some arbovirus haemorrhagic fevers, and could possibly be useful in the shock of yellow fever. Intravenous hydrocortisone may give dramatic results in encephalitis.

In the intravascular clotting which occurs in the haemorrhagic fever of the Far East, treatment with heparin has apparently been beneficial (McKay & Margaretten 1967).

Treatment of shock (WHO 1966b)

Shock is a feature of many haemorrhagic fevers, and the following treatment has been used for haemorrhagic dengue, and may be appropriate for other diseases leading to shock. Treatment is supportive, and good nursing is essential. Oxygen is useful at first. Water balance must be maintained as at near normal as possible. To restore fluids and electrolytes, infusion of 5% dextrose in half-strength normal saline, at the rate of 100 ml/kg body weight daily is recommended. Or 10–15 ml of Ringer lactate solution/kg body weight (see below) may be infused intravenously for one hour, followed by a less concentrated electrolyte replacement fluid. Plasma or a substitute may be given to combat shock. Blood transfusion is not recommended in the hypotensive phase, but may be given after recovery from shock if the patient shows signs of having had severe haemorrhage.

Hypovolaemia is usual, and haematocrit values should therefore be watched; if they remain the same, or increase during replacement, indicating loss of fluid to extracellular spaces, plasma should be given to maintain an adequate circulating blood volume, at the rate of 10–20 ml/kg/hour until the haematocrit value begins to decline.

In the hypotensive phase, hydrocortisone 50–100 mg daily, or aldosterone 0·1 mg/kg daily, in conjunction with the infusion fluid, may reduce mortality and sometimes has a dramatic effect. (Aldosterone raises blood pressure, conserves sodium and causes potassium to be excreted in the urine; it is therefore a rational treatment. The dose quoted is high.)

During recovery, when vascular fluid returns to the circulation, infusion of fluid should cease.

Ringer lactate solution for intravenous infusion (*Todd 1967*). Dissolve 1·15 grammes of sodium hydroxide in 200 ml of sterile pyrogen-free water; add 2·4 ml lactic acid; autoclave for 1 hour; cool, cautiously adding about 1·0 ml dilute hydrochloric acid (274 grammes hydrochloric acid (w/w 35–38%) mixed with 726 grammes water; this contains 10% w/w pure HCl) until a few drops of the solution give a full orange colour with one drop of phenol red solution; mix with a solution containing 6·0 grammes NaCl, 400 mg KCl and 400 mg $CaCl_2 \cdot 6H_2O$ in 700 ml sterile pyrogen-free distilled water; adjust with sterile pyrogen-free distilled water to 1000 ml; filter; sterilize by autoclaving or bacteriological filtration. pH 5–7.

This solution contains approximately (in each litre):

> 131 mEq sodium ions
> 5 mEq potassium ions
> 4 mEq calcium ions
> 29 mEq bicarbonate ions as lactate
> 111 mEq chloride ions

Some children with metabolic acidosis do not easily metabolize lactate, and should therefore receive 1–2 ml/kg of 3·75% sodium bicarbonate solution intravenously every 10–15 minutes until improvement is noted (Balankura *et al.* 1966).

To control thrombocytopenic bleeding, transfusion of fresh human platelet concentrates is valuable. One unit of platelet concentrate is obtained from one pint of blood, and the dose used in Thai children ranged from 0·176 unit to 9·998 units/kg body weight.

CONTROL OF ARBOVIRUS INFECTIONS

Vector control

Vector control has been successful in some circumstances, for instance during the construction of the Panama Canal when by strict discipline all collections of water capable of breeding *Aedes aegypti* (and vectors of malaria) were eliminated from the area. Similar methods were applied to cities and towns in South America under the threat of yellow fever. When DDT was introduced, extensive use in British Guiana and elsewhere soon eradicated *Ae. aegypti* and with it the threat of urban yellow fever. In Africa, however, *Ae. aegypti* has recently shown resistance to dieldrin, and in some areas it is exophilic in habit, so that spraying dwellings with insecticide is not likely to affect it. Forest mosquitoes, of course, are not susceptible to ordinary methods of spraying. Tick control by residual insecticides has, however, achieved some success in U.S.S.R. But the problems of vector control, especially in rural areas, are formidable.

Immunization

Vaccines have been developed for yellow fever, and are highly effective, but for most other arbovirus diseases they are either experimental, or can be used only in restricted groups of people such as laboratory workers and in face of threat of outbreaks, or in reservoir animals (e.g. pigs for JE), or are not yet available. The multiplicity of the viruses creates a difficulty, which may to some extent be reduced by the development of group vaccines where these give some cross-protection. A review of the available vaccines for man and animals is given by Smith (1969).

Many vaccines have been developed for yellow fever since Hindle and Aragão independently first used emulsions of organs from infected animals for that purpose. Hindle used a phenol–glycerin emulsion, and later an emulsion treated with formalin after reduction of virulence by freezing.

Active immunity in yellow fever is now provoked by vaccines consisting of virus selected by serial intracerebral passage in mice. Early vaccines were given along with specific immune human serum with the intention of preventing severe reactions, but some batches of the immune serum were found to carry the virus of hepatitis, and to cause that disease in the recipients; the method was therefore discontinued.

A more successful vaccine was derived from a highly virulent strain of yellow fever virus isolated from an African named Asibi, in Ghana, and cultivated *in vitro* in mouse embryonic tissue. This procedure greatly reduced the viscerotropism of the strain without altering its neurotropism. The virus was then grown in tissue culture of minced chick embryos from which the central nervous system had been removed before mincing, and after prolonged propagation in this medium it was found that neurotropism and viscerotropism were both greatly reduced, but the virus retained its antigenic properties. This was the famous vaccine 17D, still widely used and highly effective, giving protection for up to 10 years, and only very rarely causing any untoward reaction. In 120 000 persons, mostly under 12 years old, vaccinated with 17D, only 2 developed meningo-encephalitis. Like smallpox vaccine, 17D is a live vaccine. It cannot be passed from person to person by mosquitoes.

The vaccine should be given at least 4 days before primary smallpox vaccination, but if smallpox vaccine is given first, YF vaccine should not be given until 21 days later. Infants should not be given YF vaccine before the age of 9 months (6 months in the United States) unless requested in writing by the parents. If an infant under 9 months is to be given both smallpox and YF vaccines, there should be an interval of 21 days between them, no matter which is done first (Cannon 1969).

The French Dakar vaccine is a neurotropic virus which can be administered alone or with smallpox vaccine by scarification. Of 1880 000 persons vaccinated with this, 246 developed meningo-encephalitis and 23 died.

These live vaccines all provoke active immunity, not so persistent as the immunity developed after natural infection, but nevertheless extremely effective for several years.

Immunization against yellow fever is required by law before travellers are allowed into certain countries, and it has even been suggested that every traveller should be immunized, wherever bound.

An attenuated strain of Langat E5 virus has 6 markers to differentiate it from the parent strains, and is stable in tissue culture. Injected into volunteers it produced homologous neutralizing antibodies, and heterologous neutralizing antibodies against Powassan, KFD, biphasic meningo-encephalitis and RSSE, without complications, persisting at high levels for at least 2 years. It has potential value as a live vaccine against these infections.

Apart from yellow fever, vaccines have been produced against several arbovirus diseases, for use in animals (for instance horses) as well as in man.

Attenuated strains of VE, Langat, West Nile and WEE viruses (some grown on chick embryo) have been developed. Strains of chikungunya, TBE, SLE, KFD, Rift Valley and Colorado tick fever have been inactivated, some by formalin, and tested experimentally. For TBE the early brain vaccines gave meningo-encephalitis, and were superseded by cell culture vaccines. Dengue and JE vaccines have also been devised. For various reasons these vaccines are not widely used (WHO 1966).

After vaccination against SLE, HI antibody appears in the first week, to a peak in the third week. CF antibody, which is more specific, appears in the second week to a peak in the second month. CF antibody was at a low titre at 18–22 months in one Florida outbreak, but neutralizing antibodies persisted; they tend to appear early.

Immunological phenomena may play a part in the pathogenesis of haemorrhagic fever and encephalitis, and this risk needs to be carefully considered in vaccinating against some arbovirus infections. Allergic encephalitis is one such risk.

REFERENCES

BALANKURA, M., VALYASEVI, A., KAMPART-SANYAKORN, C. & COHEN, S. (1966) *Bull. Wld Hlth Org.*, **35**, 51, 75.

BOSHELL, J. (1969) *Am. J. trop. Med. Hyg.*, **18**, 67.

BOYD, J. S. K. (1961) *12th Annual Conference of the Indian Association of Pathologists,* Souvenir 118.

——— (1965) *Trans. R. Soc. trop. Med. Hyg.*, **59**, 607.

CANNON, D. A. (1969) *Trans. R. Soc. trop. Med. Hyg.*, **63**, 867.

Catalogue of Arthropod Borne Viruses of the World (1967) United States Department of Health, Education & Welfare.

CORSON, J. F. (1945) *Trop. Dis. Bull.*, **42**, 597.

HADDOW, A. J. & ELLICE, J. M. (1964) *Trans. R. Soc. trop. Med. Hyg.*, **58**, 521.

HAMMON, W. M. (1966) *Bull. Wld Hlth Org.*, **35**, 55.

McKAY, D. G. & MARGARETTEN, W. (1967) *Archs intern. Med.*, **120**, 129.

MACNAMARA, F. N., HORN, D. W. & PORTERFIELD, J. S. (1959) *Trans. R. Soc. trop. Med. Hyg.*, **53**, 202.

PINTO, M. R. (1967) *Kongressbericht über die III Tagung der Deutschen Tropenmedizinischen Gesellschaft e.V. 1967, 20–22 April*, p. 153. Munich: Urban & Schwarzenberg.

SIMPSON, D. I. H. (1968) *Symp. zool. Soc. London*, **24**, 13.

SMITH, C. E. G. (1964) *Scient. Basis Med. Ann. Rev.*, 125.

—— (1968) *Abstr. Hyg.*, **43**, 1397.

—— (1969) *Br. med. Bull.*, **25**, 142.

—— HEATHECOAT, O. H. V., HILL, M. W., BENDELL, P. J. E., SIMPSON, D. I. H. & SURTEES, G. (1970) *Trans. R. Soc. trop. Med. Hyg.*, **64**, 481.

STRODE, G. K. (1951) *Yellow Fever*. New York: McGraw-Hill.

TODD, R. G. (1967) *Martindale's Extra Pharmacopoeia*, 25th Ed. London: The Pharmaceutical Press.

TULLOCH, J. A. & PATEL, K. M. (1965) *Trans. R. Soc. trop. Med. Hyg.*, **59**, 441.

WORLD HEALTH ORGANIZATION (1966a) *Wld Hlth Org. tech. Rep. Ser.*, 325.

—— (1966b) *Bull. Wld Hlth Org.*, **35**, 17, 74.

—— (1967) *Wld Hlth Org. tech. Rep. Ser.*, 369.

ZDANOV, V. M. (1966) *Bull. Wld Hlth Org.*, **35**, 87.

15. THE POCK DISEASES

SMALLPOX (VARIOLA MAJOR)

Geographical distribution

Smallpox rarely occurs in Europe, North America, Australasia and Oceania, though there have been small epidemics originating from people who arrive from endemic areas within the incubation period, or suffering from infectious smallpox modified clinically because of previous vaccination. It is still prevalent in most hot countries, especially India, Pakistan, Indonesia, West, East and Central Africa and South America. The case mortality rate appears to be higher in Asia than in most other regions.

Epidemiology

Smallpox is spread to contacts of infectious patients through droplet infection from respiratory discharges, through direct skin to skin contact, and through infectious clothing, bed clothes etc. used by patients. The virus can be disseminated by aerial convection currents within buildings (Editorial, *Br. med. J.*, 1970a). In the endemic areas it is associated with overcrowding, poverty and ignorance, but because a person may be infectious during the late incubation period, or because his disease is modified, people in all walks of life are at risk. In Europe, hospital staffs and laundry workers have been infected from such sources.

Aetiology

The cause of smallpox is the variola virus (*Poxvirus variolae*), a member of the group which includes vaccinia virus (*P. officinale*), cowpox virus (*P. bovis*) and other viruses affecting man and animals.

It is a small (200–300 nm) ovoid DNA virus, resistant to 20% ethyl ether, 50% glycerol and (moderately) to phenol, but is susceptible to oxidizing agents such as potassium permanganate. It is present in the epithelial cells of the skin and mucous membranes, and in exudates from these lesions, surviving in skin crusts for over one year at temperatures under 25°C, and for several weeks in fluid from vesicles or pustules dried on glass slides (Wilson & Miles 1964). Experience has shown that clothing from patients can infect their contacts, and people such as hospital staffs and laundry workers.

The virus is destroyed at 55°C for 30 minutes.

It can be grown on the chorio-allantoic membrane of chick embryos 10–12 days old, on which the pocks can be distinguished from those caused by vaccinia virus. It can also be grown in tissue culture of various human and animal cells, producing cytopathic effects which can be neutralized by specific antiserum.

The animals most susceptible to this virus are monkeys.

Pathology

The virus enters by the respiratory tract, invading and multiplying in the lymphatic nodes, and thence reaching the blood, from which it invades the reticulo-endothelial cells throughout the body. After multiplying in these cells it again enters the blood, to infect the skin and mucous membranes. It invades the epidermal cells, which increase in size and proliferate; papules, vesicles, pustules and scabs form, and virus is shed from the skin. Similarly, lesions form in the mouth and pharynx and break down and ulcerate earlier than those of the skin, releasing the virus, which can be found in saliva in the first few days, and which can therefore spread by droplet as well as by skin contact.

In the skin the cells of the papules degenerate and liquefy, forming the characteristic vesicles, in which the virus can be found. At first the vesicles are bacteriologically sterile, but become invaded by polymorphonuclear cells to form pustules. These become secondarily infected. Characteristically they are umbilicated, strands of tissue holding the centre skin while the fluid swells the periphery.

The liver and spleen are enlarged, and haemorrhages may occur in the lungs and other viscera; bronchopneumonia is common in fatal cases. Areas of necrosis may occur in the liver, testes and bone marrow, and a form of osteo-myelitis of the bones around the elbow, hands, wrists, ankles and femurs. This may affect about 5% of young children with smallpox. It starts in the metaphyses as a local osteoporosis which may go on to actual destruction of bone, spread to neighbouring joints (causing effusion), and displace the epiphyses, with per-manent damage. It can be detected by X-ray (Middlemiss 1964).

Immunology

One attack of smallpox protects for life. The probable course of events is that antibodies which are formed and passed into the blood can neutralize any subsequent smallpox virus gaining access from outside. The protective mechan-isms involved in recovery from a primary attack are not clearly known; they may depend upon interferon. Virus may spread from cell to cell without meeting the circulating antibodies, and may persist within cells, probably escaping into the lymphatic system from time to time. Here they stimulate the production of antibodies, boosting the immune response.

Passively transferred antibody can protect unvaccinated persons from small-pox, but experiments suggest that delayed hypersensitivity or some other aspect of tissue immunity may be as important as circulating antibody in immunity to smallpox (Kaplan 1969).

Clinical findings

Smallpox is a biphasic disease, with a first, toxaemic, phase which is a true virus illness lasting for up to a week, and a second phase in which the charac-teristic rash appears. The incubation period is 9–15 days (usually 12).

In the toxaemic phase there is often a fugitive prodromal erythematous rash on the trunk and limbs. This is occasionally haemorrhagic, with petechiae in the groins, on the trunk or limbs (especially in flexures), and may be associated with abortion, epistaxis or haemorrhage in the bowel, conjunctivae or elsewhere. In severe cases this rash tends to persist. The temperature rises on the first day and the patient is likely to be restless, even delirious.

In the second phase the temperature rises (after a remission) and the patient becomes very ill, with general malaise and backache. This phase corresponds to the appearance of the focal rash on about the third day. The rash is distributed first mainly on the forehead and wrists, extending rapidly but always affecting chiefly the parts of the body usually left uncovered, and those most exposed to pressure and friction. It is least profuse on the abdomen and in the groins, is more marked on the chest and back, even thicker on the arms and legs—especially the distal parts and the palms and soles (i.e. is centrifugal)—and most profuse on the face. It avoids depressions, flexures, axillae, groins and flanks, but the pocks are thick over prominent bones and tendons. The rash is symmetrical. It is at full density about the third day after its appearance, and the severity of the disease is indicated by the extent of the rash.

The rash is at first papular; the papules feel shotty when pinched between the finger and thumb. They become vesicles within a day or two and by this time the toxaemic phase has generally ended. The vesicles become surrounded by areolas of inflammation, and soon become umbilicated and loculated. Within 24 hours the vesicles become purulent, the pocks soften, their tops flat, and they lose the areolas. This suppuration is accompanied by secondary fever, and the patient may become delirious. The skin shows swelling and oedema between the pocks, and is itchy and tender. The vesicles, which are now full of pus, are no longer umbilicated or loculated; they may be confluent in severe cases. They begin to dry and scab about the ninth day.

The skin rash is accompanied by an outcrop on the mucous membranes of the mouth, nose, pharynx, and even the larynx, bronchi and oesophagus may be affected. The mouth and nose are sore, and swallowing is painful. The vulva, vagina and rectum may also be affected. In severe cases skin haemorrhages appear between the pocks, and bleeding occurs beneath the conjunctiva and from mucous membranes. In such cases the fever is high and the patients may pass into the typhoid state; prognosis is grave.

Complications include septic rashes, boils and corneal ulcers which can perforate and destroy the eye, or leave opacities which impair sight. Blindness in Malawi children is commonly due to smallpox or measles. Otitis media is common and so is bronchopneumonia. The face is permanently disfigured.

Diagnosis

In epidemics diagnosis is not difficult, but in sporadic cases the initial fever may be confused with that of influenza, meningitis or other infections, and with malaria. When the focal rash appears the differentiation from chickenpox is most important in view of the implications for spread. The points of difference are as follows:

Smallpox	*Chickenpox*
Most abundant on face and back, scanty on abdomen and chest	Abdomen, chest and back as thickly covered as face
Rash present on limbs, and is centrifugal	Rash tends to avoid limbs and is centripetal
Rash favours prominences and surfaces exposed to irritation	Rash behaves indifferently
Pocks deep seated, with infiltrated base, circular, homogeneous, multilocular and umbilicated. Secondary infection usual	Pocks superficial, base not infiltrated; often oval, not homogeneous, generally not loculated, never umbilicated. Secondary infection rare
Spots appear together, and are therefore at the same stage	Spots appear in crops and are at different stages

Laboratory diagnosis. This can be most important in distinguishing smallpox from other pock diseases. A smear taken from papules or from the bases of vesicles, on a grease-proof slide, can be stained to show smallpox or vaccinia virus particles which can be distinguished from chickenpox particles; they can also be identified by electron microscopy.

Material from lesions can be inoculated on to the chorio-allantoic membrane of developing chick embryos, and can be identified in this way, and also in tissue culture.

The virus can be isolated from blood in the early stages of the disease, though viraemia probably does not last long.

Serological tests to detect virus antigen include complement fixation, for which material from vesicles or pustules or crusts is used against a potent anti-vaccinial serum. The agar-gel precipitation and fluorescent antibody tests are also used.

For detection of antibody in the patient's serum the complement fixation, haemagglutinin inhibition and neutralization tests can be used—the last involves inoculating virus and serum on to the chorio-allantoic membrane of the chick embryo, or into tissue culture. These antibodies may appear 6–9 days after the onset of illness, or even earlier in patients who have previously been vaccinated. They also develop within 10 days after vaccination, though complement fixing antibodies are not found as often as the others. Complement fixing and haemagglutinating antibodies disappear within 12 months after an attack, or after vaccination, but neutralizing antibodies may persist for years. Revaccination provokes recall of antibodies within a week or so.

Serological tests do not differentiate between antibodies to smallpox and vaccinia.

An excellent *Guide to the Laboratory Diagnosis of Smallpox for Smallpox Eradication Programmes* was published by WHO in 1969. All laboratories should possess copies.

Clinicians could with advantage send the following specimens, suitably packed, to the laboratory (Dumbell 1968):

Clinical stage	*Specimen*
Pre-eruption	Blood
Macular or papular rash	Scrapings
Vesicular rash	Vesicle fluid, scrapings
Pustular rash	Pustule fluid
Crusting stage	Crusts

Treatment

Treatment involves isolation from other patients; all attendants must have been vaccinated, and all fomites must be sterilized. There is no specific treatment, though research has been done on rifampicin, which might lead to some advance. Treatment means careful nursing and attention to the rash. The hair may need to be cut short, for access to the rash, and a mask moistened with cold water and 2% phenol solution may relieve itching. The eyes should be bathed, and the edges smeared with soft paraffin.

General effects such as higher fever, delirium and sleeplessness need cooling and sedative treatment.

Secondary pyogenic infection of the skin or respiratory tract can be treated with penicillin or sulphonamides.

When crusts form they should be allowed to dry.

Prevention

Vaccination. It is, of course, well known that vaccination with an appropriate virus provides effective protection against smallpox. The precise origin and nature of vaccinia virus used for the preparation of vaccine is obscure, but it was probably not derived directly from smallpox. It is inoculated into the thoroughly cleansed skin of the flanks and bellies of calves, on which it creates eruptions containing the 'lymph' which constitutes the vaccine. This is collected and purified, and treated with phenol to reduce the number of contaminating organisms. It is standardized and preserved in glycerol, and stored at $-10°$ to $-20°C$. Complications of vaccination due to microbial contamination are no longer a hazard when the vaccine conforms to the requirements laid down by WHO (Kaplan 1969). The vaccine can be lyophilized, and remains very stable in the dry state, to be reconstituted at the time of use. This is most important for campaigns in the tropics.

There have been many attempts to prepare vaccine from tissue culture material, but the output is small, and contamination by other viruses presents difficulties.

Vaccination is still subject to certain complications. Generalized vaccinia may occur, with successive crops of papules, vesicles and crusts, and fever, but this is rare with carefully chosen strains. It responds to treatment with antivaccinial gamma-globulin.

Babies and others with eczema or dermatitis should not be vaccinated with ordinary vaccine, because they tend to develop eczema vaccinatum, which is serious, carrying a fatality rate of 30–40% (Editorial, *Br. med. J.*, 1970b). They should also be protected from vaccinial infection from vaccinated members of the household. If eczema vaccinatum develops, it can be treated with anti-vaccinial gamma-globulin, which reduces the fatality to 7% (Editorial, *Br. med. J.*, 1970b). Moreover, a purified vaccine known as CVI-78, for which the vaccinia virus was passaged in rabbit testes, chick embryonic tissues and on chick-egg chorio-allantoic membrane, has been found effective in eczematous children, without giving rise to complications (Editorial, *Br. med. J.*, 1969).

Vaccinia gangrenosa is even more serious. In this condition the vaccination lesion spreads widely and destructively, and secondary infection occurs; it tends to appear in persons with agamma-globulinaemia, or who are being treated with corticosteroids, and, unless treated, is usually fatal. Treatment with anti-vaccinial gamma-globulin, however, can reduce the mortality to 30%. It is better to associate this with treatment with Marboran (methisazone) in a dose of 200 mg/kg, followed by 8 doses of 50 mg/kg at intervals of 6 hours. It is given as a 20% suspension in sucrose syrup (Bauer 1970); it may cause vomiting. This combination of methisazone and gamma-globulin (in appropriate doses) may prevent complications in children after primary vaccination (Kaplan 1969).

Post-vaccinial encephalitis is a serious complication of primary vaccination, reported in 6·5 per million infants vaccinated in the first year of life in the United States; rates at later ages were rather less. Although treatment of the developed disease with gamma-globulin is said to be ineffectual, the risk can be reduced by giving gamma-globulin at the time of vaccination, though this is obviously impossible on any large scale. The encephalitis is thought to be due to a cell-mediated immune reaction developing against the virus in the brain (Turk 1969); it occurs about 10 days after vaccination. Mortality is said to be about 50%. The symptoms are headache, malaise, vomiting, irritability, drowsiness or coma; there may be fits or sudden paresis, or signs suggesting meningitis, cranial nerve palsies or transient lower motor neuron weakness in the limbs. Treatment with steroids may be of some use.

Fatal generalized vaccinia has been observed in fetuses after vaccination of the mothers in the first 6 months of pregnancy. Pregnant women should therefore not be vaccinated unless the threat of smallpox is real (Kaplan 1969). Other contra-indications are eczema, leukaemia, and patients undergoing immuno-suppressive treatment.

The techniques of vaccination now advised (WHO 1968) are described below.

The multiple-pressure technique. A small drop of vaccine is placed on the skin and a series of pressures are made within the smallest possible skin area (not more than 6 mm in diameter) with the side of a sharp needle held tangentially to the skin. The pressures are made with the side of the needle, not the point; 30 strokes are completed in 5–10 seconds, with an up-and-down motion per-pendicular to the skin, with enough pressure to induce a trace of blood to appear at the vaccination site. A bifurcated needle can be used. It is dipped in the vaccine and then touched to the surface of the skin; 15 strokes of the needle are made through the droplet. Needles must, of course, be completely sterilized after each vaccination, and should be dry, to avoid dilution of the vaccine.

The scratch method. This involves a single linear scratch not more than 6 mm long through the vaccine, with a suitable instrument. The scratch should be deep enough to cause a trace of blood to appear within 30 seconds. The vaccine is then rubbed into the scratch with the side of the needle.

Jet injectors are now largely used. They inject the vaccine through a very small orifice into the superficial layers of the skin without the risk of transmitting an infection (such as serum hepatitis) from one person to another (though this has been questioned). The injected dose is 0·1 ml, but not all penetrates the skin; intradermal deposition should be confirmed by sight or touch.

No dressing should normally be applied to a vaccination site at the time of vaccination; the vaccine should be allowed to dry naturally, and vaccinated persons should not be allowed to rub off the wet vaccine.

After successful vaccination a vesicle develops in 3–5 days, becoming pustular and increasing in size up to 8–9 days, and forming a scab which separates at days 14–21.

In endemic areas primary vaccination is best performed in the neonatal period. The infant may have some immunity derived from the mother if she has been vaccinated or is immune, but vaccination of the baby will take if performed correctly; though it carries a slight risk, this is much outweighed by the risk of smallpox if the child is not vaccinated.

Smallpox vaccine can be given at the same time as other immunizing agents, but at different sites, without reduction of effectiveness, except that when given with 17D yellow fever vaccine there is some reduction in the serological response to 17D.

The frequency of re-vaccination depends upon the risk of exposure. It should be repeated every 3–5 years in the general population of endemic areas, and every year for hospital personnel and others likely to be in contact with smallpox patients. The question of deliberate campaigns of vaccination against smallpox (and measles) is discussed in WHO (1968). Results are very promising in Africa.

The overwhelming evidence of the value of vaccination is reviewed in Wilson and Miles (1964). Although vaccination is the chief preventive measure, especially for people in contact with patients, it is important to make sure that bedclothes and other fomites are sterilized, preferably by boiling.

Methisazone may have some value in preventing smallpox if given to contacts in 2 (adult) doses of 3 grammes at an interval of 8–10 hours or so. It gives temporary protection only, and does not replace vaccination (Bauer 1970).

MODIFIED SMALLPOX
(VARIOLA MINOR, ALASTRIM, AMAAS)

Variola minor is a mild variant of smallpox, clinically resembling variola major in a partially immune person, but there is a vitally important difference in that variola minor breeds true; it does not lead to outbreaks of true unmodified smallpox, whereas a mild attack of smallpox in a partially immune person can give rise to an epidemic of the fully virulent disease. Variola minor occurs in most countries where smallpox occurs.

There are usually, but not always, initial toxaemic symptoms, including fever to 39·5°C, headache, backache and other pains, nausea and vomiting and cough. Before the focal rash appears a common diagnosis is influenza.

An initial toxaemic rash is not often seen. If it occurs it may be erythematous or occasionally haemorrhagic. The focal rash appears usually on days 3–5 of illness, but sometimes earlier or later, in this not differing from variola major. It lasts 2 days as papules, one day as vesicles and 3–4 days as pustules; crusting takes place on days 6–7.

This rash usually follows the distribution of that of smallpox, appearing first on the face and last on the legs, coming out in an orderly fashion, but not in the crops characteristic of chickenpox. The pocks may be few or many. The papules are generally small and may be surrounded by areolae. The vesicles are superficial; loculation and umbilication are extremely rare. Though the pocks are generally small, occasional large 'sentinel pustules' are seen. Pigmented scars follow in a minority of patients.

Secondary fever with malaise is not common; it is found chiefly in patients in whom the focal rash is abundant, and it may last up to about 4 days; the fever is not usually high.

Complications can occur—boils, blepharitis, conjunctivitis, keratitis with ulceration; they are uncommon.

Variola minor has been diagnosed as true smallpox, chickenpox, scabies, food rash and syphilis. On the other hand patients with scabies, acne, impetigo and other skin conditions have been diagnosed as having variola minor. It is a difficult though not generally dangerous disease. In one series of 13 686 cases there were 34 deaths, in 13 of which variola minor was a possible contributory cause, in 18 a definite factor and in 3 not a factor (Marsden 1948).

Smallpox vaccination protects against variola minor.

TANAPOX

Tanapox is a virus disease described by Downie *et al.* (1971), who reported 2 epidemics in 1957 and 1962, from the Tana river area of Kenya. The outbreaks occurred in low-lying country near the Tana river after floods had isolated the people and their domestic and wild animals, on islands in the flood waters. Conditions were created in which *Mansonia uniformis* and *M. africanus* proliferated in immense numbers. The disease was discovered fortuitously during helminthological surveys of the population.

The clinical effects were mild. The incubation period is not known; it was followed by fever lasting 3–4 days, sometimes with severe headache, backache and pronounced prostration. In every case 1 or 2 (never more) pock-like lesions appeared on the skin during the fever. They resembled those of smallpox, becoming umbilicated but never going on to pustule formation. They were seen mainly on exposed parts of the body—the upper arm, face, neck and trunk, but never on hands legs or feet.

Biopsy specimens of the pocks showed cytoplasmic inclusions and yielded a virus similar to, but serologically different from, the vaccinia–variola group. Inoculation of tissue-culture virus failed to infect a calf, a lamb, 2 young pigs and a goat, but did infect a rhesus and 2 vervet monkeys, and also a human volunteer who had repeatedly been vaccinated against smallpox. In this volunteer local lesions were produced at the site of 2 inoculations, but not at the site of 2 scarifications.

Serum antibodies apparently develop slowly, and complement fixation and neutralization tests on monkey and human sera were mostly at low titre.

Tests showed not only that the virus is not related to the vaccinia–variola group of pox viruses, but that it is not inactivated by antisera to various known pox viruses of animals. Nevertheless it is a member of the pox group, as shown by the clinical and histological appearance of the lesions, and by electron microscopy; it can also reactivate heat-inactivated vaccinia virus in tissue cultures of human or monkey cells. It may be related to a mild pox infection of monkeys, and of men working with them in the United States, and it has some resemblance to yabapox virus of monkeys and man.

The epidemiological features suggest that it is an infection of monkeys transmitted by direct mechanical transfer from them to man by mosquitoes.

REFERENCES

BAUER, D. J. (1970) *Med. Today*, **4**, 50.
DOWNIE, A. W., TAYLOR-ROBINSON, C. H., CAUNT, A. E., NELSON, G. S., MANSON-BAHR, P. E. C. & MATTHEWS, T. C. H. (1971) *Br. med. J.*, **i**, 363.
DUMBELL, K. R. (1968) *Prog. med. Virol.*, **10**, 388.
EDITORIAL (1969) *Br. med. J.*, **i**, 68.
—— (1970a) *Br. med. J.*, **iv**, 127.
—— (1970b) *Br. med. J.*, **iv**, 385.
KAPLAN, C. (1969) *Br. med. Bull.*, **25**, 131.
MARSDEN, J. P. (1948) *Bull. Hyg.*, **23**, 735.
MIDDLEMISS, H. (1964) *Trans. R. Soc. trop. Med. Hyg.*, **58**, 197.
TURK, J. L. (1969) *Immunology in Clinical Medicine*. London: Heinemann.
WILSON, G. S. & MILES, A. A. (1964) *Topley and Wilson's Principles of Bacteriology and Immunity*, 5th ed. London: Arnold.
WORLD HEALTH ORGANIZATION (1968) *Wld Hlth Org. tech. Rep. Ser.*, 393.
—— (1969) *Guide to the Laboratory Diagnosis of Smallpox for Smallpox Eradication Programmes*. Geneva: WHO.

16. MISCELLANEOUS VIRUS DISEASES

MEASLES

Epidemiology

Measles is common and important in developing countries. The disastrous effects of epidemics in communities in which it had not previously been endemic, such as Fiji, Tasmania, Greenland and other places, are well known, but such communities are now rare. Nevertheless, though measles has declined enormously in severity in Europe and North America, it still remains 'the most serious of the acute infectious diseases of Nigerian children' (Morley *et al.* 1963), and the same is true of other tropical countries, in which the case mortality rate is estimated to be about 5% (or even 10% in rural areas), though much higher in children admitted to hospital with severe attacks. In village epidemics even 40% of the children have been known to die of measles. The combination of measles and whooping cough is particularly dangerous, and measles can reactivate primary tuberculosis.

Children generally show the disease at the age of 18–30 months, and in West Africa epidemics tend to occur in the dry season when festivals are held and opportunities for infection are plentiful: 'Epidemics decline with the onset of the rains and the dispersal of families to their farms' (Morley 1969), but virulent epidemics can occur at all seasons (Okojie 1969).

Pathology

Besides affecting the skin, measles attacks other epithelial surfaces: the conjunctivae, mouth, larynx, bronchial tree and intestine.

The essential lesion is catarrhal inflammation of the respiratory and alimentary tracts. The initial inflammation of epithelial cells is rapidly followed by fatty degeneration and exfoliation of dead cells. Complete resolution is the rule on recovery, but widespread denudation of epithelium in the alimentary tract may end in mucosal atrophy (Gunn, quoted by Morley *et al.* 1963).

Immunology

There is evidence that passive immunity is transferred from mother to infant; this gradually declines in the first few months of life.

Immune bodies have been found in one-quarter of older children who had not experienced overt measles, indicating inapparent infection, probably during the declining phase of maternally transmitted immunity.

Clinical findings

In developing countries measles tends to be severe; it is accompanied by loss of weight. The sequence of changes can be summarized (Morley *et al.* 1963) as in Fig. 123.

Koplik's spots are commonly recognized, and the first appearance of the rash is similar to that seen in Britain, but it tends to become confluent, dark red or purple, and to desquamate 2–4 days later, large white scales of skin sometimes separating. This may lead to patchy depigmentation lasting for some weeks, and is quite often followed by a liability to multiple small boils. A severe rash of this kind is associated with equivalent changes in the respiratory and digestive systems, and with high mortality.

The mouth becomes sore, interfering with sucking or eating, and leading to malnutrition and cancrum oris. Laryngitis is common, and may lead to laryngeal obstruction; bronchopneumonia is very common and carries a high death rate. Diarrhoea with tenesmus and mucus and blood in the stools is also common, leading to dehydration which often needs parenteral fluid replacement to prevent death. Conjunctivitis may develop, sometimes leading to permanent damage; in Malawi it is a common cause of perforation and blindness, especially in association with vitamin A deficiency. Otitis media is not uncommon. Convulsions may occur, with high mortality. A pulse rate of over 180 may indicate myocardial damage and lead to sudden death.

Of the factors leading to severe measles, malnutrition is probably the most important; measles is more severe in malnourished children because of the state of their epithelial tissues, and measles can (and does) precipitate kwashiorkor or marasmus in children on the verge of those conditions.

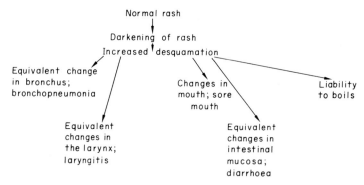

Fig. 123.—The sequence of change in measles (simplified).

Apart from the effect of sore mouth and loss of appetite in preventing a child from feeding, feeding practices in some communities are detrimental. In Mali, food, especially animal and vegetable protein, is restricted in measles. There is a conviction that measles is inevitable, and parents therefore tend not to seek medical advice. Some people believe that a child with measles should not be washed or allowed water to drink.

Many parents in Mali, and no doubt in other countries, believe that measles is due to the malevolent work of a witch, sorcerer or *marabout*, and affected children are therefore hidden because people are afraid to admit that their child has been the object of such malevolent influence. They may also be hidden from daylight so that the rash can be brought out fully, in darkness. Treatments include soaking in a solution of the bark of the wild raisin tree, covering the body with honey, bathing the child in a suspension of monkey faeces or covering it with dirt from a termite hill or with a mixture of camel faeces and sheep hair (Imperato 1969). These practices are believed to bring out the rash.

Purges are given in some communities, withheld in others. Various substances are applied to the eyes—honey, milk, tamarind juice, onion juice, peanut flour solution, soot, leaves of various plants, tannin or henna solution. Reactions to these are often mild, but occasionally severe. In general, such practices add to the risks of measles (Imperato 1969).

Treatment

No drug is known to influence the virus disease (Morley 1969). It is important to maintain the intake of food and fluid. Milk is the most suitable food, and dehydration must be countered, if necessary, with parenteral fluid. Steroids at the acute onset can be life-saving (Insley 1969).

Antibiotics do not seem to prevent bacterial complications, and the same is probably true of sulphonamides, though if the condition suggests bacterial infection—and pneumonia is the great killer—antibiotics must be given. Morley suggests a combination of long-acting penicillin and streptomycin.

A pulse rate of 180 is serious, and the child should be digitalized (Insley 1969).

Prevention

Immunization on a large scale could greatly reduce incidence. It would require deliberate vaccination campaigns every 6 months, or a continuously available service of vaccination.

Live attenuated substrains of the Edmonston strain of measles virus have been used to immunize children. These produce febrile reactions of different degrees of severity (but mostly mild) in some children, about 10 days after the injection. These reactions can be mitigated if the children are given injections of killed virus one month before the live vaccine, but killed virus does not itself give adequate protection. Gamma-globulin has been given at the same time as the live vaccine, but at a different spot, with the object of reducing reactions, but this is not now regarded as necessary. Administration of live vaccine alone is acceptable, giving 90–95% of antibody responses within 4 weeks in British children. Protection is good, but it remains to be seen how long it lasts— probably for years. Experience in West Africa strongly suggests that vaccination with live attenuated vaccine, preferably between the ages of 9 and 10 months, is a measure which will do most to reduce mortality and malnutrition in children under 5 (Morley 1969). There are few contra-indications, but children with malnutrition or known primary tuberculosis should be treated for these conditions before being vaccinated. Leukaemia is a definite contra-indication.

The jet injection technique has been used in West and Central Africa in some 15 million children, and though measles has not been controlled, it has been substantially reduced (Millar & Foege 1969).

POLIOMYELITIS

Poliomyelitis is not generally regarded as a tropical disease, and it is fully dealt with in textbooks of general medicine. It is included here as it is now recognized as a widespread infection in most tropical countries, carrying special risks for immigrants to those countries, who are not immune as a result of infection in childhood.

Epidemiology

The poliomyelitis virus (Types 1, 2 and 3) is widespread in the developing countries, most children showing serological evidence of infection in their early years. Most infections are sub-clinical and serological evidence suggests that there may be anything between 50 and 500 children infected (and mostly capable of spreading the infection for a short time) for every clinically overt case. There are therefore many opportunities for infection of susceptible people of any age. Adults tend to have more severe attacks than children, and fatalities have occurred in non-indigenous adults who could have been protected by artificial immunization.

Poliomyelitis is endemic where sanitation is poor, and the numbers of cases reported in the tropics are rising, whereas in Europe, America and Australasia they are falling.

The viruses are excreted in the faeces and the faecal–oral route of infection is usual. They can often be found in sewage and water, but efficient modern treatment of sewage and water greatly reduces them. Where sanitation, personal hygiene and food hygiene are good, infection in childhood is now rare, but epidemics can occur. Where sanitation is poor, paralytic poliomyelitis is not often seen; the incidence of paralysis varies with the degree of overcrowding, and in conditions of overcrowding children tend to be infected early. Case mortality is lowest in infancy, rising with increasing age. It is, however, possible that paralysis is rarely reported in unsanitary conditions because infection of such severity as to cause paralysis may kill children before the true nature of the disease is apparent, and they are therefore not reported as poliomyelitis. On the other hand, improvement in sanitary conditions in tropical regions will tend to reduce and delay infection. People therefore become older on first infection, and the disease is therefore more severe and obvious.

Clinical findings

The clinical course of poliomyelitis in the tropics, once acute clinical signs and symptoms develop, does not differ from the course observed elsewhere. In the early acute stage there is fever, which may be biphasic as in arbovirus infections, and signs that the nervous system is involved appear, such as loss of the patellar reflex, Kernig's sign, pain and stiffness in the neck and back, irritability and restlessness, or even stupor, and signs suggesting encephalitis.

Paralysis of the legs is more common than paralysis of the arms; the thoracic muscles may be involved, leading to respiratory failure.

In patients with these signs the disease must be differentiated from meningitis, cerebral malaria, trypanosomiasis or encephalitis due to other causes, for instance arbovirus infection. It is, therefore, important to examine blood, cerebrospinal fluid and even gland juice, to eliminate these infections.

For details of the clinical course, and of treatment, textbooks of general medicine should be consulted.

Prevention

Since opportunities for infection are so numerous in the tropics, it is extremely important that all expatriates from the more developed countries visiting the endemic areas should be immunized before entering those areas. Campaigns of vaccination are also carried out on the indigenous children. The vaccine now most generally used is the live attenuated vaccine of Sabin. It is taken by mouth and is not destroyed in the alimentary tract, since the component viruses are enteroviruses (see Immunization, page 3). This vaccine may be adversely affected by the numerous intestinal infections from which tropical children suffer, and its performance in the tropics is said to be much less good than in developed areas.

As the endemic countries become more accustomed to improved sanitation, and as the living conditions improve, natural infections in childhood will

decrease, epidemics will become more likely and the need for intensive vaccination campaigns will become pressing.

Other enteroviruses such as Coxsackie and ECHO viruses are probably
common in the tropics. They inhabit the intestine and are presumably spread
like poliovirus. One Coxsackie virus (A7) can produce paralytic disease in man,
resembling poliomyelitis. Others can cause pleurodynia or meningitis. ECHO
viruses can cause meningitis or mild gastro-enteritis.

There is no specific treatment for these infections; no doubt many of them
are symptomless. Effective vaccines are not yet available.

HEPATITIS

INFECTIOUS HEPATITIS

Epidemiology

Infectious hepatitis is found all over the world, but is especially prevalent in
hot climates, forming a risk to non-immune immigrants, for instance in West
Africa. In Accra, Ghana, it is essentially an urban disease, and fulminating
attacks are related to pregnancy, immigration, residence in shanty towns,
physically active occupation, lack of education and a low economic standing
(Morrow *et al.* 1969). Elsewhere it is especially associated with schools and
other institutions for children and mentally deficient persons, whose personal
hygiene is bad, and it is a special risk for nurses in such institutions. It was very
common in British and American troops operating in North Africa in the war
of 1939–45. Apart from an endemic distribution in countries in which sanitation
is primitive, there have been many outbreaks in more sophisticated countries,
associated with known sources of infection, including contaminated water
supplies.

Aetiology

The cause of infectious hepatitis is an enterovirus which inhabits the intestinal
tract and is excreted in the faeces of infected persons; excretion can continue for
weeks or months after infection, but is most prolific in the early stages. Numerous
experiments on volunteers have proved that infection can be acquired by
swallowing infective material, and in nature transmission of faecal matter from
one person to another probably occurs via the fingers of children and food
handlers, by flies or by water; shell-fish such as clams and oysters from water
subject to pollution, which are eaten raw, are also strongly suspected.

A particulate antigen, serologically distinct from the Australia antigen of
serum hepatitis, has been found in the faeces of hepatitis patients in the early
stages (Ferris *et al.* 1970).

Pathology

In fatal cases the liver may be shrunken and have lost its smooth contour. In
fulminating cases the microscopic appearances of the liver may be mistaken for
those of yellow fever (Boyd 1965). In yellow fever, however, the liver is not
shrunken; the epithelial cells are irregularly affected, normal and affected cells
occurring side by side; the cell lesion appears to be a coagulative necrosis, and
the contents of the affected cells stain deeply with eosin—under low power the
section looks as if red pepper has been scattered over it.

In infectious hepatitis the microscopic changes are those of toxic hepatitis.
The cells at the centre of the lobule are the first to be affected, and are usually

completely destroyed, only the stroma remaining. The necrosis spreads towards the periphery of the lobule, and may be so severe that almost all the epithelial cells disappear in some lobules. There is a varying degree of round cell infiltration, particularly near the portal tract (Boyd 1970). It should be remembered that acute hepatic necrosis can also be due to toxins in foodstuffs or herbal remedies; some plant alkaloids are known to be toxic in this way. In chronic hepatitis fibrosis may lead to cirrhosis, and carcinoma may eventually develop (Sherlock et al. 1970). (Carcinoma may also be linked with the aflatoxin content of common foods.)

Clinical findings

Infectious hepatitis may cause symptomless infection, and in one epidemic only 32 of 97 persons exposed to infection from contaminated water showed jaundice, though the rest had raised liver enzyme values (Chang & O'Brien 1970). Other authorities have put the ratio of symptomless infections to overt disease very much higher than this. The incubation period is thought to be 15–40 days.

In the overt disease there is anorexia, fever and aching pains in the limbs and back, before the onset of jaundice, which usually starts about a week after the onset of illness. Jaundice deepens, with the usual pale faeces and dark urine, and is generally more pronounced than in yellow fever. The liver is somewhat enlarged and tender, and the spleen may enlarge slightly. After a few days the temperature comes down and the jaundice diminishes, and complete recovery takes place. One features is the depression which many patients experience.

In some cases the disease is fulminating, and can be fatal even before jaundice appears. Sometimes recovery is incomplete, and this may lead to cirrhosis and even primary carcinoma of the liver.

The following list gives the main differences between infectious and serum hepatitis (after Wilson & Miles 1964):

Infectious hepatitis	*Serum hepatitis*
Contagious	Apparently not contagious
Incubation period 15–40 days	Incubation period 60–160 days
Onset acute	Onset insidious
Febrile course	Little or no fever
Affects children and young adults mainly	Affects all ages
Commonest in autumn and winter	Occurs all the year round
Virus present in stools	Virus apparently not present in stools
Disease experimentally transmissible by mouth	Disease not experimentally transmissible by mouth
One attack confers some immunity to infectious but not serum hepatitis	One attack confers some immunity to serum but not infectious hepatitis
Skin test with infectious hepatitis antigen positive	Skin test with infectious hepatitis antigen negative

Later work suggests that serum hepatitis can occasionally infect contacts (Editorial, *Lancet*, 1969), presumably by mouth.

The serum glutamic oxaloacetic transaminase (SGOT) and glutamic pyruvic transaminase (SGPT) values are much raised, especially SGPT.

Diagnosis

There is no easy differential diagnostic test, and hepatitis can be confused with jaundice from other causes, including yellow fever, leptospirosis, relapsing fever, malaria and even kala-azar. Blood should therefore be examined for parasites, and serum should be taken for diagnosis of leptospirosis.

Treatment

There is no satisfactory specific treatment. Diet should be light, and it is probably wise to abstain from alcohol for about 3 months. Corticosteroids may be valuable in fulminating cases.

It is said that injection of gamma-globulin can avert the clinical manifestations if given before the disease has become established (Wilson & Miles 1964), and this might be useful in known outbreaks.

Prevention is a matter of sanitation, and especially of personal and kitchen hygiene, including the control of flies. For persons at special risk a single intramuscular injection of human immuno-globulin (750 mg) can protect for about 6 months.

SERUM HEPATITIS

Serum hepatitis is caused by a separate though related virus, associated with the 'Australia SH antigen'. This antigen has not been found in well documented epidemics of infectious hepatitis, and is believed to be present only in the serum of patients with serum hepatitis, in which its presence is thought to be diagnostic. It is associated with particles in serum which can be demonstrated by electron microscopy, and it can be detected in serum by immunodiffusion techniques and complement fixation tests.

This virus can be present for months or years (up to 30) in blood and serum, and it is transmitted from one person to another by unsterile syringes (being a noted hazard in drug addicts); through haemodialysis units, which are at special risk of contamination; through blood or plasma transfusion; by scratches caused by thorns, barbed wire etc., which may scratch more than one person; or even by mouth.

It is not known if the Australia SH antigen can be passed across the placenta from mother to fetus, but one investigation suggested that it is not so transmitted (London et al. 1969). Complement fixation tests for this antigen have been found positive in 40% of 45 patients with hepatocellular carcinoma in Uganda, against 3% in controls, which suggests that this infection plays some part in the causation of this cancer (Vogel et al. 1970). The antigen has been found in cirrhotic livers and in primary carcinoma of the liver, and this may have a bearing on the known high incidence of primary carcinoma of the liver in Africans (Sherlock et al. 1970).

The incubation period (60–160 days) is longer than in infectious hepatitis; otherwise the differential diagnosis in individual patients depends upon a history of injections etc.

As is the case with infectious hepatitis, serum hepatitis is often present without jaundice. Though recovery is usual, the disease is sometimes fatal.

In the tropics, where drugs are so often administered by injection, it is obviously important to sterilize all injection equipment completely. Merely to change the needle after intravenous, intramuscular or even subcutaneous injection is not enough, since blood can easily enter the syringe from slight movements of the plunger. Both needle and syringe should be sterilized each time (Hughes 1946a, b; Evans & Spooner 1950).

IZUMI FEVER

This disease of children or young adults was first described in Japan by Izumi and his colleagues in 1927, and there have been many outbreaks there since then. It also occurs sporadically.

It is probably caused by an intestinal virus; Kuroya et al. (1954) isolated a virus from the faeces of a patient in the acute stage, which infected young mice on intracerebral, intranasal or intraperitoneal injection; the virus spread widely in the mouse tissues. A suspension of infected mouse brain administered by stomach tube caused the typical disease in a human subject. Neutralizing antibody has been found in human convalescent serum.

The disease is thought to be water-borne, possibly via the urine or faeces of infected rodents, or transmitted by personal contact (Nishioka & Morita 1952). Trombiculid mites have also been suspected on epidemiological grounds (Kumada et al. 1952).

The incubation period seems to be 5–13 days. Two types of illness are described, both beginning abruptly with fever and chills. In both types there is an itchy rash intermediate between scarlet fever and measles, on the trunk, face, neck and extremities, which disappears in 3–4 days and is followed by fine desquamation. The symptoms include joint and lumbar pains, nausea, vomiting and abdominal pain; the liver may be enlarged. The mild type lasts only a few days, but in the severe type, after the primary fever subsides there is a secondary attack, with the same characters, but with fever lasting up to 2–3 weeks (Nishioka & Nishioka 1952). There may even be a third febrile phase (Yanagishita et al. 1957).

Treatment with Aureomycin (chlortetracycline) or chloramphenicol is said to be effective.

LASSA FEVER

Lassa fever is a virus disease, not hitherto recognized, which was reported from the Jos area of Nigeria in 1970; serological studies suggest infection over a considerable area of that part of Africa.

The virus has been isolated from several patients, and is related to the lymphocytic choriomeningitis virus and to the Machupo and Tacaribe arboviruses; it has been placed tentatively in the Togavirus taxon. These relationships and other features of the disease suggest an animal reservoir, but this has not been proved. The virus has apparently been transmitted from one person to another in respiratory secretions; close contact is probably necessary. Patients could often be traced to a known human source of infection, and are probably infective for a long time, for the virus has been isolated from throat washings up to day 14 of illness. It has also been isolated from serum (up to day 14), urine (day 32) and pleural fluid (day 13).

Post mortem changes included small haemorrhages in the gastro-intestinal tract, focal lesions, congestion and pneumonitis in the lungs, gross haemorrhages and casts in the kidneys, necrotic areas with fatty change and congestion in the liver, congestion in the spleen and congested myocardium.

Lassa fever is one cause of haemorrhagic fever; thrombocytopenia is a feature. There may be a spectrum of clinical effects, ranging from an asymptomatic or mild infection to a fatal disease. In the known cases the onset was insidious and fever was prolonged, the illness in recovered patients lasting from 1 to over 4 weeks, with slow convalescence. There was marked lassitude and loss of weight. The main features seem to be as follows: muscular pains; vomiting, diarrhoea and abdominal pain; severe pharyngitis with white patches on the pharynx and tonsillitis; chest pain, cough and pneumonitis; renal failure with albuminuria and granular casts; myocarditis and cardiac failure; disturbance of the coagulation mechanism; diffuse encephalopathy; and leucopenia. Complement fixation tests become positive.

Of 26 suspected cases in one hospital, 10 were fatal and some were mild. Treatment with antibiotics was not helpful, but administration of plasma from a patient who had recovered apparently aborted the disease in the recipient.

(The above account of lassa fever is derived from the following articles: Buckley & Casals 1970; Frame *et al.* 1970; Leifer *et al.* 1970; Speir *et al.* 1970; Troup *et al.* 1970. The disease will also be discussed in a series of papers to be presented at the meeting of the Royal Society of Tropical Medicine and Hygiene in London, early in 1972. These papers, by some of the above and other authors, amplify the findings, and will be published in the *Transactions of the Royal Society of Tropical Medicine and Hygiene* in 1972.)

REFERENCES

Boyd, J. S. K. (1965) *Trans. R. Soc. trop. Med. Hyg.*, **59**, 607.
—— (1970) Personal communication.
Buckley, S. M. & Casals, J. (1970) *Am. J. trop. Med. Hyg.*, **19**, 680.
Chang, L. W. & O'Brien, T. F. (1970) *Lancet*, **ii**, 59.
Editorial (1969) *Lancet*, **ii**, 577.
Evans, R. J. & Spooner, E. T. C. (1950) *Br. med. J.*, **ii**, 185.
Ferris, A. A., Kaldor, J., Gust, I. D. & Cross, G. (1970) *Lancet*, **ii**, 243.
Frame, J. D., Baldwin, J. M. jun., Gocke, D. J. & Troup, J. N. (1970) *Am. J. trop. Med. Hyg.*, **19**, 670.
Hughes, R. E. (1946a) *Br. med. J.*, **ii**, 685.
—— (1946b) *J. R. Army med. Corps*, **87**, 156.
Imperato, P. J. (1969) *Trans. R. Soc. trop. Med. Hyg.*, **63**, 768.
Insley, J. L. (1969) *Br. med. J.*, **ii**, 120.
Kumada, N., Sasa, M., Miura, A. & Nishioka, K. (1952) *Jap. J. exp. Med.*, **22**, 353.
Kuroya, M., Yoshinari, Y., Ishida, N., Noda, K. & Koseki, E. (1954) *Jap. J. exp. Med.*, **24**, 105.
Leifer, E., Gocke, D. J. & Bourne, H. (1970) *Am. J. trop. Med. Hyg.*, **19**, 677.
London, W. Y., Difiglia, M. & Rodgers, J. (1969) *Lancet*, **ii**, 900.
Millar, J. D. & Foege, W. H. (1969) *J. infect. Dis.*, **120**, 725.
Morley, D. (1969) *Br. med. J.*, **i**, 297.
—— Woodland, M. & Martin, W. J. (1963) *J. Hyg.*, *Camb.*, **61**, 115.
Morrow, R. H., Sai, F. T., Edgcomb, J. H. & Smetana, H. F. (1969) *Trans. R. Soc. trop. Med. Hyg.*, **63**, 755.
Nishioka, K. & Morita, J. (1952) *Jap. J. exp. Med.*, **22**, 333.
—— & Nishioka, K. (1952) *Jap. J. exp. Med.*, **22**, 341.
Okojie, X. G. (1969) *Br. med. J.*, **ii**, 250.
Sherlock, S., Fox, R. A., Niazi, S. P. & Scheuer, P. J. (1970) *Lancet*, **i**, 1243.
Speir, R. W., Wood, O., Liebhaber, H. & Buckley, S. M. (1970) *Am. J. trop. Med. Hyg.*, **19**, 692.
Troup, J. A., White, H. A., Fom, A. L. M. D. & Carey, D. E. (1970) *Am. J. trop. Med. Hyg.*, **19**, 695.
Vogel, C. L., Anthony, P. P., Mody, N. & Barker, L. F. (1970) *Lancet*, **ii**, 621.
Wilson, G. S. & Miles, A. A. (1964) *Topley and Wilson's Principles of Bacteriology and Immunity*, 5th ed. London: Arnold.
Yanagishita, T., Ogawa, J. & Kimura, T. (1957) *Keio J. Med.*, **6**, 35.

17. RABIES; MARBURG AGENT DISEASE

RABIES is a zoonosis caused by a virus which affects many species of mammals. The urban type is propagated chiefly by dogs, less so by cats; the wildlife type is found in foxes, jackals, wolves, coyotes, skunks, stoats, civet cats, mongooses, weasels, squirrels and bats. Larger animals such as cattle (especially in Central and South America) and bears can be affected.

GEOGRAPHICAL DISTRIBUTION

Rabies in animals occurs in most parts of the world, but some countries such as Britain, Japan and Australia are free from indigenous infection, though cases in immigrants to those countries are occasionally reported, and rabid animals (including monkeys) are detected in the quarantine stations or in laboratories. The quarantine period for imported dogs in Britain has recently been extended from 6 to 8 months because of a case in a dog in which the incubation period exceeded 6 months. Macrae (1969) reported 8 human cases in Britain in recent years, all infected abroad, 7 by the bites of dogs, one by a cat; all were fatal.

EPIDEMIOLOGY AND EPIZOOTIOLOGY

The rabies virus is present in the saliva in the late incubation and early disease periods of most rabid dogs and other animals, including man; though extremely rare, man-to-man spread has been recorded, but human cases are almost all due to virus introduced through abraded skin, or through a wound made by an actual bite by a rabid animal. The saliva of an infected animal, if it contains virus during the short period of infectivity, and if it is deposited by licking on skin already abraded or cut or scratched, can transmit the disease; but if the animal remains healthy for 7–10 days after the incident, it is practically certain that no rabies virus was present in the saliva. Experimentally, virus can enter via intact mucous membranes and the digestive system, and air-borne transmission, though unlikely, is possible (Editorial, *Br. med. J.*, 1970).

In Central and South America, Trinidad and Jamaica, the main transmitters of infection are infected bats, especially vampire bats (*Desmodus rotundus*). Virus is present in the saliva of infected bats, and can persist for long periods; the bats themselves are not seriously diseased. Even insectivorous bats (*Tadarida mexicana, Dasypterus floridanus*) and other apparently innocuous frugivorous bats have been found infected. In these parts cattle are the main victims and dogs are not important. Infected insectivorous bats have also been found in Yugoslavia, Germany and Turkey.

AETIOLOGY

The cause of rabies is a virus 100–150 nm in diameter, which is inactivated by sunlight, heat at 60°C for 30 minutes and ether. It survives for only a short time at room temperature. It can be grown in chick and duck embryos and in tissue culture, and it propagates when injected into guinea-pigs, hamsters, mice and rabbits.

The street virus (*virus des rues, Strassenvirus*) is the virulent form found in rabid animals in nature. When inoculated subdurally in rabbits it causes symptoms of rabies in about 14 days, producing Negri bodies. It occurs in the saliva, central nervous system, peripheral nerves, salivary glands and (less frequently) the cerebrospinal fluid of rabid animals and in the urine and faeces of infected persons.

The fixed virus is the street virus modified by intracerebral passage through a long series of rabbits or other animals, so that the incubation period is reduced to 7 days and is constant. This is a strongly neurotropic virus but, though virulent when inoculated on to the scarified skin of a rabbit, it is not virulent on subcutaneous inoculation, nor does it produce Negri bodies.

Negri bodies are inclusions in the cytoplasm and dendrons of nerve cells, especially in Ammon's horn of the brain. They consist of acidophilic rounded masses or short rods or granules, and they contain virus particles. They can be seen in a direct smear of the brain of most rabid animals, and they are diagnostic, but they may not be found if the animal is killed before the paralytic stage of the disease is reached. Inoculation of mice with a suspension of brain tissue is a more delicate diagnostic test.

The brain of a suspected animal should be examined fresh if possible, but if not, it should be sent to the laboratory packed in ice, or half should be fixed in 10% formalin for section and half placed in 50% glycerol for inoculation.

PATHOLOGY

The virus probably travels along the nerves from the site of the original injury, to the central nervous system. It multiplies in the brain tissue and can then spread outwards along the peripheral nerves, in which interstitial neuritis has been observed. It has been found also in muscle, and reaches the salivary glands; it is therefore not strictly neurotropic. The virus can spread from cell to contiguous cell without release to the extracellular space, but in the salivary gland it can escape from the acinar cells by a process of budding from the cell membranes (Macrae 1969).

Post mortem findings in man include diffuse encephalomyelitis, particularly marked in the brain stem and cervical cord, where there is congestion, loss of cells and perivascular cuffing (Ridley 1965).

The virus may not be able to pass the placenta. Relova (1963) reports a case in which a woman 7 months pregnant was dying of rabies; 10 hours before her death a live child was delivered by caesarian section, and remained free from the disease.

IMMUNOLOGY

Antibodies are produced in infected animals. Neutralizing antibodies have been produced in horses, mules, donkeys and other animals, and the immune component, gamma-globulin, can be purified and concentrated, and even produced in powder form. The British Pharmacopoeia rabies antiserum contains not less than 80 units/ml and the dose to be infiltrated round the wound is not less than 5 ml, the parenteral dose being 2000–3000 units. Intracellular virus is not affected by circulating antibody.

The production of interferon by the rabies virus is difficult to assess, but there is no reason to suppose that it is not produced, though attempts to prevent rabies in experimental animals by treatment with injected interferon have failed, probably because the amount given has been insufficient. Recent work, however, suggests that interferon is a potent inhibitor of the virus.

Fenje (1970) states that previous injection of neuro-vaccinia virus, or of virus-free extracts of tissues from infected animals, protects against challenge with rabies street virus, presumably through the production of interferon. Certain substances, of which the double-stranded polynucleotide polyinosinic acid/polycytidylic acid (poly I/poly C) is one, are known to stimulate the production of interferon. Fenje found that a small dose of this, injected 24 or 3 hours before challenge with street virus, or at the same time, or even 3 hours after challenge, protected all the 39 rabbits tested; injected 24 hours after infection 10 of 15 rabbits survived. All controls died. The survivors withstood a second challenge 35 days later, and showed high levels of neutralizing antibody, a sign of active immunity. But though the sera showed high levels of interferon, no poly I/poly C could be detected. The conclusion is that this method of stimulating the body to produce interferon actively is successful, whereas injection of interferon is not. The prospect looks hopeful for the application of this work to human rabies.

CLINICAL FINDINGS

In animals the disease has been classified as *dumb rabies* or *furious rabies*. In dumb rabies the animal (for instance the dog) after an incubation period of 2–8 weeks, exhibits a change of character and habits, becoming morose, and dies of paralysis within a few days of the onset of symptoms. In furious rabies the change of character and habits is more dangerous as the animal tends to be aggressive. If it bites during the period (starting about 5 days before the onset of symptoms, and lasting throughout the illness) when the saliva contains virus, there is obvious risk to the person or animal bitten. But only 35–43% of people bitten by rabid dogs are thought to be infected; the proportion bitten by rabid wolves is said to be around 61%. If the bite is through clothing, the cloth may reduce the risk by wiping off the saliva. Some rabid animals are not secreting virus all the time.

In man the incubation period varies from 2 weeks to 2 years, but is usually 1–3 months. The shorter periods occur when the bite is severe or is on the hands or face, and the amount of virus introduced is important in this respect.

The two main types may not easily be recognized. In the excited (furious) type the patient shows an early rise of temperature and early psychological change, becoming anxious, melancholy, irritable and subject to strange presentiments which may be hysterical in origin. Insomnia is a prominent feature of this prodromal phase. Reflexes are increased and the pupils may dilate. The wound becomes engorged and tender.

Headache and other aches and pains (which may be shooting) occur, and paraesthesiae of the trunk and face and limbs may be marked. The patient is fully alert and orientated, but restless. Voluntary movements may be exaggerated, and there may be periods of excitement during which the patient may destroy objects near at hand, but seldom injures other persons. Sexual excitement, with priapism, is common. The face may lack expression, and squint may develop, and inability to close the eyes or mouth. The voice becomes hoarse, and mucus collects in the mouth, which the patient is unable to expel.

Extremely painful spasms of the throat and larynx occur, causing fear of food and especially drink, which may be so great that the patient cries out in terror when offered a drink. Even draughts of air or bright lights can bring on convulsive seizures, and repeated spasms of respiratory muscles lead to difficulty in breathing and cyanosis.

The convulsive seizures become more and more pronounced until the patient dies, usually during a spasm, but sometimes in coma. Death is usual 5–10 days after the onset of symptoms.

Examination of systems other than the nervous system is usually negative, but myocarditis has been reported (Cheetham *et al.* 1970).

In the paralytic form the symptoms tend to be less marked, and the diagnosis may be missed. The patient is depressed and apathetic, with fever and malaise, followed by weakness, ataxia and paralysis from acute progressive ascending myelitis, with root pains and paralysis first in the legs. Encephalitis develops later and may go on to coma. Indeed, the disease may present as encephalitis with no special neurological features, and may even resemble poliomyelitis. There may be difficulty in swallowing. Death may not take place for a month, but is inevitable. Bat-borne rabies is of this kind, and resembles the paralytic rabies of cattle (*mal de caderas*) of Central and South America.

DIAGNOSIS

This is obviously difficult, especially in countries where rabies is not indigenous, occurring in immigrants who, because perhaps of a long incubation period, may have forgotten bites of dogs, cats or other animals in their own countries before arrival. It is therefore very important, in non-endemic countries, to ask if the patient has been abroad, or has been bitten by an animal, or exposed to bats. An unusual disease of the nervous system in such patients should suggest the possibility of rabies. The symptoms may suggest hysteria, but the pyrexia and other signs indicate a more fundamental physical cause. Rabies must be differentiated from tetanus, in which the spasms are more continuous; rabies strongly affects the muscles of respiration and deglutition.

Virus can sometimes be isolated from the patient's saliva, and from specimens of tissue. Neutralization tests with known anti-rabies sera are used. Virus can also quickly be detected by the fluorescent antibody test in corneal cells of experimentally infected mice, and this technique, on corneal impression smears, has been used for diagnosis in man. In mice the corneal test becomes positive before the onset of clinical signs. The technique can also be used to detect virus in impression smears of the brain. Gel precipitation tests are also useful in detecting virus in animal tissues. Negative results in all these should be confirmed by inoculation of mice.

An animal suspected of causing rabies should be isolated and kept alive; if it does not die within 10 days it is not rabid, but if it dies or develops paralysis in this period, or was killed at the time of the bite, its brain should be examined at a laboratory. Bats, which can harbour the virus for a long time, should be killed at once on capture. Negri bodies can usually be found in about 90% of rabid animals and 70% of patients who have died from the disease.

TREATMENT

Treatment should never await the results of laboratory tests.

The introduction of anti-rabies serum and immune human gamma-globulin is the most important advance in treatment of suspected rabies. It is infiltrated round the wound and also injected intramuscularly.

Table 19a. Local treatment of wounds involving possible exposure to rabies (WHO 1966)

Recommended in all exposures

a. First-aid treatment

Immediate washing and flushing with soap and water, detergent or water alone (recommended in all bite wounds, including those unrelated to possible exposure to rabies)

b. Treatment by or under the direction of a physician

Adequate cleansing of the wound

Thorough treatment with 20% soap solution and/or the application of a quaternary ammonium compound or other substance of proven lethal effect on the rabies virus.*

Topical application of anti-rabies serum or its liquid or powdered globulin preparation (optional)

Administration, where indicated, of anti-tetanus procedures and of antibiotics and drugs to control infections other than rabies

Suturing of wound not advised

Additional local treatment for severe exposures only

a. Topical application of antirabies serum or its liquid or powdered globulin preparation

b. Infiltration of anti-rabies serum around the wound

* Where soap has been used to clean the wound all traces should be removed before the application of quaternary ammonium compounds because soap neutralizes the activity of such compounds. Benzalkonium chloride in a 1% concentration has been demonstrated to be effective in the local treatment of wounds in guinea-pigs infected with the rabies virus. It should be noted that at this concentration quaternary ammonium compounds may exert a deleterious effect on the tissues. Compounds that have been demonstrated to have a specific lethal effect on rabies virus *in vitro* (different assay systems in mice) include the following:

Quaternary ammonium compounds

0·1% (1 : 1000) benzalkonium chloride = mixture of alkylbenzyldimethylammonium chlorides

0·1% (1 : 1000) cetrimonium bromide = hexadecyltrimethlyammonium bromide

1·0% (1 : 100) Hyamine 2389 = mixture containing 40% methyldodecylbenzyltrimethylammonium chloride and 10% of methyldodecylxylylene bis(trimethyl ammonium chloride)

1·0% (1 : 100) methyl benzethonium chloride = benzyldimethyl {2-{2-[p-(1,1,3,3-tetramethylbutyl)tolyloxy]ethoxy}ethyl}ammonium chloride

1·0% (1 : 100) benzethonium chloride = benzyldimethyl{2-[2-(p-1,1,3,3-tetramethylbutylphenoxy)ethoxy]ethyl}ammonium chloride

1·0% (1 : 100) SKF 11831 = p-phenylphenacylhexamethylenetetrammonium bromide

Other substances

43–70% ethanol; tincture of thiomersal; tincture of iodine and up to 0·01% (1 : 10 000) aqueous solutions of iodine; 1–2% soap solutions

The schedule in Table 19 (WHO 1966) gives the recommended treatment, both local and general, for various degrees of exposure. The recommendations given in the schedule are intended only as a guide. It is recognized that in special situations modifications of the procedures laid down may be warranted. Such special situations include the exposure of young children and other cases where

Table 19b. Specific systemic treatment of rabies (WHO 1966)

Nature of exposure	Status of biting animal (irrespective of whether vaccinated or not)		Treatment
	At time of exposure	During observation (10 days)	
No lesions, indirect contact	Rabid	—	None
Licks			
a. Unabraded skin	Rabid	—	None
b. Abraded skin, scratches and abraded and unabraded mucosa	1. Healthy	Clinical signs of rabies or proven rabid (lab.)	Start vaccine* at first signs of rabies in the biting animal
	2. Signs suggestive of rabies	Healthy	Start vaccine* immediately; stop treatment if animal is normal on fifth day after exposure
	3. Rabid, escaped, killed or unknown	—	Start vaccine* immediately
Bites			
a. Mild exposure	1. Healthy	Clinical signs of rabies or proven rabid (lab.)	Start vaccine*† at first signs of rabies in the biting animal
	2. Signs suggestive of rabies	Healthy	Start vaccine* immediately; stop treatment if animal is normal on fifth day after exposure
	3. Rabid, escaped, killed or unknown	—	Start vaccine*† immediately
	4. Wild (wolf, jackal, fox, bat, etc.)	—	Serum† immediately, followed by a course of vaccine*
b. Severe exposure (multiple face, head, finger or neck bites)	1. Healthy	Clinical signs of rabies or proven rabid (lab.)	Serum† immediately; start vaccine* at first signs of rabies in the biting animal
	2. Signs suggestive of rabies	Healthy	Serum† immediately, followed by vaccine; vaccine may be stopped if the animal is normal on fifth day after exposure
	3. Rabid, escaped, killed or unknown	—	Serum† immediately, followed by vaccine*
	4. Wild (wolf, jackal, pariah dog, fox, bat, etc.)	—	

* Practice varies concerning the amount of vaccine per dose and the number of doses recommended for a given situation. In general, the equivalent of at least 2 ml of a 5% tissue emulsion should be given subcutaneously for 14 consecutive days. Many

a reliable history cannot be obtained, particularly in areas where rabies is known to be enzootic, even though the animal is considered to be healthy at the time of the exposure. Such cases justify immediate treatment, but of a modified nature, for example, local treatment of the wound as described in the table followed by a single dose of the serum or 3 doses of vaccine daily; provided that the animal stays healthy for 10 days following exposure, no further vaccine need be given. Modification of the recommended procedures would also be indicated in a rabies-free area where animal bites are frequently encountered. In areas where rabies is endemic, adequate laboratory and field experience indicating no infection in the species involved may justify the local health authorities in recommending no specific anti-rabies treatment.

Serum should be given as promptly as possible, in a single intramuscular dose of not less than 40 I.U./kg, followed by a course of not less than 14 doses of vaccine. Serum interferes with the production of antibody induced by vaccine, and booster doses of vaccine are therefore recommended at 10 and 20 days (or more) after the end of the vaccine schedule.

Reactions to anti-rabies horse serum often occur, and the patient should be questioned about allergy, and the usual preliminary intradermal or conjunctival test should be applied before the serum is injected. The risk of serum sickness can be reduced by giving a dose of an antihistamine drug at the time of injection and afterwards. If the patient is sensitive to horse serum, preparations from other animals may be used.

Otherwise treatment is palliative, with intravenous sodium phenobarbitone in large doses, and chlorpromazine. It has been suggested that curare, with positive pressure endotracheal ventilation, in addition to serum and vaccine, might offer a chance of survival (Editorial, *Br. med. J.* 1965).

Immunization

Vaccines have been prepared by various techniques since the original dried rabbit spinal cord vaccine devised by Pasteur. Modern vaccines are of 2 main types, one containing live virus and one containing virus inactivated by various agents. Fixed virus is used for these vaccines, and the modern trend favours the use of inactivated vaccines.

1. *Semple type*, suspension of infected brain tissue completely inactivated by incubation at 37°C in the presence of phenol; it can be freeze-dried.

---

laboratories use 20–30 doses in severe exposures. To ensure the production and maintenance of high levels of serum neutralizing antibodies, booster doses should be given at 10 days and at 20 days or more following the last daily dose of vaccine in *all* cases. This is especially important if anti-rabies serum has been used, in order to overcome the interference effect.

† In all severe exposures and in all cases of unprovoked wild animal bites, anti-rabies serum or its globulin fractions together with vaccine should be employed. This is considered by the Committee as the *best* specific treatment available for the post-exposure prophylaxis of rabies in man. Although experience indicated that vaccine alone is sufficient for mild exposures, there is no doubt that the combined serum-vaccine treatment will give the best protection. However, both the serum and the vaccine can cause deleterious reactions. Moreover, the combined therapy is more expensive; its use in mild exposures is, therefore, considered optional. As with vaccine alone, it is important to start combined serum and vaccine treatment as early as possible after exposure, but serum should be used no matter what the time interval. Serum should be given in a single dose (40 I.U./kg body weight) and the first dose of vaccine inoculated at the same time. Sensitivity to the serum must be determined before its administration.

2. *Fermi type,* suspension of infected brain tissue incubated at 22°C in the presence of phenol, and still containing residual infective virus; it can be freeze-dried, and is widely used in U.S.S.R.

3. *Duck egg type,* grown in duck embryos and inactivated by beta-propio-lactone. It was developed to eliminate factors in brain tissue responsible for paralytic accidents, but has not completely done so. A recent report (Crick & Brown 1970) indicates that this vaccine does not produce neutralizing antibodies so well as tissue culture or brain vaccines.

4. *Suckling mouse brain, or rat brain, type,* inactivated by ultraviolet irradiation, intended to eliminate the risk of encephalitis, but without complete success (WHO 1969).

Tissue culture vaccines are being developed, and attempts are being made to produce a vaccine from virus grown in primary liver cells of the golden hamster, and other tissues free from brain tissue (WHO 1969). Tissue culture vaccines may be particularly valuable (Editorial, *Lancet,* 1972).

The available vaccines are summarized in WHO (1966) (Table 20).

Table 20. Vaccines available for the immunization of man and animals against rabies

Vaccine	Strain of virus	Tissue used for preparation	For use in	Potency test
Live virus				
LEP*	Flury, 40–60 egg passage	Chicken embryo	Dog	Guinea-pig
K*	Kelev, 60–70 egg passage	Chicken embryo	Dog, cattle	Guinea-pig, mouse
HEP*	Flury, above 180th egg passage	Chicken embryo	Cattle, cat, dog	Guinea-pig, mouse
Nervous tissue	Fixed	Central nervous system	Man, dog, cattle, other animals	NIH, Habel
Inactivated virus				
Duck	Fixed virus	Duck embryo	Man	NIH, Habel
Nervous tissue	Fixed virus	Central nervous system	Man, dog, cattle, other animals	NIH, Habel

* These vaccines should not be passaged in mice or other animals at any time.

The value of vaccine treatment of persons suspected of having been at risk has always been difficult to assess. In a comprehensive review of the evidence Rhodes (1946) concluded that vaccine treatment has some value, and cannot be omitted. Since then the introduction of antiserum has greatly improved the treatment.

Complications of vaccine treatment

The prolonged series of injections of vaccine in subjects suspected of having been at risk quite commonly leads to benign systemic and local reactions, which clear up quickly. But more serious, and fortunately rare, neuroparalytic accidents may follow the use of vaccine prepared from nervous tissue of mature animals. For some unexplained reason the incidence of these accidents varies from one country to another (WHO 1966). These accidents consist of demyelinating lesions of the central nervous system, whose aetiology is similar to that of experimental allergic encephalomyelitis induced by the myelin component of nervous tissue (Turner 1969). The effects of this myelitis range from transient disturbances to permanent paralysis which may be lethal. Signs of meningo-encephalitis or encephalitis, or of polyradiculo-neuronitis, may be seen, and paralysis may extend to the cranial nerves.

This complication tends to occur after about the seventh injection of vaccine, particularly in persons who have had a previous course of vaccine treatment.

If signs of a neuroparalytic accident develop, and the amount of vaccine administered is regarded as adequate in the circumstances, further administration may be discontinued. If, however, further administration is indicated, a vaccine prepared from non-nervous tissue should be used. For treatment the use of corticosteroids should be considered whether or not the vaccine is continued.

PROPHYLAXIS

Laboratory workers, veterinarians and others who run exceptional risks of infection should be immunized by a short course of 2–3 injections of a potent vaccine, preferably of non-nervous tissue (e.g. duck egg) type, at intervals of one month, followed by a booster dose 6 months later. Serum should be tested for antibodies; if negative, further doses should be given until antibodies are found, and in any case booster doses should be given at intervals of 1–3 years.

If a person immunized up to 1 year before suffers mild exposure, a single booster dose may be enough; for moderate exposure 2 doses 24 hours apart and a booster in 7 days should be given. Severe exposure indicates 5–10 daily doses and a booster at 21 days, though some authorities advise a full course.

If more than 1 year has elapsed since the last booster, a full course should be given.

Control of rabies in animals

This is a matter for consultation with veterinary authorities. Dogs and cats may be immunized on a large scale (as was done in dogs in Malaysia with good results), but where the disease is widespread in wild animals the programme of selective reduction of proved carrier species (for instance foxes, wolves, mongooses, weasels, bats) must be carefully planned (see WHO (1966, 1969) for details).

MARBURG AGENT DISEASE
(VERVET MONKEY DISEASE)

This is an infection of vervet monkeys (*Cercopithecus aethiops*) which infected a number of persons handling them in Marburg, Frankfort and Belgrade. The agent is probably a virus belonging to the vesicular stomatitis–rabies group, and is fatal to monkeys, golden hamsters, guinea-pigs and other laboratory animals. Of 23 human cases in Marburg, 5 were fatal. The patients had worked in a factory where vaccines and sera are prepared, and all had been infected through contact with blood, organs or cultures from a consignment of monkeys from Uganda, or with patients; one was apparently infected during sexual intercourse with her infected husband.

The mode of transmission to monkeys in nature is not known.

In the Marburg series the incubation period was 5–7 days. There was acute fever with a rash of pinhead dark red papules around hair follicles on the face, buttocks, trunk and arms; this developed into a maculo-papular lesion which later coalesced into a more diffuse rash, and in severe cases into a general dark livid erythema on the face, trunk and limbs. After day 16 the patients peeled. A rash also developed on the soft and hard palate. Vomiting, diarrhoea, headache and drowsiness were common, and some patients showed mental disturbances with eventual confusion and coma. Half the patients had lymphadenopathy, and leucopenia was constant, with severe haemorrhagic tendencies in some, leading to bleeding from the gums and nose, haematemesis and melaena.

Infected experimental animals showed widespread degeneration of the liver and necrosis of the spleen, with interstitial pneumonitis. Many cells contained intracytoplasmic bodies, and from the blood of patients and animals, and from the saliva and urine of these animals, the infectious agent was isolated, and grown in tissue culture.

Patients were treated with antibiotics, but without effect. The haemorrhagic tendency needed transfusion of blood, thrombocytes, fibrinogen, epsilon-aminocaproic-acid and vitamin K. A French preparation PPSB from the Centre National de Transfusion Sanguine, Paris, containing prothrombin, proconvertin, Stuart factor and antihaemophil globulin B, was particularly useful. Electrolytes were also given, especially potassium, together with large amounts of human albumin, up to 30 grammes daily. Strophanthin and digitalis were needed. Antipyretics, especially Novalgin (dipyrone) were effective in bringing down temperatures and improving general conditions.

This seems to be a rare disease of monkeys; of 201 sera from live monkeys held in Uganda, none showed antibody to the Marburg virus, but the Marburg monkeys were apparently healthy. It is also evidently rare in man, and is mentioned here because it could occur in persons collecting monkeys for transmission as experimental animals to laboratories in various parts of the world.

This account is taken from the series of papers presented at a meeting of the Royal Society of Tropical Medicine and Hygiene in London, 20 February 1969, and from the discussions on those papers (Martini 1969; Simpson 1969; Zlotnik 1969).

REFERENCES

CHEETHAM, H. D., HART, J., COGHILL, N. F. & FOX, B. (1970) *Lancet*, **i**, 921.
CRICK, J. & BROWN, F. (1970) *Lancet*, **i**, 1106.
EDITORIAL (1965) *Br. med. J.*, **i**, 1565.
———— (1970) *Br. med. J.*, **i**, 37.
———— (1972) *Lancet*, **i**, 132.
FENJE, P. (1970) *Nature, Lond.*, **226**, 171.
MACRAE, A. D. (1969) *Lancet*, **ii**, 1415.
MARTINI, G. A. (1969) *Trans. R. Soc. trop. Med. Hyg.*, **63**, 295.
RELOVA, R. N. (1963) *J. Philip. med. Ass.*, **39**, 765 (Abstract *Trop. Dis. Bull.* (1964) **61**, 562).
RHODES, A. J. (1946) *Trop. Dis. Bull.*, **43**, 975.
RIDLEY, A. (1965) *Br. med. J.*, **i**, 1596.
SIMPSON, D. I. H. (1969) *Trans. R. Soc. trop. Med. Hyg.*, **63**, 303.
TURNER, G. S. (1969) *Br. med. Bull.*, **25**, 136.
WORLD HEALTH ORGANIZATION (1966) *Wld Hlth Org. tech. Rep. Ser.*, 321.
———— (1969) *Surveillance and Control of Rabies*. Report of a conference, Frankfurt am Main, 1968. EURO-0290. Copenhagen: WHO Regional Office for Europe.
ZLOTNIK, I. (1969) *Trans. R. Soc. trop. Med. Hyg.*, **63**, 310.

SECTION IV

DISEASES CAUSED BY BACTERIA

18. LEPROSY

GEOGRAPHICAL DISTRIBUTION

LEPROSY probably affects 12–15 million people throughout the world, but is most common in the tropics and sub-tropics. Tropical Africa has the highest disease rates, ranging from 1 to 43 per 1000 of the population in some parts of Uganda, and even more in parts of West Africa, where surveys have been made. In surveys in East Africa Ross Innes found prevalences of 12–33 per 1000, about 20% of which were lepromatous.

It is also common throughout the Far East (5·8 per 1000 in Burma, 10 in Nepal, 3·6 in Singapore) and the Pacific islands, and in South America (1·34 in Brazil; 4·25 in Surinam). It was formerly endemic in Europe, though in Biblical times and the Middle Ages the name leprosy was given to some skin conditions which were probably not true leprosy. Nevertheless, true leprosy did exist as an endemic disease, for instance in Norway and Spain, until recent times.

Figures quoted from many parts of the world may be unduly low because people are reluctant to report leprosy for fear of local ostracism, or a restraint on their movements or from natural reticence. These reactions tend to be intensified if there is any suggestion of compulsory segregation—an idea now almost universally rejected.

With modern facilities for travel, leprosy is now being introduced into Britain and other temperate countries on a considerable scale, and must be taken into account in differential diagnosis. It should be considered in any untypical or unfamiliar skin disorder in a patient from an endemic area, and in neurological practice it is important to examine for thickened peripheral nerves, particularly the great auricular nerve in the neck, the peroneal, ulnar and the terminal portion of the radial nerve as it passes round the lower end of the radius on the lateral side of the wrist, where it is easily palpable and suitable for biopsy. Thickening should suggest leprosy.

In Britain leprosy is now notifiable (in strict confidence) to the local Medical Officer of Health; there is no suggestion of compulsory segregation. At the end of 1967 there were 357 leprosy patients in England and Wales; 49 were notified in that year; 196 were known to be quiescent (MOH 1967).

AETIOLOGY

Mycobacterium leprae is now the accepted cause of leprosy and is present, usually in great profusion, in the tissues. In size, shape and staining reactions it closely resembles the tubercle bacillus. *Myco. leprae* is acid-fast; it occurs in large numbers in the lesions, chiefly in zoogloea masses within the lepra cells, often grouped together like bundles of cigars or arranged in a palisade. Chains are never seen. Most striking are the intracellular and extracellular masses, known as globi, which consist of clumps of bacilli in capsular material.

Under the electron microscope the bacillus appears to have a great variety of forms. The commonest is a slightly curved filament 3–10 μm in length containing irregular arrangements of dense material sometimes in the shape of rods. Short rod-shaped structures can also be seen (identical with the rod-shaped inclusions within the filaments) and also dense spherical forms. Some of the groups of bacilli can be seen to have a limiting membrane.

A leprotic disease of the rat, which occurs naturally throughout the world, was first observed by Stefansky in Odessa in 1903. Two types are recognized: disease of skin and muscle and disease of lymphatic glands. The bacillus is *Myco. leprae-murium*, morphologically indistinguishable from *Myco. leprae*, and the lesions resemble those of human leprosy, macroscopically as well as histologically. Attempts at cultivation have shown much the same negative results as in human *Myco. leprae*.

In spite of the general similarity of human and rat leprosy, it is generally agreed that the organisms represent two separate and distinct species and there does not seem to be any connection between this disease of the rat and human leprosy.

The most important advance in the bacteriology of leprosy has been the discovery that *Myco. leprae* can infect, and multiply in, the footpads of normal mice, and especially of mice subjected to thymectomy and total body irradiation, and that in the latter mice lepromatous lesions are found after intravenous injection of the bacilli. Inocula of 10 000 *Myco. leprae* into the footpads multiply slowly to give a 100-fold increase in 6–8 months, and during the logarithmic phase the mean generation time is 10–20 days, which is consistent with the natural history of the disease in man, and is responsible for the chronicity of the footpad test (Rees 1967). The infection spreads via the blood stream, and after 2 or more years gives rise to granulomas and neural damage at the sites of inoculation and the nose, ears and tail skin; the histological features of human leprosy in the borderline range are reproduced (Rees *et al.* 1969). Similar results have been found in the ear and footpad of hamsters and the footpad of rats.

Immunologically deficient mice are accurate models for studying the development of lepromatous leprosy. Peripheral nerves are sometimes involved, with focal damage related to the blood-vessels where they enter the nerves. This ability to cultivate *Myco. leprae* in animals, besides fulfilling one of Koch's postulates, affords an invaluable opportunity of testing and screening new drugs, and also of detecting resistance to standard drugs, which has been observed in certain strains of the bacilli. *Myco. leprae* are often found in the smooth muscle of the skin and its vessels. They have now been found in striped muscle in mice and in man, and they may be able to multiply in human muscle and smooth muscle, as well as in skin and nerve tissue at the beginning of their pathological career. Tissue culture of human skin fibroblasts may permit multiplication. These subjects are being examined.

There have been many reports of cultivation in *artificial* media of acid-fast bacilli from the skin or other tissues of leprosy patients, and many authors have claimed such bacilli to be true leprosy bacilli, but no satisfactory evidence of this has been produced. Most of the organisms were non-pathogenic, rapidly multiplying saprophytes, and similar organisms have been cultivated from the skin of persons free from leprosy.

It is now generally accepted that only leprosy bacilli which stain with carbol fuchsin as solid acid-fast rods are viable, and that bacilli which stain irregularly are probably dead and degenerating. This is not to say that all solid bacilli are viable—there must be stages at which they are dead but not yet disintegrated.

The differences are very apparent in preparations examined under the electron microscope, but can be appreciated under the light microscope. These differences are valuable pointers, in biopsy specimens, to the effects of treatment. In patients receiving standard treatment with DDS (dapsone), a very high proportion of bacilli are killed within 3 months, which suggests that many of the manifestations of leprosy, including reactions of the erythema nodosum type, which follow initial treatment, must be due in part to dead rather than living bacilli. We therefore need drugs which will help the body to dispose of dead but still intact leprosy bacilli.

Two indices (Ridley 1967), which depend on observation of *Myco. leprae* in smears from skin or nasal smears, are important in assessing the amount of infection and the viability of the organisms, and also the progress of the patient under treatment. They are:

1. *The morphological index (MI)*. This is calculated by counting the numbers of solid-staining acid-fast rods in a smear made by nicking the skin with a sharp scalpel and scraping it; the fluid and tissue obtained are spread fairly thickly on a slide and stained by the Ziehl–Neelsen method and decolorized (but not completely) with 1% acid–alcohol. Only the solid-staining bacilli are viable. It is not unusual for solid-staining *Myco. leprae* to reappear for short periods in patients being successfully treated with drugs.

2. *The bacteriological index (BI)*. This is an expression of the weight of infection. It is calculated by counting 6–8 stained smears under the 100 × oil immersion lens. The results are expressed on a logarithmic scale:

1+	At least 1 bacillus in every 100 fields
2+	At least 1 bacillus in every 10 fields
3+	At least 1 bacillus in every field
4+	At least 10 bacilli in every field
5+	At least 100 bacilli in every field
6+	At least 1000 bacilli in every field

The bacteriological index is valuable because it is simple and is representative of many lesions, but is affected by the depth of the skin incision, the thoroughness of the scrape, and the thickness of the film.

A more accurate and reliable index of the bacillary content of a lesion is given by the Logarithmic Index of Biopsies (LIB). This is mainly used in research and the details should be sought in the original paper (Ridley 1967). These indices help to assess the state of patients at the beginning of treatment, and to assess progress.

A review of modern methods of study of leprosy by laboratory techniques was published by Rees (1969b).

TRANSMISSION

Most leprologists believe that infection is contracted through the skin, but some believe that it can be contracted via the upper respiratory tract. The whole question of transmission, however, is not clear. The most important feature is the presence of, and number of, infectious persons in the community, and the risk of infection through contact with such persons.

Tuberculoid leprosy is not usually infectious in that the lesions are not open, and do not obviously shed bacilli, though there is some epidemiological evidence that secondary cases can arise from contact with patients who have tuberculoid leprosy. In lepromatous leprosy the skin lesions and nasal mucosa are loaded with bacilli, and the patients are infectious. In borderline leprosy the patients should be regarded as infectious.

EPIDEMIOLOGY

The classical view is that leprosy is an infectious disease, but that for infection to spread from one person to another, there must be close and prolonged contact, or challenge by large numbers of bacilli at one time, such as occurs within families or among close associates. On the other hand, many cases have been reported in which contact was apparently neither prolonged nor very intimate, but in which repeated contact was a factor. Sexual contact has been suggested as the source of infection, not, presumably, via the sex organs but through the close physical contact involved. Cases have also been reported in which leprosy was transmitted apparently by blood transfusion, and in the process of tattooing, and possibly that of variolation.

The mycobacteria are present in large numbers in the nasal mucosa and skin of lepromatous patients, and are presumably spread in discharges from open lesions; they may be air-borne. Whether there is a hereditary factor, a genetically controlled susceptibility, as postulated in Uganda, is a subject for research with methods of genetic study now becoming available. The study of marriage patterns may help in this. This question of genetic constitution in relation to susceptibility is difficult. Spickett (in Cochrane & Davey 1964) discusses it at length, taking the view that of the various environmental factors thought to influence susceptibility, climate is not important and nor are hygiene, the standard of living or diet. Nor does variation in the probability of contact with infectious patients provide a sufficient explanation for the distribution within populations or families. The evidence suggests that there must be some other factor, and that this factor must be genetic. It would be strange if this were not so.

The attack rate for household contacts of lepromatous patients is 6–8 times as high as for non-contacts, but the rate for contacts of tuberculoid patients is less than twice as high as for non-contacts. Nevertheless, it is probably true that most patients, whatever the form of leprosy they have, are infectious at some time or another to susceptible persons.

A high rate of conjugal leprosy (106 spouses in 1830 couples, one of whom had leprosy—58 per 1000) was reported by Mohamed Ali (1965) and somewhat higher rates have been reported elsewhere, but these may suggest an exaggerated estimate of true conjugal transmission, in that in some cases the infection was probably contracted before marriage. Nevertheless, conjugal infection has been substantiated, as in the case reported by the late Sir Philip Manson-Bahr, of leprosy in the wife of a patient who died of leprosy. She had never been out of England, but developed the disease after an incubation period of 7 years.

Age is probably a factor, and it has usually been considered that infants and children are more susceptible than adults. Browne (1965a), from a study at Uzuakoli in Eastern Nigeria, concludes that incidence of new infections increases with age for the first 4 decades. Nevertheless, there have been many reports indicating that adults are susceptible and that age is much less important than contact and the intimacy of contact. Children are likely to have more intimate contact with parents and other children than older persons have among themselves. Children have been known to infect their parents.

It has often been said that males are rather more susceptible than females, but it seems to be more likely that the difference in incidence is due rather to the fact that males have more opportunities for contact than females in many communities. Where opportunities are equal, incidence is equal. But lepromatous leprosy does seem to be more common in males than in females (1·6: 1).

Great variations have been recorded in the proportions of lepromatous and tuberculoid leprosy in different countries. Skinsnes (in Cochrane & Davey 1964) quotes 60·7% lepromatous in Brazil, 63·5% in Japan, 69·8% in the U.S.S.R., against only 21·2% in New Guinea, 12·0% in India and 7·0% in Angola; these reports were made on several thousands of observed cases in each instance. Conversely, the tuberculoid or non-lepromatous percentages were high 78·7%: in New Guinea, 88% in India and 47% (tuberculoid) and 46% (indeterminate) in Angola. Similarly, low or moderate rates were found in Brazil, Japan and the U.S.S.R. These findings suggest a racial factor in resistance to leprosy, but this may be the result of a long experience of the disease in the countries with low lepromatous rates, and vice versa; that is, a matter of natural selection.

Skinsnes distinguishes between the epidemic patterns of leprosy in fresh populations and in endemic foci. His table may be set out as in Table 21.

Table 21. Epidemic patterns of leprosy

Fresh populations	Endemic foci
Rapid spread	Slow spread
In most houses of a village	In foci and families
Endemic of tuberculoid, few macules	More lepromatous (20–25%)
Adults and children almost equally susceptible	Mostly in young adults and children
Mostly no contact with lepromatous leprosy. Not prolonged intimate contact	Most patients have contact with lepromatous leprosy, often prolonged and intimate

A sense of proportion is necessary. Thousands of doctors and nurses have attended leprosy patients without becoming infected, though there have been some tragedies. Whatever the relative importance of constitution on the one hand and opportunity for infection on the other, it is true to say that leprosy flourishes most where life is lived in primitive conditions and where over-crowding exists—not necessarily in cities, but wherever people live and sleep in close intimate contact, as in village life. Poverty and diet may be factors but, in spite of much speculation, no clear evidence has been adduced that diet has any direct bearing on susceptibility to leprosy. It is interesting to note that in spite of the occasional introduction of leprosy patients into such countries as Britain and the United States, there is no indication that the disease has spread to the communities to which they entered. This is not to say that they do not infect close physical contacts.

CLASSIFICATION

When leprosy bacilli gain access to the tissues they may quickly be destroyed by the protective phagocytes of the host; phagocytes with engulfed bacilli can sometimes be found in skin biopsies of normal contacts who do not develop overt leprosy. Genetic characters are no doubt factors in this process.

If the bacilli do obtain a foothold, the defence mechanisms of the host (varying from effective to poor) create a reaction which at first is named indeterminate because the lesion is too immature to be classifiable. This may persist for months or years, or go on to complete healing, or to one of the fairly clear-cut forms of clinical leprosy, but the indeterminate form shows no sign of the form which will emerge.

The recognizable forms of leprosy show a continuous spectrum of severity, according to the immune status of the host, from the tuberculoid form, in which resistance is high, to the lepromatous form at the other pole, in which resistance is low. Between these extremes there is a borderline (sometimes known as dimorphous) form which may show some characters of tuberculoid tendency, or some of lepromatous tendency.

This differentiation into 3 forms has been widely accepted, and is adequate for many purposes, but the general spectrum of the disease may be more usefully divided, histologically and clinically, into 5 grades (Ridley & Jopling 1966). This classification is shown in Tables 22 and 23. The initials used are:

TT   Tuberculoid
BT   Borderline-tuberculoid
BB   Borderline
BL   Borderline-lepromatous
LL   Lepromatous

Tuberculoid leprosy tends towards healing, though neural damage may be permanent.

Table 22. Histological classification of leprosy (Ridley & Jopling 1966)

Histological feature	TT	BT	BB	BL	LL
Granuloma	Epithelioid cells with or without giant cells, in foci	Like TT	Epithelioid cells but no giant cells	a. Histiocytes evolving to epithelioid cells; scanty foamy change. Lymphocytes scanty b. Histiocytes sometimes foamy; no large globi. Many lymphocytes	*Active:* Macrophages round or spindle-shaped, with very many bacilli *Regressive:* Histiocytes with fatty change; foam cells or globi often large; multinucleate
Lymphocytes	Dense zone of infiltration round foci of granuloma	Like TT	Usually scanty. If present they are diffusely spread through granuloma	a. Scanty b. Numerous, occupying whole segments of granuloma, or forming perineural cuffs	Scanty, diffuse
Nerves	Those in granuloma usually destroyed beyond recognition. Occasional caseation	Greatly swollen by Schwann cell proliferation. Perineural sheath intact	Moderate Schwann cell proliferation. Sheath intact	No cell proliferation in nerve bundle, which is often structureless. May be infiltration of histiocytes in perineurium	May show structural damage but not infiltration or cuffing
Sub-epidermal zone	Granuloma extends to basal layer of epidermis. No clear zone	Clear sub-epidermal zone, usually narrow	Clear sub-epidermal zone, broad or narrow	Like BB	Like BB
Bacilli in granuloma	None seen	0 – 3 +	3 – 5 +	5 or 6 +	5 or 6 +

Table 23. Clinical classification of leprosy (Ridley & Jopling 1966)

TT	BT	BB	BL	LL
Lesions consist of a few macules and/or plaques. Plaques tend to be large, have a rough dry hairless surface and well defined edges from which there is a gradual slope to a flattened centre	May be confused clinically with TT but differentiated by: (*a*) Lesions more numerous, surface less dry and rough, edges less well defined, and hair growth may be slight; and (*b*) Annular lesions common, the peripheral band of tissue being raised and having well defined outer and inner edges	Macules and plaques are intermediate in number and size between TT and LL. 'Punched-out' lesions are characteristic. Annular lesions occur as in BT	May be confused clinically with LL but differentiated by: (*a*) Macules and plaques not consistently small, edges less vague, and less tendency to bilateral symmetry. Some may have 'punched-out' appearance. (*b*) Papules and nodules unusual and few. Nodules may be dimpled. (*c*) Rare and less marked are iritis and keratitis, nasal ulceration, madarosis, thickened ear lobes, testicular damage and bone changes	Macules, papules, nodules and plaques may all be present. Lesions small, multiple, distributed bilaterally and symmetrically with smooth shiny surface. Macules and plaques have vague edges and and no hair loss. May be nasal ulceration, iritis and keratitis, madarosis, leonine facies, thickened ear lobes, testicular damage, oedema of legs, and bone changes in limbs and skull
Distribution of lesions asymmetrical		Distribution of lesions asymmetrical		
Lesions markedly anaesthetic	Lesions moderately anaesthetic	Lesions show mild anaesthesia	Some lesions may show slight patchy anaesthesia	Lesions not anaesthetic
Nerve thickening early, often single. First manifestations may be neural	Nerve thickening early, more numerous than in TT. First manifestations may be neural	Nerve thickening early, more numerous than in BT. First manifestations may be neural	Nerve thickening early, more numerous than in BB. First manifestations may be neural	Nerve thickening (and damage) late and tends to be bilateral and symmetrical (e.g. glove and stocking anaesthesia). First manifestations never neural
Lepromin test strongly positive	Lepromin test moderately or weakly positive	Lepromin test negative	Lepromin test negative	Lepromin test negative

The polar forms, tuberculoid (TT) and lepromatous (LL), are relatively stable, but the borderline form is unstable. Without treatment it tends to deteriorate to lepromatous. After treatment it sometimes reverts. Lepromatous leprosy, which may develop directly from indeterminate or from borderline leprosy, is less likely to revert to borderline after treatment.

PATHOLOGY

In very early infection (and in skin biopsies of some presumably healthy contacts) the fixed cells of the dermis near the acid-fast bacilli proliferate, and monocytes from the blood migrate towards the bacilli, engulfing and disintegrating them. Leprosy bacilli may also enter nerves, causing focal damage related to the blood-vessels near their site of entry into the nerves. They spread along the fine fibres of cutaneous nerve twigs and are carried centripetally, multiplying and bursting into the endoneural spaces, where they are phagocytosed by histiocytes. In this way an incipient infection may be eradicated, though this is less likely once the bacilli have gained a foothold in nerves. If a skin lesion develops, a biopsy specimen at this stage shows foci of inflammatory cellular exudate, mainly round the finest nerve fibres in plexuses in the dermis. The exudate is determined by the ability of the host to react immunologically and it consists of lymphocytes, histiocytes and other cells; clinically it is marked on the skin by weal-like papules or pink or pale macules. This is the *indeterminate* stage of infection, which usually occurs in children in whom resistance has not been determined, and which may last for months, or may resolve, or may progress to *tuberculoid, dimorphous (borderline)* or *lepromatous* leprosy, depending on the immunological response of the body.

In lepromin-negative persons (whose resistance is poor) the histiocytes gradually change into lepra cells, which in more severe cases become foamy; the ingested bacilli are not destroyed. In lepromin-positive persons (whose resistance is good) the histiocytes change into epithelioid cells after ingesting the bacilli, which they destroy.

But although the manner of evolution of these cells containing *Myco. leprae* is important, the mediators of immunity are the lymphocytes, and although the lymphocytes in skin lesions are not all immunologically active, the numbers present in tuberculoid and borderline lesions are significant indications of the degree of resistance to the infections.

Tuberculoid leprosy

The change from indeterminate to tuberculoid leprosy involves the appearance of groups of epithelioid cells (derived from histiocytes) inside fine nerve twigs and the formation of sharply circumscribed foci of these cells in the dermis, often surrounded by a zone of lymphocytes, which are fairly numerous. The epithelioid cells often coalesce to form giant cells. The epidermis is thinner than normal and there are foci of inflammatory cells reaching the epidermis without a clear space. In the dermis the granulomatous cords follow the lines of neuro-vascular bundles. The nerve bundles in the skin are swollen by proliferation of Schwann cells, which develop into epithelioid cells. The nerves become difficult to recognize; they occasionally undergo caseation, which does not occur in leprosy except in nerves.

Acid-fast bacilli are very rare in the cells of the inflammatory exudate in tuberculoid leprosy, except in reaction phases, but bacilli may be found in the active extending margin of a tuberculoid macule.

The most consistent feature of tuberculoid leprosy is the early involvement of peripheral nerves and ganglions, both somatic and sympathetic. In the upper extremity this often goes on to weakness and paralysis of the intrinsic muscles of the hand (*main-en-griffe*) and in the leg to drop foot. Damage to the sympathetic nerves leads to slow atrophy and absorption (osteoporosis) of the small bones of the hands and feet through interference with vasodilatation.

Borderline leprosy

Indeterminate leprosy often goes on to the borderline form in which large hypopigmented patches appear, often on the limbs, usually with loss of sensations of touch and temperature. Satellite macules, with varying degrees of sharpness in the edges, also appear; they are usually small. Acid-fast bacilli can always be found in these lesions by concentration techniques, or even by routine methods. The lepromin reaction is variable, but is usually weakly positive.

The histological picture shows features intermediate between those of lepromatous and tuberculoid lesions. There is an inflammatory reaction with cellular exudate in the superficial layers of the dermis; it consists of small round cells, histiocytes and clumps of epithelioid cells but no giant cells. Nerves may show large numbers of bacilli and round cells, or epithelioid cells with few bacilli, i.e. they may resemble nerves in lepromatous or tuberculoid disease. This dimorphous leprosy is unstable and tends to progress to the lepromatous form if not treated.

Lepromatous leprosy

In the skin lesions in fully developed lepromatous disease large areas of the dermis are connected into continuous sheets of chronic inflammatory tissue containing enormous numbers of bacilli in slabs of lepra (Virchow) cells (derived from histiocytes) interspersed with groups of mononuclear and plasma cells. Lymphocytes are scanty. The subepidermal zone of the dermis is clear of infiltrate. The disease is now systemic, the bacilli being transported by blood or lymph to distant parts of the body, for instance the testes, though most of them are trapped by the lymph nodes, liver, spleen and bone marrow, where miliary lepromas may be found.

The mucous membrane of the upper respiratory tract from the nose to the larynx, including the root of the tongue and the peritonsillar tissues, is heavily infiltrated in advanced lepromatous leprosy. It is oedematous, thickened and ulcerated, and the nasal cartilages may be perforated. If the disease regresses, however, either spontaneously or as a result of treatment, the skin lesions heal in a remarkable manner.

IMMUNOLOGY

Leprosy bacilli are not killed or eliminated by humoral antibodies, but are killed by cellular immune mechanisms similar to those which eliminate tubercle bacilli. But though not killed by humoral antibodies, leprosy bacilli stimulate the production of humoral antibodies against their various constituent antigens. Cell-mediated immunity (by lymphocytes) is strong in tuberculoid leprosy but weak or absent in lepromatous leprosy (Turk 1969). Humoral antibodies are plentiful, but immunologically useless, in lepromatous leprosy.

The immunity is cell-mediated by lymphocytes, which show dense infiltration round the foci of tuberculoid leprosy but are scanty and diffuse in lepromatous leprosy—the antithesis of concentrations of leprosy bacilli, which are scanty in tuberculoid leprosy but abound in lepromatous leprosy. Partial non-specific failure of cell-mediated immunity could be secondary to massive infiltration of paracortical areas of lymph nodes by histiocytes containing ingested myco-bacteria (Turk & Waters 1969). Leprosy patients can, however, resist other infections. Anergy is associated with suppression of lymphocyte production, though circulating antibodies are abundant in these patients.

Reactions associated with an increase of immunity and a movement towards the borderline form may be precipitated in experimental leprosy (in thymecto-mized mice) by injection of normal lymphoid cells.

Erythema nodosum leprosum is associated with an increase of complement and immunoglobulins, and auto-antibodies are sometimes present, though these do not differ significantly from the findings in non-reacting lepromatous leprosy. The fluorescent antibody techniques give inconstant results. Serum gamma-globulin is increased, particularly during the stage of lepra reaction, and when diffuse hepatic lesions are present. The erythrocyte sedimentation test is in accord with the albumin–globulin ratio, which is usually below unity. A modification of the haemagglutination test gives 91% positive results in lepromatous leprosy, and 70% in tuberculoid.

In lepromatous (but not tuberculoid) leprosy there are serum antibodies which react with mycobacterial polysaccharides but are not protective; this subject needs more research.

Bacillaemia

Bacillaemia occurs in leprosy. Karat *et al.* (1971) examined biopsy specimens from 240 leprosy patients in India; 21% of those with tuberculoid disease and 62% of those with lepromatous disease showed leprous granulomas in the liver; BT, BB and BL patients gave intermediate results. This indicates that bacillaemia occurs even in the so-called 'immune' group. Acid-fast bacilli were also seen in the liver in BT, BB, BL and LL groups, even when treatment had produced negative bacterial indices in the skin.

Lepromin

The lepromin test is used widely in leprosy. Lepromin is a substance derived from nodular lepromatous tissue, from which epidermis and fat are removed, and which contains masses of leprosy bacilli, or from infected lymph nodes rich in bacilli; it is autoclaved and either ground up in saline and then filtered and phenolized, or prepared by some other convenient method, and it represents a suspension of the bacilli together with much cellular matter from the host tissues. Lepromin is injected intradermally in a dose of 0·1 ml.

Lepromin may be standardized to contain about 600 million leprosy bacilli per ml, but recent work suggests that equally good results are obtained with lepromin containing only 20 million per ml.

Reactions to lepromin are of 2 kinds:

1. The early (Fernandez) reaction which becomes positive in 48 hours and shows erythema and infiltration 10–15 mm in diameter (+ reaction), 15–20 mm (+ +) or over 20 mm (+ + +).

2. The late (Mitsuda) reaction read at 4–5 weeks, positive results giving + reaction (3–5 mm), + + (over 5 mm) or + + + (with ulceration).

It is generally understood that the early, Fernandez, reaction, in which desiccated *Myco. leprae* from lepromatous tissue were originally suspended in oil, and injected intradermally in a dose of 0·1 ml, is an allergic reaction similar to the tuberculin reaction. It is positive in all forms of leprosy (unlike the Mitsuda reaction), but most strongly positive in the tuberculoid form. It is a reflection of the sensitivity of the tissues to the protein of the leprosy bacilli. The late (Mitsuda) reaction, however, which is elicited only by whole leprosy bacilli—not by separate fractions—does not reflect the allergic state, but is an index of resistance.

The suggestion has been made, with some support (Newell 1966), that most people have the capacity to react specifically to *Myco. leprae* by virtue of a constitutional factor N (natural) which they possess. A minority of people lack this factor; they are anergic, and lepromatous leprosy tends to occur in this group.

The Mitsuda reaction is strongly positive in tuberculoid leprosy, usually negative or weakly positive in borderline leprosy and almost invariably negative in lepromatous leprosy. It is sometimes positive in persons who have never been in contact with the leprosy bacillus, and the test is therefore of no diagnostic value. A positive result indicates resistance to leprosy bacilli; a negative result in a patient with the disease is a sign of poor resistance.

In lepromatous leprosy the Mitsuda reaction is negative, partly, it is thought, owing to a subnormal response of leucocytes to physical stimuli, and to antigens totally unrelated to *Myco. leprae*. These responses are suppressed by factors in lepromatous serum. Some severe lepromatous leprosy cases are associated with the delayed allergic response to skin test antigens, or delayed rejection of skin grafts (Turk & Waters 1968).

Reversal of a negative to a positive Mitsuda test in a leprosy patient is taken as a sign of increased resistance and therefore of improved prognosis; in fact this test is used to assess progress. Over-use of the test, however, is said to produce a temporary allergic sensitization to lepromin, which may have no relation to resistance and could therefore confuse the issue.

Injections of BCG in leprosy patients negative to lepromin have some effect in converting the Mitsuda reaction to positive; in patients with a positive Mitsuda reaction, BCG may increase the intensity of that reaction. How far this is related to true resistance is still a matter for conjecture.

CLINICAL FEATURES

Cochrane and Davey (1964) make an important statement: 'It should be emphasized that a diagnosis of leprosy is seldom justified unless one of two cardinal signs is present:

1. Clinical signs of nerve involvement.
2. The demonstration of *Myco. leprae* in the skin and/or in the nasal mucous membranes.'

The first definite evidence of nerve involvement is said by Cochrane to be an area of anaesthesia, which may have been preceded by vague symptoms such as tingling, or pain in a nerve trunk. A patient who complains of a patch of numbness should be examined and observed very closely, even though a definite diagnosis may not be possible for years. In such a patient the possibility of leprosy infection should be enquired into, and smears from ear lobes, forehead and buttocks should be examined for bacilli; biopsies should also be taken from the area of numbness and examined in the same way.

The initial manifestation in children is, especially, hypopigmentation with anaesthesia; no other disease produces this. Bacilli may be hard to find. Browne (1965a) from Uzuakoli described 13 patients with confluent macular lepromatous leprosy in whom, for some time, a generalized hypopigmentation was the only sign of the disease until other manifestations of lepromatous leprosy appeared. The hypopigmentation grew from the confluence of macular areas, but spared the inguinal region, the axillae and part of the lumbar region; these areas of apparently normal skin usually contained *Myco. leprae* and globi. In all the patients the confluent hypopigmentary condition had been unnoticed.

Spontaneous healing may take place after the early lesions of childhood, but though this is quite common in some communities, it obviously cannot be taken for granted; a definite diagnosis is an indication for treatment.

Incubation period

This is undoubtedly very variable, and the chief difficulty of establishing the incubation period in any given case is the fact that early symptoms and signs of the disease may be overlooked or ignored for years. Another difficulty is that patients often attempt to hide the true facts about leprosy. Although short incubation periods of a few months have been recorded in infants born of leprous parents, the average is about $3\frac{1}{2}$ years. Longer incubation periods are not unusual, especially in those who fail to observe early signs of the disease, and the late Sir Philip Manson-Bahr in London diagnosed as leprosy a case which had been regarded as seborrhoea of the face and ears in which the incubation period appeared to be as long as 31 years.

As compared with tuberculosis, one of the chief characteristics of leprosy is the absence of toxicity; enormous numbers of bacilli may be present in the body with few signs. The local inflammatory reactions to lepra bacilli vary within wide limits. Thus, in one patient the disease is so localized that it affects one small skin area or its main nerve supply. There may be acute inflammatory swelling, local pain, trophic, sensory and other disturbances. Bacilli can be demonstrated with great difficulty. In contrast, a second case may show involvement of almost the whole body, so that a preparation taken from any part of the skin may reveal numerous bacilli, though the patient is not acutely ill and is able to be about and do his work. The nerves are not noticeably thickened, and superficially the skin appears normal. At any stage during invasion sudden exanthematous reactions may appear, accompanied by fever and general symptoms.

The *chronic onset* is so gradual and insidious that the disease has advanced to a considerable extent before any abnormality is evident. There may be tenderness, tingling or thickening of a nerve, an area of anaesthesia, perhaps with some change in the appearance of the skin, insensitiveness to burning, formication, tingling or numbness of extremities. Discoloured skin patches may be mistaken for eczema or ringworm; these may at first be small, gradually increasing in size.

In the *acute onset* there are occasionally multiple lesions with less diffused margins, which tend to spread rapidly and which contain very numerous bacilli. The first noticeable sign may be an evanescent rash. The onset may be determined by some other acute disease, such as malaria or typhoid, which lowers resistance. It may also be the sequel to chronic infection, such as syphilis, ancylostomiasis or chronic disease of the gastro-intestinal tract. The period of life may also have some bearing, e.g. extra strain imposed on the body during puberty, parturition and menopause.

Lepromatous leprosy

This is the type seen in persons with a negligible resistance; leprosy bacilli are widely disseminated throughout the skin, nerves and reticulo-endothelial system. In addition, there may be bacillary invasion of eyes, testes, bones and mucous membranes of mouth, nose, pharynx, larynx and trachea; one of the earliest signs in children is swelling and tenderness of the tip of the nose, oedema and infiltration of the alar cartilages.

Skin lesions are multiple, small, symmetrically distributed, and take the form of macules, infiltrations (plaques), papules and nodules, all of which may be present in the same patient at the same time once the disease has become well established. The pure diffuse type is an exception and will be described later. The earliest skin lesions are macules; these are level with the skin and therefore cannot be palpated. They are small, circular or elliptical, are erythematous in light skins with sometimes a coppery or purple hue, and in dark skins they are coppery with sometimes a faintly hypopigmented background. They have a smooth and shiny surface, their edges are indistinct and they are not anaesthetic or anhidrotic. Owing to the fact that these macules are often difficult to see and are not associated with itching or anaethesia, they may be ignored by the patient. They may be situated on any part of the body, but are unusual in the axillae, groins, perineum, on the external genitalia or on the scalp. They are most commonly found on the face, buttocks and extremities, and on the limbs the flexor surfaces may be involved as well as the extensor, and the palms and soles as well as the backs of hands and feet.

Infiltrated lesions are raised above the level of the skin and give a sensation of thickening when gripped between finger and thumb. Their distribution and colouring are the same as those of lepromatous macules, excepting that they do not appear on palms and soles owing to the thickness and tightness of the skin. They are raised in the centre and slope away peripherally to merge imperceptibly with the surrounding skin, have a smooth and shiny surface, and do not exhibit sensory loss, unless situated in a region of skin which is already

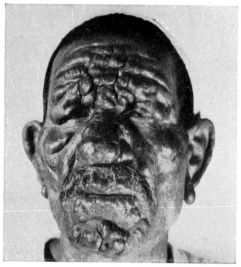

Fig. 124.—Lepromatous leprosy in an Egyptian. (*Dr H.K. Giffen*)

anaesthetic as a result of peripheral nerve damage. Papules and nodules make their appearance as the disease advances, and particularly favour the face, ears and buttocks. Ears should always be carefully examined, for the lobes are more constantly affected than any other part and appear thickened quite early in the course of the disease, such thickening being readily confirmed by palpation with finger and thumb. Advanced infiltration and nodulation of the face give rise to leontiasis, or 'leonine faces', in which the normal wrinkles on the forehead and cheeks have become deep furrows (Fig. 124). Nodules and infiltrations may undergo superficial necrosis and ulceration, and large ulcers may form on the lower legs when leprous infiltration of the skin is associated with chronic bilateral lymphoedema, secondary to massive bacillary invasion of the lymphatics. Thinning of the eyebrows is common, commencing in the lateral half and sometimes progressing to complete loss of eyebrows and eyelashes (superciliary and ciliary madarosis). Alopecia may occur, but is uncommon.

One particular variety of skin infiltration requires separate mention, namely, the pure diffuse type described by Lucio and Alvarado in Mexico in 1852 and later by Latapi in 1938. The skin of the whole body becomes diffusely infiltrated (no macular stage being observed) rendering it stiff and smooth as in sclero-derma. There is no obvious disfigurement apart from loss of eyebrows and eyelashes which always occurs, but there may be widespread small telangiectases, nasal destruction may develop and sometimes there is alopecia and loss of body hair. Laryngeal ulceration has been recorded, but cutaneous nodules and ocular involvement are absent. Mexican physicians have described, in these patients, a unique form of lepra reaction known as 'Lucio's phenomenon' in which painful, purpuric, ulcerating patches appear on the skin, becoming crusted and leaving scars (Jopling 1971).

Nerve involvement, in the absence of skin involvement, has not been described in lepromatous leprosy, but combined dermal and neural changes are a usual

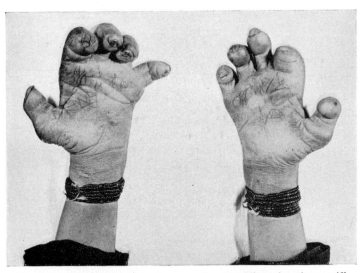

Fig. 125.—Late lepromatous leprosy, showing bilateral *main-en-griffe* and shortening of the fingers. These hands are anaesthetic. (*Dr H. K. Giffen*)

finding. Nerves do not show signs of damage as early as in the other types of leprosy, but nerve thickening and associated sensory or motor dysfunction can usually be demonstrated as the disease advances. As sensory loss is often more pronounced than muscular wasting, patients continue to use the affected limbs and the skin suffers much damage from repeated trauma owing to insensitivity to pain. Thus the hands become scarred from injuries and burns, and trophic ulcers develop on the soles of the feet. Nerve thickening, like skin involvement, tends to be bilateral and symmetrical, but there may be a difference in degree on the two sides. It is found in those peripheral nerves which are superficial in some part of their course, the thickening being localized to the superficial portion, e.g. the great auricular nerves in the neck, the supraclavicular nerves as they cross the clavicles, the ulnar nerves just above the elbows, the ante-brachial cutaneous nerves in the forearms, the radial and median nerves at the wrists, the femoral cutaneous nerves, the common peroneals as they wind round the necks of the fibulae, the superficial peroneals in front of the ankles and the

posterior tibial nerves immediately below the internal malleoli. The earliest
sensory disturbances may take the form of paraesthesia, hyperaesthesia and
hyperalgesia, to be followed later by impairment of light touch, temperature or
pain sensation. All three modalities should be tested when examining a patient,
as sometimes only one is affected (dissociated anaesthesia); in such a case it is
usually the ability to differentiate between hot and cold which is lost first.
Loss of position sense, vibration sense and tendon reflexes may occur, but not
commonly. Muscle wasting may produce deformities such as claw hand (ulnar
nerve), *main-en-griffe* (combined ulnar and median nerves), dropped foot
(common peroneal nerve) and facial palsy (facial nerve), but careful examination
of muscles will show evidence of weakness long before paralysis occurs (Fig.
125).

Involvement of autonomic nerves manifests itself, in the early stages, by
slight oedema of the hands or feet; more marked vasomotor disturbance
develops later causing the skin of hands and feet to be puffy and cyanosed.

In addition to skin and nerves the following tissues may be involved in
lepromatous leprosy:

Nails of fingers and toes. These are affected when trophic changes take place
in digits, and appear dry, lustreless, narrowed and longitudinally ridged.

Mucous membranes. The patient may complain of nasal discharge, possibly
bloodstained, and of blocking of the airway, and examination reveals hyperaemia
and swelling of the mucosa together with nodules or ulcers on the nasal septum.
Ulceration leads to septal perforation and later to cartilage destruction and
consequent 'saddle-nose' deformity. Nodules may also form on the lips, tongue,
palate and larynx, leading to ulceration. Laryngeal involvement gives rise to
hoarse cough, husky voice and to stridor. Oedema of the glottis, occurring as
part of a reactional state, used to be a dreaded complication in the precortisone
era, calling for immediate tracheotomy. Perforation of the palate may occur in
the absence of syphilis or yaws.

For the effects of leprosy on the eye, see Chapter 44.

Bones. Changes in bones in lepromatous leprosy are confined to the skull and
limbs. In the limbs the changes are almost solely concentrated in the hands and
feet and are due to a combination of factors which include: (*a*) Deposition of
bacilli; (*b*) Neurotrophic atrophy; (*c*) Repeated trauma resulting from analgesia;
(*d*) Disuse owing to paralysis and contractures; (*e*) Secondary infection from
trophic ulceration; (*f*) Generalized osteoporosis of hormonal origin. Deposition
of bacilli in the medullary cavities, the periosteum and the nutrient vessels
gives rise to bone cysts, enlarged nutrient foramina, aseptic necrosis and spindle-
shaped leprous dactylitis closely simulating that of tuberculosis or syphilis.
Leprous periostitis of the tibia, fibula and ulna have been described. Neurotrophic atrophy affecting the hands is localized to the phalanges, commencing
with shortening and gradual disappearance of the distal phalanges, followed by
gradual melting away of the middle and proximal phalanges in turn. Metacarpals
and carpal bones are spared. In the feet the atrophic changes are localized to
the metatarsals and phalanges, commencing in the proximal phalanges or in
the heads of the metatarsals. In the proximal phalanges the diaphyses become
gradually thinned by rarefying osteitis, known as 'concentric bone atrophy', so
that eventually there is but a fine needle of bone left. This may be followed by
disappearance of the affected bones, and the shortened toes are connected to
the foot by soft tissue only.

In the metatarsals absorption begins at the distal ends which become thinned
and pointed—the 'sucked candy stick' appearance. The tarsal bones are spared.

Sensory loss results in repeated trauma, both major and minor, and this is an important contributory factor to the production of bone atrophy and absorption. Brand states: 'By far the greatest proportion of finger absorption is secondary to burns and trauma which follow anaesthesia.' In addition, sensory loss can lead to the development of Charcot joints in the fingers, toes, wrists or ankles.

Muscle paralysis can lead to disuse and, in neglected cases, to fibrous or bony ankylosis of the interphalangeal, metacarpophalangeal and metatarsophalangeal joints. Disuse also results in osteoporosis owing to decreased osteoblastic activity.

Secondary infection commonly follows neglected trophic ulceration of feet or hand and can result in pyogenic osteomyelitis.

Generalized osteoporosis may follow defective production of testosterone as a result of testicular damage.

Changes in the skull in lepromatous leprosy consist of atrophy of the anterior nasal spine and the maxillary alveolar process, probably caused by a combination of aseptic necrosis—due to leprous endarteritis—and pyogenic osteomyelitis due to gross ulceration in the nose.

Reticulo-endothelial system. Lymph glands may be enlarged and painless, with the consistency of soft rubber, particularly the femoral, inguinal and epitrochlear glands, but occasionally one or more glands become very swollen and tender as part of a reactional state. The reticulo-endothelial elements of the abdominal viscera are invaded by bacilli, especially in the spleen and liver, and the red marrow is similarly invaded. Lymphoedema of the lower legs may occur, giving rise to elephantiasis in neglected cases.

Testes. Testicular atrophy may occur, resulting in sterility and gynaecomastia.

Serological tests for syphilis (Wassermann and Kahn) are usually positive in lepromatous leprosy, but the TPI test remains negative in the absence of syphilis.

Tuberculoid leprosy

This is the type seen in persons with a good resistance and may be purely neural or combined neural and dermal. The infection is never widespread but is localized to one area or to a few areas asymmetrically. Affected nerves are thickened, sometimes irregularly, and there are associated sensory or motor changes depending on the type of nerve involved. Sensory disturbance occurs as described under lepromatous leprosy except for the fact that it occurs earlier in the course of the disease and can be noted before the onset of skin lesions. If the patient complains of sensory disturbance such as paraesthesiae or anaesthesia, a search must be made for palpable thickening of the nerve responsible for the sensation of that area, e.g. face—trigeminal nerve; neck—great auricular nerve (Fig. 126); forearm—antebrachial cutaneous nerve; fifth finger—ulnar nerve; hand—median nerve at the wrist; thigh—femoral cutaneous nerve; lower leg—common peroneal nerve at the neck of the fibula; dorsum of foot—superficial peroneal nerve; sole of foot—posterior tibial nerve just below the internal malleolus. Loss of position sense, vibration sense and tendon reflexes occur rarely. Motor changes are shown by muscle weakness or wasting and must be sought in the face, in the intrinsic muscles of the hand and in the dorsiflexors of the foot. It is extremely rare for the dorsiflexors of the wrist to be affected owing to the fact that the radial nerve in the arm and forearm follows a deep course among the muscles and is therefore rarely involved. It is interesting to note that the same nerve, when it becomes superficial at the end of its course, often becomes thickened and can be palpated as a firm mobile cord as it lies against the lower end of the radius.

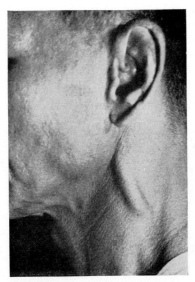

Fig. 126.—Gross thickening of the great auricular nerve in tuberculoid leprosy. (*Sir George McRobert*)

Abscesses in the course of affected nerves are not uncommon in tuberculoid leprosy.

Skin lesions take the form of macules or infiltrations (plaques) (Fig. 127). A tuberculoid macule is erythematous on fair skins and hypopigmented (not depigmented) on dark ones, has a dry and rather rough surface, its edges are

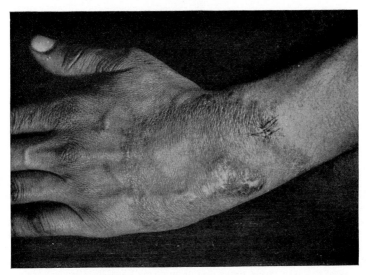

Fig. 127.—Tuberculoid leprosy in an Indian. This was a solitary lesion, anaesthetic, and with a raised red margin. The ulnar nerve was thickened. (*Sir George McRobert*)

well defined, and it is anaesthetic (except on the face) and anhidrotic. Infiltrated lesions are erythematous, whether on fair or dark skins, with sometimes a coppery, brownish or purple hue, have a dry and rather rough surface which may be irregular or pebbled, are sometimes scaly, have well marked sensory loss and have edges which are raised and clear-cut while the centres show variable flattening. In dark skins the colouring of the lesions obscures the underlying hypopigmentation. Central healing and peripheral extension give rise to annular lesions in which the *outer* edges are raised and well defined and the *inner* ones are

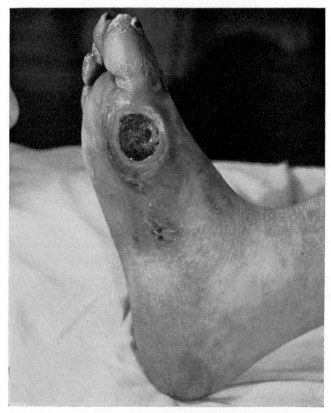

Fig. 128.—Trophic ulcer in leprosy. (*Sir George McRobert*)

flattened and indistinct. For descriptive purposes these infiltrated lesions are divided into minor and major tuberculoids (leprides), the major ones being larger, more grossly infiltrated and more deeply coloured.

Lesions of tuberculoid leprosy are usually few, large, asymmetrically situated, and favour the face, extensor surfaces of limbs, the back and buttocks, while tending to avoid the chest, abdomen, scalp, and the flexor aspects of limbs. If palms or soles are involved the lesions are not raised owing to the thickness and tightness of the skin. Sometimes one or two small 'satellite' lesions are seen in the vicinity of a large plaque and may look like nodules, but the fact that they are less elevated in the centre than at the edges can be confirmed by palpation.

Thickened cutaneous nerves may be palpated in the vicinity of the lesions, but tissues other than skin and nerves are not involved directly. The eye may suffer indirectly from corneal ulceration when there is damage to the facial nerve (exposure keratitis) and also when there is damage to the trigeminal nerve (neuropathic keratitis). Loss of eyebrows does not occur unless there is an infiltrated lesion traversing the eyebrow, and then the loss of hair is confined to that portion of the eyebrow which is actually covered by the lesion.

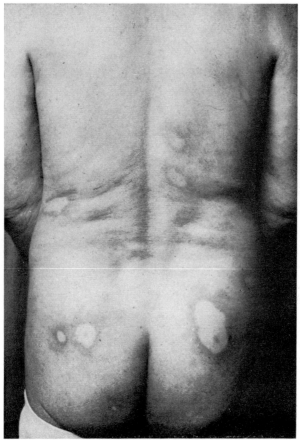

Fig. 129.—Borderline leprosy. The lesions are tuberculoid, but tend to be symmetrical. (*Dr. W. H. Jopling*)

Bone changes in hands or feet are less common than in the lepromatous type as leprosy bacilli are not deposited in the bones or their nutrient arteries; also, the early development of muscle wasting and paralysis results in disuse and therefore reduced risk of repeated trauma. However, neuropathic atrophy may occur in the phalanges of fingers or in the metatarsals and phalanges of feet, but, unlike the changes in lepromatous leprosy, they are never bilateral and symmetrical. Bone changes secondary to disuse, to loss of sensation and to trophic ulceration, may occur as described under lepromatous leprosy. Indolent ulcers of the feet are common (Fig. 128).

Borderline (dimorphous) leprosy

This is the type seen in persons with a limited or variable resistance, and usually presents with skin and nerve involvement. At the Sixth International Congress of Leprosy in Madrid (1953) the existence of a pure neural form was not accepted, but careful observation since then has proved that a polyneuritic form does exist.

The infection is neither as strictly localized as in tuberculoid leprosy nor as widespread as in the lepromatous type, but is somewhere between the two. Some patients remain dimorphous throughout, but others progress to one or

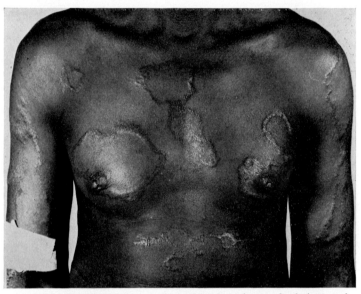

Fig. 130.—Borderline leprosy. Pin-prick blunted over the lesions and acid-fast bacilli present in moderate numbers. Note the well defined inner edges of the lesions and gynaecomastia. (*Dr Gunnar Lombolt*)

other of the two polar types depending on immunological factors not yet understood.

Skin lesions are macular, infiltrated or both, the earliest lesions being macules which are erythematous in fair skins, or hypopigmented (with sometimes an erythematous periphery) in dark skins. They may appear on trunk or limbs but have a predilection for the back, and in number and character are intermediate between the macules of the two polar types. Careful testing will reveal impairment of sensation in some if not all of the macules.

Infiltrated lesions have their own distinctive features in which the characteristics of the two polar types are merged. They are moderate in number, asymmetrical in distribution, their erythema has an admixture of purple or brown, their surface is smooth and often shiny, and they slope away peripherally from raised centres. The edges are well defined in places and indefinite in others.

Some of these infiltrations may take the form of bands, annular lesions and small nodules. Annular lesions have a characteristic form in which an oval area of normal-looking, but anaesthetic skin, is surrounded by a band of infiltrated tissue of varying width, the *inner* edge being raised and clear-cut (giving the oval area a punched-out appearance), the *outer* merging imperceptibly with the surrounding skin. These should not be mistaken for annular tuberculoid lesions for in the latter the outside edges are raised and clear-cut while the inner edges are indistinct. Sometimes there is an oval band of infiltrated tissue, even in width and more raised in the central part of the band, which has well defined outer and inner edges. Infiltrated lesions are invariably anaesthetic and may be found on any part of the body, with the exception of axillae, groins, perineum and scalp, but favour the limbs and buttocks.

Nerve involvement can always be demonstrated in borderline leprosy, and often neurological symptoms such as paraesthesiae and hyperalgesia precede the onset of skin manifestations. Nerves are involved asymmetrically and show palpable thickening and impaired function (sensory, motor or both). Other tissues are not affected directly but only indirectly as in the tuberculoid type.

Indeterminate leprosy

This is an early phase in the natural history of leprosy. At this stage the disease has not yet determined into which type it is going to evolve. Manifestations may be neural or macular (or both), macules being nondescript with uncharacteristic histology and absence of bacilli.

DIAGNOSIS

Early diagnosis is of the utmost importance, but many factors militate against it. It is, of course, easy to diagnose obvious and advanced cases. The ignorance of the patient, his dread of the disease and the fear and superstitions of the general public may hinder prompt recognition. The earlier indications are the discoloured patches on the skin, and symptoms referable to involvement of the peripheral nerves, such as tingling or numbness, formication or a feeling of woodenness in the limbs. Of fundamental importance are impairment of sensation, thickening and tenderness of nerves and demonstration of acid-fast bacilli.

To test sensation, the patient should be stripped and blindfolded. For testing anaesthesia to light touch, a feather should be used; analgesia is tested by pin-prick, using an area of normal skin as control. The two-pin test is often positive when the feather test is negative. Loss of thermal sensation is important and can be elicited by using a test-tube containing hot water and another containing iced water. Hyperaesthesia and paraesthesia may precede anaesthesia to light touch. *The possibility of leprosy should be considered in any patient presenting with a painless burn, injury or ulcer of one limb.*

Thickened nerves may be felt on palpation, and tenderness elicited by striking an area sharply with the finger or patellar hammer. The ulnar nerve is commonly affected above the elbow; the common peroneal at the head of the fibula behind the knee; the superficial peroneal in front of the ankle; the terminal branch of the radial as it passes over the lower end of the radius; the posterior tibial below the inner malleolus; the great auricular as it runs parallel to the external jugular vein; and the branches of any particular nerve supplying a tuberculoid lesion.

Bacteriological examination

This is essential in order to establish proof of the disease and to assist in correct classification and consists in carrying out a series of smears from the lesions. The scrape–incision method is recommended and is carried out as follows. The lesion is cleaned with ether and a fold is firmly held between thumb and forefinger of the left hand (to render it avascular); with a small-bladed scalpel an incision is made about 5 mm long and 3 mm deep, pressure of the fingers being maintained; the blade is then turned at right angles to the cut and the wound is scraped several times so that tissue fluid and pulp collect on one side of the blade; this is *gently* smeared on a glass slide. Smears are fixed by heat and are then stained by Ziehl–Neelsen technique. By this method acid-fast bacilli will always be found in lepromatous leprosy and frequently in the borderline form, but will usually be absent in the tuberculoid type (except in reaction) and in the indeterminate group. Nasal scrapings have been advocated in the past, but experience has shown that skin smears are far more valuable in diagnosis; not only are bacilli always readily demonstrated in the skin when they are present in the nasal mucosa, but often they are present in the skin when absent from the nose. For example, in borderline leprosy, nasal scrapings may be negative when the skin smears contain large numbers of bacilli and bacilli may disappear from the nasal mucosa long before they disappear from the skin.

Skin biopsy

Biopsy of the skin is essential for correct classification as it enables the histological changes in the skin to be studied. In addition serial biopsies carried out at regular intervals provide a valuable method of assessing prognosis and treatment. In carrying out a biopsy the most active part of the lesion must be chosen; this will be at the edge of the lesion in tuberculoid leprosy and in the centre in the lepromatous type. After ensuring local anaesthesia with 2%

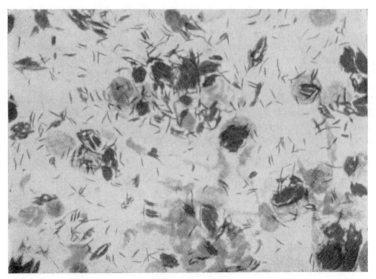

Fig. 131.—Biopsy of acute leprosy in the 'lepra reaction'. The leprosy bacilli appear as dark rods. (*After Roland Chaussinand, Institut Pasteur*)

procaine a portion of skin is removed with a scalpel or by a skin biopsy punch possessing a circular cutting edge, 5–7 mm in diameter. It is essential that the incision should reach the subcutaneous fat, otherwise the deeper layers of the dermis may not be included in the biopsy material. Paraffin sections are stained with haematoxylin and eosin to show the histological changes, and with a modification of the Ziehl–Neelsen, using pinene to demonstrate acid-fast bacilli. A nerve biopsy will be necessary in a purely neural case or where a skin biopsy has not given sufficient information, and for this purpose a thickened sensory nerve is chosen, such as the great auricular in the neck, the antibrachial cutaneous in the forearm, the radial at the lateral aspect of the wrist, the femoral cutaneous in the thigh, or the superficial peroneal on the dorsum of the foot.

In lepromatous leprosy bacilli can often be found in the sternal marrow, but this is not a practical method of diagnosis as bacilli are always readily demonstrable in the skin if present in the marrow.

Subsidiary signs

Anhidrosis, often preceded by hyperhidrosis, is characteristic of chronic cases, and is usually present in tuberculoid macules. In doubtful cases pilocarpine, 0·2 ml of 1 in 1000 solution, is injected intradermally in a suspected patch and a similar amount in adjacent healthy skin. Both areas are then painted with tincture of iodine and, when dry, powdered with starch. The control area sweats, turning the starch blue. Absence of sweat at the point of injection indicates leprosy.

A useful diagnostic aid is the intradermal mecholyl test for anhidrosis. The action of mecholyl chloride (almost identical with acetylcholine) is similar to that of pilocarpine. Denervation of sweat glands by leprous neuritis is the cause of anhidrosis, usually affecting the most distal portions of the post-ganglionic nerve fibres. In carrying out the test, equal areas of leprous and healthy skin are painted with a solution of castor oil, iodine and absolute alcohol. Then 0·05–0·1 ml aqueous solution of mecholyl chloride is injected intradermally at the border of the lesion so as to produce a weal. The whole area is lightly dusted with powdered starch. Within a few minutes sweat droplets appear on the functionally intact skin, which becomes blue from the iodine and starch combination. The response is negative when no sweat drops appear within the area tested.

The histamine test of Rodriguez is somewhat similar in slight or early cases. A drop of 1 in 1000 solution of histamine is placed within the margin of the suspected area, and a second outside. A prick is made with a needle through the drops. A red flare appears in normal skin. This test can be of great value in a purely neural case with sensory loss in one or more limbs, for it will exclude hysteria and organic disease of the central nervous system, such as syringomyelia. In all those conditions a red flare develops in the anaesthetic skin, but no flare appears if the anaesthesia is due to leprosy or other forms of peripheral neuritis.

Differential diagnosis

The characteristic marks of leprosy are sufficiently distinctive, but they have to be differentiated from psoriasis, seborrhoeic dermatitis, various forms of tinea, eczema, lichen planus, pellagra and filarial disease. Blastomycosis produces skin lesions reminiscent of leprosy. From syphilis and yaws, diagnosis may not always be so easy. Syphilitic and yaws skin lesions may often closely resemble the maculae of leprosy, but the absence of sensory changes and reaction to treatment are sufficiently distinctive. The Wassermann reaction alone cannot always be depended upon in differential diagnosis as syphilis and leprosy may co-exist; also a false positive reaction is not uncommon in lepromatous leprosy. Leprophilia is the name given for a hysterical condition with false anaesthesia developed by a peculiar kind of psychoneurotic who craves for sympathy.

The thickened skin of crab yaws on the feet may roughly resemble leprotic hyperkeratosis and may give a semblance of anaesthesia. Gangosa of yaws may be mistaken for nasal leprosy.

The early lesions of mycosis fungoides might possibly be mistaken for early nodular leprosy, and leucoderma is not infrequently associated with leprosy in the popular mind. It is extremely common, especially in India, and in Negro races, and unfortunate sufferers are sometimes to be found in leprosy institutions. Depigmentation in leucoderma, however, is more complete and sensory changes are absent. Lupus vulgaris and other tuberculides are very likely to be mistaken for leprides, and in both diseases acid-fast bacilli are difficult to demonstrate. Lupus evinces a greater tendency to scar formation and there are no sensory changes.

Cutaneous leishmaniasis and, in South America, espundia, may be mistaken for leprosy. The lesions on the skin of the face tend to concentrate round the mouth and nose and form a more raised margin than those in leprosy. Demonstration of the Leishman–Donovan body will always settle the matter, but leishmanial lupus-like lesions on the ears may cause difficulty. Burns and other injuries may leave behind anaesthetic scars. Eunuchism has been mistaken for leprosy on account of the absence of eyebrows and the smooth, shiny appearance of the skin.

Polyneuritic leprosy affecting the hands has to be differentiated from syringomyelia, in which analgesia and loss of heat sense are accompanied by retention of sense of touch and normal sweat function. The absence of nerve swelling and tenderness is important. The nerve injuries caused by trauma of the ulnar nerve or by cervical rib may possibly be called into question, but can be settled by X-ray examination. Meralgia paraesthetica (Bernhardt's syndrome) may cause anaesthesia of the anterolateral region of the thigh, and Raynaud's disease can cause trophic changes in the extremities. Familial hypertrophic interstitial neuritis (Déjerine–Sottas's disease) may cause confusion because of the characteristic thickening of peripheral nerves, together with sensory and motor changes in the limbs. Anaesthesia of the feet, leading to trophic ulceration and mutilation, can occur in diabetes, tabes, familial sensory radicular neuropathy and primary amyloidosis involving peripheral nerves. Von Recklinghausen's disease (neurofibromas) may sometimes resemble leprosy. Scarring and anaesthesia caused by extensive herpes zoster on the chest may give rise to difficulty. Scleroderma, localized or diffuse, may be compared with lepromatous leprosy, but madarosis is not present, nerves are not thickened, acid-fast bacilli are absent from smear and skin biopsy is diagnostic. The absence of fever and the presence of neural signs should differentiate tuberculoid leprosy in reaction from erysipelas. Erythema nodosum leprosum may be mistaken for other forms of erythema nodosum or for the Weber–Christian syndrome (a relapsing, febrile, non-suppurative, nodular panniculitis). Sarcoidosis can resemble tuberculoid leprosy but there is no sensory loss and no nerve thickening. Although a peripheral neuropathy has been reported complicating sarcoidosis, there is no nerve thickening. Granuloma annulare may simulate tuberculoid leprosy, but there is no sensory loss or nerve thickening, and the histological appearances are different. Granuloma multiforme may resemble tuberculoid leprosy—it appears to be localized to Nigeria. There is no sensory loss or nerve thickening, and the histological appearances are different.

REACTION

The reactional state in leprosy has been described and interpreted many times, and the subject has been much disputed, with confusing results. The following description is taken from Ridley (1969), and essentially relates the reactional state to the immune status of the patient. It is important to remember that simple extension or regression of lesions does not constitute the true leprosy reaction.

The reactions in leprosy are all acute episodes associated with alterations in the immunological balance between the bacilli and the host, and they have an allergic basis.

The reactions take place in borderline (BT, BB, BL) and lepromatous leprosy, and are described by Ridley (1969) as follows:

Borderline   Downgrading ⎱ Both associated with changes in cell-mediated
                Reversal   ⎰   immunity

Lepromatous Exacerbation nodules
                Erythema nodosum leprosum (associated with humoral mechanisms)

Reactions in borderline patients

Downgrading. Unfavourable, associated with movement towards lepromatous leprosy. Only in untreated, near tuberculoid patients.

1. Decline of immunity.
2. Increase in bacilli.
3. Extension of infection.

Reversal. Favourable. In near-lepromatous and borderline patients when the bacterial load is diminished by treatment.

1. Increase of immunity.
2. Decrease in bacilli.

Clinical features are similar in both downgrading and reversal reactions. They may appear rapidly and violently. There may be:

Fever (in severe reaction) to 37·7°–40·0°C possibly lasting several months.

Erythema and swelling of skin lesions; possibly ulceration. Hands and feet may be swollen and acutely tender.

Nerve involvement (common); lesions very tender. Gross paralysis may develop in a few days.

Appearance of new lesions (towards the tuberculoid type in reversal reactions).

Blockage of the nasal passages by swollen mucosa.

The patient may be in a miserable state.

Histological features

Downgrading

1. Increase in bacilli.
2. Dispersion of lymphocytes encompassing the lesions.
3. Infiltration through the dermis of large giant cells of foreign-body type.
4. Loss of the usual compact focalization of the granuloma.

5. Spread of the granuloma.
6. Oedema, intracellular and extracellular.
7. Dermal reaction, as in reversal reaction (below), replaced by granuloma; no heavy fibrosis.

Reversal (In marked cases. In mild cases there is little histological sign)
1. Decrease in bacilli.
2. Influx of lymphocytes usually; transient.
3. Change of host cells towards the epithelioid form.
4. Giant cell formation (foreign-body type at first, later Langhans type).
5. Necrosis in severe reactions.
6. Oedema in and around the granuloma, which enlarges.
7. Dermal reaction; influx of undifferentiated cells and fibrocytes in parts of the skin not affected by granuloma.
8. Fibrosis later.

The most severe reactions tend to occur in patients who are in the middle of the classification spectrum—a considerable shift, from BL to BT, would be associated with a heavier reaction than would a slight shift.

Reactions in lepromatous patients

Exacerbation nodules are not of great practical importance since they do not produce systemic upset. They occur in exceptionally large lesions, with excessive bacilli.

Clinical features
1. Large nodules, possibly erythematous.
2. No systemic upset.

Histological features
1. Heavy polymorph infiltration.
2. Cellular disintegration (see ENL).
3. Related to histoid lesions, which are histologically similar to hyperactive lepromatous nodules.

Erythema nodosum leprosum (ENL) may be precipitated by treatment, especially by dapsone, or by intercurrent infection etc. This is not an indication of shift in immunological status. It occurs usually when patients have been under treatment for about one year, and the bacterial load has fallen, the bacilli are disintegrating and releasing antigenic material, and are relatively numerous in the circulating blood. It is probably associated with humoral mechanisms, and represents a manifestation of the Arthus phenomenon.

Clinical features
1. Fever.
2. Transient crops of small painful red nodules lasting a few days.
3. Large painful red plaques if severe, with necrosis and ulceration.
4. Enlargement of lymph nodes, liver and spleen.
5. Iridocyclitis (allergic), orchitis and painful enlargement of nerves (neuralgia).
6. Swollen joints occasionally.
7. Nephritis (allergic) occasionally.
8. Polymorphonuclear leucocytosis.

These manifestations are found mostly where bacilli are common, except the lesions in joints, kidneys and possibly the eyes, which may be allergic. Changes in the kidneys, apparently due to deposition of protein complexes (probably antigen–antibody complexes) within the nephrons, tend to occur in patients subject to severe reactional states. The nephrons may be destroyed. The condition seems to resemble the nephrosis sometimes seen in quartan malaria.

Histological features

Mild ENL. Reaction not in the major skin lesions but in small, clinically inapparent lesions with few bacilli. Centre never in normal skin. Polymorphs present and predominant in the early stage. Cellular disintegration marked. Lymphocytes appear later. Vasculitis seen in about half the lesions.

Severe ENL. In advanced lepromatous leprosy with heavy bacillary load. Large necrotizing lesions; may be wedge-shaped like infarcts. Oedema intense. Cellular infiltration intense, often affecting the whole dermis except the fat. Lymph node and nerve involvement with polymorphs. Heavy infiltration of bacilli into walls of large vessels. Necrosis of small vessels. Dermal reaction (as in reversal reaction) can be intense. (A similar reaction is sometimes in the dermis in very mild ENL.)

TREATMENT

Although modern drugs have revolutionized the treatment of all forms of leprosy, it is essential to give them in proper doses and for long periods. The following table gives perhaps the simplest indications for the time scale; it assumes that the lepromin test was applied at the time of diagnosis, and that the bacilli were estimated in skin snips when treatment was begun (Editorial, *Br. med. J.* 1971).

Lepromin reaction	Skin smears	Length of treatment
Strongly positive	Negative	5 years
Weakly positive	Few bacilli	10 years
Negative	Moderate or large numbers of bacilli	For life

If relapses are to be prevented it is best to err on the generous side for length of treatment; not only is dapsone (see page 438) cheap and non-toxic in the doses advocated, but one can never be certain that the treatment has been taken regularly.

General

Several drugs are now known to be effective in leprosy, superseding the old preparations of chaulmoogra oil. Drug treatment, however, should not be given unless a definite diagnosis of leprosy has been made; to give these drugs merely on suspicion is quite unjustifiable. It is probably unwise to begin drug treatment in very anaemic patients; it should be delayed until the haemoglobin has been increased to 50% (Browne 1967). Once the diagnosis is established, most patients can be treated by medical auxiliaries at mobile or static clinics, but patients who are undergoing reaction, or who are sensitive to drugs, are better treated in hospital.

The modern era of chemotherapy was started when the sulphones, originally introduced for the treatment of tuberculosis, were used in leprosy and found to be effective. The early preparations—promin, diasone, solapsone—had disadvantages, and were superseded by the parent substance, 4:4'-diaminodiphenyl sulphone (DDS, dapsone, diaphenylsulphone) which is effective by mouth. It was soon found that treatment must not only be regular, but must also be continued for very long periods, and that if this is done, and treatment is begun early, the results, especially in tuberculoid and borderline cases, can be excellent, and even in lepromatous cases the improvement is impressive.

The sulphones, however, though astonishingly better than chaulmoogra and any other drugs previously used, are slow in action. Moreover, drug treatment of any kind is only one part of the general care of the patient; physiotherapy, attention to the hands, feet and eyes, and general measures of health, are essential.

Dapsone. This remains the drug of choice. The routine treatment for all forms of leprosy is (Browne 1967):

Adult dose by mouth

First month	25 mg once each week
Second month	50 mg once each week
Thereafter	100 mg once each week

Though the weekly dose of 100 mg may be as effective as larger doses, and does not provoke so many acute exacerbations, some authorities give up to 200 mg each week. Indeed, the WHO (1970) expert committee concluded that the standard dose is 6–10 mg/kg body weight/week, for both adults and children, which for a person of 50 kg works out at 300–500 mg each week. It seems obvious, however, that doses should be small if they are found to be effective, and the *British Medical Journal* (1971) advises 100–200 mg each week. The doses are scaled down for children in the usual way, but they take dapsone well. In borderline cases the increments are made cautiously.

Recent experimental work, and pilot trials in man, indicate that even smaller doses may be effective. In mice the bacilli have been inhibited by serum concentrations of dapsone of 0·02 μg/ml, corresponding to a daily dose of only 1·0 mg for man. Whether this will prove effective generally remains to be seen, but preliminary trials suggest that it might (Rees & Weddell 1970), though the possibility that small doses may lead to drug resistance in the bacilli should be remembered.

Dapsone should be suspended if signs of reaction appear, and it should not be started again until 1–2 weeks after all signs of reaction have disappeared, and then in smaller doses than before, increased only gradually, and perhaps to no more than the dose at which reaction took place.

Side-effects of dapsone are rare (about 1 per 1000 patients treated), but it can cause haemolytic anaemia, methaemoglobinaemia, hepatitis or skin conditions including dermatitis, fixed eruptions (blackish macules or diffuse hypermelanosis) in dark skins, together with systemic symptoms, slight or severe. These may occur with large doses; they may disappear without withdrawal of the drug, or they may need desensitization by standard methods for dapsone dermatitis (Browne 1964). In large doses dapsone can probably cause acute psychosis (Garrett 1971).

Drug resistance to dapsone has been observed but is extremely rare (about 1 in 1000 patients). Apparent resistance should be carefully investigated. Some patients do not follow instructions, and do not take the drug—possibly even selling their tablets. In some such cases it has been shown that dapsone given by injection is perfectly effective. True resistance is apparently developed by a stepwise process; it may particularly be a risk in patients treated with very low doses (5–10 mg each week) of sulphone, which is an argument for maintaining relatively high serum levels with the doses advocated above. There may thus be a dilemma. Very small doses may lead to resistance, but may be indicated in some lepromatous patients who cannot tolerate higher doses.

Dapsone may be given by injection. For this it is suspended (20–25%) in various oils (chaulmoogra, arachis) and is intended for intramuscular injection in initial (adult) doses of 0·2 ml (50 mg dapsone in 25% suspension) once each week, rising to a maximum of 0·8 ml.

Another preparation for injection consists of 5 grammes dapsone dissolved in 40 ml absolute alcohol, to which 55 ml propylene glycol is added, and 5 ml benzyl alcohol is incorporated to reduce discomfort on intramuscular injection (French 1968).

Other injectable preparations of dapsone are also available. No advantage is apparent for the injectable preparations except, perhaps, that the doses are known to be given, whereas a patient given a supply of tablets to be taken at intervals, for a week or more, by mouth, may fail to take them regularly.

DADDS (acedapsone, 4,4'-diacetlydiaminodiphenyl sulphone) is a repository sulphone, suspended in a mixture of benzyl benzoate and castor oil, which releases dapsone slowly. In intramuscular doses of 225 mg every 75–77 days, it is as active as dapsone in patients with lepromatous leprosy. It does not seem to lead to drug resistance, as it releases dapsone at a rate of 2·4 mg daily, but some patients have experienced erythema nodosum leprosum in some degree (Shephard *et al.* 1968). This dosage, together with 1 mg dapsone daily by mouth, has also been effective in short-term trials in lepromatous leprosy. DADDS is an excellent prophylactic in some communities (see below).

Sulphonamides have been used in special circumstances. They are no better than dapsone, and are much more dangerous and more expensive. They include sulphadimethoxazine (Madribon), sulphamethoxypyrazine (Sultirene, Kynex), acetyl Kelfizine, sulphormethoxine (Fanasil) and sulphamethoxydiazine (Kiron).

Thiambutosine (diphenylthiourea; DPT; SU 1906 (CIBA)). This drug is active in all types of leprosy; it is given by mouth twice daily because it is rapidly excreted after being poorly absorbed.

Browne (1967) suggests for adults:

> 250 mg daily for 1 month
> 500 mg daily for 1 month
> 1000 mg daily for 1 month
> 2000 mg daily thereafter

An alternative scheme (WHO 1966) is 500 mg daily gradually increased to 1500 mg daily.

Thiambutosine is less effective than dapsone, but can be useful if dapsone is badly tolerated. During the second half of the second year the dose of thiambutosine should be gradually reduced, and dapsone cautiously introduced so that by the end of the second year thiambutosine is abandoned. It should not be continued beyond 2 years because its activity diminishes, probably owing to drug resistance, which has been observed in some patients.

Thiambutosine is now available as a 20% suspension in arachis oil, for deep gluteal intramuscular injection; 10 ml (i.e. 2 grammes) of this are injected each week or fortnight, and the active product is released slowly from the depot thus formed. An alternative schedule (WHO 1966) is 200 mg in 1·0 ml arachis oil once each week, gradually increasing to 1000 mg in 5·0 ml once each week.

Clofazimine (Lamprene; B663 (Geigy); G30·320). This is a rimino compound derived from phenazine dye. It appears to have a remarkable action on erythema nodosum leprosum, and on the course of lepromatous leprosy itself.

It is indicated:

1. In lepromatous leprosy, particularly if the patient is liable to severe and prolonged exacerbation.
2. In lepromatous leprosy with long-standing erythema nodosum leprosum severe enough to necessitate continuous corticosteroids.
3. In patients harbouring dapsone-resistant *Myco. leprae*.
4. In patients responding only slowly to dapsone, or who are intolerant of, or hypersensitive to dapsone.

Clofazimine has been given by mouth in doses of 100–300 mg daily for long periods to patients in reaction, formerly dependent on corticosteroids, and the steroids have been reduced gradually, and eventually abandoned completely, with good clinical and bacteriological results. Once reaction is controlled the dose can be reduced (Browne 1966). If reaction does break through, the dose should not be reduced, but should be increased. Clofazimine has now been found effective in previously untreated lepromatous leprosy in doses of 100 mg 2–3 times each week; this treatment is as effective as the standard dapsone regimen. Monthly administration has been used in lepromatous leprosy, with success, after a loading dose. In reactional states larger doses are needed.

Clofazimine is slowly eliminated from the body. The main adverse reaction is deep and persistent redness followed by pigmentation of the skin, which is resented by patients with light skins, but not by others who appreciate its therapeutic value. It not only controls erythema nodosum leprosum, but also improves the clinical condition, the bacillary index, and the morphological index. It may rarely cause abdominal pain and diarrhoea.

Thiosemicarbazone (thiacetazone; amithiozone; TB 1/698). Originally used for tuberculosis, this has been used with success in non-lepromatous leprosy, and with less success in lepromatous leprosy. It is now largely superseded but may be useful in cases in which dapsone is not tolerated. The dose is 12·5 mg daily for 2 weeks and 25·0 mg daily for the next 2 weeks, increased by 25 mg daily every 2 weeks until the dose of 100 mg daily is reached. This is given for 4 weeks and can be increased by 25 mg each week to 150 mg daily, which is given for $1–1\frac{1}{2}$ years. It is better, however, to keep the maximum dose at 100 mg daily. Toxic reactions include depression of bone marrow activity and even (though rarely) agranulocytosis. Resistance is likely to develop after 2–3 years.

Two other drugs—vadrine and ditophal (Etisul)—in use some years ago, have now been discarded.

Rifampicin. This is a recent and promising addition to the anti-leprosy drugs, which was originally introduced for tuberculosis. It is bactericidal to the tubercle bacillus, whereas other anti-leprosy drugs are bacteriostatic to that organism. In experimental leprosy it is even more active than dapsone, against both dapsone-sensitive and dapsone-resistant strains. It has proved as effective as dapsone in a preliminary trial in human leprosy.

The dose is 450–600 mg daily, by mouth, in a single dose *on an empty stomach* (this is important). It may produce a reddish-brown colour in urine, sputum or sweat, but no important side-effects have been proved (Ross & Horne 1969; Rees & Weddell 1970). Six lepromatous patients treated with 600 mg daily for $4\frac{1}{2}$–12 months showed satisfactory clinical, bacteriological and histological responses, especially in the morphological index (Rees *et al.* 1970). A few cases of acute thrombocytopenia have been observed in tuberculous patients on high dosage (see Tuberculosis, page 452).

For the treatment of eye conditions associated with leprosy and with the reactional state, see Chapter 44.

Treatment of reactional states

Erythema nodosum leprosum. This reactional state occurs in lepromatous leprosy, and may be precipitated by smallpox vaccination, intercurrent infection (for instance malaria), physical or emotional stress, injury or pregnancy. Treatment should take such features into account.

If the reaction is mild the only treatment is to reduce temporarily the dose of the anti-leprosy drug by 50%, explaining to the patient that his tissues have been destroying the bacilli too quickly. He may need a tranquillizer if there is mental depression.

If the reaction is moderately severe the anti-leprosy treatment should be stopped for a time, and the patient may need an analgesic such as aspirin or indomethacin for pain (but habit-forming drugs must be avoided) and a tranquillizer. Empirically, antimony compounds have been found useful, but should be used with caution, for instance stibophen injection (Fouadin) in intramuscular doses of 1·0 ml on alternate days and increasing to 3·0 ml every other day to a total of not more than 15 ml. Other antimonials are Anthiomaline intramuscularly (0·5 ml increasing on alternate days) or sodium (or potassium) antimony tartrate (20 mg in 10 ml sterile water intravenously every second day, increasing to 40 or 60 mg). There is a disadvantage in intravenous administration.

Chloroquine 200 mg twice daily for 2 weeks sometimes relieves the condition.

When the acute phase has subsided, anti-leprosy drugs may be started again, but in very small doses (e.g. 12·5 mg dapsone twice each week). Even this small dose can produce satisfactory results when larger doses would cause reaction. An alternative is to give clofazimine or one of the long-acting sulphonamides.

Clofazimine has definite anti-inflammatory action, and also a definite action on the leprosy itself. Thalidomide has also been used for its anti-inflammatory effect in doses of 100–400 mg daily, reduced as recovery takes place. Side-effects are numerous and usually transient. It has no anti-leprosy effect. Dapsone can be given at the same time. The use of thalidomide during pregnancy, especially the earlier stages, must be absolutely prohibited. Indomethacin is said to have an anti-inflammatory action and to be valuable in lepromatous leprosy.

For pain and swelling in the motor nerve, with weakness or paralysis, an injection of 1500 units of hyaluronidase in 1·0 ml of 2% procaine solution, mixed with 1·0 ml hydrocortisone suspension (25 mg/ml) may be given slowly into or around the nerve through a size 14 needle—for instance, just above the elbow for the ulnar nerve and the neck of the fibula for the common peroneal nerve. The solution should be freshly made each time. Nerve stripping is not now in vogue. If surgery is necessary it suffices to incise the epineurium.

For severe reactions treatment with corticotrophin or corticosteroids is indicated if other measures fail. It is important to give only the smallest dose which will control the condition. For corticotrophin a gel preparation can be given intramuscularly in daily doses of 40 units, gradually increasing the intervals to one injection every second day, or twice each week, and then reducing the dose; for cortisone a 5-day course by mouth (in divided dosage) as follows: 100 mg the first day, decreasing each day to 75 mg, 50 mg, 25 mg and 12·5 mg. With these courses the patient should reduce dietary salt, and take a daily dose of a potassium salt equivalent to 3–5 grammes of potassium chloride.

Prednisone, prednisolone and dexamethasone are suitable alternatives, but their doses are much smaller (20 or 30 mg daily in divided doses). Prednisone is important for acute epididymo-orchitis; it causes less electrolyte disturbance than cortisone. Another suggested course is to give an injectable preparation of cortisone—75 mg daily for 3 days, 50 mg daily for 3 days, 25 mg daily for 3 days, and 12·5 mg daily for 3 days (Browne 1967). If this does not abort the reaction, larger doses and more gradual tapering off may be needed. Some authorities, however, think that injected cortisone is not necessary, and prefer corticotrophin gel.

One advantage of corticosteroids is that anti-leprosy treatment can be continued; but the steroids should be withdrawn as soon as possible. The danger that the patient may become accustomed to bed rest and habituated to corticosteroids is real and must be avoided. Graded physical exercises, passive at first, are valuable in this connection.

One point about treatment with corticosteroids is that when such patients complain of abdominal pain or diarrhoea, trophozoites of *Entamoeba histolytica* can often be found in their stools. These exacerbations of amoebic colitis respond to standard anti-amoebic treatment and do not indicate cessation of steroid treatment (Goodwin 1969).

In tuberculoid and dimorphous leprosy the reactionary state is less severe, but the lesions may become painful, or ulcerate, and a peripheral nerve may be involved, with pain and weakness.

In general no special treatment is needed, but if pain and ulceration are present, the doses of anti-leprosy drugs should be halved. If a motor nerve is involved, anti-leprosy treatment should be stopped, weakened muscles should be splinted, and steroid treatment should be started in doses higher than for erythema nodosum leprosum. Intraneural injection may be called for. If a nerve abscess develops it should be aspirated or even dealt with surgically. Lesions which ulcerate require appropriate dressings.

Surgical treatment

The results of nerve involvement in leprosy so often lead to ulceration, paralysis and deformity of the limbs, that the prevention or correction of the deformities involves a multitude of special techniques up to full orthopaedic surgery. A discussion of these complicated treatments is outside the scope of this book, and surgeons who wish to study the subject are referred to the relevant chapters in Cochrane and Davey (1964), and to Brand (1966).

Primary deformity is due to the activity of the disease—for instance to erosion of the phalanges due to lepromatous granulomas. Secondary deformity is due to damage which the patient inflicts on himself as a consequence of anaesthesia or paralysis.

It is important to keep the hands under constant examination for swelling, sensation and function, and to ensure as far as possible that the hands are protected from trauma during the period when decalcification of the bones may be taking place. Examination by X-ray is essential for complete assessment. The same is true of the feet, but in the feet deep plantar damage may occur before anaesthesia is complete, and nerve damage must therefore be recognized when loss of localization of light touch occurs on the sole. In England, lepromatous leprosy is far more important than tuberculoid or borderline leprosy as a cause of plantar ulceration. Plantar damage and ulceration can be prevented, partly by provision of footwear with rigid wooden soles and soft insoles, and by the use of Plastazote insoles placed inside orthopaedic shoes (Jopling 1969). It is important to scrape away, regularly, the callus which forms over a healed ulcer. Dry cracked skin can be treated by soaking in water for several hours each day and then covering with soft paraffin. Ulcers can be treated by rest, dressings and antibiotics; a plaster cast may obviate the need for more than a few days' bed rest.

Foot drop and other signs of damage to nerves need special apparatus or surgical measures such as tendon transplantation.

In all cases the need for physiotherapy must be borne in mind; it can do much to help the patient. The same is true of occupational therapy, which should satisfy the patient's need to be a useful member of the community in which he can do productive work, mental or physical. Occupational therapy is limited because many manual skills involve the risk of damage to the hands, for instance carpentry. But some form of satisfactory occupation should be sought; the mental effect of enforced idleness can be disastrous to the personality of the patient.

PROGNOSIS

Leprosy in its milder forms is a self-healing disease; it is also curable. Of those who become infected, only a small proportion develop overt signs. Its old terrible reputation is justifiable only in extreme cases.

In *macular tuberculoid leprosy* the prognosis after treatment is excellent, though with severe hypopigmentation the pigment may not return to completely healed lesions, and if anaesthesia is extensive, sensation may not be restored completely, even after complete cure.

In *infiltrated tuberculoid leprosy* also the prognosis is excellent after treatment, but if nerves have been grossly enlarged there may be some permanent anaesthesia, and the patient should be warned not to damage hands and feet because of the risk of permanent ulceration or deformity.

In *lepromatous leprosy* the prognosis, though now much better than ever before, must be guarded. The earlier the treatment is instituted, the better the prognosis, but cure must not be promised lightly. If the patient suffers from acute erythema nodosum leprosum, especially if this goes on to progressive reaction, the prognosis becomes more grave. No estimate of prognosis can be given until the patient has been treated for at least 2 years, possibly 5 years or even longer. In advanced lepromatous leprosy permanent sequelae—deformity, paralysis or paresis from nerve injury, damage to the eyes—may occur, though modern treatment can do much to prevent these.

In *infiltrated borderline* leprosy the prognosis should be guarded at first; there is a tendency to severe deformity after reactional borderline lesions; careful physiotherapy is needed, with avoidance of trauma, for instance accidental burns. Moreover, this form may go on to lepromatous leprosy. This borderline group is particularly prone to lead to serious deformities, and to relapse; the patients need careful attention.

With modern treatment, including drug treatment, surgery and physiotherapy, much deformity can be avoided or relieved, but treatment must be continued for a long time (see page 437).

Relapse may occur, especially when full courses of treatment are not observed. Even after 5 years of treatment Cochrane and Davey (1964) found that 11 of 98 lepromatous patients relapsed, and in Nigeria Browne (1965b) reported 6% of relapses in treated patients, mostly with lepromatous or borderline disease. The commonest cause of relapse appeared to be insufficient treatment in conditions prone to relapse.

PREVENTION

For prevention Cochrane and Davey (1964) suggest certain factors:

1. A well informed and educated public opinion (including medical and para-medical personnel).
2. Reasonable measures for controlling infective persons to prevent infection of healthy persons.
3. Successful treatment.
4. A rise in the standard of living, resulting in reduction of overcrowding.

They make the points that the public should realize that leprosy is an infection, not a hereditary disease, to be controlled on that basis, and that control of infective persons must depend upon their willingness to accept restrictions, which should not be excessive—otherwise, as so often in schemes of compulsory segregation, the disease will be concealed.

Persons suffering from bacilliferous leprosy should avoid skin-to-skin contact with others, particularly children—pus from ulcerating succulent lesions or from skin which is the seat of chronic diffuse lepra reaction contains large numbers of bacilli (Browne 1967).

Treatment has not yet become available to most persons suffering from leprosy in remote areas, and has not yet made a great impact on the prevalence of the disease, but with more extensive organization and more money it can become much more widespread. Prevention therefore depends upon knowledge of prevalence, and this in turn depends upon deliberate surveys of whole populations, such as have been done in Africa and elsewhere. The layout and amenities of settlements for isolation of patients must obviously be attractive.

Where children are in close contact with infective parents or siblings the one obvious preventive measure is to treat the infective persons, but this is slow. The question whether to give healthy children prophylactic half doses of sulphones has been raised; this can be successful, as in an investigation in India. Prophylactic DADDS is allowable if there is proper supervision. It has shown remarkable prophylactic effects in a long trial in a small, highly infected community in Micronesia (Sloan et al. 1971), but is probably not suitable for this in the widely scattered African and Asian regions where infection is not so intense. The dose is 225 mg (in suspension) every 75 days.

BCG

The one active measure that has been suggested to protect uninfected members of a community is to use BCG. This has been done on a large scale, sometimes in very carefully supervised campaigns, as in Uganda where over 16 000 children, all relatives or contacts of known leprosy patients but all free from signs of leprosy, were tested with tuberculin. Those who were tuberculin-negative, or only slightly positive, were divided at random into 2 groups, one receiving BCG and the other not. After 3 years the incidence of leprosy in the unvaccinated was 11·0 per 1000, and in the BCG group only 2·2; BCG apparently protected 80% in this period. Results at 3½ years show protection in 87% (15·8 per 1000 cases in the unvaccinated against 2·1 per 1000 in the vaccinated). In the unvaccinated children the incidence varied with the initial tuberculin sensitivity—those with the strongest reactions having the lowest incidence. Some, at least, of the mild reactions to tuberculin are apparently due to infection by atypical mycobacteria, but these infections do not affect the results of vaccination with BCG.

It remains to be seen whether the protection will last. In some of the un-vaccinated children the early indeterminate or tuberculoid lesions will probably resolve spontaneously. In New Guinea BCG protected 56% and in Burma no benefit was found from its use. Further experience is therefore obviously needed, especially in an area with a high proportion of lepromatous cases, and in 1971 the World Health Organization considered it premature to recommend BCG for this purpose. It is, of course, used in the prevention of tuberculosis.

In this work a point to be borne in mind is that in Uganda (and most of Africa) about 90% of cases of leprosy are tuberculoid, and the same is true of New Guinea, but in Burma the incidence of lepromatous leprosy is 3–4 times as high as in Uganda and New Guinea (Rees 1969b).

The different results in these various countries cannot be attributed to differences in technique or planning of the experiments. There may be differences in strains of *Myco. leprae*, and these can now be tested. But the general im-pression from experimental work and from these experiments in man strongly suggests that BCG is to some significant degree protective against leprosy (Rees 1969a).

Personal protection for physicians and others who are in contact with infective patients is not difficult. Hands should be washed with soap and water, but gloves should be worn if there is prolonged contact or in taking smears or skin specimens. A protective gown should be worn. They need not take pro-phylactic sulphones (Cochrane & Davey 1964).

REFERENCES

BRAND, P. (1966) *Insensitive Feet: A Practical Handbook on Foot Problems in Leprosy.* London: The Leprosy Mission.
BROWN, S. G. (1964) *Br. med. J.*, iii, 664.
———— (1965a) *Leprosy Rev.*, 36, 157.
———— (1965b) *Int. J. Leprosy*, 33, 267, 273.
———— (1966) *Leprosy Rev.*, 37, 141.
———— (1967) *Trans. R. Soc. trop. Med. Hyg.*, 61, 265, 601.
COCHRANE, R. G. & DAVEY, T. F. (1964) *Leprosy in Theory and Practice.* Bristol: Wright.
EDITORIAL (1971) *Br. med. J.*, iii, 174.
FRENCH, T. M. (1968) *Leprosy Rev.*, 39, 171.
GARRETT, A. S. (1971) *Br. med. J.*, iv, 300.
GOODWIN, C. S. (1969) *Br. med. J.*, iii, 174.
INTERNATIONAL CONGRESS OF LEPROSY (1953) *Int. J. Leprosy*, 21, 484.
JOPLING, W. H. (1969) *Leprosy Rev.*, 40, 175.
———— (1971) *Handbook of Leprosy.* London: Heinemann.
KARAT, A. B. A., JOB, C. K. & RAO, P. S. S. (1971) *Br. med. J.*, i, 307.
MINISTRY OF HEALTH (1967) *Annual Report*, p. 42. London: HMSO.
MOHAMED ALI, P. (1965) *Int. J. Leprosy*, 33, 223.
NEWELL, K. W. (1966) *Bull. Wld Hlth Org.*, 34, 827.
REES, R. J. W. (1967) *Trans. R. Soc. trop. Med. Hyg.*, 61, 581.
———— (1969a) *Br. med. Bull.*, 25, 183.
———— (1969b) *Bull. Wld Hlth Org.*, 40, 785.
———— PEARSON, J. M. H. & WATERS, M. F. R. (1970) *Br. med. J.*, i, 89.
———— & WEDDELL, A. G. M. (1970) *Trans. R. Soc. trop. Med. Hyg.*, 64, 31.
———— ———— PALMER, E. & PEARSON, J. M. H. (1969) *Br. med. J.*, iii, 216.
RIDLEY, D. S. (1967) *Trans. R. Soc. trop. Med. Hyg.*, 61, 596.
———— (1969) *Leprosy Rev.*, 40, 77.
———— & JOPLING, W. H. (1966) *Int. J. Leprosy*, 34, 255.

Ross, J. D. & Horne, N. W. (1969) *Modern Drug Treatment in Tuberculosis*, 4th ed. London: Health Horizon.
Shepard, C. C., Tolentino, J. G. & McRae, W. H. (1968) *Am. J. trop. Med. Hyg.*, **17**, 192.
Sloan, N. R., Worth, R. M., Jano, B. & Shephard, C. C. (1971) *Lancet*, **ii**, 525.
Turk, J. L. (1969) *Immunology in Clinical Practice*. London: Heinemann.
—— & Waters, M. F. R. (1968) *Lancet*, **ii**, 436.
—— —— (1969) *Lancet*, **ii**, 243.
World Health Organization (1966) *Wld Hlth Org. tech. Rep. Ser.*, 319.
—— (1970) *Wld Hlth Org. tech. Rep. Ser.*, 459.

Tuberculosis

TUBERCULOSIS has recently been much reduced in Europe, North America and Australasia, and in the more affluent parts of Asia and Africa, but it is still rife in most parts of Africa, in India and South-east Asia generally and in South America. Indeed, in some areas it is one of the commonest killing diseases.

It is estimated that there are perhaps 20 million cases of active tuberculosis in the world, that every year more than 2 million new cases occur and 1–2 million people die of it. More than three-quarters of these cases are found in the developing countries. Various reports suggest that the incidence of active disease, mostly pulmonary, reaches 10 or more per 1000 in parts of tropical Africa, 13–32 or more per 1000 in some cities of Asia, and even more in other crowded parts of the Far East.

Annual death rates have been estimated to reach over 2 per 1000 population in Latin American cities, 2–3 in parts of Africa and 2–5 in Asian cities. In Malaya tuberculosis has been described as the largest single cause of death, responsible for 7% of all deaths, but the rate has fallen considerably in Singapore in recent years. In Uganda it is probably the commonest cause of death in young adults (Hutt 1971).

These facts indicate how important it is for the clinician and the public health administrator alike, to bear tuberculosis in mind.

AETIOLOGY

Mycobacterium tuberculosis of the human type is the common organism, especially in developing countries, but there are areas of Africa (Ankole in Uganda) and Asia (parts of India) where cattle are infected with the bovine organism, and in which cases of human infection with this organism occur. Milk should therefore be suspect, and either pasteurized or boiled. It is also, of course, suspect as a vehicle for brucellosis and other infections.

Other acid-fast organisms are met occasionally in the tropics—for instance, *Myco. ulcerans*, the cause of skin ulcers in Australia and quite commonly in tropical Africa (see Buruli ulcer, page 454). Similarly, skin ulcers may be due to *Myco. balnei*, which infect abrasions due to contact with the rough walls of swimming baths.

Mycobacteria of the Runyon group, sometimes known as anonymous mycobacteria, have been found in man. A classification has been suggested:

1. Photochromogens producing yellow pigment in cultures in the light.
2. Scotochromogens producing yellow pigment in cultures even in the dark.
3. Non-chromogens—no colour produced (avian Battey type).

The photochromogens (*Myco. kansasii*) can cause pulmonary disease resembling mild tuberculosis, usually resistant to isoniazid and PAS; the scotochromogens behave like saprophytes in man.

The Battey organisms have been found in patients with lymphadenitis, or pulmonary disease, including pneumoconiosis (with cavitation in 78%), in the southern United States and Britain, and may be found elsewhere. Of the cases reported in Florida 17% were fatal, drug treatment was disappointing and almost half of the patients were discharged with active disease. This infection is obviously serious. The avian type of tubercle bacillus is responsible for a substantial proportion of these cases (Schaefer *et al.* 1969); the tuberculin reactions cannot be relied upon to differentiate these infections from tuberculosis.

EPIDEMIOLOGY

Tuberculosis has notoriously been associated with poverty, which means malnutrition, overcrowding and industrial stress. But it has been associated also with transition from a rural, pastoral life to an urban, industrial life, in which people from remote country areas living on adequate diets migrate for social and financial reasons to cities where they find work in mines and factories, and live in organized communities in which conditions are good (as on the gold mines of South Africa), or in private uncontrolled dwellings where cheap carbohydrate food is the rule and lodging is expensive. In these cheap shanty-town lodgings a healthy immigrant from pastoral life can within a few months become a moribund malnourished skeleton infected with amoebiasis, venereal disease and tuberculosis of the lungs, which is likely to kill him. This type of epidemiological picture, which is by no means confined to the tropics, suggests that rural communities do not possess the degree of immunity which has developed over the centuries in urban communities, and that their immunity is less effective because in their rural surroundings they have not been subjected to intense infection and selection, they have lived on a better diet and stress, overcrowding and poverty have not been so oppressive as in towns (Wilcocks 1962).

This view is supported by the results of tuberculin tests which, in general, are much less commonly positive in rural than in urban areas, and less intense. But the fact that some persons, even in remote places, are tuberculin-positive shows that the infection is not absent. In crowded towns, however, the tuberculin rates and intensities and the rates for active disease are very much higher than in rural areas.

It is obvious that in this epidemiological situation the opportunity for contact with a sputum-positive person is a major factor, and as usual elsewhere, the incidence of infection and overt disease is much higher in house contacts than in non-contacts; 'tuberculosis in the East African is a family catastrophe' because of this contact (Gordon 1962). School and other contact is also sometimes important. A school or class in which the tuberculin rates and intensities are unduly high may include a sputum-positive teacher or pupil—or even bus driver. The corollary is that contacts of tuberculous patients should be sought out and examined.

Pneumoconiosis, especially silicosis, is another factor. Much work has been done in evaluating and controlling the dust hazard in mines, particularly in the Johannesburg area. Figures from Rhodesia show how vulnerable to tuberculosis is a man with silicosis; 'the attack rate of pulmonary tuberculosis in established silicotics has been found to be thirty times greater than in non-silicotics' (Girdwood 1962).

Behind these factors are the beliefs held in some communities that disease of any kind is due, not to natural causes, but to the working of evil spirits or the wrath of the gods. In such a background treatment, especially if it entails injections, is easily accepted (but may not be persisted with); prevention by environmental control is not.

PATHOLOGY

The pathology of tuberculosis in tropical countries does not differ from that seen in developed countries, except in degree. In primitive communities the lesions of established disease tend to resemble those found in susceptible laboratory animals—widespread caseating adenopathy, pulmonary cavitation without much fibrosis, bronchogenic spread, miliary disease and tuberculous meningitis. In Uganda, even in the absence of miliary disease, tuberculous granulomas are common in the liver, often with necrosis and only minimal cellular infiltration (Hutt 1971). But there are always some patients in whom a fibrotic reaction is present, indicating resistance, though such patients are not so common as in Britain.

In Nigeria tuberculosis of the urinary tract is uncommon, but the genital tract is more often affected.

Glandular tuberculosis (apart from the glands in the hilum of the lungs, which are often affected) is particularly common, especially affecting the cervical, axilliary, inguinal and abdominal glands, and tuberculosis of the bones and joints is occasionally seen. In India the elbow is often affected, and local glands (which should always be examined, even by biopsy) are enlarged. These forms are mostly caused by the human type of *Myco. tuberculosis.*

CLINICAL FEATURES

These do not differ from those found in other parts of the world, except that in tropical countries pulmonary tuberculosis tends to be more acute and destructive of tissue, with less fibrous reaction, than elsewhere. The usual signs of cough, haemoptysis, fever, wasting and asthenia are common and marked, and physical signs are prominent.

Non-pulmonary tuberculosis, of glands, bones, joints, meninges, pericardium and kidneys, is often seen, with the usual consequences.

Atypical forms are common. In Indians, localized tuberculous lesions of the bowel often occur, which resemble Crohn's disease and may produce signs of intestinal obstruction. In Africans, primary abdominal glandular tuberculosis is common, often affecting the mesenteric and para-aortic glands, with or without tuberculous peritonitis. Partial haematogenous spread may take place, giving lesions in the liver and spleen, in which the lesions vary in size from miliary tubercles to quite large tuberculomas. This form may present as pyrexia without localizing signs; it can be diagnosed by liver biopsy. Tuberculoma of the brain, with signs of a space-occupying lesion, has been found in Africans.

DIAGNOSIS

In tropical countries the problems of diagnosis relate more to geography and money than to anything else. The physical signs of pulmonary tuberculosis are generally more easily recognized than in the developed countries because most of the patients suffer from relatively acute disease with early cavitation and profuse mucopurulent sputum.

X-ray facilities are now common in big tropical hospitals, and examination of sputum by culture is also common. But in rural areas the diagnosis is likely to rest on stethoscope examination and direct microscopy of sputum.

Sputum most likely to be positive is that containing mucus alone or, better, mucus and pus, and which comes from patients with cavities, but sputum containing saliva only or saliva with mucus, or from patients with little X-ray evidence of the disease, is sometimes positive. Moreover, as by far the most specimens received contain only saliva with mucus, in spite of the low proportion of positive sputa, the total of positive sputa is high—up to 70% of all positives coming from this group.

Ideally of course, the bacilli from each patient should be tested for resistance to the standard drugs, but this may be difficult or impossible.

The tuberculin test has a bearing on diagnosis since it is accepted that patients with strong reactions (over 10 mm) to small doses of tuberculin, especially if accompanied by other signs, yield many more positive sputa than patients with slight reactions. A strong positive tuberculin reaction in a child, and more especially in several children of a single family or school group, should lead not only to further examination of the strong reactors, but also to examination of all contacts—parents, siblings, teachers and even bus drivers etc.—who may have been spreading the infection. It is, of course, necessary to know if the children have recently had BCG.

There has been much controversy on the question whether tuberculosis of the adult form, with destruction of lung tissue accompanied by a fibrotic reaction of varying degree, but without general spread to the lymphatic glands, is the result of superinfection from outside, or of extension from a primary focus which has broken down, possibly owing to some temporary reduction of resistance, for instance in malnutrition. Both processes probably occur. Infection in families seems undoubtedly to be related to heavy and persistent infection from the index case, and states of extreme malnutrition (as in concentration camps) are associated with widespread and extensive disease, though in these circumstances the crowding offers abundant opportunities for superinfection.

Whatever the explanation, there is no doubt that a first infection which is well resisted results in enhanced immunity, accompanied by an allergic state which may be deleterious in that the allergic process in the lung leads to destruction of tissue.

TREATMENT

Modern drugs have revolutionized the treatment of tuberculosis; they are particularly active in the acuter forms of the disease such as are often seen in the tropics.

Provided that the tubercle bacilli are not resistant to any of the standard drugs the recommended regimen for previously untreated adult patients is:

Streptomycin 1·0 gramme daily by intramuscular injection (750 mg is probably enough if given with the other drugs).
Sodium PAS 5–6 grammes twice daily (or 10–12 grammes once daily).
Isoniazid 200 (3 mg/kg) to 300 mg once daily.

All these are taken each day until sensitivity tests have been made on the bacilli. If they are sensitive to PAS and isoniazid the streptomycin can be omitted after 8 weeks.

For children the doses are scaled down as usual.

Single preparations containing PAS and isoniazid are available, for instance:

Sodium aminosalicylate and isoniazid cachets (BP, BNF) containing sodium aminosalicylate 1·5 grammes and isoniazid 33 mg.
Inapaside granules, containing sodium aminosalicylate 6·0 grammes and isoniazid 150 mg. Dose: 2 granules daily.

Pasinah D, containing sodium PAS 6·0 grammes and isoniazid 150 mg. Dose: 2 daily.

Streptomycin may rarely affect the auditory nerve if given at 1·0 gramme daily, but this is almost unknown at 750 mg daily.

Isoniazid is rarely toxic at 200 mg daily, but at 800 mg daily there may be peripheral neuropathy and other neurological effects, which may be prevented by giving pyridoxine (vitamin B_6), 10 mg daily.

Oral PAS is often associated with gastro-intestinal disturbances, diarrhoea being not uncommon; steatorrhoea has been reported (Coltart 1969). Hypersensitivity reactions may occur, and PAS may have an effect on the kidneys and thyroid (producing goitre with features of myxoedema). Reactions are especially common in persons of Indian descent.

The regimen quoted above should be continued until the susceptibility of the tubercle bacilli to the drugs has been determined in each case (if this is possible); if tests cannot be made it may be modified after 3 months by giving streptomycin 1·0 gramme 3 times each week instead of once each day. Streptomycin (1·0 gramme) plus isoniazid (14 mg/kg) can be given twice each week in suitable cases.

If the bacilli are sensitive to all three drugs the treatment can be continued without streptomycin, by giving PAS and isoniazid daily in the same doses as before, or with a schedule of:

Streptomycin	1·0 gramme	
Isoniazid	14 mg/kg	} twice each week
Pyridoxine	10 mg	

This is recommended for patients who may not cooperate well on the standard treatment.

On this kind of treatment, carried out for at least 2 years, cure can be expected in 90–100% of patients. There is, however, the formidable difficulty of educating and persuading people, especially in scattered villages, to persist with treatment.

If PAS cannot be used, ethambutol (15–25 mg/kg daily) is valuable instead, or thiacetazone may take its place in the regimen:

Isoniazid	300 mg	} as a single oral dose daily, preferably with
Thiacetazone	150 mg	streptomycin 1·0 gramme daily for the first 8 weeks

Combined preparations of these two are available, for instance Thiazina (Smith & Nephew), tablets of which contain the above doses, or half those doses; they are available with methylene blue as an indicator, which colours the urine and shows whether the tablets have been taken. This preparation can be supplemented with streptomycin (1·0 gramme daily) for the first 2 months, with advantage. Thiacetazone is cheap, but in the Far East and Africa some strains of tubercle bacilli may be resistant. Side-effects of thiacetazone include gastro-intestinal troubles, flushing, anaemia and vertigo; it may also increase the deleterious effect of streptomycin on the auditory nerve. Toxicity has caused it to be discontinued in advanced countries.

In developing countries money is the problem. The treatment outlined above is desirable where funds are adequate, but where they are not, Fox (1964) considers that it is more justifiable to give modified treatment to all patients with active pulmonary tuberculosis, than to give full treatment to only a few. If streptomycin is available it can be given together with isoniazid for about 2 months, followed by isoniazid alone for the rest of the year. Or isoniazid can be given with PAS or with thiacetazone, for a year, followed if possible by isoniazid alone for the second year, even at the risk of development of isoniazid resistance.

If absolutely necessary, isoniazid can be used alone, in doses of 8–10 mg/kg, but there is a great risk of emergence of resistant tubercle bacilli. Pyridoxine should be added if possible to reduce the incidence of side-effects. Two drugs are always better than one.

For tuberculous meningitis isoniazid at 10–12 mg/kg is advocated.

Other drugs include cycloserine, ethionamide and pyrazinamide, which, though relatively expensive, can be recommended in cases in which the bacilli are resistant to 2 of the standard drugs. Doses are:

Cycloserine   1·0 gramme daily, in 2 halves, by mouth
Ethionamide   1·0 gramme daily, in 2 halves, by mouth
Pyrazinamide   40 mg/kg daily, in 2 halves, by mouth

A combination of ethionamide 500 mg with isoniazid 500 mg daily, 6 days each week, has been recommended as a result of a controlled test in Morocco.

Drug resistance is common in many developing countries. A promising new reserve drug is rifampicin (also useful in leprosy). The usual adult dose is 450–600 mg orally once daily. The drug must be taken fasting, and this is important. It produces reddish-brown or orange colouring of urine or sputum, and of sweat, but is apparently well tolerated (Ross & Horne 1969). It should not be given within 12 hours of a dose of PAS, since PAS tends to delay and reduce blood levels of rifampicin.

Several cases of thrombocytopenia with purpura due to rifampicin have been reported. One patient had been treated with ethambutol 1200 mg and rifampicin 1200 mg, twice each week. Severe thrombocytopenia (with nose bleeding, haemorrhagic spots on the tongue, and headaches) developed after 7 months of this treatment, and recovered quickly when rifampicin was discontinued. It was apparently due to an immune reaction to rifampicin; ethambutol was not a factor (Blajchman et al. 1970). Jaundice, rising transaminases and liver cell damage have been reported a few weeks after beginning rifampicin treatment. Biochemical observation is important. Other temporary features are fever, flushing, nausea, dyspnoea and renal failure.

Ethambutol has been used in tuberculosis resistant to other drugs, the usual dose being 25 mg/kg daily. Visual impairment has been reported in about 10% of patients after prolonged courses. It can be used along with rifampicin in resistant cases.

For tuberculous meningitis in children, diagnosis can be confirmed by examination of not less than 10 ml cerebrospinal fluid by smear, culture or guinea-pig inoculation. Treatment should include intrathecal streptomycin (10 or more injections of 10–50 mg/dose according to age) to which isoniazid (10–50 mg/dose) and hydrocortisone (10–20 mg/dose) should be added in special circumstances such as relapse or if spinal block is threatened, or if the bacilli are suspected of resistance to streptomycin.

It may be necessary to test the patient's urine to make sure that he is taking the treatment properly. The following tests are used for PAS and isoniazid.

PAS. To 1·0 ml of urine add a few drops of N HCl and then drop by drop a 10% solution of ferric chloride. If PAS is present a colour change takes place, varying from blue-black to reddish purple according to the amount of PAS. Other salicylates also give the colour change.

The Phenistix reagent strips are also used. The reagent strip is dipped into the urine; if PAS is there a reddish-brown colour develops. A dose of 5 grammes PAS continues to produce the colour for about 12 hours. Sulphonamides and salicylates may also produce the colour.

Strips can also be made by soaking strips of filter paper in 5% ferric chloride and leaving them to dry. When dipped in urine containing PAS or salicylates they turn blue.

Isoniazid. A porcelain or plastic plate with circular wells is used. In each well 4 drops of urine are placed, and then 4 drops of 10% potassium cyanide solution and 4 drops of chloramine T are added without shaking. A red or pink colour indicates a positive result, which follows if isoniazid has been taken within 12 hours, though after 12 hours the colour is only pink.

Drug prophylaxis with isoniazid has its advocates for people at special risk, such as children of sputum-positive parents or other contacts; the daily dose is 300 mg for adults, and in the United States it is estimated that this has reduced the incidence of tuberculosis by 75% in controlled trials.

One of the most remarkable features of modern drug treatment of tuberculosis is that it has eliminated the necessity of bed rest, extra food and isolation of the patient. Experience in Madras and elsewhere has shown that the treatment can successfully be carried on in even the poorest and most crowded homes, without risk of spread of the disease. The bacilli soon become non-viable and therefore non-infective. Obviously, however, the better the conditions and the more nutritious the diet, the better for the patient in general, who may have malaria or other parasitic disease such as hookworm infection. And there still remains the fact that tuberculosis, in the absence of treatment, spreads more widely in conditions of crowding, fatigue and under-nutrition than in more favourable circumstances. The social aspect of prevention should not be obscured by the successes of chemotherapy.

BCG

BCG (Bacille de Calmette et Guérin) is an attenuated strain of the bovine type of *Myco. tuberculosis*, used as a live vaccine. When injected into people with a negative or only slightly positive tuberculin reaction (i.e. who have not been infected with virulent tubercle bacilli) it produces a degree of cellular (not humoral) immunity which has been estimated at 14–18% over periods of 2–20 years. Nobody claims that the protection is complete or universal, but most agree that it is substantial. BCG replaces 'the natural and potentially harmful primary infection with virulent tubercle bacilli by an artificial and innocuous infection with avirulent bacilli, on the assumption that this artificial infection will similarly enhance resistance to subsequent infection with *Myco. tuberculosis*' (Rees 1969).

Substantial protection can last for $7\frac{1}{2}$–10 years. BCG is now widely used in the tropics, and has had a great effect. In Singapore, for instance, tuberculosis was the chief killing disease around 1960, but in 1970 was reduced to the eighth place largely as a result of BCG.

A BCG campaign must be conducted carefully. Children and others should first be tested with tuberculin, either 5–10 T.U. of Old Tuberculin or PPD in solution, injected intradermally, or by the Heaf multiple puncture technique through a stronger solution. In Britain it has been recommended that BCG can be given to children whose reaction to the Heaf test is either completely negative, or shows 4 or more discrete papules at least 1 mm in diameter (Heaf grade 1).

The assumption is that weak sensitivity to tuberculin is due, not to previous infection with *Myco. tuberculosis*, but to infection with other antigenically related mycobacteria. Children with this weak reaction are less likely to develop tuberculosis than children with a negative reaction, but the protection afforded by BCG is greater than that afforded by infection with atypical mycobacteria (Newham Health Department 1969). Whether this applies to other countries is perhaps a matter for research.

A positive intradermal tuberculin test shows induration over 5 mm in diameter, or in the Heaf test, papules forming a ring with normal skin in the middle, or a plateau of induration, or vesiculation or ulceration.

Freeze-dried BCG vaccine should be used, and must be injected within 2 hours of reconstitution; sunlight kills it. 0·1 ml is injected intradermally into the upper arm or leg; no dressing is needed.

However, in some countries it is difficult to carry out the complete programme of tuberculin testing, with BCG for negative or slight reactors, and BCG has therefore been given indiscriminately without previous tuberculin tests. The results show that BCG does not cause undue local, focal or general reactions in those already tuberculin-positive, and WHO advocates this direct and universal vaccination where preliminary tuberculin tests would considerably reduce the numbers of people returning for BCG. In developing countries BCG and smallpox vaccination have been given together, with success, without preliminary tuberculin tests.

BCG gives some protection against infection with *Myco. ulcerans* and leprosy (see Chapter 18).

Buruli Ulcer

Buruli ulcer (named after the part of Uganda where it has been studied) is an ulcer of the skin and deeper tissues. It has also been observed in Nigeria, Malaysia, New Guinea, Mexico and other countries. In some series of cases the patients have come from very limited geographical areas (Editorial, *Br. med. J.* 1970).

It is caused by an acid-fast bacillus, *Mycobacterium ulcerans*, first described in Australia (MacCallum *et al.* 1948), which can be isolated from the bases and edges of the lesions, and cultivated on media at 33°C, though the growth on Petragnani or Loewenstein–Jensen medium is slow, taking 8–14 weeks or more (Clancey 1964).

It is not clear how the infection is acquired. There may or may not be a history of local injury; but the infection is often associated with riverine areas, and is probably acquired while bathing in infected water, for instance, in swimming pools. Barker *et al.* (1970), however, now think that the organism may be a saprophyte on grass (from which they have cultivated a strain with the same characteristics) and that man becomes infected through scratches.

The lesion begins as a small subcutaneous nodule attached to the skin, and the pathological process is a spreading non-caseous necrosis of the subcutaneous tissue. The epidermis is not at first affected (Dodge 1964). There is little inflammatory reaction, though foci of polymorphs may be present where the necrosis approaches the epidermis. The core of the necrotic mass may be surrounded by epithelioid cells, fibroblasts and lymphocytes. When ulceration occurs the necrosis may involve subcutaneous fat, connective tissue, nerves and blood vessels. Granulations in the ulcer bed tend to have a gelatinous appearance, and calcification may occur (Gray *et al.*, 1967).

There may be desquamation over parts of the indurated area, and pitting oedema of the leg down to the ankle has been observed when the leg is extensively ulcerated. The area is not tender, but movements of neighbouring joints may be restricted and painful.

Large numbers of *Myco. ulcerans* can be found at the base of the ulcer, and in clumps at the edges.

Most patients are young, aged 5–15, though some are 50 or more. The initial lesion is a single, firm, painless nodule, mostly on a leg or arm—never on the scalp. Multiple lesions are not common. The lesion may itch. It is attached to the skin, and may extend slowly (during several months), though in some cases it can be fulminating, spreading widely in 2–3 weeks. In uncomplicated cases it

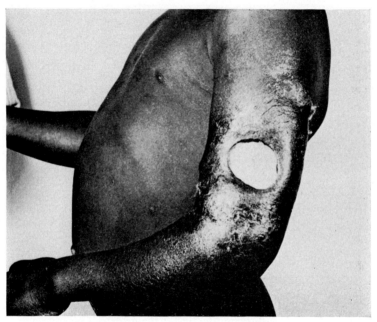

Fig. 132.—Buruli ulcer before preparation for grafting. (*H. F. Lunn, Makerere University College*)

is not tender, and there are no constitutional disturbances or lymphadenopathy. It breaks down to form an ulcer with undermined edges, which may become very large. In fulminating cases the limb is not hot or tender, but becomes tense and shiny owing to massive oedema, which must be differentiated from cellulitis (in which there is inflammation and fever). Secondary infection may occur to complicate the picture. In general the ulcer tends towards natural healing after months or years, but may leave severe scarring, possibly with contracture of neighbouring joints.

The lesions should be differentiated from foreign-body granulations (usually with a history of trauma); nodular fasciitis, fibroma or low-grade fibrosarcoma; phycomycosis (by excision and histological examination); injection abscess; boils or panniculitis; sebaceous cysts or skin accessory tumours; and acute cellulitis (with inflammation) (Uganda Buruli Group 1970).

TREATMENT

The small pre-ulcerative lesions can be excised completely under local anaesthesia in an outpatient department, and the wound usually heals by first intention. Somewhat larger lesions can often be excised and grafted (Figs 132, 133), but they are usually more extensive than pre-operation examination suggests (Uganda Buruli Group 1970).

In very large lesions the object is to excise non-viable skin and skin bridges, and to cut flaps to gain access to diseased fascia; it is usually not possible to remove all the diseased tissue initially, and repeated operations may be needed, but the diseased tissue should be removed completely as soon as possible. If

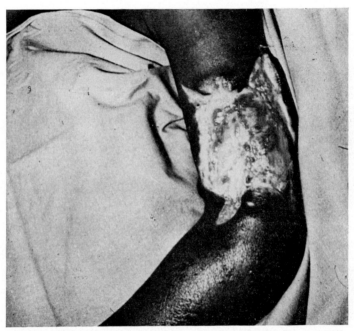

Fig. 133.—Buruli ulcer on the upper arm after removal of irreparably damaged skin and fat. The granulated area is awaiting grafting. (*H. F. Lunn, Makerere University College*)

healthy granulations do not appear and skin flaps do not stick down in 1–2 weeks after operation, the disease is still present, and if further operation is delayed the discharge and organization of necrotic material take months, leaving considerable fibrosis which limits the final result.

In one series of cases (Gray *et al.* 1967) wet dressings of 0·25 or 0·5% silver nitrate were applied to the ulcers, repeatedly, after they had been surgically cleaned up. This arrested and cleaned them so that pinch grafts could be applied in due course. If the lesions are large before treatment, fibrosis tends to be extensive, and may affect joint movement, for instance by contracture near the knee.

Treatment by drugs is disappointing, though clofazimine (Lamprene, B663) and rifampicin have been suggested because of their actions in leprosy. But the important treatment is surgical.

BCG seems to give some protection—18% in high-incidence areas and 74% in low-incidence areas (Uganda Buruli Group 1969).

REFERENCES

BARKER, D. J. P., CLANCEY, J. K., MORROW, R. H. & RAO, S. (1970) *Br. med. J.*, **iv**, 558.
BLAJCHMAN, M. A., LOWRY, R. C., PETTIT, J. E. & STRADLING, P. (1970) *Br. med. J.*, **iii**, 24.
CLANCEY, J. K. (1964) *J. Path. Bact.*, **88**, 175.
COLTART, D. J. (1969) *Br. med. J.*, **i**, 825.
DODGE, O. G. (1964) *J. Path. Bact.*, **88**, 167.
EDITORIAL (1970) *Br. med. J.*, **ii**, 378.
FOX, W. (1964) *Br. med. J.*, **i**, 135.
GIRDWOOD, M. I. (1962) *Transactions of the Sixth Commonwealth Health and Tuberculosis Conference*, p. 62. London: Chest and Heart Association.
GORDON, C. G. I. (1962) *Transactions of the Sixth Commonwealth Health and Tuberculosis Conference*, p. 38. London: Chest and Heart Association.
GRAY, H. H., KINGMA, S. & KOK, S. H. (1967) *Trans. R. Soc. trop. Med. Hyg.*, **61**, 712.
HUTT, M. S. R. (1971) *Trans. R. Soc. trop. Med. Hyg.*, **65**, 273.
MacCALLUM, P., TOLHURST, J. C., BUCKLE, G. & SISSONS, H. A. (1948) *J. Path. Bact.*, **60**, 93, 102, 110, 116.
NEWHAM HEALTH DEPARTMENT (1969) *Lancet*, **ii**, 537.
REES, R. J. W. (1969) *Br. med. Bull.*, **25**, 183.
ROSS, J. D. & HORNE, N. W. (1969) *Modern Drug Treatment in Tuberculosis*, 4th ed. London: Health Horizon.
SCHAEFER, W. B., BIRN, K. J., JENKINS, P. A. & MARKS, J. (1969) *Br. med. J.*, **ii**, 412.
UGANDA BURULI GROUP (1969) *Lancet*, **i**, 111.
—— (1970) *Br. med. J.*, **ii**, 390.
WILCOCKS, C. (1962) *Aspects of Medical Investigation in Africa*. London: Oxford University Press.

Plague

AETIOLOGY

THE specific cause of plague is the bacillus which was discovered by Yersin and Kitasato in 1894. It occurs in great profusion in the characteristic buboes, generally in pure culture, and is also present in great abundance in the spleen, intestines, lungs, kidneys, liver and other viscera and, though in smaller numbers, the blood, while in the pneumonic type it is found in the sputum in profusion. It may be found also in the urine and faeces. Towards the termination of rapidly fatal cases it occurs in great numbers in the blood.

Pasteurella pestis as seen in a blood-film or in preparations from any of the other tissues, is a short, thick cocco-bacillus ($1 \cdot 5$–$2 \times 0 \cdot 5$–$0 \cdot 7$ μm) with rounded ends, very like the bacillus of chicken cholera. A capsule, or the appearance of one, can generally be made out, especially in bacilli in the blood. The organism is readily stained by aniline dyes, especially by Romanowsky stains, the extremities taking on a deeper colour than the interpolar part, giving a bipolar appearance.

Bhatnagar states that virulent strains of *P. pestis* can be recognized by the abundance of the envelope substance.

It is non-motile, Gram-negative, indole-positive and gives nitrite reaction with sulphanilic acid and α-naphthylamine.

Cultural characters. When sown on blood-serum and kept at body-temperature in from 24 to 48 hours an abundant moist, yellowish-grey growth is formed without liquefaction of the culture medium. On agar, but better on glycerin agar, the growths have a greyish white appearance. On agar plate cultures they show a bluish translucence, the individual colonies being circular, with slightly irregular contours and a moist surface; on mannite neutral red bile salt agar the colonies are bright red, but are colourless on a similar medium in which lactose is substituted for mannite. Litmus milk and glucose broth are rendered slightly acid; lactose broth is unchanged. Young colonies are glass-like, but older ones are thick at the centre and more opaque; they are singularly coherent and may be removed *en bloc* with a platinum needle. Stab-cultures show after one or two days a fine dust-like line of growth. Cultivated on broth in which clarified butter or coconut oil is floated, *P. pestis* usually presents characteristic stalactite growths which gradually fall off, forming a granular deposit. Examined with the microscope, these various cultures show chains of a short bacillus, presenting large bulbous swellings here and there. In gelatin the bacilli sometimes form fine threads, sometimes thick bundles made up of many laterally agglomerated bacteria, and involution forms are common. The bacillus does not produce spores.

The most favourable temperature for culture is 28°C. Jackson and Morris (1961) state that when *P. pestis* is cultivated on human serum, growth is enhanced by the addition of iron.

Three varieties of *P. pestis* are recognized (Pollitzer 1960). They can be distinguished by their ability to acidify glycerol and reduce nitrites.

	Glycerol acidifying	Nitrite reducing
P. pestis var. orientalis or oceanica		
(adapted to rats)	−	+
P. pestis var. antiqua	+	+
P. pestis var. mediaevalis		
(adapted to Meriones)	+	−

There is a fourth subgroup which is of a mixed nature.

A distinction between the varieties of P. pestis can be epidemiologically important, since if the P. orientalis variety is found in both wild and domestic rodents, the original source of infection for both was the same, and plague was imported into the area and passed from domestic to wild rodents. If, however, as in Kenya, two varieties have been found coexisting, this would indicate two separate sources of infection, one ancient and the other more recent and imported.

The plague bacillus can be modified by artificial methods and it is well known that some process of this kind takes place in nature for as a plague epidemic decreases so the case mortality falls. There is difficulty in producing virulent mutants from an avirulent strain.

IMMUNOLOGY

P. pestis has a complicated antigenic structure. The antigens so far defined are Fraction I (envelope substance), which is stable, initiates a strong antibody response and provides the main protective effect against wild strains of plague bacilli, Fraction II (murine toxin), Fractions V, W, L, PF, antigen 4, Ph6 and the specific polysaccharide (Chen 1965). Three of these antigens are held in common with P. pseudotuberculosis: the PF antigen, which has been shown to protect guinea-pigs against plague, and the V and W antigens, which enable organisms to survive and multiply within monocytes (i.e. determine virulence).

The main mechanism of immunity to plague is the formation of antibodies which neutralize the antiphagocytic properties of the Fractions I, V and W antigens (Pollitzer 1954). Protective immunity does not depend upon antitoxins to murine toxin (Fraction II).

Complement fixing and haemagglutinating antibodies are found in both man and rodents and appreciable antibody levels against Fraction I can be found for months in the sera of persons recovered from plague. The passive haemagglutination test (WHO 1970), which is widely used for epidemiological studies on plague, is especially useful for detecting plague foci in rodent populations. Antitoxin is found in the sera of patients with pneumonic plague and of convalescent patients but does not persist for long; vaccinated individuals who contracted plague showed both antibodies and antitoxins for months or years (Pollitzer 1960).

When purified, Fraction I is used as antigen for the CF and HA tests, which are sensitive and specific. The HA test is useful in rodents, and the CFT will demonstrate antibodies in immunized or infected hosts. The presence of Fraction I can be detected in animal tissues by immunofluorescence and microtechniques, which can be used to determine the presence of P. pestis in small amounts of tissue (Chen & Meyer 1966).

Vaccination against plague

Although both live and inactivated vaccines are available, their effectiveness is not well established. The use of vaccines may reduce the morbidity and mortality in bubonic but not in pneumonic plague (WHO 1970). The immunity conferred is of short duration, not longer than 6 months, so that revaccination is necessary to maintain immunity and must be spread over a period and reinforced by booster injections (Ehrenkrantz & Meyer 1955). Mass vaccination cannot be recommended for general plague control, but under highly endemic conditions or for high-risk groups vaccination may be given for individual protection.

To be effective against plague a vaccine must contain an adequate amount of Fraction I antigen or in the case of live vaccines they must produce sufficient Fraction I *in vivo*. Two types of vaccine are available: inactivated highly virulent cultures of *P. pestis*, originally prepared by Haffkine, and live avirulent cultures of the EV strain, available from the Pasteur Institute, Paris.

Inactivated vaccine. Meyer's modification of Haffkine's vaccine consists of *P. pestis* grown for 3 days at 37°C and killed by formaldehyde. The adult dose is 0·5 ml (containing 1500 million organisms) subcutaneously followed by 1·0 ml 10–28 days later and then 0·5 ml every 6 months to persons at risk.

Live vaccine. An avirulent culture of smooth *P. pestis* has been used in Madagascar. In experimental animals this vaccine gives a better immunity than that obtained with dead cultures. The immunity is long lasting, of high degree and protects them against any form of plague (Ehrenkrantz & Meyer 1955). This method was used in Java in 1935–9 when up to 9286 000 people were inoculated, and the present decline of plague in Java is attributed chiefly to this vaccine.

No stable reference vaccine is at present available and countries desiring to use live plague vaccine should produce it from the original EV strain (WHO 1970).

TRANSMISSION

Plague is transmitted between rodents and to man by fleas. Less common methods of transmission are droplet spreads (pneumonic plague), direct contact from handling infected animals and laboratory infection. Aerosol transmission of plague is one of the suggested forms of bacterial warfare.

Role of the flea in plague

Plague is readily communicated from rat to rat by fleas, principally by *Xenopsylla cheopis* (Fig. 461, page 1130), the rat flea of the tropics, *Ceratophyllus fasciatus*, the rat flea of temperate climates, and *Ctenocephalus canis* and *C. felis* which bite man, dogs and cats indifferently. *Pulex irritans*, the human flea, though important in the Middle Ages, does not often act as carrier now, although in Manchuria it may convey the bacillus directly from one patient to another without the intervantion of the rat. Wild rodent fleas transmit infection in a similar manner in wild rodent plague. The Indian Commission showed that if fleas were excluded, healthy rats would not contract the infection from diseased rats and young rats suckled by infected mothers remained healthy in the absence of fleas. The transfer of fleas to a healthy animal or placing them in jumping range of fleas (about 4 cm above the floor) permitted infection.

The capacity of a flea's stomach is about 0·5 mm³ and in most cases of bubonic plague there are not sufficient bacilli in the peripheral blood to infect fleas except in the terminal stages of fatal cases. After the ingestion of infected blood, *P. pestis* multiplies in the flea's stomach and is then passed out in the faeces so that the flea serves as a multiplier of the bacillus. The life span of an infected flea is about 3·2 days and a proportion become 'blocked', a condition in which the stomach and oesophagus become obstructed with a pure culture of *P. pestis* (Fig. 134). Blocked fleas die rapidly in a warm dry atmosphere. When such a flea feeds the culture is regurgitated and communicates infection. The flea transmits infection either by fouled mandibles, regurgitation in the act of feeding or by provoking scratching and the inoculation of infection via the faeces.

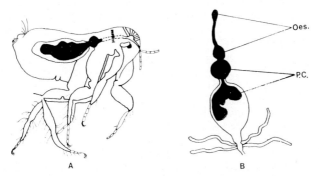

Fig. 134.—A, The flea viewed as a transparent object. The proventriculus and stomach contain a mass of plague culture. B, The flea's stomach, obstructed by growth of plague culture.

Oes., Distended oesophagus containing fresh blood. *P.C.*, The obstructing mass of plague culture. This figure illustrates the method of transmission of *P. pestis* by *Ceratophyllus fasciatus*. (*By permission of Sir C. J. Martin*)

Species of flea

It has long been known that some areas of India remained free of plague although in direct contact with other plague infested areas. Rat fleas in India belong to 3 related species, *X. cheopis*, *X. brasiliensis* and *X. astia*. It was discovered that where plague was uncommon *X. astia* replaced *X. cheopis* as the common rat flea. It is now known that *X. astia* is unable to transmit *P. pestis* to the same extent as *X. cheopis* and the '*cheopis* index' (i.e. the number of fleas per rat) is of considerable importance; an index of over 5 is thought likely to produce an outbreak of plague.

Bionomics of the rat flea

The rat flea ordinarily completes its developmental cycle in from 14 to 21 days but in warm damp weather this may be shortened to 10 days. The average life of a flea separated from its host is about 10 days but it is capable of remaining alive without food for 2 months at low temperatures. In temperate climates fleas are most numerous during the warmer months and summer and autumn are the plague seasons. In warm climates plague is likely to become epidemic at temperatures between 10° and 30°C but over 30°C is unfavourable. *X. cheopis* can flourish in northern countries in superheated houses and factories even during the winter months.

Persistence of infection in the absence of fleas

The Plague Commission has shown that floors of cowdung contaminated with *P. pestis* do not remain infective for more than 48 hours and that floors of 'chunam' cease to be infective in 24 hours.

EPIDEMIOLOGY AND GEOGRAPHICAL
DISTRIBUTION

Plague is a disease of 'natural foci' (Pavlovsky 1966) and a typical zoonosis (Fig. 135). It exists in two forms: sylvatic or wild rodent plague, existing in nature independent of human populations and their activities, and domestic plague, intimately associated with man and rodents living with man.

Wild rodent plague

Plague exists all over the world, in wild rodents, among the marmots (tarabagan) of Siberia and Manchuria, the susliks, mice and jerboas of the desert region of South-east Russia, the gerbils and muridae of the African veld and high regions, the chipmunks and ground squirrels of California and in South America the cavies ('cuis', wild guinea-pigs) and other rodents of the pampas. In these areas the infection is maintained permanently by hosts which are relatively resistant, termed 'permanent reservoir hosts' (Table 24). They pass the infection to less resistant animal hosts and cause epizootics (murine plague) which affect some domestic rodents, and thus cause outbreaks of plague in man. Certain wild rodents, such as *Arvicanthus* and *Otomys* in Africa, are relatively resistant and form permanent foci of plague. Rodents which are highly susceptible to plague during the active period of their lives become less so as hibernation approaches, and may be quite refractory whilst in hibernation (Zhigilev & Otdelskaya 1956) and thus serve as a source of permanent infection in a natural focus. Epizootics, which usually begin in northern regions after hibernation, attack rodent colonies and wipe out the susceptible population. The infection then dies out, only to return when the population builds up again. Baltazard et al. (1963) have shown that in Iran, plague bacilli can survive in the soil of burrows in the absence of rodents and fleas for a long time and thus maintain a permanent focus of plague in the rodents of that region. Serological testing with the haemagglutination test has shown the persistence of rodent plague in the foothills of Kenya (Davis et al. 1968). Rodent fleas play a part in transmission and proventricular blocking with plague bacilli occurs in the gerbil fleas (*Ceratophyllus tesquorum* and *C. laeviceps*), and also in *Oropsylla silantievi*, the flea of the tarabagan (*Arctomys bobac*), which sticks in the fur and is found in pelts. It is also found to occur in *Ceratophyllus tesquorum* and *Neopsylla setosa* which infest 'susliks'. A large number of species of wild rodent fleas have been found to be naturally infected with *P. pestis* (Pollitzer 1960).

Infection is also transmitted by the intestinal tract, and carnivores such as mongoose are susceptible to plague from feeding on dead and dying rodents. In South Africa the discovery of gerbil remains in the faeces of the suricate and yellow mongoose is a valuable indication of the existence of rodent plague, as these animals do not normally eat them unless they are sick. When epizootics occur in the wild rodents the infection is passed on to rats commensal with man and outbreaks of human plague occur. Man can acquire plague directly by inhalation from wild rodent skins such as the tarabagan (*Marmota sibirica*) in Manchuria and Siberia or indirectly via semi-domestic rodents as in parts of Africa. Foci of wild rodent plague may be very ancient, as in Iran and Africa, or may follow from the introduction of plague by the brown rat, as occurred in California after the San Francisco outbreak in 1903.

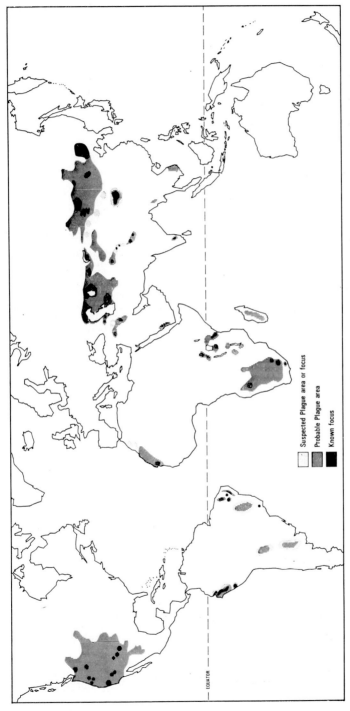

Fig. 135.—Known and probable foci of plague in 1969. (*Reproduced from Wld Hlth Org. tech. Rep. Ser.* (1970) 447).

Table 24. Permanent wild rodent reservoirs of plague (after Pollitzer 1960)

Focus	Host
U.S.S.R.	
The Caspian Region—steppes	*Citellus pygmaeus* (suslik)
The Caspian Region—sandy stretches	*Meriones meridianus*
	Meriones tamaricinus
Central Asiatic focus—desert lowlands	*Rhombomys opimus*
	Meriones erythrourus
Central Asiatic focus—high mountains	*Marmota barbacina*
	Marmota caudata
Transcaucasian area	Gerbils
Transbaikalia	*Marmota sibirica* (tarabagan)
Mongolia	
Central part	*Marmota barbacina*
	Marmota sibirica
Southern part	*Meriones meridianus*
	Rhombomys opimus
	Meriones unguiculatus (Mongolian gerbil, jerd)
	Citellus pallidicauda
	Citellus dauricus
Kenya (Davis *et al.* 1968)	*Acomys* spp.
	Arvicanthus
	Rattus natalensis (commonly called multimammate mouse)
	Otomys angoniensis (Swamp rat)
	Tatera spp.
	Aethiops kaiseri
South Africa	*Tatera brantsi* (gerbils, source of infection of *Mastomys,* the multimammate mouse)
Iranian Kurdistan	*Meriones persicus*
	Meriones libycus
Northern India	*Tatera indica* (primary reservoir)
	Millandia ⎱ (susceptible and secondary
	Bandicota ⎰ reservoirs)
Java	*Rattus exulans* (Polynesian rat, permanent reservoir)
U.S.A.	*Citellus beecheyi* (ground squirrels)
	Microtus
	Peromyscus
New Mexico and Mexico	*Cynomys mexicanus* (prairie dog)
South America	
Argentine	*Microcavia australis*
	Microcavia galea
	Graomys griseoflavus
	Holochilus balnearum
Venezuela	*Heteromys anomalus*
	Sigmodon hirsutus

Other animals are susceptible to plague and may die during an epidemic. Dogs are said to be insusceptible. Camels are often infected but are not important in the maintenance and spread of plague.

Rat plague (bubonic plague)

The brown or sewer rat (*Rattus norvegicus*) is the prime originator and main means of spread of bubonic plague. Originally the infection is picked up from susceptible secondary reservoirs of plague (murine plague), the commensal semi-domestic rodents which come into contact with permanent reservoirs, which initiate the epizootic in the commensal rodents. The brown rat is a great traveller but does not come into direct contact with man. It frequents cities, sewers and docks and when it dies the fleas leave the dead rat and in some circumstances infect the black rat (*Rattus rattus*), the domestic rat, which lives in close contact with man in his houses. Rat plague is seasonal, and spreads during the period when fleas are most numerous. The first sign of plague is the

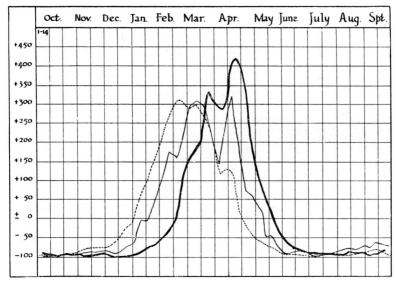

Fig. 136.—A chart showing the progress of plague in rats and in man.
.... Infected *R. norvegicus*. ———— Infected *R. rattus*. ————
Human deaths from plague. (*Indian Plague Commission*)

appearance of dead rats, and dead sewer rats first appear in the region of docks and grain stores. When the black rat becomes infected dead rats appear in houses and the phenomenon of 'rat fall' occurs when rats fall from the rafters and die on the floor. This is a sign of the imminent outbreak of epidemic bubonic plague in man (Fig. 136). The sewer rat also lives on ships, spreading the infection from one port to another, and was responsible for the spread of plague around the world during the great pandemics. Rats also accompany certain trade goods, such as wool and cotton, which in olden times spread plague along the trade routes (Hirst 1953).

Rattus rattus, Linn. The black rat (Fig. 137). Build slender; muzzle sharp; ears large, translucent, cover eyes when folded down; tail usually long, never much shorter than head and body; coarse hair on rump; hind foot (heel to tip of longest toe, without claw) 35–40 mm; weight of adults rarely more than 225 grammes. Indigenous, wild, more or less arboreal in Indo-Burmese countries.

In tropics generally dominant domestic rat in houses and ships. The chief domestic races are distinguished as follows:

A.   Back reddish or greyish brown.

     a.   Under parts pure white or pale lemon. *R. r. frugivorus* Raf. (= *tectorum*) common in Mediterranean region. *R. r. kijabius* in Uganda.

     b.   Under parts darkened.

         (i) Ventral hairs with rusty tips. *R. r. rufescens* Gray. Common rat of Indian houses.

         (ii) Ventral hairs without rusty tips. *R. r. alexandrinus* Geoff.

B.   Back black; under parts dusky or slate-grey. *R. r. rattus* Linn. Essentially a domestic form which has been evolved in cold temperate countries.

N.B.—The black rat tends to be brown in the tropics.

The forms *frugivorus*, *alexandrinus*, and *rattus* have now acquired an almost world-wide distribution; *frugivorus* is the least, *rattus* the most modified race. These are climbing rats, common on ships; frequent in dwellings in warm countries, and not shunning man; they are of especial importance as plague-

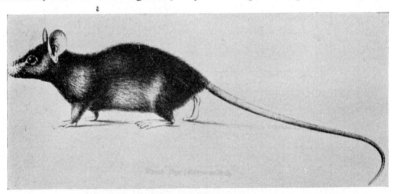

Fig. 137.—The black rat, *Rattus rattus*. (*London School of Hygiene and Tropical Medicine*)

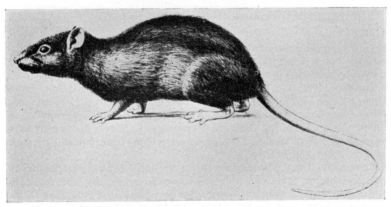

Fig. 138.—The common sewer rat, *Rattus norvegicus*. (*London School of Hygiene and Tropical Medicine*)

carriers; attain sexual maturity early (min. weight sex-mature, 70 grammes); breed throughout the year; gestation about 21 days, but with concurrent lactation about 31 days; litter of from 4 to 11; average litter 5 or 6.

Rattus norvegicus, Berkenhout (= *decumanus*). The brown, grey or sewer rat (Fig. 138). Robust; muzzle blunt; ears small, opaque; tail noticeably shorter than head and body; fine hairs on rump; hind foot 40 to 45 mm; weight of adults commonly 460 grammes, often much more; colour brown or grey above, silvery below. A melanic form (often confused with *R. rattus*) quite common.

Human plague

Man can become infected directly from wild rodents by handling them during skinning or trapping. Under these conditions plague is sporadic and

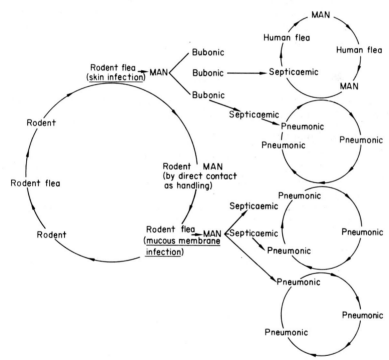

Fig. 139.—Transmission cycles of plague. On the left, the enzootic cycle, and on the right, the potential epidemic cycles in man. (*Reproduced from Faust & Russell* (1964) *Craig and Faust's Clinical Parasitology*)

only a few cases occur every year. Under some circumstances semi-domestic rodents which have become infected may introduce the infection to rural houses or villages and cause small outbreaks. This occurs in Kenya and India, in the mountain foothills, but not on the plains below. In Mongolia and Siberia outbreaks of pneumonic plague occur when trappers, who have become infected from tarabagans, in which there is an intestinal infection, spread the infection directly by inhalation in crowded tents and huts during the Siberian winter.

Plague was once common in Eastern Europe, occurring as great epidemics such as the Black Death in the fourteenth century and the Plague of London in the seventeenth century. These ceased shortly after and the reason is thought to be that the brown rat (*R. norvegicus*) ousted *R. rattus* from Europe. As *R. norvegicus* is a sewer or stable rat, contact with man was greatly reduced.

During the least great pandemic, which started in 1896, plague spread from Hong Kong to Bombay, and then rapidly to other parts of India, as well as to Mauritius, whence it was introduced to East Africa causing outbreaks in Mombasa, Zanzibar, Delagoa Bay, Capetown, Port Elizabeth and Durban. Alexandria and the Nile Delta were invaded from the same source as was Australia, with outbreaks in Sydney and Brisbane. In 1903 plague appeared in the New World in San Francisco and spread later to Brazil and Argentina. Plague appeared in Colombo, Ceylon, in 1914 and in Java in 1910, where for the next 40 years there were some 3000 to 4000 cases each year.

Sometimes human plague spreads rapidly from point to point, but more generally it creeps slowly from one village to another from one street or house to another. Sometimes it skips a house or a village.

PATHOLOGY

The toxin of *P. pestis* causes vascular damage and leakage of fluid into the tissues, with haemoconcentration and shock.

Experimental plague

In the guinea-pig, within a few hours of the introduction of the bacillus, a considerable amount of oedema appears around the puncture, and the adjacent gland is perceptibly swollen. At the end of 24 hours the animal is very ill; its coat is rough and staring; it refuses food, and presently becomes convulsed and usually dies on the third or fourth day. If the body is opened immediately after death a sanguineous oedema is found at the point of inoculation, with haemorrhagic inflammatory effusions around the nearest lymphatic gland which is much swollen and full of bacilli. The intestines are hyperaemic; the adrenals, kidneys and liver are red and swollen. The much enlarged spleen frequently presents an eruption of small whitish granulations resembling miliary tubercles. All the organs, and even any serous fluid that may be present in peritoneum or pleura, contain plague bacilli. In the blood, besides those free in the liquor sanguinis, bacilli are found in the mononuclear, though not, it is said, in the polymorphonuclear leucocytes.

Human plague

After death from plague the surface of the body very frequently presents numerous ecchymotic spots or patches. Buboes are characteristic; they are enlarged, congested lymphatic glands with haemorrhagic points, and later necrosis. Plague bacilli are numerous. The glands are hard and can be moved under the skin. Occasionally there are also furuncles, pustules and abscesses.

The characteristic appearance of plague in a necropsy is that of engorgement and haemorrhage, nearly every organ of the body participating more or less. There is also parenchymatous degeneration in most of the organs. The brain, spinal cord and their meninges are markedly congested, and there may be an increase of subarachnoid and ventricular fluid.

Ecchymoses are common in all serous surfaces; the contents of the different serous cavities may be sanguineous. Extensive haemorrhages are occasionally found in the peritoneum, mediastinum, trachea, bowel, stomach, pelvis of kidney, ureter, bladder or in the pleural cavities. The lung frequently shows evidence of bronchitis and hypostatic pneumonia; sometimes haemorrhagic infarcts and abscesses are found. The right side of the heart and the great veins are usually distended with feebly coagulated or fluid blood. In pneumonic plague the superficial lymphatic glands are not enlarged; the pleural cavities contain blood-stained fluid; the infected lungs are deeply congested and oedematous, and at a later stage pneumonic consolidation is found. The bronchi contain blood-stained mucus, and the bronchial glands are swollen and haemorrhagic.

The liver is congested and swollen, its cells are degenerated and may be the seat of miliary plague abscesses. The spleen is enlarged to 2 or 3 times its normal size. The kidneys are in a similar condition.

The lymphatic system is always involved; around the glands there is much exudation and haemorrhagic effusion, with hyperplasia of the gland-cells and enormous multiplication of plague bacilli.

CLINICAL FEATURES

Incubation period. Symptoms of plague begin to show themselves after an incubation period of from 2 to 8, rarely 15 days.

The average case of plague: prodromal stage. In a certain but small proportion of cases there is a prodromal stage characterized by physical and mental depression, anorexia, aching of the limbs, feelings of chilliness, giddiness, palpitations and sometimes dull pains in the groin at the seat of the future bubo.

Pestis minor, or ambulatory stage. Abortive or ambulatory cases of bubonic plague have been reported in connection with almost every true outbreak of the disease, and in some constitute a high proportion. Clinically these cases present mild, general febrile symptoms with a bubo, and when that suppurates the temperature falls, and the patient recovers. The diagnosis may be difficult because the plague bacilli may be scanty in the pus. The differential diagnosis has to be made from climatic bubo (lymphogranuloma venereum).

Marshall et al. (1967) have isolated *P. pestis* from throat swabs of patients with plague, as well as from healthy contacts. This suggests that healthy carriers of plague can be found. Treatment with streptomycin did not hasten clearing of the carrier state.

From the clinical aspect, plague in man can be divided into the following varieties: (*a*) Bubonic; (*b*) Septicaemic; (*c*) Pneumonic; and (*d*) Meningeal.

Bubonic plague (zootic plague)

This is the most common form and constitutes about three-quarters of the total number. The incubation period is usually very short; A small vesicular primary lesion has been described at the site of the infective flea bite. The characteristic bubo or buboes develop within 24 hours. It is possible to distinguish three varieties of bubonic plague: (*a*) well marked bubonic infection not leading to secondary septicaemia; (*b*) bubonic affection followed by secondary septicaemia; (*c*) serious general septicaemia combined with slight affection of lymph glands. Generally (in 70%) the bubo appears in the groin, especially on the right side and affecting one or more of the femoral glands; less frequently (20%) the axillary; more rarely still (10%, especially seen in children) the submaxillary lymphatic gland may be the seat of the bubo. In rare cases the tonsil may be the primary focus of infection. Buboes are usually single, but in about one-eighth of the cases they form simultaneously on both sides of the body. Very rarely buboes form in the popliteal, epitrochlear or clavicular glands. Occasionally they develop simultaneously in different parts of the body. A curious point, noted in North-west America, is that in plague conveyed by squirrels axillary buboes are more common than in plague conveyed by rats. Plague buboes vary very much in size. Sometimes they are not as large as a walnut; in others again they may be as large as a goose's egg. Pain may be very severe, but sometimes it is hardly felt. Besides the enlargement of the gland there is, in most instances, considerable pericellular infiltration and oedema.

Stage of fever. The stage of invasion may last for a day or two without serious pyrexia, but usually it is much shorter, or it may be altogether absent. The disease usually develops abruptly, without a definite rigor or other warning, the thermometer rising rapidly to 39.4 or $40°C$, or even to $41.7°C$, with corresponding acceleration of temperature and pulse. Sordes form on the teeth and about the lips and nostrils. Thirst is intense, prostration extreme, and from utter debility the voice is reduced to a whisper. Sometimes there is wildly fatuous delirium, or it may be of the low muttering type.

Coma, convulsions, sometimes tetanic retention of urine, subsultus tendinum and other nervous phenomena ensue. Vomiting is in certain cases very frequent. Some patients are constipated, but in others there is diarrhoea. The spleen and liver are usually enlarged. Urine is scanty, but rarely contains more than a trace of albumin. The pulse at first is full and bounding; in the majority it rapidly loses tone, becoming small, frequent, fluttering, dicrotic and intermittent. There is usually a polymorphonuclear leucocytosis.

Stage of recovery. In favourable cases, sooner or later, after or without the appearance of the bubo, the constitutional symptoms abate with the onset of profuse perspiration. The tongue begins to moisten, the pulse-rate and temperature to fall and the delirium to abate. The bubo, however, continues to enlarge and to soften. After a few days, if not incised, it bursts and discharges pus and sloughs—sometimes very ill-smelling. Owing to contracture and fibrosis of lymphatic tissue, oedema of the leg on the affected side usually supervenes.

Skin affections. In a very small proportion of cases what are usually described as carbuncles, in reality small patches of moist gangrenous skin that may gradually involve a large area, develop on different parts of the integument. These occur either in the early stage or late. Sometimes they slough and lead to extensive gangrene.

A generalized papular rash on the hands, feet and pectoral region has been described. Should life be continued sufficiently long, the vesicles become converted into pustules resembling smallpox. These observations confirm in a remarkable manner, as MacArthur has pointed out, the old writers who described manifestations, in the Plague of London of 1665, as 'blains'.

Complications. Occasionally a pyaemic condition, with boils, abscesses, cellulitis, parotitis or secondary adenitis, succeeds the primary fever. During convalescence fatal sudden cardiac failure is not uncommon. Secondary pneumonic plague with blood-stained sputum may supervene, but the patient may recover.

Septicaemic plague (pestis siderans)

In this type there is no special enlargement of the lymphatic glands during life, although after death they are somewhat enlarged and congested throughout the body. The high degree of virulence and the rapid course of the disease depend on the entry of large numbers of the bacilli into the blood, where they can be readily found during life. The patient is prostrated from the outset; he is pale and apathetic; there is generally little febrile reaction (37·8°C). Great weakness, delirium, picking of the bed-clothes, stupor and coma end in death on the first, second, or third day, or, it may be, later. Frequently in these cases there are haemorrhages.

Pneumonic plague (demic plague)

This occurs frequently in epidemic form among the marmot-trappers of Northern China, who live under very insanitary conditions, but may occur spontaneously wherever the bubonic form is found. It is especially dangerous to the patient's attendants and visitors, because of the multitude of bacilli which are scattered about in the patient's expectoration, because the clinical symptoms are unlike those of typical plague and are apt to be mistaken for some ordinary form of lung disease. The illness commences with rigor, malaise, intense head-ache, vomiting, general pains, fever and intense prostration. In the early stages there may be little to suggest pneumonic plague, except the marked discrepancy between the almost negligible physical signs and the gravity of the patient's condition. Cough and dyspnoea set in, accompanied by a profuse, watery, blood-tinged sputum. The sputum is not viscid and rusty, as in lobar pneumonia. From the outset clouding of consciousness is very marked. Moist râles are audible at the bases of the lungs, the breathing becomes hurried; other symptoms rapidly become worse, delirium sets in and the patient usually dies on the fourth or fifth day. This is the most fatal as well as the most directly infectious form of plague. Epidemics of 50 000 and more cases have occurred in Manchuria, where the plague bacillus exists as an intestinal infection in the marmot which acts as a reservoir. Pneumonic plague has been recorded from Nigeria, Ghana, Ecuador, New Orleans and elsewhere. In these countries haemorrhage into the intestinal canal occurs in about 8% of plague-infected rats and the organism is passed out in the faeces; in this manner the plague bacillus can be disseminated in dust and inspired by man directly into the lungs.

It has been pointed out that, whereas in rat-borne plague pneumonia is rare, in wild rodent plague it is the reverse.

Meningeal plague

Primary plague meningitis has been found in Dakar, the Congo, East Africa (Williams 1934), Chuanchow, South China (Landsborough & Tunnell 1947), Southern California and South America. In most cases meningeal involvement was a complication of the bubonic form from the ninth to the seventeenth day. In clinical features it rather resembles cerebrospinal meningitis with painful headaches, stiff neck and Kernig's sign. Special symptoms are meningeal irritation, convulsions, vestibulo-cerebellar symptoms and coma. The cerebro-spinal fluid is under pressure and yellow in colour, closely resembling that of acute suppurative meningitis; *P. pestis* may be obtained by lumbar puncture. The initial infection is probably due to droplet spread. The brain shows congestion and flattening of sulci and is covered with a thick fibrinopurulent exudate.

MORTALITY

The mortality is usually greatest at the beginning and height of the epidemic. The death-rate may be anything from 60 to 95% of those attacked. Much appears to depend on the social condition of the patient and the attention and nursing available. Thus, in a Hong Kong epidemic, while the case mortality among the indifferently fed, overcrowded, unwashed and almost unnursed Chinese amounted to 93·4%, it was only 77% among the Indians, 60% among the Japanese and 18·2% among the Europeans—a gradation in general correspondence with the social and hygienic conditions of the different nationalities. Modern treatment has greatly reduced the mortality.

DIAGNOSIS

Fever and adenitis during a plague epidemic must invariably be viewed with suspicion, particularly if the fever rapidly assumes an adynamic character. Blood culture was recommended by Onoto, by inoculating blood into broth containing 1% of sodium citrate. Rosier stated that in Java splenic puncture is valuable in establishing a diagnosis and is not opposed by the local population. Junior and de Albuquerque described an allergic skin test for which an emulsion of infected guinea-pig lymph gland was used. In Western America the differentiation of mild cases of plague from tularaemia is important (page 493), but the discovery of the bacillus in the glands, blood, sputum or discharges is the only thoroughly reliable test. Should a coccobacillus be found with the characteristic bipolar staining, it should be cultivated by Haffkine's method in broth on which clarified butter (ghee) or coconut oil is floated. In case of doubt, animal inoculation should be used; infective material from the patient or a culture is rubbed into a shaven area (2·5 mm square) on the abdomen of a white rat or a guinea-pig. P. pestis inoculated in this way kills the guinea-pig in 7 days, the rat sooner and white mice in 48 hours. The latter may be inoculated at the root of the tail.

Post mortem indications of plague in the rat. Before rats suspected of being plague-infected are handled, they should be immersed in disinfectant to destroy ectoparasites.

The lymphatic glands should be first exposed. If the rat is infected, subcutaneous injection around the glands is generally recognizable. If the glands are inflamed, this is almost diagnostic of plague; the liver will be yellow, sprinkled with innumerable pinky-white granules. The spleen is enlarged, congested and occasionally granular. The serous membranes are of dull lustre with petechial or diffuse haemorrhages. Serous or blood-stained serous effusions are present in 72% of such rats; if, on microscopical examination of scrapings from glands or spleen, bipolar-staining bacilli are detected, the case is probably plague.

P. pestis, P. pseudotuberculosis rodentium, P. suiseptica and *P. aviseptica* closely resemble each other and are scarcely distinguishable by the usual cultural methods, but the last two have no 'envelope substance', though they have a common antigen with *P. pestis*. None coagulates milk, but on agar *P. pestis* produces a more glistening membranous growth. *P. pseudotuberculosis rodentium* produces a clear, yellowish growth on potato. On Drigalski medium it produces blue colonies and *P. pestis* reddish ones. *P. pseudotuberculosis* readily associates itself with the production of smooth and rough colonies with all degrees of transition between them. The smooth colonies show closest association to *P. pestis* and are the most virulent. *P. aviseptica* produces indole and does not reduce methyl red. In cases of doubt some assistance is afforded by the fact that *P. pseudotuberculosis* has not been found in Central Africa, China, Indo-China and Madagascar.

The most satisfactory means of differentiation is animal inoculation. Rabbits, guinea-pigs and white mice are susceptible to *P. pseudotuberculosis*, but white rats are not. The Indian Plague Commission laid stress on the latter point, as these animals are quickly killed by *P. pestis*. Some strains of *P. pestis* from Brazil, however, do not affect guinea-pigs; they depend on asparagine, and guinea-pigs possess circulating asparaginase (Burrows & Gillett 1971).

P. pestis can be identified by serological methods (see Immunology, page 459) and by bacteriophage.

Rodent plague and fleas. In the investigation of rodent plague the inoculation into animals of pooled fleas is important. Cyanide gas is the best method of collecting fleas from rodents. The long bones of rodents and finger-bones from human cadavers may be sent to the laboratory for culture tests of marrow.

Differential diagnosis

Bubonic plague has sometimes to be distinguished from other affections associated with enlarged glands, such as streptococcal infections, lympho-granuloma venereum, filarial adenitis and occasionally from an anthrax pustule.

In filarial and streptococcal infections lymphangitis tracks are usually visible, but in bubonic plague there is usually no visible sign of the primary infection. In glandular fever the cervical glands are as a rule primarily affected and there is an excess of heterophil antibodies in the serum (Paul-Bunnell test).

Generalized pustular plague has to be differentiated from chickenpox or smallpox; carbuncular plague may be mistaken for anthrax; septicaemic plague may be confused with typhus and subtertian malaria. In the United States, North Europe and Russia, tularaemia may resemble plague.

Pneumonic plague differs from other forms of pneumonia in three main characteristics:

1. The patient is extremely prostrated, although his critical state can hardly be accounted for by such physical signs as are present in the chest; but by the time definite involvement of the lung can be demonstrated, he generally dies.

2. The sputum is watery, never thick, and soon becomes very blood-stained.

3. Pleural effusion is usually present in plague pneumonia.

TREATMENT

Sulphonamides

Bubonic plague can be cured by the administration of sulphonamides alone, but these should be used only when effective and safe antibiotics are not available. 12 grammes of sulphadiazine daily for 4–7 days appreciably reduce mortality from bubonic plague. In less severe cases after an initial dose of 4 grammes, 2 grammes may be given every 4 hours until the temperature is normal. Thereafter 500 mg is given every 4 hours until 7–10 days after the initial dose. The usual precaution of alkalinizing the urine should be taken, using 2–4 grammes of sodium bicarbonate with each dose of sulphadiazine. This schedule of treatment is ineffective against pneumonic plague.

Antibiotics

Streptomycin is very effective but severe intoxication can occur because of its highly bactericidal effect and the massive destruction of the plague bacilli in some cases. Tetracycline is the preferred antibiotic for both bubonic and pneumonic plague (WHO 1970).

Tetracycline. This should be given in large doses of 4–6 grammes daily during the first 48 hours. Intravenous therapy is essential in severely ill patients.

Streptomycin. This should be given intramuscularly in a dosage of 500 mg every 4 hours for 2 days and then 500 mg every 6 hours until clinical improvement occurs. Under field conditions the total daily dose may be given in two equal injections.

Chloramphenicol. This can be given orally at the rate of 50–75 mg/kg daily to a total dosage of 20–25 grammes.

PREVENTION

Chemoprophylaxis

Chemoprophylaxis is recommended for persons in contact with plague and for individuals contaminated in laboratory accidents. In selected populations it may also be used as a short-term measure in small explosive outbreaks until other measures can be instituted. Tetracycline should be used wherever possible in a dose of 250 mg every 6 hours for 1 week or, failing this, sulphonamides, 6 grammes daily for 3 days or 3 grammes daily for 1 week.

Personal prophylaxis

The attendants on pneumonic cases should provide themselves with masks of muslin, three- or four-fold, changed when at all damp, and also with goggles to protect the eyes. In Mukden a mask of absorbent cotton-wool (16 × 12 cm) enclosed in muslin, and retained in position by a many-tailed gauze bandage, together with goggles, rubber gloves and cotton uniform, proved thoroughly effective.

General prevention

Quarantine. Modern systems of land or sea quarantine directed against plague take cognizance of the facts that the incubation period of the disease may extend to 10 days, and that plague may affect certain of the lower animals as well as man.

Eradication of rats from ships requires special measures. At present Cyanogas, $Ca(CN)_2$, is employed as a fumigant. It is a fine greyish-white powder which is dusted or pumped into rat burrows and harbourages, where it liberates HCN. In disc or granular form it is used in the treatment of rooms, ships' holds and enclosed spaces. For rat holes on land a sturdy and powerful pump or blower should be available, usually with a cut-out device which renders it possible to blow in air after the required amount of dust has been delivered. The pump is adjusted so as to clear a known amount of dust with a given number of strokes (e.g. 28 grammes with 30 strokes), the exact delivery being ascertained beforehand. Before, or during, pumping all openings of burrows, except one, should be blocked and care must be taken that no unblocked holes lead into rooms in houses. 28 grammes suffice for average burrows, but under Indian conditions, 450 grammes suffice for 60 burrows.

For fumigation the ship is divided into sections each of which is measured by volume. Water-bottles and cabin water-tanks are emptied, moist food removed and mattresses turned on edge. All apertures are sealed. Danger boards are prominently displayed. Ships may be fumigated loaded or unloaded. A plague-infected ship should be treated before unloading.

In an outbreak in a town, it must be borne in mind that plague, once established in human beings, is communicable to others and to rats by expectoration, and by discharges from the buboes or glandular swellings; and that plague in rats usually precedes plague in human beings. The main efforts should be directed towards destruction of rats by methods detailed below.

After death the rat is treated with Flit or soaked in lysol. Smears are made from lymph glands, liver and spleen, and stained by Leishman. Broquet's medium (calcium carbonate 2; glycerin 20; distilled water 80 parts) is a good preservative for fleas and permits isolation of *P. pestis* after 6 days.

In India the compulsory inspection of all dead bodies before burial has been found a valuable measure.

Destruction of vermin and other measures in anticipation of the introduction of plague bacilli. The campaign against rats is usually carried on by rat-traps and rat-catchers, and the cautious laying down of poisons. The pumping of sulphur dioxide gas under pressure is useful for warehouses. So long as the sulphurous acid gas is dry, and not used on damp articles, no damage is done to merchandise. Care has to be taken with damp things, as they may get discoloured.

Where possible, houses and warehouses should be made rat-proof—not an easy measure, considering the burrowing and climbing habits of the rat. *R. norvegicus* can penetrate ordinary lime-mortar or soft brick, but is stopped by cement and concrete. Its burrows may attain a depth of 46 cm, but *R. rattus* is not so active in this respect. Simpson recommended that walls should be at least 15 cm thick, when made of hard brick or concrete, and that they should extend to not less than 46 cm below the level of the ground floor, and the latter should be paved with concrete 8 cm thick, covered with 1·25 cm of cement. All ventilators should be protected with iron gratings, and all openings around wires and pipes cemented. In New Orleans some warehouses are elevated, leaving a clear open space beneath: in others an impervious wall is built around the ground floor, penetrating 60 cm into the ground. In a third, and a most effective type, the ground floor is laid out in concrete with a protective wall round the edges sinking 60 cm into the ground. The mooring cables of ships should be shielded in such a way as to prevent egress or ingress of rats, and all gangways should be taken up at night or when not in use. Village food-stores are, sometimes set out on poles and can be protected from rat-invasion by suitable wooden discs.

Rodenticides

All rodenticides should be handled with great care; they can affect man.

Warfarin is an anticoagulant derived from coumarin; it easily takes first place for combined safety and effectiveness. Water-soluble warfarin can be used in addition to the solid bait. Warfarin-treated oats are prepared as follows:

Warfarin 0·025%, white mineral oil 11·0%, *p*-nitrophenol 0·25% and rolled oats 88·73%.

Sorexa warfarin (3 (2-acetyl-1-phenylethyl)-4-hydroxy-coumarin) has fewer disadvantages than other poisons. It acts slowly and creates no suspicion in rats; it kills without pain. Sorexa (1% warfarin in fine oatmeal) kills rats by drastically reducing the clotting power of the blood and by causing leaks in the small capillary vessels. This leads to extensive internal haemorrhages which are rapidly fatal. It inhibits the formation of prothrombin which is produced in the liver.

Initial clearance is readily achieved by making available to rats sufficient bait to satisfy the appetites of the whole population. Reinfestation can be controlled by the use of permanent baiting points which attract the migratory rats. Perimeter defence of premises is by use of permanent or semi-permanent bait containers.

Bait. Any bait that causes rats to feel ill is immediately suspect and the entire colony is warned against the bait. No prebaiting is necessary with Sorexa. Ground cereals are used as a basis for bait. In the U.K. it is medium oatmeal; in the U.S.A. yellow corn meal and in South Africa maize meal. Palatability is increased by the addition of 2–10% fine sugar or 1–2% refined vegetable oil. Good results are obtained if Sorexa is dusted on to soft egg shells. When conditions are dry and warm and foodstuffs available with low moisture content, increased bait-take can be achieved only if water is placed near the dry bait.

Table 25. Rodenticides

Rodenticide	Recommended strength by weight	Relative safety	Relative effectiveness
Warfarin	0·025%	2	2
Red squill*	5–10%	1	7
ANTU	2–3%	3	6
Zinc phosphide	1%	4	5
Arsenic trioxide	3%	5	4
Thallium sulphate	0·5%	6	3
Sodium fluoroacetate (1080)	—	7	1

* The Cruel Poisons Act prohibits the use of red squill in Great Britain.

Rules of bait replacement

1. Lay many baits (116–168 grammes), wherever rats are known to run.
2. Inspect baiting points and replenish where bait is being taken.
3. Replenish bait as long as there are signs of feeding (7–14 days).
4. Maintain permanent baiting points to destroy any rats which may come into the cleared area.

The quickest clearance of rats is obtained where enough attractive bait is laid in the correct places. Mix 1 part Sorexa to 19 parts of bait base.

Siting of the bait: Rats are particular where they feed and while preferring quiet corners, they do not like feeling hemmed in. Rats like a quick and easy 'get-away', but feed in a draught or any open space. It is generally accepted that for every rat seen there are at least 10 living in the area and enough bait must be laid for the whole colony. Rats will not eat food which is mildly rancid or made unpalatable.

Control of wild rodent reservoirs of plague

Wild rodent reservoirs of plague have been successfully controlled and eradicated in some areas in the U.S.S.R., California and South Africa. There are three main methods of control:

a. Complete clearing principle. Rodent extermination is carried out over a number of years. No anti-flea measures are necessary.

b. Current prophylaxis. This is more of an emergency method and is undertaken when an epizootic of plague is occurring in the rodents. Rodent destruction must be accompanied by disinfestation of the burrows.

c. Long-term prophylaxis.

Methods of rodent destruction. Gassing with chloropicrin and black cyanide. Poison bait of oats impregnated with 10–20% zinc phosphide.

Flea control. Effective flea control is achieved by dusting burrows with 5% DDT dusting powder but some fleas are more resistant to insecticides. Benzene hexachloride is also effective.

Surveillance of wild rodent plague. The passive haemagglutination test is widely used in detecting plague foci in rodent populations. A routine programme of testing rodent sera for plague antibody should be incorporated into any epidemiological survey and effective control of rodent plague should be reflected in the disappearance of plague haemagglutinating antibody from the sera of the rodent population.

Melioidosis

Synonyms

Stanton's disease; pneumoenteritis; pseudocholera.

Definition

A rare glanders-like disease endemic in South-east Asia, mainly in Burma, Malaysia, Vietnam and Ceylon.

AETIOLOGY

Loefflerella whitmori (*Pfeifferella whitmori* or *Pseudomonas pseudomallei*) resembles *Loefflerella mallei*, the cause of glanders in horses. It is a small bacillus about the same size and shape and occurs in very large numbers in all acute lesions of the disease. In films stained with Leishman bipolar staining is common. On culture it resembles the glanders bacillus closely but is more actively motile and liquefies gelatin more rapidly. It grows luxuriously upon peptone agar, forming a dense wrinkled culture especially when the medium contains glycerin. A peculiar aromatic odour reminiscent of truffles is given off though on repeated subcultures this feature is lost. On broth cultures a pellicle is formed. *L. whitmori* can be distinguished from *L. mallei* by its behaviour on a peptonized medium containing 1% sodium fumarate. The organism is pathogenic for most laboratory animals and, for guinea-pigs at any rate, the infection is more rapidly fatal than glanders, but in each case acute orchitis is produced by intraperitoneal injection (Strauss reaction). There may be difficulty in distinguishing *L. whitmori* from *Ps. pyocyanea*. Susceptible animals can be infected by scarification, by feeding or by simple application of cultures to the nasal mucosa. A characteristic feature in infected laboratory animals is discharge from the nose and eyes and the organism is excreted in the urine and faeces.

TRANSMISSION

The route of infection is uncertain. It has been considered that the bacillus enters through open skin lesions, a view supported by the fact that all the patients described by Thin *et al.* (1970) had scars and lacerations received during outdoor activities, and in addition 2 patients showed some evidence of an associated leptospiral infection which is waterborne and enters through the skin and mucous membranes. Pulmonary lesions which preceded septicaemia were present in 8 cases (Thin *et al.* 1970), which suggested that inhalation was a likely source of infection.

EPIDEMIOLOGY AND GEOGRAPHICAL DISTRIBUTION

The infection was first recognized by Whitmore in Rangoon in 1911 (Whitmore 1913), Malaysia in 1921 (Stanton & Fletcher 1921), Vietnam in 1925 (Pons & Advier 1927), in Ceylon in 1927, in Singapore in 1931 and in Indonesia in 1932.

Melioidosis occurred during the Second World War in Burma, Malaysia and Thailand and several human cases have been reported from Queensland. Melioidosis has also been described in patients who have never visited a known endemic area or had contact with a case. Three cases have been reported from the U.S.A., 2 from Panama, 1 from Ecuador, 1 from Central India and 1 from Turkey (Thin et al. 1970).

Source of infection

Several cases of natural infection have been observed in rats, cats and dogs and for many years it was thought that this disease was spread by rats, but extensive surveys have shown only a few infected rats. After the Second World War the disease appeared in sheep, horses, pigs, cattle and goats in Queensland, suggesting that it had been brought back by servicemen returning from Southeast Asia. *L. whitmori* has been isolated from surface water in Vietnam and Australia (Ellison et al. 1969) and the bacillus is most prevalent in rice growing areas; surface water from a housing development contained *L. whitmori*.

Serological surveys among healthy people have shown that subclinical infections may be commoner than is realized (Strauss et al. 1969)

PATHOLOGY

The lesions vary very considerably. Numerous small pulmonary abscesses, roughly resembling those of miliary tuberculosis, are produced. Nodules which coalesce and break down into abscesses are found in the spleen and liver; they somewhat resemble those of portal pyaemia, and have to be distinguished from amoebic abscesses. The organisms have been recovered from the blood, urine, sputum, and fluid from cutaneous vesicles of patients dying from the disease. In laboratory animals, artificially infected, small nodules form in the internal organs.

CLINICAL FEATURES

The clinical features are very variable and are well described by Thin et al. (1970). Cases can be divided into acute, subacute and chronic (Alain et al. 1949) and a fourth group who have experienced subclinical infections. The first three types are rare, but the fourth is probably not uncommon. It is possible that the acute form develops only in debilitated persons and that previously healthy people develop the subacute and chronic disease.

Acute septicaemic form

The acute septicaemic form usually occurs only in persons debilitated from alcoholism or diabetes, or who are extremely obese (Thin et al. 1970). The onset is gradual and the intestinal and pulmonary systems are usually involved.

Fever is high, remittent and often irregular. There is commonly a generalized pustular rash and *L. whitmori* can be isolated from the pustules. Vomiting and diarrhoea, which may be so severe as to cause collapse and resemble cholera, are common. Pneumonia is usual, with other signs of septicaemia, and *L. whitmori* can be isolated from the sputum. Often there is a synovitis, with effusion into a large joint, from which the organism can be cultured. The spleen is soft and enlarged. The cerebral system may be involved, and death invariably occurs after a few days or weeks, with delirium or mania.

Subacute form

The subacute form starts as an intestinal infection with diarrhoea, and pulmonary signs develop, with consolidation of part of one lung and rapid cavitation, closely resembling tuberculosis. The sputum is profuse and often

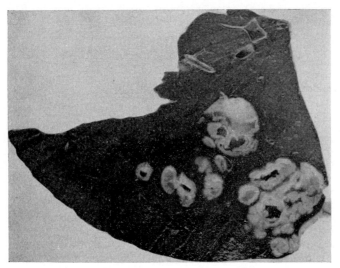

Fig. 140.—The characteristic appearance of liver abscesses due to melioidosis. (*Sir A. T. Stanton*)

blood-stained, and *L. whitmori* can be isolated from it. Fever is usual and there are widespread abscesses in the subcutaneous tissues, liver (Fig. 140) and spleen. Recovery can occur in this form after antibiotic treatment.

Chronic form

This is very variable; lesions occur in the skin and subcutaneous tissues, leading to subcutaneous abscesses and collections of pus in the liver, lungs and spleen. The initial signs may be those of acute parotitis. In 1 case (Grant & Barwell 1943) there was a latent period of 3 years between possible infection and the development of parotid swelling, abscesses, osteomyelitis of the frontal bone, perispinal abscesses and bronchopneumonia. An afebrile case with cervical adenitis and recovery was reported in an Indian (Green & Mankikar 1949). Ten cases of all 3 types have been reported from Malaysia (Thin *et al.* 1970). Localized cutaneous melioidosis has been described (Fournier & Chambon 1958). Few cases have been described in women, in whom the bladder and kidneys are chiefly involved.

DIAGNOSIS

This is best carried out by isolation of the bacillus from urine, blood or pustules in the skin. Isolations are not usually made from faeces. *L. whitmori* has been isolated from cerebrospinal and synovial fluid.

Serological tests

These are useful in the subacute and chronic cases in which isolation of the organism is extremely difficult. The procedures available are agglutination, haemagglutination and complement fixation tests.

Agglutination. Formolized suspensions of a smooth strain are used and readings are made after 4 hours' incubation at 37°C or 18 hours on the bench. Agglutination is the O granular type. Cross-reactions may be found with glanders, *Escherichia, Aerobacter* and *Salmonella*.

Haemagglutination (Strauss *et al.* 1969). This a more specific test. Antibodies appear early in the infection and titres of 1/40 are considered diagnostic. A rising titre is very significant.

Complement fixation test. This is less sensitive. Antibodies appear much later and rise more slowly.

TREATMENT

In acute cases treatment is usually without avail; subacute and chronic cases respond to treatment. The treatment of choice is a combination of tetracycline and chloramphenicol. Very large doses are necessary and they must be continued for a long time. Up to 6·0 grammes each of tetracycline and chloramphenicol have been given intravenously in 24 hours to a total dosage of 112 grammes of chloramphenicol and 107 grammes of tetracycline. Careful watch must be maintained for pancytopenia and the drugs stopped if this supervenes (Thin *et al.* 1970). Two cases of melioidosis have been treated with the prolonged administration of sulphonamides (Magee *et al.* 1967). One case recovered after 10 months of Triple Sulpha and another after 16 months of oral sulphonamide.

The susceptibility of the organisms to various drugs and antibiotics gives a lead for treatment.

REFERENCES

ALAIN, M., ST ETIENNE, J. & REYNES, V. (1949) *Med. trop.*, **9**, 119.
BALTAZARD, M., BAHMANYAR, M., CHAMSA, M., MOSTACHFI, P. & POURNAKI, R. (1963) *Bull. Soc. Path. éxot.*, **56**, 1108.
BURROWS, T. W. & GILLETT, W. A. (1971) *Nature, Lond.*, **229**, 51.
CHEN, T. H. (1965) *Acta trop.*, **22**, 97.
—— & MEYER, K. F. (1966) *Bull. Wld Hlth Org.*, **34**, 911.
DAVIS, D. H. S., HEISCH, R. B., McNEILL, D. & MEYER, K. F. (1968) *Trans. R. Soc. trop. Med. Hyg.*, **62**, 838.
EHRENKRANTZ, N. J. & MEYER, K. F. (1955) *J. infect. Dis.*, **96**, 138.
ELLISON, D. W., BAKER, H. J. & MARIAPPAN, M. (1969) *Am. J. trop. Med. Hyg.*, **18**, 694.
GRANT, A. & BARWELL, C. (1943) *Lancet*, **i**, 119.
GREEN, R. & MANKIKAR, D. S. (1949) *Br. med. J.*, **i**, 308.
HIRST, L. F. (1953) *The Conquest of Plague. A Study of the Evolution of Epidemiology.* Oxford: Clarendon Press.
JACKSON, S. & MORRIS, B. C. (1961) *Br. J. exp. Path.*, **42**, 363.
LANDSBOROUGH, D. & TUNNELL, N. (1947) *Br. med. J.*, **i**, 4.

MAGEE, H. R., MITCHELL, R. M., FITZWATER, J. J., CHRISTIE, D. G. S. & RAO, A. (1967) *Med. J. Aust.*, **23**, 1180.
MARSHALL, J. D. jun., QUY, D. V. & GIBSON, F. L. (1967) *Am. J. trop. Med. Hyg.*, **16**, 175.
PAVLOVSKY, E. N. (1966) *Natural Nidality of Transmissible Diseases with Special Reference to the Landscape Epidemiology of Zooanthroposes.* Urbana, Ill.: University of Illinois Press.
POLLITZER, E. N. (1954) *Monograph Ser. W.H.O.*, 22.
—— (1960) *Bull. Wld Hlth Org.*, **23**, 313.
PONS, R. & ADVIER, M. (1927) *J. Hyg., Camb.*, **26**, 28.
STANTON, A. J. & FLETCHER, W. (1921) *Studies from the Institute of Medical Research.* Kuala Lumpur: FMS Government Printing Office.
STRAUSS, J. M., ALEXANDER, A. D., RADMUND, G., GAN, E. & DORSEY, A. E. (1969) *Am. J. trop. Med. Hyg.*, **18**, 703.
THIN, R. N. T., BROWN, M., STEWART, J. B. & GARRETT, C. J. (1970) *Q. Jl Med.*, **39**, 115.
WHITMORE, A. (1913) *J. Hyg., Camb.*, **13**, 1.
WILLIAMS, A. W. (1934) *E. Afr. med. J.*, **11**, 229.
WORLD HEALTH ORGANIZATION (1970) *Wld Hlth Org. tech. Rep. Ser.*, 447.
ZHIGILEV, D. S. & OTDELSKAYA, A. A. (1956) *Coll. Pap. Anti-plague Inst. Rostov*, **10**, 20 (quoted by Pollitzer 1960).

Brucellosis

Synonyms

Undulant fever (melitensis type); Febris undulans; Malta fever; Mediterranean fever; Gastric remittent fever.

Definition

The brucelloses are caused by organisms of the genus *Brucella* of which 3 species may infect man: *Br. melitensis, Br. abortus,* and *Br. suis,* of each of which there are a number of biotypes.

AETIOLOGY

Brucella organisms measure 0·6–1·5 μm in length and 0·5 μm in width and occur generally singly, often in pairs and sometimes in fours but never in nature in longer chains. They are Gram-negative, are readily stained by a watery solution of gentian violet and are best cultured in a 1·5%, very feebly alkaline, peptonized beef agar on which some time after inoculation they appear as minute clear pearly specks. After 36 hours the cultures become transparent amber and later they are opaque. No liquefaction occurs in gelatine. The individual colonies are small, round somewhat raised discs growing 2–3 mm in diameter about the ninth day. The optimum temperature for growth is 37°C.

Species identification

The conventional methods of species differentiation of brucellae are the need for CO_2 for growth, production of H_2S, differential growth on liver agar containing basic fuchsin and thionin and agglutination by monospecific sera (Table 26). Only *Br. abortus* is lysed by phage.

Table 26. Identification of *Brucella* species

	Br. melitensis	*Br. abortus*	*Br. suis*
CO_2 requirement	—	+	—
H_2S production	—	+ 4 days	+ 5 or more days
Growth on thionin	+	—	+
Growth on basic fuchsin	+	+	—
Monospecific agglutination			
abortus	—	+	+
melitensis	+	—	—

Brucellosis in animals

Brucellosis is a zoonosis and is in the main an infection of animals, many species of which can be parasitized in nature.

Brucellosis in goats. The Mediterranean Fever Commission demonstrated that the goat was the reservoir of brucellosis on the island of Malta, the infection being transmitted to man through the milk. Goats are infected in many parts of the world. Under natural conditions the goat harbours only *Br. melitensis* and the most susceptible animal is the young goat, especially during the first pregnancy. Little illness is caused and the most healthy animals may shed large numbers of organisms in the milk for a considerable time. The organisms are located in the reticulo-endothelial tissues of the pregnant uterus, kidney and mammary gland and infection of man is from the milk and products of conception.

Brucellosis in sheep. Natural infections of sheep are caused by *Br. melitensis*, but *Br. abortus* has also been recovered from them. They are more resistant than goats but the pregnant young female is quite susceptible. Organisms are rarely excreted in the urine or for longer than one or two months in the milk.

Brucellosis in cattle (Bang's disease). Brucellosis in cattle is primarily due to *Br. abortus*, but *Br. melitensis* can also infect them under normal conditions. The most susceptible animal is the pregnant heifer and the organism lodges in the uterus and causes abortion. Organisms also lodge in the supramammary lymph glands and are shed in the milk for a long time. Man is infected from milk and the products of conception.

Brucellosis in pigs. All species of *Brucella* can infect pigs. There are 2 strains of *Br. suis*: the American strain, which produces abundant H_2S and is highly infective for man, and the Danish strain which produces little or no H_2S and is not infective for man. Natural infections with *Br. melitensis* and *Br. abortus* have also been found. The pregnant sow is not especially susceptible and the infection is spread by the boar in the semen. Infection of man is mainly by handling pig meat.

Brucellosis in other animals. Brucellosis has been found in horses and rarely in dogs. Strains have been isolated from reindeer and susliks (rodents) in the U.S.S.R. and from caribou in North America. Camels are not uncommonly infected and serological evidence of infection has been found in eland and wild rodents in East Africa. Guinea-pigs may be used to isolate *Brucella* from suspected material in the laboratory. Strains of *Brucella* differing from the classical strains have been isolated from the desert wood rat (*Neotoma lepida*) and called *Brucella neotomae*.

TRANSMISSION

Viability of organisms

Br. melitensis remains viable for up to 37 days in both fresh and salt water, in dried soil for 43 days and in damp soil for 72 hours. Exposure to the sun greatly reduces the survival time.

The processing of ice-cream and cheese does not destroy *Br. melitensis*.

Br. abortus can survive in butter up to 142 days and has been isolated from ice-cream which had been frozen for 1 month.

Br. suis has been isolated from hog carcases after 21 days of refrigeration.

Transmission to man

As far as the evidence is concerned direct interhuman transmission is minor and might only occur via the urine or blood transfusion. No case of brucellosis in nursing infants has been recorded. *Brucella* infection is transmitted to man from animals by ingestion, direct or indirect contact or via the respiratory or ocular route.

Ingestion. Br. melitensis is acquired mainly by the ingestion of goats' milk or fresh goats' cheese; rarely food and drinking water may be contaminated by dust, by products of abortion or by the urine of infected goats.

Br. abortus is acquired by the ingestion only of raw cows' milk. No proved cases have been traced to cheese, ice-cream, butter or contaminated water.

Direct contact. Direct contact is important in the transmission of *Br. suis* to man and to a lesser extent *Br. melitensis.* Farmers and meat-packing employees contract the infection in North America through abrasions in the skin coming into contact with infected hog carcasses.

In dry areas of the world *Br. melitensis* is contracted by handling the products of abortion and manure of infected animals. *Br. abortus* is contracted by veterinarians who handle infected animals.

Respiratory tract and ocular mucosa. Circumstantial evidence occasionally favours the respiratory tract as the route of infection but it is of minor importance. Accidental laboratory infections have been acquired through the eye, and it is known to be a particular laboratory risk.

Insect vectors. Mosquitoes and blood-sucking flies have been found experimentally to be able to carry *Brucella* organisms for 4–5 days, and *Brucella* have been isolated from wild caught mosquitoes in the southern U.S.S.R. Transmission by this method is, however, not proved and is only of minor importance.

EPIDEMIOLOGY AND GEOGRAPHICAL DISTRIBUTION

Brucellosis, which was originally investigated in Malta by Sir David Bruce, is widely distributed in both the temperate and tropical areas of the world. *Br. melitensis* occurs mainly in those countries where the goat is extensively used, usually the hotter and drier areas: the shores of the Mediterranean, Southern France, Italy, Spain, South, East and West Africa and Somalia.

Br. abortus is commoner in the temperate countries where cattle are raised more extensively, especially North and South America (New Mexico and Texas), and Mexico but also in other dairying areas of the world.

Br. suis infection in man is confined mainly to North America.

Age and sex distribution

Brucellosis is predominantly a disease of adult males, which suggests a connection with occupation. Unlike animals, children show a comparative resistance to the disease and, although the infection rate in children may be high, the morbidity rate is low. The physiological and metabolic factors responsible for this resistance are not known.

OCCUPATION

Brucellosis is a disease of farmers, dairy-men, herdsmen, meat-packers, veterinary surgeons and laboratory workers. Not more than 10% of the cases of brucellosis in North America are due to drinking unpasteurized milk (Spink 1956). In the Mediterranean area the greatest prevalence of *Br. melitensis* is the season of lowest rainfall, explained by the birth of kids in the spring and the greater consumption of goats' milk during the summer months.

Veterinarians show a high incidence of infection, though they do not necessarily manifest illness, but may exhibit an extreme degree of hypersensitivity to *Brucella* antigen.

Meat-packers may acquire both *Br. abortus* and, in the U.S.A., *Br. suis* infection which appears intermittently, involving several patients at a time, suggesting intermittent exposure to a contaminated environment.

Among farmers and ranchers it is a common practice for families to drink unpasteurized milk. In areas of high endemicity, such as parts of the Mediterranean and Africa, a considerable proportion of the inhabitants show serological evidence of past infection.

IMMUNOLOGY

Some immunity results from an attack of brucellosis but second attacks do occur. The immune response of the host is both humoral and cellular.

Humoral immunity

Agglutinin, precipitin and opsonin antibodies appear in the blood towards the end of the first two weeks and persist for a long time. The primary response is an increase in IgM (agglutination reaction) followed later by a secondary response with an increase in IgG and IgA (anti-human-globulin, Coombs test). In primary acute infections the IgM (agglutination) antibodies are present in high titre and a prozone phenomenon seen when there is no agglutination below 1/100, although agglutination occurs at higher dilutions. This is due to the presence of 'blocking' antibodies. In chronic infections and in persons with past exposure to infection only IgG and IgA antibodies are present.

Cellular immunity

A well marked cellular immunity is found with delayed hypersensitivity, a positive brucellin reaction of the skin and a granulomatous reaction in the tissue to the presence of intracellular *Brucella*, which is responsible for the pathological changes found in the liver, spleen, lymph glands and bone marrow.

PATHOLOGY (Spink 1956)

A significant feature of brucellosis is the location of the organism intracellularly. The brucellae enter the body and localize in the regional lymph glands where they proliferate and may cause necrosis. The bacteria invade the blood stream and are carried in leucocytes to those areas where there is abundant reticulo-endothelial tissue, the liver, spleen, lymph glands and bone marrow, where they become localized, mainly in the mononuclear cells. The basic and characteristic tissue response consists of monocytes and large phagocytes which form granulomas, especially in the liver, spleen marrow and lymph glands, which consist of collections of epithelioid cells, lymphocytes and giant cells of the Langhans and foreign body type. These granulomas, which disappear rapidly with recovery from the infection, have been used in diagnosis especially by liver and bone marrow biopsy. Rarely is there necrosis and abscess formation.

Spink (1956) believes that *Brucella* endotoxin is responsible for most of the signs and symptoms of brucellosis but that tissue hypersensitivity is responsible for the granulomas. The *Brucella* organisms are responsible directly for the metastatic lesions which may cause abscesses in the bones (especially the vertebrae), bacterial endocarditis and meningitis.

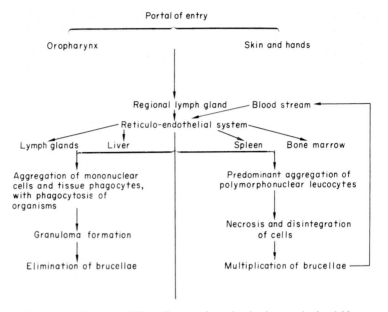

Fig. 141.—The fate of *Brucella* organisms in the human body. (*After Spink 1956*).

CLINICAL FEATURES

Incubation period

The incubation period is usually 1–3 weeks, although several months may elapse between exposure to infection and the appearance of symptoms. The onset may be sudden, as in the malignant or undulating type, or insidious, as in the intermittent type.

Symptoms

Weakness associated with fatigue is the commonest symptom. Chills and sweats are a conspicuous feature, with profuse nocturnal sweating so that the night-clothes and bed-linen have to be changed several times during the night.

Anorexia, loss of weight and headache are common, and pain in the back of the neck is sometimes associated with *Brucella* spondylitis. There may be pain in the back and abdominal pain associated with a tender enlargement of the liver and spleen. Pain in the right iliac fossa may resemble appendicitis and is caused by mesenteric gland involvement.

Joint pains are a prominent feature and usually involve one or more of the larger joints. The pain is an arthralgia and there is sometimes no evidence of inflammation of the joints.

There may be nervousness and mental depression associated with insomnia.

Signs

Patients with brucellosis present with a multitude of complaints but show a paucity of signs, the most prominent of which is fever.

Fever. Fever is almost invariably present in an active case and bacteriologically proved disease rarely occurs without fever. The most characteristic feature of the fever of brucellosis is the peculiar behaviour of the temperature chart (Fig. 142). In a mild case there may be a ladder-like rise through a week or 10 days to 39° or 40°C and then through another week or so a gradual fall to normal. In mild cases, which are the exception, the fever which is of continued or remittent type disappears without complication in about 3 weeks. Usually after a few days of apyrexia the fever returns and runs a similar course, the relapse being in its turn followed by an interval of apyrexia, and so on during several months. This is the 'undulant' type of fever, from which Hughes (1897) derived the name he gave to the disease, undulant fever. The fastigium of the temperature curve occurs towards midday or early afternoon, which distinguishes it from typhoid and other continued septic fevers, in which this takes place towards night time.

In other cases a continued fever persists for 1, 2 or more months—the 'continued' type of Hughes (1897).

Usually remittent or continued in type, the fever exhibits in a proportion of cases distinct daily inter-missions, the swinging temperature chart suggesting septic endocarditis or malaria. This is the inter-mittent type of Hughes (1897) (Fig. 143). In some patients 2–3 months may elapse before the fever subsides. According to Bassett Smith (1903) the average duration of the untreated case is 4 months but it may last 2 years. The shortest period is about 3 weeks and cases of all degrees of severity may be met with. Bassett Smith (1903) recognized 6 types:

(a) Ambulant. The patients have no symptoms but excrete *Br. melitensis* in their urine.

(b) Mild cases last about a fortnight and are apt to be mistaken for typhoid.

(c) The ordinary type already described.

(d) The malignant type with hyperpyrexia and toxaemia. This may be fatal and death has occurred as early as the twenty-seventh day.

(e) An intermittent type with hectic fever and sweats, apt to be mistaken for tuberculosis (Fig. 143).

(f) A chronic type with symptoms related to the central nervous system with headache and nuchal rigidity.

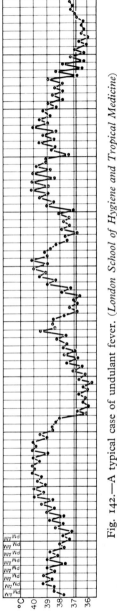

Fig. 142.—A typical case of undulant fever. (*London School of Hygiene and Tropical Medicine*)

Splenomegaly. This is found in almost half the patients (Spink 1956) and is a good index of the continuing activity of the disease. The spleen is tender and firm and seldom extends beyond 5–6 cm from the costal margin. Occasionally in

Br. melitensis infection the spleen may be greatly enlarged and *Brucella* can be isolated in pure culture from it.

Lymphadenopathy is a common sign. The cervical and axillary glands which are most often involved are soft, discrete and slightly tender.

Hepatomegaly is much less frequent than splenomegaly. When enlarged the liver is tender. Jaundice occurs rarely.

Tenderness over the spine is common and cases of suspected brucellosis should always be examined by heavy percussion over the spine.

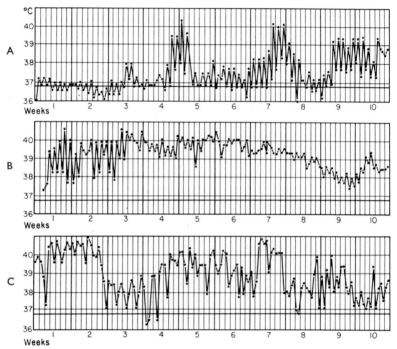

Fig. 143.—Various types of temperature charts in undulant fever. A, Intermittent. B, Remittent. C, Irregular.

Course of the disease

Brucellosis is essentially a self-limiting disease and 50% of cases recovered their health in 1 year (Spink 1956). The death rate of untreated brucellosis overall is about 2%. Death usually occurs from bacterial endocarditis.

Chronic brucellosis

Of patients with *Br. abortus* 80% recover completely within a year with antibiotic therapy (Spink 1956). A minority of patients who have continued ill health will show definite evidence of localized disease, such as spondylitis, meningo-encephalitis, cholecystitis, bone lesions or radiculoneuritis. A smaller number show persistent ill health without any signs of disease and are subject to severe headaches, mental depression, nervousness and vasomotor dysfunction. It is probable that these individuals have a psychopathic or hypochondriacal background and brucellosis accentuates this instability and causes further symptoms.

Clinical differences between *Br. abortus*, *Br. melitensis* and *Br. suis*

On the whole *Br. abortus* infections are much milder and run a shorter course than *Br. melitensis* and prolonged pyrexial cases lasting many months are not as common as in *Br. melitensis*. On the other hand *Br. abortus* infection may be very persistent, lasting over a year or more. *Br. suis* infections may be severe and fatal, suppurating complications are more frequent and a chronic state of debility ensues more frequently if proper treatment is not given (Spink 1956).

COMPLICATIONS

Complications involving bones and joints (surgical brucellosis)

Spondylitis. *Brucella* spondylitis is very painful and incapacitating (Lowbeer 1948). Bones and discs are invaded, causing osteomyelitis with destruction of bone which is replaced by granulation tissue. The symptoms are similar to those of a herniated disc with root pain and it may be difficult to distinguish *Brucella* spondylitis of the spine from tuberculosis, except that in brucellosis repair proceeds along with bone destruction which can be seen on the X-ray as osteoporosis with osteosclerosis. Rarely an epidural abscess may form.

Bones and joints. Suppuration may occur in the larger joints, especially the hip-joint. Osteomyelitis of the long bones is occasionally seen.

Cardiovascular complications

Bacterial endocarditis usually develops on a congenital or acquired valvular lesion.

Hepatic complications

The great majority of patients develop granulomatous lesions in the liver parenchyma. When hepatic enlargement is accompanied by jaundice there is some degree of liver failure (Rossmiller & Ensign 1948) and cirrhosis may follow severe necrotizing hepatitis (McCullough 1951). Cholecystitis may appear in association with hepatitis.

Hypersplenism

Hypersplenism with leucopenia, thrombocytopenia and haemorrhage is a rare complication. Haemolytic anaemia has also been recorded in association with splenomegaly and *Brucella* were recovered from the spleen (Weed *et al.* 1952).

Genito-urinary

Orchitis and epididymitis are not uncommon. *Brucella* are excreted in the urine over a long period of time and chronic pyelonephritis has been reported.

Neurobrucellosis

Neurological complications of brucellosis may appear at the onset of the illness, during convalescence or long after the fever (Nelson-Jones 1951), and may be caused by *Br. melitensis*, *Br. abortus* or *Br. suis*.

A meningomyelitis may occur with spinal features; leptomeningitis is an early feature and may lead to an adhesive arachnoiditis with signs of spinal block and xanthochromic cerebrospinal fluid (Sahadevan *et al.* 1968).

Diffuse progressive encephalitis, often associated with optic, VI and VIII nerve lesions, may occur and Fincham *et al.* (1963) have described meningo-encephalitis as well as subarachnoid haemorrhage, neuritis and myelopathy.

Transient episodes including aphasia, dysarthria, paralyses, tinnitus, deafness and visual disorders can all occur (Spink & Hall 1949). The organisms are not usually recovered from the CSF in which agglutination tests are negative.

A neuropsychiatric form of the disease is well known (Spink 1959).

Hypersensitivity reactions

Veterinary surgeons who are especially exposed to infection may become sensitized to the products of *Brucella* and develop hypersensitivity reactions, such as skin rashes and fever, when exposed to infected animals and their excretions.

DIAGNOSIS

Differential diagnosis

The differential diagnosis of brucellosis may be difficult in the early stages when it has to be distinguished from typhoid, tuberculosis and other causes of prolonged fever such as reticulosis.

Chronic *Br. melitensis* infection can closely resemble kala-azar with fever, splenomegaly and hypersplenism and where both infections are endemic both can coexist in the same patient.

Brucella spondylitis of the spine closely resembles tuberculous or typhoid osteitis and may only be distinguished by the evidence of repair (osteosclerosis) which is present alongside destruction (osteoporosis) and can be seen on radiological examination.

Other localized manifestations of brucellosis may be confused with a multitude of conditions and brucellosis should be considered in the diagnosis of uveitis, acute choroiditis, orchitis and epididymitis.

Blood changes

Anaemia is not usual in uncomplicated brucellosis, but in areas of the world where *Br. melitensis* is common and there are other parasitic infections, a moderate iron deficiency anaemia may be found.

The white cell count is usually normal with a relative lymphocytosis, and abnormal lymphocytes are frequently present, such as are found in infectious mononucleosis. Some cases show a leucopenia. Only occasionally does the count rise above 10 000/mm³ (Spink 1956).

Isolation of *Brucella*

Blood culture. The organism may be recovered from the blood as early as the second day of fever. 5–10 ml should be drawn and distributed into several flasks of broth. The broth should be incubated for at least 24 hours and for as long as 26 days. Subcultures should be made on trypsin agar slopes. Cultures of blood clot sometimes give better results. The clot is macerated and transferred to crystal violet tryptose broth (bactotryptose 20 grammes, bactodextrose 1 gramme, sodium chloride 5·0 grammes, *p*-aminobenzoic acid 100 mg, crystal violet 0·1% aqueous solution 1·4 ml, distilled water 1000 ml) in a screw capped vial. The medium is adjusted to *p*H 6·9. Incubate at 35°C under CO_2 tension for 4–7 days. The culture is then streaked on to a solid medium consisting of bactotryptose agar containing 1·0 ml of 0·1% aqueous crystal violet. Inoculations are made once a week for 3 weeks and the plates incubated for 4 days.

Isolation from urine. This is much more difficult to achieve. The urine must be a catheter or mid-stream specimen obtained after the fifteenth day.

Isolation from bone marrow. *Br. abortus* has been isolated from the bone marrow when blood cultures are sterile.

Isolation from tissues. *Brucella* may be isolated from excised lymph glands, bone and lung but not from liver. Material can be inoculated into guinea-pigs whose blood is then examined for a rise in agglutination titres to *Brucella*.

Biopsy of liver and marrow may show granulomas which are not specific but may be suggestive of brucellosis.

Immunodiagnosis

Antibodies can be demonstrated by agglutination, complement fixation, and anti-human-globulin (Coombs) tests.

Agglutination. Agglutinating antibodies appear in the blood after the second week of the disease and persist for a long time.

Specificity. Cross-reactions occur with *Br. tularensis* and *Vibrio cholerae*. Heterologous titres are lower than homologous and heterologous antibodies can be removed by absorption. Persons immunized with cholera vaccine will show a raised titre of *Brucella* agglutinins, especially if they have had previous *Brucella* infection, and these decrease rapidly with time. A properly standardized antigen may be prepared from any species of *Brucella* and the test can be carried out by tube or rapid slide agglutination, using Castaneda's antigen (Spink & Anderson 1952).

Prozone phenomenon. Blocking antibodies may prevent agglutination in dilutions below 1/100, and may be obviated by testing dilutions up to 1/10 240. Blocking antibodies may be found in the sera of patients who have had active disease for a number of years and patients whose sera show either a low titre or no agglutination should be tested with anti-human-globulin serum.

Interpretation of the test. Low titres of 1/20 to 1/80 are most likely to be found in patients without evidence of brucellosis or in healthy persons. Active brucellosis is most likely to be associated with a titre of above 1/100. When a properly standardized antigen is used the great majority of patients with bacteriologically proved disease will have titres of 1/160 to 1/320. However, a diagnosis of brucellosis cannot be established on the titres alone since many people connected with animal husbandry may show a significant titre of *Brucella* agglutinins in their blood.

Rapid slide agglutination test. A rapid slide agglutination test using standard antigens as supplied to veterinarians has been used very successfully in the field for the diagnosis of brucellosis, and compared very favourably with the standard agglutination test (Cox 1968).

Complement fixation test. The complement fixation test measures IgG antibodies and should be performed in combination with the anti-human-globulin test.

Anti-human-globulin (Coombs) test (Kerr *et al.* 1966). *Brucella* organisms which have absorbed their specific antibodies are washed free of serum and exposed to anti-human-globulin (Coombs) reagent prepared in the rabbit. Agglutination follows. The advantages of this test are that blocking antibodies are overcome and that the test measures only IgG antibodies so that differentiation can be made in association with the agglutination test between acute (IgM and IgG) and chronic (IgG and IgA only) cases. Two types of antibody response can be distinguished: chronic cases and those persons regularly exposed to *Brucella* antigen, such as veterinary surgeons, where the direct agglutination test is either weakly positive or negative but the anti-human-globulin test is positive to a high titre, and acute cases, where the direct agglutination test is positive to a high titre but who show later a marked reduction in all types of antibody over a period as long as 12 months or more (Coghlan & Weir 1967).

Brucellin (Melitine) test. A polyvalent antigen prepared from all 3 species of *Brucella* and standardized by the nitrogen content has been used to measure delayed hypersensitivity. A positive reaction denotes exposure to or infection with brucellosis at some time in the past and is useful only for epidemiological purposes. A negative reaction may be useful in individual cases to exclude infection.

TREATMENT

On the whole *Br. abortus* infection is more amenable to treatment than *Br. melitensis.*

Tetracycline

Tetracycline is the antibiotic of choice and chlortetracycline or oxytetracycline should be given in a dose of 500 mg 4 times daily by mouth for 21 days. Using this régime 90% of 32 cases of acute brucellosis recovered (Spink 1956). The temperature approaches normal by the fourth or fifth day. This course should be repeated within 6–8 weeks if a relapse occurs.

Streptomycin and tetracycline

A combination of streptomycin 1·0 gramme daily intramuscularly with 500 mg tetracycline 4 times daily by mouth for 21 days is the most widely recommended therapy. It can be supplemented by moderate doses of sulphonamide.

Sulphonamides

Sulphonamides alone are not so effective and have no effect on the course of bacterial endocarditis due to *Brucella.*

Trimethoprim and sulphamethoxazole

Four patients were treated with trimethoprim and sulphamethoxazole (Lal *et al.* 1970). The treatment was successful in 3 of 4 cases, the fourth case developing trimethoprim resistance. The dose was 3 courses of 4 tablets of Septrin daily for 4 weeks, the courses being separated by 4 weeks. Septrin contains 80 mg trimethoprim and 400 mg sulphamethoxazole in each tablet.

Steroids

Steroids administered in combination with antibiotics to acutely ill patients have a dramatic effect and improvement may be noticed in 24 hours. The mechanism of this favourable action is not understood but is similar to the effect of steroids on patients severely ill with typhoid fever.

Steroids may be administered in the form of ACTH gel 25 I.U. intramuscularly every 6 hours, or 100 mg hydrocortisone intravenously every 8 hours for 72 to 96 hours.

Hypersensitivity reactions may be treated by desensitization with Castaneda's antigen in gradually increasing doses.

PREVENTION

In endemic areas all milk and milk products should be sterilized by boiling or pasteurization. Unfermented goat-milk cheese must be forbidden.

Meat-packers must be protected by gloves when handling carcases. Farmers should be suitably garbed when dealing with the products of conception, which must be destroyed.

The eradication of brucellosis from herds is a major problem and must be tackled on a government scale.

Prophylactic vaccination

Vaccination of man against *Brucella* infection using killed vaccines has proved a complete failure (WHO 1964).

The most widely used live vaccine is 19-BA, which has been used on a large scale in the U.S.S.R. Skin tests for hypersensitivity must be employed before vaccination and revaccination, and the vaccine should only be used in workers at high risk (WHO 1964).

Tularaemia

Synonyms

Deer-fly fever; Pahvant Valley plague; Rabbit fever; Ohara's disease; Yato-byo (Japan); Lemming fever.

Definition

Tularaemia is a specific infectious disease of rodents, caused by *Brucella (Pasteurella) tularensis* and is transmitted from these animals to man by the bite of infected blood-sucking insects, by the handling of infected animals or by the ingestion of infected water.

AETIOLOGY

Br. tularensis is a small non-motile Gram-negative organism measuring 0·3–0·7 μm in length; when stained in the tissues it gives the appearance of being surrounded by a capsule. Though normally occurring as a rod-like structure, it frequently assumes a coccus shape. It stains best in tissue preparations with Giemsa's stain, but in smears from cultures it shows up well with aniline gentian violet. On account of their small size some of the organisms pass through the coarser bacterial filters.

Cultural characteristics

The organism is difficult to culture. It will not grow on plain agar or in bouillon but will produce an abundant growth on serum–glucose–cystine agar. The cystine medium is inoculated with the heart blood of an infected animal or a small piece of the liver or spleen is rubbed on the surface and allowed to remain in contact with the medium. Growth appears about the third day and flourishes luxuriantly in subcultures without the addition of fresh animal tissue. To ensure the primary growth it is necessary that a piece of animal tissue be added to the medium. Fermentation of glucose, laevulose, maltose and glycerine occurs with acid formation.

Composition of cystine agar. Cystine agar consists of beef infusion agar, having a *p*H of 7·6, to which 0·02% of cystine is added. It is then sterilized for 15 minutes in a steam sterilizer and subsequently incubated for 24 hours to ensure sterility. Cultures of *Br. tularensis* are very infectious and should be handled with great care.

Natural infections

Br. tularensis occurs as a natural infection of wild rodents, especially rats, field mice, hares and rabbits. It has an extremely wide spectrum of infection and many other species of animals as well as birds can be infected. A complete list of natural infections has been given by Burroughs *et al.* (1945). Natural infections occur in the following:

1. In the U.S.A.: Wandering shrew, grey fox, dog, cat, various ground squirrels (Pirote, Wyoming, Beechey's and Columbian), chipmunk, beaver, woodrat, white-footed mouse, meadow mouse and varieties (Sawatch and Tule), muskrat and brown rat (*R. norvegicus*), varying hare, jack rabbit, black-tailed jack rabbit, cotton-tail rabbit, sheep, calves, ruffed grouse, sharp-tailed grouse, bobwhite quail and horned owl.
2. In Canada: Richardson's ground squirrel, Osgood's white-footed mouse, Drummond meadow mouse, varying hare, white-tailed jack rabbit and Franklin's gull.
3. In Sweden: Lemming and varying hare.
4. In Central Europe: Rabbit and hare.
5. In U.S.S.R.: Introduced muskrat, little ground squirrel, steppe lemming, water rat, continental vole, large water vole, house mouse and long-tailed field mouse.
6. In Asia Minor: Continental vole, house and harvest mouse.
7. In Japan: Local rabbit.

TRANSMISSION

Br. tularensis is transmitted in nature by a large variety of routes of which there are 3 main ones: among rodents by water, to carnivores by ingestion from eating rodents and to birds and larger animals by ticks, biting flies and mosquitoes. Man acquires the infection by direct contact from skinning rabbits, by ingestion from eating them as food and from tick and horsefly bites. It can also be easily acquired as a laboratory infection. It is predominantly a disease of rural populations.

Water-borne infection

The infection is maintained among rodents mainly by water. The water is contaminated by dead animals and excreta and large numbers of rodents may be infected and die in this way.

Ingestion

Carnivora are infected chiefly from the consumption of sick infected rodents which are easy to catch.

Insects

Ticks can act as vectors and are very suitable, since the nymph stages feed on small rodents and when they become adult feed on larger mammals including man, thus transmitting the infection from rodents in an efficient manner. The infection is also transmitted through the egg, and this is a method by which the infection is maintained in nature through the winter.

Dermacentor andersoni (wood tick), *D. variabilis*, *D. occidentalis*, *Ixodes ricinus* and *Haemaphysalis leporis palustris* (rabbit tick) can all transmit the infection. *Dermacentor andersoni* is particularly important in the U.S.A. and *Br. tularensis* is found in the intestinal lumen in the cells of the gut wall in the body fluids and in the faeces. The organism can also be transmitted by biting flies, *Chrysops discalis*, the deer fly, as well as *Stomoxys calcitrans*, the stable fly. The bedbug (*Cimex lectularis*), the squirrel flea (*Ceratophyllus acutus*), the rabbit louse, (*Haemodipsus ventricosus*) and the mouse louse (*Polyplax serratus*) can all transmit the infection, and maintain it in rodents. Four species of mosquito, *Aedes* and *Theobaldia*, have been shown to transmit *Br. tularensis* under experimental conditions, and in Sweden *Aedes cinereus* does so in nature. Mosquitoes are the agent whereby infection is transmitted to birds.

GEOGRAPHICAL DISTRIBUTION AND EPIDEMIOLOGY

Tularaemia occurs as a human infection in three main geographical areas: North America, Europe and the U.S.S.R., and to a less extent in Japan. In each area the epidemiology is distinct. There are 9 main types of outbreak of human infection (Pavlovsky 1966).

a. Vector-borne by ticks and tabanid flies.

b. Trapping, from the skins of infected rodents, muskrats and rabbits.

c. Hunting, from the consumption of rabbit meat.

d. Water-borne from the water of streams infected by dead rats, well water infected by mice and field voles.

e. Agricultural, from working in haystacks contaminated by field voles and mice.

f. Domestic laboratory infections.

g. Use of grain and other products contaminated by mice.

h. Processing of agricultural products.

i. Trench and foxhole outbreaks in wartime.

North America

In North America the most important reservoir of infection is the jack rabbit and its congeners. The infection is found in Wyoming and Montana in streams contaminated by dead beavers, which have been found in large numbers. Man acquires the infection as a hunter from skinning rabbits, and preparing carcases for cooking and also after tick and deer fly bites (*Chrysops discalis*). Occasionally contact with sheep is the source of infection. The disease is most prevalent during the months of June, July and August (Cumming 1937).

Europe

In Sweden the lemming and varying hare are the main reservoirs, and tularaemia is known as 'lemming fever' which is caused by contact with infected water contaminated by the bodies and excreta of lemmings. Outbreaks have occurred in peasant women who go barefoot in summer and are bitten by numerous mosquitoes. In Austria, Czechoslovakia and Poland the rabbit and hare are the main reservoirs and in France the infection has become much more common since the introduction of hares from Central Europe for sporting purposes. In Northern Europe cases occur from July to October, and in Southern Europe from June to August.

U.S.S.R.

In Russia the water rat and introduced muskrat, which spread widely in the Ukraine after the disturbance caused by the great tank battles of the Second World War, are the main reservoirs, and there was a great increase in the number of human infections after the war.

PATHOLOGY

Br. tularensis can enter the body by one of 3 main routes:

a. The respiratory route via the tonsil.
b. Intestinal canal from ingestion.
c. Cutaneous route by insect bite or direct contact.

Since the disease is rarely fatal the pathology is best seen in infected animals. The pathological appearances of infected guinea-pigs and rabbits at autopsy much resemble those of plague. In an experimentally infected guinea-pig there is haemorrhagic oedema at the site of inoculation, with blood-stained peritoneal exudate and diffusely enlarged spleen in which characteristic small necrotic foci can be found. Similar lesions may be detected in the liver. On microscopic section of these organs a dense infiltration with polymorphonuclear cells can be found but the organisms can only be detected with difficulty. In the spleen of the mouse, on the other hand, little or no leucocytic response occurs and when stained with Twort's light-green neutral red stain *Br. tularensis* can be demonstrated in large numbers. In the few recorded cases in man nodules have been found in the lung and spleen.

IMMUNOLOGY

There is apparently a long lasting immunity in man and there is no record of a second generalized attack, though a local reinfection may occur. Agglutinating antibodies appear in the serum in the second week and reach their maximum between the fourth and eighth weeks, when there is a gradual fall, but they may persist for up to 11 years. Serum antibodies can be used in diagnosis but cross-reactions occur with *Br. melitensis* and *Br. abortus* (23% of tularaemia sera cross-react with *Br. melitensis* and *Br. abortus* and 35% of *Br. melitensis* and *Br. abortus* with tularaemia). In 13% of cases of tularaemia the serum agglutinates *Proteus* OX 19 in a dilution of 1:80 or over.

Skin sensitivity can be demonstrated by an intradermal test employing a suspension of killed organisms.

CLINICAL FEATURES

The disease in man presents in a number of ways dependent upon the route of infection. The incubation period is 1–10 days.

Cutaneous (ulceroglandular) form

Local cutaneous disease results from infection from the bite of an infected tick or fly or direct contact of the skin with an infected source. An inflamed papule develops at the site of infection, which becomes pustular with a necrotic centre. This separates, leaving a punched-out ulcer which is replaced by a scar on healing. There is a painful enlargement of the local lymph glands, which may suppurate after 1–2 months and may remain enlarged for 2–3 months. There are general signs of infection with fever and prostration.

Ophthalmic (oculoglandular) form

The site of entry of infection is the conjunctival sac, which is usually involved unilaterally and only rarely bilaterally. There is itching, lacrimation, photophobia and pain in the eye with swelling of the pre-auricular, parotid, submaxillary and cervical lymph glands. The eyelids become swollen and the conjunctiva red and covered with small discrete nodules and grey exudate. Punched-out ulcers develop and last for 2–3 weeks, after which there is recovery. Suppuration of the glands is common. Dacrocystitis, corneal ulcers, and permanent impairment of vision may be found.

Oral and abdominal form

This follows infection by ingestion of infected meat. There is a necrotizing pharyngitis with abscesses on the roof of the mouth, fever, enlargement of local lymph glands and sometimes abdominal pain, vomiting and diarrhoea. Peritonitis may develop.

Typhoidal (septicaemic) form

This form may arise primarily from infection via the respiratory route or as a late result of a local infection. The onset is sudden with severe headache, vomiting, chills and fever. Myalgia and arthralgia are common. The initial rise in temperature is above $40°C$, with generalized weakness, aching, prostration, sweats and loss of weight. The fever may show an initial rise followed by remission and a secondary rise or a continuous course lasting usually 10–15 days, and rarely 3–4 weeks. Petechial, roseolar, papular and pustular rashes may appear. In one-half of the cases pulmonary symptoms develop. A slightly tender enlargement of the spleen is found in one-third of cases. There is a moderate polymorphonuclear leucocytosis of 12 000–15 000/mm^3.

Pleuro-pulmonary form

Pulmonary symptoms develop secondarily to the other forms. There are dyspnoea, malaise, chills and pleuritic pain. Milder forms resemble atypical pneumonia and may last up to 1 month. There may be pleurisy, effusion, pneumonic consolidation or lobular bronchopneumonia with abscess, gangrene and cavitation in severe cases. There is an associated enlargement of the bronchial and mediastinal glands.

Subclinical infections

Subclinical infections are commoner than is supposed, and serological tests recently showed that in Sweden up to 23% of the population has been infected, the infection being subclinical in as many as 32% of those with positive reactions (Dahlstrand et al. 1971).

Complications

Complications have been reported: peritonitis, persistent ascites, appendicitis and intestinal haemorrhage in the oral and abdominal forms. Pericarditis, osteomyelitis and meningitis have all been recorded.

Course

Except in the severe forms the disease is not usually fatal. In one-third of cases recovery is slow, the debilitating effect may be very marked and lassitude may persist for months. The mean duration of fever in untreated cases is 26 days and adenopathy may last for 3–4 months.

Although tularaemia is not usually fatal, in a series of severe untreated cases there was a mortality rate of 62% in pulmonary and 20% in typhoidal forms of the disease.

Br. tularensis may remain dormant intracellularly in the body for years.

DIAGNOSIS

The differential diagnosis of the local form must be made from plague, tick typhus and rat bite fever. The diagnosis is made by isolation of the organism from the patient's ulcer or gland juice obtained by aspiration and inoculated into guinea-pigs, mice or rabbits, from whose tissues the organism may be isolated on special media as described. The organisms are rarely present in the blood. Serological diagnosis may be made using agglutination tests with cultures of *Br. tularensis* or the spleens of infected mice in a formalinized citrate suspension. Cross-reactions with undulant and typhus fevers may occur as described previously.

TREATMENT

Streptomycin is specific for the infection and of all infections of man in which streptomycin has been tried the maximal effect is found in tularaemia; 1 gramme intramuscularly daily for 7 days will terminate the infection. The patient should be kept in bed for a time after subsidence of the fever and convalescence should be prolonged. More recently tetracycline 250 mg 4 times daily for 2 weeks has been preferred. The inflamed glands should be dressed with a saturated solution of magnesium sulphate and incision must be avoided.

PREVENTION

Prevention depends upon avoidance of the circumstances leading to infection in the various endemic areas. Rabbits should not be skinned without gloves and sick rabbits should not be eaten. Cooking destroys the infection, as does prolonged freezing. Experimental work in the laboratory with *Br. tularensis* must be undertaken with great caution.

REFERENCES

BASSETT SMITH, B. W. (1903) *Br. med. J.*, ii, 1589.
BURROUGHS, A. L., HOLDENFELD, R., LONGANECKER, D. S. & MEYER, K. F. (1945) *J. infect. Dis.*, **76**, 115.
COGHLAN, J. & WEIR, D. M. (1967) *Br. med. J.*, ii, 269.
COX, P. S. U. (1968) *Trans. R. Soc. trop. med. Hyg.*, **62**, 521.
CUMMINGS, H. S. (1937) *Bull Off. int. Hyg. pub.*, **29**, 2532.
DAHLSTRAND, S., RINGERTZ, O. & ZETTERBURG, B. (1971) *Scand. J. infect. Dis.*, **3**, 7.
FINCHAM, R. W., SAHS, A. L. & JOYNT, R. J. (1963) *J. Am. med. Ass.*, **184**, 269.
HUGHES, M. L. (1897) *Mediterranean, Malta or Undulant Fever*. London: Macmillan.
KERR, W. R., COGHLAN, J., PAYNE, J. D. H. & ROBERTSON, L. (1966) *Lancet*, ii, 1181.

LAL, S., MODAWAL, K. K., FOWLE, A. S. E., PEACH, B. & POPHAM, R. D. (1970) *Br. med. J.*, **iii**, 256.

LOWBEER, L. (1948) *Am. J. Path.*, **24**, 723.

McCULLOUGH, N. B. (1951) *Pub. Hlth Rep. Wash.*, **66**, 205.

NELSON-JONES, A. (1951) *Lancet*, **i**, 495.

PAVLOVSKY, E. N. (1966) *Natural Nidality of Transmissible Diseases.* Urbana, Ill.: University of Illinois Press.

ROSSMILLER, H. R. & ENSIGN, W. G. (1948) *Cleveland Clin. Q.*, **15**, 184.

SAHADEVAN, M. G., MAHINDER SINGH, JOSEPH, P. P. & NOOR, R. S. (1968) *Br. med. J.*, **iv**, 432.

SPINK, W. W. (1956) *The Nature of Brucellosis.* Minneapolis: University of Minnesota Press.

—— (1959) in *Textbook of Medicine* (ed. Cecil, R. L. & Loeb, R. F.), 10th ed., p.226. Philadelphia: Saunders.

—— & ANDERSON, D. (1952) *J. Lab. clin. Med.*, **40**, 593.

—— & HALL, W. H. (1949) *Trans. Am. Clin. Climat.*, **61**, 121.

WEED, L. A., DAHLIN, D. C., PUGH, D. G. & IVINS, J. I. (1952) *Am. J. clin. Path.*, **22**, 10.

WORLD HEALTH ORGANIZATION (1964) *Wld Hlth Org. tech. Rep. Ser.*, 289.

22. CHOLERA

Synonym

Cholera asiatica.

Definition

Cholera ($\chi o \lambda \eta \rho o \iota a$ = flow of bile) is an acute infectious epidemic disease characterized by profuse purging and vomiting of a colourless watery material, by muscular cramps, suppression of urine, algidity and collapse, the presence of the cholera vibrios in the intestines, and by a high mortality.

AETIOLOGY

Discovery of *Vibrio cholerae* (the comma bacillus)

The cholera vibrio was first discovered by Koch in Egypt in 1883; this he confirmed in Calcutta in 1884 by finding it in every case of the disease examined. His observations have since been abundantly confirmed. Rogers recounted that in India, many years before Koch, Surgeon-Major Macnamara suggested that cholera was due to living organisms spread by water.

Description of the cholera vibrio

The cholera vibrio (Fig. 144) is a very minute organism, 1·5–2 μm in length by 0·5–0·6 μm in breadth—about half the length and twice the thickness of the tubercle bacillus. It is generally curved like a comma, hence its name. After appropriate staining, flagella can be distinguished at each end or at one end only—sometimes 1, sometimes (though less frequently) 2. These flagella, though of considerable length—from 1 to 5 times that of the body of the bacillus—are difficult to see in ordinary preparations owing to their extreme tenuity. They are not always present during the entire life of the parasite. They impart very active spirillum-like movements. The individual bacilli, when stained, show darker parts at the ends or at the centre. Sometimes in culture 2 or more bacilli are united, in which case an S-shaped body is the result; several bacilli may thus be united producing a spirillar appearance. The cholera vibrio is easily stained by watery solutions of fuchsin or by Löffler's method, dried cover glass films being used. It is Gram-negative. The vibrio grows best in alkaline media at a temperature of from 30° to 40°C. Growth is arrested below 15° or above 42°C; a temperature over 50°C kills the vibrio. Meat broth, blood serum, nutrient gelatin and potato are all suitable culture media. It multiplies rapidly without curdling in milk; it dies rapidly in distilled water; it survives longer if salt is added to the water and survives for up to 285 days in sea water.

Culture by enrichment. For the isolation of vibrios from stools the value of enrichment is recognized. The first method is inoculation into a weakly alkaline solution containing 1% peptone and 0·5% sodium chloride. Minor alterations have been employed and highly selective media, such as Read's modification of Wilson and Blair's medium, bismuth sulphite medium, have been evolved. Panja's method is as follows. Suspected cholera faeces are placed in a L3 candle fitted inside a test-tube containing peptone water to which boric acid has been added in concentration of 0·08%. The vibrios grow through the candle after

24–48 hours' incubation. Potassium tellurite media have also been used with some success in suppressing the growth of coliform and other organisms. Dieudonné's alkaline blood agar and a number of modifications such as Kabeshima's, in which haemoglobin is employed instead of blood, have been widely used. A modification of Endo's medium is highly reliable. Bile salt media such as desoxycholate citrate agar are widely used.

In gelatin plates cholera vibrios grow readily as minute white colonies, irregular in shape and granular, with surrounding liquefaction, into which colonies of vibrios sink as into funnel-shaped depressions. Rough and smooth colonies are recognized. In gelatin stab cultures the growth at first is most active near the surface; later as growth proceeds along the needle track a finger-shaped liquefaction results, which in time extends to the sides of the tube. In older cultures involution forms are common and they may die out after 5 or 6 weeks.

The preservation of *V. cholerae* in stools is based upon the favourable action of a suitable salt concentration along with its ability to survive at high alkalinity.

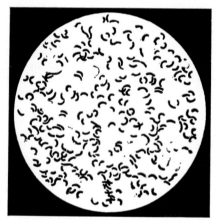

Fig. 144.—The cholera vibrio grown on an agar culture after 24 hours' growth. ×1000. (*Muir & Ritchie*)

A small quantity of cholera stool is added to a medium consisting of a boric acid buffer solution at *p*H 9·2 to which 2% salt is added, from which the vibrio can be recovered up to 2 months or longer.

Haemolytic reaction. As a rule the cholera vibrio does not produce haemolysis if blood is added to the medium such as agar after 24 hours' incubation. The test is best performed in a fluid medium by adding varying amounts from 1 ml downwards of a 3-day culture in alkaline broth to 1 ml of a 5% suspension of sheep or goat corpuscles and then thoroughly mixing. After incubation for 2 hours the tubes are placed in the ice-chest overnight and read the next day.

Sugar reactions. With the solutions of sugars (1%) usually employed, the true cholera vibrio produces acid without gas-formation in glucose, mannose, saccharose and maltose but not from arabinose. Fermentation of lactose with acid production occurs 2–3 days later.

Cholera red reaction. This is obtained by the addition of pure sulphuric acid to a culture in 1% peptone solution. The peptone must be of a brand which contains tryptophan as this is necessary for the production of indole. The true cholera vibrio gives positive cholera red and negative Voges–Proskauer re-actions. It does not produce early haemolysis of erythrocytes (non-haemolytic).

The El Tor vibrio and many other vibrios produce haemolysis and also give a strongly positive Voges–Proskauer reaction.

Isolation from water

Vibrios have been isolated from water by collecting 200 ml in screw-capped bottles to which 20 ml of a solution of 10% peptone and 5% sodium chloride were added. The pH was raised to 9·0 with $N/1$ NaCl, thymol blue being the indicator. After incubation overnight 2 ml amounts were added to 10 ml quantities of peptone water and after 6 hours 1 drop was placed on Aronson's medium. Several litres of water can be filtered through kieselguhr-impregnated filter paper. This is subsequently folded and placed in bismuth sulphite enrichment medium and incubated. Chibrikova et al. (1962) have suggested that the fluorescent antibody technique could be used for the rapid detection of V. cholerae in water after concentrating the vibrios on membrane filters in the usual way.

Classification of vibrios

Certain organisms known as the paracholera or inagglutinable vibrios (NAG vibrios) resemble the cholera vibrio minutely. Organisms found in fowl cholera and in river water also resemble it closely; they behave differently in serological reactions. The vibrios possess H and O antigens. All vibrios having the same H antigen are classified into group A and include V. cholerae. This group is further divided into subgroups I–VI, each having a different O antigen. V. cholerae and most El Tor vibrios fall into subgroup I and may be characterized within this group as Ogawa (A/B), Inaba (A/C) and Hikojima (AB/C) (Felsenfeld 1964). Groups II to VI are not all pathogenic. Group B contains vibrios inagglutinable by sera which agglutinate those of group A and are NAG vibrios.

Identification of cholera vibrios

The only fully reliable method for identification of the vibrio is the use of serological reactions which will demonstrate the characteristic O antigen of V. cholerae. Along with this, haemolysis tests should be employed to identify El Tor vibrios.

Agglutination test. The method used is an agglutination test with a pure O high-titre serum against a living or formolized suspension of the vibrio. A boiled suspension must not be used since for the preparation of pure O sera suspensions of V. cholerae are used from which the H antigen has been removed by prolonged boiling. Sera are prepared in rabbits against O antigens of the Inaba, Ogawa and Hikojima subgroups which will contain agglutinins not only against the main O antigen but also against the subsidiary antigens characteristic of each of the subgroups. Formol suspensions are satisfactory and for pre-liminary diagnosis rapid slide agglutination with O sera of a titre of 1/4000 diluted to 1:50 or 1:100 can be used, but results should be confirmed by tube agglutination. Agglutination tubes should be placed in a water-bath at 52°C and a preliminary reading made at the end of 2 hours. For the confirmation of rough or partially rough variants of V. cholerae a high-titre serum prepared against a rough strain should be employed. Tests should be carried out with suspensions in 0·4–0·5% NaCl.

Haemagglutination reaction. The technique of a haemagglutinating test for the identification of cholera vibrios has been described by Felsenfeld *et al.* (1955). The O antigens of vibrios are absorbed on to human, rabbit or sheep red cells and are tested against increasing dilutions of homologous sera. Incubation at 36°C for 1 hour and standing for 1 hour at room temperature gives the best results when the slide method is used. One drop of each serum dilution and 1 drop of antigen are mixed on excavations on a slide and then rocked. Visual clumping appears rapidly with homologous antigens and agglutination is complete within 15 minutes.

Pfeiffer's reaction. Serum obtained from guinea-pigs or rabbits immunized by repeated injections of killed cultures of cholera vibrios is protective when injected with live vibrios into the peritoneal cavity of a young guinea-pig. When this happens active bacteriolysis takes place.

A loopful of a young agar culture of the vibrio is added to 1 ml of broth containing 0·001 ml of anticholera serum and is injected into the peritoneal cavity of a young guinea-pig. By means of capillary tubes inserted into the peritoneum the peritoneal fluid is examined every few minutes. If the original culture was a true cholera vibrio the organisms break up into globules; if not no change takes place.

El Tor vibrio

In 1905 a haemolytic vibrio was isolated from the dead bodies of Mecca pilgrims at the quarantine camp at El Tor in Egypt. In 1961 this variety of cholera spread from an endemic focus in the Celebes and by 1965 had invaded 23 countries, among them countries from which cholera had been absent for many decades. In 1970 El Tor cholera had spread to the Middle East, the U.S.S.R. and Africa south of the Sahara.

The El Tor vibrio belongs to the same serological group as *V. cholerae*, but many strains show antigenic instability. It is haemolytic but this is not a constant feature. There are several biochemical and physical differences, haemagglutination and resistance to a specific kind of bacteriophage. El Tor biotypes are resistant to group IV cholera phage and to polymixin B. They agglutinate chicken erythrocytes and may produce haemolysin. They survive longer in water than *V. cholerae* and survive well on prepared foods.

Bacteriophages

About 14 races of bacteriophage which lyse the cholera vibrio have been isolated. They are known as A–N. Of these only A and N are selective and act upon the true cholera vibrios only.

TRANSMISSION

Cholera is transmitted by the oral route. Cultures of cholera vibrios have been swallowed many times by way of experiment and, although in some instances diarrhoea has resulted, in only 1 case has true cholera been produced. Probably, for the production of cholera, several conditions are necessary, of which the cholera vibrio is only one. Gastric acidity is an important factor in determining infection. When vibrios are ingested they are quickly killed in undiluted gastric juice. There is no record of natural infection in animals and no animal reservoir is known. Cultures administered in an alkaline medium have produced cholera-like symptoms in animals, and infection of the isolated rabbit intestinal loop is used as an important experimental tool.

Since the source of infection is always a human case or a carrier of the vibrio the natural history of clinical cases and carriers of infection is important. There are two types of human infection—the clinical case and the chronic or true carrier, who has been defined as any person with a positive stool for more than 3 weeks (Bart & Mosley 1970).

Clinical or asymptomatic case

This is traditionally considered to be the principal source of transmission of the disease. The index case, the symptomatic infection and the asymptomatic infection are all newly acquired infections and are usually transitory, rarely excreting cholera vibrios for more than 1–2 weeks. In El Tor infections the carrier state lasts longer (up to 3 years). Asymptomatic cases occur 5–10 times as frequently as cholera cases, regardless of whether the infecting biotope is a classical or El Tor type. The key role of symptomless cases as a reservoir of infection is now being more generally realized and young children may play an important part (Sen *et al.* 1968). In Calcutta a single sampling has revealed 1·5% of excretors of vibrios in the general population.

Chronic carriers

These carriers may shed organisms intermittently for an indefinite period and the infection, which is in the biliary tract, can be detected by culturing duodenal fluid obtained after the administration of a cholagogue. One carrier excreted vibrios intermittently for 329 days and the well known carrier in the Philippines, Dolores M., who suffered cholera in August 1962, was still positive for vibrios on duodenal intubation in April 1968.

Carriers might be recognizable by their high level of persisting antibodies but serological screening of large populations is not feasible. Evidence from Hong Kong, Taiwan and the Philippines indicates that the true carrier often serves as the source of infection and can be of great importance in the persistence of the disease and in its transmission within or between neighbouring countries.

Environmental factors

Cholera can occur if vibrios are introduced in any part of the world where overcrowding and poor sanitation exist. Water is an important source of infection; vibrios can live in reservoir water for 2 weeks but contaminated water is unfavourable for their survival. Stools kept in the dark remain infective for 8 days but the vibrios survive for only a few hours in dry conditions.

Certain foods—milk, milk products and boiled rice—are important vectors since laboratory studies have shown that vibrios multiply readily in them. The addition of salt to fish, meat, watermelon and boiled rice makes them excellent propagating material.

International spread

The presence of relatively large numbers of asymptomatic infections makes wide dissemination of the organism possible within 1 or 2 weeks. Chronic carriers who cannot be detected prolong the duration of possible spread. Uncontrolled migration and pilgrimages introduce infection into a country. In some countries widespread smuggling has contributed to the international spread of cholera.

EPIDEMIOLOGY AND GEOGRAPHICAL DISTRIBUTION

Endemic areas of cholera

The true endemic cholera centres are found in Lower Bengal and in the Yangtse valley in China. These endemic foci are related to certain water systems near the coast at a low level and are densely populated (Swaroop & Pollitzer 1954). There are other large areas in India and China which suffer from epidemics but are often free in inter-epidemic periods and are therefore not endemic zones. An endemic area is one in which the total number of months with absence of cholera does not exceed 30 in 32 years or one in which a break of 5 or more months in cholera incidence does not take place. It has not been possible to trace the manner in which infection is maintained in the endemic zones or the method of infection from patient to patient especially in the inter-epidemic periods. In the endemic areas temperature and relative humidity are the main determining factors. In Bengal in January, when the relative humidity is low and the temperature relatively so, cholera is at its lowest ebb. As the temperature rises so does the cholera incidence, until May or June when the monsoon sets in. Then the humidity rises but the temperature falls, although it shows a minor rise in October as the monsoon subsides. It was found in Shanghai that cholera tends to occur when the vapour pressure exceeds 10 mg Hg. Rogers believed that the condition necessary for the spread in India of cholera is a relative humidity of over 40% and that by watching the climatic conditions which influence the annual incidence of cholera, increased or epidemic prevalence should usually be foreseen in time for steps to be taken to lessen its spread and that the combined study of periodicity of epidemics and humidity renders forecasting of epidemics possible.

Epidemic cholera

Periodically in the past cholera has broken out of the endemic areas in the East and has spread all over the world in pandemics.

Spread of cholera

Cholera follows the great routes of human intercourse and is conveyed by man from place to place. In India and Arabia during religious gatherings hundreds of thousands of people used to be collected together under highly insanitary conditions, as at the Hardwar and Mecca pilgrimages (Fig. 145). Cholera broke out among the devotees who, when they separated and proceeded home, carried the disease along with them, infecting the people of places they passed through. The Hedjaz has for the past 100 years been the point of relay of cholera in its progress from the Far East towards the West. During that period there have been more than 27 outbreaks. In India cholera spreads from its home in lower Bengal over the northern, western, central and southern provinces in a series of waves of 2–4 years' duration. Cholera never travels faster than a man can travel, but in modern times, owing to the increased speed of locomotion and the increased amount of travel, epidemics advance more rapidly and pursue a more erratic course than they did formerly. On the other hand isolated countries such as the Andaman Islands, Australia, New Zealand and the Pacific islands have so far escaped. An epidemic of considerable virulence occurred in Celebes (Indonesia) in 1938. Cholera broke out in Bengal in 1947 and in the autumn

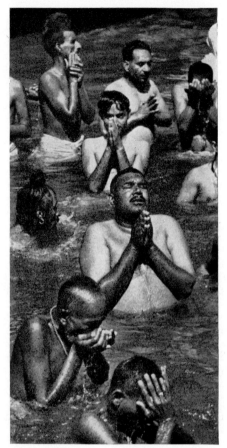

Fig. 145.—Pilgrims bathing in the Ganges during the Kumbh Mela. These festivals were formerly followed by cholera epidemics. (*By courtesy of Life Magazine*)

months an epidemic of considerable proportions raged in the Delta of Egypt. Centres of less importance are Burma and the Philippines.

Pandemics

From a study of the great pandemics it can be concluded that cholera has reached Europe by three distinct routes: (1) Via Afghanistan, Iran, the Caspian Sea and the Volga River; (2) Via the Persian Gulf, Syria, Asia Minor and Turkey in Europe; and (3) Via the Red Sea, Egypt and the Mediterranean. Swaroop and Pollitzer (1954) have given an account of the world incidence since 1923.

El Tor cholera

The cholera of the great pandemics of the past was caused by the classical *Vibrio cholerae*. In 1961 El Tor cholera spread from an endemic focus in the Celebes and by 1965 had invaded 23 countries, among them countries from which cholera had been absent for many decades. El Tor cholera spread as far as Iran and the U.S.S.R. In 1970 El Tor cholera spread again as far as the southern part of the U.S.S.R. and North Africa, and appeared for the first time in the twentieth century in Africa south of the Sahara. El Tor cholera was spread by land, often by smugglers, over uncontrolled routes and by sea by small coastal ships. It has now been reported as far south as the Southern Sudan, Uganda and Kenya, and also in West Africa. It has reached Europe.

IMMUNOLOGY

Immunity following cholera infection

Well documented reports on second attacks of cholera are virtually non-existent. The mechanism of immunity to cholera is not understood. Some persons develop cholera despite the presence of serum antibody levels generally associated with resistance to cholera. Reinfection with cholera vibrios is common in endemic areas but recurrent disease is rare.

Humoral immunity

As far as is known immunity in cholera is entirely humoral. Cholera vibrios live in the intestinal canal where they produce enterotoxin; they do not circulate in the body. However, humoral antibodies are produced along with copro-antibodies. The antibodies may be of importance in the defence of the body against multiplication of the vibrios in the gut if they come into contact with them after being produced in the intestines (coproantibodies) or excreted into the intestinal lumen from the circulation.

The antibodies which are formed are both antitoxic and antibacterial.

Enterotoxin (exotoxin, choleragen) (Finkelstein et al. 1966; Carpenter 1971). Enterotoxin, which results from the destruction of vibrios within the lumen of the gut, is responsible for the symptoms of cholera. Enterotoxin is a 7-S globulin with a molecular weight slightly greater than 90 000; it is heat-resistant and acid-labile, and trypsin-resistant but destroyed by pronase. It is antigenic and toxin neutralizing antibodies develop during clinical cholera which have been shown to be IgG. A method of detecting them has been developed (Felsenfeld 1959), which uses the power of these antibodies to neutralize enterotoxin. The supernanant fluid of a culture of vibrios serves as the antigen which is standardized and matched against test sera by double diffusion agar technique.

Antibacterial antibodies. These include agglutinins, vibriocidal antibodies and coproantibodies. Agglutinins are responsible for Pfeiffer's reaction, page 503. Vibriocidal antibodies appear early and persist for many weeks (Finkelstein et al. 1966) and require complement for their demonstration. They increase in the serum of man during exposure to cholera and after immunization. Copro-antibodies appear in the absence of serum antibody and are present along the entire gut. They decline soon after they are formed and could be of importance in immunization against infection, since they could be induced by live avirulent oral vaccines.

Immunoglobulins

Felsenfeld et al. (1966) described changes in the immunoglobulins in 12 patients with classical cholera, 10 with El Tor and volunteers given cholera lipo-polysaccharide (LPS) or phenolized vaccine. All cholera patients showed an increase in IgA and IgM. All sera gave precipitation reactions and showed neutralizing activity. There were higher precipitin titres in the cholera patients. IgG is involved in antitoxic activity, and IgM and IgG in vibriocidal activity in which IgM predominates. IgA and IgG are found in the stools of monkeys infected with cholera and IgA may play a part in the mechanism of immunity within the lumen of the bowel (WHO 1969).

Serological tests

There are many laboratory tests for cholera (Felsenfeld 1964). Serological tests at present are useful only for retrospective diagnosis and may be of little value in a vaccinated or exposed population. They are, however, useful in measuring the results of vaccination.

Antibodies may be measured by a vibriocidal test, agglutination or haemolysis inhibition.

The vibriocidal test (Finkelstein 1962) is the most sensitive and has been used on paired sera of patients suspected of cholera and in surveys to determine the level of past experience and the current immune status of a community.

Antitoxin levels may be determined by a mouse protection test or by agar gel double diffusion technique against the supernatant of a vibrio culture.

Neutralizing antibodies may be determined by inoculating an isolated rabbit intestinal loop with the test sera and cholera enterotoxin.

PATHOLOGY

Cholera is not a systemic infection and vibrios are confined to the intestinal canal. The clinical syndrome of cholera is produced by hypovolaemia, hyponatraemia and hypokalaemia, which are the result of a rapid loss from the gut of an isotonic fluid very low in protein with a mean bicarbonate concentration approximately twice and a potassium concentration four times that of normal plasma. Cholera enterotoxin (exotoxin, choleragen) is responsible for the fluid and electrolyte loss (Carpenter 1971), and when introduced to isolated gut loops causes severe electrolyte and water loss unaccompanied by any histological evidence of damage to the intestinal mucosa. Glucose and sodium absorption are not interfered with and intraluminal glucose enhances sodium absorption, an observation which has been made use of in the treatment of cholera (Cash et al. 1970).

Increased capillary permeability plays no significant part in this abnormal movement of electrolytes across the gut wall, but enterotoxin stimulates the production of adenyl cyclase in the mucosal cells, which increases adenosine $3'5'$-cyclic monophosphate (cAMP), which is responsible for the abnormal fluid and electrolyte movement. In future it should be possible to institute an effective biochemical mechanism to counteract the effect of this potent bacterial toxin (enterotoxin).

Rigor mortis occurs early and persists for a considerable time. Curious movements of the limbs may take place in consequence of post mortem muscular contractions. On dissection, the most characteristic pathological appearances in cholera are those connected with the circulation and with the intestinal tract.

If death occurs during the algid stage, the surface presents a shrunken and livid appearance. All the tissues are abnormally dry. The muscles are dark and firm; sometimes one or more of them are ruptured—evidently from the violence of the cramps during life. The right side of the heart and the systemic veins are full of dark, thick and imperfectly coagulated blood which tends to cling to the inner surface of the vessels. Fibrinous clots, extending into the vessels, may be found in the right heart. The lungs are usually anaemic, dry and shrunken, occasionally congested and oedematous. The pulmonary arteries are distended with blood, the veins empty. The liver is generally loaded with blood; the gall-bladder full of bile; the spleen small. Like all the other serous cavities, the peritoneum contains no fluid, its surface being dry and sticky. The inner surface of the bowel has generally a diffuse rosy-red, occasionally an injected appearance. It contains a larger or smaller amount of the characteristic rice-water material, occasionally blood. The mucous membrane of the stomach and intestine is generally pinkish from congestion, or there may be irregular arborescent patches of injection here and there throughout its extent.

On microscopical examination of the contents of the bowel during the acute stage of the disease the cholera vibrio, in most cases, may be demonstrated. Usually it is in great abundance, occasionally in almost pure culture in the upper part of the small intestine and duodenum. but it may be very scarce in the large gut. Sections of the intestine show the vibrio lying on and between the epithelial cells of villi and glands.

The vibrios are confined almost entirely to the gastro-intestinal canal, mainly to the lumen. The tissue changes could possibly be explained by dehydration of the tissues and by haemo-concentration and low blood pressure, which results in temporary ischaemia.

De (1961) and his associates have paid special attention to the renal and suprarenal changes of those who have died in the stage of shock. The kidneys show patchy ischaemia of the cortex with medullary congestion, and there may also be necrosis of the cortical tubules. It is thought that cortical vasospasm is responsible for the complete cessation of urinary secretion. In a histochemical examination of the suprarenal glands it was concluded that depletion of the lipoid material from the cortex may be associated with increased liberation of cortical hormones, so that the suprarenals may play an active part in the symptomatology of cholera.

CLINICAL FEATURES

The incubation period is 3–6 days. Most infections are asymptomatic or present as a simple self-limiting diarrhoea.

Description of the average case

When true cholera sets in, profuse watery stools usually associated with griping pains, and at first faecal in character, pour, one after the other, from the patient. Quickly the stools lose their faecal character, becoming colourless, or rather like thin rice or barley water, later containing small white flocculi in suspension. Enormous quantities—pints—of this material are generally passed. Presently, vomiting, also profuse, at first perhaps of food, but very soon of the same rice-water material, supervenes. Agonizing cramps attack the extremities and abdomen; the implicated muscles stand out like rigid bars, or are thrown into lumps from the violence of the contractions (due to depletion of chlorides and hypocalcaemia affecting the neuromuscular junction). The patient may rapidly pass into a state of collapse. In consequence, principally, of the loss of fluid by the diarrhoea and vomiting, the soft parts shrink, the cheeks fall in, the nose becomes pinched and thin, the eyes sunken, and the skin of the fingers shrivelled like a washerwoman's (Fig. 146). The surface of the body becomes cold, livid, and bedewed with a clammy sweat; the urine and bile are suppressed; respiration is rapid and shallow; the breath is cold, and the voice is sunk to a whisper. The pulse soon becomes thready, weak and rapid, and then after coming and going and feebly fluttering, may disappear entirely.

The surface temperature sinks several degrees below normal—33·9° or 34·4°C —whilst that in the rectum may be several degrees above normal—38·3° to 40·6°C. The blood pressure is low. The systolic may register 50 mm Hg, but is frequently unregistrable. The patient is now restless, tossing about uneasily, throwing his arms from side to side, feebly complaining of intense thirst and of a burning feeling in the chest and racked with cramps. Although apathetic, the mind generally remains clear, but sometimes the patient may wander or may pass into a comatose state.

This, the 'algid stage' of cholera, may terminate in one of three ways—in death, in rapid convalescence or in febrile reaction.

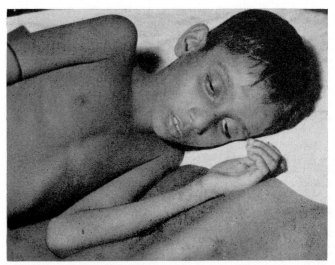

Fig. 146.—Dehydration and collapse on the first day of cholera. Note the sunken orbits. (*Dr C. J. Hackett*)

When death from collapse supervenes, it may do so at any time from 2 to 30 hours from the commencement of the seizure, usually in from 10 to 12. On the other hand, the gradual cessation of vomiting and purging, the reappearance of the pulse at the wrist, the increase of blood pressure and the return of some warmth to the surface may herald convalescence. In such a case, after many hours' absence, secretion of urine returns, and in a few days the patient may be practically well again. Usually, however, a condition known as the 'stage of reaction' gradually supervenes on the algid stage.

Anuria. This is accompanied by congestion of the mucous membranes and conjunctivae, malar flush, delirium and gradual increase in depth and rate of respiration. Recovery is marked by the passage of a few ounces of turbid, highly coloured urine and this is followed by a 'critical diuresis' resembling that seen in some cases of acute glomerulo-nephritis.

Renal failure in cholera has been compared to anuria following crush injuries. The blood urea is invariably raised and may reach 350 mg. Anuria may persist for 50 hours, and the patient may yet recover. When the patient passes 2 pints of clear urine in 24 hours the danger of relapse has usually passed. According to the modern school of physiological thought the main factor is *renal anoxia*.

The importance of charting the amount of urine, hour by hour, day by day, in the reactionary stage of cholera cannot be over-emphasized. These data are essential if threatened anuria is to be successfully combated.

Reaction or *cholera typhoid*. When the patient enters on this stage the surface of the body becomes warmer, the pulse returns, the face fills out, restlessness disappears, urine is secreted, and the motions diminish in number and amount, becoming bilious at the same time. Coincidently with the subsidence of the more urgent symptoms of the algid stage and this general improvement in the appearance of the patient, a febrile condition of greater or less severity may develop. Minor degrees in this reaction generally subside in a few hours; but in more severe cases the febrile state becomes aggravated, and a condition in many respects closely resembling typhoid fever, 'cholera typhoid', ensues.

Hyperpyrexia is an occasional, though rare, occurrence in cholera. In such cases the axillary temperature may rise to 41·7°C and the rectal temperature perhaps to 42·8°C. These cases also are almost invariably fatal.

In cholera there is a considerable variety in the character of the symptoms and in their severity, both in individual cases and in different epidemics. It is generally stated that the earlier cases are the more severe, those occurring towards the end of the epidemic being on the whole milder.

Ambulatory cases occur during all epidemics, characterized merely by diarrhoea and malaise.

Cholera sicca

A very fatal type is known as 'cholera sicca'. In these cases, though there is no, or very little, diarrhoea or vomiting, collapse sets in so rapidly that the patient is quickly overpowered as by an overwhelming dose of some poison.

For the effects of cholera on the eye, see Chapter 44.

Complications

The common complications are persisting enteritis, diarrhoea, corneal ulcers, cholecystitis and abortion in pregnant women. Pneumonia is common in the older countries, but rare in hot ones. Gangrene of the extremities, penis and scrotum, formerly observed, is seldom seen nowadays.

These changes disappear on rehydration.

CLINICAL PATHOLOGY

Loss of fluid and salts

The total loss of fluid may amount to as much as 5 litres in 24 hours. The salt content of the stools in the rice-water stage is about 0·5 to 1·0%. There is considerable loss of alkaline bases in stools which disturbs the osmotic balance and leads to acidosis. The vomits are usually less in volume than the stools and in contrast they are acid and contain a lesser amount of salt.

Blood changes

The loss of fluid may be more than 60% in fatal cases. The plasma specific gravity is elevated. There is haemoconcentration with red cell counts of 6 million and over. Leucocytosis is constant in cholera, the counts being 20 000/mm³ in some. The percentage of neutrophil leucocytes is increased to 80% or over, compared with the normal of 68%, while the number of lymphocytes is diminished. This increase is more than can be accounted for by the concentration of the blood. The protein content of the blood is increased in the acute stage of cholera.

Blood urea

There is a definite rise of blood urea in all patients from the time of onset of the attack. The urea increases progressively, but falls fairly rapidly in patients during recovery. In the acute stage it varies from 28 to 125 mg/100 ml with an average of 62 mg (compared with the normal of 15–35 mg).

Circulatory failure

The profound circulatory failure which is such a feature of cholera is not of central, but of peripheral nature. The loss of body fluid is of course a factor, but the distribution of the blood plays a much more important role in the circulatory changes which occur. The arteries and capillaries are empty and the veins engorged in the splanchnic area. The effective circulatory volume of the blood is very much reduced. There is a fall in blood pressure as the result of loss in circulating fluid, the systolic pressure being often 70 mm or lower on admission to hospital. In severe cases there is no measurable diastolic pressure. The circulation time is lengthened owing, partially, to the increased viscosity of the blood.

Sequelae

These are unusual. Recovery is generally complete. Occasionally there are minor sequelae, such as anaemia, mental and physical debility, insomnia, a diphtheritic inflammation of the mucous membranes of the intestines, fauces and genitalia, nephritis, different forms of pulmonary inflammation, parotitis apt to end in abscess, ulceration of the corneae, boils, bedsores and gangrene of different parts of the body. Jaundice occurs at times and is said to be of the gravest import. An interesting, but unusual, sequel is bradycardia. Pregnant women almost invariably miscarry, the fetus showing evidences of cholera.

The prognosis of cholera is especially bad in opium addicts.

DIAGNOSIS

During the height of the epidemic the diagnosis of cholera is generally easy; the profuse rice-water discharges, shrivelled fingers and toes, feeble husky voice, cold breath, cramps and suppression of urine, together with the high rate of mortality, are generally sufficiently distinctive. But in the first cases of some outbreaks of diarrhoea, which may or may not turn out to be cholera, and the true nature of which, for obvious reasons, it is important to determine, correct diagnosis may not be so easy. Control measures should be applied if the clinical evidence is suggestive, without waiting for bacteriological confirmation.

In the first place stools should be examined microscopically. If vibrios are present in large numbers they may be detected by their scintillating rotatory movements in hanging-drop preparations, or by their characteristic shape in faecal films stained by carbol fuchsin. Diagnosis may be made in as follows:

1. Inoculate several loopfuls of stools into a tube of peptone water (1% peptone, 0·5% sodium chloride, adjusted to pH 8·4). Incubate for 8 hours. Take a loopful and examine fresh or stained for Gram-negative motile vibrios.

2. Take a loopful from the peptone culture and streak on Vedder and Van Dam (haemoglobin–peptone–glycerin and KOH, pH 8·4), Dieudonné's or

Aronson plates for 12 hours. Pick out greenish colonies in the first two, red in the third, and confirm that they are vibrios.

3. Carry out agglutination tests with standard high-titre and anti-O subgroup I cholera serum to exclude all but El Tor and true cholera vibrios.

4. In order to show whether haemolytic (El Tor) or non-haemolytic (true cholera vibrio) add an equal quantity of vibrio emulsion of a 5% sheep blood corpuscular suspension in saline.

Bandi's method consists in inoculating the suspected faeces into peptone water containing agglutinating serum of such strength as to clump the cholera

Table 27. Differential diagnosis of cholera and food-poisoning

Symptom	Cholera	Food-poisoning
Diarrhoea	Often associated with griping. Precedes vomiting	Associated with some intestinal pain. Follows vomiting
Vomiting	Causes no distress. Watery and projectile; follows diarrhoea	Often violent and distressing. Vomit consists of food and is never watery, copious or projectile. *Generally precedes diarrhoea*
Nausea	Absent	Common
Retching	Rare	Common, often severe
Abdominal pain	Not usually severe	Constant
Tenesmus	Absent	Common
Stools	Watery and copious	Liquid, faecal, and offensive. Never colourless and copious
Urine	May be completely suppressed	Never suppressed
Muscular cramps	Constant and severe	In very severe cases, confined to extremities
Collapse	Frequent. Chiefly from loss of fluid	Faintness and syncope from toxaemia
Fever	Surface temperature below normal, but rectal temperature may be raised	Axillary temperature 37·2°–42·8°C
Headache	Absent	Frequent

bacillus in high dilution. Within as short a period as 3 hours' incubation agglutination is said to be visible to the naked eye. This method, when employed in a large number of cases, naturally consumes a large quantity of immune serum. Rectal swabs are useful for diagnosis, especially in an epidemic.

In an autopsy on a suspected case of cholera at least 2 sections of the small gut, each about 13 cm in length—one just above the iliocaecal valve and the other in the middle of the ileum—should be ligatured, cut off, dropped into sterile saline and sent to a bacteriological laboratory for examination as soon as possible.

Differential diagnosis

True cholera may have to be differentiated from mushroom poisoning, which may simulate it very closely, though in this case there is usually a history of several persons being attacked at the same time. Leucocytosis is absent in food-poisoning, though usually found during the early stages of cholera. Differential diagnosis of food-poisoning from cholera is based upon the violent and distressing vomiting which precedes the diarrhoea of food-poisoning, the severity of the pain and the greenish, offensive nature of the stools. The urinary flow is never suppressed, whilst the axillary temperature is raised. Salient points of differential diagnosis are set out in Table 27.

Algid or choleraic subtertian malaria may simulate true cholera very closely (see page 57); acute bacillary dysentery may occasionally be so sudden and severe in its onset as to resemble cholera; acute trichinosis is distinguished by leucocytosis and pronounced eosinophilia; in arsenical or antimony poisoning vomiting, continuous, mucous and often freely streaked with blood, is more usually the most urgent commencing symptom. Children suffering from cholera are apt to develop hyperpyrexia with cerebral manifestations, which may be mistaken for meningitis.

TREATMENT

The aim of treatment is to restore the fluid and electrolyte balance of the body and remove the vibrios from the intestinal canal (WHO 1967).

Antimicrobial drugs

The administration of antimicrobial agents to which vibrios are sensitive shortens the duration of diarrhoea and the excretion of vibrios in the stools.

Good results were obtained with a mixture of dihydrostreptomycin, sulphadiazine and sulphamerazine, but streptomycin-resistant vibrios appeared shortly after the massive application of the drug.

Tetracycline and chloramphenicol are equally effective whether administered orally or intravenously, causing a very rapid reduction in the number of vibrios in the stools. To ensure freedom from bacteriological relapses 500 mg of the drug should be administered about 3 hours after admission and then every 6 hours for 3 days. Tetracycline is valuable in the treatment of subclinical cases and carriers. Purging with magnesium sulphate has disclosed that some persons continue to harbour *V. cholerae* after such treatment.

Erythromycin is also effective, but should be held in reserve in case tetracycline-resistant vibrios appear.

A combination of trimethoprim (10 mg/kg) and sulphamethoxazole (50 mg/kg), to a daily maximum of 390 mg trimethoprim and 1600 mg sulphamethoxazole (4 tablets), in 2 equal doses for 4 days (not less), eliminated the vibrios (Gharagozloo *et al.* 1970).

Dehydration and electrolyte replacement

Cholera patients require immediate replacement of fluid and electrolytes and correction of the acidosis, even, if possible, before admission to hospital. Thereafter the fluid balance is maintained by replacing the fluid lost during treatment. Fluid replacement may be by the oral or the intravenous route.

Intravenous route. In the adult 2 units of isotonic saline should be followed by

1 unit of isotonic (1·39%) sodium bicarbonate, or 3 units of isotonic saline followed by 1 unit of 2% sodium bicarbonate.

Isotonic sodium lactate solution (0·16 M, 1·87%) can be used instead of the sodium bicarbonate. Sterile sodium lactate can be obtained in 40 ml ampoules of molar strength, which when diluted with 200 ml of water or 5% dextrose gives 0·16 M sodium lactate solution. Sodium acetate can be used instead of sodium lactate; it is cheaper and more stable.

Oral route. This is being used increasingly instead of the intravenous route. Since glucose can enhance sodium absorption by the small bowel, Cash *et al.* (1970) have used an electrolyte and glucose solution orally to correct the acidosis and dehydration of cholera. Patients are given nothing by mouth except the oral solution and tetracycline, which is continued for 5 days—250 mg every 6 hours for adults, 125 mg every 6 hours for children. The solution used contains sodium 120 mEq/litre, bicarbonate 48 mEq/litre, chloride 87 mEq/litre and potassium 15 mEq/litre, together with 110 mmoles glucose per litre. The solution is given by mouth at a rate of 750 ml/hour for 6 hours (250 ml for children) at a temperature of 45°C. For children the potassium is increased to 25 mEq/litre. Vomiting takes place in the first hours, but the loss of fluid is soon made up in this way. The fluid can be administered by nasogastric drip, which allows the patient to sleep, and is often necessary for children. Three hundred patients have been treated by this method, with 100% recovery.

Oral medication. Potassium losses may be replaced orally. Green coconut water, which contains 70 mEq/litre potassium, is very palatable. A 10% potassium citrate solution may be given by mouth in 15 ml doses diluted in water, 3 or 4 times a day.

Correction phase. The plasma specific gravity (normal 1·027–1·029) is measured to determine the degree of dehydration, which is then corrected by the necessary amount of fluid, estimated as follows by the copper sulphate method: Prepare a saturated solution of copper sulphate by placing 1800 grammes of copper sulphate ($CuSO_4 \cdot 5H_2O$, Analar) in a 4 litre bottle and adding 2500 ml of distilled water. Shake vigorously and decant the supernatant fluid through loose-textured filter paper. Take 587 ml at 10°C or 527 ml at 15·5°C or 453 ml at 25°C and make up to 1 litre with distilled water. This will make a solution of copper sulphate of specific gravity 1·100 at 25°C. To prepare solutions of specific gravity from 1·025 to 1·035 make up the following amounts of the 1·100 solution to 100 ml with distilled water:

Specific gravity	Volume of copper sulphate solution to be made up to 100 ml with water
1·025	24·14 ml
1·026	25·12 ml
1·027	26·10 ml
1·028	27·08 ml
1·029	28·06 ml
1·030	29·04 ml
1·031	30·00 ml
1·032	31·00 ml
1·033	32·00 ml
1·034	33·00 ml
1·035	34·00 ml
1·036 onwards	add 1·0 ml for each point

Place 100 ml of each solution in a numbered bottle. To measure the plasma specific gravity drop 1 drop of citrated plasma in each bottle and note the one in which the drop remains suspended and neither sinks nor rises. This is the specific gravity of the specimen.

The amount of intravenous fluid required can be calculated according to the formula

(Estimated plasma specific gravity $-$ 1·025) $\times$ 200 000 $=$ ml

If the estimated specific gravity is 1·037 then 1·027 $-$ 1·025 $=$ 0·012, which multiplied by 200 000 gives 2400 ml.

Fluid is given as rapidly as possible until a full pulse returns and the general condition of the patient becomes essentially normal. An indwelling polyethylene catheter may be used for measuring the central venous pressure, and should be kept 1–2 cm below the sternal angle.

Maintenance phase. The measurement of the excreta is facilitated by the 'cholera cot', which is a bed with a hole in the middle under the patient's buttocks and a calibrated plastic bucket placed underneath to collect the excreta. The total fluid lost is replaced, plus 500 ml daily. Anuria often occurs and every effort must be maintained to re-establish the blood pressure. Pitressin in doses of 0·5–1·0 ml subcutaneously or intramuscularly 2–4 times a day or noradrenaline should be given. Avomine (promethazine chlorotheophyllinate) 1–2 tablets of 25 mg checks the vomiting.

Treatment of cholera in children

The treatment of cholera in children is more difficult. The initial fluid requirement cannot be calculated on the basis of plasma specific gravity and body weight so that the initial fluid requirement must be judged clinically. Acidosis and potassium deficiency may be of greater importance. A single replacement solution with which acidosis is corrected at the same time is used.

Potassium is included in the intravenous solution at a level of 13 mEq/litre. This is provided for by an isotonic solution containing 5 grammes sodium chloride, 4 grammes sodium bicarbonate (or an equivalent amount of sodium lactate) and 1 gramme potassium chloride per litre. This is called the 5–4–1 solution.

Mortality rate

The death rate for cholera was always high. In former days in India it was seldom less than 70%. In the decade ending 1908, it was 54·2% in Indian and 78·5% in British troops in India. With improved methods of treatment it has declined considerably and cholera has now become one of the most effectively treated diseases. When treatment procedures are properly applied deaths are extremely rare. In children case fatality rates remained at 15–20% until the single replacement solution was used, when the rate fell to 0·6% in a series of 300 children under the age of 10 years.

Convalescence

A patient should not be discharged from treatment control unless there have been 3 negative stools or at least 3 days of treatment with an effective antibiotic at a dosage of 500 mg every 6 hours. Neither procedure guarantees the absence of vibrios in the body.

Treatment of carriers

Oral streptomycin has been found to be the best treatment for carriers (Forbes *et al.* 1968). Streptomycin was given orally and the course completed in

24 hours. Dosage was 1 gramme at hourly intervals for 8 doses in patients over 10 years, from 500 mg at hourly intervals for patients aged 2–9 and 250 mg for 2-year-olds and under. Resistance can develop in 24 hours but did not prove a problem. Rectal swabs were examined after treatment and any persons found to be excreting vibrios were given a 5-day course of chloramphenicol.

Recently in Kenya the main weapon has been rapid identification of clinical and asymptomatic cases and immediate treatment of all contacts with tetracycline. This has been very successful.

PREVENTION

Quarantine prevention

Quarantine can never be an efficient protection against the introduction of cholera since convalescent patients pass vibrios in their stools, and it is necessary to examine the stools of all contacts to detect the carrier state. The tendency of cholera caused by the El Tor vibrio to create endemic foci in various parts of the world is of great importance. It is due to the existence of carriers, some of whom may excrete vibrios over a long period of time, and to the fact that vaccines in use at present do not confer a sufficient degree of immunity to protect a community in the absence of adequate environmental sanitation and other anti-cholera measures. Early and reliable reporting of cholera is a moral and legal obligation for every state.

Sanitation

Control of cholera can only be obtained by the investigation and surveillance of all enteric and diarrhoeal diseases, the construction of sanitation facilities to keep pace with social and industrial development and with the growth of tourism and trade. During the great religious festivals the sanitary condition of the devotees must be looked after as far as possible, special care being given to provide them with good drinking and bathing water.

Water supplies

For chlorination the usual residual free chlorine is 1–2 parts in 5 million or 2·7–5·4 kg of bleaching powder per 5 million litres. Potassium permanganate at a dilution of 1 : 500 000 (faint purple colour) kills cholera vibrios in a short time. This dilution is obtained by adding 454 grammes to each 250 000 litres. In a well of 9000 litres the amount would be 15 grammes. The mixture should be made in a bucket first and thoroughly mixed with the well water.

Food supplies

Only certain foods under special circumstances and for a limited period of time may be effective vehicles of vibrios.

Prophylactic vaccination

The immunity produced by vaccination does not seem to be very persistent, lasting at the maximum for 3 or 4 months.

Epidemics of cholera are readily controlled by vaccine when inoculation is made compulsory. When cholera was introduced into Korea from China in 1926 the outbreak was promptly brought to a close by the inoculation of more than 1 million persons. The outbreaks of cholera in Egypt in 1947 offered an opportunity of estimating the prophylactic value of cholera vaccine. It was shown that villages in which inoculation was carried out before cases of cholera had occurred showed a lower incidence and case mortality than those in which inoculation was commenced after the outbreak. Six controlled field trials of cholera vaccines have been carried out since 1963 in India, Pakistan and the Philippines. Six of 13 vaccines given in a single dose provided statistically significant protection with an effectiveness ranging from 40 to 80%.

Rogers has long advocated compulsory inoculation for the control of cholera in pilgrims in India and has quoted figures in relation to this measure since 1940. There has been an unprecedented and rapid decline of cholera mortality among 20 million pilgrims. During 15 years (1941–55) about 300 million people have been inoculated in India. Formerly the pilgrims became infected and carried the disease back to their villages. It is relevant to add that the sanitary arrangements for the great Indian pilgrimages have been greatly improved in recent years, and the same is true for the Hedjaz pilgrimages. There are areas where cholera is endemic at all seasons of the year because of the monthly absolute humidity, such as Burma, Thailand and Indo-China which are contiguous with endemic areas of Assam and East Bengal from which cholera epidemics spread over North-west and Central India. To strike at the root of the problem it is essential that the endemic regions of Burma, Thailand and Indo-China should adopt the successful Indian plan of enforcing compulsory inoculation every year of all pilgrims within their territories (Rogers 1957).

Three main types of vaccine are used:

1. Agar grown phenol killed (Kasauli).
2. Formol killed freeze-dried (Walter Reed).
3. Phenol killed grown on casein hydrolysate (Haffkine).

Vaccines prepared with classical vibrio strains are effective against both classical and El Tor biotypes. WHO requirements for cholera vaccine are 4000 million organisms/ml, but it has been recommended that no vaccine should contain less than 8000 million per ml.

The initial dose is 0·5 ml of a strength of 4000 million/ml followed 7–10 days later by a second inoculation of 1·0 ml of 8000 million/ml. Undesirable reactions have been observed among adults from endemic areas who have circulating antibodies and among those who have had repeated booster doses. Intradermal injections of 0·1 ml should be considered for boosters as they are less reactogenic. Cholera may be combined with TAB vaccine as TAB/Chol vaccination. Since vaccination can hardly be considered as satisfactory with the vaccine employed at present, oral vaccination has again become of interest, especially after its success in poliomyelitis. If an organism with strong immunogenicity could be found with no tendency to become virulent, oral vaccination might well become an efficient form of control using live vaccines.

On the ground that cholera toxin is the pathogenic agent, it has recently been suggested that a toxoid might give better protection than a bacterial vaccine.

REFERENCES

Bart, K. J. & Mosley, W. H. (1970) *Lancet*, **ii**, 47.
Cash, R. A., Forrest, J. H., Nalin, D. R. & Abrutyn, E. (1970) *Lancet*, **ii**, 549.
Carpenter, C. J. (1971) *Am. med. J.*, **50**, 1.
Chibrikova, E. V., Schurkina, I. I., Tabakov, P. K. & Mosolova, O. N. (1962) *Zh. Mikrobiol. Epidem. Immunobiol.*, **33**, 9.
De, S. N. (1961) *Cholera, Its Pathology and Pathogenesis*. Edinburgh & London: Oliver & Boyd.
Felsenfeld, O. (1959) *Abstr. Rep. 1st Sci. Sess. Ass. Microbiol. India*, 8.

FELSENFELD, O. (1964) *Bact. Rev.*, **28**, 72.
———— FELSENFELD, A. D., GREER, W. E. & HILL, C. W. (1966) *J. infect. Dis.*, **116**, 329.
———— FREEMAN, N. L. & MOORIG, V. L. (1955) *Am. J. trop. Med. Hyg.*, **4**, 318.
FINKELSTEIN, R. A. (1962) *J. Immunol.*, **89**, 264.
———— SOBOCINSKI, P. Z., ATTHASAMPUNNA, P. & CHARUNMETHEE, P. (1966) *J. Immunol.*, **97**, 25.
FORBES, G. I., LOCKHART, J. D. F., ROBERTSON, M. J. & ALLEN, G. L. (1968) *Bull. Wld Hlth Org.*, **39**, 381.
GHARAGOZLOO, R. A., NAFICY, K., MOUIN, M., NASSIRADEN, M. H. & YALDA, R. (1970) *Br. med. J.*, **iv**, 281.
ROGERS, L. (1957) *Br. med. J.*, **ii**, 1193.
SEN, R., SEN, D. K., CHAKRABARTY, A. N. & GHOSH, A. (1968) *Lancet*, **ii**, 1012.
SWAROOP, S. & POLLITZER, R. (1955) *Bull. Wld Hlth Org.*, **12**, 311.
WORLD HEALTH ORGANIZATION (1967) *Wld Hlth Org. tech. Rep. Ser.*, 352.
———— (1969) *Wld Hlth Org. tech. Rep. Ser.*, 414.

23. SHIGELLOSIS AND DIARRHOEA

BACILLARY DYSENTERY (SHIGELLOSIS)

BACILLARY dysentery is a diarrhoeal disease, usually of the large intestine, caused by bacteria of the genus *Shigella*; the terminal portion of the small intestine may be involved in particularly severe infections.

Bacillary dysentery has a long history. It has always been associated with conditions of overcrowding and poor sanitation, and has always been a major feature in military campaigns, for instance in the Gallipoli campaign of World War I, where it was a main cause of illness and death, and the Middle East campaign of World War II. It is prevalent throughout the developing countries, particularly in the tropics, but it also occurs epidemically in temperate climates when, for some reason, the sanitary barriers to intestinal infection break down, as in the water-borne Montrose outbreak in Scotland reported in 1968. Mental hospitals and institutions for children are particularly prone to outbreaks.

In temperate climates the incidence was formerly highest in late summer and early autumn, but the periodicity has changed in Britain, where the peak has recently tended to occur in winter or spring. In the tropics and subtropics the peak is expected during or after the period of heavy rains, when houseflies are most abundant (see page 521).

Aetiology

The *Shigella* group comprises 4 subgroups:
- A. Mannitol not fermented. *Shigella dysenteriae* Types 1–10 (including types formerly known as *Sh. shigae* and *Sh. schmitzii*, and the Large-Sachs group).
- B. Mannitol usually fermented. Types antigenically interrelated. *Shigella flexneri*, Types 1–6, and X and Y variants.
- C. Mannitol usually fermented. Types antigenically distinct. *Shigella boydii*, Types 1–15.
- D. Mannitol usually fermented. *Shigella sonnei*, a late lactose fermenter.

For details of biochemical reactions textbooks on bacteriology should be consulted.

Shigella dysenteriae 1 (Shiga) causes the most severe form of dysentery. It is rarely encountered outside the tropics and Eastern Asia, though in 8665 cases of dysentery in troops in North Africa and the Middle East in World War II the following figures of incidence were found by Fairley and Boyd (1943):

Entamoeba histolytica	12·3%
Shigella dysenteriae Type 1 (Shiga)	15·8%
Shigella dysenteriae Type 2 (Schmitz)	5·2%
Shigella sonnei (Sonne)	6·3%
Shigella flexneri and *Sh. boydii* (Flexner-Boyd)	52·3%
Other non-mannitol fermenters	3·6%
Other mannitol fermenters	4·5%

Sh. dysenteriae 1 (Shiga) produces (unlike the other shigellae) a specific soluble exotoxin which is destroyed by heat. This exotoxin is very powerful; it affects rabbits but not guinea-pigs, producing paralysis; it gives rise to a specific antitoxin. The organism also produces an endotoxin which is insoluble and which is present in bacterial bodies and is fatal to rabbits and guinea-pigs.

The other shigellae are not nearly as virulent as this, though the Schmitz bacillus is more virulent than *Sh. flexneri, Sh. boydii* and *Sh. sonnei*. The disease provoked by *Sh. sonnei* is the least severe.

Dysentery bacilli, other than *Sh. sonnei*, are delicate organisms which do not thrive and multiply in the intestinal contents, and can only be recovered from stools which contain mucus from the dysenteric lesions in the bowel. *Sh. sonnei*, however, can survive for many days on lavatory seats, at low temperatures and high humidities, and in subdued lighting, features which encourage transmission in institutes for children and mentally subnormal persons.

Epidemiology

Dysentery bacilli are excreted in the faeces of patients in the acute stage of the disease, and in those of patients whose intestinal lesions have not completely healed. Infection takes place through the mouth, and many of the ingested bacilli are probably destroyed by the gastric juice; large numbers may be required for experimental infection (Rowland 1967), and Christie (1968) conjectured that the decreased incidence of *Sh. flexneri* in Britain is due to the fact that the large doses needed for infection do not occur where sanitation is efficient, whereas the common *Sh. sonnei* may be able to infect with a small dose, persisting where personal hygiene is poor.

In hot countries bacillary dysentery tends to break out during the early summer, but as the heat increases the sun may sterilize exposed human faeces and kill fly maggots, and the disease may decline. In temperate countries Sonne dysentery tends to be most prevalent in winter.

There is abundant circumstantial evidence that houseflies (*Musca domestica*), where they are numerous, are important carriers of shigellae from the faeces of infected persons (especially in the acute stages of the disease) to other people, perhaps largely by contaminating food. Shigellae have been isolated from the intestines of flies and from flies crushed in fluid media. The infection, however, seems to be conveyed mainly on the feet of flies, though also probably via their vomit and faeces.

Apart from flies, shigellae are probably transferred from infective material to other people, or to food (blancmange, pies, watercress, cheese, etc.) by direct contact of unwashed fingers soiled with faeces. This is important, especially in children playing together, but also in the tropics where the mothers generally feed their young children by hand after weaning. Acute diarrhoeal disease is a very common cause of illness in infants in the tropics.

Water can be the vehicle of infection, and many outbreaks of this kind have been reported, for instance in Java. Some have been explosive outbreaks associated with hepatitis, which has occurred in waves following the dysentery after a delay of days or more usually weeks, and thus reflecting the different incubation periods of the two diseases. Sometimes the sanitary control of the water-supply breaks down, for instance when wells are contaminated from nearby cesspools, or when chlorination fails.

Carriers of shigellae are either convalescent patients who remain infective for short periods, usually a week or two, or chronic carriers (a minority) who may be infective for several months, excreting shigellae intermittently. Carriers of the Shiga bacillus tend to persist much longer than carriers of the Flexner group, and the Shiga carriers tend to be ill, with chronic dysentery and relapses, whereas the Flexner carriers are more normal. The carrier state may exist in persons who do not give a history of actual dysentery.

These long-term carriers are important in the epidemiology of the disease, especially if they are cooks or food-handlers. The faeces of kitchen staffs should be examined more than once, especially during outbreaks. The presence of the characteristic microscopic features of bacillary dysentery and mucus in the stools is diagnostic, and the pathogens can usually be recovered from such mucus *if the specimen is fresh.*

Pathology

Shigellae invade the mucosa of the large bowel, and the resulting pathological process affects chiefly the lower part of the colon, but may spread to the last few feet of the small intestine.

In Shiga and Flexner infections the primary lesions are in the solitary follicles of the large intestine, which may go on to 'snail track' ulceration of the mucous membrane, which is acutely inflamed. In mild cases (Sonne) there is general catarrhal inflammation without ulceration and usually without haemorrhage beyond a few flecks of blood in the stools. Mucus is exuded, with some plasma and polymorphonuclear cells.

In Shiga and some Flexner infections, however, the process is much more severe. The mucosa and submucosa are widely and intensely inflamed, and there is early excoriation of the tops of the mucosal ridges. Blood vessels are congested and thrombosed, and there are large areas of haemorrhage with blood-stained mucus or mucopus. The bowel wall is oedematous and inelastic, and there may be a large greyish membrane consisting of necrosed mucosa infiltrated with fibrin. The mucosa bleeds on sigmoidoscopy, which is painful and should not be performed early in these severe cases.

Coagulation necrosis occurs, with a greyish or green membrane, and large patches of the mucosa may slough, leaving raw ulcerated areas exuding pus. Bleeding takes place, giving the 'red currant jelly' appearance of the stools, or it may be even more copious. Other lesions include small discrete nodular lesions with yellow crusts, punched-out pock-like ulcers and small clean-cut ulcers with well defined edges like those found in amoebic dysentery.

The mesenteric glands may be enlarged, and shigellae have been isolated from them in severe infections.

In prolonged cases the bowel wall may become paper-thin, but perforation is unusual. A late result may be patchy chronic ulceration of the large bowel. Such ulcers must be differentiated from the ulcers of tuberculosis, schistosomiasis and ulcerative colitis.

Immunology

In World War II, in North Africa, dysentery always broke out in troops newly arrived from Britain, but thereafter the incidence was never more than sporadic. It seems, therefore, that some degree of immunity was acquired, in spite of the fact that so many types of dysentery bacilli were identified there (Boyd 1957). Infection with any one of these apparently gave some protection against the others, but it could not have been produced by the O antigen (somatic). The immunity was not solid. Attempts at immunization have been made but have hitherto been unsuccessful, and vaccination with the preparations tried plays no useful part in prevention.

Sh. shigae (*Sh. dysenteriae* 1), unlike other dysentery bacilli, produces a soluble exotoxin, which provokes a neutralizing antitoxin when inoculated into horses. This antitoxic serum has been used in treatment of Shiga dysentery, and has a value, but its action is transient, since it has no antibacterial action. It should be used only in fulminating or severely toxic cases immediately on admission to hospital, or if chemotherapy has failed. The dose is not less than 200 000 I.U. intravenously, repeated in 12 hours if necessary (Fairley & Boyd 1943). The usual precautions to avoid serum reaction should be taken. Antitoxic sera prepared against Flexner or Sonne bacilli have no therapeutic action.

Clinical findings

The effects of bacillary dysentery may range from mild diarrhoea to fulminating, toxic and fatal illness, with collapse and dehydration. In peace time the milder forms predominate, but in war time, or when widespread disasters or famine occur, epidemics of severe dysentery are to be expected.

The incubation period is short, under 7 days, mostly about 2.

Mild cases are commonly associated with infection by *Sh. sonnei* or *Sh. flexneri*. The main sign is diarrhoea, the stools being at first watery and later more mucoid. There is some straining and griping, but there is little or no rise of temperature, and the illness is over in a few days.

In more severe cases the onset is more abrupt, and the stools soon come to consist of little save blood-stained mucus. Griping and tenesmus may be severe, with distressing dysuria. Fever is high and there may be a rigor. The face is pinched and the expression anxious; the patient may even become delirious and mentally confused. There is marked thirst.

Fulminating and gangrenous attacks are almost invariably due to *Sh. shigae* (*Sh. dysenteriae* 1). The onset is abrupt, with chills or smart rigor, vomiting and rapid rise of temperature. The stools soon become excessively frequent, 20–60 in the day, and are mucoid or mucopurulent, with blood and occasionally sloughs of mucous membrane. Toxaemia is a feature as a result of absorption of the Shiga exotoxin. The cheeks are flushed, the expression anxious, the pulse rapid and the tongue coated and yellow or dry and brown. Abdominal distension and hiccough occur. Muscular cramps and oliguria may develop as a result of dehydration due to loss of fluid, with dry shrivelled skin, collapsed veins, low blood pressure and peripheral failure of circulation. The urine contains albumin and granular casts and there may be retention of nitrogen. The patient is restless and may die in uraemic coma.

If the intestinal mucosa is extensively ulcerated there may be such loss of protein that hypoproteinaemia develops; this is always serious and may be fatal (Fairley 1961).

Perforation with peritonitis may occur, though it is rare. It demands immediate laparotomy. On the other hand chronic peritonitis may occasionally develop, with effusion of serum into the peritoneal cavity, and distension of the abdomen, tenderness and perhaps dullness in the flanks, flatulence, vomiting and colicky abdominal pain. This is accompanied by polymorphonuclear leucocytosis. The treatment is not surgical.

A choleraic form has been described, in which the onset is acute, with collapse and profuse watery stools later containing blood. This form is usually fatal.

Bacillary dysentery may relapse, and in many severe cases the condition, though it improves, becomes chronic, the faeces do not become normal for a long time, continuing to show blood and mucus. Any indiscretion can lead to an attack of diarrhoea.

Granular rectitis, with excoriation of the lowest part of the rectum, and the passing of blood and mucus, has been described as a sequel of Shiga dysentery.

Complications

Perforation may occur, but as the inflammation is generally confined to the mucosa, it is rare. If it is a terminal process the prognosis is bad. Chronic peritonitis is described above.

Haemorrhoids are common as a result of straining, and rectal prolapse has been recorded—it is a common and persistent feature in malnourished African children who also have dysentery or diarrhoea, for instance when they are caught up in civil war.

Toxic arthritis is fairly common during convalescence after severe dysentery. It affects the larger joints, especially the knee and ankle, and there is some fever. The articular fluid is usually sterile, and may agglutinate dysentery bacilli.

Conjunctivitis may occur, but is usually mild; iritis occurs, but is rare.

Pneumonia is quite common in fatal cases; tachycardia, peripheral neuritis and parotitis may also be found. The effort syndrome may persist.

In children intussusception of the small intestine has been reported, and may be fatal in acute cases. Sequelae include stenosis of the large intestine, abdominal adhesions and megacolon, but they are not common.

The relationship of bacillary dysentery and Reiter's disease is debated. It is a non-specific urethritis, with conjunctivitis or iritis, lesions of the mouth and penis, and keratodermia blenorrhagica of the hands and feet.

Diagnosis

Mild attacks are difficult to diagnose from other forms of diarrhoea, and laboratory tests may be needed.

The cellular exudate in the stools is a help. In typical cases an early specimen shows a preponderance of swollen polymorphonuclear leucocytes, which constitute over 90% of the total cells. There are numerous discrete red cells intermingled with the leucocytes. Macrophage leucocytes are also seen, and often lead to confusion because, being large phagocytes and often containing red cells, they are misdiagnosed as trophozoites of *Entamoeba histolytica*. They are hyaline, containing vacuoles, fatty granules, red cells and even occasionally leucocytes, and they are non-motile. The late Sir Philip Manson-Bahr drew attention to this common cause of misdiagnosis 50 years ago, and described the characteristics of the bacillary dysentery stools which differentiated them from the amoebic dysentery stools, but these mistakes are still common, leading to incorrect and unnecessary drug treatment. The red currant jelly appearance of the stools and the cell content in bacillary dysentery are characteristic.

Dysentery bacilli are delicate organisms which die quickly in stools. Specimens should therefore be taken at once to the laboratory for bacteriological examination. If this cannot be done they can be collected in buffered 30% glycerol saline solution for transport. Rectal swabs should also be cultured while fresh. Cultures can be made on Leifson's deoxycholate citrate agar or on the S-S medium. The Sonne bacillus grows more easily than the others. Colonies are differentiated by serological methods.

For diagnosis of the disease the serological tests have not been very useful, though agglutinins may appear in the serum 6–12 days or more after onset, but in some cases they fail to appear. Haemagglutinating (HA) antibodies appear in over 60% of *Sh. dysenteriae* 1 (Shiga) infections within 10 days of infection, and persist for several months.

Sigmoidoscopy is useful in the chronic stages, but is not justified in the acute stage, when the bowel is highly inflamed and the operation is extremely painful, and can be dangerous. When it is used, the patient should be prepared by clearing the bowel with a warm water enema. In severe cases necrosed mucous membrane shows as a greyish membrane, or a greyish or green membrane due to coagulation necrosis, with areas of haemorrhage and intense inflammation. Blood-stained mucus or mucopus is also present. In subacute cases the mucosa bleeds on sigmoidoscopy, and there are irregular superficial ulcers, with mucopus.

Table 28. Diagnosis between bacillary and amoebic dysentery

Bacillary dysentery	*Amoebic dysentery*
Acute disease with tendency to epidemic spread. 'Lying-down dysentery'	A chronic endemic disease. 'Walking dysentery'
Incubation period short; 7 days or less	Incubation period long; 20–90 days or more
Onset acute	Onset insidious
Pyrexia common	Pyrexia rare unless complicated
Complications: toxic arthritis, eye complications	Complications: hepatic and other abscesses, amoebiasis of skin, perforation
Tenderness over whole abdomen, more marked over sigmoid	Tenderness local, mostly over sigmoid, thickening of sigmoid, transverse colon and caecum
Ulcers on free edge of transverse folds of mucous membrane, distributed transversely to long axis of gut	Ulcers begin as small abscesses of submucosa in long axis of gut; flask-shaped
Ulcers serpiginous with ragged undermined edges communicating with other ulcers; bases of granulation tissue. Rarely perforate	Ulcers oval, regular, involving all coats; bases of black necrotic tenacious sloughs (dyak-hair sloughs). Not uncommonly perforate
Mucous membrane hyperaemic and inflamed. Bowel wall not thickened	Mucous membrane not inflamed. Bowel wall thickened
Stools scanty in quantity but very frequent; bright blood red, gelatinous viscid mucus, odourless, 'red currant jelly'	Stools, faeces mingled with blood and mucus, offensive, smelling of decomposing blood. Generally copious
Tenesmus very severe	Tenesmus not usual
Stools, microscopic picture: numerous discrete red cells; polymorphs abundant, some macrophages. Few bacteria visible	Stools, microscopic picture: red cells numerous and in clumps; polymorphs and macrophages scanty. Large numbers of motile bacilli. *E. histolytica* trophozoites containing ingested red cells present
Leucocytosis present in early stages	Leucocytosis 10 000–25 000, with 70% polymorphs

The mucosa is inflamed (perhaps patchily), pitted and ulcerated, oozing pus, or there may be small discrete nodular lesions with yellow crusts, pock-like ulcers or small clean-cut defined ulcers. In chronic cases the ulcers resemble those of ulcerative colitis, scattered over apparently normal mucosa.

Treatment

General. Except in the mildest cases the patient should be confined to bed. For the first day or so no food should be given, but water or dilute normal saline must be freely available because thirst develops rapidly as fluid is lost. Potassium chloride 2 grammes every 4 hours may be given by month. Later the diet should be light, and food should be taken in small amounts at short intervals until the patient's hunger demands satisfaction.

The patient may need a sedative—chloral hydrate to a maximum of 1·0 gramme for adults, scaled down for children. For severe abdominal pain tinct. opii (0·6 ml) gives great comfort (Rowland 1967), but should perhaps be used sparingly in case it delays passage along the bowel. A hypodermic of morphine may be needed.

Tenesmus and dysuria may be relieved by an enema of a wineglassful of thin starch containing 40–50 drops of tinct. opii, or by suppositories of morphine and cocaine.

Pain and incessant desire to defaecate can sometimes be alleviated by washing out the colon with a pint of warm water. Bismuth carbonate 8 grammes, tincture of opium 2 ml and thin starch 56 ml make a good sedative enema.

If signs of dehydration appear, which are not corrected by oral fluid, intravenous infusion may be necessary (Christie 1968). For babies a fluid containing 4·3% glucose in 1/5 normal saline is satisfactory and intravenous administration may not be necessary after 24 hours, but in the tropics a careful watch must be kept for signs of dehydration as long as diarrhoea is profuse. Elderly patients with tetany usually respond to the intravenous infusion of a litre of isotonic saline. Calcium gluconate may also be added to this, the dose being 10–20 ml of a 10% solution.

For severe forms, prolonged intravenous administration of fluid may be needed, as in cholera (page 514), controlled if possible by estimations of electrolytes, but care must be taken not to overload the circulation—too much fluid is dangerous. An infusion of 1–2 litres in the first hour, maintained at a lower rate thereafter until the patient's condition is satisfactory, may be suitable.

Many patients with mild Sonne dysentery are quite effectively treated with chalk and opium mixture or other non-specific remedy alone, and sulphonamides are not needed in such cases.

Sulphonamides. Treatment of more serious attacks was revolutionized when the sulphonamides were introduced. The first great successes were achieved with the 'insoluble' sulphaguanidine and succinylsulphathiazole, which may be given in doses of 10–20 grammes daily (divided) for 5 days, or 9–12 grammes daily for 3 days followed by 6–10 grammes daily for 4 days. Phthalylsulphathiazole in doses of 5–10 grammes daily for 5 days is also successful. These compounds were thought to act directly in the bowel without being absorbed, and therefore without the risk of crystallization in the kidneys such as was possible with large doses of the more soluble sulphonamides, but in fact both succinylsulphathiazole and phthalylsulphathiazole release sulphathiazole in the bowel, and this is soluble; as much as 40% of sulphaguanidine may be absorbed. The dissolved drugs presumably attack dysentery bacilli in the tissues of the bowel wall, which could hardly happen with insoluble compounds.

In recent years sulphadimidine in doses of 1 gramme every 6 hours for 5 days, or 2 grammes followed by 1 gramme every 4 hours, has been favoured. It is safe and is highly soluble in urine, so that it does not form crystals in the urinary passages. Trimethoprim–sulphamethoxazole has also been used in tablets containing 80 mg and 400 mg respectively.

If these compounds are not available, sulphadiazine or sulphathiazole can be used in their own appropriate doses, but a watch must be maintained to detect crystalluria, and plenty of fluid must be given to dilute the urine.

Sulphonamides can also be given as retention enemas (7–10 grammes in water and mucilage) of 250 ml.

Antibiotics. The sulphonamides are generally successful, non-toxic and cheap. Sometimes, however, the organisms are resistant to them, and other drugs must be used. In Britain most strains of *Sh. sonnei* are resistant to sulphonamides (Christie 1968) and antibiotics (Carpenter 1970). Where the bacilli are sensitive to antibiotics, oral streptomycin in doses of up to 2 grammes every 6 hours (babies 0·5 gramme every 6 hours) can be given until the patient improves, or for 5 days. Neomycin (1 gramme every 6 hours for adults) or nalidixic acid (in the same doses) for 5 days are useful, but nalidixic acid should not be given to women in the first 3 months of pregnancy, and care should be exercised in patients with damage to the central nervous system or hepatic function. It may also give false positive urine tests for sugar.

Tetracycline (250–500 mg every 6 hours) can be used if the organism is sensitive to it, though resistance is quite common. But resistance *in vivo* may not correspond with resistance *in vitro*, and patterns of resistance and sensitivity in cultures can be confusing (Christie 1968).

Chloramphenicol should never be given (Christie 1968).

Though these treatments are usually effective, however, Levine *et al.* (1970) refer to a very serious epidemic in Central America of dysentery due to *Sh. dysenteriae* I (the classical Shiga organism) which proved to be highly virulent, and resistant to the sulphonamides, tetracycline, chloramphenicol, streptomycin and low doses of penicillin, but sensitive to ampicillin, kanamycin, gentamicin, cephalothin and high doses of penicillin G. It is thought to have caused 120 000 cases and 13 000 deaths in Nicaragua alone during one year, 1968–9. Attack rates are highest in children under 2, and in infants death rates have reached 20%. An important point is that at first the disease was thought to be due to *Entamoeba histolytica* because this amoeba was found in the bloody mucus of many patients, and no bacterial pathogen was consistently isolated until later. But emetine was useless, and the true nature of the infection became apparent when the Shiga organism was isolated. This reinforces what has been said before, namely that the finding of *E. histolytica* does not necessarily mean that it is the cause of the disease. Nevertheless, in Nicaragua there is evidence that where *E. histolytica* trophozoites and abscesses are found the disease is sometimes much more serious, often with severe haemorrhage, and does not respond to treatment until anti-amoebic drugs such as emetine or metronidazole are used (Vijil 1971). The sudden emergence of this virulent variant of *Sh. dysenteriae* I is evidently most serious.

In bacillary dysentery, bacteriological tests of cure include 3 negative rectal swabs or specimens of faeces, examined a few days after the end of treatment, and examined fresh. For food-handlers, nurses and others who may spread the infection, 6 or even 12 negative bacteriological examinations are desirable before return to work after an attack (Christie 1968).

For the use of antitoxic serum in fulminating Shiga dysentery, see Immunology, page 522.

Granular rectitis is best treated with suppositories of succinylsulphathiazole (3 grammes in 7 grammes cocoa butter). They are longer than ordinary suppositories.

Prevention

Personal prevention consists in avoiding food (cooked or uncooked) which may have been contaminated by flies or the hands of infected persons, and in strict attention to kitchen hygiene and personal hygiene such as washing the hands in clean water after defaecation. In homes and public lavatories fresh clean water should be available alongside the lavatory pan, and in kitchens washing facilities should be close at hand. Cooks and food-handlers should be fully instructed, and subject to discipline. They must be suspended from work if suffering from diarrhoea, and examined before returning to work.

Public prevention is the responsibility of the public health, hospital, military or other authorities, who should supply wholesome water, supervise food and markets, provide for disposal of human and animal wastes and suppress flies.

ACUTE GASTRO-ENTERITIS OF YOUNG CHILDREN

This common disease of young indigenous children in the tropics is one of the two most common causes of death; the other is respiratory infection. Gastro-enteritis of this kind may occasionally be caused by salmonellae, but in 80% of cases no definite organism has hitherto been identified, and the cause is still unknown. In this respect the disease resembles traveller's diarrhoea; in each the cause is probably some infection, but the aetiology is obscure.

Gastro-enteritis of young children appears to be related to weaning, poor sanitation and uncleanliness, and is often associated with malnutrition and perhaps with unsuitable food after weaning.

It can be a sudden medical emergency. Young children easily become dehydrated, and require immediate replacement of fluid lost in the diarrhoea and vomiting. This may entail intravenous infusion of suitable fluid, and this is more important than treatment with antibiotics during the critical stage.

TRAVELLER'S DIARRHOEA (TURISTA)

It is painfully well known that visitors to the tropics and subtropics usually suffer attacks of diarrhoea within a week or two after arrival (Kean & Waters 1958). The attacks later become much less frequent, as if some degree of immunity is acquired. No country with a warm climate is exempt, and many local names have been given to the condition; in Mexico it is known as *turista*, and this name has recently become popular.

Aetiology

The cause is not known, in spite of the many attempts that have been made to isolate pathogenic organisms from the stools (for instance by Varela *et al.* 1959). Nevertheless, it is widely believed that some infective agent is responsible, and the reported value of prophylactic sulphonamides and antibiotics tends to confirm this opinion. Some cases are probably due to mild infections with dysentery bacilli. Other theories blame changes of climate or unusual types of food but, though contamination of food may well be a factor, it is unlikely that the food *per se* is responsible, and no proof that climate causes the disease has been produced. An unaccustomed intestinal flora is the most likely explanation, including infection with pathogenic strains of *Escherichia coli*.

The diarrhoea is probably the result of a general inflammation of the lower bowel, and the stools, which are watery and mucoid but may contain some blood, show some of the characters of bacillary dysentery, including large numbers of polymorphonuclear leucocytes. Difficulty in diagnosis occurs when trophozoites of *Entamoeba histolytica* are found in the stools; they may be harmless commensals prevented from encysting by rapid transit through the bowel, in which case they are not the cause of the disease.

Clinical findings

The attack usually begins abruptly, with mild abdominal colic and diarrhoea, but in more severe cases there may be fever, chills, vomiting and pains in joints and muscles. The profuse diarrhoea and consequent loss of fluid leads to thirst and dehydration, and this must be prevented by liberal fluid by mouth, Diarrhoeal diseases in general can lead to water depletion heat exhaustion, or heat stroke, and this possibility should always be borne in mind when babies, who cannot express their needs for fluid, are concerned. This water depletion is particularly important in hot climates, where so much fluid is lost by sweating as well as by the bowel.

The attack is usually over in a day or two, but may last a week. The patient is little the worse for it, regaining intestinal stability and appetite very quickly.

Treatment

For mild cases and those in which no pathogenic organisms can be found in the stools, the following treatment may be enough. An initial purge of magnesium sulphate, followed by tinct. chlorof. et morph. (Chlorodyne) in doses of 0·3–0·6 ml every 4 hours for as long as required (Hill 1961), or kaolin and morphine mixture (B.P.C.) in doses of 15 ml. Mist. cret. c. opio. (B.N.F.) in doses of 15 ml or aromatic chalk powder with opium (B.P.C.) in doses of 0·6–4·0 grammes can also be used. There is no doubt that the morphine of these preparations is very soothing. There is also some risk of addiction if these remedies are used too often.

For more severe cases the sulphonamides are effective. Sulphatriad, for instance, in doses of 500–1000 mg every few hours, or succinylsulphathiazole 10 grammes daily in divided doses. Ampicillin with sulphadimidine and kaolin (Penbritin KS) in doses of 20 ml 3 times each day, is also successful (Roantree 1969). Streptotriad can also be used, 1–2 tablets every few hours.

Thirst, indicating the loss of fluid by diarrhoea, should be relieved by weak tea or other sterile drinks.

Diarrhoea can be caused by salmonellae and such organisms as *Giardia intestinalis*, the schistosomes and other helminths. Diagnosis of such conditions is therefore important, the patients needing specific treatment.

Prevention

The stools of patients must be disposed of with every care, and attendants must be watchful not to become infected. Hand-washing in clean water, or water containing a disinfectant, is important.

As in bacillary dysentery, personal prevention is paramount, resting on personal and kitchen hygiene, and on care in the choice of food and drink, avoiding or thoroughly cooking those which may be contaminated. All meat must be cooked, milk and water boiled, fruits without thick skins should not be eaten raw unless their growth is impeccable—they may have been grown in soil fertilized with animal or human faeces.

In general, drug prophylaxis is not recommended, but in special circumstances, such as short visits of athletic teams to international games, when physical fitness is essential, the participants may be given prophylactic Streptotriad, 2 tablets daily (each containing sulphadiazine 100 mg, sulphathiazole 100 mg, sulphadimidine 100 mg and streptomycin (as sulphate) 65 mg). They may also be given bottles of hexachlorophane for routine hand-washing after defaecation and before meals (Owen 1968). They should not eat any food not sponsored by their managers.

Bloss (1964), however, thinks that preparations of 3 sulphonamides with streptomycin should not be used for prophylaxis, partly because bacteria soon become resistant to streptomycin, and partly because some sulphonamides are slowly excreted and may produce toxic symptoms. He prefers phthalylsulphathiazole, whose toxicity is low, and whose effect is significant (Kean et al. 1962).

Other drugs have been suggested for prophylaxis, particularly neomycin sulphate (0·375 gramme night and morning), which has some apparent effect (Kean & Waters 1959), and furazolidone (200 mg daily), which also has a definite effect but also has undesirable side-effects in some people after the consumption of even small amounts of alcohol.

REFERENCES

BLOSS, J. F. E. (1964) Trans. R. Soc. trop. Med. Hyg., **58**, 278.

BOYD, J. S. K. (1957) Trans. R. Soc. trop. Med. Hyg., **51**, 471.

CARPENTER, K. P. (1970) Br. med. J., **ii**, 225.

CHRISTIE, A. B. (1968) Br. med. J., **ii**, 285.

FAIRLEY, N. H. (1961) in Recent Advances in Tropical Medicine (ed. Fairley, N. H., Woodruff, A. W. & Walters, J. H.), 3rd ed. London: Churchill.

—— & BOYD, J. S. K. (1943) Trans. R. Soc. trop. Med. Hyg., **36**, 254.

KEAN, B. H., SCHAFFNER, W., BRENNAN, R. W. & WATERS, S. R. (1962) J. Am. med. Ass., **180**, 367.

—— & WATERS, S. R. (1958) Archs indust. Hlth, **18**, 148.

—— —— (1959) New Engl. med. J., **261**, 71.

LEVINE, M. M., DUPONT, H. L., FORMAL, S. B. & GANGAROSA, E. J. (1970) Lancet, **ii**, 607.

OWEN, J. R. (1968) Br. med. J., **iv**, 645.

ROANTREE, W. B. (1969) Lancet, **ii**, 799.

ROWLAND, H. A. K. (1967) Med. Today, **1**, 29.

VARELA, G., KEAN, B. H., BARRETT, E. L. & KEEGAN, C. J. (1959) Am. J. trop. Med. Hyg., **8**, 353.

VIJIL, C. (1971) Lancet, **ii,** 823.

24. SALMONELLOSES

Salmonella infection in man is caused by the 'enteric fever' group—*Salmonella typhi*, *S. paratyphi* A, *S. paratyphi* B, *S. paratyphi* C—and the *Salmonella* group which causes bacterial enteritis or food poisoning.

Enteric Fevers

Synonyms

Typhoid fever; Paratyphoid fever.

AETIOLOGY

The enteric group of fevers are caused by four organisms:

Salmonella typhi (*S. typhosa*)
Salmonella paratyphi A
Salmonella paratyphi B (*S. schottmülleri*)
Salmonella paratyphi C (*S. hirschfeldii*)

S. typhi is the cause of typhoid fever, *S. paratyphi* A and B are the cause of paratyphoid fever, which is essentially similar to typhoid fever but is clinically milder and of shorter duration. *S. paratyphi* C has a somewhat different symptomatology.

Morphology

The *salmonellae* are Gram-negative non-sporing bacilli about 2–4 × 0·5 µm, actively motile, with numerous long peritrichous flagellae. They do not possess a capsule and most strains are fimbriate.

Cultural characteristics

They grow well on ordinary media and form 'pale' or colourless colonies on MacConkey's medium, since they do not ferment lactose. Typhoid and para-typhoid organisms may be identified by biochemical reactions, antigenic characters and phage typing.

Biochemical reactions. The biochemical reactions used are the fermentation of glucose, mannitol, xylol, D-tartrate, and mucate (Table 29).

Table 29. Cultural characteristics of *Salmonella* species

Species	Glucose	Mannitol	Xylose	D-Tartrate	Mucate
S. typhi	A	A	V	A	V
S. paratyphi A	+	+	—	—	—
S. paratyphi B	+	+	+	—	+
S. paratyphi C	+	+	+	+	—

A, Acid, no gas. +, Acid and gas.
V, Variable reaction. —, No reaction.

Antigenic characters. The enteric bacilli have flagellar (H) and somatic (O) antigens. The H antigens differ from one another, but the O antigens are group specific and are more conveniently considered in relation to other salmonellae (page 543).

Vi antigen. Freshly isolated strains of *S. typhi* possess a somatic antigen designated 'Vi'. The Vi antigen renders the organism relatively inagglutinable by an O antiserum, so that serological identification with an O antiserum must be made on a fresh saline suspension of *S. typhi*, from which the Vi antigen has been removed by boiling for an hour and washing by centrifugation. The Vi antigen is used in the detection of carriers.

Phage typing. Vi strains of *S. typhi* may be differentiated into types by means of an anti-Vi phage which on serial cultivation with one of these types acquires an increased activity to strains of this type. There are 72 phage types of *S. typhi*, so that freshly isolated strains possessing Vi antigen can be classified, and epidemiological studies of typhoid have been greatly helped in correlating cases, the source of an outbreak and the mode of spread (Anderson & Williams 1956). Phage typing of *S. paratyphi* A and B is also used and 8 types of A and 43 types of B have been recognized.

Animal pathogenicity

S. typhi and *S. paratyphi* show a strong host specificity for man and do not infect animals under natural conditions. When they are given to laboratory animals no infection results unless massive doses are used, when the illness is quite unlike that of typhoid fever. This is in contradistinction to the other salmonellae, which infect animals naturally and where epizootic spread will follow the introduction of *S. typhi-murium* into a mouse colony.

TRANSMISSION

Transmission is from one infected person to another either directly or indirectly through the water supply, by flies or by contamination of food by food-handlers.

Typhoid Fever

EPIDEMIOLOGY

Prevalence

Typhoid fever is world-wide in distribution and is particularly prevalent throughout the tropics where it is one of the commonest causes of 'fever'.

In Africa mainly typhoid is present. Paratyphoid A occurs in Eastern Europe, the U.S.A., the Far East and India. Paratyphoid B occurs in Europe and is responsible for 20% of the cases in North America. Paratyphoid C is widespread in Guyana and is also found in Eastern Europe.

Source of infection

Since there is no animal host, the sources of infection are patients suffering from the disease, including mild and ambulatory cases and carriers.

Patients. The typhoid patient excretes bacilli in the faeces and urine for about a month. Infected vomit and pus from abscesses are also sources of infection.

Carriers. There are three types of carrier, convalescent, chronic faecal and chronic urinary:

1. The convalescent carrier passes bacilli in the excreta for up to 6 months after an attack of typhoid.

2. The chronic carrier continues to pass bacilli intermittently in the excreta at least one year after infection (faecal carriers). Chronic faecal carriers are more often women than men, the gall-bladder and bile ducts being the seat of chronic infection; gall-stones and chronic cholecystitis may occur. The renal pelvis may also be infected (urinary carriers) and bacilli are passed in the urine. In *S. haematobium* areas there is a connection between that infection and urinary carriers of *S. typhi.*

Spread of infection

The carrier is a danger to the community unless there is an efficient water carriage system of sewage disposal. Bacilli present on the hands of the carrier can be transferred by many vehicles—ice-cream, milk (in which the bacilli multiply)—and in the preparation and distribution of food. Water sources, shellfish harvested from sewage-contaminated sea water, vegetables, salads, watercress contaminated with human excreta and canned meat cooled with contaminated water which penetrates improperly sealed cans, the meat in which acts as a culture medium, have all caused epidemics.

S. typhi is spread mainly by water and *S. paratyphi* A and B by foodstuffs. All the enteric group are spread by ice-cream.

IMMUNOLOGY

An attack of typhoid confers some immunity, although second attacks can occur. Marmion *et al.* (1953) described an outbreak in which 11 men who had suffered typhoid 5 months before had second attacks. There was, however, a significant diminution in the attack rate in previously infected persons.

Antibodies appear in the blood as early as the fifth day, usually about the seventh to tenth day, but may be delayed until after recovery, especially in children.

Both H (IgG) and O (IgM) agglutinating antibodies develop, but in some cases only one may be detected, especially in the early stages of the illness. The titre rises from the time of first appearance of the agglutinins and reaches its maximum about the end of the third week. For determining the type of infection H agglutination is much more reliable than O; however, the presence of O (IgM) agglutinins usually reflects recent infection.

Widal reaction

The H and O agglutinins are measured by the Widal agglutination test.

Interpretation of the Widal test

1. The usual limits of agglutination with normal sera are *S. typhi* and *S. paratyphi* B, H 1/30, O 1/50 and *S. paratyphi* A, O and H 1/10.

2. Non-specific antigens, such as fimbrial antigens, may be present in the test suspensions employed, which must be known to be free from such antigens.

3. Persons inoculated with TAB also show specific agglutinins in their sera. In previously vaccinated cases a rising titre may be regarded as significant of active infection. However, non-specific factors, such as non-enteric febrile conditions, may cause an anamnestic rise in titre.

4. In persons previously vaccinated the agglutinins are mainly of the H type, and if over 6 months have elapsed since the date of vaccination an O agglutinin titre higher than 1/100 which rises on repeated testing may be considered significant of an active infection.

5. The presence of Vi agglutinin shown by testing with a Vi-containing strain of *S. typhi* has considerable value in recognizing carriers of *S. typhi* and a titre of 1/10 is regarded as significant. However, TAB vaccinated individuals may possess Vi agglutinins and in highly endemic areas the presence of Vi agglutinins is of little use in the detection of carriers. A haemagglutination test using red cells sensitized with a stable Vi extract is easier and equally reliable, although false positives are found in areas where typhoid is endemic (Anderson 1970).

PATHOLOGY

Infection is by ingestion. The organisms pass from the small intestine via the lymphatics to the mesenteric glands whence, after a period of multiplication, they invade the blood stream via the thoracic duct. The liver, gall-bladder, spleen, kidney and bone marrow become infected during this bacteraemic phase in the first 7 days of the disease. From the gall-bladder a further invasion of the intestine results, and lymphoid tissue—Peyer's patches and lymphoid follicles— are particularly involved in an acute inflammatory reaction and infiltration with mononuclear cells (typhoid cells) followed by necrosis, sloughing and the formation of characteristic typhoid ulcers.

The main pathological changes are found in the gastro-intestinal tract. The Peyer's patches show hyperplasia during the first week, necrosis during the second and ulceration during the third week. Healing takes place without scarring during the fourth week. The ulcers are oval in shape and are situated in the long axis of the lower ileum. There is exudate on the peritoneal surface. Separation of the sloughs may lead to haemorrhage and perforation. Healing takes place usually without scar formation. The incidence of ulcers bears little relationship to the clinical severity of the infection.

The liver shows cloudy swelling and typhoid nodules, which are small lesions consisting of collections of macrophages and lymphocytes with or without central necrosis.

The gall-bladder and bile ducts, which maintain the source of infection, may be unaffected, but the carrier state may be associated with chronic cholecystitis and gall-stones. Chronic cholecystitis is not common in most tropical areas and the gall-bladder carrier is rare in the Chinese in Hong Kong (McFadzean & Ong 1966).

The reticulo-endothelial system shows hyperplasia and the mesenteric glands and spleen are enlarged. The spleen is enlarged with the appearance of an acute septic spleen, but in areas where there is holoendemic malaria the picture is complicated by the presence of pigment in children and the colour is grey. There is marked proliferation of the histiocytes and typhoid nodules may be present.

The mesenteric lymph glands are swollen and hyperaemic, and the sinusoids are filled with histiocytes and monocytes from the blood.

The kidneys show cloudy swelling and perinephric abscesses. Pyelonephritis and pyleitis have been described in kidneys with persistent structural damage (Belzer 1965). Acute nephritis and the nephrotic syndrome may occur (Huckstep 1962). Chronic infections occur in the kidney in *Salmonella* infections.

The lungs show bronchitis and pneumonia occurs in many patients. Lung abscess and empyema are not unusual. A true typhoid granulomatous pneumonia may be found.

The myocardium shows fatty degeneration, but pericarditis is rare. Venous thrombosis used to be common in Europe but is rare in tropical areas. A pyogenic meningitis may occur (Vaizey 1959). Osteomyelitis of the long bones occurs years after infection. The vertebrae may be affected with the development of typhoid spine. Osteomyelitis due to *Salmonella* organisms is a complication in children with sickle cell disease. Typhoid nodules may be present in the marrow. Zenker's degeneration is a focal hyaline degeneration occurring in the rectus abdominis and diaphragm and thigh muscles.

Differences between *S. typhi* and *S. paratyphi* infections

In paratyphoid fever the small intestine may be acutely inflamed throughout its length, although more commonly there is no change. There may be ulceration of the large intestine. Paratyphoid C is in most instances a septicaemia and deep metastatic abscesses are found (Giglioli 1930).

The organism may be recovered by culture post mortem from the intestinal lesions, enlarged lymphatic glands, spleen, gall-bladder, heart blood and other tissues.

CLINICAL FEATURES

Symptoms

The usual incubation period for all the enteric infections is about 14 days but may be shorter than 7 or longer than 21 days. There is a wide range in the severity of the infection from the mildest to the most severe cases.

The typical onset is gradual, but it may be sudden, especially in paratyphoid, with shivering or even a rigor. Headache is the most constant early symptom and is usually accompanied by malaise, anorexia, pains in the body and limbs and insomnia. Epistaxis is commoner in typhoid than paratyphoid. There may be pain or general uneasiness in the abdomen but this is absent in mild cases of paratyphoid. There may be diarrhoea at the commencement or diarrhoea followed in a few days by constipation or there may be constipation from the beginning. Slight nerve deafness is common during the first week (Huckstep 1962).

Signs

The tongue is coated, the mouth dry and uncomfortable and the patient thirsty. There is a characteristic moist facies with flushed cheeks and general apathy. Meningism is not uncommon. Slight jaundice is common in the more toxic patients.

Fever (Figs 147–9). The temperature is invariably raised. It may mount step ladder during the first week or it may rise suddenly to reach its highest point in the first 24–28 hours, and after a period of continued fever begin to remit in the morning and terminate by lysis. A highly characteristic feature of all the enteric infections is the pulse, which is usually soft, often dicrotic and relatively slow. Normally the pulse rate rises 18 beats to every degree C in the temperature. In enteric fever the pulse is as a rule 20–30 or 40 beats/minute slower than thus indicated.

Abdomen. The abdomen may be found more or less distended in typhoid but there may be little or no distension in paratyphoid. The spleen is enlarged in

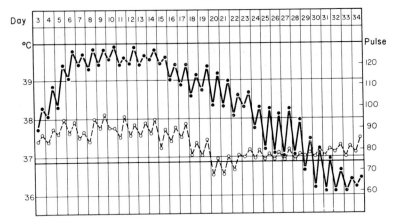

Fig. 147.—Temperature chart of typhoid fever, with a graph of the pulse rate. *Salmonella typhi* was isolated from the blood on the sixth day; on the ninth day rose spots were present and the spleen was palpable.

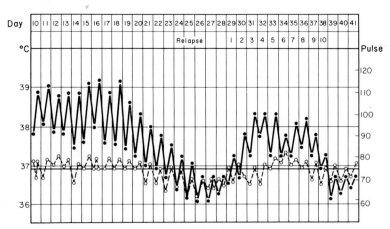

Fig. 148.—Temperature chart of paratyphoid A fever, with a graph of the pulse rate. *Salmonella paratyphi* B was isolated from the blood on the tenth day and *S. paratyphi* A on the thirty-first day.

20–70% of cases (Marmion 1952) at some stage in the illness, sometimes as early as the second or third day, in others not until the second or third week or even later. Rarely it may be palpable for the first time only after the fever has settled. Splenomegaly is of little use in diagnosis in a holendemic malarious area where the spleen tends to be enlarged and firm in a high proportion of the population.

Rose spots appear usually about the seventh to tenth day. They vary considerably in number, shape, size and distribution. There may be only 2 or 3 on the abdomen or the body and limbs may be covered from the soles of the feet to the scalp. In 90% or more the rash is on the trunk between the iliac crests and the nipples. The spots are of a pale rose colour, slightly raised, round or lenticular and fade on pressure. They are darker than the surrounding skin in coloured patients and are hardly ever seen in Negroes. The more profuse eruptions occur in paratyphoid, especially paratyphoid A.

The *stool* is characteristic in about 25% of the cases, being loose and pale, resembling 'pea soup'.

The *chest* almost invariably shows evidence of bronchitis.

The *mental* condition is one of apathy (typhoid facies) and meningism is common.

The *white cell count* shows a leucopenia with a relative lymphocytosis. A leucocytosis rules out the diagnosis of typhoid except when there are complications.

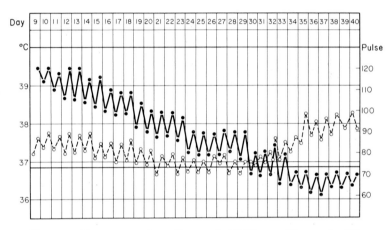

Fig. 149.—Temperature chart of paratyphoid B fever, with a graph of the pulse rate. *Salmonella paratyphi* B was isolated from the blood on the ninth day.

Atypical cases

Mild cases may be met with in tropical countries, especially in children with a simple diarrhoea. A patient with a perforated intestinal ulcer may present as an ambulant case.

Medical complications

Typhoid lobar pneumonia is a rare complication seen in the second to third week of illness. There are signs of lobar consolidation, but the typical symptoms and rusty sputum of pneumonococcal pneumonia are absent. The incidence is 1–2% (Huckstep 1962). A haemorrhagic pleural effusion which grew *S. typhi* has been reported, as has empyema.

Venous thrombosis appears commonly as a minor thrombosis of the calf vein. Major thromboses occur (rarely) in the femoral and subclavian veins.

Haemolytic anaemia is a well recognized complication. In Hong Kong it is often associated with G-6-PD deficiency or haemoglobinopathy (McFadzean & Choa 1953). Severe haemolytic anaemia occurred in 2% of cases (Huckstep 1962) but despite detailed investigation the cause may not be found, although in some cases the Coombs test is positive and the haemolysis may be the result of an auto-immune phenomenon.

Nephrotyphoid resembles the nephrotic form of nephritis, with gross albuminuria, oedema and haematuria. It should be suspected in any case of nephrosis with fever. Treatment with chloramphenicol relieves the condition promptly.

Typhoid meningitis. Meningitis is rare and occurs in 1% of cases (Huckstep 1962). The picture is that of a typical pyogenic meningitis and typhoid may not be suspected until a bacteriological investigation shows *S. typhi* in blood culture. Sometimes but not always *S. typhi* can be recovered from the C.S.F., which is otherwise typical of a pyogenic meningitis.

Peripheral neuropathy of the 'burning feet' type may occur, which responds to large doses of vitamin B complex after 2–3 weeks.

Pharyngitis and *suppurative parotitis* are found in 1–3% of cases.

Surgical complications

The two main surgical complications are intestinal perforation and haemorrhage.

Intestinal perforation. Intestinal perforation occurs in 3–4% of cases and is responsible for 25% of the deaths. The classical signs of perforation are rare. Much commoner is the atypical variety which occurs in the seriously ill toxic patients. The first signs may be the appearance of free fluid in the peritoneal cavity, the disappearance of bowel sounds and vomiting. Diminished liver dullness and the demonstration of gas in the peritoneal cavity by X-ray are valuable signs. A pelvic abscess may form. Perforation may occur in a patient on chloramphenicol therapy, in which case the bowel contents are sterile, producing only a localized area of adherent bowel and pus.

Treatment of perforation is conservative with gastric suction and intravenous fluid and electrolyte replacement in conjunction with antibiotic treatment. In one series the mortality rate after conservative treatment was 27% (Huckstep 1962) in contrast to an 80 and 100% mortality in surgically treated cases. Surgical intervention may be necessary in sudden perforation in an otherwise convalescent patient or where there are adhesions leading to obstruction.

Intestinal haemorrhage. This occurs in 2–8% of cases and is usually seen between the fourteenth and twenty-first days of illness. There may be several small bleeds or a massive silent haemorrhage. This complication is signalled by an increase in pulse rate, a fall in blood pressure and the development of shock. Treatment is by immediate transfusion.

Acute cholecystitis is commoner in women than men and may occur in patients who have never had a clinical attack of typhoid. Severe upper right-sided abdominal pain with jaundice may develop with a positive Murphy's sign. Treatment should be conservative, on the same lines as intestinal perforation. Other intestinal complications occur, such as paralytic ileus, acute intestinal obstruction from adhesions and adherent and twisted loops of bowel.

Genito-urinary complications include typhoid orchitis in convalescence. Pyelitis is common in typhoid and is rarely recognized.

The skeletal system is affected by typhoid arthritis, which may affect the ankle- and hip-joints. Typhoid osteomyelitis of the long bones is rare. Typhoid spine is rarer than is thought and is usually confused with brucellosis and tuberculosis. It may occur many years after an attack of typhoid although rarely after chloramphenicol. Zenker's degeneration of muscle affects especially the muscles of the abdominal wall and the thighs.

DIAGNOSIS

There is something very characteristic in the general appearance, facies and decubitus of the enteric fever patient. He has a dull, heavy, toxin-laden appearance in the early acute stage, which is different from the toxaemia of malaria, relapsing fever or tuberculosis. In the mildest infections there is little or no toxic appearance. The splenic enlargement is acute so that when super-added to a spleen enlarged from malaria there are features of diagnostic signifi-cance; the enlarged spleen of typhoid is tender.

Rose spots may not appear until the temperature is normal and in tropical climates many European skins are apt to show spots more or less like those of enteric fever as the result of mosquito bites or a sweat rash.

Every undiagnosed fever in the tropics should be regarded as a possible case of enteric fever and closely observed and even treated as such while bacterio-logical and serological investigations are being carried out. The 5 cardinal signs are fever, low pulse–temperature ratio, characteristic toxaemia, splenic enlarge-ment and rose spots. The presence of the first 3 should raise strong suspicion, and occasional signs such as epistaxis, pea-soup stools, abdominal distension and haemorrhage from the bowel may provide strong support.

Bacteriological diagnosis

The organisms may be isolated from the blood, stool, urine and bile.

Blood culture. In the early stages of the illness blood culture is the most con-clusive diagnostic method and should be employed in all suspected cases during the first 7–10 days and in relapses. However, a positive blood culture can be obtained at any stage in the illness. The blood should be cultured in bottles containing bile salts (0·5% sodium taurocholate).

Clot culture (Thomas *et al.* 1954). This method is superior in the isolation of *S. typhi* from early cases since the use of normal serum instead of the patient's serum enhances the chances of isolating the organism. Positive cultures may be obtained in less than 24 hours by culturing clots free from the patient's serum in streptokinase broth (15 ml of 0·5% bile salt broth containing 100 units of streptokinase per ml) put up in 100 ml bottles containing slopes of Wilson and Blair's medium.

Faecal culture. S. typhi and the paratyphoid bacilli can be isolated from the faeces throughout the illness but most frequently during the second and third weeks. Cultivation of the organisms from the faeces in all stages of the disease is now successful in about 75% of cases by employing the brilliant green enrichment method, tetrathionate broth or Wilson and Blair's agar medium for concentrating the bacilli. Stools may be sent through the post in meat broth in which the organisms remain viable for many days.

Some positive findings from stool culture are open to fallacy and the case may be one of an enteric carrier suffering from some other illness.

Urine. Bacilluria occurs after the fourteenth day in about 25% of cases. Since it may be intermittent the morning urine should be examined daily for a week when other methods have proved unsuccessful.

Bile. By means of a duodenal tube bile may be aspirated and cultured. This technique is of value in the later stages of the illness and in carrier detection.

Marrow culture. Culture of material obtained by sternal puncture (medulla culture) has been shown to be useful in paratyphoid B infections and in China has proved to be more practical and reliable than blood culture.

Serological diagnosis

This has been dealt with under Immunology (page 533).

Diazo reaction in the urine (Huckstep 1962)

In the absence of laboratory facilities the diazo reaction of the urine is of great value. The test is a red coloration given by the froth of the urine of typhoid patients when mixed with the diazo reagent and is caused by the presence of a substance containing a phenol ring formed by the putrefaction of protein in the intestine.

The diazo reagent is made up from two stock solutions, A and B. Stock solution A: sulphanilic acid 0·5 gramme, conc. HCl 5 ml and distilled water 100 ml. Stock solution B: sodium nitrite 0·5 gramme, distilled water 100 ml. Mix 40 parts of A with 1 part of B. Solution A is stable. Solution B must be made up fresh every 3 weeks and kept at 4°C.

A quantity of diazo reagent is mixed with an equal quantity of an early morning specimen of urine and a few drops of 30% ammonium hydroxide are added. The mixture is shaken and a positive reaction is a red or pinkish coloration of the froth. The diazo reaction is positive in typhoid in 80% of the cases between the fifth and fourteenth day of illness, not usually as early as the second or later than the twenty-first day of clinical illness. False positive reactions in non-typhoid patients are about 5% and positive reactions may also be found in pulmonary tuberculosis, measles and typhus.

Diagnosis of carriers

The diagnosis of a carrier depends on the isolation of *S. typhi* or *S. paratyphi* from the faeces or urine and in view of the intermittent nature of excretion at least 6 consecutive examinations should be made before the result is declared negative. Examination of the aspirated bile is invaluable, or the stool may be examined after 200 mg of calomel followed by a saline purgative.

The presence of Vi agglutinins in a dilution of over 1/10 is valuable as a screening measure.

TREATMENT

Chloramphenicol

Chloramphenicol, introduced by Woodward *et al.* (1948), is bacteriostatic and not bactericidal so that early exhibition of the drug does not lead to eradication of the infection since the immune response of the patient does not develop to a sufficient extent. Hence the use of chloramphenicol has led to an increase in the relapse rate and an increased carrier rate unless the drug is given in adequate doses and for a sufficient length of time.

Dosage. A loading dose should be omitted in view of the danger of toxic crises. In a severe case chloramphenicol should be given, 1·0 gramme 6-hourly for 3 days and then 500 mg 6-hourly for 12 days. There is a lag period of 36–48 hours before the effects of chloramphenicol become apparent. With this dosage Huckstep (1962) found that the duration of pyrexia was 4·6 days. Marmion (1952) found that the duration of pyrexia varied with the severity of illness from 2·8 days in the milder to 4·3 days in the severe cases, the maximum duration of fever is just over 7 days. Another dosage schedule in milder cases is 500 mg 6-hourly until defervescence of the fever, followed by 500 mg 8-hourly for 4 days and 500 mg 12-hourly for 10 days. If chloramphenicol is given for less than 10 days there is a marked increase in the relapse rate. A smaller dose was found satisfactory by Rowland (1962). Those not seriously ill were given 7·9 mg/kg 4-hourly for 5 days (500 mg 4-hourly or 3 grammes daily for a 70 kg man); 90% recovered completely, 5% relapsed and 5% developed complications. Seriously ill patients were given 7·9 mg/kg 6-hourly for 10 days (2 grammes daily for 10 days); 97% recovered completely and there were fewer relapses and complications in only 7%. Combined treatment with chloramphenicol 500 mg and tetracycline 500 mg 6-hourly for 3 days followed by 250 mg chloramphenicol and 250 mg tetracycline 6-hourly for 12 days may reduce the carrier rate and can be used in cases of typhoid fever where there are no complications or severe toxicity.

Toxic crises. In severe cases a toxic crisis with central and peripheral circulatory failure and mental derangement may develop, probably due to a large-scale destruction of typhoid bacilli and release of large amounts of typhoid endotoxin. This complication may be eliminated by using a combination of steroids and chloramphenicol. For the other toxic effects of chloramphenicol see Chapter 45.

Resistance. Resistance to chloramphenicol has only rarely been described. Wright (1961) has recorded a case in a schoolboy with persistent fever in spite of chloramphenicol in whom a culture of *S. typhi* taken during treatment showed resistance to chloramphenicol *in vitro* but moderate sensitivity to streptomycin, which cleared up the infection.

Ampicillin

This has been used in the treatment of typhoid but is considered inferior to chloramphenicol, except that side-effects are lacking. The dose is 1·0 gramme 6-hourly until the fever settles and then 750 mg 6-hourly for 7–10 days. With this régime the temperature fell to normal in from 2·5 to 3 days (Sanders 1965) but in 6 of 10 cases the condition worsened while under treatment and chloramphenicol had to be substituted. Ampicillin should be reserved for the milder cases, and for carriers.

Trimethoprim plus sulphamethoxazole

This preparation (Septrin, Bactrin) has been used successfully in the treatment of typhoid (Kamat 1970; Farid *et al.* 1970). The period to defervescence of the fever is the same as with chloramphenicol but there are no toxic crises and the relief of symptoms is more rapid. Dosage is 2 tablets (each tablet contains 80 mg trimethoprim and 400 mg of sulphamethoxazole) twice daily until defervescence and for 7 days after. In one trial (Farid *et al.* 1970) there was clinical improvement in 48 hours and there were no relapses or carriers.

Furazolidone

Furazolidone, a nitrofuran derivative, has been used with encouraging results in India and elsewhere (Masood 1970).

Steroid therapy

The immediate effect of steroids is dramatic in very toxic and ill patients. Steroids can be given early in the infection and where there are minimal intestinal symptoms. They should be avoided during the third week of the illness. 200 mg hydrocortisone should be given at once parenterally followed by 15 mg prednisone 3 times daily for the first day, 10 mg t.d.s. the second day, 5 mg t.d.s. the third day, 5 mg b.d. the fourth day and 5 mg on the fifth day.

Relapses

Relapse accompanied by a return of fever and a positive blood culture can occur on the average 5 days after recovery from an attack but rarely later than 2 weeks. Rarely a chronic relapsing form may be found lasting for many months, especially following treatment with insufficient doses of chloramphenicol. Relapses are seldom more severe than the original attack (Marmion 1952) but can be of the utmost severity. The general relapse rate is higher after chloramphenicol and is over 50% in cases treated for 8 days or less. A relapse rate of only 4% was found in patients who had chloramphenicol for 12 days after defervescence of the fever (El Ramli 1950). A relapse is treated in the same way as the primary attack.

Treatment of carriers

Faecal carriers. The convalescent carrier is easier to treat than the chronic carrier. Six of 9 convalescent carriers were cured by a combination of tetracycline and chloramphenicol used as in treatment of a normal case (Huckstep 1962). Chronic carriers must be treated with a prolonged course of treatment.

Ampicillin has been used successfully in massive doses (Whitby 1964), 500 mg 6-hourly for at least 14 days, and a course for as long as 6 weeks has been necessary.

Trimethoprim with sulphamethoxazole given for one month as in treatment of a case of typhoid cleared one out of four carriers, but the remaining 3 cases had chronic cholecystitis (Brodie *et al.* 1970).

Surgical treatment of carriers. Since either the gall-bladder or the biliary tract may be the source of the chronic infection, where there are gall-stones or a lesion of the gall-bladder the only chance for successful eradication of the typhoid infection is cholecystectomy. Since the deep bile passages are often involved the common bile duct should always be drained.

Urinary carriers. These should be treated in the same way as chronic faecal carriers, and if *S. haematobium* infection is present this must also be treated.

PROPHYLACTIC INOCULATION

Evidence accumulated in two world wars and subsequently shows that TAB vaccination provides protection against enteric infection. A well controlled trial in Guyana showed that a phenolized vaccine gave significant protection against typhoid fever and that an acetone-killed vaccine was better (Ashcroft *et al.* 1964). Three types of vaccine are available: heat-killed phenol preserved (phenolized), alcohol-killed and acetone-killed acetone-dried (acetone) vaccine. It is now agreed that an acetone vaccine is definitely superior to a phenolized vaccine (Cannon 1969).

TAB vaccine contains 1000 million *S. typhi*, 750 million *S. paratyphi* A, 750 million *S. paratyphi* B and an equal dose of *S. paratyphi* C is added if necessary. There is a growing feeling that vaccine of *S. typhi* alone would be preferable to TAB since paratyphoid vaccines are ineffective and may increase the incidence of reactions (Kline 1968). At present however pure typhoid vaccines are not generally available.

Dosage

Usually TAB is given subcutaneously as 2 doses (0·5 and 1·0 ml) with an interval of 4–6 weeks in between and a third dose of 1·0 ml 6–12 months later.

Intradermal inoculation is just as effective and reduces the incidence of reactions. Vaccine should be administered in double strength as 3 doses each of o·1 ml intradermally at the same intervals as for subcutaneous inoculation.

A single injection of vaccine has been found to confer a substantial degree of immunity not significantly different from that obtained with two doses (WHO 1966; Ashcroft *et al.* 1967). Immunity develops 10–21 days after vaccination so that this period should be allowed before immunizing travellers who require one injection of TAB only when going abroad for a short period. It may be desirable to give a second dose to those going abroad for a period of more than 6 months. TAB may be combined with tetanus vaccine as TABT/Vac either subcutaneously or intradermally, but should not be used for annual booster injections (Cannon 1969). TAB may also be combined with cholera as TABCho/ Vac and given either subcutaneously or intradermally and for primary immuniza- tion against enteric infection. The third dose should be given 6 months after the second and acts as a reinforcing dose against cholera.

PARATYPHOID FEVERS A AND B

Paratyphoid organisms are seldom transmitted by water. Meat pies and ice- cream are the usual vehicles.

The paratyphoid A and B organisms are less invasive and more irritant to the intestinal tract, so that there is usually an initial attack of diarrhoea and vomiting before the invasive stages. The incubation period is shorter and the disease milder. Ambulant cases are commoner than in typhoid but the carrier stage is shorter. In paratyphoid A the pyrexia is longer, although there are less likely to be complications; relapses are commoner.

In paratyphoid B lymphoid follicles of the whole of the intestinal tract may be involved including the stomach, colon and rectum. Jaundice, venous thromboses and suppurative lesions are commoner.

PARATYPHOID C

Paratyphoid C as observed by Giglioli (1929) in Guyana is a septicaemia in which the intestinal tract may not be specially involved. Complications such as arthritis, abscess formation and cholecystitis are common, whilst fixation abscesses from intramuscular injections may occasionally contain a pure culture of the bacillus. The mortality of Giglioli's (1929) series of 92 patients was 38%.

BACTERIAL ENTERITIS OR FOOD POISONING

Aetiology

More than 400 *Salmonella* serotypes have been recognized which are identical with the paratyphoid bacilli morphologically and in their cultural and bio- chemical characteristics. The majority of epidemics investigated bacteriologically are caused by one of the following: *S. typhi-murium, S. enteritidis, S. thompson, S. newport* or *S. dublin. S. typhi-murium* accounts for more than 70% of the outbreaks.

Antigenic structure. Identification of the O (somatic) antigen provides a means of placing any one member of the genus in one of a number of groups designated A–I. Organisms are tested by diagnostic sera which have been absorbed to remove all antibodies except that for the group specific O antigen. The species of organism is typed by identifying the H (flagellar) antigen structure of the specific phase.

Epidemiology

Source of infection. Salmonella food poisoning usually originates from animal sources. Cows, sheep and pigs may be infected and foodstuffs have been incriminated as the source of animal infection. Birds, particularly hens, ducks and turkeys, suffer from *Salmonella* infections. Animal and bird carcases and duck eggs, fresh or dried, are important sources of infection. The eggs are infected in the process of being laid through contamination of the shell by the duck's cloaca.

Transmission

Even if not infected at source, meat and poultry may be infected during handling and packing, and the preparation of meat pies. Cows' milk, milk products and food contaminated by rodents are other sources.

Pathology

The organisms multiply in and are ordinarily confined to the intestine but bacteraemia and septicaemia may occur. Cholecystitis and meningitis may occur. *Salmonella* osteitis occurs commonly in persons with homozygous sickle cell disease.

Clinical features

The history is of an acute gastro-enteritis following the ingestion of made-up food and usually a number of cases occur together in patients who have attended the same picnic or restaurant.

The incubation period is 10–30 hours. The onset is abrupt, with diarrhoea, vomiting and abdominal pain. There may be moderate fever, seldom over 38 °C. The symptoms abate over a period of 1–4 days but very occasionally death may ensue owing to dehydration and electrolyte imbalance.

This is to be differentiated from staphylococcal food poisoning, where the vomiting is more profuse and the incubation period shorter. The vomit may be bile- or blood-stained. The stools are watery without obvious blood, although microscopic blood may be present.

Complications are (rarely) a generalized illness with septicaemia similar to typhoid fever or a chronic illness in which attacks of abdominal pain and diarrhoea may continue for several months. *Salmonella* osteitis occurs in children with sickle cell disease and in bartonellosis. *Salmonella* abscesses may develop at the site of intramuscular injections. *Salmonella* septicaemia and meningitis have occurred.

Treatment

Unless there is severe illness or septicaemia, treatment is essentially symptomatic and antibiotics should be avoided because there is evidence that they prolong the carrier stage (Dixon 1965). If antibiotics must be administered tetracycline should be given in a dosage of 500 mg 6-hourly until the symptoms abate.

Treatment of carriers. This is difficult. Jafary and Burke (1970) treated all of 7 carriers successfully with 2 tablets of Septrin 3 times daily for 7 days.

REFERENCES

ANDERSON, E. S. & WILLIAMS, R. E. O. (1956) *J. clin. Path.*, **9**, 94.

ANDERSON, K. (1970) *Guy's Hosp. Rep.*, **119**, 111.

ASHCROFT, M. T., RITCHIE, J. M. & NICHOLSON, C. C. (1964) *Am. J. Hyg.*, **79**, 196.

—— SINGH, B., NICHOLSON, C. C., RITCHIE, J. M., SOBRYAN, E. & WILLIAMS, F. (1967) *Lancet*, **ii**, 1056.

BELZER, M. (1965) *J. Urol.*, **94**, 23.

BRODIE, J., MACQUEEN, I. A. & LIVINGSTONE, D. (1970) *Br. med. J.*, **iii**, 318.

CANNON, D. A. (1969) *Trans. R. Soc. trop. Med. Hyg.*, **63**, 873.

DIXON, J. M. S. (1965) *Br. med. J.*, **ii**, 1343.

EL RAMLI, A. H. (1950) *Lancet*, **i**, 618.

FARID, Z., HASSAN, A., WASHAB, M. P. A., SANBORN, W. A., KENT, D. C., YASSA, A. & HATHOUT, S. E. (1970) *Br. med. J.*, **ii**, 323.

GIGLIOLI, G. (1929) *Trans. R. Soc. trop. Med. Hyg.*, **23**, 235.

—— (1930) *J. Hyg., Camb.*, **29**, 273.

HUCKSTEP, R. L. (1962) *Typhoid Fever and Other Salmonella Infections*. Edinburgh & London: Livingstone.

JAFARY, M. H. & BURKE, G. J. (1970) *Br. med. J.*, **ii**, 605.

KAMAT, S. A. (1970) *Br. med. J.*, **ii**, 320.

KLINE, S. A. (1968) *J. occup. Med.*, **10**, 285.

McFADZEAN, A. J. S. & CHOA, G. H. (1953) *Br. med. J.*, **ii**, 360.

—— & ONG, G. B. (1966) *Br. med. J.*, **i**, 1567.

MARMION, D. E. (1952) *Trans. R. Soc. trop. Med. Hyg.*, **46**, 619.

—— NAYLOR, G. R. E. & STEWART, I. D. (1953) *J. Hyg., Camb.*, **51**, 260.

MASOOD, A. (1970) *Lancet*, **ii**, 1365.

ROWLAND, H. A. K. (1962) *Pakistan med. J.*, **13**, 19.

SANDERS, W. L. (1965) *Br. med. J.*, **ii**, 1226.

THOMAS, J. V., WATSON, K. C. & HEWSTONE, A. S. (1954) *J. Clin. Path.*, **7**, 50.

VAIZEY, J. M. (1959) *E. Afr. med. J.*, **36**, 65.

WHITBY, J. M. F. (1964) *Lancet*, **ii**, 71.

WOODWARD, T. E., SMADEL, J. E., LAY, H. L., GREEN, R. & MANKIKAR, D. S. (1948) *Ann. intern. Med.*, **29**, 131.

WORLD HEALTH ORGANIZATION (1966) *Bull. Wld Hlth Org.*, **34**, 211.

WRIGHT, F. J. (1961) Personal communication.

TETANUS

Aetiology

Clostridium tetani is a straight, slender, rod-shaped organism 2–5 × 0·4–0·5 μm. It is spore-bearing and Gram-positive, an obligatory anaerobe and grows well on ordinary nutrient media. Tetanus is common throughout the tropics and is an important cause of morbidity and death in some areas. Neonatal tetanus is an important cause of neonatal mortality.

Transmission

Any major or minor wound may act as the portal of entry for tetanus. Tetanus can also follow vaccination or occur postoperatively after intramuscular injections, such as quinine.

Pathology

Cl. tetani multiplies in the wound and produces an exotoxin *tetanospasmin* which reaches the central nervous system by passing along the motor nerves to the anterior horn cells of the spinal cord where it acts as an excitant and then diffuses to involve the whole central nervous system.

Clinical features

The incubation period varies from 7–8 days up to several weeks. The shorter the incubation period the worse the prognosis and it is unusual for a case with an incubation period of a week or less to survive.

The first symptom is usually the onset of painful trismus due to spasm of the masseter muscle. The spasms then spread to involve the muscles of the neck, vertebral column and abdominal wall, following which generalized spasms typical of tetanus occur. During a spasm the muscles contract in an exaggerated fashion giving rise to the risus sardonicus and opisthotonos. The paroxysms are initiated by some stimulus such as light or touch but sometimes occur spontaneously.

Examination shows board-like rigidity which is best seen in the abdominal muscles.

Course. Respiratory distress is due to the interference with respiration and there is anoxia. Death may occur often quite suddenly from asphyxia. Hyperpyrexia is common and is a sign of poor prognosis. There is often severe electrolyte imbalance.

Recurrent tetanus. An attack of clinical tetanus does not confer any lasting immunity once the effect of the protection given has worn off. It is difficult to distinguish between relapses and recurrent attacks. When several months have elapsed with freedom from symptoms, then a second attack is probably responsible; the mortality rate in second attacks is low. Active immunization with tetanus toxoid should be performed in all cases of tetanus after recovery.

Atypical tetanus. A chronic ambulant form is not uncommon, lasting for some weeks with some stiffness of the jaw and rigidity of the muscles; recovery is usual. Localized tetanus may occur, especially in the cervicofacial region, following a wound of the face.

Neonatal tetanus. This is a highly lethal form of the disease due to infection of the umbilical stump with spores usually conveyed by the application of cow dung dressing.

The incubation period is between 3 and 10 days. The onset is gradual and the first symptom is inability to suck the breast, due to trismus. This is followed by constipation and rigidity of the abdominal muscles, and then by tetanic spasms which occur at first infrequently but increase in number until they become almost continuous. The mortality rate was 100% before the introduction of assisted respiration.

Diagnosis

The diagnosis of tetanus is clinical and bacteriological proof is usually unnecessary. It is difficult to isolate *Cl. tetani* from the wound, which may be so small as to be indistinguishable.

Treatment (Laurence 1966)

Surgical treatment of the wound must be carried out. The wound must be excised and any foreign bodies present removed. Antibiotics must be administered to treat the infection in the wound and to stop the further production of toxin.

Anti-tetanic serum. If the patient has had horse serum before or is sensitive to it, then larger doses of ATS will be necessary than usual since the antibodies to the horse serum will neutralize some of the antitoxin. 0·2 ml (600 units) of a test dose of ATS must be given intracutaneously. If there are no local or systemic reactions after 30 minutes then 20 000 units of ATS may be given intravenously. If there is no history of the administration of or sensitivity to horse serum then 10 000 units of ATS will be sufficient. If there is a reaction to the test dose and ATS must be given, then antihistamine 50 mg orally or 25 mg intravenously may be given together with 100 mg hydrocortisone intravenously. To desensitize the patient a test dose is given every 30 minutes, doubling the dose each time until there is no reaction, when the full dose may be given.

Cortiscosteroids have proved useful (Sanders *et al.* 1969). Repeated small doses of ATS, 1500 units intravenously daily for 2–5 days with betamethasone intravenously reduced the mortality of adult tetanus from 61% to 37% in a large series of cases over one year. Betamethasone 8 mg with promazine 50 mg and ATS 1500 units is given intravenously immediately on arrival. The ATS is given for 2–5 days and the betamethasone is given intravenously daily for 10–18 days. The mode of action of the steroid drug is not understood but possible modes of action are thought to be antihistaminic, anticholinergic or antitoxic.

Supportive treatment. Convulsions may be controlled by barbiturates, paraldehyde (5 ml intramuscularly) or bromethol. Chlorpromazine is useful in mild cases but may fail in the most severe cases. In large centres artificial respiration with positive pressure respiration after curarization has proved life saving. Tracheostomy is useful but should only be used where adequate facilities are available to provide nursing and tracheal toilet.

Immunization

Tetanus toxoid containing an aluminium adjuvant will prevent tetanus. A complete course comprises 3 doses of alum precipitated toxoid with about 6 weeks between the first and second and 6–12 months between the second and third. The dose is 0·5 ml intramuscularly for all ages. All patients with tetanus treated in hospital should be given the first dose of toxoid while in hospital, to be followed by a second and third after discharge. Neonatal tetanus may be prevented by immunization of pregnant women. Two doses of alum-precipitated toxoid are given at least one month apart, the first at the first antenatal visit and the second between the seventh and eighth months of pregnancy (McLennan *et al.* 1965).

Prevention of tetanus in the wounded

Antitetanic serum is now no longer necessary since it can cause severe reactions and it may fail to protect some patients. For wounds that are clean and less than 6 hours old, one booster dose of 0·5 ml of toxoid should be given if there has been recent immunization. Where there has been no previous immunization then a complete course of toxoid must be given. Other types of wound should receive one dose of toxoid as for previously immunized patients, but patients who have not been previously immunized should receive a complete course of toxoid plus antibiotic with or without antitoxin. Antitoxin should be used only if there is thought to be a high risk of tetanus and 1500 units should be given.

Clostridium welchii INFECTION

Synonyms

Enteritis necroticans; Pigbel; Struck.

Definition

A diffuse sloughing enteritis of the jejunum, ileum and colon caused by the toxin of *Clostridium welchii* Type C.

Aetiology

Clostridium welchii Type C has been isolated from a significant portion of resected bowel segments in enteritis necroticans. This organism is associated with a similar enterotoxaemic disease of sheep, known in Kent as 'struck'.

Clinical features

Pigbel occurs in the Highlands of New Guinea (Murrell *et al.* 1966) where it is both epidemic and sporadic and is related to pig-feasting which is an integral part of the indigenous cultures of the highland tribes. Males are affected more than females. The disease follows the ingestion of a large meal of pork, cooked at a feast and is characterized by anorexia, severe upper abdominal pain, bloody diarrhoea and vomiting. The mortality rate varies considerably from nil in some cases up to 85% in others. Large segments of the bowel become necrotic and the only form of treatment is resection of the affected portions of the bowel.

ANTHRAX

Aetiology

Bacillus anthracis is a non-motile Gram-positive sporing capsulated bacillus which is both an aerobe and facultative anaerobe, growing readily on agar. The vegetative form produces a toxin which causes gelatinous oedema and haemorrhage in animal tissue. There are 3 distinct antigenic components: a somatic protein, a capsular polypeptide and a somatic polysaccharide. The protein somatic antigen (toxin) stimulates immunity in most animals, is present in the oedema of anthrax lesions, and is neutralized by the antitoxic activity of anthrax antiserum. The spores of *B. anthracis* are very resistant and will resist dry heat at 140°C for 1–3 hours and 100°C moist heat for 5–10 minutes.

Transmission

The anthrax bacillus causes an epizootic disease in herbivorous animals, particularly sheep and cattle, but no species is immune. In animals the portal of entry is the mouth and intestinal tract by the ingestion of spores on vegetation.

In man infection is acquired from animal sources through the skin, cutaneous anthrax (malignant pustule), or by the inhalation of spores into the lungs (pulmonary anthrax) or by the intestinal route from using infected animals as food.

Epidemiology

In the tropics cutaneous anthrax is the commonest form and occurs anywhere where the people are predominantly cattle-owners and prepare the hides for sale.

Intestinal anthrax occurs not uncommonly in epidemics when cattle which have died from anthrax in heavily infected areas may be eaten by large numbers of people. These outbreaks are explosive and many people are involved. Anthrax spores resist the action of gastric juice.

Intestinal anthrax is very common in parts of Africa (Fendall & Grounds 1965).

Clinical features

The malignant pustule forms at the site of infection, sometimes on the head but more usually on the arm. It starts as a papule, becomes a blister within 12–48 hours and then a pustule with a surrounding area of inflammation. Coagulation necrosis of the centre results in the formation of a dark-coloured eschar which is later surrounded by a ring of vesicles containing serous or serosanguineous fluid and outside this an area of oedema and induration which may become very extensive. There is fever and general toxaemia. Septicaemia with haemorrhagic meningitis may occur and may be found in the absence of skin lesions. Numerous *B. anthracis* are found in the cerebrospinal fluid.

After the consumption of an animal which has died of anthrax a large number of people are taken ill suddenly with vomiting and sometimes diarrhoea, fever and general malaise. The incubation period is 12–18 hours. The stools do not contain blood. The mortality rate is low and the great majority recover in a few days. At autopsy there is a severe haemorrhagic infiltration of the ileum and caecum with submucosal abscesses. In fatal cases the disease has usually proceeded to septicaemia.

Diagnosis

Anthrax is easily diagnosed by the presence of the typical bacilli in smears of the pustule or in the faeces in intestinal cases.

Treatment

Anthrax responds readily to penicillin, 1 mega unit 6-hourly for 7 days. Tetracyclines are also effective, as is sulphadimidine.

Prevention

Animals that have died of anthrax must be promptly buried in quicklime or burnt. A protective vaccine has been used for workers especially at risk. Alum-precipitated protective antigen is very safe but the immunity does not last as long as that made from live spore vaccine, which is not considered safe enough for use in man.

TROPICAL PYOMYOSITIS

Synonyms. Tropical myositis; bung pagga.

Aetiology

The cause of tropical pyomyositis is a haemolytic *Staphylococcus*, usually *S. albus* but also *S. aureus. Streptococcus pyogenes* is occasionally found. Secondary streptococcal and staphylococcal infection in filaria-infected subjects has also been considered as a cause.

Pathology

The site of entry is uncertain but dissemination takes place by the bloodstream and the lymphatics and lymph glands show no sign of inflammation. Pyomyositis is apt to occur in persons who are debilitated as the result of some long-standing infection. In 50% of one series of cases the Wassermann reaction was positive.

Clinical features

First there is an acute non-suppurative stage when an indurated, tender, ill-defined mass can be felt in the affected muscles where the patient complains of pain. There is slight pyrexia with surrounding inflammatory reaction and slight superficial pitting oedema. On incision the tissues are oedematous.

This stage may then proceed to an acute suppurative stage with all the signs of a deep-seated abscess and on incision the evacuation of large collections of pus. The abscess cavity is loculated and usually requires wide incision with the breaking down of septa in the cavity. These abscesses occur in widely separated sites, the thigh muscles, pectoralis major, serratus magnus, latissimus dorsi, gastrocnemius, flexor muscles of the arm, iliopsoas and internal oblique. Generalized septicaemia may result.

Diagnosis

Pyomyositis must be distinguished from filarial abscesses which are usually sterile, glanders, melioidosis, rheumatic nodules, osteomyelitis, tuberculous abscesses of the sacroiliac joint, septic mastitis, perinephric abscess and fibrosarcoma.

Treatment

Treatment consists of surgical incision and the administration of antibiotics.

RHINOSCLEROMA

Rhinoscleroma is a disease in which spontaneous painless chronic inflammatory growths caused by *Klebsiella rhinoscleromatis* develop anywhere in the respiratory passages.

Aetiology

The cause of rhinoscleroma is *Klebsiella rhinoscleromatis* described by Frisch in 1882, which is a Gram-negative organism closely related to *Klebsiella pneumoniae* or Friedländer's bacillus, from which it can be distinguished by its growth as well as by its reactions in media containing bile. It is easily cultivated, and forms knob-like colonies on gelatin or agar, greyish on the whole and less conspicuous than *K. pneumoniae*. In sections it is found in hard fibrotic swellings in the nose, scattered throughout the mucosa and submucosa. It exhibits a very low order of pathogenicity for laboratory animals with the exception of mice and has to be differentiated from other capsulated pneumococcus-like organisms in the nose.

Immunology

Klebsiella rhinoscleromatis has both somatic and capsular antigens. Antibodies to the capsular antigens are more specific and are used for complement fixation and haemagglutination tests. The complement fixation test is most usually used in diagnosis, but the Middlebrook–Dubos, a haemagglutination test, is more specific and sensitive (Hencner & Tuszkiewicz 1958).

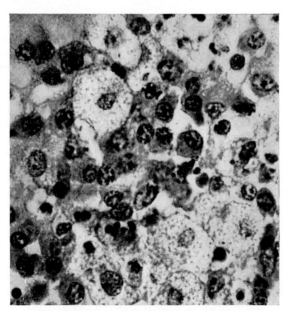

Fig. 150.—Rhinoscleroma. A photomicrograph of tissue, showing Mikulicz cells and general histological picture. (*Dr H. K. Giffen*)

Geographical distribution

Rhinoscleroma is spread over widely distributed regions in special nests or foci and occurs all over the world. According to Kouwenaar (1956) between 3000 and 4000 cases have been recorded. Small foci exist in Switzerland and Italy. The most extensive area of infection is in Eastern Europe, Hungary, Poland, Galicia, the Ukraine and the northern shores of the Black Sea and Caspian Sea. Other foci have been noted in Tomsk in Siberia, Turkestan, Bengal, Java, Sumatra, Central and Southern France, Morocco, Egypt, New England, Argentina, Cuba, Mexico, Panama, Colombia, Brazil, Peru, Chile, El Salvador and Costa Rica.

Pathology

Rhinoscleroma is characterized by a peculiar form of plasma-cell infiltration of great density and by gaps or 'foam cells' which consist of swollen cells with foamy cytoplasm ('foam cells' or 'Mikulicz cells') (Fig. 155). Very frequently there are also hyaline drops or Gram-positive 'Russell's bodies' which occur in all kinds of degenerative tissue and are probably derived from the plasma cells. The rhinoscleroma nodule is known as a plasmoma. It never breaks down but becomes progressively sclerosed. The scleromatous process may spread, and via the paranasal sinuses may grow into the upper lip and infiltrate the alveolar process of the maxilla, involve the pharynx by direct extension from the nose and may affect the lacrimal duct. In rare cases it may spread through the cribriform plate and invade the brain, giving rise to a tumour affecting the base of the brain. The nasal septum and the alveolar border of the maxilla may show local destruction. The cervical glands are often enlarged.

Clinical features

Rhinoscleroma causes spontaneous painless chronic inflammatory growths occurring at any place in the respiratory passages from the nostrils to the hilum of the lung. Gross deformity of the nose or distortion of the respiratory passages

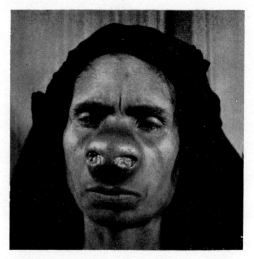

Fig. 151.—Rhinoscleroma of 2 years' duration in an Egyptian woman. (*Dr H. K. Giffen*)

results. The typical splayed out nasal organ is known as the 'Hebra nose' (Fig. 151) and is most commonly found in Sumatra but is rare elsewhere. Sometimes there is perforation of the nasal septum with total destruction of the uvula. The process extends along the respiratory passages with little change in the surrounding tissues. On the whole it tends to form metastases with enlargement of the neighbouring lymphatic glands but in spite of this the general health and condition remain unaffected.

Diagnosis

The appearance of the patient is suggestive. A portion of tissue is teased out and a smear is made and stained by Pappenheim's method. Characteristic foam cells can be demonstrated within 30 minutes.

Treatment

The treatment is mainly surgical, by plastic operation to remove the unsightly growths. Intramuscular streptomycin is effective in some cases in doses of 1 gramme daily intramuscularly for a month. More extended courses may be necessary (Kouwenaar 1956).

REFERENCES

FENDALL, N. R. E. & GROUNDS, J. G. (1965) *J. trop. Med. Hyg.*, **68**, 77.
HENCNER, Z. & TUSZKIEWICZ, M. (1958) *Annls Univ. Mariae Curie-Skłodowska*, **13**, 129 (Quoted in *Trop. Dis. Bull.* (1960) **57**, 73).
KOUWENAAR, W. (1956) *Documenta Med. geogr. trop.*, **8**, 13.
LAURENCE, D. R. (1966) *Clinical Pharmacology*, 3rd ed., pp. 175–81. London: Churchill.
McLENNAN, R., SCHOFIELD, F. D., PITTMAN, H., HARDEGREE, M. C. & BARILE, M. F. (1965) *Bull. Wld Hlth Org.*, **32**, 683.
MURRELL, T. G. C., ROTH, L., EGERTON, J., SAMUELS, J. & WALKER, P. H. (1966) *Lancet*, **i**, 217.
SANDERS, R. K. M., STRONG, T. N. & PEACOCK, M. L. (1969) *Trans. R. Soc. trop. Med. Hyg.*, **63**, 746.

26. CEREBROSPINAL MENINGITIS

CEREBROSPINAL meningitis is endemic throughout the tropics and sub-tropics, as in the temperate zones. It is usually sporadic, but occasionally breaks out into devastating epidemics.

The meningococcus (*Neisseria meningitidis*) is antigenically divisible into 4 groups, of which Group A is the most important in Africa; Group B has been responsible for outbreaks in Europe. The disease is essentially the same wherever it occurs, and the prognosis is also the same if patients are treated with modern drugs.

EPIDEMIOLOGY

Meningococci are spread from one person to another via the nasopharynx and the nasal and buccal discharges. In general the epidemiology is that of a respiratory infection in which the numbers of patients who become ill are very much less than the numbers of healthy carriers in the general population. In closed communities, such as military units living in barracks, the proportion of carriers may reach 50% within the first 3 months of barrack life, but only a small proportion are ill. In these conditions the proportion of carriers is influenced by the inflow of new recruits, most of whom are not infected before arrival.

The proportion of carriers to the numbers diseased is inverse—those who get meningitis do so early in their exposure, when the numbers of carriers are increasing; when the carriers are at their peak the numbers of clinical cases fall off.

The disease often tends chiefly to affect children. In Delhi, India, an epidemic in 1966 did so, with a case mortality rate of 37% below the age of 1 year. In other outbreaks the incidence may be highest at age 15–19. Like other epidemics, the Delhi outbreak was most severe in congested areas.

Special conditions exist in Africa which favour the occurrence of epidemic waves. In a wide belt of country between the Sahara to the north and the equatorial forest to the south, stretching from the Sudan westwards through Chad, Northern Nigeria, Dahomey, Ghana and Upper Volta, there are some 10 000 cases of meningitis each year with an average case mortality of around 12% (WHO 1969), and the incidence is seasonal. The feature of this area which probably determines the epidemic waves is that between January and March the weather is dry and the nights are very cold. The people therefore sleep inside their houses at this time, though at other seasons they tend to sleep outside or on the roofs. In this dry weather the mucous membranes of the nasopharynx tend to be dry, ceasing to act as an efficient barrier to infection. Conditions for transmission from carriers are favourable, and cases of meningitis occur. This cycle tends to end in about 3 months, when a degree of immunity has been established.

At other times of the year in this area, carriers maintain the infection at a low rate, and actual disease is sporadic. There seems to be no evidence that disease is provoked solely by organisms of increased virulence, but lack of immunity in individuals is probably a factor. Subclinical infections may provide some immunity.

Nasopharyngeal carriers can be detected by taking swabs, but the technique needs care. Metal rods (for instance bicycle spokes) are better than wooden sticks since wood releases harmful substances. The toxicity of cotton-wool swabs can be reduced by rolling them in finely powdered vegetable charcoal before sterilization. The swabs can be dipped in 0·1 M phosphate buffer solution at pH 7·4, boiled in this for 10 minutes and then dried and sterilized (WHO 1969). Meningococci can be isolated in Thayer-Martin medium, but this is a task for the specialist.

Meningococci are delicate organisms. They are sensitive to heat, not surviving more than $1\frac{1}{2}$ hours at 40°C, which is quite usual in the epidemic season. They are very sensitive to sunlight, and to changes in temperature, and although they survive freezing, they suffer badly at the usual temperature found in a refrigerator (WHO 1969). Specimens of cerebrospinal fluid or throat swabs should therefore not be kept in a refrigerator or in sunlight, but should be taken at body temperature at once to the laboratory, and inoculated on to culture medium as soon as possible.

PATHOLOGY

In fatal meningitis there is usually suppurative inflammation of the pia-arachnoid, especially at the base of the brain, with foci of haemorrhage; the ventricles are distended with fluid or pus. Minute foci of encephalitis without obvious meningitis may be found, especially in fulminating cases. Meningococcal septicaemia is common, and may become chronic, even without meningitis.

IMMUNOLOGY

Various antibodies have been detected in serum, some of which have some protective action, and have been used in treatment, though now abandoned. The fact that only a few carriers become diseased indicates a protective mechanism, but its nature seems to be far from clear.

CLINICAL FINDINGS

In the meningitic form of the disease the incubation period is 2–5 days. The illness starts suddenly with a rigor and fever, severe headache and vomiting; convulsions are common in children. The neck muscles soon become rigid, and Kernig's sign is positive. In pale skins a macular rash develops, which becomes purpuric.

Acute fulminating cases sometimes occur, and the Waterhouse–Friderichsen syndrome (in which there is bleeding into the suprarenals, with vomiting and collapse) may develop quickly; these severe forms are usually fatal.

In infants posterior basal meningitis is common, with insidious onset, head retraction and opisthotonos; lumbar puncture may be dry owing to closure of the foramen of Magendie. The patient may become deaf, mentally deficient or spastic.

A chronic form of meningococcal septicaemia is also described, in which meningococci can, by appropriate though difficult techniques, be isolated from the blood.

DIAGNOSIS

This can usually be made by lumbar puncture, the cerebrospinal fluid becoming turbid and containing pus cells and meningococci, which can often be demonstrated by microscopy of the centrifuged deposit or by culture.

Various serological tests have been investigated. Agglutinins and complement fixing antibodies are often present, and Edwards and Devine (1968) have obtained an antigen from various strains of meningococci which reacts well with sera from patients and carriers. An indirect haemagglutination test is described by Vandekerkove et al. (1968) which becomes positive in 40% of cases on days 2–3, and in over 90% on days 10–15. These tests could be useful in doubtful cases, for instance in 'aseptic' meningitis in which meningococci have been suppressed by drug treatment, and as epidemiological tools.

Differential diagnosis in epidemics is usually easy, but sporadic cases may be more difficult. They must be differentiated from cerebral malaria, the encephalitic forms of virus diseases (especially those due to arboviruses), and leptospirosis. Examination of the cerebrospinal fluid is obviously important, but blood should also be examined for parasites, and if leptospirosis is suspected, serum should be sent for the appropriate tests.

Other forms of meningitis occur, usually as isolated cases, particularly pneumococcal meningitis, or forms due to *Haemophilus influenzae* and other bacteria. Pneumococcal meningitis is not uncommon in West Africa, particularly in the cold dry season, and is dangerous, with a case mortality reaching 45% in spite of high doses of penicillin (Pirame et al. 1968).

TREATMENT

The sulphonamides are the standard drugs, and are very successful. A warning must be given, however, that if malaria is present it must also be treated, because malaria interferes seriously with the effect of sulphonamides on the meningococcal infection.

In recent years sulphonamides have been very successfully used, in various schedules. Sulphadimidine may be given by intramuscular injection of a 33% solution, in adult doses of 6 ml (2 grammes) every 8 hours until the patient can swallow tablets, when sulphaphenazole can be given in doses of 500 mg every 12 hours up to the fifth to seventh day of treatment. For less severe cases sulphaphenazole can be used alone by mouth in doses of 1500 mg twice in the first 24 hours, followed by 500 mg every 12 hours for 5–7 days. Minimum doses for infants should be: sulphadimidine injection 2 ml; sulphaphenazole by mouth, 500 mg as initial dose, followed by 250 mg every 12 hours (Thomson 1970; Waddy 1970).

Sulphamethoxypyridazine (Lederkyn), which is excreted slowly, has been used as a single intramuscular injection of a 25% solution as follows (Lapeyssonnie et al. 1961):

Age (years)	Dose
0–1	0·5 gramme (2 ml)
1–3	1·0 grammes (4 ml)
3–6	1·5 grammes (6 ml)
6–15	2·0 grammes (8 ml)
over 15	2·5 grammes (10 ml)

Fanasil (sulphormethoxine) has also been used; it has a more prolonged action than Lederkyn, and can be given by intramuscular injection in single doses of

500 mg for infants, to 2·5 grammes for adults, or by mouth in (adult) doses of 1–2 grammes, repeated if necessary after a few days.

Other sulphonamides such as sulphathiazole and sulphadiazine can be used in doses of 5–10 grammes (divided) by mouth on each of the first 2 days, reduced on subsequent days, to a total period of 6–8 days. But recently there have been indications of cross-resistance to sulphonamides which, if it becomes general, will seriously affect treatment. The meningococcus, however, is sensitive to penicillin and other antibiotics. A dose of 1–5 mega units of penicillin, possibly in addition to sulphonamide, may be enough, and tetracycline in doses of 50 mg/kg daily has been effective.

Trimethoprim (Syraprim) may be given in doses of 200 mg every 4 hours.

In inter-epidemic periods meningitis is often due to pneumococci or *H. influenzae*, and if the causal organism cannot be identified it is wise to give treatment effective against all likely bacteria. Chloramphenicol with the sulphonamides may be the treatment of choice, but intrathecal and massive intramuscular doses of crystalline penicillin may be more effective against pneumococci (Thomson 1970; Waddy 1970).

PREVENTION

In organizing campaigns against epidemics of cerebrospinal meningitis, speed in the administration of sulphonamides is all-important. Camps should be organized for the sick, and precise instructions should be issued to dispensers in fixed and mobile units on the methods and doses to be used in the administration of these drugs. In the past sulphonamide tablets have been distributed to village chiefs in remote parts, for use as directed by the medical staffs, but it is difficult to prevent abuse. Even under the best circumstances many persons are likely to be dosed on ungrounded suspicion.

In any campaign mobile treatment and vaccination units should be organized, and an effective system of information developed. Fixed dispensaries, hospitals and tribal authorities also play an important part. If any healthy or convalescent carriers are detected, they must be given a course of sulphonamides, but detection is difficult and unlikely.

In communities under close control, such as military units, drug prophylaxis by sulphonamides may be justified. A single dose of 2–4 grammes of sulpha-dimidine, or a comparable dose of some other sulphonamide, may be given, or even a 3-day course of sulphadiazine, but before such prophylaxis the sensitivity of the local strain to sulphonamides must be determined. In one field experiment in Nigeria Vollum and Griffiths (1962) gave nasal snuff containing 1 gramme of sulphadimidine daily for 2 days to a population of almost 100 000, with a rapid fall of incidence of disease in one area, and a slower fall in another.

If the meningococci are resistant to sulphonamides, penicillin may be used for prophylaxis—for instance, aqueous procaine penicillin, 600 000 units every 12 hours for 4 doses.

Drug prophylaxis may be demanded by contacts of patients, and can hardly be refused, but it may fail, and overuse of sulphonamides can lead to resistance.

Vaccines have been developed, and extensive vaccination campaigns have recently been carried out in West Africa, in which much successful use has been made of the Dermo-Jet injector. The fear of meningitis is so vivid in those parts that there is no difficulty in inducing the people to be vaccinated. It remains to be seen how effective the vaccines are.

Prevention in general is difficult, as with any respiratory infection in which living conditions and aerial spread are so important, and climate is so great a factor.

REFERENCES

EDWARDS, E. A. & DEVINE, L. F. (1968) *Proc. Soc. exp. Biol. Med.*, **122**, 1168.

LAPEYSSONNIE, L., CHABBERT, Y., BONNARDOT, R., LEFÉVRE, M. & LOUIS, J. (1961) *Bull. Soc. Path. éxot.*, **54**, 955.

PIRAME, Y., PATACQ-CROUZET, J., N'GUYEN TRUNG LUONG, DUJEU, G., HERAUT, L. & SAWADOGO, R. (1968) *Méd. trop.*, **28**, 165.

THOMSON, K. B. D. (1970) Personal communication.

VANDEKERKOVE, M., BIDEAU, J., NICOLI, J. & FAUCON, R. (1968) *Ann. Inst. Pasteur*, **115**, 212.

VOLLUM, R. L. & GRIFFITHS, P. W. W. (1962) *J. clin. Path.*, **15**, 50.

WADDY, B. B. (1970) Personal communication.

WORLD HEALTH ORGANIZATION (1970) *WHO Chron.*, **23**, 54.

SECTION V

DISEASES CAUSED BY SPIROCHAETES

27. TREPONEMATOSES

THE treponematoses include:
Venereal syphilis (*Treponema pallidum*)
Non-venereal syphilis (endemic syphilis, bejel, njovera) (*T. pallidum*),
Yaws (buba, pian, framboesia) (*T. pertenue*)
Pinta (carate, mal del pinto) (*T. carateum, T. herrejoni*)

ORIGIN

Two opinions are held about the origin of the treponematoses. Hackett (1963) considers that the progenitor of the group was pinta, which probably arose from an animal infection about 15 000 B.C., spreading throughout the world but later becoming isolated in the Americas. Yaws arose from mutants of the pinta treponeme, and by about 10 000 B.C. had spread throughout much of the world, but did not reach the Americas, which were then isolated by the flooding of the Bering Strait as a result of the melting of the polar ice caps. Endemic syphilis arose from yaws about 7000 B.C. when arid climates followed the retreat of the last glaciation, favouring the selection of suitable treponemes. Venereal syphilis evolved from endemic syphilis about 3000 B.C., when big cities developed in South-west Asia, favouring the selection of suitable mutants. Venereal syphilis spread through Europe after the first century A.D. as a mild disease, until a mutation to the present form took place towards the end of the fifteenth century. It was carried throughout the world with the European expansion which has taken place since then.

Hudson (1958), however, thinks that the group of diseases probably originated in Africa, possibly from spirochaetes living on decaying vegetable matter, which in the course of time became parasitic in man. The infection was then non-venereal (like yaws) and existed, again like yaws, in conditions of heat, humidity and naked human skin. About 100 000 years ago people migrated from Africa to as far as Australia and Oceania, and may have taken yaws with them—it could even have reached the Americas. Pinta probably developed from yaws as a result of some environmental factor, and, although there are more cases of pinta in Central and South America than anywhere else, Hudson holds that 'pinta' cases can be found constantly, but in varying degree, in association with yaws and syphilis all over the world. Disturbance of pigmentation, the prominent feature of pinta, is a constant characteristic of infection with *T. pallidum*, and Hudson does not recognize pinta as a separate disease.

With migration to dry areas there was a change from yaws to endemic syphilis, which now flourished in desert conditions, the parasite finding suitable situations in the sheltered moist areas of skin, neck, limbs, groins and round the orifices. With the rise of city civilizations, and their relatively high standards

Table 30. Primary lesions of treponematoses

Character of the lesions	Sporadic syphilis	Endemic syphilis	Yaws (*framboesia*)	Pinta
Incidence	Very common. May be absent if infection is by blood transfusion or needle prick (i.e. *syphilis d'emblée*). May be multiple	Very rare. Occurs as a 'throwback' from child to non-immune mother; and in rare cases of venereal transmission	Common. Sometimes not noted (? overlooked; ? '*d'emblée*'). More than one, occasionally	Common. ?
Common sites	Genitalia (95%); may be overlooked if intraurethral (male), in vagina, or on cervix. Extra-genital (5%); lips, mouth, fingers, nipples (female)	Nipple(s) of woman suckling child with oral lesions. Genitalia in rare cases of venereal transmission	Exposed parts: legs, arms, face. Breast or hip, in women, occasionally	Exposed parts: legs, arms, face
Type(s) of lesion	(i) Papule which undergoes superficial, indolent, ulceration. Sometimes, but not always, indurated (i.e., Hunterian chancre) (ii) Often an erosion; may resemble an abrasian or fissure (iii) Extra-genital forms are more ulcerative; may be painful	Papule becomes papulo-ulcerative	Papule, grows into a papilloma	Erythematous papule becoming a papulo-squamous (i.e., raised and scaly) patch
Regional adenitis	Very common. May be contralateral	—	Frequent	Uncommon
Duration (untreated)	2–6 weeks	?	2–9 months; rarely as long as 2 years	Months

Table 31. Secondary lesions of treponematoses

Lesions	Sporadic syphilis	Endemic syphilis	Yaws (framboesia)	Pinta
	(Syphilides)	(Syphilides)	(Framboesides)	(Pintides)
I. Skin, generally				
1. Macular	+(= roseola)	+	Rarely noted	Early phase
2. Maculo-papular	+	+++		Later phase
3. Papular	+	+++	+	(later)
4. Papillomatous	Very rare	?	Usual	No
Condylomatous	Uncommon	Common	Very common	No
Erosive	Rare	?	+(in malnourished)	No or 'never'
Rupial	+++	+++	+	No
5. Papulo-pustular	+++		+	No
6. Papulo-squamous	+++	+++	+++	Usual type; coloured
Pleomorphism				+
Itching	Rare	Rare	Occasional	Quite common
II. Oral				
1. 'Split papules'	±	Very commonly the first sign of disease	Rare, seldom noted	No
2. 'Mucous patches' (also occur in vagina)	+	+	+	No, but buccal lesions have been reported
III. Plantar, palmar skin lesions				
1. Papulo-squamous	+	Never	Very common	Only in Cuban series
2. Papillomatous	Never		Common	Never
IV. Generalized lymph-node enlargement	Common	Common	Fairly common	Fairly common
V. Skin appendages				
1. Hair (alopecia)	++	++	Never	Never
2. Nails (onychia)	++	±	+	? never
VI. Bones				
1. Osteochondritis	+(congenital)	Not reported	Never	Never
2. Osteoperiostitis		+	Common	Never
3. Goundou	Not reported	Not reported	In some areas	Not reported
VII. Joints (hydrarthrosis)	±	±	±	Never
VIII. Laryngitis, pharyngitis	±	Common	Very rare	Never
IX. C.N.S.				
1. C.S.F. abnormality	Common	?	±10%	In some series
2. Meningeal symptoms	++	?+	Rare and mild	Never (?)
X. Ocular: uveitis	+	?	Never	Never
XI. Visceral: hepatitis, nephrosis	Rare		Never	Never

+, Occurs. ±, Has been recorded.

Table 32. Tertiary lesions of treponemotoses

Lesions	Sporadic syphilis	Endemic syphilis	Yaws (framboesia)	Pinta
I. Skin (+ subcutaneous tissues):				
1. Gummas				
Nodular	++	Common	Common	No
Ulcerative	++	Common	Common	No
Spreading nodulo-ulcerative	+	Common	Occasional	No
2. Hyperkeratosis	Uncommon	In some (*bejel*)	Occasional/common	? occasional
3. Leucoderma	Uncommon	Occasional	Occasional	Common
4. Juxta-articular nodes	Rare	Occasional	Quite common	Rare
II. Oronasal: (gangosa) Rhinopharyngitis mutilans	Uncommon	Occasional	Common in some series	No/never
III. Bones:				
Gummas; periostitis	Occur	Quite common	Quite common	No
IV. Joints, destruction	Charcot type (trophic)	Rare	Interphalangeal	No
V. Other systems/viscera:				
1. Cardiovascular (aortitis, aneurysm)	Common	Uncommon, but do occur in some communities affected	Never proved	Aortitis reported in few cases
2. C.N.S.	Tabes, GPI, gumma	Uncommon, but do occur in some communities	Never proved	Not reported
3. Viscera	Gummas, not common	? rare	No	No
4. Eyes; (iritis, keratitis, choroido-retinitis, papillitis and optic atrophy) i.e. ophthalmic or ocular and neuro-ocular	+	?	Not reported	Not reported

+, Occurs.

of living, about 10 000 years ago, non-venereal syphilis tended to die out in them, but gave rise to venereal syphilis from sores on the genitalia.

The arguments on which these opinions are based cannot be given in detail here. Both accept the influence of environment on the kinds of disease encountered in various parts of the world. Both accept mutational change in the organisms in the course of evolution. Hackett recognizes 3 species of treponemes infecting man—*T. pallidum* of syphilis and endemic syphilis, *T. pertenue* of yaws, and *T. carateum* of pinta—largely on the evidence of experimental infections in animals. Hudson recognizes only *T. pallidum*, of which the others are intra-specific strains, which cannot be distinguished. The nomenclature recognized by Hackett is used for convenience in this book.

Whatever the truth of these interpretations, the fact remains that, clinically and epidemiologically, there are differences between the various diseases, and that although treatment is the same for all, prevention is not.

T. pallidum, *T. pertenue* and *T. carateum* are all highly motile organisms. They are morphologically identical and serological tests fail to differentiate them. They have not been cultivated in artificial media. In experimental work complete cross-protection has been demonstrated between different strains of *T. pallidum* from venereal syphilis and non-venereal syphilis, and between different strains of *T. pertenue*. There is less cross-protection between strains of venereal *T. pallidum* and strains of *T. pertenue*, and least between strains of venereal *T. pallidum* or *T. pertenue* and the animal parasite *T. cuniculi* of rabbits.

A comprehensive list of the distribution of primary, secondary and tertiary lesions is given in Tables 30–32, which are reproduced by permission of the Institute for Medical Research, Kuala Lumpur, from *Notes on the Treponematoses with an Illustrated Account of Yaws* (1959) by L. H. Turner.

The basic tissue reactions in the treponematoses are (Turner 1959):

1. An exudate with infiltration of lymphocytes, plasma cells and macrophages.
2. Proliferation of fibroblasts.
3. Endarteritis.

In primary (local) and secondary (blood-borne) lesions exudation is prominent, with little or no fibrosis; these lesions can resolve with little or no permanent trace. Treponemes are present in most of them, especially in the primary and early secondary stages. The primary lesion may be associated with enlargement of the lymph nodes draining the area; this constitutes the primary complex.

In the tertiary stage the notable feature is tissue loss, of 2 main types (Turner 1959):

1. Chronic degeneration and atrophy, with replacement of the specialized cells of the affected part by fibrous tissue. These changes are permanent. Treponemes are scanty in these lesions except in the brain in general paresis.
2. Gummas, which are localized necrotic processes surrounded by fibroblasts, capillaries, cellular infiltrations and occasional giant cells. Healing is by fibrosis. Treponemes are seldom seen.

All the treponemes of these diseases almost certainly become blood-borne early in the infection, and therefore reach all tissues of the body, but they exhibit affinities for certain tissues, as shown in Table 33.

In pinta the early lesions remain active, and contain treponemes for many years, before they become inactive and depigmented. They are therefore infective for long periods (which is unique among the treponematoses). Palmar and plantar lesions do not occur, and there are no bone lesions or late destructive lesions.

In the early stages of non-venereal syphilis and yaws, skin, palmar, plantar and bone lesions occur; later there are destructive skin and bone lesions.

In the early stages of venereal syphilis there are skin lesions and not infrequently bone lesions. In the late stages there are destructive lesions of skin, bone and other tissues, and lesions of the heart and brain (Hackett 1963).

Table 33. Tissues generally affected in treponematoses

Tissue	Venereal syphilis	Non-venereal syphilis	Yaws	Pinta
Placenta, fetus	+	+ or —*	—	—
Cardiovascular	+	±	—	+?
C.N.S.				
Parenchyma	+	±	—	—
Meningo-vascular	+	+	±?	—
Viscera	+	—	—	—
Bone	+	+	+	—
Skin	+	+	+	+
Lymph nodes	+	+	+	+
Mucosa	+	+	+	—

Modified from Turner (1959).

* Congenital infection occurs in some foci of non-venereal syphilis, but not in others.

+, Certainly occurs.   ±, Recorded but uncommon.
—, Not recorded.

In the secondary stages of venereal syphilis and yaws the lesions may be of 2 kinds (Turner 1959):

1. *Minor.* More or less symmetrical generalized eruptions, profuse or sparse. They are either macules or tiny papules, often grouped, and they seldom increase in size; they are short-lived and benign, and never ulcerate. Prognosis is good. Treponemes are very scanty, or cannot be demonstrated. These lesions have the characteristics of '-ides'.

2. *Major.* The major lesions in yaws and pinta often resemble the primary lesions. Treponemes are present in large numbers.

The differences can be set out as in Table 34 (Turner 1959).

Table 34. Major and minor lesions in venereal syphilis and yaws

	Major	Minor
Size	Large	Small
Morphology	Papillomatous	Macular, micropapular
Treponemes	Numerous	Scanty or none
Tendency to exude serum	Great	Slight
Infectivity	Great	Slight
Duration	Comparatively long	Short

Venereal syphilis is not described in detail in this book; it is a large subject for which textbooks on venereology or general medicine should be consulted.

The other treponematoses, however, are common in hot climates and are therefore included here.

Non-venereal Syphilis

Synonyms

Endemic syphilis; bejel (Near East); njovera (Rhodesia); skerlievo (Bosnia); dichuchwa (Botswana); siti (Gambia).

Geographical distribution

This extends across Saharan and Rhodesian Africa, through the Near East and parts of the Balkans, to Central Asia, and appears in Central Australia.

TRANSMISSION AND EPIDEMIOLOGY

It is transmitted by contagion from infectious lesions on skin and mucous membranes, often by the use of common feeding utensils, tobacco pipes, etc.; venereal transmission is uncommon. It is essentially a disease of hot, dry countries.

Children are the chief reservoir of infection, which is favoured by over-crowding, primitive hygiene and sanitation, and, of course, by low standards of education. It is mainly a rural disease, accepted by the people, like other afflictions, as inevitable.

Existing diseases of the mucous membrane of the mouth, for instance the stomatitis associated with deficiency of vitamin B_2, predispose to infection by affording suitable sites for the treponemes to enter; vitamin deficiency is common in primitive rural communities.

Warm weather and relatively high humidity are associated with increase of infectious cases.

CLINICAL FEATURES

Primary

Primary chancres are rarely seen, but have been found on the mouth and lips, the nipples of women, and on the genitalia. But in Bosnia less than 1% of early cases show a primary lesion.

Secondary (Hudson 1958)

Characteristic secondary lesions (which are usually the first manifestations) include mucous patches on the lips and tongue, and papules or macules favouring the warm and moist areas (e.g. the flexures), especially round the genitalia and anus, neck, axilla, elbows and knees, though the eruption may be generally distributed over the whole body. The eruption is florid and luxuriant, and the picture is clinically unmistakable (Hudson 1958). The lips, tongue, palate, tonsils, nasal septum (sometimes with collapse) or larynx may be involved, going on to dysphagia and dysphonia. There may be ulcers on the skin, which is usually itchy.

Adenitis of the groin and cervical, axillary and epitrochlear lymph nodes is marked, but the nodes do not break down—they remain discrete, elastic and not tender. Periostitis, usually of the tibia, but also of the humerus, radius and bones of the hand, can occur at this stage.

Untreated early endemic syphilis usually resolves in about one year, followed by a period of latency, though relapses may occur. Late (tertiary) lesions may follow.

Tertiary (Hudson 1958)

In the late stage lesions include occasional erosions and ulcers of the mouth, the nasal structures (gangosa) and larynx. On the skin gummatous ulcers are characteristic, and may persist for years. Hyperkeratosis of the soles of the feet occurs, causing great thickening of the skin, with fissures, and disability. Juxta-articular nodules are also seen. Depigmentation of the skin can be extensive, but is not common.

Periostitis, with bone pain, and arthritis (especially of the knee), gummas of various bones, and even osteomyelitis, have been reported. Sabre tibia indistinguishable from the same condition in yaws is reported by Hudson (1958).

It is noticeable that in endemic syphilis, as in yaws, the cardiovascular and central nervous systems escape serious damage, except in very rare cases.

SEROLOGY AND IMMUNOLOGY

On the whole the serology of endemic syphilis does not differ from the serology of venereal syphilis, in which the fluorescent antibody absorption test and the passive haemaglutination test, both highly sensitive and simple, have taken their place beside the older tests. Experimental cross-immunity is described above (page 563).

TREATMENT

As in the other treponematoses modern treatment with penicillin and other antibiotics is successful. Dosages are shown on page 577. A mass campaign in Bosnia in 1948–53 has apparently ended transmission.

Yaws

Synonyms

Framboesia (French *framboise*, a raspberry), pian, buba.

A disease caused by *Treponema pertenue* and characterized by granulomatous primary skin lesions, generalized spread in the secondary stage, and chronic disease of the skin, bones and joints in the tertiary stage.

Geographical distribution

Yaws is found in the Caribbean and South America, throughout tropical Africa, the Far East, Northern Australia and the tropical Pacific islands. It is, however, now much less common than it was before the introduction of antibiotics, yet it still occurs, and the diagnosis could easily be missed by doctors unfamiliar with the clinical effects.

EPIDEMIOLOGY AND TRANSMISSION

Yaws is essentially a disease of primitive rural people living in hot, humid climates.

Congenital transmission does not occur. The infection is transmitted by direct contact of the skin with an infective lesion in the skin of another person. The treponemes probably enter through a breach in the epidermis, which may not even be visible.

The treponemes are present in the skin wherever there are lesions, and the lesions remain infective for a few months. There are latent periods after the primary or secondary manifestations, but relapses tend to occur, when infective lesions appear and may last 3–5 years.

Transmission often occurs from mothers to their infants, or vice versa. Early cases are much more common in children than in adults, possibly because adults tend to be immune through previous infection, or because they do not have such close physical contact with infective persons and such a propensity to minor skin injuries.

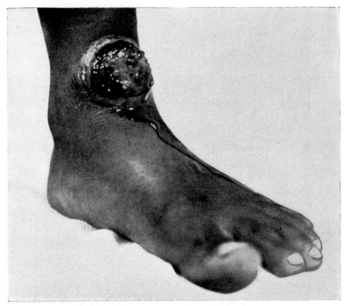

Fig. 152.—Primary yaws chancre on the foot. (*Dr L. A. Leon, Quito*)

Transmission is particularly likely in hot and humid conditions, where little clothing is worn, the skin is constantly moist (and therefore the lesions tend to be open) and bodily cleanliness is not generally stressed. It has been said that an adequate supply of soap and water would go a long way towards eradicating yaws (and trachoma and no doubt many other diseases).

Transmission by non-biting flies (especially *Hippelates pallipes*), which are attracted to raw surfaces, has been suggested but not satisfactorily proved. If it does occur it is probably of minor importance.

There is some serological evidence that a reservoir of yaws may exist in baboons in West Africa; treponemes have also been found in a number of these animals (Mollaret & Fribourg-Blanc 1967).

It is to be noted that as rural yaws dies out, men from rural villages who visit cities, for instance to attend fairs, are likely to acquire venereal syphilis and to return to their villages with secondary syphilitic sores, and from them to infect children via the skin. The result is syphilis, not yaws, in the children, though the infection is by the skin.

PATHOLOGY

Primary

The primary lesion is a granular papilloma, raised above the skin and usually covered with a scab. There is oedema of the epidermis, and infiltration with polymorphs, plasma cells and lymphocytes; there may be an irregular fungating mass of granulation tissue. Sometimes the initial lesion takes the form of an ulcer with a granulating base, which is rarely indurated (Figs 152, 153).

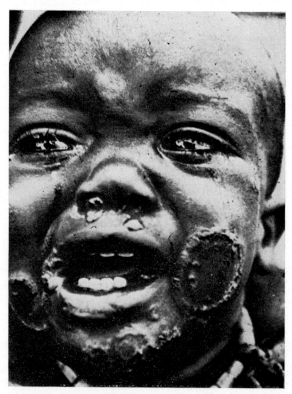

Fig. 153.—Typical facies with secondary yaws. The lesion is circinate. The child has the characteristic miserable expression, tearfulness and running nose. (*Dr C. J. Hackett*)

Healing takes place by scab formation and epithelialization from the periphery (Hill *et al.* 1951; Turner 1959).

Treponemes are most numerous in the tips of the dermal papilli and in the foci of polymorphs.

Secondary (Hackett 1946; Hill *et al.* 1951; Turner 1959)

The secondary lesions resemble the primary lesions in degree rather than in character. They are often very prominent, coming in crops all over the body (Fig. 154).

The histological picture of the papillomatous framboeside shows acanthosis and fusion of some of the rete pegs, giving an appearance of islands of dermal papilli. There is hyperkeratinization and thickening of the epidermis, infiltration with polymorphs and focal necrosis (micro-abscesses), oedema and reduction of melanin, but without ulceration. The papules are granular but there is no true granulation tissue—they consist of greatly proliferated epithelium, and there is little scarring. Small papules often occur in groups.

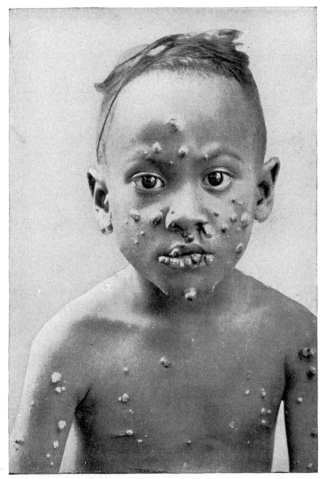

Fig. 154.—Secondary yaws in a Malay boy. (*Sir W. Le Gros Clark*)

Infiltration with plasma cells and lymphocytes occurs; there is some swelling of the capillary endothelium, but there is little change in the larger vessels.

Macular framboesides show increased keratinization but only slight thickening of the epidermis; there is little cellular infiltration; treponemes are relatively scanty. There are other framboesides intermediate between papillomas and macules.

Atypical secondary lesions include pigmented macules, localized serpiginous areas of fine desquamation. Onychia is sometimes present. Enlargement of lymph glands is common, possibly as a result of breaches of the surface.

Tertiary (Hackett 1946; Turner 1959)

Tertiary skin lesions include gummas in which the centre consists of hyalinized fibrous tissue which may go on to necrosis. Capillaries may be blocked by epithelioid cells, but there is no destruction of the vessel walls. Healing takes place by replacement of the necrotic mass by scar tissue. Ulcers occur, with fibrous tissue in the depths (Fig. 155).

Hyperkeratosis of the palms and soles is seen mostly in the later stages, but can occur in all but the very earliest stage. The stratum corneum may be 5–10 times its normal thickness. Contractures may affect the fingers.

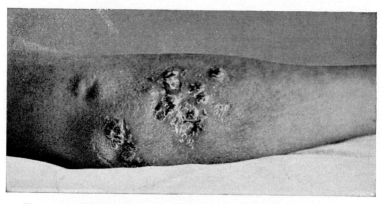

Fig. 155.—Tertiary yaws ulceration on the forearm of a European. (*P. H. Manson-Bahr*)

Bone lesions consist of periosteal thickening with small foci of lymphocytes and plasma cells, vascular sclerosis, decalcification, osteoclasis and absorption of lamellae, with increase in fibrous tissue and plasma cell infiltration in the medullary spaces. Fluid may form in the knee-joints.

Gangosa is an ulcerating gummatous lesion (Fig. 156).

Juxta-articular nodes are composed of subcutaneous fibrous tissue, which is loose on the outside and more dense in the middle, with hyaline material going on to softening. They are freely moveable and rubbery, painless, and usually multiple, occurring in several sites—over the ankle, head of the fibula, olecranon, great trochanter and sacrum. They are usually found in adults, and may be related to trauma, which provides a nidus for treponemes. Though usually thought of as tertiary, they may perhaps originate at an earlier stage.

IMMUNOLOGY

Serological tests such as are used in the diagnosis of syphilis (Wassermann, Kahn, etc.) become positive 3–4 weeks after appearance of the primary lesion of yaws, and rapidly increase in titre; they are strongly positive in the secondary stage, continuing into the tertiary stage. The same is true of pinta, except that positive reactions are less common in the primary stage.

Tests with treponemes (TPI etc.) and fluorescent antibody tests are difficult to carry out in field conditions, but are positive in yaws as in syphilis (Hackett 1967).

How far the antibodies detected in these serological tests reflect resistance or immunity is problematical, since C-F and flocculating antibodies are not necessarily protective. Susceptibility to infection, however, does seem to increase in a community as the proportion of seroreactors falls, and we assume that a seronegative person is susceptible to infection.

A few actual experiments have been made in man to test immunity to re-infection with *T. pertenue,* and these indicate that resistance to homologous treponemes develops early, but that resistance to heterologous treponemes (such

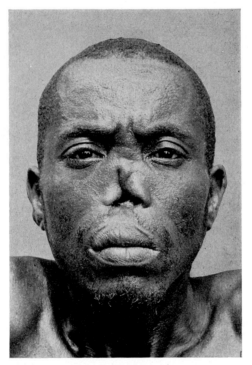

Fig. 156.—Gangosa. (*Dr C. J. Hackett; by courtesy of the Wellcome Museum of Medical Science*)

as would reflect actual field conditions) develops slowly over a period of years. Immunity is more evident in patients who maintain a latent state for 2 years or more than in those who have had treatment for active lesions within the previous year.

Cure, with gradual loss of acquired immunity, may occur at any stage during a latent phase, and during the secondary stage reinfection may then occur, though the lesions may be modified as a result of residual immunity. The same is true of the tertiary stage.

Immunity to yaws probably carries cross-immunity to syphilis, and vice versa, though in some areas of the world the two diseases apparently coexist, and primary chancres have developed in subjects with old latent yaws who were subsequently inoculated with *T. pallidum*.

CLINICAL FEATURES

The course of yaws may be divided into primary, secondary and tertiary stages (Fig. 159), with latent periods between them. It may go on to spontaneous cure without treatment, or it may lead to extremely painful and destructive lesions of skin and bones. Hackett (1951) sets out the course diagrammatically, and this may be interpreted as in Fig. 160.

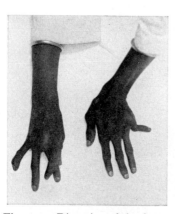

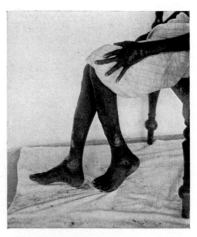

Fig. 157.—Distortion of the fingers in tertiary yaws.

Fig. 158.—Tibial periosteal nodes, ulcers and deformity of the phalanges in yaws.

Primary (Hackett 1946; Turner 1959)

The incubation period varies from about 10 to 45 days. The primary lesion or chancre develops at the site of inoculation, though a few patients may not notice this. The lesion is proliferative, developing to a papilloma exuding serum rich in treponemes, and therefore highly infectious. Local lymph nodes are usually enlarged but do not suppurate.

This primary papilloma persists usually for 6–9 months, sometimes up to 12, resolving spontaneously and leaving a scar. Occasionally it ulcerates, as a result of bacterial infection.

Primary lesions of the soles of the feet are uncommon, but may occur on the outer edges or between the toes.

Secondary

General (Hackett 1946; Turner 1959). The secondary stage usually erupts 6–16 weeks after the appearance of the primary lesion, but may do so at any time from 3 weeks to 2 years; the 2 stages may therefore overlap. Lesions of secondary type may develop years after the earliest manifestations of infection have healed.

The secondary stage may be ushered in with pains in the bones, joints, loins

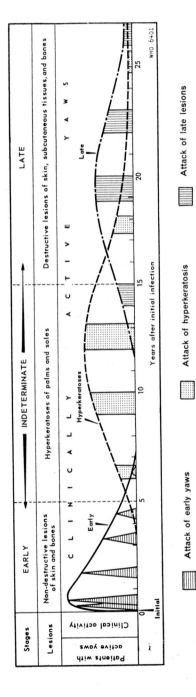

Fig. 159.—The clinical course of untreated yaws. The diagram attempts to show what types of lesion might be expected in patients from the time of infection onwards. Adequate data based on long periods of observation of individual patients are not available. The time relations of this diagram are based on observations for 1–2 years of patients at various times after infection. The relapsing of clinical manifestations is clearly indicated. When no clinical manifestations are present in an infected person, that person's infection is in the latent stage: the diagram stresses how such cases may relapse with active lesions during the first few years of infection and later with hyperkeratosis or late lesions. For each person with active yaws, there are probably 2–4 persons without active lesions who are seroreactors and thus latent cases. (*After Hackett & Guthe 1956*)

and head, and fever. Secondary lesions of the skin are usually multiple, disseminated and proliferative, containing many treponemes; they heal without permanent trace.

The early disseminated lesions are due to treponemes carried in the blood from the primary lesion, or to local spread by lymphatics. These lesions are usually exudative, but may be dry. The serum exuding from them contains treponemes, and even non-exudative lesions, especially papules, contain them. Secondary lesions are therefore infectious.

There is no definite evidence of involvement of the eyes, cardiovascular system or central nervous system, in spite of the fact that treponemes at this stage are blood-borne. At this stage generalized enlargement of the lymph nodes is not notable.

Secondary skin lesions (cutaneous early yaws). These may be divided into 2 groups, major and minor framboesides.

The major framboesides are large raised papillomas and papules, in which exudation of highly infectious serum is a feature. They are discoid, annular, crescentic or irregular in shape. They occur on any part of the body—limbs, face, body and anogenital region (which should always be examined in children).

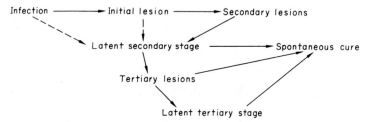

Fig. 160.—The course of yaws.

The anal condylomas are often large and bilaterally contiguous; they ooze serum containing many treponemes. In debilitated patients shallow ulcers may form and become covered by crusts resembling oyster shells (rupia).

The papular form consists of much smaller lesions about the size of a small grain of rice. They may be very numerous, simulating the rash of chickenpox or smallpox, and they may be umbilicate.

The minor framboesides are less obvious, and are easily missed. They are small and dry. They may occur as small papules or collections of small pale buff-coloured lesions, slightly raised, with flat tops. They are scattered over the trunk, and may itch.

Squamous macular framboesides are 12·5–25 mm in diameter, and are sometimes confluent. The edges may be pigmented and desquamating. Erythematous macular framboesides are rare; the erythema is transient.

Secondary lesions of the buccal mucous membrane and of the vagina have been reported.

Secondary plantar lesions. Plantar lesions are common and often painful; the sole is the commonest site of infectious recurrences.

In communities accustomed to walking barefoot, the foot is constantly subject to trauma, and hyperkeratosis is the normal response. There may also be cracks, pitting, erosions and maceration. The plantar and palmar skin may develop diffuse non-ulcerative dermatitis, with permanent sequelae.

Secondary plantar papillomas are quite common as part of a generalized eruption, but they are most important as the commonest infectious lesions to reappear later, possibly appearing up to 20 years after the main eruption. They take longer to erupt than elsewhere on the skin. They are constantly disturbed by trauma, and scabs are rare. Papillomas of long duration tend to develop a firm dry centre, but with a gap between the hard core and the margin. On healing there is a flat-bottomed crater in which the skin appears to be normal.

Lesions which could appear as macules on the skin elsewhere may occur on the soles; they have a papular element.

Squamous macular framboesides are flat or slightly raised areas, firmer and paler than the unaffected parts. They are dry, and measure 6–30 mm across, but may be confluent. They eventually desquamate, leaving erythematous patches in the soft soles of young people.

Hyperkeratotic macular framboesides are similar to squamous macular framboesides but are exaggerated because of the abnormally thick skin of the soles; they are rare in young people but common in older people. They crack and become fissured. They often involve the sides of the feet and the clefts between the toes. They may be painful. Spontaneous healing occurs, but treatment helps.

Secondary bone lesions. Bones are commonly affected in yaws; 15–20% of patients voluntarily attending clinics may have obvious lesions. Bone pain is a common complaint; it is a deep-seated ache, worse at night and aggravated by damp conditions. It may be present in the absence of radiographic changes, but is commonly associated with such changes.

Bone lesions are common in the stage of active secondary skin lesions. The changes consist fundamentally of osteoperiostitis with cortical rarefaction and periosteal deposits, going on to cortical thickening and bony expansion. Spontaneous healing occurs within a few months, without ulceration.

The bones involved, in order of frequency, are the ulna, the hand bones, tibia and fibula, the foot bones and the radius. Polydactilitis is not uncommon in children. Goundou may occur. There may occasionally be ganglion of the wrist.

In the secondary stage the tibiae are commonly bowed, with thickening and expansion of the cortex, and periosteal deposits.

Tertiary

Tertiary skin lesions (Turner 1959). These are gummas, which pass through 4 stages—nodule, central necrosis and abscess formation, rupture and ulceration and healing with scarring. The gummatous process may be superficial, or may involve the subcutaneous tissues as well as the skin.

The localized gumma begins as a small painless nodule, enlarging to about 2·5 cm across. There are no signs of acute inflammation though softening is present. The skin above this abscess ultimately gives way and the contents are discharged, leaving an ulcer with a yellowish slough, later showing irregular granulations becoming indurated. The gummas are often grouped, and may coalesce; they can persist for years. Secondary infection may involve deeper structures, tendons and joints. When they ultimately heal they leave thin depigmented scars.

A localized gumma may arise secondary to underlying osteitis, particularly on the skull, face, sternum and superficial bones of the extremities.

Serpiginous (spreading) gummas start as small nodules tending to coalesce and break down, resulting in an area of affected skin which spreads centrifugally, and may be enormous. The centre of the area tends to heal while the edge is still spreading. Keloid formation is common. Scars from these processes may produce contractures of joints, crippling or disfigurement, even a form of elephantiasis.

Epithelioma formation has been observed in a yaws ulcer.

Tertiary plantar and palmar lesions (Hackett 1946; Turner 1959). Tertiary palmar lesions are much less common than plantar lesions. Tertiary lesions tend to be diffuse, the margins are often ill defined, and the pathological processes affect deeper tissues. They may appear within a few years of first infection. Lesions of secondary and tertiary yaws are never observed in the same patient at the same time, nor is the initial lesion present when tertiary lesions have developed.

The outstanding feature of tertiary lesions is hyperkeratosis. The lesions are probably due to a diffuse chronic inflammatory process which tends to affect all layers of the skin. These lesions may persist for months or years, but eventually spontaneous arrest occurs, leaving permanent changes due to fibrosis. The skin is thin but stiff and smooth, and there may be contractures of the fingers.

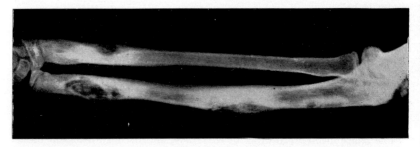

Fig. 161.—Gummatous osteitis of the radius and ulna in yaws. (*Dr C. J. Hackett*)

Depigmentation (leucoderma) is common, especially of the hands and feet, often bilateral. The Kahn reaction is positive.

Tertiary bone lesions (Hackett 1951; Turner 1959). The bone lesions of this stage are due to periostitis, gummatous osteitis (Fig. 161) or a combination of the two. Gummas may become necrotic and involve overlying tissues, going on to ulceration. These changes lead to well defined rarefied areas in the cortex, either large or small. Pathological fractures are not uncommon.

There are tender swellings, and the skin over some bony swellings is tense and shiny, with induration of the soft tissues. Bone pain is common.

The earliest change is cortical thickening, with multiple rarefied foci, especially in the tibia, but also in all bones of the leg and arm. A characteristic result of cortical thickening due to organizing periosteal deposits is the condition known as sabre tibia, and, in Australia, boomerang leg (Hackett 1936). Nodular swellings are sometimes found on the skull, and swelling of the hand bones is not rare (the foot bones are less frequently involved), and the sternum and clavicles may be affected. Ulceration may occur over these bony lesions.

Fluid may be found in some joints, especially the knees (hydrarthrosis).

Lesions of the hand may consist of minor thickening and expansion of the metacarpals and phalanges, or of destructive focal rarefactions with periosteal deposits, which sometimes result in shortening of the bones, or even complete destruction of a phalanx. There may be sinus formation, spontaneous fracture and deformity.

Bone lesions of the foot resemble those of the hand, but extensive damage is not common. Pain and swelling are constant. The tarsal bones may be affected, and sinuses may form. Metatarsals and phalanges may also be involved.

In the skull there are localized thickenings of the calvarium. These nodes are rounded swellings 40 mm or more in diameter and raised. The centre is usually fluctuant, with an indurated rim attached to the bone. They may resolve or ulcerate. The bone may be rarefied in the area.

Gangosa is sometimes seen, or collapse of the nose with perforating ulceration of the palate. It usually starts as a painful ulcer on the palate or nasal septum, spreading to perforation and destruction of the turbinates, and to the pharynx, causing dysphagia. A dirty nasal discharge may be due to gangosa of parts inaccessible to direct examination in the field, and a voice suggesting cleft palate may have a much more serious cause. Gangosa, however, often responds to penicillin or arsenicals.

Goundou involving the nasal processes of the maxillae bilaterally, is one form of yaws osteitis. It is not found in some areas (such as the Far East) where yaws is endemic, and doubt has been expressed as to its aetiology. It usually begins in childhood, though adults may be attacked. There is a discharge from the nostrils and the formation of small bony swellings on either side of the nose, not involving the cartilages. The swellings persist and can grow to a large size, tending to obstruct the nostrils, and sometimes involving the hard palate. In the early stages goundou may respond to medical treatment, but in the later stages the bone may have to be removed surgically.

Apropos of the bone lesions of yaws and syphilis, Hackett (1951) states that 'apart from the absence of osteochondritis in yaws, there are probably no bone lesions that occur in one disease that may not be observed in the other'.

TREATMENT

The treatment of yaws has been revolutionized by penicillin to which, like *T. pallidum*, *T. pertenue* is very sensitive; the early stages of yaws respond to a single intramuscular injection of PAM.

The minimum total dosage of PAM recommended by WHO (1960) is:

Age-group	Early and late active cases	Latent cases and contacts
Under 15	0·6 mega unit	0·3 mega unit
15 and over	1·2 mega units	0·6 mega unit

These doses can be given in a single intramuscular injection.

For mass campaigns, when the prevalence of clinically active cases in a community is over 10%, total mass treatment (TMT) should be given, i.e. all patients with clinically active yaws should be given the full dose; the remainder of the population should be given half doses.

In areas of lower incidence of active cases (5–10%), in addition to the actual patients (at full doses), all children under the age of puberty, and contacts, are treated with half doses (juvenile mass treatment, JMT).

If the incidence of active yaws is under 5%, selective mass treatment (SMT) may be given. In this only those with active disease (full doses), and their contacts (half doses) are treated.

Late yaws may require longer treatment, and a dosage of 0·6 mega unit of

PAM, given daily or twice weekly for 15–20 doses has been suggested, corresponding to the treatment of late syphilis.

In all mass campaigns, re-surveys at various intervals are important. These treatment policies have been widely adopted with great success, but they depend on careful organization and supervision to detect cases, assess conditions, and ensure acceptable response on the part of the people.

Similar treatment schedules may be used for endemic syphilis where the prevalence of clinically active disease is 3% or more.

For pinta a single dose of 1·2 mega units is satisfactory.

Penicillin, as is well known, may give rise to reactions, sometimes fatal. The fatalities have been estimated at slightly more than 1 per million injections

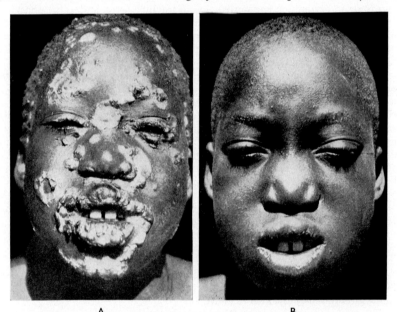

A.   B.

Fig. 162.—Secondary yaws. A, Papillomas in various stages of activity. B, After penicillin treatment. The absence of scarring is well shown. (*Dr C. J. Hackett*)

(WHO 1960); non-fatal anaphylactic reactions probably number 10 times as many.

For the treatment of these reactions, immediate and repeated injections of adrenaline are essential, and prolonged administration of anti-histamine drugs. An emergency kit of suitable anti-shock drugs, portable oxygen and steroids should be available for immediate use (WHO 1960). The procedure recommended is:

1. Immediately on the appearance of signs of reaction, the patient should be made to lie down (head down, feet up).
2. 0·5–1·0 ml of adrenaline (1 in 1000) should be injected subcutaneously into the upper arm.
3. If there is no immediate response the adrenaline should be repeated, or 25–100 mg cortisone should be given by intramuscular injection, or the same dose of hydrocortisone intravenously.

4. In angioneurotic oedema, urticaria or conjunctivitis, antihistamines should be given intramuscularly or intravenously.
5. If there is cough, dyspnoea, respiratory distress or substantial discomfort, a slow intravenous injection of 0·25–0·5 gramme aminophylline can used (WHO 1960).

Apart from penicillin, other antibiotics can be used: chlortetracycline (Aureomycin), oxytetracycline (Terramycin), tetracycline (Achromycin), chloramphenicol (Chloromycetin) and others.

Dosage (for adults) is:

Chlortetracycline 2·0 grammes (divided) daily for 5 days.

Oxytetracycline, 3·0 grammes (divided) on the first day, 2·0 on the second and third days.

Other antibiotics are given on similar lines.

Old treatments with bismuth preparations and neoarsphenamine have now been superseded.

PREVENTION

The prevention of yaws (and also of endemic syphilis and pinta in their endemic areas) depends upon deliberate treatment campaigns to eliminate infectious lesions and relapses. These can be conducted from existing hospitals and dispensaries or by travelling teams. Contact tracing is important.

Medical officers and other personnel, and heads of village communities (and school-teachers) should be alert to the possibility of new cases arriving in areas in which the incidence is thought to be low. If such cases are found, the SMT programme of treatment should be instituted.

In the long term, much can be done by raising the standard of living and of education of the people. The provision, for instance, of adequate and safe water supplies—and of soap—by promoting skin cleanliness, would help enormously in yaws and perhaps in pinta, as it does in so many unrelated diseases, such as trachoma. These treponematoses are diseases of relatively primitive rural communities, and would disappear in better conditions—to be replaced, perhaps, by venereal syphilis picked up in towns where prostitution is likely to be rife.

Pinta (Carate, Mal Del Pinto)

Pinta is endemic only in the Americas, from Mexico and Cuba, through Central America, to parts of sub-tropical South America down to the upper Amazon basin, where the incidence in some areas is high. Conditions resembling pinta reported from the Pacific areas are likely to be 'pintoid' yaws (Fig. 163).

AETIOLOGY

As stated above, *T. carateum* cannot be differentiated from *T. pallidum* and *T. pertenue*; like them, it has not been cultivated in artificial media, but it has successfully been inoculated into chimpanzees. See also pages 561 and 581.

TRANSMISSION

Congenital transmission does not occur.

T. carateum is present in the skin lesions, especially early lesions, wherever

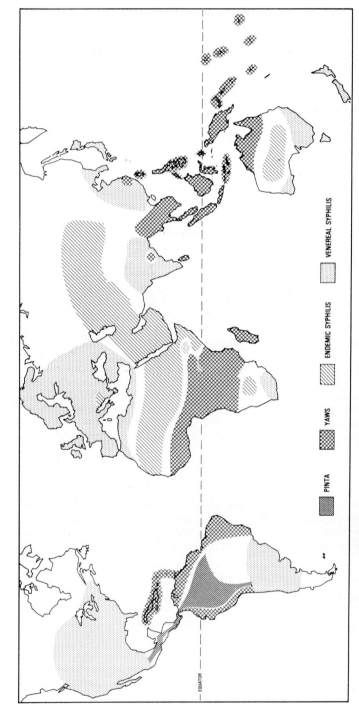

Fig. 163. Probable geographical distribution of the treponematoses about A.D. 1900 (*After Hackett 1963*)

they are. The lesions tend to be dry and scaly, rather than exudative, but the papules are itchy, and scratching can cause excoriation and fissuring of the skin, releasing serum to the surface; in this serum the treponemes are abundant, and if it finds its way to the skin of another person, especially if abraded, transmission is possible. Treponemes can be found in fluid expressed from the lesions on examination with dark ground illumination. They have also been found in abrasions of the skin of infected persons, and in material obtained by puncture of lymph nodes.

Direct contact is therefore the route of transmission, but venereal transmission via the genitalia is not a feature, since lesions of the genitalia are unusual. Pinta is often a house disease.

Individual lesions remain infectious for many years; there are no latent, non-infectious periods, such as occur in the other treponematoses.

PATHOLOGY

The treponemes are chiefly located in the Malpighian cells, especially in small areas of acanthosis in the epidermis. They are present in primary lesions and in fluid from such lesions.

The initial lesions in pinta are never moist, or necrotic, and the epithelium is intact unless broken or excoriated. The earliest papule begins with acanthosis and diffuse round cell infiltration of subepithelial tissues and the rete malpighii. The involvement of the epidermis never proceeds to intradermal abscess formation such as is seen in secondary yaws. The blood vessels and lymphatics are dilated but the intima and media of the vessel walls are not affected even in long-standing lesions.

In the secondary pintid the localization of the infiltration (often rich in plasma cells) about the vessels of the cutis is characteristic. The elastic tissue is rarefied and stretched.

In later pintids a hyperkeratosis may develop which, together with existing local oedema of the cutis, leads to progressive atrophy and flattening of the rete malpighii. There is diffuse infiltration of the corium, and perivascular nodulation of the deeper cutis. In the later lesions the inflammatory changes recede, pigment is reduced or atrophied and may collect and clump in the deep cutis. In this stage depigmented leucodermic areas coexist with blue, red or copper-coloured lesions. Eventually there may be accumulations of epithelioid cells, but no changes occur in the walls of the blood vessels (Hasselmann 1955).

IMMUNOLOGY

Léon y Blanco (1940) has successfully inoculated *T. carateum* into persons with advanced syphilis, and a patient with pinta may develop an unmodified syphilitic chancre. Yaws can develop in a pinta subject, and pinta can develop in persons who have had yaws. There seems, therefore, to be no protection in pinta against the other treponematoses, though sera from pinta patients react to the same antigens as sera from subject with yaws, venereal and non-venereal syphilis. The tests reveal no differences between the treponemes causing these conditions.

In pinta the total prevalence of clinically active disease approaches that of the seroreactors, which might be as high as 80%, because latency apparently does not occur. Yet one attack of pinta does not protect against reinfection.

CLINICAL FEATURES

Primary

Primary lesions are almost always found on uncovered parts of the body— leg or dorsum of the foot (common), thigh, buttock, forearm or dorsum of the hand (common), arm, face, neck. The lesion appears as an itchy erythematous papule after an incubation period of 7–20 days, becoming in 30–50 days an erythematous raised squamous patch, round which other papules may develop and spread.

Secondary

In the secondary stage there are skin rashes or multiplication of papules described as pintids and seen 5–12 months after the primary lesions, which themselves continue to develop. These lesions are widespread. Hyperchromic patches may appear in the mouth. Generalized lymphadenitis is fairly common.

Tertiary

In the third stage pigment changes occur, with coloured or blanched spots, keratoderma or superficial atrophy. The lesions may be grey, with bluish tones, or almost black, red or copper-coloured. They are round, oval or irregular, not elevated, but always strikingly visible. Pruritus is marked.

Hyperkeratosis has been said to occur on the palms and soles in the late stages, but Hackett (1963) does not accept the diagnosis, considering that they may have been confused with hyperkeratosis due to yaws. There are no lesions of bone, heart, brain or other viscera.

DIAGNOSIS

Treponemes can be found in fluid expressed from the early lesions especially, but even from those of all stages, and examined under dark ground illumination. Fungi from the surface of the skin have often been seen and wrongly considered to be the cause of the condition. They should be ignored. The appearance of the patient with developed pinta is striking.

The characteristic colour, or depigmentation, of the skin gives the clue to diagnosis in endemic areas, but depigmented patches of skin are occasionally found in tertiary yaws, and may resemble those of pinta. Pinta is also to be differentiated from leprosy, vitiligo and other skin conditions.

Serological tests of the reagin type become positive 2–4 months after onset, and are usually positive at high titre thereafter.

TREATMENT

Treatment rests on penicillin and other antibiotics, in the same dosages as for yaws.

REFERENCES

HACKETT, C. J. (1936) *Boomerang Leg and Yaws in Australian Aborigines*, Monograph 1. London: Royal Society for Tropical Medicine and Hygiene.
—— (1946) *Trans. R. Soc. trop. Med. Hyg.*, **40**, 206.
—— (1951) *Bone Lesions of Yaws In Uganda*. Oxford: Blackwell.
—— (1963) *Bull. Wld Hlth Org.*, **29**, 7.

HACKETT, C. J. (1967) *Trans. R. Soc. trop. Med. Hyg.*, **61**, 148.
—— & GUTHE, T. (1956) *Bull. Wld Hlth Org.*, **15**, 869.
HASSELMANN, C. M. (1955) *Arch. klin. exp. Derm.*, **201**, 1 (Abst. *Trop. Dis. Bull.* (1957) **54**, 295).
HILL, K. R., KODIJAT, R. & SARDADI, M. (1951) *Monograph Ser. W.H.O.*, 5.
HUDSON, E. H. (1958) *Non-venereal Syphilis: A Sociological and Medical Study of Bejel*. Edinburgh & London: Livingstone.
LÉON Y BLANCO, F. (1940) *Revta Med. trop. Parasit.*, Habana, **6**, 13, 21, 39, 43, 47, 49.
MOLLARET, H. H. & FRIBOURG-BLANC, A. (1967) *Méd. Afr. noire*, **14**, 397
TURNER, L. H. (1959) *Bull. Inst. med. Res. Malaya*, 9.
WORLD HEALTH ORGANIZATION (1960) *Wld Hlth Org. tech. Rep. Ser.*, 5.

Relapsing Fever

Synonyms

Recurrent fever; spirillum fever; famine fever; tick fever; tick-bite fever.

Definition

A febrile disease caused by organisms of the genus *Borrelia*, characterized by febrile relapses, and transmitted by lice or ticks. In some parts of the world tick-borne relapsing fever is a zoonosis; louse-borne relapsing fever is not.

GEOGRAPHICAL DISTRIBUTION

The two forms—louse-borne and tick-borne—are found in conditions where lice and soft ticks respectively are prevalent.

The louse-borne form is largely a disease of people living in squalor where clothing (in which lice thrive) is worn continuously and where bodily cleanliness is poor. It is specially prevalent in conditions of famine where people tend to crowd together in the search for food; in such conditions lice travel easily from one person to another. In the past it has often been associated with louse-borne typhus. It is still prevalent in Ethiopia where over 5000 cases per annum have recently been reported, though the true incidence is probably much higher.

Tick-borne relapsing fever is prevalent in the Near East and southern U.S.S.R., the Mediterranean basin including Spain, North Africa and Israel, Africa south of the Sahara, southern U.S.A. and Central and South America.

AETIOLOGY

The genus *Borrelia* includes:

Louse-borne
   B. recurrentis

Tick-borne

B. duttoni	Africa
B. latychevi	Iran
B. persica	Asia
B. hispanica	Spain (south), Spanish Africa
B. parkeri	
B. turicatae	North America
B. hermsi	
B. venezuelensis	Central and South America

B. recurrentis does not infect ticks, but there is evidence that *B. duttoni* can infect lice. The others are distinguished by their antigenic structure, virulence for laboratory animals, and specificity for ticks.

They are spiral organisms, actively motile, some 6–10 μm in length, with 5–10 fairly regular but loose waves; they multiply by transverse fission. They can be found in blood smears, lying among the red cells, and they stain easily with Giemsa and Leishman. They are best seen by dark-ground illumination, in which their motility can be demonstrated. They are most likely to be found during the first paroxysm of fever, less so in subsequent paroxysms. They are more easily detected in louse-borne than in tick-borne relapsing fever.

These organisms are difficult to cultivate either in the test-tube or in the fertile egg, and are best conserved by animal inoculation (Wilson & Miles 1964). But *B. duttoni* has been grown on the chorioallantoic membrane of fertile eggs, and this has provided the antigen for a complement fixation test.

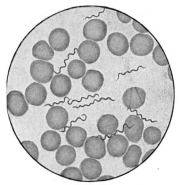

Fig. 164.—*Borrelia recurrentis* in a blood film. × 500. (*Dr John Bell*)

TRANSMISSION

The louse-borne form is transmitted from man to man by *Pediculus humanus* var. *corporis* and can be transmitted by *P. h.* var. *capitis*. The organisms are taken up when the louse feeds on the host's blood, passing through the louse stomach into the haemocoele and thence to all the tissues of the louse body, including the legs, where they multiply. Within 6 days they are numerous in the haemocoele. They do not return to the feeding apparatus, and infect man only when the louse is crushed on the skin. They are not transmitted from lice to their offspring.

In human beings transplacental transmission (and abortion) is not uncommon in louse-borne relapsing fever.

The tick-borne form is different. It is transmitted by soft ticks of the genus *Ornithodorus*. Soon after a blood meal the organisms disappear from the tick digestive tract, but are found in the haemocoele and various organs, including the coxal glands, salivary glands (in nymphs) and ovaries, where they multiply. They are not found in tick faeces.

Infection of a susceptible animal can take place through the bite of an infected tick, which is a relatively large puncture, into which infected saliva is pumped, or which may be the portal of entry of coxal fluid, secreted while the tick is feeding. The organisms can also penetrate intact mucous membranes or skin. Infection can also be caused in drug addicts who use unsterilized syringes.

A tick remains infected for many years, and transmits the organisms to its offspring; the organisms therefore perpetuate themselves enzootically in the ticks without need for other hosts, to the extent of at least 5 generations of ticks. The organisms can also infect and survive in lice, without change.

Tick-borne relapsing fever is carried from certain animals to man, or from man to man, and is therefore a zoonosis. The ticks live in warm climates, and the disease is found in southern Europe, the Near East, Asia, Africa and the Americas.

In Central, East and South Africa man is the reservoir, but in North Africa, the Eastern Mediterranean region, Central Asia, tropical and subtropical America and many parts of the United States it is primarily a disease of rodents, transmitted only incidentally to man. The rodents live in open country, in holes, caves and burrows; they do not tend to infest human dwellings.

Animal hosts also include monkeys, squirrels, chipmunks, rats, hedgehogs and possibly bats and other cave-dwelling mammals.

Ticks concerned in transmission include:

Ornithodorus marocanus	Spain, Morocco
O. erraticus	Portugal, North Africa
O. tartakovskii	Iran
O. verrucosus	Iran
O. crossi	Asia
O. lahorensis	Asia
O. tholozani	Asia
O. moubata	Africa
O. porcinus domesticus	Africa
O. hermsi	North America
O. parkeri	North America
O. savignyi	Africa
O. talaje	Central America
O. turicata	Central America
O. rudis (venezuelensis)	South America

Walton (1957) points out that in East Africa *O. moubata* is of two kinds, one of which prefers to feed on chickens and is therefore abundant in houses in which chickens are kept, and the other feeds preferably on man, and is therefore more prominent in houses in which chickens are not kept. The chicken feeders are associated with hotter conditions, the man feeders with cooler, wet climates. Relative humidity appears to be more important than temperature in the biological differentiation of these ticks.

O. porcinus domesticus (which belongs to the *O. moubata* complex) is primarily a parasite of man and is found at all altitudes; it is favoured by high rainfall and high relative humidity. It is a better vector than *O. moubata* (Walton 1961). It is widely distributed in African dwellings at all altitudes in eastern Africa.

In human beings transplacental infection has been reported in tick-borne relapsing fever.

EPIDEMIOLOGY

The epidemiology of relapsing fever depends on the mode of transmission and the habits of the arthropod vectors.

Louse-borne

Man is the only host, apart from lice, which are prevalent in conditions of poverty and uncleanliness of body and clothing. Once the infection is introduced into lice, it can spread as an epidemic in human communities where people are crowded together. Lice leave the bodies of dead persons and seek their blood meals among the living. The epidemiology of louse-borne relapsing fever differs from that of louse-borne typhus in that typhus can be (and often is) contracted through inhaling dried, infected louse faeces in dust from clothing, whereas relapsing fever is not, because louse faeces do not contain infective *Borrelia*. In combined epidemics (as in Ireland in the nineteenth century) doctors attending the sick in their homes often contracted typhus through inhalation, but did not contract relapsing fever, because they themselves were free from lice.

Tick-borne

Tick-borne relapsing fever, on the other hand, does not usually spread in epidemic form; it is a disease of places normally inhabited by soft ticks which, unlike lice, do not live in clothing or on the bodies of people, but in crevices of walls and floors of houses, in animal burrows and in caves. They feed on animals or man at long intervals, transmitting the infection as they do so. This disease is therefore a disease of places, associated particularly with rest houses, caves (for instance in Cyprus and dry river beds in the Jordan valley) and animal burrows in bush country. Travellers, hunters, trappers and campers are at risk.

Man can be infected through contamination of a wound, or even of the conjunctival sac or nasal mucosa, by the blood of an infected animal; laboratory infections of this kind are not uncommon (Wilson & Miles 1964).

PATHOLOGY

The borreliae circulate and multiply in the body fluids, producing toxic metabolites which mainly affect the parenchyma cells of the liver, the spleen cells and the endothelial cells of the blood vessels.

The general features found post mortem are jaundice, congestion of the organs and petechial haemorrhages in the pleura, lungs, heart, brain, kidneys, stomach and intestines.

In the liver borreliae accumulate and multiply, causing focal necrosis of the parenchyma cells, which they invade. The fixed phagocytes do not respond to live borreliae, but do ingest dead ones. Shortly before the crisis the borreliae roll up and are taken in by the endothelial cells of the liver, spleen and bone marrow. Surviving borreliae remain in these organs and in the brain until the next relapse (Felsenfeld 1965).

In the spleen the borreliae accumulate and multiply in the sinuses, causing cellular infiltration; they may enter the endothelial cells and cause infarcts and necrosis; they can be demonstrated in the infarcts. The spleen is large, soft and red, and perisplenitis is common. Borreliae may also be found in the kidneys.

In the blood vessels the damage to the endothelium tends to cause haemorrhage, which may show as petechiae on the skin.

The bone marrow is hyperaemic. There is polymorphonuclear leucocytosis, and borreliae may sometimes be seen within the polymorphs. Lymph glands may be involved.

The heart shows cloudy swelling. Bronchopneumonia is common.

The borreliae are distinctly neurotropic, affecting the meninges and central nervous system. In infected animals they may be found in the brain and cerebellum as much as a year after infection. In the brain they are found in capillaries. There are no changes in the nerve cells, but there is intense microglial reaction in the cortex. Meningitis is sometimes found.

IMMUNOLOGY

Borreliae appear in the peripheral blood, and are often numerous, at the height of the first bout of fever, though they may even then be scanty in some patients. This blood infection is heavier in louse-borne than in tick-borne fever, especially during the first bout of fever.

After the fever subsides the organisms can be found microscopically in the blood in only a small proportion of patients, but at the onset of a relapse they again appear, though not always in such numbers as in the first attack. This cycle is repeated in subsequent relapses. During the intervals between relapses the organisms remain latent, probably especially in the central nervous system (Felsenfeld & Wolf 1969).

During the infection antibodies are formed by the immunologically active cells of the lymph glands, chiefly agglutinins, immobilizing antibodies, spirochaeticidins and lysins. They are apparently able to overcome the blood infection but not to eliminate the organisms from the tissues. There are also leucotactic serum bodies which promote phagocytosis. Relapse occurs when these antibodies decrease in the blood, allowing the tissue borreliae to emerge. The borreliae are antigenically unstable, and the relapse forms are antigenically different from the original forms, provoking new and different antibodies, which then can eliminate them from the blood. After one or more relapses the active immunity developed is enough to prevent further invasion of the blood, but the organisms may remain alive in the tissues, and this latent infection may, in some conditions, break through, to give further impetus to the production of immune globulins.

In *B. turicatae* infection of experimental animals, IgG, IgA, IgM and IgD immunoglobulins have been found; IgM responses were the earliest and strongest, and most adhesin–lysin activity was associated with this immunoglobulin. Later, IgG production replaced initial IgM responses in many infections (Felsenfeld & Wolf 1969).

Of the antigenic factors analysed, 2 were strain- and relapse-specific. Human sera had strong immobilizing and lytic activity, the lytic activity depending on complement (Felsenfeld *et al.* 1965).

CLINICAL FEATURES

Louse-borne (epidemic cosmopolitan type) (Bryceson *et al.* 1970)

After an incubation period of 2–10 days (usually 4–8) the onset is sudden, with chill and fever to 40–40·5°C (104–105°F), or even higher (when the patient may become delirious). He sits or lies on the ground, silent, with glazed expression, apathetic manner, mentally dull or confused. There is dizziness, severe headache and pain in the back, chest, abdomen, legs (especially the calves) and joints. Nausea and vomiting, dysphagia, cough and dyspnoea are fairly common. The sputum may contain borreliae. The spleen is often enlarged, sometimes very enlarged, and has been known to rupture spontaneously. The liver is also often enlarged, and jaundice is common—laboratory tests indicate extensive hepatocellular damage. Relapsing fever should therefore be remembered in the diagnosis of jaundice. There may be albuminuria.

The blood may show polymorphonuclear leucocytosis of 15 000–30 000. Bleeding often occurs into the skin (petechiae), especially over flanks and shoulders, and into mucous membranes, and epistaxis is quite common, indicating a haemorrhagic type of infection. Conjunctival vessels are congested and may bleed. Clumps of adherent borreliae become impacted in capillaries and enmesh red cells, causing rupture of the capillaries and bleeding. There may possibly be widespread intravascular coagulation. Secondary anaemia develops.

Complications include pneumonia, which may be a leading feature (pneumonic type), nephritis, parotitis, meningism, meningo-encephalitis, diarrhoea (pseudo-dysenteric type), arthritis, neuritis, ophthalmia and iritis.

The attack commonly lasts 5–7 days, and the temperature then drops by crisis to 36°C (96·8°F), or even lower (when there may be a state of collapse), with profuse sweating, diarrhoea, weakness and relief from pain.

In Ethiopian cases myocardial damage is not uncommon on the day of crisis, with prolonged QTc, altered T waves, pulse over 100, systolic blood pressure of 90 or less, gallop sounds and reversed splitting of the second sound in the pulmonary area. There may be a phase of critically low cardiac output, due to myocardial damage. These effects mostly disappear after treatment.

Relapse occurs 5–9 days after the first attack in two-thirds of the patients, and is rather less severe—there is no rash; a second relapse tends to occur in one-quarter of the patients. Relapses are fewer than in the tick-borne form, and it is said that there are never more than 4. Case mortality is usually around 2–9%,

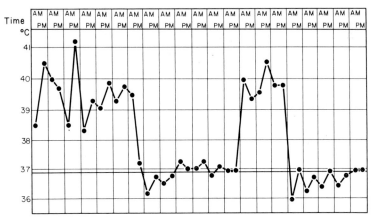

Fig. 165.—Temperature chart of relapsing fever, cosmopolitan louse-borne type.

but 12% has been recorded. Death occurs in the first attack, whereas in the tick-borne form it occurs later. The causes of death are haemorrhage due to prothrombin deficiency, hepatic coma, myocarditis and disseminated vascular coagulation. In the crisis (see above) death may be due to hyperpyrexia with convulsions, heart failure, shock or cerebral oedema. Death is usually sudden and unexpected, and may occur shortly after treatment has been given.

In areas where louse-borne relapsing fever occurs it is as well to remember that louse-borne typhus is also likely to occur. The two have been known to be present in the same patient.

Tick-borne

The incubation period may be quite short (1–2 days has been reported in the Spanish form), but more usually is longer, up to 14 days.

The primary attack begins abruptly with severe headache and the usual symptoms and signs of fever up to 40°C (104°F). The attack may be fulminating, leading to coma and death in a day or two; on the other hand it may take the form of a chronic low fever.

During this attack the spleen often (up to 45%) becomes enlarged and may develop infarcts and haemorrhage. The liver also enlarges (11%) and jaundice is quite common, and may be intense. The patient may have diarrhoea, and bronchitis and pneumonia may develop. Massive haematuria and mild nephritis have been recorded in Israel (Eisenberg *et al.* 1968).

There is polymorphonuclear leucocytosis, and slight microcytic anaemia.

The organisms are not as numerous in the blood as in the louse-borne form; they are neurotropic, having a distinct affinity for the nervous system. They may be present in the cerebrospinal fluid, detected either microscopically or by inoculation of animals. Lymphocytic meningitis sometimes occurs, and even subarachnoid haemorrhage; the fluid is under pressure and shows pleocytosis. This meningitic form is common in Europeans in the Dakar area, where Africans are more prone to pulmonary and hepatic affections.

The cranial nerves are sometimes affected; optic atrophy occurs very occasionally, but more often there is ophthalmoplegia and facial paralysis (in 22% of one series in North Africa). In the central nervous system there may be serious complications, with aphasia and hemiparesis; signs of encephalitis have been noted. Iritis and iridocyclitis are not uncommon. Arthritis is also not uncommon.

It has been noticed that tick-borne relapsing fever, which is an endemic rather than an epidemic disease, is considerably more severe in newcomers to the endemic areas than in the indigenous people, who have probably acquired some resistance as a result of earlier infection.

The primary attack may last 4–5 days (rather less in the African form), ending in crisis. Sometimes the crisis leads to collapse, in which adrenaline may be called for. Relapses tend to occur at intervals which may be as short as a day or two, or as long as 3 weeks. In untreated patients there are usually 3–6 relapses, but there may be as many as 11 in the African form.

DIAGNOSIS

The primary attack can be mistaken for malaria and other acute fevers, including the virus infections (particularly the arbovirus infections), leptospirosis, typhus, pneumonia, meningitis and even plague. The first essential is to keep the disease in mind in any patient who has been to the endemic areas.

Sometimes in the tick-borne form diagnosis is helped by the presence of a black pock at the site of the tick bite (as in an outbreak in Kashmir).

The most satisfactory diagnosis is the finding of *Borrelia* in the blood by microscopic examination. A thick drop should be taken during the period of high fever, and stained either with Leishman or Giemsa, or examined under dark-ground illumination. But the organisms are by no means always to be found by microscopic examination (only 15·2% were positive in an outbreak in Kashmir); many more positives can be detected by inoculating blood or cerebrospinal fluid into young rats or white mice, in which blood becomes positive in 2–3 days. Guinea-pigs, rabbits and dogs are relatively refractory. Blood infection is much heavier in louse-borne than in tick-borne relapsing fever, especially in the primary attack.

Other means of diagnosis include serological tests. In a complement fixation test with an antigen of *B. duttoni* prepared from the allantoic fluid of infected chick embryos, fixation of complement at a titre of 1 in 25 is probably diagnostic (Wolstenholme & Gear 1948), but it has been said that this test is not very reliable. The Wassermann reaction may be positive, and in the louse-borne form the Weil–Felix reaction (*Proteus OXK*) may also be positive.

Agglutinin tests have been used with antigens derived from the blood of animals at the peak of infection. They tend to give cross-reactions between borreliae, and also with treponemes.

Immobilizing antibodies can be found in animals; they are highly strain-specific and persist for long periods. Lysins are also important; they vary with relapses, but persist for 10 months or more.

The indirect fluorescent antibody test with the agglutinin antigen has proved sensitive, though not as specific as the immobilization test. There was some cross-reaction with *Treponema pallidum* and some non-specific fluorescence.

TREATMENT

The old treatment with neoarsphenamine was generally successful, leading to a crisis and recovery. The dose was calculated as 0·01 gramme/kg body weight (0·15–0·6 gramme in all, as a single dose) intravenously, best given at the beginning of a paroxysm. A combination of arsenic and prednisolone has proved useful. Better results have been obtained with antibiotics. Penicillin is usually effective, injections being given daily until the temperature falls. But certain strains are said to be resistant to penicillin (and neoarsphenamine), and penicillin does not easily clear residual brain infection. The tetracyclines are very effective, as is novobiocin.

For shock adrenaline may be called for in addition to the usual forms of treatment.

A Jarisch–Herxheimer reaction quite commonly occurs after the administration of tetracycline or penicillin. The patient is restless and there is a rigor lasting 10–30 minutes, with a quick rise of temperature, pulse rate, breathing and blood pressure, and intense shivering. This is followed by a phase of flushing and profuse sweating, and the blood pressure falls; the patient becomes more comfortable and falls asleep, the temperature being normal the next day. Borreliae disappear from the blood about the time of the peak of this reaction (Bryceson et al. 1970).

Dehydration may be a factor in hypotensive collapse, and careful attention should be paid to fluid intake, by mouth if possible. Patients should be confined to bed for at least 24 hours after treatment, to avoid collapse, which can be fatal.

PREVENTION

This means eliminating or avoiding the louse and tick vectors. In epidemics of louse-borne relapsing fever the usual steps should, if possible, be taken to destroy lice. Insecticide powder blown into the clothing of the population at risk soon eliminates body lice, and louse eggs can be dealt with by time-honoured methods of heat sterilization of clothing. There is no danger from inhalation of dried louse faeces.

The endemic tick-borne relapsing fever is more difficult to control. It is a zoonosis, and some of the vector ticks haunt caves and animal burrows in open country. These should therefore be avoided in endemic areas, particularly by campers. In Africa, the U.S.S.R. and other places, some ticks of the genus *Ornithodorus* haunt human dwellings, particularly rest houses (in Africa), coming out to feed at night from the crevices in walls and floors in which they live. They are particularly active in seeking blood meals in spring and autumn in the middle Asian republics, and cattle sheds are favourite haunts because the ticks obtain their blood meals from these animals, though the cattle themselves are not infected by the borreliae. These ticks are best controlled by BHC, but large doses are needed (4 grammes/m² for houses, 6 grammes for cattle sheds). This should be applied to the lower part of the walls and to the floor near the walls, and especially to cracks and crevices (Pospelova-Shtorm 1968).

Travellers using rest houses should sleep in beds raised from the floor, and if possible under mosquito nets (for instance in tropical Africa). Shoes and slippers, luggage, carpets, etc. left overnight on the floors should be shaken and inspected to make sure that ticks have not been caught up in them.

It is said that the normal processes of agricultural development of land destroy the habitations of field rodents in which the disease is enzootic. Better hygiene and better house design are basic factors in control.

Rat Bite Fevers

Two forms of fever have been ascribed to infection through the bites of rats: Sodoku (Sokosha) named by Japanese workers and caused by *Spirillum minus* (*S. morsus-muris*), and Haverhill fever (infectious erythema), named by American workers and caused by *Actinobacillus muris* (formerly known as *Streptobacillus moniliformis* and other names).

These are not strictly tropical diseases, but are included here because they are relapsing diseases which may be confused with other similar infections.

SODOKU

Sodoku is usually caused by the bites of brown or black rats, though it can also be caused by the bites of cats, or even bandicoots or ferrets. It has been reported from Japan, Australia, Africa, the Americas and Europe.

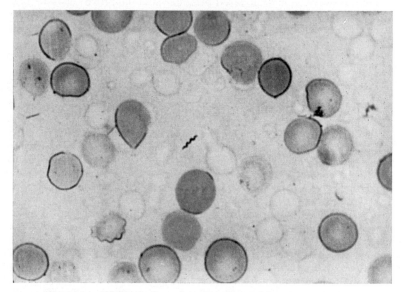

Fig. 166.—*Spirillum minus* of rat bite fever in the mouse. × 2500.

Aetiology

Spirillum minus is a short spiral organism (2–4 μm long), rather thick, with regular rigid spirals, and pointed ends continued into one or more flagella. It moves rapidly, like a vibrio. It is easily stained by methylene blue or Giemsa.

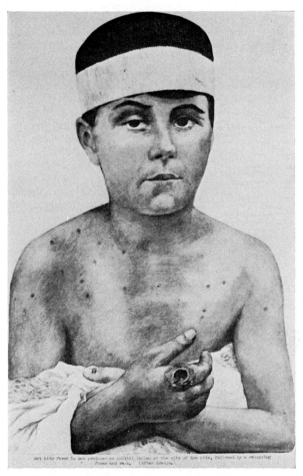

Fig. 167.—Rat bite fever in man produces an initial lesion at the site of the bite, followed by relapsing fever and rash. (*By courtesy of the Wellcome Museum of Medical Sciences*)

Symptoms

The incubation period varies from 5 to 30 days, the average being from 5 to 10 days, during which time the wound heals. Then the cicatrix itself, and sometimes the surrounding tissues, becomes inflamed, with the formation of blebs and even necrosis. The lymphatics draining the area are implicated and the glands themselves become swollen and tender. The onset of fever is characterized by rigors and malaise; the temperature gradually rises in 3 days to a

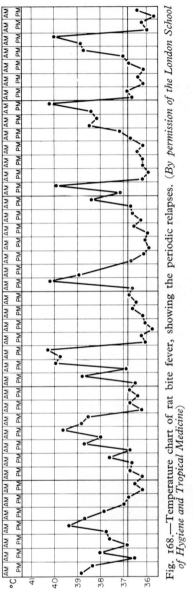

Fig. 168.—Temperature chart of rat bite fever, showing the periodic relapses. (By permission of the London School of Hygiene and Tropical Medicine)

maximum of 39·4–40°C (103–4°F) and after a further period of 3 days ends in crisis with profuse sweating.

After the primary attack a quiescent interval of 5–10 days ensues. One or more relapses associated with the same symptoms and a characteristic purple papular exanthem, or urticaria, on the chest and arms, have been noted. The eruption is sometimes nodular. With each bout of fever the cicatrix at the site of the original bite becomes inflamed.

In most cases the reflexes are increased; there may be pains in the muscles and joints, hyperaesthesia and oedema of various parts of the body. In some cases arthritis has been reported. The death-rate is about 10%. In fatal cases the end is ushered in by delirium, often lapsing into coma. Some cases subside spontaneously, others go on for months.

As in relapsing fever, the organism can be demonstrated in the blood during the fever only, disappearing during the apyrexial intervals. The serum agglutinates the *Spirillum* in low dilutions. There is an eosinophilia during the paroxysm and a moderate leucocytosis of about 15 000. It is said that the serum in this disease gives weak positive Wassermann and Kahn reactions. *Proteus OXK* may be agglutinated.

Diagnosis

In many cases the diagnosis of rat bite fever can be fully established from the history, the infiltration at the seat of the bite, the typical temperature curve, the rash, and the effects of the administration of neoarsphenamine or penicillin. This diagnosis can be confirmed either by dark-ground illumination, when spirilla may be seen in the exudate obtained from the site of the bite, or in the serous fluid from the papule, or by Giemsa-stained smears. It is seldom possible to demonstrate spirilla in a thick blood film. If a number of relapses have occurred, probably the best examination to make is for the presence of lytic antibodies. Absolute proof of the clinical diagnosis may be obtained by inoculating the patient's blood, lymph gland, or a piece of excised wound into guinea-pigs and mice.

Differential diagnosis. This has to be made from the different forms of relapsing and trench fevers, with which the temperature chart has much in common. In tropical countries the possibility of a co-existent malaria has to be taken into account. The puffiness of the face accompanying the urticarial eruption may simulate Bright's disease.

The reaction occurring around the site of the scar is apt to be confused with erysipelas or cellulitis.

S. minus is not easily found in the blood, though it does invade the blood after a few days, but it can be found in the exudate near the bite, and in juice from the local lymph nodes. Inoculation of infected material into mice and rats produces blood infection, and in guinea-pigs a febrile disease. Dogs can be infected, but remain symptomless. Monkeys and rabbits are also susceptible. The spirilla appear to be present in the muscles of the rat tongue, and rats, mice and guinea-pigs may be healthy carriers.

S. minus can be cultivated, but subcultivation has not been successful (Wilson & Miles 1964).

Pathology

There have been few post mortem examinations in man, but degenerative changes have been seen in the liver and kidneys, and hyperaemia of the cerebral cortex with increase in the cerebrospinal fluid. There is polymorphonuclear leucocytosis and secondary anaemia.

The area of the bite tends at first to heal, but later breaks down to an ulcer.

Treatment

Penicillin, streptomycin and the tetracyclines are effective within a few days, as is neoarsphenamine, of which one injection (0·4–0·6 gramme) may be enough. Rat bites should always be cauterized.

HAVERHILL FEVER

This has been described from the United States, Europe and elsewhere.

Aetiology

Actinobacillus muris is a natural parasite of the nasopharynx of rats. It forms slender branching filaments which break up to be replaced by chains of bacillary or coccoid bodies. It is non-motile. It grows on serum agar, Loeffler's serum, egg, and in the developing chick embryo. It is pathogenic for mice on intra-peritoneal or subcutaneous injection (Wilson & Miles 1964).

Transmission

This is a more common cause of rat bite fever than *Spirillum minus*, but though infection can often be traced to a rat bite, outbreaks have occurred as a result of the consumption of raw milk. It is not known how the milk became infected in these outbreaks—possibly from the urine of infected rats.

Pathology

Little is known of this, but ulcerative endocarditis and subacute myocarditis have been reported. The liver may be enlarged.

Clinical findings

After an incubation period of 3–10 days, during which there may be gastro-intestinal upset, there is chill and fever. The local wound heals. There is extreme prostration, severe generalized muscular pain and tenderness, headache, and a widespread morbilliform rash or petechial eruption, with general enlargement of lymph nodes. Non-suppurative shifting arthritis is characteristic. There is polymorphonuclear leucocytosis.

The fever may be prolonged, with night sweats, or the temperature may fall by crisis after a few days, but relapses occur at irregular intervals, for weeks or months (Sprecher & Copeland 1947; Brown & Nunemaker 1942).

Case mortality is about 10%.

Table 35. Differentiation of sodoku and Haverhill fever

	Sodoku	*Haverhill fever*
Transmission	Bite of rat	Bite of rat or other animal. Possibly contaminated food
Incubation period	5–30 days	3–10 days, average 5
Wound from bite	Apparent healing, followed by chancre-like ulceration	Heals promptly
Lymph glands	Regional lymphadenitis	Not involved
Systemic manifestations	(a) Regularly relapsing type of fever	(a) Intermittent, but not regularly relapsing type of fever
	(b) Generalized maculo-papular rash	(b) Macular, pustular and petechial eruption
	(c) Varying degrees of prostration and debility	(c) Varying degrees of prostration
	(d) Arthritis very rare	(d) Metastatic arthritis fairly common
Laboratory findings	Polymorphonuclear leucocytosis	Same
	Secondary anaemia	Same
	Kahn test, usually +	Negative
	Isolation of *Spirillum* by animal inoculation of blood or infected gland	Isolation of *A. muris* by blood culture and from pustules on veal infusion broth enriched with rabbit serum
	Agglutination test negative	Agglutination tests with *A. muris* positive. Serum agglutinates a polyvalent antigen of the bacillus
Treatment	Responds to arsenicals and to penicillin	Arsenicals of little or no value. Curable with penicillin

Diagnosis

Blood culture may be positive. After a few weeks of illness the patient's serum may agglutinate *A. muris*. It is difficult to distinguish this fever from sodoku on clinical grounds alone.

Treatment

Penicillin and streptomycin are effective; arsenicals are not.

Leptospirosis

Leptospirosis (Turner 1967, 1968, 1969) is a zoonosis caused by highly motile spiral organisms of the genus *Leptospira*. It has been known by many names—mud fever, slime fever (*Schlammfieber*), swineherd's disease (*maladie des porcheurs*), swamp fever, 7-day fever, autumnal fever, infectious jaundice, field fever and cane-cutter's disease.

Geographical distribution

Leptospirosis is found throughout the world when it is looked for.

EPIDEMIOLOGY

Leptospirosis affects domestic animals (dogs, cattle, pigs and other livestock, in which it is often mild) and wild animals (rodents, mongooses, skunks, marsupials and others). Infected animals shed leptospires in their urine, and man becomes infected through contact with fresh water, soil, mud and foodstuffs contaminated with virulent leptospires from these hosts, and through contact with the animals themselves. Stagnant water (as in late summer in temperate climates) or slow-flowing water is important in transmission, but infection can be contracted from rapidly flowing water in jungle and other foci.

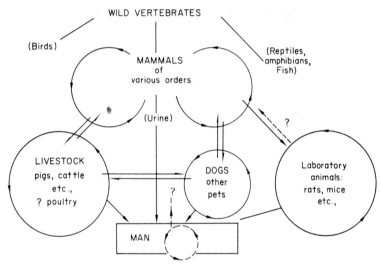

Fig. 169.—Relationships of the principal reservoir hosts of *Leptospira*. (*Adapted from Turner 1967*)

For pathogenic leptospires in the free-living state the optimum conditions are moisture, warmth (about 25°C) and pH values of soil and surface water around neutrality. These conditions are often found throughout the year in the tropics, and in summer and autumn in temperate climates, and in them leptospires can survive for weeks. Desiccation, excessive sunlight, pH outside the range 6·2–8·0, salinity and chemical pollution tend to kill the organisms. The pathogenic strains do not survive more than a few hours in sea water, but strains of the saprophytic *L. biflexa* complex have been isolated from this source.

Leptospires may enter through the skin (especially if wounded or macerated), nose, mouth or conjunctiva. Man may also become infected through bites when handling infected animals. Though there is no evidence that leptospires are secreted with saliva, bites can become infected by leptospires which the handler may have picked up from the animal.

People working in sewers, abattoirs, farms, rice fields, sugar plantations, mines, ditches and other environments infested by rats and other animals, where there is a possibility of infected material or water, are at special risk. The same is true of veterinarians and others in contact with cattle, pigs, dogs (including pets), poultry, fish and other animals. Outbreaks of human disease have occurred, which have been linked with epizootics in wild or domestic animals.

In Malaysia leptospirosis has been associated with troops operating in swampy jungle areas, and elsewhere with people camping near, and bathing in, lakes and streams, and with fishermen and boatmen.

Man is usually a dead end in the chain of infection.

AETIOLOGY

The genus *Leptospira* consists of 2 complexes, one of which, the *L. interrogans* complex, is pathogenic for man and animals, and the other, the *L. biflexa* complex, is *mainly* non-pathogenic (Turner 1967; 1968).

The *L. interrogans* complex comprises some 16 serogroups, of which those isolated from man incorporate too many serotypes to be included here. Serogroups connected with human disease include:

L. icterohaemorrhagiae	*L. ballum*	*L. australis*	*L. bataviae*
L. javanica	*L. pyrogenes*	*L. pomona*	*L. tarassovi*
L. celledoni	*L. cynopteri*	*L. grippotyphosa*	*L. andamana*
L. canicola	*L. autumnalis*	*L. hebdomadis*	

In addition, strains belonging to serogroups *L. panama*, *L. shermani* and *L. semaranga* have been isolated from animals or surface water.

The serogroups include some 119 serotypes, but the numbers of both serogroups and serotypes grow as investigations continue. Serogroups and serotypes are not regarded as species; they are distinguished serologically. A list of each was published by WHO (1967).

Some serotypes tend to cause severe, even fatal, illness with jaundice (*L. icterohaemorrhagiae* in man, dogs, guinea-pigs); some tend to cause moderately severe but seldom fatal illness (*L. australis*, *L. pyrogenes*, *L. bataviae*); others cause mild anicteric illness in man (*L. canicola*, *L. ballum*, *L. grippotyphosa*, *L. hebdomadis*, *L. pomona*, *L. hyos* etc.). There are, however, exceptions to these generalizations, and differences in pathogenicity of strains may be related to geographical distribution.

PATHOLOGY

Leptospires probably enter the blood soon after penetrating the epithelium, and probably multiply in the blood, from which they can reach any organ or tissue. In most tissues they are removed by phagocytosis and other non-specific defence mechanisms, but their numbers diminish more rapidly as they are exposed to the increasing concentration of specific antibodies. In most tissues they are eradicated, and the tissues return to normal function. In the kidneys, however, some leptospires tend to reach the convoluted tubules in the cortex, and to settle, forming colonies in the lumen, and therefore appearing in the urine. They may continue to be shed in the urine (after about 8 days from infection) for several weeks (in the convalescent state) or even for months or years (Turner 1967). The leptospires in the tubules seem to be unaffected by serum antibodies and by antibodies which have been detected in the urine. They may be present in the urine even if the animal is seronegative. Exceptionally the kidneys are apparently liable to permanent nephritic damage.

The infection can also cause uveitis, 'aseptic' (i.e. non-bacterial) meningitis, and jaundice from involvement of the liver, which is then enlarged.

CLINICAL FEATURES

The clinical manifestations (Turner 1967) range from mild, transient fever, either not noticed or disregarded, or diagnosed as influenza or PUO, to severe and fatal infections such as Weil's disease—though these are rare. Most of the infections do not cause severe illness, and the old conception that leptospirosis is synonymous with (the severe) Weil's disease is highly misleading.

After an incubation period of 2–20 days (commonly 7–10) the onset is often sudden, with fever, malaise and muscular pain and tenderness. The fever commonly lasts for 2–12 days. Headache and meningism, with increased pressure and cellular content of the cerebrospinal fluid, indicate invasion of the meningeal space. Leptospires are present in the cerebrospinal fluid. There may be a macular or maculo-papular rash; enlargement of lymph nodes is not uncommon. The lungs may be congested and oedematous, with basal râles, blood-tinged sputum, and X-ray signs of pneumonitis. There may be haemorrhages into muscles, skin, kidneys, lungs, stomach or intestines; epistaxis is not uncommon. The conjunctivae are often injected, sometimes with haemorrhages. There may be cardiac arrhythmia.

The erythrocyte sedimentation rate is increased, and there is often leucocytosis, though the count may be normal or subnormal; neutrophils usually predominate, and if this occurs with a subnormal count, leptospirosis is likely.

Albuminuria and casts in the urine are common, but may occur early and persist for only a short time; blood urea may be raised. Renal failure may go on to uraemia. Jaundice is not the rule; if tests of liver function are abnormal they suggest hepatocellular rather than obstructive dysfunction (Turner 1967).

Adrenal failure and the Waterhouse–Friderichsen syndrome have been observed.

The general condition of the patient may affect the severity of the disease—immaturity and pre-existing dysfunction of the liver, for instance.

Convalescence is often protracted.

Weil's disease, with jaundice, is severe, but is not as common as is generally supposed. It will be remembered that when Noguchi was investigating the cause of yellow fever, he was assured by the physicians that the patients from whom he took material for culture were suffering from that disease, yet it is now clear that they were suffering from severe leptospirosis, and that the organism he isolated and named *Leptospira icteroides,* in the belief that it was the cause of yellow fever, was *L. icterohaemorrhagiae.* Noguchi later admitted this; it was a tragedy for him. He died of true yellow fever while still investigating it, in West Africa.

DIAGNOSIS

Whenever leptospirosis is suspected, a specimen of blood should be taken as early as possible after the onset of illness and *before* treatment with antibiotics. This should be sent to a laboratory for serological diagnosis; it may be negative at this stage, but the specimen can be very useful for comparison with later specimens. A rise in titre in a second specimen taken 7 or more days after the first is a most important finding. Some of the requisite serological techniques are well within the capacities of general purpose laboratories, and should be included in the routine battery of such examinations. Otherwise cases will be missed (Ross & Ives 1970; Turner & Mohun 1970).

Leptospiral agglutinins may be detected in serum as early as day 6 of illness, more generally day 10, and persist in diminishing but detectable concentrations for 1–20 years. For routine diagnosis the microscopic or macroscopic agglutination reactions with living or formalin-killed organisms are usual, but in critical experimental investigations living cultures are used. The tests can be set up by using the depressions of a porcelain palette with a drop technique to make a range of final dilutions of serum 1:10, 1:30 and so on, or four-fold. If the test serum has a high antibody content, agglutination may be incomplete in low dilution (prozone effect).

These tests are read by examining for agglutinated leptospires, and comparing them each time with a negative control. There are many technical difficulties and careful technique is therefore needed.

With formalin cultures a titre of 1 in 300 is strongly suggestive, and 1 in 1000 is probably conclusive in suspected cases.

Complement fixation tests are also used with individual antigens, but for routine screening a reliable 'genus-specific' antigen is required, capable of detecting infection irrespective of serotype. These antigens are easily prepared, and the tests are valuable for the general diagnosis of leptospirosis. Turner and Mohun (1970) have distributed an antigen prepared from the Patoc I strain of the *L. biflexa* complex and serotype *L. wolffii* for use in laboratories in Britain. Other antigens suitable for other countries are under investigation.

Other genus-specific tests are the sensitized erythrocyte lysis (SEL, HL) test and an indirect immunofluorescence (IF) test.

For a full description of the serology of leptospirosis readers are referred to Turner (1968).

Blood can also be sent to a laboratory for microscopical examination (leptospires being visible under dark-field illumination at low magnifications) though this is not reliable. However, leptospires can be isolated from blood during the febrile period, but rarely after 8–10 days. Venous blood collected aseptically before antibiotics have been given, can be inoculated, preferably at the bedside, in small volumes (2–3 drops) into several tubes of a suitable culture medium (5–7 ml each). Larger volumes of blood are less satisfactory because antibodies may have been formed. If blood cannot be inoculated at once, an oxalated specimen (5·0 ml blood to 0·5 ml of 1·0% sodium oxalate solution) should be prepared for despatch to the laboratory. Leptospires may also be isolated from cerebrospinal fluid 3–11 days after onset.

Culture from urine is less easy. Leptospires cannot tolerate an acid reaction. They may be present in human urine on days 8–30, but are usually scanty. In the urine of infected animals, however, they may be abundant, and be excreted throughout life. From any urine they may be cultivated after dilution with buffered saline, Stuart's medium, or 0·2% peptone broth. This also dilutes contaminants.

Leptospires can be cultivated in Fletcher (semisolid) medium, or in the media of Korthof or Stuart, details of which should be sought in textbooks of bacteriology. Cultures should be incubated at 28–30°C, but if this is not possible they may be kept in the dark at room temperature. They should be examined by dark-ground microscopy on days 3, 7, 10 and 14 after inoculation. The morphology and movements of leptospires are characteristic.

For a full discussion of the maintenance, isolation and demonstration of leptospires, see Turner (1970). It is important that material for culture must be collected in well rinsed vessels completely free from detergents and antiseptics, and in sterile conditions.

Diagnosis can also be made by inoculation of material into animals—weanling hamsters and guinea-pigs, gerbils, deer mice, chinchillas or 1-day chicks. White mice and albino rats should not be used unless they are known to be free from leptospirosis; the infection may be present in animal colonies without any sign of ill health. Some serotypes do not produce obvious signs of infection in laboratory animals. Inoculated animals should therefore be weighed daily (loss of weight or failure to gain weight being suggestive). Their peritoneal fluid should be examined by dark field for leptospires, and heart blood taken for culture. Post mortem examination is also important, liver and kidneys being examined by the dark field method, fluorescent antibody techniques or silver impregnation and by culture. Experience is needed in detecting leptospires in fixed or stained preparations, because artefacts may be mistaken for them.

Leptospires can usually be detected in centrifuged urine, and may be present up to day 63, though generally disappearing by day 40. Their numbers are somewhat inconstant, and they may disappear altogether in acid urine. Negative results mean nothing.

Differential diagnosis

Leptospirosis should be considered in patients with:

Pyrexia of uncertain origin (PUO)
Influenza-like illness, especially if sporadic
'Aseptic' meningitis (i.e. non-bacterial)
Other acute diseases of the nervous system
Rickettsial diseases
Dengue-like illnesses
Enteric-like illnesses
Glandular fever
Brucellosis
Jaundice with fever (yellow fever, infectious hepatitis)
Atypical pneumonia

Occupation is also obviously a factor to be taken into acount, as are recreations which may lead to contact with an environment where infectious urine is likely to be present (i.e. the habitats of animal hosts).

TREATMENT

Treatment fortunately does not depend on the serotype with which the patient is infected. Antibiotics are indicated, especially penicillin, and should be given when the first blood sample has been obtained for laboratory examination. They are the more effective the earlier treatment is started: days 1–3 very good; 4–6 less good; 7 onwards probably useless.

The adult dose of penicillin should be high, at least 2·0 mega units daily, increased to 8·0 or even 12·0 mega units (which may be given with intravenous fluids) in severe cases, or if treatment starts after day 4. WHO (1967) suggest 6–12 mega units daily from the beginning. This may produce an exacerbation of signs and symptoms for a short time, but these can be dealt with by supporting measures without interrupting treatment. The course of penicillin may be repeated if there is a febrile relapse.

Impairment of renal function may need peritoneal dialysis or the artificial kidney, and these measures should not be delayed, because death is usually due to renal failure, and they may be life-saving (Turner 1967). (For peritoneal dialysis see page 67.)

PREVENTION

Persons engaged in work which brings them into contact with water contaminated with the urine of infected animals (sewer workers, mine workers, pig keepers, abattoir workers, rice field and sugar-cane field workers, etc.) should be warned to avoid contact and to maintain careful personal and environmental cleanliness, and to wear protective clothing (which is often discarded if uncomfortable). Campers and bathers are not likely to pay much attention, but should be warned. Laboratory workers (and others) should wash down flat surfaces—benches etc.—with sodium hypochlorite (1 in 4000) or detergents (Turner 1967). Troops, surveyors, forestry workers etc., operating in swampy areas are at risk, and leptospirosis should be borne in mind in differential diagnosis.

The ordinary treatment given to public water supplies—filtration and chlorination—is enough to render them safe from the point of view of leptospirosis.

Vaccines of local strains have been used. They may be useful where leptospirosis is a hazard in certain occupations. If properly prepared, they are potent and safe, and give good protection against clinical illness.

Abortive treatment (2·0 mega units of penicillin daily for 5 days, intramuscularly) may be given to a laboratory worker or animal handler thought to have been contaminated by a virulent strain. Blood should be taken at the beginning of treatment and again if the patient develops fever within 6–7 weeks. If this happens another course of penicillin is indicated.

REFERENCES

BROWN, T. M. & NUNEMAKER, J. C. (1942) *Bull. Johns Hopkins Hosp.*, **70**, 201.
BRYCESON, A. D. M., PARRY, E. H. O., PERINE, P. L., WARRELL, D. A., VUKOTICH, D. & LEITHEAD, C. S. (1970) *Q. Jl Med.*, **39**, 129.
EISENBERG, S., GUNDERS, A. E. & COHEN, A. M. (1968) *Trans. R. Soc. trop. Med. Hyg.*, **62**, 679.
FELSENFELD, O. (1965) *Bact. Rev.*, **29**, 46.
——— DECKER, W. J., WOHLHIETER, J. A. & RAFYI, A. (1965) *J. Immun.*, **94**, 805.
——— & WOLF, R. H. (1969) *Acta trop.*, **26**, 156.
POSPELOVA-SHTORM, M. V. (1968) *Eighth Int. Congr. trop. Med. Malar.*, 888.
ROSS, C. A. C. & IVES, J. C. J. (1970) *Br. med. J.*, i, 433.
SPRECHER, M. H. & COPELAND, J. R. (1947) *J. Am. med. Ass.*, **134**, 1014.
TURNER, L. H. (1967) *Trans. R. Soc. trop. Med. Hyg.* **61**, 842.
——— (1968) *Trans. R. Soc. trop. Med. Hyg.*, **62**, 880.
——— (1970) *Trans. R. Soc. trop. Med. Hyg.*, **64**, 623.
——— & MOHUN, A. F. (1970) *Br. med. J.*, i, 433.
WALTON, G. A. (1957) *Bull. ent. Res.*, **42**, 669.
——— (1961) *Symp. zool. Soc. Lond.*, **6**, 83.
WILSON, G. S. & MILES, A. A. (1964) *Topley & Wilson's Principles of Bacteriology and Immunity*. London: Arnold.
WOLSTENHOLME, B. & GEAR, J. H. S. (1948) *Trans. R. Soc. trop. Med. Hyg.*, **41**, 513.
WORLD HEALTH ORGANIZATION (1967) *Wld Hlth Org. tech. Rep. Ser.*, 380.

SECTION VI

DISEASES CAUSED BY
RICKETTSIAE AND BARTONELLAE

29. RICKETTSIAL FEVERS

Definition

Febrile diseases caused by organisms of the genus *Rickettsia* and transmitted by lice, fleas, ticks and mites. All are zoonoses, with the exception of louse-borne typhus and trench fever.

AETIOLOGY

The rickettsial fevers have a world-wide distribution and are divisible into a number of local forms which have become adapted to local conditions in some way connected with those intermediate arthropod hosts which convey the infection. Classical typhus is called 'louse-borne', true or exanthematic or epidemic typhus, and the local varieties are known by their descriptive pseudonyms, murine typhus, scrub typhus, Rocky Mountain spotted fever, *fièvre boutonneuse* etc., and may be classified according to their vectors (Fig. 170).

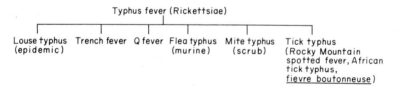

Fig. 170.—Classification of typhus fevers.

Rickettsiae are classified mainly into the following groups: the typhus group (*R. prowazeki, R. canada, R. prowazeki* var. *mooseri*); the spotted fever group (*R. rickettsi rickettsi, R. rickettsi conori, R. rickettsi conori* var. *pijperi*); and the tsutsugamushi group (*R. orientalis*). They are Gram-negative, bacteria-like bodies, usually less than 0·5 μm in diameter. There are 8 named species and several varieties. The *Rickettsia* of louse-borne typhus was named *R. prowazeki* by Rocha-Lima in 1916 in honour of 2 investigators, Ricketts and Prowazek, who both succumbed to rickettsial fevers they were investigating.

The cause of flea-borne typhus is *R. prowazeki* var. *mooseri* (*R. muricola*). The cause of mite-borne typhus was distinguished by Sellards in Japan as *R. orientalis* (*R. tsutsugamushi, R. nipponica*). The causal agent of Rocky Mountain spotted fever is known as *R. rickettsi*, first described by Ricketts in 1911 and originally named *Dermacentroxenus rickettsi* by Wolbach. The cause of *fièvre boutonneuse* is *R. rickettsi conori* and of African tick typhus is *R. rickettsi conori* var. *pijperi*. The cause of trench fever is *R. quintana*. The cause of Q fever is *Coxiella burneti* and of rickettsialpox is *R. akari*.

TRANSMISSION

Rickettsiae are found commonly in the alimentary tract of blood-sucking and non-blood-sucking insects but probably they were primarily parasitic in the cells lining the intestinal canal as is the case with *R. prowazeki*. *R. pediculi* is an extracellular organism which is an inhabitant of the gut of the louse and is harmless to its host as well as to man. *R. quintana* develops in the same manner and situation.

Louse typhus

The cycle of development of *R. prowazeki* in the louse consists primarily of great multiplication in the epithelial cells of the gut, which become distended. After a few days they rupture and rickettsiae appear in large numbers in the faeces. This rickettsial invasion kills the louse if it is infected up to the tenth day of the patient's illness, occasionally later when the patient is afebrile. The disease is conveyed to man mainly by louse faeces through abrasions in the skin or even through the conjunctivae or from inhalation from fomites. Louse faeces kept dry at room temperature have been proved to be infective for 66 days. It is possible that it can be transmitted by infected louse saliva. There is no hereditary transmission and louse eggs do not contain the organism. Clean lice may possibly infect themselves by eating the excreta of other typhus-infected lice. Man was thought to be the only reservoir of infection until Reiss-Gutfreund (1956) produced evidence suggesting the *R. prowazeki* could be isolated from sheep and goats and that ticks could convey the infection. This suggested that an animal as well as a human reservoir existed in nature.

Flea typhus (murine typhus)

R. prowazeki var. *mooseri* is normally transmitted from rat to rat by the rat louse (*Polyplax spinulosa*) and by the tropical rat mite (*Bdellonyssus* (*Liponyssus*) *bacoti*). The cycle in these insects is similar to that described in the louse.

The infection is transmitted from rat to man by the flea *Xenopsylla cheopis* which is not harmed by the infection. *X. astia* may also act as a vector. The rickettsiae remain alive and virulent in the faeces of the flea for 40 days in the dark and 100 days *in vacuo*.

Tick typhus

The cycle of development of rickettsiae in ticks follows on much the same lines but in a more widespread manner. The rickettsiae invade the cells and their nuclei and are found in all the tissues including the ovaries of the female tick, so that the infection is transmitted hereditarily. Rickettsiae are also found in the salivary glands, so that the infection is conveyed by bite. Zinsser has pointed out that the hereditary factor in tick transmission indicates a very ancient host–parasite relationship with a mutual tolerance so adjusted that the well-being of neither the animal reservoir nor the tick intermediary is impaired.

Mite typhus

Rickettsia orientalis is normally a parasite of forest rodents and is transmitted chiefly by larval mites of the genus *Leptotrombidium* (*Trombicula*). The rickettsiae have been found in the body cavity of the adult mite and are transmitted by the larval stages in their salivary glands which are infective. The rickettsiae persist from one generation to the next, about 30 days, and so infection is hereditary.

The mode of transmission of the rickettsiae from animals to man or from man to man and the relationship of the various forms of typhus can be expressed as follows:

Epidemic louse-borne typhus	Man–Louse–Man (Sheep–Tick–Goat possible)
Murine typhus	Rat–$\begin{bmatrix}\text{Rat Flea}\\\text{Rat Louse}\end{bmatrix}$–Rat Rat–Flea–Man Rat–Flea–Man–Louse–Man (possible)
Scrub typhus	Rat or field rodent–Mite–Man
Spotted fever	Rodent–Tick–Rodent Rodent–Tick–Man
Fièvre boutonneuse; African tick fever	Rodent–Tick–Rodent Rodent–Tick–Dog–Tick–Man
Rickettsialpox	Mouse–Mite–Mouse–Mite–Man
Q fever	Usually direct spread, sometimes tick

The different species of rickettsiae may develop in other than their usual vectors. *Rickettsia quintana, R. prowazeki, R. mooseri, R. conori, R. rickettsi, R. akari, R. orientalis* and *Coxiella burneti* all multiply in the haemolymph of the body louse (*Pediculus*), and can be passaged through lice by intracoelomic inoculation, though after a certain number of passages *R. orientalis* ceases to multiply in the coelom, and all except the latter can multiply in the stomach of the louse. All the rickettsiae except *R. orientalis* and *R. quintana* multiply or survive in the haemolymph of the mealworm (*Tenebrio molitor*) and in the tick *Ornithodorus moubata*. All except *R. orientalis* and *R. rickettsi* can be passaged repeatedly from louse to louse by rectal inoculation. *R. conori* is pathogenic to lice and causes severe damage to the mucosa of the stomach and death within 3–7 days (Weyer 1953).

MORPHOLOGY

In their morphology in human tissues rickettsiae appear as small bacilli or cocci, very variable in arrangement. Diploid forms and also coccoid forms in dense masses are common (Fig. 171). With the possible exception of *R. orientalis* they stain well by Giemsa's method and blue with Castaneda's stain (Fig. 172); with Macchiavello's stain they are red and the containing cell blue.

Isolation and culture

All rickettsiae grow readily on the chorio-allantoic membrane of fertile egg or preferably in the yolk sac, and duck eggs are highly suitable. The rickettsiae do not kill the embryo but produce round prominent foci 5 days after inoculation and develop completely in 7–8 days. They also grow in tissue culture and in a medium of minced chicken embryo with a mixture of guinea-pig or rabbit serum and Tyrode's solution. Rickettsiae may be isolated by inoculation of material into animals. Guinea-pigs are used for murine, epidemic typhus and spotted fevers, mice for *R. akari* and North Queensland tick typhus and monkeys for *R. conori*.

Ground or whole blood clot is used for intraperitoneal inoculation of animals. The animals are killed later and the peritoneal exudate examined for rickettsiae. The sera are examined for the development of antibodies to the specific rickettsiae. Rickettsiae may be adapted to mice by intranasal passage or to eggs by yolk sac inoculation to allow for the study of the morphology and the preparation of antigens. None of the species can readily be cultivated on solid media. Practically pure strains of *R. prowazeki* can be obtained by intrarectal injection of lice (Weigl's method).

Differentiation of rickettsiae

Rickettsiae may be differentiated by their behaviour in guinea-pigs and by serological reactions.

Neill–Mooser reaction. This is a distinctive reaction in guinea-pigs inoculated with blood or material infected with rickettsiae. In a positive reaction a redness and swelling of the scrotum appears and typical typhus lesions are found in the scrotum in the endothelial lining of the tunica vaginalis, whose cells are swollen and filled with rickettsiae. Some strains of rickettsiae give this reaction more strongly than others. It is nearly always positive with *R. rickettsi* and *R. mooseri* but in only 70% of cases with *R. prowazeki* and is usually negative with *R. conori.*

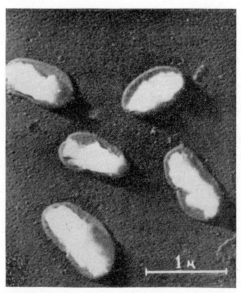

Fig. 171.—Electron micrograph of chromium-shadowed *Rickettsia prowazeki. (Wisseman et al. 1951)*

Serological reactions. Specific rickettsial antisera are prepared in guinea-pigs and used to identify unknown strains by agglutination, complement fixation and fluorescent tests.

Pathological differences. Rickettsiae conveyed by lice and fleas are characterized by invasion of the endothelium and mesothelium, producing distension of the cytoplasm of the host cells without affecting the nuclei, while in guinea-pigs they cause proliferative endangiitis without thrombonecrosis. In typhus-infected lice and fleas the rickettsiae are intracytoplasmic, inhabiting the lining cells of the gut and are not hereditarily transmitted. The spotted fever group conveyed by ticks is characterized by thrombonecrosis of arterioles and venules. In human tissue rickettsiae invade smooth muscle cells as well as endothelium, mesothelium and histiocytes. In tissue cultures a massive infection of nuclei takes place. In infected ticks the rickettsiae are intranuclear as well as intracytoplasmic and invade nearly all types of cells, features which serve to distinguish the spotted fever group. They are hereditarily transmitted.

IMMUNOLOGY

Serum antibodies appear in typhus fevers as in other infections. There is the usual primary response of IgM antibodies followed by a secondary response of IgG antibodies. These different responses can be used to differentiate between primary epidemic typhus and a recrudescence of typhus as shown in Brill–Zinsser disease (Murray *et al*. 1965), since in a primary attack of epidemic typhus only IgM antibodies will be seen: in Brill–Zinsser disease both IgM and IgG antibodies will be found.

There is immunity to reinfection in epidemic typhus and Rocky Mountain spotted fever which lasts for up to 1 year. In scrub typhus there is immunity

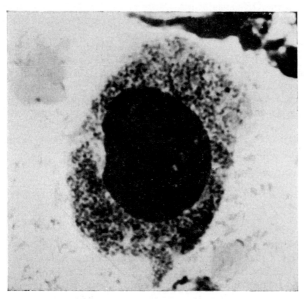

Fig. 172.—*Rickettsia prowazeki* var. *mooseri* (Mooser cell). Tunica vaginalis of the guinea-pig infected with murine typhus from wild rats. Cytoplasmic rickettsiae invading a mononuclear cell. Giemsa. × 4000 approx. (*Anigstein & Bader, Galveston, Texas*)

against homologous strains but there are a number of antigenic variants of *R. orientalis*. In nature second attacks of scrub typhus are uncommon since all strains tend to be a mixture of antigenically distinct types.

Weil–Felix reaction

The Weil–Felix reaction uses the strains of *Proteus* known as $OX2$, $OX19$ and OXK, which are agglutinated by the sera in rickettsial fevers. The typhus fevers can be classified serologically as follows:

$OX19$ type	Vectors: Louse and flea
OXK type	Vector: Mite
Indeterminate	Vector: Tick

Cross-reactions may occur with undulant fever, relapsing fever, tularaemia and rat bite fever, especially with the *OXK* strain.

Specific rickettsial agglutination and complement fixation tests

Rickettsiae are obtained as antigenic material from yolk sac cultures treated with ether or from mouse lung suspensions centrifuged and treated with kieselguhr. Agglutination tests are left at $37–40°C$ for 18 hours and read by the naked eye. Complement fixation tests are done in the usual manner. Rickettsial agglutinins appear earlier than *OX19* antibodies. Complement fixing antibodies appear later.

Specific rickettsial tests are of value in the diagnosis of laboratory infections in previously vaccinated individuals in whom the Weil–Felix agglutinin response is less vigorous. Specific rickettsial antigens are also needed for the differential diagnosis of murine and epidemic typhus and the spotted fever group, which all show a rise in the *OX19* agglutinins. With highly purified washed antigens from yolk sac cultures it is possible to differentiate epidemic from murine typhus and Rocky Mountain spotted fever.

Specific toxin–antitoxin tests in mice can also be used to demonstrate a protective effect with homologous immune sera.

Indirect fluorescent antibody tests can be used to diagnose typhus cases retrospectively since they show a group specific response in the sera of patients convalescent from typhus fevers. Specific serological and active immunization tests have shown antigenic differences in *R. orientalis* in contrast to the antigenic homogeneity in *R. prowazeki*. There are 3 main antigenic variants of *R. orientalis* and there is no cross-immunity relationship with the other rickettsiae. These differences are important in the preparation of vaccines.

Vaccination in typhus infections

Vaccination has been used for the prevention of epidemic typhus, Rocky Mountain spotted fevers and Q fever, but is of no use for the prevention of scrub typhus, owing to the antigenic variations between the different strains of *R. orientalis*.

Two general types of vaccine have been used, killed and live. Killed vaccines can be prepared from rickettsiae grown in the yolk sacs of embryonated eggs killed with formalin and extracted with ether. These are known as Cox-type vaccines, and are used in epidemic typhus and Q fever. Killed vaccines prepared from the tissues of infected ticks treated with formalin are known as 'tick' vaccines, and are used in the Rocky Mountain spotted fever group. Cox-type and tick-type vaccines are protective for a period from 6 months to 1 year.

The only living vaccine at present in use is the E strain of *R. prowazeki* used in epidemic typhus, the protective effect of which may last for 5 years (Wisseman 1967).

EPIDEMIC OR LOUSE-BORNE TYPHUS

Synonyms. True exanthematic, historic, or classical typhus; tabardillo (Mexico). Chronic form: Brill's (Brill–Zinsser) disease; recrudescent epidemic typhus.

Geographical distribution

The classical form of typhus was world-wide and constituted the most important disease in world history. In the Middle Ages it was widespread in

Europe and was especially prevalent in Ireland during the Great Famine of 1845–7. Between 1917 and 1923 there were 30 000 000 cases with over 3000 000 deaths in Russia and Europe. It has been reported from every country in Europe and the last great wave was in 1933–4 in the Soviet Union and throughout Europe, including Spain and Portugal. During World War II typhus occurred in Eastern Europe and Italy, where an epidemic was halted in 1943 for the first time with DDT and other insecticides. Epidemic typhus can be found in the temperate highlands of the tropics over 1600 m. It has been found in the North-west Frontier province of Pakistan, the Himalayas, Afghanistan, China, Manchuria, Mongolia, Indonesia, the Philippines, Hawaii, North-east Australia and Japan. Typhus is endemic in Ethiopia; epidemics have crossed the Sahara and occurred south of it. In America typhus is still endemic in Mexico, Peru and some other areas of South America.

Epidemiology

Formerly it was considered that man was the only reservoir of infection, which was conveyed from man to man through the louse faeces, which are rubbed into abrasions when the louse is crushed during scratching. Infection may also enter through the conjunctiva. Epidemics would occur whenever a population became louse-infested and the source of infection was either a case from another infected area or cases of Brill–Zinsser disease. R. prowazeki is present in the blood plasma, especially the platelets, during the first 5 days of the disease. In Ethiopia it has been found that sheep and goats may act as reservoirs of infection (Reiss-Gutfreund 1956) and the isolation of a closely related Rickettsia from ticks in Canada, R. canada, supports the view that epidemic typhus may be maintained in the absence of a man-louse-man cycle (McKiel et al. 1967).

During World War I so many physicians died of typhus that methods of transmission other than by lice were suggested. It is certain that the rickettsiae may be spread by air-borne infection, especially through inhalation of dried infected louse faeces in dust from clothing. There are German reports that infection has been acquired by attendants taking blood for examination. Typhus can also be contracted in laboratories working with rickettsiae, and it has also been conveyed by blood transfusion when the donor was in the incubation period of the disease.

Classical typhus is a disease of dirt and poverty and its presence denotes low economic standards. In Europe and North Africa it was most frequent in the winter and spring months when heavy clothing affords an excellent opportunity for lice breeding. During the last twenty years it has almost disappeared from these areas.

Brill–Zinsser disease

A mild or larval form of typhus was originally described in New York by Brill in 1898 among the Jewish population. The infection was introduced by immigrants from South-east Europe who were all born abroad. Brill's disease is a late recrudescence of a long-dormant infection and has been described in persons free from lice. Rickettsia-infected glands have been excised from 2 asymptomatic patients who had emigrated from Poland 20 years previously.

Brill's disease probably constitutes the main reservoir of infection in inter-epidemic periods in Eastern Europe (Gaon & Murray 1966).

Pathology

The basic lesion is the result of invasion of the endothelial cells of the smaller blood-vessels by rickettsiae with necrosis and a local infiltration of lymphocytes and plasma cells in the adventitia forming 'typhus nodules' (Fig. 173) which resemble miliary tubercles and were described by Frenkel and subsequently by Aschoff, Wolbach and others.

The essential lesion is due to phagocytosis by cells of the vascular endothelium followed by necrosis of these which contain rickettsiae and their toxins. Typhus nodules are found in the skin, myocardium and viscera and in the brain where the basal ganglia, medulla and cerebral cortex are specially affected.

The rash is visible after death and there are conjunctival haemorrhages and as a rule areas of skin necrosis and gangrene. The spleen is moderately enlarged with hyperplasia of the lymph follicles.

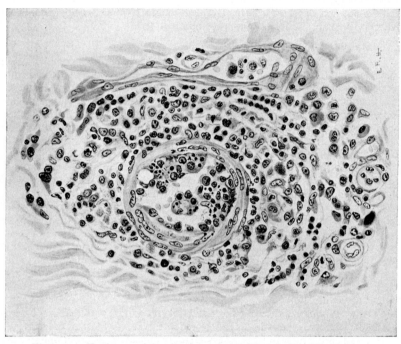

Fig. 173.—Typhus nodule. Section of arteriole of skin, showing an attached mural thrombus, composed almost wholly of phagocytic endothelial cells, with early proliferative perivascular reaction. (*After Wohlbach & Todd*)

A rickettsial pneumonia can result and organisms may be seen in sections of the lung. The peripheral circulatory failure seen in typhus is caused by damage to the capillaries and injury to the vasomotor centres. A myocarditis may also be responsible.

Clinical features

The incubation period varies between 5 and 23 days, the average being 12. The period of onset lasts about 2 days, during which the patient has rigors, headaches, pains in back and limbs, nausea and giddiness and vomiting. Occasionally, fulminant cases (typhus siderans), with general convulsions and delirium, are met. On the third day the temperature rises suddenly to 39·4° or

40°C, the face becomes congested, with general suffusion of the eyes. The headache is very severe (German—*Kopfwehkrankheit*) and with it goes a peculiar stuporose, drunken look not seen in any other disease except perhaps, plague. The patient is drowsy, often delirious (coma vigil), usually with insomnia.

The mouth is foul, the tongue coated with a dense brown fur and the breath offensive. Epistaxis is frequent in the early stages and vomiting may be distressing. For twelve to fourteen days the temperature remains raised with slight, sometimes scarcely perceptible, morning remissions (Fig. 174). The urine is concentrated, offensive, with a cloud of albumin, urea and chlorides initially increased in amount. In severe cases there is often haematuria. The spleen is usually enlarged and palpable.

The rash so characteristic of typhus may appear as early as the third day, but more usually on the fifth or sixth, upon the abdomen, inner aspect of the arms, spreading over the chest, back and trunk, usually pleomorphic, involving

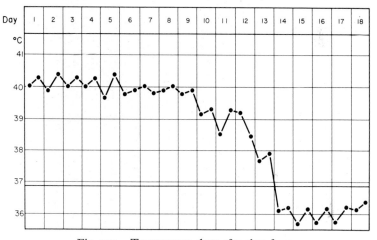

Fig. 174.—Temperature chart of typhus fever.

the face only in severe cases. It may be absent in about 10%. The term 'mulberry rash' is usually employed to describe it, but essentially it consists of roseolar macules, with fine, irregular dusky mottling underlying the epidermis, best described in the words of Murchison as 'subcuticular mottling'. Usually it becomes petechial and may then be seen especially on the hands and soles of the feet.

Rarely, it is bright red, instead of a mingling of copper and purple; sometimes, too, it may be haemorrhagic. The rash fades very slowly and may remain visible for 10 days. A fine branny desquamation towards the end of the third week has been described.

In dark-skinned people the typhus rash is necessarily very difficult to discern. To make the subcuticular mottling visible, a thorough cleansing of the skin and a good light are necessary. Congestion of the upper arms by a tourniquet, such as the band of a blood pressure apparatus, usually renders the petechiae more easily visible. In such people the rash is usually more pronounced around the umbilicus.

On the appearance of the rash there are usually signs of bronchitis and in severe cases sometimes icterus; prostration and cardiac weakness become more pronounced, and with increase of the mental lethargy the patient sinks into the 'typhus state'. The expression becomes dull and vacant, the face flushed, with a peculiar earthy hue (facies typhosa). The skin at this stage sometimes emits an odour which has been compared to that of 'gun-washings', or that emanating from a cupboard containing well-blackened or mouldy boots.

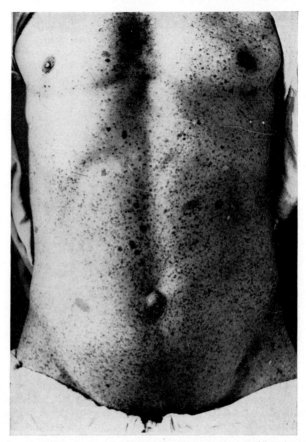

Fig. 175.—Typhus rash in the second week, showing the typical distribution. The dark coloured areas are petechial; the lighter coloured, less discrete areas disappear on pressure.

During the second week a low muttering delirium usually supervenes. Meningism is not uncommon. The secretion of urine may then be diminished or even suppressed. Often symptoms of cortical irritation, such as muscular twitchings, and incontinence of urine and faeces may be observed. The cerebrospinal fluid is under pressure and there is usually an increase in the cell content. It is estimated that 80% suffer from some degree of deafness. Especially common are septic infections of the middle ear which usually appear from the sixth to eighth day.

In severe cases the pupils become pinpoint and the eyes 'ferrety'. As the fourteenth day approaches, signs of improvement may set in; the temperature falls by crisis, or sometimes by rapid lysis. Death generally occurs on the twelfth or fourteenth day, or it may be later, when the temperature is subnormal, from exhaustion or cardiac failure. The blood picture usually shows nothing very definite, but a moderate leucocytosis of 12 000 to 15 000/mm^3, mostly of large mononuclear cells, is not unusual. The blood is concentrated so that the haemoglobin and red blood count are abnormally high.

Among indigenous populations terrible complications due to sepsis and neglect may ensue. Terminal bronchopneumonia is common. Hemiplegia or paresis of the limbs due to typhus nodules in the brain has been reported. Parotitis and noma are frequent. Abortion in pregnant women is common. Constipation rather than diarrhoea is the rule. The mouth becomes very foul, with the lips and teeth covered with sordes. Bedsores are frequent. Thrombosis of the femoral vein is not uncommon, while gangrene of the extremities, especially of the toes or scrotum, due to arterial thrombosis, is frequently seen in wartime epidemics. One of the most distressing features is gangrene of the lung as a termination of typhus bronchopneumonia.

Convalescence is usually slow and prolonged, and during this period great care should be taken not to excite the heart. Snapper pointed out that thrombocytopenia is not infrequent in typhus and some cases, even after the typhus infection is over, show a typical anaphylactoid, sometimes even a thrombocytopenic, purpura. Loss of hair on the head and legs is said to be common.

Relapsing fever and typhus frequently co-exist and this superadded infection is serious. Mild forms of typhus, lasting some ten days, are frequently seen in children; it is usually the aged and the ill-fed who most readily succumb.

In the absence of modern treatment, case mortality is negligible in children. It is 10–15% up to the age of 40, but 50% at 50; over that age few survive. Relapses of typhus have been recorded.

Diagnosis

Rickettsiae may be isolated from the blood most easily in the first 5 days of fever by inoculating ground blood clot intraperitoneally into male guinea-pigs which are then observed for fever 6–10 days afterwards. The Neill–Mooser reaction is slightly positive, but less so than in murine typhus (page 607). Rickettsiae may also be isolated by inoculating blood into the yolk sacs of embryonated eggs.

Serology. The Weil–Felix reaction is highly diagnostic. The titre of agglutination against the *OX19* strain rapidly rises to 1 in 500 towards the end of the fever and maximum titre is reached in the third or fourth week. During convalescence it remains about 1 in 50 or 100 for weeks and even months. The type of titre curve is generally related to the clinical course. Moderately severe cases show high titres, and this indicates a good prognosis, but some severe cases have very low titres, and the mildest cases either very low or very high titres.

In countries where typhus is endemic the titre of normal persons may be above 1 in 100, and after antityphus inoculation agglutinins aften appear in low titre. Specific rickettsial agglutinins appear at the same time and follow the same course. Complement fixing antibodies appear a little later. Skin biopsy for the identification of the rash has proved particularly useful. Sections show the typical lesions resembling periarteritis nodosa. The petechiae in the skin are due to thrombosis of the smaller vessels.

Differential diagnosis. This has chiefly to be made from typhoid fever. The difference is based upon the onset and course of the fever and in the time of appearance and character of the skin rash. Typhus is of quicker onset and the temperature climbs quickly to a high level.

The differential diagnosis from septic meningitis may be difficult and is determined by the cerebrospinal fluid and Weil–Felix reaction. Diagnosis must be made from measles, especially the malignant variety found in the tropics. In measles there are Koplik's spots and the rash is brighter, the edges more marked and it is more profuse on the face.

The distinction from dengue and other forms of haemorrhagic fever may be difficult but in dengue the patient is not so ill nor is the suffusion of the face so marked. In severe smallpox the prodromal rash may be confusing. Purpura, cerebrospinal meningitis and relapsing fever have also to be considered. Other forms of typhus can be distinguished by the specific rickettsial serological tests.

Brill–Zinsser disease is usually milder and IgG antibodies are present from the start, as distinct from primary attacks of epidemic typhus in which the IgM antibodies are increased in the early stages (Murray *et al.* 1965).

Treatment

On admission the patient should be bathed with soap and water or a 1% solution of lysol. His clothes should be promptly disinfested by heat. The patient and hospital garments should be carefully dusted with 10% DDT delousing powder on admission and once a week until discharge. After these measures no quarantine is required. Nursing is of great importance. Stuporose patients and those in coma should be moved from side to side to prevent bedsores. If the temperature rises above 40°C cold sponging is indicated. Fluids should be administered in adequate quantities, at least 1500 ml/day. Barbiturates must be avoided and delirium or restlessness treated with paraldehyde and chloral hydrate. In severely ill and toxic patients steroid therapy should be given concurrently with antibiotics, prednisone 40 mg at once followed by 20 mg at intervals of 6 hours for 12 hours.

Where there is circulatory collapse, fluid and electrolyte balances must be restored by saline infusions.

Antibiotics. Chloramphenicol and the tetracyclines are highly specific. Chloramphenicol is given as a loading dose of 2–3 grammes and continued as 1–2 grammes every 24 hours in 4 divided doses. Chlortetracycline (Aureomycin) or oxytetracycline hydrochloride (Terramycin) is given in similar doses. The antibiotics must be continued for 3 days after the temperature has become normal.

Treatment of complications. Where there is gangrene the sloughs must be allowed to separate and the areas of gangrene should be protected from infection and kept cool to prevent extension. Gangrenous limbs must be packed in ice until the typhus infection has been brought under control.

Prevention and control

The basis for the control of epidemic typhus is louse control and immunization. In dealing with epidemics where case reporting has been good and the number of cases small, residual insecticides should be applied to all contacts. Where the infection is known to be widespread the application of residual insecticides to all persons in the community is indicated. 10% DDT powder for delousing can be applied by a powder duster which can operate 10 guns simultaneously. The DDT powder is sprayed down the opening of the neck and up the trousers in men and skirts in women. The lethal effect of DDT on lice lasts for more than 2 weeks, and if it is impregnated as an emulsion on clothes for more than 4 weeks. Where resistance to DDT has been developed by the lice then other residual insecticides must be employed.

Immunization. Killed vaccine probably reduces the incidence of the disease in exposed persons and definitely reduces the mortality to practically zero. Cox-type vaccine should be administered subcutaneously in two doses each of 1 ml separated by an interval of 10–14 days, followed by a booster dose of 1 ml at the beginning and in the middle of the typhus season. The use of egg yolk vaccine should be avoided in persons sensitive to egg protein. Living vaccine of the E strain will produce immunity for up to 5 years but febrile reactions are common.

Laboratory personnel working with epidemic typhus rickettsiae should be immunized regularly with killed vaccine, as should doctors, nurses and health personnel working with typhus patients.

MURINE TYPHUS (FLEA TYPHUS)

Synonyms. Endemic typhus; shop typhus.

Geographical distribution

Murine typhus is of world wide distribution. It is especially endemic in certain areas such as North America, Mexico, India, Pakistan, Darling Downs in Queensland, and Malaya (shop or urban typhus). Infected rats have been found in the Mediterranean basin, Malaya, North and West Africa and the Congo.

Epidemiology

Nicolle and Zinsser took the view that murine typhus is the more primitive disease and that it is a disease of rodents. The brown rat, *Rattus norvegicus*, is mainly concerned in temperate climates. The infection is transmitted from rat to rat by the rat louse (*Polyplax spinulosa*). The most important factor in the occurrence of murine typhus is the residence of human beings in areas where rats abound, such as grain stores and breweries. The infection is transmitted from rat to man by the rat flea (*Xenopsylla cheopis*), and *R. mooseri* seems to have undergone two mutations, changing both its vertebrate and invertebrate host, to evolve into *R. prowazeki*. In Mexico a type of typhus exists which may be regarded as intermediate between the murine and louse-born types. The more recent origin of epidemic typhus is shown by the fact that *R. mooseri* is harmless to the flea, whereas *R. prowazeki* causes death of the louse to which it is less well adapted. It is probable that endemic typhus may be converted into the epidemic and that typhus may be maintained in interepidemic periods by rats in this manner. Raynal *et al.* (1939) have adduced evidence that in Shanghai under certain conditions rickettsiae can be converted from the rat–louse–rat cycle via the rat flea to man–louse–man cycle. The armadillo and field rats in South America are susceptible to murine typhus and intracellular strains of rickettsiae virulent for mice sometimes become non-virulent and extracellular after passage through the mouse flea (*Leptopsylla segnis*) which is susceptible to *R. mooseri*.

Trombiculid mites, *Schöngastia indica*, have been found naturally infected with murine typhus (Gispen 1950) in Malaya. The mites were taken from house rats and sewer rats (*Rattus norvegicus*).

The seasonal incidence remains constant and the majority of cases occur in the summer and autumn. The incidence is twice as high in males as females and Negroes are less susceptible than Europeans.

Clinical features

The symptoms resemble those of epidemic typhus but are much milder in every respect. The mortality rate is very low, about 1·5%.

Treatment

The treatment is the same as for epidemic typhus.

Prophylaxis

The flea populations should be reduced by the application of 10% DDT to rat runs, burrows and harbourages. After this rodent populations should be controlled by Warfarin and the rat proofing of large grain stores.

TRENCH FEVER

Synonyms. Wolhynian fever; five-day fever.

Aetiology

Trench fever is caused by *Rickettsia quintana* which Weyer (1949) has suggested is a transformation from mild interepidemic typhus to a milder labile type resulting from certain environmental conditions which affect both the human and louse hosts.

Transmission

Rickettsia quintana live and multiply in the cuticular margin of the epithelium of the midgut of lice and not intracellularly as does *R. prowazeki*. Lice become infected by feeding on infected humans and remain infected for a year. It is not certain whether human infection is caused by the bite or by faecal contamination.

Geographical distribution and epidemiology

Trench fever occurred in epidemic form in Europe in the 1914–18 war. In 1942–3 again it appeared among soldiers on the eastern front. *R. quintana* has been isolated from human lice in an experiment in which healthy lice were found infected with *R. quintana* after feeding on humans previously inoculated with infected louse faeces (Varela *et al.* 1954). Human infection is found in louse-infested people living in confined quarters. No animal reservoir has been demonstrated although rhesus and spider monkeys can be experimentally infected.

Clinical features

The incubation period is 10–30 days, following which there is a sudden onset of severe headache, prostration and hyperaesthesia of the skin and pain in the back and lower extremities ('shin bone fever'). The fever is intermittent every 4 or 5 days ('febris quintana'). In the majority of cases there is a macular eruption of rose coloured spots lasting for a variable period. No lasting immunity develops and rickettsiae may persist in the blood of carriers for months or even years (Mohr & Weyer 1964). The disease is never fatal.

Diagnosis

Rickettsiae can be demonstrated by feeding clean lice on the patient and transmitting the infection to laboratory mice or monkeys. Specific rickettsial agglutination tests are positive.

Treatment

Chloramphenicol and tetracyclines are specific as in epidemic typhus.

MITE TYPHUS

Synonyms. Scrub typhus; tsutsugamushi; shimamushi; Japanese river fever; Kedani mite disease; 'K form'.

Aetiology

Mite typhus is caused by *Rickettsia orientalis* (*tsutsugamushi*), which is a parasite of rodents and is transmitted by a larval mite of the *Leptotrombidium* genus, the adult of which is non-parasitic.

Transmission

The adult mites (*Leptotrombidium*) are non-parasitic and live on vegetation; they lay their eggs on the ground where they hatch; six-legged larvae (Kedani mite or 'patau') emerge and then attach themselves to birds, reptiles, rodents or man upon which they feed and extract lymph and tissue fluids but not blood. In the larval mite the rickettsiae pass through the intestinal wall and enter the haemocoele and extra-intestinal tissues including the salivary glands in which they multiply, remaining viable through the nymph and adult stages until they are passed on to the larval mites of the second generation via the egg. The larval mites do not cling to their animal hosts for more than 3 or 4 days, when they drop off. Rickettsiae are inoculated repeatedly into the same patch of skin upon the ears of rodents and this facilitates the uptake of rickettsiae by uninfected mites, which always tend to feed upon the same place.

Seven species of *Leptotrombidium* transmit infection to rodents and man. The two main vectors are *L. akamushi* in Japan and *L. deliense* in Malaya and South-east Asia. Other known or suspected vectors are *L. scutellare*, *L. pallidum*, *L. palpale*, *L. intermedium*, and *L. torosum*. Because of transovarial transmission a site can remain infected for long periods, at least 1 year in the absence of an infected host.

Geographical distribution and epidemiology

Scrub typhus is indigenous in Japan, South Korea, Formosa, the Pescadores, the Philippines, Hong Kong, Yunnan Province in China, extensive areas in Indochina, Northern Thailand, Burma, Malaya, India (Madras, Simla Hills, Bombay, Bihar, Punjab), Ceylon in the south-east province, the Maldive Islands, the Andaman and Nicobar Islands, Sumatra, Java, Borneo, Northern Celebes, New Guinea and islands off the coast, New Britain, Bougainville, New Georgia, the northern New Hebrides, Queensland and North-eastern Australia. The geographical range also extends from South-eastern Siberia to west of the Indus river and possibly also Tibet, Nepal, Afghanistan and eastern Iran. There are also pockets in the Pakistan Himalayas. Scrub typhus may occur anywhere where the ecological factors for its presence are operative, namely the presence of rodent hosts and the trombiculid mites. The larval mites live and feed upon 'maintenance' hosts which, in the case of *L. akamushi* in Japan, are rice field rats and quail, in a biocoenose. The rickettsiae passage between the 'reservoir' hosts (rodents) and the mites. The numbers of mites are built up by successive generations infected with rickettsiae in 'mite' or 'typhus' islands until there is a spillover into man, who is an 'incidental' or casual host.

There is a wide variation in infection rates and mortality in man, which is not dependent on the virulence of the local strain of rickettsiae but on the number of organisms in the mites. It is recorded that in South Bat Island in the Purdy group off New Guinea, which is uninhabited by man, there is a saturated population of rats saturated with *R. orientalis* and infested with larval mites (*L. deliense*). In 1944, 26 of 41 sailors contracted scrub typhus there in 46 days and 2 died.

Scrub typhus occurs in scrubby terrain associated with man's modification of the vegetation and also in forest, glacial slopes and semi-desert. In the Pakistan Himalayas there are ecological islands of appropriate fauna of rodents and ectoparasites in some of which scrub typhus has been demonstrated and from which, in spite of isolation, the infection may have spread to form new endemic areas (Traub *et al.* 1967). In endemic foci the infection evolves slowly and different species of mites and rodents are concerned over a period of years. Man-made activities may introduce scrub typhus to new areas or increase its endemicity if already present. In Malaya and South East Asia the areas of highest endemicity have been largely man-made by deforestation, as in abandoned rubber plantations overgrown with rank kunai grass known as 'lalang' (Malaya and New Guinea) and in weed-covered waste patches on the outskirts of large towns, such as Calcutta, Bombay, Rangoon, Mandalay, Singapore and Kuala Lumpur, where scrub typhus is a backyard disease.

Endemic areas may also be developed on the edges of virgin forest, where they form the hedgerow type of endemic centre.

In Japan man acquires mite typhus in 'yudokuchi', which means poisonous places. These areas, which have been known for centuries, occur chiefly along the banks of big rivers in the southern island of Honshu.

There is a seasonal incidence of scrub typhus carried by *T. akamushi* from May to October, but an epidemiological variant known as 'winter scrub typhus' or 'shichito fever' carried by *L. scutellare* is also found. Outbreaks of scrub typhus may be of various types. It is explosive in people who visit a 'yudokuchi' for the first time, when all the cases will occur in 10–12 days, or the outbreak may be followed by a rapid decline consequent upon occupation and clearance of the site. Sporadic cases may occur following occasional visits to a 'yudokuchi' from an uninfected site. There may be a delayed epidemic consequent upon subsequent use of a 'yudokuchi' as a latrine or recreation area. Lastly cases may occur repeatedly following upon occupation, abandonment and reoccupation of an infected camp site (Audy 1968).

Maintenance hosts comprise some 20 species of rats, tree shrews and several species of birds which can disseminate the infected mites. In Upper Burma the Yunnan buff-breasted rat (*R. flavipectus yunnanensis*) and Assamese tree shrew (*Tupai belangeri versurae*) have been found naturally infected with rickettsiae (Mackie *et al.* 1946). Larval trombiculae are also found in large numbers on the ears of the maintenance hosts, the field vole (*Microtus montebelloi*), *Mus jerdoni*, *R. rattus rufescens*, *R. norvegicus*, *R. agrarius*, *R. jalorensis* and in the Imphal district *R. bullocki*. In the forests around Kuala Lumpur the main hosts are 3 giant rats, *R. mulleri*, *R. sabanus* and *R. bowersi*. In Jarak Island in the Malacca Straits

R. r. jaraki and *R. argentiventer* form the main hosts. The rat–mite cycle is kept up in these rodents and in towns in Malaya, for instance Kuala Lumpur, the infection is transmitted from the jungle rats to the Malayan house rat (*R. r. diardi*).

Pathology

The rickettsiae multiply locally at the site of inoculation, from which they disseminate. A local lesion forms an eschar with coagulation necrosis affecting the epidermis, corium and surrounding tissues, well delineated by a surrounding line. The lymph glands in the area become enlarged and show central necrosis. There is general lymph gland enlargement. The rickettsiae have a predilection for the vascular endothelium and cause intravascular and perivascular lesions in the smaller blood vessels, especially in the skin, myocardium, lungs and brain.

Endovascular lesions with thrombosis and haemorrhage are marked in the lungs and there is a perivascular infiltration with monocytes, plasma cells and lymphocytes with focal oedema. In the myocardium there is an interstitial invasion of monocytes, and focal necrosis; in the lungs the walls of the alveoli become thickened and the alveolar spaces are filled with serum and red cells.

In the brain there is a focal perivascular reaction with neuroglial proliferation, monocytic infiltration and focal necrosis. The 'typhus nodules' in mite typhus differ from those of the louse-borne form in that the chief change is the perivascular infiltration and the intima of the blood vessels is only secondarily involved. The spleen is enlarged and shows septic changes with focal necrosis. The liver is enlarged and congested and shows focal necrosis. The kidneys show pale swelling of the cortex and a narrow zone of congestion. There is an effusion of fluid into the tunica vaginalis and generalized oedema with haemorrhage into the tissues.

Clinical features

The person attacked by the mite does not usually notice the bite, but later feels a pricking sensation when he happens to touch the spot. The mite, or mites, can easily be seen through a strong magnifying glass, with their heads buried in the skin, but only when they are carriers of the disease do any definite changes take place round the lesions they inflict. After an incubation period of from 4 to 10 days or longer, the disease begins with severe frontal and bitemporal headache, anorexia and chills alternating with flushes of heat. Presently the patient becomes conscious of pain and tenderness in the lymphatic glands of the groin, armpit or neck. On inspection of the skin there is sometimes discovered—usually about the genitals or armpits—a small (2–4 mm), round, dark, tough, firmly adherent eschar with necrotic centre surrounded by a painless livid red areola of superficial congestion. This is the initial ulcer (Fig. 176). Sometimes it may be merely a papule, which develops and disappears during the incubation period and therefore is seldom visible. Occasionally 2 or 3 eschars are discovered. Although a line of tenderness may be traced from the sore to the swollen, hard, and sensitive glands, no well defined cord of lymphangitis can be made out. The superficial lymphatic glands of the rest of the body, especially those on the side opposite to the glands primarily affected, are also, but more slightly, enlarged.

Clinical observers in Burma describe adenopathy as present in 90%. The glands are most noticeably palpable in the posterior triangles of the neck. In a few cases this is so pronounced as to give a bull-neck appearance. The enlargement of the posterior occipital glands may be the cause of occipital pain in association with neck rigidity.

Fever of a continued type now sets in, the thermometer mounting in the course of 5 or 6 days to 40° or 40·6°C. The conjunctivae become injected; the eyes are half-closed, watery and faintly glistening. Photophobia is invariable. At the same time, a considerable bronchitis gives rise to harassing cough. The pulse is full and strong, ranging rather low (80–100) for the degree of fever present. The spleen is moderately but distinctly enlarged, and there is marked constipation.

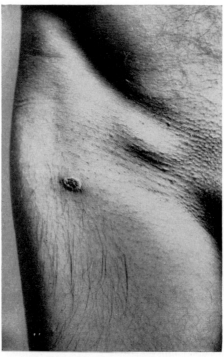

Fig. 176.—Mite typhus. Eschar with enlarged satellite lymph node. (Dr T. J. Danaraj, Singapore)

About the sixth or seventh day the eruption of large dark-red papules appears. It is usually maculopapular, sometimes papular or macular. It lasts 3–4 days, mainly on the trunk, upper arms and thighs. It sometimes extends to the face, hands and feet.

During the height of the fever the patient is flushed and at night may be delirious. He complains incessantly, probably on account of a general hyper-aesthesia of skin and muscles. Deafness is also a constant feature.

As the disease advances, the symptoms become more urgent; the conjunctivitis is intensified, the cough becomes incessant, the tongue dries, the lips crack and bleed, and there may be from time to time profuse perspiration. By the end of the second week—sooner or later according to the severity of the case—the fever begins to remit by lysis, the tongue to clean and, after a few days, temperature falls to normal and the patient speedily convalesces. There is a well marked leucopenia; if the leucocytes are increased some extraneous infection may be suspected. The red cells are normal, but there is a decrease in the coagulability of the blood. Bronchitis, diarrhoea or diuresis may occur during the decline of the fever. The circular, sharp-edged, deep ulcer left after the separation of the primary eschar—usually during the second week—now begins to heal, and the enlargement of the glands gradually to subside. The urine contains albumin and gives a positive diazo-reaction.

Such is the course of a moderately severe case. In some instances, however, the constitutional disturbance is very slight, although the primary eschar may be well marked and perhaps extensive. On the other hand, the fever may be much more violent, and complications, such as parotitis, melaena, coma, mania, cardiac failure or oedema of the lungs may end in death. Similarly, the duration of the disease varies according to severity from 1 to 4 weeks, 3 weeks being about the average. Relapses do not occur in the untreated case.

Eye sequelae are found in 98%, especially subjective retinal findings consisting of enlargement of blind spots, contraction of visual fields and scotomas. Minor non-specific involvement of the cochlear system of the ear was found in only 11% during convalescence.

Pregnant women contracting scrub typhus mostly abort and die.

Complications. An important complication is myocarditis, and myocardial failure may occur during the second week. Inversion of the T-wave is an important sign of myocardial involvement. Death may occur from broncho-pneumonia or exhaustion. A defibrination syndrome, caused by intravascular coagulation, has been described (Chernof 1964).

Immunity

There is immunity to reinfection with the homologous strain of R. orientalis, which lasts for about 1 year. Second attacks may occur after infection with heterologous strains from other areas, but these are not important, since most areas have a mixture of 2 of the 3 main antigenic strains of Rickettsia.

Diagnosis

The diagnosis must be made from other fevers: malaria, typhoid, haemorrhagic fever, smallpox and cerebrospinal meningitis. Points in diagnosis are lympha-denopathy and splenomegaly in typhus. Rickettsiae may be isolated from the blood in the early stages by grinding up blood clot with normal saline and centrifuging at low speed. 0·3 ml of supernatant fluid is inoculated intraperi-toneally into mice. The mice die 10–16 days later, when rickettsiae can be demonstrated in peritoneal smears. Antibodies appear during the second week and last until cure. Serologically the reactions are of the OXK type and the Weil–Felix shows agglutination of the OXK strain. Specific agglutination, haemagglutination and complement fixation tests are positive to R. orientalis antigens.

Treatment

Chloramphenicol, chlortetracycline and oxytetracycline hydrochloride are specific. These antibiotics are given orally in a loading dose of 3·0 grammes followed by 500 mg 6-hourly until the temperature is normal. Usually 5·0 grammes in the first 24 hours are sufficient but more seriously ill patients may require this dosage for another day or two. Since the antibiotics are rickettsio-static a cure is obtained with the immunity which begins to develop during the second week of the illness. Relapses are not seen in patients in whom treatment is begun on the seventh day of disease or later. Recrudescences may occur in half the patients treated from the fourth to sixth day of illness but can be prevented by administration of 3·0 grammes of antibiotic on the sixth day after termination of the original dose.

Treatment of complications. Falciparum malaria and scrub typhus may coexist in the same patient, and the possibility should be considered in patients with falciparum malaria who are not responding to antimalarial therapy. Severe cases of scrub typhus should be carefully watched and electrocardiograms taken for signs of myocardial failure. Where inversion of the T-waves has occurred then a prolonged convalescence must be ensured. Myocardial failure must be treated with complete bed rest and digitalization and diuretics. Patients showing ECG changes should be kept in bed for 6 weeks after treatment.

Prophylaxis and control

Control is based upon regulation of the environment and antimite measures. Chemoprophylaxis can be used but immunization is of little value. The environmental features which produce infection must be identified in different districts, and known endemic areas, which are often localized to relatively small geographical regions such as second degree growths in deforested areas, should be avoided. Prospective camp sites may be prepared by cutting all vegetation level with the ground and burning it. After thorough clearing the ground dries in 2–3 weeks, killing the mites. More immediate occupation can be achieved by spraying with dieldrin or gammexane (BHC). Antimite measures consist in the use of miticides and repellents.

Dibutyl phthalate (DBP) is lethal to mites which are killed when walking on impregnated cloth. 58 grammes of DBP or dimethyl phthalate (DMP) will treat two sets of tropical uniform. Fingers are dipped into the fluid and rubbed lightly over the cloth. DBP and DMP will resist up to 8 washes in cold water and wading through rivers. 5% emulsion of DBP or DMP in 2% soap emulsion is effective as a repellent. A mixture of benzyl benzoate and dibutyl phthalate is effective.

Chemoprophylaxis. Chloramphenicol has been tested as a prophylactic by giving 1·0 gramme daily by mouth during exposure to infection and for 13 subsequent days. 70% of a control untreated group were attacked by scrub typhus whereas in the treated group the disease was suppressed until 8 days after the cessation of treatment (Smadel et al. 1952). In another régime 3·0 grammes of chloramphenicol are given once a week when the drug must be continued for 4 weeks after leaving the endemic area, otherwise clinical disease can occur after withdrawal of the chloramphenicol. A similar result could be expected with tetracyclines.

AMERICAN TICK TYPHUS

American tick typhus is also known as Rocky Mountain spotted fever, and is caused by *R. rickettsi rickettsi*.

Geographical distribution and epidemiology

Spotted fever occurs in the New World in both North and South America. In North America it is found in two main forms, Western and Eastern.

Western Rocky Mountain spotted fever. Western Rocky Mountain spotted fever is found in the Western States of the U.S.A., Idaho, Montana (Bitter Root Valley), Wyoming, Utah, Nevada, Oregon, Colorado, New Mexico and Washington. It is confined principally to the valleys near the foothills in sharply defined limited zones. It is transmitted by the woodtick, *Dermacentor andersoni*, of which the natural maintenance hosts are the Rocky Mountain goat, sheep, black bear, coyote, badger and lynx. The larval stages of the ticks develop on ground squirrels and the woodchuck, from which they become infected with rickettsiae, which they pass on to man in the adult stages.

Eastern Rocky Mountain spotted fever. This form is spreading rapidly and has now been reported from east British Columbia, Alberta and Saskatchewan, and has spread as far east as Maryland. It is transmitted by the dog tick, *Dermacentor variabilis*, the larval stages of which are found on the meadow mouse (*Microtus pennsylvanicus*), from which rickettsiae have been isolated. Infected adult ticks are carried by dogs into suburban gardens where they infect man and spotted fever is a 'backyard' disease. In Virginia rickettsiae have been found in cottontail rabbits and antibodies in grey and red foxes, opposums, raccoons and deer.

Attacks of spotted fever tend to occur in North America in the spring when the ticks are most numerous. After feeding on infected blood there is a period of 12 days during which the rickettsiae multiply and all stages of the tick, larva, nymph and adults of both sexes, are efficient intermediary hosts. The proportion of infected ticks is about 1 in 296 and transovarial transmission takes place.

In Oklahoma the natural reservoir of infection is the pocket gopher (*Geomys breviceps dutcheri*) and the vector *Amblyomma americanum*. In Texas the vectors are *Rhipicephalus sanguineus* and *Amblyomma americanum*.

South American tick typhus. In South America spotted fever is found in Colombia on the Tobia River, a tributary of the Rio Negro, in a narrow valley of the Magdalena basin at an altitude of 700–1400 m. A second endemic zone exists north-west of the Villeta River at 500–1500 m. The tick vectors are *Amblyomma cajennense* and *Dermacentor nitens*. Tick typhus is common in Minas Geraes in Brazil. The natural reservoirs of infection are the opossum, domestic and wild dog, wild rabbits and the agouti. The tick vectors are species of *Amblyomma*, *A. cajennense*, *A. striatum* and *A. braziliense*.

From north to south there is a clinical transition from the spotted fever of North America without an eschar to the form found in Brazil where there is an eschar and the infection resembles *fièvre boutonneuse*.

Pathology

R. rickettsi, in contrast to other rickettsiae, invades the nuclei of the endothelial cells of the blood vessels, where they may be found in considerable masses, as well as the cell cytoplasm and other tissues. The endothelial cells are destroyed and the rickettsiae escape into the blood-stream and establish other foci. This vascular damage results in mural thrombi (Fraenkel's nodules), perivascular infiltration and gangrene. There is usually a well marked skin rash, bronchopneumonic consolidation and subserous petechial haemorrhages. Similar lesions are found in the brain. The myocardium shows cloudy swelling and the spleen is enlarged and firm. The lymphatic glands are generally enlarged. Focal necrosis of the hepatic cells and congestion of the renal cortex are found. Constant lesions in man and animals are haemorrhages in the genitalia and gangrene of the prepuce and scrotum.

Clinical features

The incubation period is 3–7 days. There may be a history of a tick bite but except in Brazil there is no eschar. The attack is ushered in by the sudden onset of chills, rigors and fever. By the second day the temperature rises to 39·4–40°C and by the fifth to 40·6–41·7°C. A typhus condition supervenes, with intense headache, photophobia, irritability and meningeal irritation.

The rash appears from the fourth to the seventh day. It is seen as small rose coloured spots resembling measles but soon becomes petechial, spreading so as to become confluent, especially on the more dependent parts, though it may occasionally be seen on the forehead.

During the third week desquamation sets in and the eruption gradually fades (Fig. 177). The liver is usually enlarged, the spleen enlarged, firm and tender. The highly coloured urine contains albumin and casts. Death may occur between the seventh and tenth days, often with symptoms of cardiac failure. Bronchopneumonia is a serious complication. Jaundice and vomiting may occu during the second week in severe cases. A defibrination syndrome has been described in spotted fever (Chernof 1964). Mortality varies considerably and has

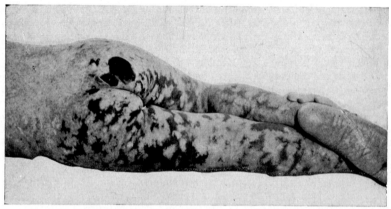

Fig. 177.—Rocky Mountain spotted fever on the tenth day, showing confluent haemorrhagic areas and a necrotic pressure area of skin over the buttock. A Texas outbreak, conveyed by *Amblyomma americanum*. (Dr L. Anigstein)

been as high as 70–90% in untreated cases. Until the use of antibiotics became widespread the general death rate was 19·6% for the Western and 18·1% for the Eastern form.

Diagnosis

The diagnosis must be made from other forms of typhus fever, haemorrhagic fevers, smallpox, cerebrospinal meningitis and septicaemia.

The serological reactions belong to the indeterminate group. The Weil–Felix shows positive agglutination against the *OX19* and *OX2* strains and differentiation from epidemic and murine typhus is made by specific rickettsial agglutination and complement fixation tests. These become positive during the second week. Rickettsiae, which can only be isolated from the blood very early in the infection, can be identified by the universal presence of a positive Neill–Mooser reaction in infected guinea-pigs and by specific rickettsial antisera.

Treatment

No quarantine measures are necessary. The broad-spectrum antibiotics, chloramphenicol and the tetracyclines, are all highly effective in treatment.

These antibiotics, which should be given as early in the infection as possible, are rickettsiostatic and suppress the growth of rickettsiae until the patient overcomes the disease by developing immunity. After recovery the individual may harbour rickettsiae for some time. Chloramphenicol is given as a loading dose of 3·0 grammes followed by 500 mg 4-hourly. Chlortetracycline hydrochloride and oxytetracycline hydrochloride are given as 2·0–3·0 grammes daily in divided doses. The antibiotics must be given until the patient's temperature has been normal for 48–72 hours and the period of drug administration usually lasts for 4–6 days. If there is a relapse a further course must be given.

A combination of specific antibiotic therapy with steroids will modify the severe effects and shorten the course of the illness. Prednisone 40 mg followed by 2 further doses of 20 mg at 6-hourly intervals is the usual course. In severely ill and comatose patients intravenous chloramphenicol 500 mg in glucose with 100 mg cortisone intramuscularly is given every 6 hours for 3 doses. Improvement will be noticed in 6 hours.

Control

Control measures are based upon tick control, prevention of tick bites and immunization. Tick control may be obtained in some areas by spraying the woodsides and pathsides with DDT once or twice a month during the tick season. Tick bites may be prevented by avoiding notorious areas in spring and summer and wearing protective clothing. The shirt must be tucked inside the trousers, and socks or high boots should be worn outside over trousers. An important precaution is to remove the clothes and search for ticks twice daily since ticks will only transmit the infection after 1 or 2 hours *in situ*.

Vaccination is an effective method of prevention. Formalin killed 'tick' vaccine or Cox vaccine may be used subcutaneously in 3 injections each of 1·0 ml at 5–7 day intervals. Vaccination must be performed in winter or early spring and should be repeated once a year.

TICK TYPHUS

Synonyms. Fièvre boutonneuse; Marseilles fever; eruptive fever; *fièvre exanthe matique*; *escharo nodulaire*; tick bite fevers, South African and Indian forms.

Aetiology

Tick typhus, first described by Conor and Bruch in Tunis in 1910, is caused by *Rickettsia rickettsi conori* in Southern Europe and the Mediterranean area and by *Rickettsia rickettsi conori* var. *pijperi* in South and East Africa.

Geographical distribution and epidemiology

Fièvre boutonneuse (*R. rickettsi conori*). This disease occurs throughout the Mediterranean littoral and many other districts in Southern France, Italy, Portugal, Spain, Greece, Romania and the Crimea. The rickettsiae are transmitted by the dog tick, *Rhipicephalus sanguineus,* and the dog constitutes the reservoir, since these animals have been shown to be susceptible and their blood infective for man and monkeys. A rodent reservoir has not been excluded, however. The rickettsiae pass from one generation of ticks to another by transovarial transmission.

African tick typhus (*R. rickettsi conori* var. *pijperi*). This was first described by McNaught in 1911 and Pijper and Dan in 1934. It occurs in South,
West and East Africa, the Sudan, Eritrea, Somalia and Ethiopia. In South
Africa the rickettsiae are transmitted by ixodid ticks, *Rhipicephalus appendiculatus* and *Amblyomma hebraeum*, and the dog tick, *Haemaphysalis leachi* (Gear
1969).

In Kenya the rickettsiae are transmitted by *Haemaphysalis leachi, Rhipicephalus
simus* and *Amblyomma variegatum*, all of which are found on dogs (Heisch 1957).
The natural reservoir may well be small rodents, since brain emulsions of
Otomys angoniensis and spleen emulsions of *Lemniscomys* have produced
rickettsiae when inoculated into guinea-pigs (Heisch *et al.* 1957) and serological
studies have shown the presence of rickettsial antibodies in rodents caught on
the Kenya coast. In Africa the disease is contracted in the bush or on the veld in
uninhabited areas, but in Nairobi in Kenya the disease is a backyard infection
and is acquired from ticks brought into the house by dogs. In Ruanda a
rickettsia has been found transmitted by *Ornithodorus moubata* (Jadin & Panier
1953).

Clinical features

The distinguishing features of this form of typhus are the presence of a
primary sore or eschar and secondary adenitis. Two forms occur: one mild and
abortive with the occurrence of an eschar and secondary adenitis, and the second
a fully developed form, in which a primary sore forms at the site of the tick bite
which becomes gangrenous and is known as 'tache noire', varying in size from
a pin's head to a pea, and painless. These lesions are situated in the axilla or on
the leg, or are sometimes hidden in the hair on the scalp. There is a secondary
lymphadenitis and enlargement of the local lymph glands. There is accompanying fever with headache, neck stiffness and a mild petechial rash appearing on
the fifth day. This form of typhus is much milder than spotted fever and the
mortality rate is practically negligible. In some cases an inverted T-wave
develops in the E.C.G. with accompanying breathlessness. Gangrene of the
scrotum has been described in Africans.

Diagnosis

The diagnosis must be made from cerebrospinal meningitis, measles and
typhoid fever, and in the abortive cases from an infective adenitis. Serologically
the disease gives an indeterminate reaction and in most cases the Weil–Felix
shows a higher titre of agglutination to the *Proteus OXK* strain than the *OX19*.
Specific rickettsial antibodies can be demonstrated against the homologous
strain of rickettsiae by agglutination and complement fixation tests.

Treatment

Treatment is the same as for other forms of typhus, and chloramphenicol or
tetracycline should be administered until the temperature has been normal for
48 hours.

Prophylaxis

Avoidance of sleeping on the ground in endemic areas, regular deticking and
the exclusion of dogs from the house all help in avoiding infection.

OTHER FORMS OF TICK TYPHUS

Indian and Southern Asian tick typhus

A mild sporadic form of typhus has been found in the Kumaon Hills in the North-west Frontier of Pakistan and other cases have been reported from Lucknow and the Simla Hills. Hoogstraal (1967) states that tick typhus in Asia includes *boutonneuse* fever and Siberian tick typhus, but there is also evidence that mite-borne typhus exists in parts of India.

Siberian tick typhus

A tick-borne rickettsial disease has been reported from East and Central Siberia. It is a mild form with a primary eschar, headache and rash, and is transmitted mainly by *Dermacentor nuttalli* but also by *Dermacentor silvarum* and *Haemaphysalis concinna*. Rickettsial complement fixing antibodies have been found in farm animals (Yastrebov *et al.* 1968).

North Queensland tick typhus

A mild form of rickettsial disease has been described in North and to a lesser extent in South Queensland. It causes a syndrome resembling *boutonneuse* fever. Although it is related to this group it can be differentiated by specific rickettsial serological tests; the *Rickettsia* has been provisionally named *R. australis*. The vector is probably *Ixodes holocyclus* and rickettsial complement fixing antibodies have been found in bandicoots, kangaroo rats and bush-tailed opossums. There is an eschar with regional adenopathy, a rash and a typhus-like course.

Q (QUERY) FEVER

Synonyms. Nine mile fever; Balkan grippe; Red River fever of the Congo.

Aetiology

Q fever is caused by *Coxiella burneti*, a *Rickettsia* widely spread in small wild mammals and ticks in nature and a common infection of domestic animals, goats, sheep and cows. *Coxiella burneti* is morphologically similar to *C. diaporica* (Fig. 178), is the smallest of the rickettsiae and is filterable. In nature it exists in the 'smooth form' of Phase 1 and changes on adaptation to chick embryos to the 'rough form' of Phase 2. It causes characteristic pathological effects in monkeys, mice and guinea-pigs. There is a well defined febrile reaction, during which the blood is infective for guinea-pigs. Mice inoculated intraperitoneally show enlargement of the liver and spleen with characteristic histological changes. In sections and smears of infected mouse liver and spleen large numbers of rickettsiae occur in relatively large intracytoplasmic colonies (Fig. 178). Fluorescent microscopy is of special value in estimating the number of rickettsiae in yolk sac cultures.

C. burneti can be cultivated on minced chicken embryo, reaching its maximum growth during the second week. When 8- or 9-day embryos are inoculated numerous rickettsiae are visible in membranes removed after 6 days and incubated at 34°C.

Immunology

C. burneti of Australia and America are identical. Both Montana and Australian Q strains are agglutinated to the same titre by sera of animals infected with one or other strain. There is no cross-immunity in guinea-pigs to Rocky Mountain spotted fever. Protective immunity may develop in man and animals without febrile response, but the subsequent complete immunity of the animal indicates that infection has taken place. A well marked immunity develops in man, which is taken advantage of in vaccination. Agglutinating and complement fixing antibodies appear in both animals and man. Both appear early in the infection and last for some months after recovery or cure and can be used retrospectively to diagnose past infections and to determine the incidence of the disease in a human community and farm animals. Neither the sera of patients nor those of infected animals agglutinate *Proteus OX19, OXK* or *OX2*. Cross-reactions have been described with the complement fixing antibodies of adenovirus 7 infections (Grist & Ross 1968).

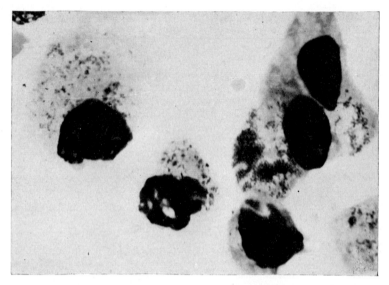

Fig. 178.—*Coxiella burneti* (*diaporica*). American Q fever (Wyoming). Slide prepared from peritoneal scrapings of infected guinea-pig. Giemsa. × 1500. (*Dr L. Anigstein*)

The antigen is prepared from yolk sac cultures of *C. burneti* purified with ether, differentially centrifuged and stained with a modified Harris haematoxylin stain. Stock preparations may be lyophilized and kept indefinitely. Capillary tubes 9 cm × 0·4 mm are filled one-third with antigen and the remainder with dilutions of sera. The end point is easy to read.

History

Q fever was first reported by Derrick as an obscure illness among abattoir employees in Brisbane in 1937 and the organism was isolated and described by Burnet and Freeman as *Rickettsia burneti*. In 1939 it was established that the organism was the same as *R. diaporica*, spread by the ticks *Dermacentor andersoni* and *Ornithodorus turicata* in the West U.S.A. *R. burneti* has now been renamed *Coxiella burneti* and is becoming increasingly common in almost every country in the world and numerous laboratory infections have been reported.

Transmission

C. burneti is maintained in nature in small wild animals by ticks which introduce the infection into domestic flocks and herds, in which further dissemination is direct from one animal to another as well as by ticks. Since *C. burneti* is excreted in milk, placental tissues and amniotic fluid, it is transmitted by milk, placental products, faeces and air dust. Man may be infected by ticks (in the Western U.S.A.) or more usually by air-borne infection from infected animals and by handling meat products, milk or placentae, or by drinking infected milk.

Geographical distribution and epidemiology

Because of the many and varied methods of transmission Q fever has a widespread distribution throughout the world and a varied epidemiology.

Reservoir in nature. It has been suggested (Marmion *et al.* 1954) that *C. burneti* originated as a commensal inhabitant of ticks and that they may constitute a permanent reservoir since transovarian passage of the organism has been demonstrated in *Dermacentor andersoni* and *Ornithodorus* and *Hyalomma* species. Natural infections of rodents have been found in nature and *C. burneti* has been isolated from a gerbil (*Meriones*) in Morocco, a rabbit in North Africa and from the brown rat, house mouse, vole and marmot (*Spermophilus leptodactylis*) in Transcaspia. In East Africa Heisch has found it in a rodent, *Lemniscomys striatus*. In the Salt Lake City region the rabbit and chipmunk have been found infected. In Australia the natural reservoir in Queensland is the bandicoot (*Isoodon torosus* or *I. obesulus*) and rickettsiae have been isolated from a tick, *Haemaphysalis humerosa*, an ectoparasite of the bandicoot and opossum. In Russia it is claimed that infection is also found in birds such as field sparrows, redstart, wagtail, pigeon, domestic hen, swallow, buzzard and magpie, and in their mites. The infection is maintained in nature by ticks and *C. burneti* has been demonstrated in the following ticks: *Rhipicephalus sanguineus* in Arizona, *Hyalomma savignyi* in Spain, *Hyalomma mauritanicum* in Algeria, *Haemaphysalis excavatum* in Morocco, *Haemaphysalis punctata* from sheep in Rhodesia and *H. dromedarii* from bulls in Egypt. The cattle tick, *Boophilus annulatus microplus*, maintains the infection in cattle in Australia and transmits it to man.

Human infection. When ticks are involved in human transmission, cases are few and sporadic. Farm workers are commonly affected by direct transmission when they are in contact with sheep at lambing time or with sheep which abort. There is a high incidence in those whose work takes them to farms where they are exposed to direct infection, rural postmen, agricultural machinery salesmen and those in contact with agricultural workers, such as village barbers and grocers. Where direct transmission is involved outbreaks may be explosive and involve a number of individuals. Abattoir workers are at risk.

Pathology (Whittick 1950)

Coxiella burneti is a cytoplasmic parasite and develops in the histiocytes of the spleen and the Kupffer cells of the liver. The infected cells swell and cause enlargement of these organs. In some cases liver biopsy has shown focal lesions where there is eosinophilic necrosis of the sinusoid walls with a granulomatous appearance and occasional multinucleate giant cells. A frequent finding in fatal cases is interstitial pneumonitis. In cases of endocarditis there are vegetations on the affected valves.

Clinical features

Q fever may present as a variety of clinical syndromes: fever, pneumonitis, endocarditis, pericarditis (Grist & Ross 1968) and a condition resembling glandular fever (Eshchar *et al.* 1966).

Fever. This fever is known in America as 'nine mile fever' from the Nine Mile Creek in the Rocky Mountains. The course and duration vary considerably. There may be a rapid defervescence after 6–9 days or the course may be protracted to the third or fourth week and the temperature falls by lysis. There is no rash except in the form described as Red River fever of the Congo. There is severe headache, shivering and even rigors, photophobia, anorexia and pain in the back and legs. There is often splenomegaly and a tender enlargement of the liver.

Pneumonitis. Q fever characteristically causes an interstitial pneumonitis with physical signs developing in the lungs during the first week. There is coryza and a non-productive cough with transitory infiltrations of the lung resembling an atypical virus pneumonia seen on X-ray, but there are no cold agglutinins in Q fever.

Endocarditis. Q fever endocarditis is being increasingly reported, especially in cases where artificial heart valves have been inserted. It should be suspected in cases with unexplained aortic regurgitation, fever and heart failure. It is very resistant to treatment.

Glandular fever. Syndromes occur with pharyngitis, headache, an absolute lymphocytosis and occasionally cervical lymphadenopathy and splenomegaly. Signs of pericarditis and myocarditis may supervene.

Subclinical infection. In many cases the infection is asymptomatic and serological surveys have shown evidence of past infection in farm workers and in persons associated with farming who have had no previous illness.

Diagnosis

Q fever has to be differentiated from typhoid, atypical virus pneumonia, influenza, ornithosis, glandular fever and toxoplasmosis.

The diagnosis is made by serological studies. The agglutination test is highly specific and a complement fixation test is available. Rickettsiae may be isolated from the blood early in the infection by inoculating blood into guinea-pigs and demonstrating rickettsiae in peritoneal smears or the development of specific antibodies in guinea-pig serum.

Treatment

Chloramphenicol and tetracyclines are specific when given as 2–3 grammes daily by mouth and continued for several days after the temperature falls to normal. Endocarditis is very resistant to treatment and streptomycin and sulphonamides should all be exhibited. It may respond to tetracycline and Septrin (Freeman & Hodson 1972).

Prevention and control

Control of the infection on a community basis rests upon the control of the disease in domestic animals either by immunization or treatment. Milk from goats, sheep and cows must be pasteurized. Calving and lambing in endemic areas should be confined to an enclosed area which can be decontaminated. Immunization is the most effective control measure for the individual.

Vaccination. Vaccination should be performed on high-risk laboratory workers and heavily exposed groups, such as farm workers in endemic areas and workers handling farm products such as meat and milk. Inactivated formolized Cox vaccine prepared from Phase 1 *C. burneti* is more effective than Phase 2. A standard vaccine Q-34, containing 10 complement fixing units/ml is given in 1·0 ml doses as 3 weekly subcutaneous injections. Preliminary skin testing with 1·0 ml of a 1/50 dilution of the vaccine should be performed to avoid reactions. Successful vaccination is shown by the development of a positive skin reaction after 40 days. Live Phase 2 rickettsiae have been used as a live vaccine but there is a danger of the development of endocarditis, especially in persons with cardiac lesions.

RICKETTSIALPOX

Synonyms. Vesicular rickettsiasis; Kew Gardens spotted fever.

This curious infection was described (Huebner *et al.* 1946a, b) in inmates of an apartment house in New York with a pox-like rash. Within the next 3 years nearly 500 cases had been reported—all in New York City. The initial lesion resembles that of mite typhus and the rash is similar to that of other members of this group, except that vesicles occur. A case has been reported from former French Equatorial Africa (Le Gac & Giroud 1951) as rickettsiose vesiculeuse.

The incubation period is about 7 days and the temperature rises on the tenth day after infection. The lesion starts as a small erythematous patch and soon a vesicle appears with centre developing into an eschar with enlargement of the corresponding lymph glands. Malaise and headache are invariably present. Fever lasts 1–7 days. The rash appears on the second day in the form of discrete erythematous, maculo-papular spots, 2–10 mm in diameter, all over the body. The mucous membranes are seldom involved and the hands and soles of the feet escape.

At a later stage the vesicles are replaced by blackish crusts which drop off leaving pigmented spots. This disease has no mortality. The lesions of smallpox, though initially similar, in their deeper and firmer character, have a different maturation (Rose 1949).

The causal agent is *R. akari* which is transmitted by the mouse-mite, *Allodermanyssus sanguineus* (Huebner *et al.* 1946b). *Bdellonyssus bacoti*, another murine parasite, is also capable of transmission under laboratory conditions. The rickettsiae are extracellular or intracytoplasmic and intranuclear.

The domestic mouse is undoubtedly the reservoir and mice have been found carrying infected mites, while they themselves have been proved to be immune to infection. The Weil–Felix reaction is negative, but complement fixation tests, with ether extracted soluble antigens, are reliable, giving a rising titre response. Reactions with Rocky Mountain fever antigens are positive also.

Treatment with Aureomycin, 2–4 grammes daily, has been successful; oxytetracycline (Terramycin) is also effective.

REFERENCES

AUDY, J. R. (1968) *Red Mites and Typhus.* University of London Heath Clark lectures. London: Athlone Press.

CHERNOF, D. (1964) *New Engl. J. Med.,* **270,** 1042.

ESHCHAR, J., WARON, M. & ALKAN, W. J. (1966) *J. Am. med. Ass.,* **195,** 390.

FREEMAN, R. & HODSON, M. E. (1972) *Br. med. J.,* **i,** 419.

GEAR, J. H. S. (1969) *Br. med. Bull.*, **25**, 171.

GAON, J. A. & MURRAY, E. S. (1966) *Bull. Wld Hlth Org.*, **35**, 133.

GISPEN, R. (1950) *Documenta neerl. indones. Morb. trop.*, **2**, 23.

GRIST, N. R. & ROSS, C. A. C. (1968) *Br. med. J.*, **i**, 119.

HEISCH, R. B. (1957) *Trans. R. Soc. trop. Med. Hyg.*, **51**, 287.

—— MCPHEE, R. & RICKMAN, L. R. (1957) *E. Afr. med. J.*, **34**, 459.

HOOGSTRAAL, H. (1967) *Ann. Rev. Ent.*, **12**, 337.

HUEBNER, R. J., JELLISON, W. L. & POMERANZ, C. (1946a) *Pub. Hlth Rep. Wash.*, **61**, 1677.

—— STAMPS, P. & ARMSTRONG, G. (1946b) *Pub. Hlth Rep. Wash.*, **61**, 1605.

JADIN, J. & PAINIER, E. (1953) *Ann. Soc. belge Med. trop.*, **33**, 119.

LE GAC, P. & GIROUD, P. (1951) *Bull. Soc. Path. exot.*, **44**, 413.

MACKIE, J., DAVIS, G. E., FULLER, H. S., KNAPP, J. A., STEINACKER, M. L., STAGER, K. E., TRAUB, R., JELLISON, W. L., MILLSPAUGH, D. D., AUSTRIAN, R. C., BELL, E. J., KOHLS, G. M., WEI HSI & GIRSHAM, J. A. U. (1946) *Am. J., Hyg.*, **43**, 195.

MCKIEL, J. A., BELL, E. J. & LACKMAN, D. B. (1967) *Can. J. Microbiol.*, **13**, 503.

MARMION, B. P., STEWART, J., BARBER, H. & STOKER, M. G. P. (1954) *Lancet*, **i**, 1288.

MOHR, W. & WEYER, F. (1964) *Dt. med. Wschr.*, **89**, 244.

MURRAY, E. S., O'CONNOR, J. M. & GAON, J. A. (1965) *J. Immunol.*, **94**, 734.

RAYNAL, J. H., FOURNIER, J. & VELLIOT, E. (1939) *Chin. med. J.*, **56**, 11.

REISS-GUTFREUND, R. J. (1955) *Bull. Soc. Path. exot.*, **48**, 602.

ROSE, H. M. (1949) *Ann. intern. Med.*, **31**, 871.

SMADEL, J. E., LEY, H. L. jun., DIERKS, F. H., PATERSON, P. Y., WISSEMAN, C. L. jun. & TRAUB, R. (1952) *Am. J. trop. Med. Hyg.*, **1**, 87.

TRAUB, R., WISSEMAN, C. J. & AHMAD, N. (1967) *Trans. R. Soc. trop. Med. Hyg.*, **61**, 23.

VARELA, G., FOURNIER, R. & MOOSER, H. (1954) *Revta Inst. Enferm. trop. Méx.*, **14**, 39.

WEYER, F. (1949) *Zentbl. Bakt. ParasitKde*, **153**, 115.

—— (1953) *Z. Hyg. InfektKrankh.*, **137**, 419.

WHITTICK, J. W. (1950) *Br. med. J.*, **i**, 979.

WISSEMAN, C. L. jun., (1967) *First International Conference on Vaccines against Viral and Rickettsial Diseases in Man*, pp. 532-7. Pan-American Health Organization.

YASTREBOV, V. K., MIKHAILOV, A. K. & SHPYNOV, N. V. (1968) *Zh. Mikrobiol. Épidem. Immunobiol.*, **45**, 98.

30. BARTONELLOSIS

Synonyms

Carrión's disease, Oroya fever, guaitara fever, verruga peruana.

DEFINITION

Bartonellosis is an infection caused by *Bartonella bacilliformis*, which invades primarily the red cells and secondarily the reticulo-endothelial cells, causing Oroya fever and verruga peruana.

AETIOLOGY

Bartonella bacilliformis occurs in 2 forms: one is a rod-shaped slightly curved Gram-negative bacillary organism, 2 × 0·5 µm, staining well with Giemsa, often in branching rods and chains but never crossed, which occurs in a large proportion of the red cells (Fig. 179) during Oroya fever. The other is a rounded body about 1 µm or less in diameter, usually oval or pear-shaped and containing chromatin granules. Some occur singly or end-to-end in pairs or chains. V forms probably represent dividing organisms; Y-shaped forms are also not uncommon.

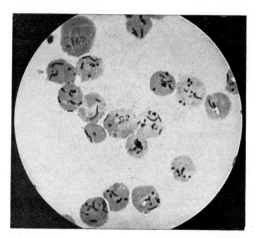

Fig. 179.—Blood smears with numerous *Bartonella bacilliformis* (human Oroya fever). (*Kikuth*)

They are difficult to detect in fresh blood and Peters and Wigand (1952) using phase contrast microscopy have shown that they are feebly motile in fresh blood. When dried films are 'shadowed' with palladium and examined by bright field microscopy it is found that the organisms lie in depressions; by electron microscopy lashing flagella are visible, each with a diameter of 20 nm, in bundles of up to 10 flagellae for each organism.

Intravenous injection of *Bartonella bacilliformis* into Macaca monkeys causes irregular fever and anaemia, while the organisms can be demonstrated in the blood cells. Intradermal inoculation into the supraorbital tissues gives rise to verrugous nodules. From the morphological point of view *Bartonella* and *Rickettsia* have resemblances, since both are minute, pleomorphic, Gram-negative and intracellular. Barton considered them protozoal but Noguchi regarded *Bartonella* as a bacillus.

Cultural characteristics

Noguchi and Battistini (1926) first cultured *Bartonella* on solid media from citrated blood of patients with Carrión's disease sent in cold storage from Lima to New York. It is an obligatory aerobe and grows best at low temperatures on blood agar media. Battistini's method of culture is simple. A small drop of blood from the finger of the patient is withdrawn into serum-agar or Noguchi's *Leptospira* medium. The end is sealed in flame and the whole placed in the incubator at 28°C. Colonics are visible in 5–6 days. *B. bacilliformis* is also readily cultivated in the allantoic fluid of the developing chick embryo at 25°–28°C. The growth is rapid and abundant and the cultivated bodies are 0·6–1·6 μm in length. Weinman and Pinkerton (1938) preferred the agar slant method devised by Zinsser for cultivation of rickettsiae.

HISTORY

It is probable that this disease existed in certain Andean valleys in Northwest South America in pre-Columbian days. Many thousands died of this fever during the reign of the Inca Huayna Capac and it is possible that Pizarro's men also suffered from it.

The earliest account of this disease was that of Gago de Vadilla in 1630. In the 1870's, when the central railway was being constructed from Lima to Oroya in Peru, a severe epidemic broke out among the construction workers, resulting in 7000 deaths. In 1906 out of 2000 men employed on tunnel work 200 perished. In 1885 a medical student Carrión inoculated himself with blood from a verruga nodule and died from Oroya fever, from which experiment Peruvian physicians concluded that verruga and Oroya fever were different stages of the same disease.

TRANSMISSION

The transmission between vertebrate hosts is by sandflies (*Lutzomyia*).

Animal reservoir

Although *Bartonella* can be transmitted experimentally to monkeys and grey squirrels (*Citellus tridecemlineatus*), no animal reservoir has yet been demonstrated in nature. After inoculation of grey squirrels the organism could only be recovered for the first 24–48 hours and the animals were asymptomatic (Herrer 1953).

Bartonella-like (*Haemobartonella muris*) bodies are found in the blood of healthy mice and certain rodents; they cannot be cultured and exist as a latent infection. They are transmitted by rat lice and after splenectomy cause an acute fatal anaemia resembling Oroya fever. A similar anaemia occurs in the dog after splenectomy when infected with *Bartonella canis*. Verruga can be conveyed by inoculation to puppies and rabbits and according to Townsend (1913) *Bartonella* occurs as a natural infection in native American Indian dogs.

Human reservoir

It is probable that the main reservoir consists of a number of asymptomatic human cases in whom the blood contains *Bartonella*. Herrer (1953) cultured *Bartonella* from 7 of 81 students and 3 of the 7 were completely asymptomatic. *B. bacilliformis* can be seen in the endothelial cells of cutaneous verruga nodules so that cases of verruga can act as a source of infection.

Sandfly transmission

Townsend (1913) conjectured that the vector was a sandfly, *Lutzomyia* (*Phlebotomus*) *verrucarum*, and further evidence incriminating *L. noguchii* and *L. verrucarum* was obtained by Pinkerton and Weinman (1937) when insects were collected in a verruga district of Peru and sent to New York, where they were ground up in saline and injected intradermally into monkeys. Only sand-flies were found to contain *Bartonella* and *L. verrucarum* is now regarded as the only proved vector, though Herrer *et al.* (1959–60) have described an outbreak of Oroya fever in the Mantaro valley of Peru in the absence of *L. verrucarum*. In the Narino department of south-western Colombia the habits of *L. colombianus* are so nearly like those of *L. verrucarum* that it may be a vector in this area. *L. noguchii* and *L. peruensis* are also suspected as vectors.

EPIDEMIOLOGY AND GEOGRAPHICAL DISTRIBUTION

The disease occurs between the ninth and sixteenth parallels of south latitude at an elevation of 800–3000 m in certain narrow valleys (quebradas) of the western slopes of the Andes. It is therefore found in Peru, Ecuador, Bolivia, Colombia and Chile, and probably in Guatemala. A considerable outbreak occurred in the Guaitara valley in southern Colombia near the Ecuador boundary in 1936 mainly in the valleys of the Mayo, Sambingo, Pacual and Juanambu tributaries of the Rio Patia. The latest outbreak, with 200 deaths, was in 1959 and occurred between January and April in the city of Anco which lies at 2400 m above sea level in the valley of the Mantaro river in the Peruvian Andes (Herrer *et al.* 1959–60).

The range of the infection is singularly limited and is confined to certain narrow valleys and ravines, the inhabitants of neighbouring places being exempt.

The disease is acquired only at night and a single night's residence in an endemic area may be sufficient. During the outbreak in the 1870's on the central railway in Peru, infection could be avoided by leaving the endemic area before nightfall. The disease is most prevalent from January to April when the streams are in flood, the air hot, still and moist, malaria epidemic and insect life abundant.

IMMUNOLOGY

Recovery from the disease in any of its forms confers lasting immunity and Howe (1943) has shown that immunity to *Bartonella* infection is rapidly acquired but bears no relation to the presence of specific agglutinins in the blood. Passage from the Oroya fever to the verruga stage, which is a change in the host–parasite relationship resulting from the development of immunity, is accompanied by a diminution of symptoms. Pinkerton and Weinman (1937) showed that graduated inoculation of verrugous material induces an artificial immunity. In monkeys infected with verruga, splenectomy reverses the process and produces Oroya fever.

Serum antibodies which agglutinated the organism in titres from 1/10 to 1/80 were found by Howe (1943) in the sera of patients in both the Oroya and verruga stages. Cross-reactions occurred with *Proteus OX19, OXK* and *OX2*. A strong agglutinating serum can be prepared for testing cultures of *B. bacilliformis*.

Prophylactic inoculation with formolized suspension of *B. bacilliformis* was introduced by Howe (1943), and resulted in partial immunity so that any subsequent attacks of Oroya fever were modified.

PATHOLOGY

Red blood cells

The aetiological agent invades red blood cells in which it multiplies, causing destruction of the cells with a rapid and extreme blood destruction. In severe cases the blood count may drop in 3 or 4 weeks to 500 000/mm^3. The anaemia is usually normocytic and hypochromic but may be macrocytic. This destruction of the red cells is due to an intravascular haemolysis since 50% of labelled erythrocytes were found to have a half-life of 6 days. Those red cells, however, which survived this period had a normal survival rate. Normal erythrocytes injected into patients in the febrile anaemic phase behaved similarly, but red cells from a patient with verruga peruana survived normally, suggesting that they had acquired the property of resistance to the haemolytic process after cessation of the febrile stage.

There is an associated polymorphonuclear leucocytosis with an absence of eosinophils.

Reticulo-endothelial system

The organisms invade the cells of the reticulo-endothelial system, causing reticulo-endothelial hyperplasia in the lymph glands, Kupffer cells of the liver and histiocytes in the spleen, bone marrow, kidneys, adrenals, pancreas, thyroid and testes. They also parasitize the endothelial lining cells of the blood and lymph vessels, which may be so distended by clusters of the parasites that the infected cells may be detected on low-power microscopic examination (Pinkerton & Weinman 1937). Marked changes are present in the liver, spleen and bone marrow. In the liver, areas of degenerative and central necrosis are found around the hepatic veins. In the centre of the necrotic areas a yellow pigment resembling haemosiderin is present in abundance. The spleen is invariably enlarged and contains necrotic areas with pigment.

The Malpighian bodies are not affected. The lymphatic glands contain large macrophage endothelial cells studded with rod-shaped bodies. *B. bacilliformis* is found in closely packed masses in swollen endothelial cells, especially those of the lymphatic glands, spleen, liver and intestines. The bone marrow shows proliferation, necrosis and marked phagocytosis of the large endothelial cells.

Verruga stage

The verrucous eruption is a sequela to the lesions in the reticulo-endothelial system. Primarily the pathological changes consist in proliferation of the endothelium of the lymphatic channels which become obstructed by plasma cells and fibroblasts, but the structure is much more vascular than that of yaws which it otherwise resembles. The capillary blood vessels become dilated so that the granulomatous tumours are vascular, almost cavernous and apt to bleed profusely. A feature of the pathological histology is the formation around the blood vessels of nodules of angioblasts characteristic of the disease. *B. bacilliformis* is seen in considerable numbers in the endothelial cells of cutaneous verruga nodules, but distension of the cells is less than that seen in Oroya fever cases. *Bartonella* bodies may be found in blood corpuscles after prolonged search.

CLINICAL FEATURES

Oroya fever

The incubation period of Oroya fever is about 3 weeks. Its onset is insidious and is marked by malaise, soon followed by a rapidly developing anaemia and an irregular remittent pyrexia, associated with very severe pains in the head, joints and long bones. The bone pains are probably connected with disturbances

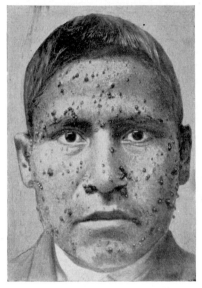

Fig. 180.—Verruga peruana. Miliary form from Equador. (*Odriazola*)

in the haemopoietic system. Very often the initial fever is like that of malaria. The most severe types resemble fulminating typhus and are known as 'the severe fever of Carrión'. The liver and spleen are enlarged and tender and the anaemia develops with great rapidity. The death rate varies from 10 to 40%, the end coming within 2–3 weeks of the onset of the disease. A terminal delirium is often noted. In those cases which proceed to the verruga stage the fever may last 3–4 months. Often there is a secondary infection with *Salmonella typhimurium*, which may prove fatal.

Verruga peruana stage (localized bartonellosis or eruptive stage)

The period of incubation subsequent to the development of Oroya fever is 30–40 days, but where the initial fever is absent it is at least 60 days. Although verruga is usually a sequel of Oroya fever it may arise spontaneously and independent of Oroya fever. The initial stages are characterized by peculiar rheumatic-like pains together with fever, the pains being like those of yaws only more severe. As in yaws the constitutional symptoms subside on the appearance of the skin lesions. The eruption (Fig. 180) may be sparse or abundant, discrete or confluent. Some granulomas may fail to erupt, others may subside rapidly and others may continue to increase and then, after remaining stationary for a time, gradually wither, shrink and drop off without leaving a scar.

Two types of eruption are seen, miliary and nodular. The miliary eruption, not exceeding the size of a small pea, is found most abundantly on the face and extensor aspect of the extremities, less commonly on the trunk (Fig. 180). A pink macule first appears, later darkening and becoming nodular. The verruga artificially produced in monkeys by injection of *Bartonella* bodies is bright cherry pink. These nodules, which are flat or somewhat pedunculated, are vascular and may develop on mucous surfaces in the mouth, oesophagus, stomach, intestine, bladder, uterus and vagina; hence the dysphagia, which is a common symptom, and occasional haematemesis, melaena, haematuria and bleeding from the vagina.

The Oroya and verruga stages frequently coexist and relapses of both the fever and the eruption may occur.

The nodular eruption, which is rarer, is more chronic than the miliary. Individual lesions may grow to the size of a pigeon's egg and may become strangulated and a source of danger from haemorrhage. This type does not invade the mucous membranes and is usually confined to the regions of the knees and elbows. It appears in crops and lasts 2–3 months.

The mortality rate from verruga is practically nil.

DIAGNOSIS

The Oroya fever stage must be distinguished from malaria, typhus, typhoid and acute haemolytic anaemia of various causes. The verruga stage is hardly likely to be mistaken for any other disease, but most closely resembles yaws. It may also be simulated by multiple warts, molluscum contagiosum and multiple fatty tumours (Dercum's disease). Individual tumours may resemble fibrosarcoma or angioma.

TREATMENT

Urteaga and Payne (1955) used chloramphenicol successfully. The fever subsided within 48 hours and *B. bacilliformis* assumed a coccoid form in 24 hours. There was a marked reticulocytosis and a rapid return of the blood to normal. As well as having an action on the *Bartonella*, chloramphenicol is most effective against the secondary infection with *Salmonella* especially *S. typhimurium*. The average dose is 17 grammes in divided doses over 5 days. Other drugs effective against *Salmonella*, such as trimethoprim and sulphamethoxazole or ampicillin, would also be effective.

CONTROL

Control of the vector sandflies is easily obtained with DDT and Hertig and Fairchild (1948) have demonstrated the remarkable effect of DDT in eradicating sandflies from human habitations.

REFERENCES

HERRER, A. (1953) *Am. J. trop. Med. Hyg.*, **2**, 645.
——— BLANCAS, F., CORNEJO-UBILLUS, J. R., LUNG, J., ESPEJO, L. & FLORES, M. (1959-60) *Revta med. exper.*, **13**, 27.
HERTIG, M. & FAIRCHILD, G. B. (1948) *Am. J. trop. Med.*, **28**, 207.
HOWE, C. (1943) *Archs intern. Med.*, **72**, 147.
PETERS, D. & WEIGAND, R. (1952) *Z. Tropenmed. Parasit.*, **3**, 313.
PINKERTON, H. & WEINMAN, D. J. (1937) *Proc. Soc. exp. Biol. Med.*, **37**, 587.
TOWNSEND, C. H. T. (1913) *J. Am. med. Ass.*, **19**, 1717.
URTEAGA, B. & PAYNE, E. H. (1955) *Am. J. trop. Med. Hyg.*, **4**, 507.
WEINMAN, D. J. & PINKERTON, H. (1938) *Proc. Soc. exp. Biol. Med.*, **37**, 596.

SECTION VII

TROPICAL VENEREAL DISEASES

31. LYMPHOGRANULOMA VENEREUM; GRANULOMA INGUINALE

LYMPHOGRANULOMA VENERUM

Synonyms

Climatic bubo; lymphopathia venereum; esthiomène; lymphogranuloma inguinale; inguinal poradenitis; poradenolymphitis; Nicolas-Favre disease.

Definition

A generalized virus infection usually transmitted by venereal infection and associated with a self-healing primary sore and changes in the lymph nodes draining the area where the primary sore is situated. In addition to these lesions the virus may give rise to a genito-anorectal syndrome with inflammatory stricture of the rectum, to meningo-encephalitis and to eye lesions.

Aetiology

The causative agent, which was first isolated in 1930 by Hellerström and Wassen (1930), was formerly described as a large virus and is a typical member of the group of organisms causing psittacosis, trachoma, inclusion conjunctivitis and enzootic hepatitis of sheep. This group has been called *Bedsonia* (Meyer 1953) or *Chlamydia* (Andrewes 1967).

The virus, which is an obligatory intracellular parasite, is found in leucocytes and consists of minute particles which can be stained by Victoria blue, Giemsa (bluish purple), or Castaneda's method (reddish purple). Both large and small forms of the parasite can be demonstrated outside the cells, lying close to cell debris in compact colony-like masses which may attain considerable size forming cyst-like spaces. Later the cyst wall may rupture. These resemble similar bodies found in psittacosis, in which large morula-like particles break up to form the small virus or elementary bodies. When they are within cells the elementary bodies may be found in the cytoplasm of either mononuclear or polymorphonuclear leucocytes.

Cultural characteristics. The most reliable methods of isolation are by inoculation into the yolk sac of eggs and the intracerebral inoculation of white mice (Wassen test). The virus can also be cultivated in the yolk sac of chick embryos.

In inoculated mice a characteristic train of symptoms is evolved in 5–70 days, in which weakness, paresis, opisthotonos and convulsions occur. Dilutions greater than 1/1000 fail to give positive results.

Intraglandular injection of guinea-pigs with the virus will produce inguinal buboes.

Immunology

There is a marked increase in serum globulin and the total protein content of the serum lies between 8·1 and 10·3 grammes/100 ml. The globulin varies between 3·9 and 5·6 grammes/100 ml so that a positive formol gel test may be given. Combes et al. (1945) found that 38 out of 42 cases gave a positive formol gel reaction and concluded that hyperglobulinaemia is of value in diagnosis and in delineating the activity of the disease since it reverts to negative with cure.

There is a well marked delayed hypersensitivity reaction which can be demonstrated by the Frei–Hoffmann test (Frei & Hoffmann 1928). Antigenically lymphogranuloma venereum closely resembles the psittacosis/trachoma group of viruses but tests with virucidal antibodies have shown that these viruses are not antigenically identical.

Frei–Hoffmann test. Frei originally prepared antigen from the pus withdrawn from a suppurating bubo which had not burst. At present antigen is prepared from the virus grown in the yolk sac of developing chick embryos (Rake et al. 1940) and is commercially available under the trade name of Lygranum. 0·1 ml of antigen is injected intradermally into the skin of the forearm and 0·1 ml of control material made from egg yolk into the other. The test is read at 48–72 hours. If the test is positive a raised red papule at least 6 mm across appears at the site of the injection and a hardness of indurated skin may persist for a few days. The test becomes positive at varying intervals after infection, from 1 week to 6 months but usually within 2–3 weeks, and remains positive for many years, perhaps for life. False positive reactions may occur, and cross-reactions occur with trachoma, psittacosis and virus pneumonitis, but Barwell (1952) has shown that an acid extract of the virus is specific for lymphogranuloma.

Complement fixation test. Complement fixing antibodies appear earlier in the serum and the test is a more sensitive and reliable method of diagnosis than the intradermal reaction, but is of little use in assessing the results of treatment. The same antigen, Lygranum, is used and a positive titre of 1 in 16 or above means recent or active infection in a patient with clinical manifestations of the disease; when acute and convalescent sera are available a rising titre of up to 1 in 40 is diagnostic (Annamunthodo 1962). Low titres may persist for a long time in past infections. Cross-reactions occur with psittacosis and an antigen made from this organism gives equally satisfactory results.

Mouse protection test. Test serum diluted 1 in 5 with normal saline is mixed with infected mouse brain and kept overnight at 4°C; 0·5 ml of the suspension is inoculated intracerebrally into another mouse and sera containing virucidal antibodies will protect the second mouse against encephalitis.

Transmission

In every instance infection is acquired by sexual intercourse, either normal or abnormal.

Epidemiology and geographical distribution

Lymphogranuloma is world-wide in distribution and has been called the 'sixth venereal disease'. This disease is found especially among Negroes of both sexes in West Africa and North and South America and in seaports throughout the world. More recently it has been described in Europe and there are numerous reports of its occurrence in France, England, Italy, Romania, Scandinavia and the whole of Europe.

Sex incidence. Lymphogranuloma inguinale is commonest in the male but it is now recognized that this infection does occur in women, although inguinal buboes are comparatively rare on account of the different anatomical disposition of the lymphatic system in the female. Typical inguinal buboes have been found in prostitutes in Singapore and inguinal buboes with a positive intradermal reaction have been reported among prostitutes by French writers. Definite evidence of infection of the wife by her husband has been obtained in an English case.

Pathology

The primary lesion consists of an ulcer surrounded by plasma cells and histiocytes containing the cone or dumb-bell shaped basophilic inclusion bodies which can be found in Giemsa-stained smears of pus. Occasionally eosinophils are prominent.

The secondary lesions are found in the lymph glands, where there is a proliferation of monocytes and plasma cells, with a few neutrophils, poly-morphonuclear leucocytes and eosinophils present. There is a granulomatous reaction with a proliferation of macrophages and epithelioid cells and sometimes central necrosis with giant cells which may simulate tuberculosis. These granulomas are scattered in a pin-point manner all through the gland and a Giemsa-stained preparation may show intracytoplasmic inclusion bodies. In the late stages a central area of necrosis may be surrounded by a palisade of epithelioid cells merging with a wall of acellular hyaline material which may be of diagnostic significance.

Pathological changes in the spleen, liver, heart and central nervous system have been described, and generalized lymphadenopathy may occur.

Clinical features

The incubation period is short, usually less than 1 week, but periods of 3–5 weeks and longer have been reported.

Inguinal syndrome. *Primary sore.* Hanschell (1926) described a small herpetiform ulcer on the prepuce, which usually heals in a few days, though it may ulcerate; the adenitis proper does not start until after the primary lesion has healed. Hanschell (1926) believed that the disease does not usually occur in the circumcised. The primary lesion is an erosion with clean edges, surrounded by a reddened zone, but with only slight infiltration and induration. The base of the ulcer is usually whitish-grey.

Adenitis. The incubation period of adenitis is 3–4 weeks after coitus, but it may be as long as 6 weeks to 2 months. The disease generally commences with remittent pyrexia, which may precede the actual localizing signs and may be mistaken for typhoid. Soon, subacute inflammatory swellings of the groin glands are noted. The inflammation may be unilateral or bilateral; though the inguinal glands are most frequently affected, at times the crural glands are attacked. Sometimes one groin is affected after the other. In well marked cases the internal iliac glands, sometimes the lumbar glands also, can be felt enlarged and tender on deep palpation. Signs of intoxication from absorption may be widespread, producing prolonged intermittent or remittent fevers, sometimes even pyrexia of 39·4°–40·6°C. Rigors, vomiting, cyanosis, even slight jaundice and considerable pain have been noted. Rheumatic-like pains in joints and painful effusions into joint cavities may also occur as a result of absorption. The affected glands slowly enlarge to the size of a hen's egg, or even larger, and after several weeks, it may be months, the swelling gradually subsides (Fig. 181). Usually, the periglandular connective tissues inflame, and the integuments become adherent until suppuration ceases. At other times fistulous tracks form, and continuously exude a clear sticky fluid. The most striking clinical feature in the male is the extensive inflammation of the periglandular tissues with comparatively little pain and suppuration. The following stages are recognized:

1. A firm solitary gland, with no apparent causative lesion other than a recently healed ulcer on the genitalia.
2. A firm solitary gland adherent to overlying skin and deeper tissues. Adjacent glands are enlarged, including external iliac glands, palpable as a mass above Poupart's ligament. The affected glands tend to coalesce.
3. The glands in the groin soften and fluctuate. If incised, a cavity is disclosed, trabeculated by coarse, fibrous strands.

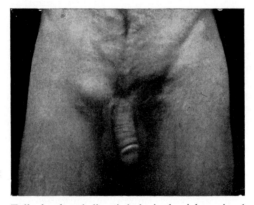

Fig. 181.—Fully developed climatic bubo in the right groin, showing also a small primary lesion on the corona penis. (*A. H. Walters*)

Genital syndrome. Genital elephantiasis (esthiomène) is an ulceration of the vulva associated with elephantiasis of the labia and is the counterpart of lymphogranuloma in the male.

The primary lesion is probably hidden in the posterior wall of the vagina and the anorectal lymph gland is the first to be attacked. The infiltration of this gland extends via the lymph flow to the anterior part of the vulva, and posteriorly to the rectum, resulting in the genito-anorectal syndrome, which is more common in women than in men.

There is swelling due to chronic lymphatic oedema of the vulva. The male genitalia may be affected by the same process, but less commonly. Vegetations and polypoid growths develop on the skin surface, and fistulas may form and break down to destructive ulceration. The oedema may extend from the clitoris to the anus, and in the male elephantiasis may involve the penis and the scrotum.

Urethral syndrome. Involvement of the urethra with infiltrative lesions in the posterior part, followed by stricture and fistula formation may follow, and the disease can present as non-gonococcal urethritis.

Anorectal syndrome. The virus spreads from the initial site of implantation by the lymphatics to the inguinal and pelvic glands and later, in the female, the lymphatics of the anus and rectum become involved, producing at first proctitis and later stricture of the rectum. In the male stricture of the rectum follows the occurrence of a primary lesion in the rectum.

The earliest symptom is bleeding from the anus, followed by purulent anal discharge. Proctoscopy may reveal proctitis, rectal ulceration or rectal stricture, or a combination of these. Severe proctocolitis resembling ulcerative colitis may develop. Fistula-in-ano, perirectal abscesses and rectovesical and rectovaginal fistulas may develop, and tumour-like swellings may be seen at the anal orifice. Stricture formation will cause rectal discharge and bleeding associated with constipation, and finally complete obstruction may occur. Several varieties of rectal stricture are recognized: anal stricture in women associated with esthiomène; annular rectal stricture; tubular rectal stricture, which may extend to the sigmoid or even the descending colon and may cause skip lesions seen on radioscopy (Middlemiss 1961); rectal communicating strictures from ulceration between the rectum, bladder, vagina, prostate and seminal vesicles; strictures associated with carcinoma of the rectum, in some cases causing a tender, fixed and palpable ileum resembling Crohn's disease.

Extragenital infections. Extragenital infections have been recorded on the tongue with glandular enlargement in the neck and axilla and on the foot. A few cases of meningo-encephalitis due to the virus of lymphogranuloma venereum have now been recorded.

Ocular lymphogranuloma. This was described by Macnie (1941). The whole globe may be covered with granulation tissue and the washings of the conjunctival sac will infect monkeys. A number of cases of uveitis and kerato-conjunctivitis have given positive intradermal tests, and fundus changes have been reported with peripapillary oedema and dilatation and tortuosity of the veins.

Complications. If too much lymphatic tissue is removed by excision of the glands elephantiasis of the scrotum and leg on the affected side may develop and secondary sepsis may ensue. Rupture of lymphatics with lymphogranulomatous suppuration into the bladder has been recorded.

Malignant changes have been described as a sequel to genital elephantiasis and the anorectal syndrome (Levin *et al.* 1964). In 220 cases diagnosed as rectal stricture the Frei test became negative in 5 and carcinoma became apparent after a period of 14 years.

Blood changes. There is usually a leucocytosis accompanying the suppuration and the leucocyte count varies between 8000 and 27 000/mm³.

Diagnosis

The disease must be differentiated from soft sore, filarial adenitis, ambulant plague (pestis minor), tularaemia and femoral hernia. The diagnosis is made by isolation of the virus, the Frei skin test, the complement fixation test and gland biopsy.

The virus may be demonstrated in a smear of the lesion stained with Giemsa, showing intracytoplasmic inclusion bodies, and may be isolated by the inoculation of pus from buboes intracerebrally into the yolk sac of an embryonated hen's egg. The Frei skin test and complement fixation test are described under immunology.

Gland biopsy will show the characteristic histological changes described on page 642.

The formol gel test is positive in active cases and will return to normal after clinical cure.

Treatment

Drug treatment. *Antimony drugs* have been used in the past but are now largely superseded. Anthiomaline 2 ml on alternate days intramuscularly for 4–5 doses has been recommended (Willcox 1952).

Sulphonamides give good results in early cases. Sulphathiazole, sulphadiazine or sulphadimidine may be given in a dose of 5 grammes daily in divided doses for 7 days (Willcox 1952). Sometimes it is necessary to prolong the course for as much as 2–3 weeks or give another course of the same or another sulphonamide drug.

Long-acting sulphonamides, sulphamethoxypyridazine 1·5 grammes first, followed by 500 mg daily, may be of use.

Genital elephantiasis and the anorectal syndrome should be treated first with sulphonamides but the results are disappointing.

Antibiotics. Penicillin and streptomycin are ineffective (Greenblatt *et al.* 1950). Tetracycline, chlortetracycline and oxytetracycline should be used when sulphonamides have failed. The main effect is probably on the secondary infection. Greenblatt *et al.* (1950) gave 75–100 grammes of chlortetracycline (Aureomycin) over 37–60 days and sinuses, proctitis and inflammatory strictures showed marked improvement, but ulcers showed a poor response. Oxytetracycline (Terramycin) has been given successfully in doses of 15–36 grammes over a period of 15–30 days.

Surgical treatment. Surgical treatment should only be undertaken after adequate antibiotic therapy has been given. Fluctuant abscesses in the groins should be aspirated and incision avoided. The lymphatic glands should not be removed because of the danger of elephantiasis developing subsequently in the lower limbs.

Rectal stricture. Palliative measures consist in dilating with graduated bougies. Operative measures may be necessary and include internal proctotomy, excision of the rectal stricture, or colostomy. Local vulvectomy may be indicated in genital elephantiasis.

GRANULOMA INGUINALE

Synonyms

Ulcerating granuloma of the pudenda; Donovanosis.

Definition

An infective and granulomatous condition of the pudenda, widespread in some parts of the tropics.

Aetiology

The cause of granuloma inguinale is a bacterium, *Donovania granulomatis* (*Calymmatobacterium granulomatis*), which can be seen in mononuclear cells of the lesion as a small Gram-negative pleomorphic bacillus (1–2 μm in length). It may show bipolar staining and appears to be capsulate. Extracellular forms may also be observed.

Cultural characteristics. It is difficult to cultivate on the ordinary media but it can be grown readily at 37°C in the yolk sac of chick embryos when, after adaptation, growth can be obtained on enriched artificial media. Laboratory animals are not susceptible to inoculation but the disease has been reproduced in man by inoculation with yolk sac cultures.

Immunology

The organism has morphological resemblances to *Klebsiella* and cross-reacts serologically with *Klebsiella rhinoscleromatis*. Sterilized cultures will give an allergic skin reaction in infected persons and a positive complement fixation with the serum. The capsular material also fixes complement in patients' serum, but intradermal and serological tests are of little use in diagnosis because of frequent false positive reactions.

Transmission

Transmission is by sexual intercourse and auto-inoculation.

Epidemiology and geographical distribution

Granuloma inguinale is widespread in India, Guiana, Brazil, the West Indies, Puerto Rico, the Pacific Islands and Northern Australia. It occurs sporadically in the Southern United States, on the West Coast of Africa and in Southern China. One case has been described from Scotland (Ferguson & Roberts 1953). It is extremely common in New Guinea, where in 1925 one-quarter of a population of 20 000 were affected and in 1946 422 cases were found in 8761 persons examined (Maddocks 1967).

Age and sex. Ulcerating granuloma has only been found after the age of 13 or 14 and up to 40 or 50. It occurs in both sexes, twice as common in males as in females. It may be more common in women where polyandry is practised.

Pathology

Histologically this disease is allied to rhinoscleroma and the close association between these two diseases in Sumatra has been emphasized by Snijders. It is a reticulo-endotheliosis and on microscopical examination the new growth at the margins of the sores is found to be made up of nodules, or masses of nodules, consisting of round cells having large and, usually, badly-staining nuclei. These cell-nests of Malpighian cells are embedded in a delicate fibrous reticulum. The predominating cells are plasma and endothelial cells forming small poly-morphonuclear micro-abscesses. An important feature in the histopathology is a peculiar pathognomonic cell described by Pund and Greenblatt (1937) (Fig. 182). It is a large mononuclear varying from 25 to 90 μm in diameter, probably derived from a plasma cell. The specific cell, laden with the so-called Donovan bodies, can be shown best by the Dieterle silver impregnation method in which these bodies appear as dark brown or black elongated ovoid masses with intense bipolar staining. The nodular masses are, for the most part, covered by epithelium, their under-surfaces merging gradually into a thick, dense, fibrous stroma in which small clusters of similar round cells are here and there embedded. The growths, though very vascular, contain no haemorrhages, and there are no signs of suppuration or of caseation, no giant cells and no tubercle bacilli. In vertical sections of the small nodules the round cell mass will be found to be wedge-shaped, the base of the wedge being towards the surface; the deep lying apex is usually pierced by a hair or two. The growth is found around sebaceous follicles, blood vessels, lymphatics and sweat glands, but it is most abundant and most deeply situated around hair follicles.

Clinical features

The incubation appears to be relatively short, from 2 to 8 days after sexual contact, but it may be as long as 12 weeks. In experimental infections it was 50 days. The disease commences in the great majority of cases somewhere on the genitals, usually on the penis or labia minora, the pubes or the groin, as an insignificant, circumscribed, nodular thickening and elevation of the skin. The affected area, which on the whole is elevated above the surrounding healthy skin, and is covered with a very delicate pinkish membrane which is easily rubbed off, excoriates easily, exposing a surface which tends to break down and bleed, although rarely ulcerating deeply. The disease advances in two ways: by continuous eccentric peripheral extension, and by auto-infection of an opposing surface. It exhibits a distinct predilection for warm and moist surfaces, particularly the folds between scrotum and thighs, the labia and the flexures of the thighs. Its extension is very slow, years elapsing before it covers a large area.

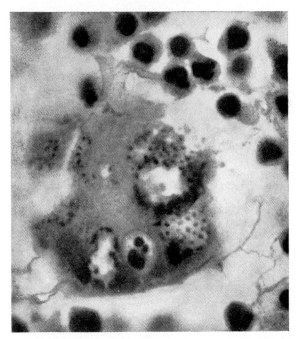

Fig. 182.—Granuloma inguinale, showing the pathognomonic cell and contained Donovan bodies. (*Pund & Greenblatt*)

Concurrently with peripheral extension, a dense, contracting uneven scar, which breaks down readily, forms on the surface travelled over by the coarsely or finely nodulated elevated new growth which constitutes the peripheral part of the diseased area. Occasionally islands of active disease spring up in this scar tissue, but it is at the margin of the implicated patch that the special features of the affection are best observed. In cases of long standing the partially healed areas are covered with thin depigmented skin and thus show up as white patches (Fig. 183).

In the female (Fig. 184) the disease primarily attacks the crura of the clitoris, thence extending into the vagina, over the labia and along the flexures of the thighs. The women thus affected are rendered sterile. In the male the disease may spread over the penis, involve the glans, scrotum, and upper part of the

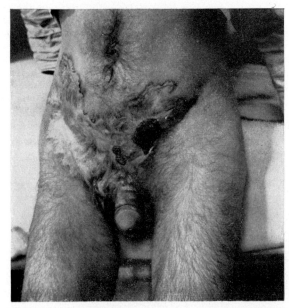

Fig. 183.—Healing and extensive scar tissue in granuloma inguinale with superimposed non-haemolytic streptococcal infection. (*Dr Butterfield*)

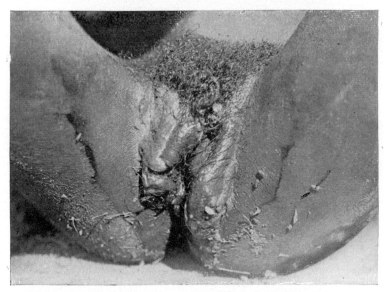

Fig. 184.—Granuloma inguinale in the female, an Australian aborigine. (*Dr H. Basedow, Adelaide*)

thighs (Fig. 185). Occasionally, the glans penis is not involved. In either sex it may spread in the course of years to the pubes, over the perineum, and into the rectum, the rectovaginal septum in the female ultimately breaking down. At times, a profuse watery discharge exudes, and even drips from the surface of the new growth, soiling the clothes, soddening the skin, and emitting a peculiarly offensive odour. In this condition the disease, slowly extending, continues for years, giving rise to inconvenience and perhaps seriously implicating the urethra, vagina or anus, but not otherwise materially impairing the health. In neither sex do the lymphatic glands become affected. The disease continues entirely local,

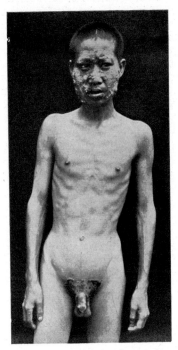

Fig. 185.—Granuloma inguinale of the face and penis in a Chinese. (*Dr B. Hawes*)

but in the process of cicatrization the lymph-channels may become blocked, and pseudo-elephantiasis of the genitalia may occur. Impassable strictures of the urethra may result, and rectovaginal fistulas are common. It may even cause death by eating its way into the bladder, causing septic cystitis.

Gross secondary infection may occur, even leading to phagedaenic ulceration, with much destruction of tissue and constitutional symptoms.

General dissemination has been described in which there were metastases in the bones and Donovan bodies were cultured from the blood (Packer *et al.* 1948). Carcinoma may be associated with the disease in India (Rama Ayyangar 1961) and a pseudocarcinomatous proliferation in association with the disease in the rectum has been described (Sluis 1966).

Diagnosis

Malignant and syphilitic ulcerations of the groin are common enough; the disease under notice, however, differs widely from these—clinically, histologically, and therapeutically. It is characterized by extreme chronicity—10 or more years—by absence of cachexia or of a tendency to cause death and by non-implication of the lymphatic system as a whole.

The disease which it most resembles is lupus vulgaris. From this it differs inasmuch as it is usually confined to the pudendal region, tends to follow in its extension the folds of the skin and is not associated with the tubercle bacillus, giant cells, caseation or other evidences of tuberculous disease. Unless complicated by a coincident syphilitic infection, the Wassermann reaction is negative. The inefficiency of antisyphilitic treatment soon convinces the physician that the ulceration is not due to this disease. Its characteristic mode of spread suffices to distinguish it from epithelioma and carcinoma. The discharges from ulcerating granuloma have, moreover, a peculiar acrid smell. Pund and Greenblatt described a fungating form affecting the cervix uteri in Negro women, which greatly resembles the ulcerative and vegetative type of carcinoma of the cervix. It has also to be distinguished from gonorrhoeal endocervicitis and from simple erosions, and in New Guinea from amoebic infection of the genitalia. The characteristic Donovan bodies may be demonstrated by biopsy.

Treatment

Streptomycin is specific in most cases (Greenblatt et al. 1947). The optimum dosage is 4 grammes/day by intravenous injection for 5 days in divided doses. Healing commences in 2–3 days and is complete in 1–2 weeks. Resistance can develop and 10% of cases relapse, half of which fail to respond to a second course.

Good results can be obtained with Aureomycin (Greenblatt et al. 1948). The maximum curative dose is 20 grammes given in doses of 500 mg 6-hourly for 10 days. Chloramphenicol in the same dosage cured 32 out of 34 cases (Greenblatt et al. 1948), but because of its toxic effects it should be avoided if possible (King & Nicol 1969). Triacetyloleandomycin was successful in one case (Kerdel Vegas et al. 1961).

Some aspects of venereal syphilis are discussed in the section on treponematoses (page 559).

REFERENCES

ANDREWES, G. H. (1967) *Viruses of Vertebrates*, 2nd ed., p. 365. London: Baillière, Tindall & Cassell.
ANNAMUNTHODO, H. (1962) *W. Indian med. J.*, **11**, 73.
BARWELL, C. F. (1952) *Br. J. exp. Path.*, **33**, 268.
COMBES, F. C., CANIZARES, O. & LANDY, S. (1945) *Am. J. Syph.*, **29**, 611.
FERGUSON, A. G. & ROBERTS, G. B. S. (1953) *Br. med. J.*, **i**, 1257.
FREI, W. & HOFFMANN, H. (1928) *Arch. Derm. Syph.*, **153**, 197.
GREENBLATT, R. B., DIENST, R. B., CHEN, C. & WEST, R. (1948) *Sth med. J.*, *Nashville*, **41**, 1121.
————— ———— KUPPERMAN, H. S. & REINSTEIN, C. R. (1947) *J. vener. Dis. Inf.*, **28**, 183.
———— WAMMOCK, V. S., CHEN, C. H., DIENST, R. B. & WEST, R. M. (1950) *J. vener. Dis. Inf.*, **31**, 41.
HANSCHELL, H. M. (1926) *Lancet*, **ii**, 276.

HELLERSTRÖM, S. & WASSEN, E. (1930) *VIII ème Congres Internationale de Dermatologie et de Syphilographie*, Copenhagen.

KERDEL VEGAS, E., CONVIT, J. & SOTO, J. (1961) *Archs Derm.*, **84**, 248.

KING, A. & NICOL, C. (1969) *Venereal Diseases*, p. 219. London: Baillière, Tindall & Cassell.

LEVIN, I., ROMANO, S., STEINBERG, M. & WELSH, R. A. (1964) *Dis. Colon Rect.*, **7**, 129.

MACNIE, J. P. (1941) *Archs Ophthal.*, **25**, 255.

MADDOCKS, I. (1967) *Papua New Guinea med. J.*, **10**, 49.

MEYER, K. F. (1953) *Ann. N.Y. Acad. Sci.*, **56**, 545.

MIDDLEMISS, H. (1961) *Tropical Radiology*, pp. 229–231. London: Heinemann.

PACKER, H., TURNER, H. B. & DULANEY, A. D. (1948) *J. Am. med. Ass.*, **136**, 327.

PUND, E. R. & GREENBLATT, R. B. (1937) *Archs Path.*, **23**, 224.

RAKE, G., MCKEE, C. M. & SHAFER, M. F. (1940) *Proc. exp. Biol. Med.*, **43**, 332.

RAMA AYYANGAR, M. C. (1961) *J. Indian med. Ass.*, **37**, 70.

SLUIS, I. V. D. (1966) *Dermatologica*, **133**, 325.

WILLCOX, R. R. (1952) *Trans. R. Soc. exp. Biol. Med.*, **46**, 658.

SECTION VIII

DISEASES CAUSED BY FUNGI

32. SUPERFICIAL MYCOSES

DHOBIE'S ITCH (TINEA CRURIS) AND PITYRIASIS VERSICOLOR

Aetiology and nomenclature

By the lay public all epiphytic skin diseases in the tropics—more especially all forms of intertrigo—are spoken of as dhobie's (washerman's) itch, in the belief, probably not very well founded, that they are contracted from clothes which have been contaminated at the washerman's. There are many sources of ringworm infection in warm climates besides the much-maligned dhobie.

In the tropics, local children often exhibit dry, scurfy patches of ringworm on the scalp, and the skin of the trunk and limbs of adults is not infrequently affected with red, slightly raised, itching rings, or segments of rings, of *Trichophyton* infection. In some cases these rings enclose areas that are many centimetres in diameter.

Pityriasis versicolor (tinea versicolor) is also very common in the tropics. It is the usual cause of the pale, fawn-coloured, slightly scurfy patches so frequently a feature of the dark-skinned bodies of the people. On the dark-pigmented skins of Negroes, Indians and dark-complexioned Chinese, the patch of pityriasis—unlike that in Europeans and light-skinned Chinese—is usually paler than the healthy integument surrounding it. The pigment in the fungus and the profuse growth of the latter conceal, as a coat of paint might, the dark underlying natural pigment of the skin, which, moreover, in certain cases seems to be affected (either increased or decreased) by the action of the fungus. The disease is most commonly seen in young adults, is favoured by excessive perspiration, and especially by flannel underwear, and is rarely seen in the aged. Pityriasis versicolor is caused by *Malassezia furfur*.

The mycelium and spores are refractile with slow budding. The hyphae are 2–3 μm, the spores 3–8 μm. Fluorescence can be demonstrated in scaly patches by Wood's light. Treatment by daily thorough washing, or by application of benzoic acid compound ointment, salicylic acid and sulphur ointment or liquid iodine compound is usually successful.

The expression 'dhobie's itch', although applied to any itching, ringworm-like affection of any part of the skin, most commonly refers to some form of epiphytic disease of the crutch or axilla. This infection has now become widespread in Great Britain and endemic in many English public schools, where it is spread by infected clothes and water-closet seats. The infection has also been found in hedgehogs in England and in New Zealand (Marples 1961). The causative fungi are *Epidermophyton floccosum* (syn. *E. cruris*, *E. inguinale*, etc.), *Trichophyton mentagrophytes* (syn. *T. gypseum*, *T. asteroides*, etc.), *T. rubrum* (syn. *T. purpureum*, *E. rubrum*, etc.). *Trichophyton verrucosum*, the commonest cause of ringworm in cattle, is occasionally transmitted to man. *T. quinckeanum* (of mouse favus) and *T. equinum* of horses may also be involved.

E. floccosum is peculiar to man only; it is easily cultivated, but grows slowly. On Sabouraud's agar medium it takes a week to develop, and appears first as a yellowish glabrous growth with a powdery surface in which masses of the characteristic pyriform spindles are found. Subcultures tend to be cottonous and show fewer spindles.

Symptoms

The suffering to which certain forms of dhobie's itch give rise is often severe. In hot damp weather, especially, the fungi proliferate actively, producing, it may be, acute dermatitis. The affection begins usually as slightly raised, rounded and elevated papules which spread peripherally, producing a raised festooned border covered with thick scales. The excessive irritation thus set up leads to

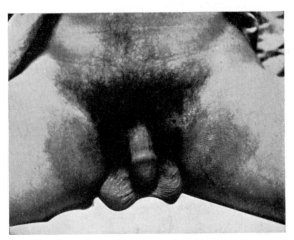

Fig. 186.—Symmetrical lesions of dhobie's itch in the groin.

scratching and, very likely, from secondary bacterial invasion, to boils or small abscesses. The crutch, scrotum or axillae are sometimes rendered so raw and tender that the patient may be unable to walk or even to dress (Fig. 186). It commonly extends backwards on the perineum and into the natal cleft about the anus. It often affects the skin under pendulous breasts and occasionally forms patches resembling tinea circinata on the thighs. The irritations thus produced are usually worse at night, and may keep the patient awake for hours. Even without treatment, when the cold season comes round, the dermatitis and irritation subside spontaneously. The affected parts then become dry, pigmented and scurfy, and the fungus remains quiescent until the return of the next hot weather.

Diagnosis

The diagnosis of mycotic dermatitis is usually easily made; the festooned margin is almost conclusive. If doubt exists, the microscope (especially phase-contrast) may be necessary; but, owing to the inflamed condition of the parts, there may be much difficulty in finding fungous elements, even when the case is certainly epiphytic. A negative result is, therefore, not always conclusive against ringworm. The mycelial elements can be distinguished in epidermal scales soaked in liquor potassii. It has to be distinguished from seborrhoeic dermatitis, intertrigo, flexural psoriasis and dhobie mark dermatitis.

Treatment

The patient should get 2 pairs of running shorts, which should be worn on alternate days, the pair not in use being boiled. After a thorough use of soap and water, a preliminary soothing treatment by lead lotion or an ichthyol or witch hazel cream (Hazeline) is desirable.

Chrysarobin may be prescribed in the following form with gutta-percha, and should be painted on with a brush on alternate nights:

Chrysarobin	1·3 grammes
Chlorof.	3·5 ml
Liq. gutta-percha	28·4 ml

Griseofulvin is absorbed from the intestinal tract and reaches the skin by the blood-stream. It is an oral fungicide which offers a new approach in treatment, and should be given in doses of up to 1·5 grammes daily for adults for 2–4 months. For children half this dose is appropriate. Clinical improvement can be expected in 8 weeks and the skin is normal by the sixteenth (Russell *et al.* 1960).

In America undecenoic and propionic acids have been found effective in all forms of tinea infections. Undecenoic acid is used in the form of 10–20% cream of the Carbowax or Lanette wax types; a dusting powder containing 2% undecenoic acid and 20% zinc undecenoate is also employed. Mixtures containing them are also effective:

Undecenoic acid	5%
Zinc undecenoate	20%
Vanishing emulsion base up to	100%

For the ringworms of thick-skinned persons, linimentum iodi of double strength, freely applied, is the best, speediest and most efficient remedy, but it is too irritating and painful for the European skin.

As tinea cruris is often associated with tinea pedis, treatment for the latter is essential.

Prophylaxis

The various forms of crutch dhobie's itch may be avoided by wearing next the skin short cotton bathing-drawers and changing them daily, at the same time powdering the axillae and crutch with equal parts of boric acid, oxide of zinc, and starch after the daily bath.

RINGWORM OF THE FEET (HONGKONG FOOT; ATHLETE'S FOOT; MANGO TOE; BROCQ'S ECZEMA; TINEA PEDIS); TINEA OF THE HANDS

A peculiarly intractable infection of the feet, occurring especially among Europeans, is commonly observed in China and is known locally as 'Hongkong foot', but now has a world-wide distribution; is found in schools, athletic clubs, coal mines and the services, where communal bathing facilities are provided and the organisms are picked up by the feet, and is associated with conditions which produce hot, sweating feet. Gentles (1957) has clearly shown that the dermato-phytes do not live as saprophytes on the floors of bath-houses, but the spread of infection takes place by transfer of infected skin fragments which contain stable parasitic fungi, sometimes in large numbers. This mycotic infection is believed to be due to a variety of *Epidermophyton floccosum* or *Trichophyton interdigitale*, *T. mentagrophytes* or *T. rubrum*. It occurs especially during the summer months and appears as deep-seated vesicles about the inner margin of the hollow of the sole, or on, or between, the toes at their proximal extremities; or as a macerated condition of the skin of the interdigital clefts and of the contiguous surface. Scaling of the skin with persistent and intolerable itching is a marked feature, and it often becomes secondarily infected (Fig. 187). Often a mycotic infection of the nails and the palms of the hands is associated with it,

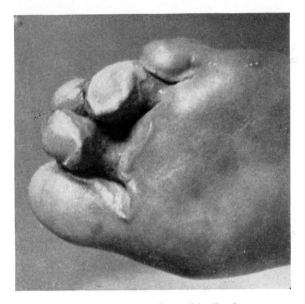

Fig. 187.—Ringworm of the foot, with allergic eczema.

resembling Hebra's eczema marginatum, which is said to be due to *E. floccosum* and shows itself by closely set vesicles on the palms. Hyperkeratoses of the palms of the hands or soles of the feet, especially of the heel, are also common. Isolation of the fungus presents difficulties owing to contaminating bacteria and moulds, but can be overcome by using potassium tellurite or penicillin to inhibit bacterial growth and by adjusting the reaction of the culture media to pH 10.5 to discourage the growth of moulds. A similar condition has been described in Turkish baths in England and in swimming pools in the Southern United States, as well as among bathers in Holland. Tinea of the big toe or 'Mango toe' is prevalent in the mango season in India and is also due to infection with *E. floccosum* and to transference from one person to another chiefly by bath mats.

Sulfo-Merthiolate dusting powder (Lilly) should be dusted into socks after bathing.

Care must be taken to distinguish dermatophytids or allergic reactions which are superimposed upon foot ringworm, especially in *T. gypseum* infections. Where such reaction is present treatment must be directed on other lines; trichophytin skin sensitivity tests are useful in differentiation; treatment should be directed to the relief of inflammation and fungicides should be avoided till the acute stage has subsided. Potassium permanganate 1:4000 should be used in cases with much vesiculation and applied before and after evacuation of the vesicles.

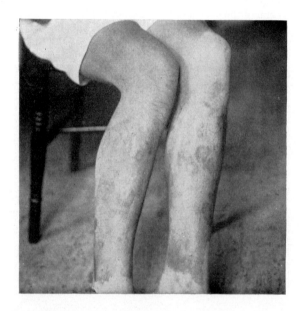

Fig. 188.—Extensive tinea circinata of the legs in an Indian. (*Philip Manson-Bahr*)

Treatment

The application of Whitfield's ointment, after the feet have been soaked in hot water, is recommended: salicylic acid 1, benzoic acid 1, coconut oil 12, soft paraffin 16 parts. This ointment must be persisted with for 3 weeks or more. Castellani's 1% fuchsin paint is widely recommended. Tineafax ointment and powder contain zinc undecenoate, and are very satisfactory in treatment.

Mycil dusting powder is chlorphenesin 1%, talc, zinc oxide, boric acid and starch. Sopronol ointment is composed of sodium propionate, propionic acid, sodium octoate, zinc octoate and dioctyl sodium sulphosuccinate and is recommended. Asterol (Roche) and Mersagel (Glaxo) are fungicide jellies containing phenyl mercuric acetate (1 in 750). Another is Merthiolate cream, and also tincture of Merthiolate, a solution of Merthiolate in alcohol, acetone and water, which sinks deep into the affected skin and thereby kills off the spores of the fungus.

For eczematous complications the toes should be separated by strips of gauze, and the foot should be covered with it and kept constantly wet with glycerin of lead subacetate 2·8 grammes, glycerin 2·8 grammes and water to 0·5 litre. This lotion can be later replaced by Lassar's paste. If a staphylococcal infection is present, dressings of acriflavine, 1 in 20 000, should be applied. Griseofulvin, the oral fungicide, is not so effective as in other skin fungus infections. The toe-web variety is especially resistant and treatment must be continued for months (Russell *et al.* 1960).

Infected patients should take careful precautions against the spread of the fungus, and should wear special slippers in the bathroom, and the feet should be dusted with 1% salicylic acid in talc. Loofah soles are recommended as they can be sterilized by washing.

As a measure against reinfection the patient may wear cotton toe-caps, which must be boiled, and he should also have a rubber bath-mat for exclusive personal use. Shoes may be swabbed out with 2% formaldehyde.

Tinea circinata (Fig. 188), with its characteristic papilliferous rings, is the most common ringworm of the tropics and may assume many different shapes and forms. They may be raised above the level of the normal skin or may be slightly elevated, particularly at the border, which is more usually inflamed and more scaly than the central portion. In some cases concentric circles develop or rings form upon one another making various patterns. The fungi whose spores and mycelial element can be seen in scrapings are *Trichophyton rubrum*, *T. mentagrophytes*, *T. sulphureum* or *T. violaceum*.

RINGWORM OF THE NAILS (TINEA UNGUIUM)

This is a mycotic infection of the nails and is a comparatively common and extremely intractable condition in Europeans, especially in India and China; it may last for 20 years or more. It may occur as an independent affection, or secondary to ringworm of the skin, scalp or beard, and is often found in association with tinea cruris. One or all of the nails of both hands and feet may be attacked. The fungus is a trichophyton, usually *T. rubrum* or *T. mentagrophytes*. English (1957) has shown that the first signs of this serious infection are scaling or macerated areas between the toes indistinguishable from tinea pedis.

The fungus first attacks the epidermis of the nail-bed and gradually invades the nail matrix. In doing so it causes considerable discoloration, ridging and fissuring of the nail itself, which becomes opaque, with a brittle, frayed edge. The fungus may pass from the skin over the nail-fold and in this manner reach the matrix. It is apt to be a conjugal infection and children are specially liable to contract it.

Diagnosis

The appearance of the affected nail is not sufficiently characteristic to be distinguished without microscopic examination. The disease is generally well advanced before it can be recognized. For microscopic diagnosis, scrapings of the nail are boiled in liquor potassii, or left to soak for 24 hours. The scrapings themselves should be made as thin as possible with a piece of glass. The fungus can then be recognized in the softened nail debris, especially in small dark haemorrhagic spots. For culture nail scrapings are first examined in 15% potassium hydroxide solution and cultured on Sabouraud's glucose agar with added penicillin and streptomycin. The diseases liable to confusion with ringworm of the nails are eczema, syphilis and, especially, psoriasis.

Treatment

In the early stages, when the lunule is attacked, the disease may be stamped out by softening the affected portion with solution of potash, and painting with tincture of iodine or with a 2% solution of corrosive sublimate in alcohol, twice daily. When the nail is completely involved, cure is almost impossible save by extirpation or by avulsion. The result is, however, disappointing, as the new nail usually becomes infected in turn. After removal, the thickened nail-bed should be scraped, and the matrix dressed with a parasiticidal ointment. Griseofulvin (Grisovin) tablets in doses of 1·5 grammes daily are strongly recommended in this distressing condition. The antibiotic griseofulvin orally, endows newly formed keratin with the power to resist fungal attack. Russell and colleagues (1960) treated their cases for as long as 3 months to 1 year. Those with infected toe-nails are more refractory and only a small percentage of these can be cured by this method.

The shedding of the nails by application of X-rays is unsatisfactory. Less severe cases are treated by softening the nail-plate by wearing rubber finger-stalls containing soft soap for a few days; the softened nail is then scraped down as far as possible with glass, followed each time by the application of lint soaked in Sabouraud's iodine (iodine 5, potassium iodide 1, water 100), which should be kept in position by a loose rubber finger-stall.

TINEA TONSURANS (RINGWORM OF THE SCALP)

This is very common in children, but rarely found in adults. It appears first as a small, greyish scaly patch, covered with broken hairs. The patches increase in size and number and may involve the whole scalp. It may be associated with tinea circinata.

It occurs all over the world and has been identified in England. The organism is *Microsporum audouini*, but *M. ferrugineum*, first isolated in Japan, Manchuria and the Far East, is more characteristic of the true tropics and is found commonly in the Congo. It is an ectothrix. *M. canis* and *M. gypseum* may also be involved.

On most mycological media the colony appears as a yellow to orange glabrous colony. On microscopic examination the cultures usually show only chlamydo-spores and swollen hyphae. In treatment griseofulvin (Grisovin) tablets, 1 gramme daily, have been found most effective.

FAVUS (WITKOP)

Favus is a severe type of chronic ringworm which can be caused by any one of three fungi, *T. schoenleinii*, *T. violaceum* and *M. gypseum*, which can occur in countries bordering on the Mediterranean, South-eastern Europe, Southern Asia and the Far East. It also occurs in South Africa. It is a clinical entity characterized by the formation of a dense mass of mycelium and arthrospores originating in a hair follicle, taking the form of a lozenge or inverted cone, the favus 'scutulum' or 'godet'. Removal of this leaves a moist scarlet base. When adequate treatment has destroyed the crusts the lesions heal with dense scarring and permanent alopecia (witkop). Lesions may also occur in the nails. Treatment with griseofulvin tablets (strength not stated) 4 times a day and undecenoic acid ointment is successful if carried on for 4-6 months (Van Beukering 1968).

MYCOSIS OF THE EAR (OTOMYCOSIS)

Mycosis of the external auditory meatus is popularly known as 'Panama ear', 'surfer's ear', 'hot weather ear', or otitis externa diffusa, and more descriptively as 'desquamative external otitis'. It was of frequent occurrence in U.S. Army in World War II, especially in Guam. There is a racial predisposition especially in Caucasians and natives of temperate climes. The infection declares itself by soreness and redness of the external auditory meatus, with tenderness on contact and pain on chewing. Itching and pain may be intolerable. The external canal is coated with a moist, soft, sebaceous-like detritus. In the third stage the walls become swollen so that the canal is obliterated. The pain produced is worse at night and there is moderate pyrexia. Fungous mycelium and spores can be demonstrated in the detritus. Some authorities think that *Ps. pyocyanea* is the chief factor. *Candida albicans*, *Malassezia furfur* and other fungi have been found.

In treatment the meatus is washed out with 4% boric acid solution through a straight attic cannula attached to an all-rubber irrigating syringe. After washing, the ear is gently dried. When the canal is free from debris a length of 1 cm (or 0·5 in) gauze ribbon, soaked in 1·5% hydrocortisone with neomycin sulphate, should be inserted into the meatus and kept there for 24 hours. For otomycosis 2% salicylic acid in 70% alcohol should be used as drops.

TINEA IMBRICATA (TOKELAU RINGWORM)

Geographical distribution

The affection is principally met in the Eastern Archipelago and in the islands of the South Pacific, where it affects a large proportion of the population. It has been found to extend westwards as far as Burma, and northwards as far as Formosa and Foochow on the coast of China. Cases have been reported from Central Africa and the interior of Brazil. Once introduced, it spreads very rapidly in countries with a damp, equable climate and a temperature of 26·7°–32·2°C. Very high or very low temperatures and a dry atmosphere are inimical to its extension.

Aetiology

On detaching a scale and placing it under the microscope, after moistening with liquor potassae, a *Trichophyton*-like fungus can be seen in enormous profusion. The parasite evidently lies between the stratum corneum of the epidermis and rete, and by its abundance causes the former to peel up. As the fungus does not die out in the skin travelled over, it burrows under the young epithelium almost as soon as the latter is reproduced. Hence the peculiar concentric scaling and the persistence of the disease throughout the area involved. When the scales are washed off by the vigorous use of soft soap and hot water, the surface of the skin is seen to be covered with brownish parallel lines— evidently the slightly pigmented fungus proliferating and advancing under the young epidermis.

The parasite, *Trichophyton concentricum* (syn. *Endodermophyton concentricum*), can be cultured by immersing the scales in alcohol for 5–10 minutes and then placing them, one scale to each tube, in glucose broth. After 5 or 10 days the scales, if uncontaminated, are transferred to solid media, and growth takes place in 3 or 4 weeks.

Symptoms

Tinea imbricata may at first be confined to one or two spots on the surface of the body; usually, in a short time it comes to occupy a very large area. It does not generally affect the soles and palms, although it may do so; nor is the scalp a favourite site. Baker remarked that it avoids the crutch and the axillae. With these exceptions it may, and commonly does, sweep over and keep its hold on almost the entire surface of the body, so that after a year or two a large part of the body is covered with the dry, tissue-paper-like scales, arranged in more or less confused systems of concentric parallel lines. This arrangement of the scales is absolutely characteristic of the disease (Fig. 189).

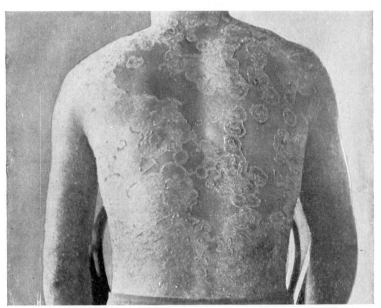

Fig. 189.—Tinea imbricata. (*By permission of the Medical Department of the former Sarawak Government*)

An inoculation experiment readily explains the production of the scales, their concentric parallel arrangement, and the mode of extension of the patches. About 10 days after the successful inoculation of a healthy skin with tinea imbricata, the epidermis at the seat of inoculation is seen to be very slightly raised and to have a brownish tinge. Presently the centre of this brownish patch—perhaps 0·6 cm in diameter—gives way, and a ring of scaling epidermis, attached at the periphery, but free, ragged, and slightly elevated towards the centre of the spot, is formed. In a few days this ring of epidermis has extended so as to include a larger area.

The scales, if not broken by rubbing, may attain considerable length and breadth; but, of course, their dimensions are in some degree determined by the amount of friction to which they are subjected. Usually, they are largest between the shoulders—that is, where the patient has a difficulty in scratching himself. The lines of scales are from 0·3 to 1·25 cm apart.

Diagnosis

From oidinary ringworm, tinea imbricata is easily distinguished by the absence of marked inflammation or congestion of the rings, by the abundance of the fungus, by the large size of the scales, by the concentric arrangement of the many rings or systems of rings, by the non-implication of the hair, and by the avoidance of crutch and axillae. From ichthyosis it is distinguished by the concentric arrangement of the scaling, by the peripheral attachment of the scales and by the presence of an abundance of fungus elements.

Prophylaxis

Daniels related that tinea imbricata is a comparatively rare disease in Tonga, and the people attribute this to their custom of oiling the body with coconut oil. Since the Fijians adopted this practice the disease has become somewhat less prevalent among them. Personal cleanliness, and the immediate and active treatment of any scaling spot, should be carefully practised in the endemic countries. Among certain Central African tribes it has never been observed in women, who oil their bodies, whereas the men, who do not adopt this custom, are subject to the disease.

TRICHOSPOROSIS (PIEDRA)

The black piedras are found in South America, chiefly in Brazil, Paraguay, Ecuador, Argentina, Uruguay, Colombia, etc. The small black nodule on the hair shaft is the ascostioma of the fungus *Piedraia hortai* belonging to the

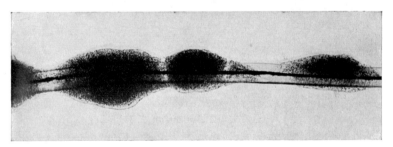

Fig. 190.—A human hair (magnified) affected with *Trichosporon beigelii*.

Asterineae, a family of fungi parasitic on the leaves of trees in very humid climates. The nodules consist of tightly packed stroma of dark-brown hyphae 4–8 μm in diameter; when crushed, asci containing fusiform curved ascospores are revealed. The white piedras are more widely distributed, being found in various countries of South America, Africa, Southern Asia, Japan and parts of Europe. The multiple white nodules on the hair are formed of sclerotial masses of the mycelium of the fungus *Trichosporon beigelii* and other species, which are related to the common fungi known as *Geotrichum*, *Oidium* or *Mycoderma*. In contrast to black piedra this white form attacks chiefly the coarse hairs of the body (Figs 190, 191).

Microscopically, the nodules, which are not so discrete as in black piedra, consist of a mass of polygonal cells, yellowish-green to brown, with a definite cell wall. The cells of a mycelial thread are separated from one another by thick black cell walls, between which there is little intercellular substance.

The hyphae tend to be perpendicular to the surface of the hair and segment into round or oval cells, 2–4 μm in diameter. Budding cells (blastospores) are also seen in the mycelial mass. Colonies of *T. beigelii* on Sabouraud's medium develop at room temperature and appear first as a cream-coloured, slimy growth which is soft in consistency.

Treatment

The affected hair should be bathed twice daily with a lotion consisting of 4 ml of formalin to 150 ml of rectified spirit, reinforced by 2% sulphur ointment. The affected surrounding skin should be rubbed with mercurial ointment.

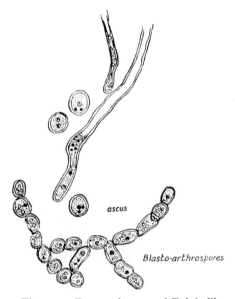

ascus

Blasto-arthrospores

Fig. 191.—Fungus elements of *T. beigelii*.

TROPICAL CHEIROPOMPHOLYX

This name is given to vesicular eruptions on the hands, fingers or feet usually known as dysidrosis. In the majority of cases these are due simply to eczema; others are signs of dermatitis due to external irritants, or are toxic eruptions due to ringworm infection of the toes. It is an example of interepithelial vesicular formation and is therefore similar to the eczema vesicle. Owing to the thickness of the horny layer on the hand, the vesicles cannot rupture as they would elsewhere, and remain in the skin for days like grains of boiled sago. The best treatment is calamine and lead lotion with coal tar solution, and sometimes with the addition of weekly doses of a quarter of a pastille of X-rays, not more than 4 in all.

It is claimed that a distinct form, endemic in tropical Africa and India, is caused by an anaerobic bacterium which attacks the palmar and interdigital aspects of the hands and the plantar aspects of the feet. A protective or pellanthum paste is soothing for the irritation. The following ointment is suitable:

Ichthyol	1 gramme
Zinc oxide	15 grammes
Olive oil	15 grammes
Anhydrous lanolin	4 grammes
Water	15 ml

To be applied night and morning

The ointment is rubbed well into the affected parts, and cotton gloves or socks are worn. In conjunction with this, resorcin soap should be used.

REFERENCES

ENGLISH, M. P. (1957) *Br. med. J.*, **i**, 744.
GENTLES, J. C. (1957) *Br. med. J.*, **i**, 746.
MARPLES, M. J. (1961) *Trans. R. Soc. trop. Med. Hyg.*, **55**, 216.
RUSSELL, B., FRAIN-BELL, W., STEVENSON, C. J., RIDDELL, R. W., DJANAHISZWILI, N. & MORRISON, S. L. (1960) *Lancet*, **ii**, 1141.
VAN BEUKERING, J. A. (1968) *Trop. geogr. Med.*, **20**, 240.

Mycetoma

Synonyms

Madura foot; pseudoactinomycosis; maduromycosis.

Definition

Mycetoma is a clinical syndrome caused by any one of many species of fungi. It may affect any part of the body exposed to trauma and occurs most frequently in the foot or hand. It can also affect the skull. Madura foot is the term applied to the disease as it affects the foot. True visceral mycetoma must be distinguished from aspergillosis, and actinomycosis is not a mycetoma.

Table 36. Fungi and Actinomycetes capable of causing mycetoma

Organism	Colour	Grain Size (mm)	World distribution	Favoured rainfall (cm/year)
Fungi				
Madurella mycetomi	Black	ca. 1·0	Africa, S. America, Madagascar, India, Indonesia	25–50
Madurella grisea	Black	ca. 1·0	Mainly N. and S. America	—
Leptosphaeria senegalensis	Black	ca. 1·0	Senegal and Chad	—
Pyrenochaeta romeroi	Black	ca. 1·0	Seldom seen	—
Allescheria boydii	White or yellow	ca. 1·0	Europe, America, Africa	100–200
Cephalosporium species	White or yellow	ca. 1·0	S. America, Africa, Europe, India	—
Corynespora cassiicola	Black	> 0·5	Sudan	—
Actino-mycetes				
Nocardia species	White or yellow	Tiny < 0·5	Cosmopolitan	100–200
Streptomyces somaliensis	Yellow	ca. 1·0	Africa, N. and S. America, Israel	5–25
Streptomyces madurae	Yellow	Large > 2·0	Africa, N. and S. America, Vietnam	—
Streptomyces pelletieri	Red	Tiny < 0·5	Africa, S. America	25–100

Modified from Murray (1966).

AETIOLOGY

Mycetoma is caused by 2 main groups of organisms:

1. Maduromycetoma caused by true fungi, species of *Madurella*.

2. Actinomycetoma caused by various species of aerobic and anaerobic bacteria which are species of *Nocardia* and *Streptomyces*.

In the Sudan the commonest aetiological agents are *Madurella mycetomi* (70%), *Streptomyces somaliensis* (20%) and *Streptomyces madurae* and *S. pelletieri* (10%). In Mexico most of the mycetomas are caused by *Nocardia brasiliensis*. The causative micro-organism of mycetoma is seen in the lesion as a small compact colony or 'grain' of various sizes and colours according to the species.

Table 37. Characters of grains of mycetoma

Organism	Naked eye			Microscopically	
	Colour	Diameter (mm)	Intrinsic colour	Diameter of filaments (μm)	Staining affinities
M. mycetomi ⎫ M. grisea ⎬ L. senegalensis ⎪ P. romeroi ⎭	Black	ca. 1·0	Brown	> 2·0	None in particular
A. boydii ⎫ Cephalosporium ⎬ species ⎭	White or yellow	ca. 1·0	None	> 2·0	PAS positive*
Nocardia species	White or yellow	< 0·5	None	< 1·0	Acid-fast†
S. somaliensis	Yellow	ca. 1·0	None	< 1·0	Eosinophilic** Not acid-fast
S. pelletieri	Red	< 0·5	Not pronounced	< 1·0	Stain deeply and uniformly with haematoxylin** Not acid-fast
S. madurae	Yellow	> 1·0	None	< 1·0	Margin stains deeply with haematoxylin** Not acid-fast

Modified from Murray (1966).

* Periodic-acid-Schiff stain.
† Decolorize with 1% sulphuric acid.
** Standard haematoxylin and eosin stain for tissues.

The mycelium in the grain is arranged in radial formation and in the case of some fungi the peripheral part is formed of large thick walled cells usually known as chlamydospores. Surrounding the grain in many species is a layer of hyaline eosinophil material often drawn out into club-like bodies forming a kind of corona on the grain which is more or less characteristic of the species of micro-organism. These hyaline formations which are common also in most other species of fungi, notably *Sporotrichum* and *Aspergillus*, represent a reaction by the host which is probably defensive. The maduromycoses which are caused by true fungi possess grains composed of coarse septate mycelium, whereas the grains of the actinomycoses show only very slender non-septate hyphae, usually not exceeding 1 μm in diameter, which represent the characteristic bacillus-like thallus of the actinomyces (Fig. 192).

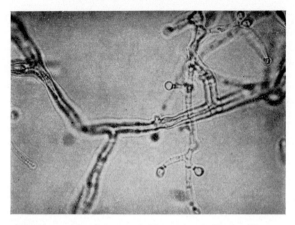

Fig. 192.—Aleurospores of *M. mycetomi*. (*Peter Abbott*)

CARTER'S BLACK MYCETOMA (*M. mycetomi*)

This is found mainly in tropical Africa, India, other Asiatic countries and also in parts of North and South America. There and perhaps also in India the geographical distribution of *M. mycetomi* and *M. grisea* may overlap.

The parasitic grains of *M. mycetomi* consist of a radially spreading septate and branching mycelium, measuring 1–5 μm in diameter with chlamydospores up to 25 μm. The actual grains are dark brown or black and measure 1–2 mm diameter. They are also hard and brittle. This fungus grows readily on Sabouraud's medium. Abbott (1956) has shown that the grains remain viable for 3 months or longer. In culture *M. mycetomi* can utilize glucose, maltose and galactose, but not sucrose, as sources of carbon; as sources of nitrogen it makes use of potassium nitrate, ammonium sulphate, asparagine and urea.

Madurella grisea may be the predominant form in the geographical range of mycetoma in S. America.

The parasitic grains of this species differ from those of *M. mycetomi* in the unpigmented central part surrounded by a blackish, cortical zone. In this marginal zone the mycelium is embedded in a brown cement. On culture *M. grisea* is unable to utilize sucrose, in addition to other sugars already mentioned.

The colonies on glucose-agar are hard, creased and folded, almost black in colour, and covered with greyish-white pulvescence.

In Czapek's medium puff-ball colonies are formed with dark centres.

Hyphae are either cylindrical, measuring 2–3 μm in diameter, or moniliform and thicker, 3–4 μm. They are branched and septate and give rise to more slender, almost colourless hyphae.

MADURA FOOT—VINCENT'S WHITE MYCETOMA
(*Streptomyces madurae*)

The organism is *Streptomyces madurae* (formerly *Actinomyces madurae* (Vincent) 1894). It has been found in Algeria, Ethiopia, Somalia, Cyprus, India, Argentina and Cuba. The species is monomorphic and constant. The grains may reach a size larger than that of any other species. They are whitish-yellow, sometimes with a pink tinge. The central part of the grain may be hollow and contain scant, loosely and irregularly packed filaments which radiate. Clubs are usually observed. They are elongated, up to 25 μm, tape-like and sometimes branched. The ends may be pointed and they usually stain pink with eosin. (*S. madurae* is synonymous with *Actinomyces brumpti* and *Discomyces bahiensis.*)

YELLOW-GRAINED MYCETOMA
(*Streptomyces somaliensis*)

The fungus is *Streptomyces somaliensis* (or *Nocardia somaliensis*) Brumpt, 1906, and has been extensively studied by Abbott (1956) in the Sudan. It occurs also in Ethiopia, Egypt, commonly in the Sudan and Somalia, West Africa and São Paulo. (The fungus appears to be identical with *Indiella somaliensis* of Brumpt and at one time the disease was called Bouffard's white mycetoma.) On Krainsky's medium it forms a thin, smooth pellicle and a short, light, ochreous aerial mycelium. On glucose peptone agar, cream coloured pellicles are produced and the culture may become brownish or blackish.

The mycelium is non-segmented with some chlamydospores about 1 μm in diameter. The aerial conidia are 1·25 μm typical of the genus *Streptomyces*.

Peptone and asparagine are assimilated, but ammonium sulphate, potassium nitrate and urea are not. The grains are yellowish, 1·25 mm in diameter, round, oval and compact. They are composed of a matrix of amorphous material showing slits and embedded on this the filaments of actinomyces are easily observed. Inoculations of mice and guinea-pigs have proved unsuccessful.

RED-GRAINED MYCETOMA (*Streptomyces pelletieri*)

This form has been shown by Abbott to be widespread in the Sudan. In its gross pathology it is similar to the others, but it is of greater virulence.

The organism is *Streptomyces pelletieri* (Laveran 1906) or *Nocardia pelletieri*. It is found in the Sudan, Senegal, Nigeria, India, Arabia and other countries. It produces (according to Mackinnon) slow growth in all media. On Krainsky's medium it forms hard red, purple, adherent colonies. There is a poor growth on Czapek's medium.

Non-segmented branched vegetative mycelium is produced with some swellings up to 1 μm in diameter. No conidia are observed. The organism is not acid-fast and stains well by Gram's method. On basal medium with asparagine only glucose favours growth. Peptone and asparagine are utilized; urea and potassium nitrate are not.

The parasitic grains are deep red in colour, rather small, and rarely reach 1 mm in diameter. They are very irregular in shape and have smooth or denticulate edges. Some are seen to be enveloped by a refringent hard pellicle.

Nocardia brasiliensis (Lindenberg 1909)

The general term *Nocardia* is reserved for the semi-acid-fast species. This species is found in Mexico, Brazil and Venezuela.

It is a rapid growing actinomycete and on Krainsky's medium forms heaped-up colonies with membranous consistency and marked furrows. The colour varies from pale ochre to orange or red ochre. Scarce aerial mycelium is formed on Krainsky and more abundantly on Czapek's media. The cultures produce an earthy odour.

A non-pigmented mycelium prevails. All strains are semi-acid-fast and stain well by Gram's method.

On basal medium with asparagine, glucose and galactose are utilized, but maltose, sucrose and lactose are not.

The parasitic grains are irregular, of moderate size, built up by lobules without clubs. Mice inoculated in the peritoneum developed abscesses, 1–3 mm in diameter, in pancreas, omentum and in between the liver and diaphragm.

Nocardia asteroides (Eppinger 1891)

This species was isolated by Fonseca in Rio de Janeiro and in Montevideo. On Krainsky's medium it produces a soft, inconsistent, creamy growth which acquires some orange and rose colour. On liquid media an inconsistent veil is formed.

The cultures are similar to those of *N. brasiliensis*. The mycelium may be segmented.

This fungus has no proteolytic activities and does not hydrolyse starch and can utilize all the nitrogenous compounds.

When inoculated into mice it produces small abscesses similar to those described above.

Leptosphaeria senegalensis n.sp.

Baylet *et al.* (1959) found this organism in maduromycosis in Senegal and Mauritania, isolating it in pure culture.

Culture. Cultures can be made, as in actinomycosis, both under aerobic and anaerobic conditions on glucose or glycerol-agar plates, in shake cultures or in Löffler's serum, as well as on Krainsky's and Czapek's media. Media are as follows: glucose peptone (1% Difco bactopeptone) agar, Krainsky medium (glucose 10 grammes, asparagine 0·5 gramme, bipotassium phosphate 1 gramme, agar 15 grammes, water 1 litre). Czapek's agar (sodium nitrate 2 grammes, bipotassium phosphate 1 gramme, magnesium sulphate 0·5 gramme, potassium chloride 0·5 gramme, ferrous sulphate 0·01 gramme, glucose 30 grammes, agar 20 grammes and water 1 litre). Some workers recommend keeping cultures in an atmosphere of CO_2. The medium should be inoculated directly with colonies from the pus, but, owing to slow growth of the actinomyces, pure cultures are somewhat difficult to obtain, unless the pus is free from contamination with other organisms.

Allescheria boydii

Allescheria boydii (*Monosporium apiospermum*) is widely distributed and causes a mycetoma with yellowish white grains in the Congo (Courtois *et al.* 1954). It grows well on Sabouraud's medium.

Cephalosporium falciforme has been isolated from cases of mycetoma in Puerto Rico, and *C. acremonium*, *C. recifei* and *C. granulomatis* have been isolated from human and animal cases of mycetoma (Baylet *et al.* 1961).

Corynespora cassiicola has been isolated from mycetoma in the Sudan (Mahgoub 1969) and is a true cause of that condition.

TRANSMISSION

Mycetoma is not contagious. Transmission is probably by puncture of the skin by infected thorns. Abbott (1956) found thorns embedded in the tissues at operation in 7 subjects of yellow and 2 of black mycetoma.

IMMUNOLOGY

The serology of mycetoma is in an experimental stage. Skin sensitivity, specific agglutinins and complement fixing antibodies to *Allescheria boydii* were found in 1 case (Seeliger 1956). There was no overlapping with other causes of maduromycosis although with complement fixation tests there was some cross-reaction with *Trichophyton*.

Specific precipitating antibodies have been demonstrated in the sera of 14 patients with actinomycetoma and 9 with maduromycetoma (*M. mycetomi*) (Baxter *et al.* 1966), and there was no cross-reactivity between the two groups.

Skin sensitivity tests on patients with *Nocardia brasiliensis* infection produced specific positive Type 4 reactions using purified protein antigens (Bojalil & Zomora 1963). Positive skin reactions were obtained with *Streptomyces* antigens in actinomycetoma and in some cases of maduromycetoma with *Madurella* antigens (Murray & El Moghraby 1964).

EPIDEMIOLOGY AND GEOGRAPHICAL DISTRIBUTION

Mycetoma occurs round the world in tropical and temperate regions. In India where mycetoma was first described it is an important disease and is endemic in widely scattered districts, although whole provinces, such as Lower Bengal, enjoy an almost complete freedom.

Africa is the chief home of mycetoma, extending from the east across the Southern Sudan and Equatorial Africa to the West Coast and down through Nigeria to the Congo. Cases are commonly seen in Mexico, Central America and adjacent areas and it has been described from Italy and South Vietnam.

Mycetoma is not contagious and man is infected by the accidental implantation by thorns or splinters of one of the causative agents. There is no evidence that the organisms are saprophytic but the grains of mycetoma can withstand drought for prolonged periods and it is probable that they can remain dormant but viable until the rains fall. With the moistening of the ground they may develop with the production of numerous aleurospores which may transmit the infection to man.

Environment

Mycetoma is a disease of semi-arid climates, and in the Sudan there is a close correlation between the incidence of the disease and rainfall and most patients come from an area where almost no rain falls for 7 months.

In a 2½-year period in the Sudan 1231 cases of mycetoma were admitted for hospital treatment (Abbott 1956).

In Senegal it has been suggested (Baylet *et al.* 1959) that black grain mycetoma is connected with the annual flooding of the valley of the Senegal river. Mycetoma occurs most frequently in males, reflecting a greater exposure, and in farmers and others in rural areas who are exposed to minor but penetrating wounds caused by thorns or splinters.

PATHOLOGY

On cutting into a mycetomatous foot or hand the knife passes readily through the mass, exposing a section with an oily, greasy surface, in which the anatomical elements in many places are unrecognizable, being, as it were, fused together, forming a pale, greyish-yellow mass. The bones have in parts entirely disappeared; where their remains can still be made out, the cancellated structure is very friable, thinned, opened out and infiltrated with oleaginous material. Of all the structures, the tendons and fasciae seem to be the most resistant.

The most remarkable feature revealed by section is a network of sinuses and communicating cyst-like cavities of various dimensions, from a mere speck to a cavity 2·5 cm or more in diameter (Fig. 193). Sinuses and cysts are occupied by a material unlike anything else in human morbid anatomy. In the black varieties this material consists of a black or dark-brown, firm, friable substance which, in many places, stuffs the sinuses and cysts; manifestly it is from this that

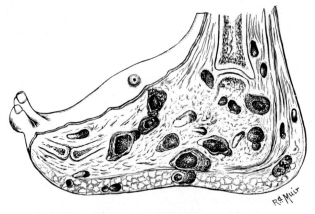

Fig. 193.—Section of a Madura foot. (*T. R. Lewis*)

the black particles in the discharge are derived. In the white varieties the sinuses and cysts are also more or less filled with a white or yellowish roe-like substance, evidently an aggregation of particles identical with those escaping in the corresponding discharge. In the very rare red variety the colour of the accretions is red or pink.

Under the microscope the mycotic elements can be readily recognized in the concretions. In microscopic sections of the tissues, evidences of extensive degenerative changes, the result of a chronic inflammatory process, can be made out. There are differences in the pathology of different types of mycetoma.

Black mycetoma shows a marked tendency to spread along tissue planes and through fibrous tissue in the foot where numerous fibrous septa pass between the muscles and tendons. In the earlier stages of this deeper growth it may be possible to remove the tumour and it will be found enclosed in a capsule of fibrous tissue and may be dissected out.

Muscle tissue is resistant to invasion. A black mycetoma in a sheet of muscle on the back or buttock will grow for years without penetrating the muscle fibres. Nerves and tendons are also resistant.

Neurological complications and trophic changes are conspicuously absent in mycetoma. Yellow mycetoma caused by *S. somaliensis* shows an insidious growth. The edges blend imperceptibly with surrounding tissues. From the first these tumours infiltrate the underlying muscles. Yellow mycetoma is harder than the black. The fibrous stroma is more compact and in it the yellow grains may be embedded. Red mycetoma due to *S. pelletieri* is similar in gross pathology to the yellow. The sinuses are more numerous and active.

CLINICAL FEATURES

Whatever the colour of the grains or species of fungus, the clinical course remains remarkably uniform. The first sign noticed is a painless swelling, usually, but by no means invariably, on the sole of the foot. Abbott has shown

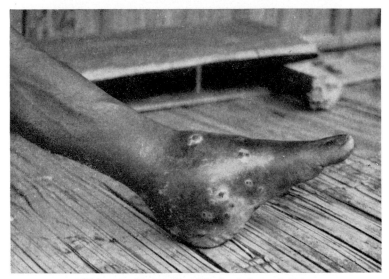

Fig. 194.—Madura foot. (*Dr L. A. Leon, Quito*)

that in yellow mycetoma it is ill-defined, while in black mycetoma it takes the form of a clearly defined, painless nodule in the subcutaneous tissues. The concept of an incubation period can hardly be applied.

Probably the fungus commences to develop as soon as it is implanted— sometimes, too, it may happen that a period of 10 years may elapse before the patient has been sufficiently incommoded to seek treatment. In the meantime, the growth continues slowly and inexorably. It may be a very long time before the deeper tissues are invaded, but the granuloma spreads inwards, invading the bones. Nodules, at first paler than the surrounding skin, form on the surface, revealing the mouths of the sinuses. From there a purulent fluid is discharged, containing the characteristic coloured grains of the fungus (Fig. 194). With all this the relative lack of pain is most remarkable and it is only when the foot or leg has been rendered quite useless that the patient suffers appreciably. No fever or other systemic effects accompany mycetoma, however long-standing, large or destructive the lesion may be, unless secondary bacterial infections supervene.

The regional glands may sometimes be involved and the causal fungus has been found in them by Abbott in 6 cases. The visible lesions are situated in less disabling sites. Back, buttocks or thigh may remain well-nourished and in good condition. In the majority of cases it is the effects of inactivity and economic loss which lowers the patients' vitality.

An important feature, not sufficiently emphasized in text-books, is the fact that sinuses that are diagnostic may be late in appearing. The interval may be as long as 6 years. As the foot enlarges, the leg commences to atrophy from

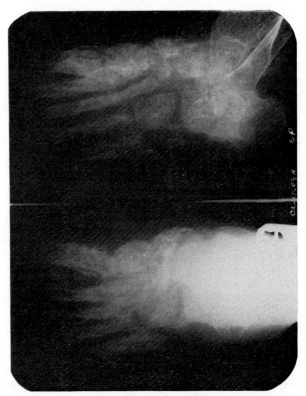

Fig. 195.—X-ray of a Madura foot.

disuse, so that in advanced disease, an enormously enlarged and misshapen foot, flexed or extended, is attached to an attenuated leg consisting of little more than skin and bone.

The intra-osseous mycetoma is primarily a fungous tumour occurring in the metaphysis of a long bone, usually the upper end of the tibia. All the cases of this variety have been in boys under 13 and all were caused by *M. mycetomi*.

The patient usually complains of dull, aching pains in the affected part. Examination reveals widening of the bone at the site of infection without involvement of the skin. It is probable that in these cases the infection is blood-borne. Periosteal tumours appear in all varieties. When a periosteal tumour forms on a long bone it presents itself as a hard, painless, smooth swelling without sinuses. It is probable that this type is due to direct inoculation of the organism into the periosteum of the tibia.

Cranial maduromycosis caused by *Streptomyces somaliensis* Hickey (1956) is not very uncommon and causes enlargement and distortion of the skull with loss of vision, proptosis and headache. The X-ray appearances are characteristic; there is expansion of the bone, periosteal new bone formation and punctate areas of osteoporosis without sequestrum formation. The picture may be confused with that of a neoplasm.

DIAGNOSIS

Direct examination of pus reveals the presence of the granules which are diagnostic. With knowledge of the usual mycetomas of the area, the fungus can be identified by the size, shape, colour and consistency of the granules. Direct examination is made by placing the granules in a drop of 10% sodium hydroxide and crushing under a coverslip to examine the hyphae. The granules should be crushed in the pus in which they have been obtained for staining (Gram's stain).

Direct culture from a biopsy of deep tissues should be performed on Sabouraud's modified agar (2% glucose, 1% neopeptone, pH 6·5–7·0), at room temperature and at 35°–37°C. If granules are to be cultured they must first be washed in saline to remove contamination.

TREATMENT

Actinomycetoma may be treated with antibacterial substances such as antibiotics, sulphones and even sulphonamides. 8 of 18 cases of mycetoma in the Sudan responded to treatment with broad-spectrum antibiotics and dapsone (Cockshott & Rankin 1960). Maduromycetoma cannot be treated by any other method than amputation. Actinomycetoma caused by species of *Nocardia* frequently responds to dapsone (100 mg 3 times daily) over a period of 6–24 months. Actinomycetoma caused by species of *Streptomyces* responds in only a proportion of cases and surgery is often necessary.

Nocardia brasiliensis infection has been treated successfully with amphotericin B but treatment must be continued for 1 year after clinical cure where the bones are involved.

Surgical treatment

The effective treatment is amputation well above the seat of the disease, since the long bones may be implicated as well as the small and unless the entire disease is removed it will recur in the stump. Complete removal is not followed by relapse. If a toe or a small portion of the foot or hand alone is involved this may be excised. Surgical removal of as much tissue as possible combined with injection of 1–2 ml of tincture of iodine every 10 days for at least 2 months into any suspicious area remaining has been found useful.

Chromoblastomycosis

Synonyms

Verrucous dermatitis; chromomycosis; mossy foot.

Definition

Chromoblastomycosis is a chronic mycosis of the skin and subcutaneous tissues characterized by verrucous ulcerated and crusted lesions which may be nearly flat, or raised and irregular, presenting a cauliflower-like appearance. Lesions are usually localized to the lower leg but may occur anywhere. Satellite lesions arise by auto-inoculation, by lymphatic spread and very rarely by haematogenous spread to the brain.

AETIOLOGY

Chromoblastomycosis is caused by several fungi: *Phialophora verrucosa*, *P. pedrosoi*, *P. compacta* and *Cladosporium carrionii*. The first 3 species produce spores of 2 diverse types in proportion which may vary with the species. *P. verrucosa* produces mainly phialospores (cup-shaped) and rarely arborescent sporeheads typical of abbreviated *Cladosporium* sporulation. *P. pedrosoi* and *P. compacta* sporulate predominantly by lateral production of conidia, and terminal arborescent spore heads, but rarely produce phialospores. *Cladosporium carrionii* sporulates only by branching chains of spores.

IMMUNOLOGY

Precipitins have been found to antigen prepared by ultrasonic destruction of fungal cells of *P. pedrosoi* which showed some cross-reaction with *P. compacta* and *P. verrucosa* but none with a wide range of other fungi including *Cladosporium* (Buckley & Murray 1966).

Precipitation, agglutination and fluorescent antibody tests have been used to separate the various organisms which cause chromoblastomycosis (Seeliger *et al.* 1959; Gordon & Al-Doory 1965).

EPIDEMIOLOGY

Chromoblastomycosis is seen more often in males than females and in rural than urban workers, in those people who are exposed to thorn and puncture wounds while working without shoes.

It is suspected that *Phialophora* are saprophytes in soil or timber and *P. verrucosa* has been isolated in a few instances from the soil and is responsible for the blue discoloration of wood pulp. *P. pedrosoi* has been isolated from saprophytic sources only rarely but probably occurs commonly in decaying vegetation in the soil.

Spores of *Cladosporium* can be identified in surveys of air-borne spores and perhaps sometimes causes respiratory allergic disease.

PATHOLOGY

Lesions of chromoblastomycosis show pseudoepitheliomatous hyperplasia associated with keratolytic micro-abscesses in the hyperplastic epidermis and must be distinguished from epithelioma. The deeper dermis contains confluent granulomatous nodules composed of pale, irregularly distributed epithelioid cells bordered by lymphocytes, plasma cells and other inflammatory cells. The centres may contain large foreign body giant cells. When ulceration ensues there is accompanying acute or chronic pyogenic infection. Brown hyphae may occasionally be demonstrated in the superficial crusts, but the characteristic findings are in the dermis where the yeast form is seen as round thick walled *brown* septate fungus cells. Owing to the brown colour special stains are of little use. Six or 7 fungus bodies may be found crowded in a giant cell, resembling peas in a pod.

CLINICAL FEATURES

The patient may be able to describe a minor wound preceding by months or years the fully developed lesion.

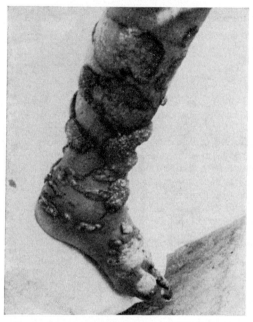

Fig. 196.—Chromoblastomycosis of the leg. (*By permission of the Mycology Department of the London School of Hygiene and Tropical Medicine*)

The primary lesion is minimal, persisting for months as a papule or pustule which finally ulcerates. The ulcer spreads slowly laterally and is replaced by a chronic dry crusted or verrucous violaceous lesion with a raised border (Fig. 196). It may remain flat or extend 1–3 cm above the normal skin surface. After many years the lesion becomes pediculated with a stalk producing a cauliflower-like tumour.

The lesions may heal at the centre while spreading marginally but spontaneous cure does not occur. There is little pain but considerable irritation. There may be spread by the lymphatic channels to remote areas and a few cases have been recorded of brain abscesses from which *P. pedrosoi* has been isolated. Secondary infection may cause considerable lymph stasis with lymphoedema.

DIAGNOSIS

Direct examination

Superficial crusts removed from the lesion contain long brown branching hyphae 2–5 μm wide which can be seen after digestion in sodium hydroxide.

Biopsy

Brown rounded bodies are found within giant cells or extracellularly among the polymorphs in the suppurative areas.

Culture

Culture of material should be on media containing chloramphenicol or other antibiotics and incubated at 30°C.

Differential diagnosis

Lymphostatic verrucosis and filarial elephantiasis must be distinguished, as must diffuse cutaneous leishmaniasis.

TREATMENT

Although the organisms which cause chromoblastomycosis are sensitive to amphotericin B *in vitro*, most drugs are unsuccessful in treatment of the disease. Local infiltration of the lesions with 15 mg amphotericin B dissolved in 3 ml of 2% procaine solution repeated weekly or at longer intervals for 4–8 injections has proved successful in some cases (Costello *et al.* 1959).

Local infiltration with amphotericin B and excision thermocoagulation of the small lesions and grafting of healthy skin in the large ones has been helpful but relapses occur often (Whiting & Cloete 1968).

5-Fluorocytosine by mouth and by local infiltration of the lesions has given good results (Lopes *et al.* 1969).

Heat treatment

Since the maximum temperature of growth of these fungi lies between 35° and 39°C, heat has been used in treatment. Cases caused by *P. verrucosa* have been cured with infra-red radiation (Conti Diaz *et al.* 1966).

Coccidioidomycosis

Synonyms

Posada's disease; coccidioidal granuloma; valley fever; desert rheumatism.

Definition

Coccidioidomycosis is an inapparent and benign or severe and fatal mycosis. It is respiratory in origin and in benign forms limited to the lung. In disseminated cases the infection spreads to other visceral organs, and to the skin and sub-cutaneous tissues (Fiese 1962).

AETIOLOGY

Coccidioidomycosis is caused by *Coccidioides immitis*, which is a dimorphic organism. The parasitic form is a spherical cell 30–60 μm in diameter (spherule) which does not bud but divides internally forming numerous endospores (2–5 μm in diameter) creating a multinucleate cell. The endospores are freed by rupture of the cell walls.

The mycelial form, which grows rapidly in culture on Sabouraud's and other media, grows readily in soil, producing great numbers of arthrospores which are easily disseminated by air currents.

TRANSMISSION

Coccidioidomycosis is not contagious, and infection is from exogenous sources. Man is infected via the respiratory route by the inhalation of arthrospores from the soil disseminated by air currents in endemic areas. Laboratory infections are common.

IMMUNOLOGY

Coccidioidomycosis is in the main an asymptomatic infection in which there is a primary infection followed by delayed hypersensitivity and recovery with permanent immunity. The recovered persons show hypersensitivity to coccidioidin. In white females allergic-type lesions of erythema nodosum and multiforme may develop but these are rare in dark skinned males. In a very small percentage of cases no resistance develops and there is disseminated spread.

Delayed hypersensitivity is measured by a skin reaction and circulating antibodies by complement fixation, immunodiffusion and fluorescent antibody tests. The most valuable tests are the skin test, complement fixation and precipitin tests. Coccidioidin is prepared from a pool of cultures of *C. immitis* grown under carefully standardized conditions (Smith *et al.* 1948) and is used as antigen for both skin hypersensitivity tests and circulating antibody.

Skin hypersensitivity is a delayed type (Type 4) reaction and a positive reaction is manifested by an area of induration 5 mm or more at the site of intradermal injection of 0·1 ml coccidioidin. Reactivity develops 2–21 days (80% within a week) after the appearance of symptoms and persists for at least 20 years in persons who have left the endemic zones. The test is relatively specific, although a few patients react mildly to histoplasmin, blastomycin and para-coccidioidin. The degree of hypersensitivity is very great in patients with erythema nodosum. Reactivity to coccidioidin may decrease or disappear at the time of dissemination of the infection only to reappear with recovery. The coccidioidin skin test is of great diagnostic value and positive serological tests were not obtained in patients with primary coccidioidomycosis or with impending dissemination in the absence of a positive skin test (Smith *et al.* 1956).

Complement fixing antibodies (Smith *et al.* 1956) are of the IgG type and appear late in the infection, not until 3 months after symptoms, and may never be detectable in asymptomatic and mild cases. When present they disappear in 6–8 months. They are best used to detect disseminated disease in which they persist until death or after recovery, and a high and rising titre of complement fixing antibodies indicates a poor prognosis.

Positive titres of 1 in 2 or 1 in 4 can be significant but have occasionally been obtained in patients not known to have coccidioidomycosis. Negative serological tests do not exclude the disease.

Precipitins are of the IgM type and appear 50% within the first week and 90% by the third week. They disappear from 12 to 16 weeks after infection, even in disseminated disease. An immunodiffusion test has now been perfected and gives a 95% accuracy (Bailey *et al.* 1965).

With a combination of complement fixation and immunodiffusion tests 90% of primary cases with clinical symptoms can be confirmed (Smith *et al.* 1956).

Fluorescent antibody inhibition tests can be used for the rapid detection of antibodies to *C. immitis* (Kaplan & Clifford 1964).

Immunization

The use of a vaccine is being investigated (Converse 1965). Suspensions of killed spherule walls and endospores have conferred a high level of immunity in mice and monkeys (Levine & Kong 1966).

EPIDEMIOLOGY

Coccidioidomycosis is endemic in the Lower Sonoran life zone in the United States, including areas of Southern California, Arizona, New Mexico, South Texas and Northern Mexico, which is characterized by low rainfall, high summer temperature and a characteristic association of certain plants, cacti and creosote bushes, with certain species of rodents, *Perognathus, Dipodimys* and *Citellus.* Similar areas also occur in the Chaco of Northern Argentina and Paraguay.

Cases in other areas can be explained on the basis of fomites brought in from an endemic area. Many of the rodents have pulmonary lesions caused by *C. immitis* and play an important part in the maintenance of endemic infection and *C. immitis* can be isolated from both the soil and rodents (Emmons 1942).

The greatest endemic focus is in the San Joaquin Valley, where skin tests have shown that 75–97% of children react positively to coccidioidin. No age-group is immune and the condition is a mild disease of early childhood, most apparent in the adult migrant population. There is no evidence of sex or racial differences in susceptibility to infection but there is a marked difference in the occurrence of progressive and disseminated disease. About 1 in 400 adult white males develop granulomatous disease. In white females the rate is one-fifth of this and in male Negroes the rate is 10–15 times greater than in white males.

PATHOLOGY

Primary coccidioidomycosis is a benign self-limiting respiratory disease in the majority of cases. Progressive coccidioidomycosis is a relatively malignant disseminated infection involving cutaneous, subcutaneous, visceral and osseous tissues.

Primary lesion

The early lesions of coccidioidomycosis are indistinguishable from focal pulmonary pyogenic pneumonitis of bacterial origin except that spherules with endospores may be obtained in the lesions. The pyogenic reaction may be attributed to the released endospores, while the delayed hypersensitivity cellular response to the spherules is a granulomatous exudate with giant cells. Small developing spherules are seen intracellularly in histiocytes and giant cells; small released endospores are smaller than neutrophils and are difficult to identify with H. & E. stains. Both forms are readily seen with PAS.

Coccidioidal granuloma (coccidoidoma) is a solitary circumscribed pulmonary granuloma which closely resembles the solitary lesions found in tuberculosis and histoplasmosis. Calcification is not so pronounced and the diagnosis can only be made by identification of the causal agent.

Disseminated coccidioidomycosis

At autopsy lesions are widespread, involving lymph glands, spleen, skin, subcutaneous tissue, liver, kidney, bones, joints and meninges. The lesions may be miliary or extensive and the histological picture is a combination of suppuration and granulomatous cellular reaction in which many spherules may be demonstrated.

Central nervous system

The characteristic lesion is that of a diffuse granulomatous meningitis which encases the brain and may cause obstruction to the flow of C.S.F. Small granulomatous lesions occur within the brain substance. In rapidly progressive cases the meningeal exudate is more suppurative in character. In some cases a fatal meningitis has been found in persons without any evidence of a pulmonary lesion.

CLINICAL FEATURES

Inapparent infections

In 60% of infections there is no history of anything which can be diagnosed as coccidioidomycosis. In these persons the diagnosis of past infection is based upon a positive skin reaction to coccidioidin. The remaining 40% develop a mild upper respiratory infection, primary pulmonary coccidioidomycosis, and less than 0·5% disseminated infection.

Primary pulmonary coccidioidomycosis (Richardson et al. 1967)

The incubation period is between 7 and 28 days. The onset is with fever, varying from a few hours (valley fever) to months in duration, which may be remittent, when eventual dissemination is more probable. The fever exhibits diurnal variation and sweats are common.

Pulmonary symptoms are frequent, with pleuritic pains which may be severe, dyspnoea and cough, which may be productive with white purulent or blood-stained sputum. There may be no cough, however, even in the presence of pulmonary disease. The lungs may show pneumonic spread or pleural effusion with râles, signs of consolidation or pleural friction rub. There may be associated pericarditis. Later pulmonary cavitation may occur.

X-ray appearances are not specific but show patches of consolidation as nodular lesions 2–3 cm in diameter and widening of the hilar shadows although there is no peripheral lymphadenopathy. Calcified lesions may be found later after recovery.

Dermal lesions

Dermal lesions are caused by hypersensitivity. An early generalized macular erythematous rash in 10% of cases may precede the onset of sensitization.

Erythema nodosum and erythema multiforme (desert rheumatism) occur in about 20% of symptomatic cases, are observed most frequently in adult white females and denote a good prognosis. Erythema nodosum occurs as crops of bright red nodules on the anterior surface of the tibia and lasts a few days. Erythema multiforme on the thighs may be associated with joint pains. They are both accompanied by a pronounced eosinophilia.

Healed or residual coccidioidomycosis

Chronic pulmonary cavitation occurs in 2–8% of symptomatic infections, the chronic cavity is solitary, has a thin wall with little surrounding reaction and may contain fluid. It may be almost symptomless or associated with chest pain, cough and haemoptysis, and may persist for many years without dissemination. Coccidioidoma (coccidioma) is a benign residual granulomatous lesion in the lungs, varying in size, usually discovered by accident as a 'coin lesion', and is difficult to diagnose from carcinoma.

Cutaneous coccidioidomycosis

The skin lesions which have been described may be determined by local trauma but are almost certainly of primary pulmonary origin. The lesions

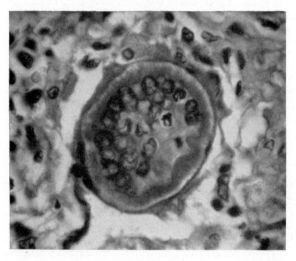

Fig. 197.—Sporangium of *Coccidioides immitis.* × 2000. (*W. St C. Symmers*)

ulcerate, exuding pus (Fig. 198) in which the organisms can be found, and after a few weeks become papillomatous. A scrofulodermic type of lesion is associated with the superficial cervical glands. Progressive coccidioidomycosis of the skin (Fig. 199) is found in the disseminated form of the disease.

Disseminated coccidioidomycosis

Massive dissemination following immediately after the primary infection occurs most often in Negroes and Filipinos. In other groups the dissemination is preceded by primary disease characterized by pneumonia, pleural effusion and high eosinophilia. There may be a remission but this is followed after a few days or weeks by recurrence of fever and a rise in titre of complement fixing antibodies. Disseminated lesions may be found in skin, subcutaneous lesions, bones, joints and all visceral organs. The course of the disease is marked by remission and exacerbations with recovery or a slow or rapid progression. Acute miliary dissemination and meningitis are always fatal.

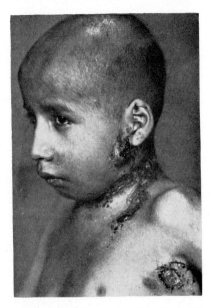

Fig. 198.—Cutaneous coccidioidomycosis (Wernicke or Posada's disease).
(*Dr L. A. Leon, Quito*)

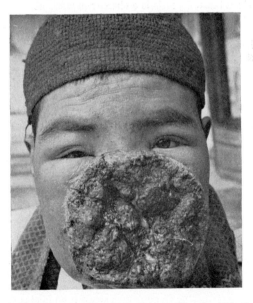

Fig. 199.—Coccidioidomycosis of the face in Ecuador. (*Dr L. A. Leon, Quito*)

DIAGNOSIS

Direct examination of exudates may show the sporangia of *C. immitis* in sputum or pus prepared with sodium hydroxide and examined both with and without ink under the low-power microscope. Heat fixed stained films are of no value.

Culture of the organism may be made on Sabouraud's medium incubated at 25–30°C and kept for 1–2 weeks.

Animal inoculation of material into mice may be useful.

TREATMENT

Treatment is indicated in the disseminated disease. Amphotericin B is active against *C. immitis* when given by the intravenous route (Section XVI) (Baker & Kemberling 1960), but relapses occur frequently. Surgical resection may be necessary for chronic residual pulmonary lesions.

South American Blastomycosis

Synonyms

Brazilian blastomycosis; Lutz–Splendore–De–Almeida's disease; paracoccidioidal granuloma.

Definition

South American blastomycosis is a chronic mycosis characterized by ulcerative granulomas of the buccal and nasal mucosa with extension to the skin, by regional and generalized lymphadenopathy and by metastases to the lungs, spleen and other viscera.

AETIOLOGY

South American blastomycosis is caused by a dimorphic fungus *Paracoccidioides brasiliensis* which grows in tissue cells (and often in giant cells) in the yeast form of spherical or oval cells which reach diameters of 30 μm and reproduce by budding; the distinctive feature is the cell which bears buds (gemmules) 1–5 μm in diameter over the external surface (ectosporulation). This budding type of growth can be maintained *in vitro* by incubation at 37°C on blood agar. In culture at room temperature the mycelial form grows slowly on Sabouraud's medium.

TRANSMISSION

Clinical records and epidemiological studies suggest that this mycosis is not transmitted from person to person. The organism has been isolated from soil, and primary lesions are usually on the buccal mucosa, suggesting the introduction of the fungus to these tissues by fragments of wood used in cleaning the teeth. It is also possible that primary infection of the lung occurs through inhalation.

EPIDEMIOLOGY AND GEOGRAPHICAL DISTRIBUTION

No animal reservoir is known and the organism probably lives saprophytically in the soil. This type of blastomycosis is confined to South America. Most of the reported cases have been from the state of São Paulo, Brazil, but it occurs not uncommonly elsewhere in Brazil and has been reported from all South American countries. It occurs at all ages but with the highest incidence between 30 and 50 years of age.

IMMUNOLOGY

Although benign cases of the disease are not known, patients who develop some resistance after a primary infection show delayed hypersensitivity, but disseminated cases are anergic.

Skin tests of delayed hypersensitivity (Type 4) have been developed, using a wide variety of culture filtrates and cellular antigens which have produced confusing results. A polysaccharide antigen (Fava Netto 1965) gave positive results in 87% of patients with confirmed disease. A positive result produced a small granuloma of foreign body type beneath the epithelium after 10–15 days (De Brito *et al.* 1961). Positive tests may be expected in clinically well people living in endemic areas and the test can distinguish between blastomycosis, cutaneous leishmaniasis and sporotrichosis.

Complement fixing antibodies (IgG) after using the polysaccharide antigen are present in the highest titre in disseminated disease, and in low titre or negative in localized disease (Fava Netto 1965). A combination of complement fixation and precipitin tests demonstrated antibodies in 98·4% of patients. Complement fixing antibodies persist for a long time but decrease in titre in cured patients. Cross-reactions occur with histoplasmosis but higher titres are found with the homologous antigen.

Precipitating antibodies (IgM) demonstrated by agar gel precipitation using a concentrated culture filtrate of the yeast phase as antigen are the first antibodies to appear and disappear (Restrepo 1966). No cross-reactions occur with North American blastomycosis, histoplasmosis, coccidioidomycosis, sporotrichosis, tuberculosis or healthy individuals.

PATHOLOGY

A characteristic feature is a tendency to involve lymphoid tissue, first in the lymph glands draining the lesions in the skin or mucous membranes and later by widespread involvement of lymphatic tissues including the spleen. Lesions of the intestinal tract are common. In the disseminated form of the disease granulomas are found in most organs, including the liver, heart, pancreas and kidney. Occasionally the caseous necrosis of the suprarenal glands resembles histoplasmosis. Osteomyelitis may occur. The central nervous system is rarely involved; there is a granulomatous basal meningitis with large numbers of giant cells containing *P. brasiliensis*.

CLINICAL FEATURES

The incubation period is usually very prolonged, between 5 and 9 years (Scarpa *et al.* 1965). There are 4 main clinical types.

Oral lesions

The primary lesion is usually in the nasal or oral mucosa (gums), but may be in the conjunctiva or the anorectal mucosa. A severe ulcerative painful stomatitis develops which may extend to the tonsils. Laryngeal lesions are usually secondary to the pulmonary lesions, and may cause great diagnostic difficulty because of the close resemblance to tuberculosis. The appearance is that of hyperaemia, oedema, ulceration and granulations on the epiglottis and vocal cords. Gingival lesions are accompanied by ulceration and spontaneous loss of teeth, and lesions may develop on the tongue.

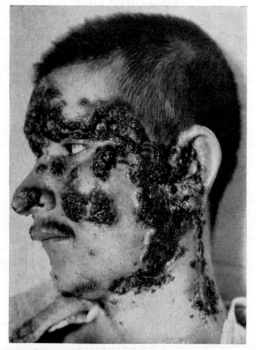

Fig. 200.—South American blastomycosis. (*Lacoz & Pupo, São Paulo*)

Cutaneous lesions

The typical lesions are an ulcerative and crusted granuloma of the skin arising by direct extension from the mucosal lesions or by autoinoculation (Fig. 200). Spread to the skin may also take place via the blood and lymph channels. Occasionally a solitary pustular lesion may represent a primary implantation of the fungus.

Lymphatic lesions

The lymphatics draining the primary lesion are invariably involved. The cervical lymph glands are involved early. They are painlessly enlarged, adherent and may suppurate, forming sinuses. Massive enlargement of the lymph glands of the neck is an early sign. Visceral lymphadenopathy is common.

Visceral lesions

The lymphatic system, spleen, intestines, lungs and liver are the organs chiefly affected. The spleen is almost always affected. The intestines always contain lesions which begin in the submucosal lymphoid tissue and erode into the lumen. The lesions in the lungs resemble those of pulmonary tuberculosis and involve chiefly the apex. Diffuse hilar lesions also occur.

X-ray appearances are those of nodular lesions, patchy infiltration, fibrosis and emphysema. Ventilatory studies show an obstructive form of respiratory insufficiency.

The adrenals may be affected. Osteolytic lesions of the bones may be found and lesions of the central nervous system may predominate with a high protein content in the C.S.F. caused by basal meningitis.

Anal, rectal and penile lesions also occur.

DIAGNOSIS

South American blastomycosis differs from North American blastomycosis in its predilection for the mucosal tissues, in the frequency of gingival lesions, in a tendency to central healing and in regional and generalized lymphadenopathy. It must also be differentiated from tuberculous adenitis, cutaneous tuberculosis, syphilis, yaws, sporotrichosis and leishmaniasis.

The diagnosis is made by examination of fresh sputum and other discharges for the typical spherical or oval cells with external buds.

The fungus may be cultured on blood agar incubated at 37°C or as the mycelial form on Sabouraud's medium.

Serodiagnosis

The skin test is of little use. The complement fixation test is satisfactory (see Immunology, page 683).

Although a benign form of the disease is suspected, clinical cases of the disease as actually known are fatal unless effective treatment is given.

TREATMENT

Most clinical forms of the disease except lymphoidal and central nervous system disease may be kept in remission by maintaining a serum level of 5 mg/100 ml of sulphonamide. This is achieved by the use of long-acting sulphonamides. However, relapse follows cessation of therapy.

Sulphormethoxine (Fanasil) 1 gramme daily for 10 days followed by 2 grammes weekly gave the best results (Lopes et al. 1966) and should be continued for 1 to 2 years. Resistance to sulphonamide therapy may develop.

Trimethoprim (Ro 5–6846) has been used in conjunction with sulphonamides as Septrin, especially in the treatment of sulphonamide resistant cases (Lopes & Armand 1968).

Amphotericin B gives good results and should be used in all severe forms of the disease especially where the C.N.S. is involved. It is given in the usual way (Section XVI) to a total dosage of 2 grammes.

Complications

Complications of treatment can occur from sensitivity to the organism developing during treatment of pulmonary disease, with asthma which may necessitate the use of steroids to control it.

The results of treatment are followed by observations on the presence of the fungus in sputum and tissue, radiological appearances of the lungs and the titre of complement fixing antibodies.

KELOIDAL BLASTOMYCOSIS (LOBO'S DISEASE)

Keloidal blastomycosis is a localized cutaneous benign process observed primarily in the Amazon and Orinoco river areas (Dias *et al.* 1970), but also in Surinam and Costa Rica. About 69 cases have been observed to date. Clinically it is a mycosis characterized by keloidal skin lesions without lymphangitis or visceral dissemination. The disease is probably distinct and not a clinical variant and the fungus is called *Loboa loboi*.

North American Blastomycosis (Gilchrist's Disease)

Definition

North American blastomycosis is a chronic granulomatous and suppurative disease which originates as a respiratory infection and disseminates, usually with pulmonary, osseous and cutaneous involvement predominating.

AETIOLOGY

The cause of North American blastomycosis is *Blastomyces dermatitidis*, a dimorphic fungus which grows in mammalian tissues as budding cells 8–15 μm in diameter (rarely reaching 30 μm) and in culture as a dry white mould, bearing spherical or ovoid conidia 2–10 μm in diameter or short slender conidiophores. The parasite grows *in vitro* by incubation at 37°C on blood agar. Budding is usually single and *Blastomyces* differs from *Histoplasma* and *Cryptococcus* by its multinucleate condition.

TRANSMISSION

The exact form of transmission is unknown. There is no evidence of transmission to patient contacts. Occasional cases have been attributed to fomites.

IMMUNOLOGY

Four basic antigens have been used, culture filtrates of a broth supporting the mycelial phase (blastomycin), extracts of mycelium, suspension of yeast phase cells and extract of yeast phase cells. There is considerable antigenic overlap with *Histoplasma capsulatum* and *Coccidioides immitis*. From the diagnostic point of view serological results have proved disappointing owing to the large percentage of negative reactions and the incidence of cross-reactions. Blastomycin has been used in skin tests but is frequently associated with histoplasmin reactivity and has been regarded as useless. Using a heat-killed yeast phase antigen, positive reactions were obtained in 84% of active cases (Balows 1963).

The complement fixation test is unsatisfactory, confirmed diagnosis being obtained in only 46% of tests with blastomycin (Busey 1964). An antigen from yeast phase cells gave a positive result in 71% of affected patients but cross-reacted with *H. capsulatum*.

Precipitins against blastomycin were present in the sera of 14 of 22 patients with blastomycosis and could be distinguished from the cross-reactions occurring with coccidioidomycosis and histoplasmosis (Abernethy & Heiner 1961).

EPIDEMIOLOGY

This mycosis is almost entirely American in distribution, extending southwards from North America to Mexico and Central America, with a few cases in South America. Recently verified cases have been reported from the Congo, South Africa, Tunisia and Uganda (Ajello 1967). The occurrence of benign respiratory forms of North American blastomycosis has not yet been proved. Cases of the established disease are sporadic in incidence and when groups of cases have occurred these have been small. Natural infection has been recorded in dogs and the infection is probably saprophytic from the soil, yet the fungus has never been isolated from soil. Blastomycosis occurs at all ages, with a slightly higher incidence in the third and fourth decades; males are affected 9 times as frequently as females.

PATHOLOGY

There are two main types of blastomycosis, systemic and cutaneous. The primary lesions occur in the lungs. The characteristic response to *Blastomyces dermatitidis* is a combination of suppuration and epithelioid cell granulomatous reaction with giant cells. The reaction closely resembles tuberculosis or histoplasmosis with extensive caseous necrosis. The fungus can be demonstrated as a rounded intracellular body 8–15 μm in diameter with the protoplasm shrunk away from the cell wall leaving a clear space. Budding is difficult to demonstrate.

CLINICAL FEATURES

Pulmonary blastomycosis

Primary pulmonary blastomycosis begins as a mild respiratory infection which progresses with dry cough, hoarseness and low grade fever. The symptoms and signs closely resemble those of pulmonary tuberculosis with increasing blood-stained sputum, dyspnoea, loss of weight, fever and night sweats.

X-ray examination of the chest shows widespread miliary lesions, homogeneous consolidation, solitary or multiple nodular shadows or abscesses or fibrotic lesions. Cavitation is rare (Boswell 1959).

Systemic blastomycosis

In the systemic infection there is involvement of the skin, subcutaneous tissues, respiratory organs, bones, urogenital canal and central nervous system. The gastro-intestinal tract is rarely involved. Dissemination to the skin is common.

Cutaneous blastomycosis

The presenting complaint of many patients is in the skin. The infection may start as a papule or pustule, which ulcerates and develops into an ulcerated or warty granuloma. Characteristic organisms can be demonstrated in the pus. The lesions spread slowly over a period of months or years, leaving their atrophic scars in the centre. Cutaneous lesions associated with bone lesions are sinuses.

Course of the disease. Cutaneous blastomycosis is very chronic and indolent, and the lesions may clear up with antifungal treatment, without cure of the deep mycosis.

In the widely disseminated disease the prognosis is poor in spite of treatment.

TREATMENT

Hydroxystilbamidine isethionate has been used successfully in some cases in intravenous doses of 150–200 mg daily for 30 days at a time. Courses may be repeated. Many cases relapse.

Amphotericin B is preferable, and should be given in standard doses (page 705) up to a total of 2 grammes. A smaller percentage of patients relapse.

Experimentally, 81 cases were treated with diamidines and 30 with amphotericin B; 15 were treated with both drugs; 54 (67%) were arrested by diamidines and 5 (6%) died; 27 (90%) were arrested by amphotericin B and 2 (7%) died. Using both drugs 12 of 15 were arrested and 2 died (Furcolow 1963).

Cryptococcosis

Synonyms

Torulosis; European blastomycosis; Busse-Buschke's disease.

Definition

Cryptococcosis is an acute, subacute or chronic pulmonary, systemic or meningeal mycosis caused by *Cryptococcus neoformans*.

AETIOLOGY

Cryptococcus neoformans is seen as a thick-walled spherical cell surrounded by a wide capsular structure of mucoid character which is less refractile than the cell wall. Mounted in a suspension of China ink or nigrosin the cell is seen to measure 5–15 μm in diameter, occasionally up to 20–30 μm, and the entire parasite with its capsule 15–45 μm in diameter. The young cryptococci are easily stained by Gram's stain but the best differentiating stain is mucicarmine with haematoxylin, which colours the cell wall an intense red and the contents and capsule a faint pink. The parasite multiplies by gemmation, does not produce endospores or mycelium and can be cultivated in glucose broth or Sabouraud's medium at 37°C. The colonies are honey coloured and semi-fluid.

TRANSMISSION

Cryptococcosis is not contagious and *C. neoformans* cannot be isolated easily from the skin, mucous surfaces or faeces of man. *C. neoformans* grows frequently in accumulations of pigeon droppings, and inhalation of cells of cryptococci and infection of the respiratory tract from this source is probably the usual method of infection.

IMMUNOLOGY

Although there is some evidence that man can be resistant to infection there is no evidence that an initial benign exposure immunizes man against subsequent exposure. Most mammals have a high degree of innate resistance to infection and there is a relatively high incidence of cryptococcosis in people with disorders of the reticulo-endothelial system, which suggests that a humoral mechanism is involved in this resistance.

C. neoformans has been divided into a number of serotypes (Evans 1950); the capsular polysaccharides are antigenic and cross-reactions are found with *Candida albicans* and other fungi as well as Types II and XIV pneumococci.

The serological diagnosis of cryptococcosis has not yet been developed to a level of routine reliability.

The presence of cryptococcal antigens has been demonstrated in spinal fluid, blood and urine of a patient by precipitin and complement fixation tests using *C. neoformans* antisera. A slide test with antibody-coated latex particles (Gordon & Vedder 1966) has been used to detect antigen in cerebrospinal fluid as a diagnostic measure. Significant titres of serum antibodies have also been reported in a passive haemagglutination test with human type O red cells coated with *C. neoformans* Type A capsular polysaccharide (Pollock & Ward 1962). Fluorescent antibody techniques have been used to detect the presence of cryptococcal polysaccharide lining the bronchial epithelium and in alveolar exudate and macrophages in a granulomatous reaction (Kase & Marshall 1960).

Fluorescent antibodies have been demonstrated in the sera of 7 of 8 proved cases of cryptococcosis but false positive reactions were obtained with *C. albicans* sera (Vogel *et al.* 1961) and positive reactions were reported in 18 of 23 patients with proved cryptococcosis (Kaufman 1966).

Skin tests of delayed hypersensitivity type have not yet proved of any use in the diagnosis of infection.

EPIDEMIOLOGY

Cryptococcosis is world-wide in distribution and all ages, sexes, races and occupations may be affected.

Reservoirs of infection

Soil reservoir. Emmons (1955) found a frequent saprophytic association of *C. neoformans* with pigeon manure; it has been isolated frequently from old nests and excreta under roosting sites of pigeons in the upper floors of buildings in cities and in stables in rural areas. Accumulations of pigeon droppings are the most important source of the fungus.

Animal reservoir. Cryptococcosis has been described in the horse, rat, mouse, dog, cat, tiger, cheetah, marmoset monkey, cow, koala and domestic pigeon. Extensive outbreaks of cryptococcal mastitis have been reported in dairy herds in the U.S.A. (Pounden 1952). The infection was transmitted through the suction cups of milking machines and the disease was generally confined to the udder. Nevertheless there is no evidence that the disease in lower animals is a source of direct infection of man.

Susceptibility

Cryptococcosis occurs as a sporadic infection. Although many people must be exposed benign infections are rare. It is possible that individual suscepti-bility plays a part in determining infection since important predisposing factors are a pre-existent Hodgkin's disease, lymphosarcoma, leukaemia, and other malignant disease of the reticulo-endothelial system. Cryptococcosis is also an 'opportunist' infection, occurring with immunosuppresive treatment, but anti-biotic therapy does not aid this infection as it undoubtedly does candidiasis.

PATHOLOGY

The portal of entry is most likely the lung with haematogenous spread to the skin, bones, abdominal viscera and especially the central nervous system.

Benign pulmonary cryptococcosis

A few sporadic cases of a pneumonic form of cryptococcosis have been reported. Benign pulmonary cryptococcosis may be found only at autopsy by finding a small encapsulated healed granuloma.

Pulmonary cryptococcosis

The histological reaction in the lung may be a marked cellular reaction indistinguishable from those of other granulomatous diseases. Where the cellular reaction is slight the cryptococci are numerous and there is a mucoid quality of the lesion suggesting a myxomatous condition.

The 'primary' pulmonary lesion, a solitary cryptococcal granuloma, may be seen as a nodule 1–7 cm in diameter near the pleural surface. It is sharply circumscribed but does not have a thick or calcified wall.

Cryptococcus lesions present histologically as pure histiocytic granulomas with large mono- or multinucleate histiocytes supported by a delicate vascular stroma containing spherical or oval bodies without visible internal structure but a clear halo 3–5 μm in thickness separating the fungus wall from the cytoplasm of the histiocyte. In actively growing lesions budding cells are found. In progressive infection there are miliary granulomas, small abscesses or large solid or mucoid lesions varying from granulomatous to pure mucoid reaction involving one or more lobes of the lung.

Central nervous system

Gross changes are usually minimal. The arachnoid space contains adherent mucoid exudate. A coronal section shows numerous gelatinous or myxoid foci predominantly located in the grey matter. Tumour-like granulomas may be found. Microscopically the lesions contain great numbers of thickly capsulated cryptococci and the almost total absence of any inflammatory reaction.

Cryptococci reach the brain through the blood stream or from the sub-arachnoid space along the perivascular lymph channels or the cortical branches of the pial vessels. The cryptococci multiply in these channels within endothelial and multinucleate cells and also extracellularly and form a gelatinous nodule around the little vessels. These nodules usually multiply and increase in size and coalesce, causing pressure atrophy of the surrounding and intervening brain tissue.

CLINICAL FEATURES

Cryptococcosis most frequently presents as meningitis.

Pulmonary cryptococcosis

Pulmonary cryptococcosis may be accompanied by cough and scanty mucoid or blood-tinged sputum. Low grade fever, malaise and weight loss may occur in some cases. There may be signs of bronchitis, consolidation râles or pleural effusion, all closely resembling pulmonary tuberculosis.

X-ray appearances are not diagnostic. Spherical or oval tumour-like masses may resemble a neoplasm. There is no hilar gland enlargement or caseation or calcification. These changes may be obscured by surrounding cavitation (Donnan 1959).

Central nervous system cryptococcosis

This closely resembles tuberculous meningitis. The onset is usually insidious and the course chronic. The first symptom is intermittent headaches increasing in frequency and severity without any previous pulmonary symptoms associated with the development of granulomatous lesions of the meninges. More rarely there is a sudden severe onset indicating the presence of rapidly spreading cerebral lesions. The signs are those of chronic meningitis with low grade fever and neck stiffness. There are general signs of meningitis with changes in personality and local signs which may include papilloedema, amblyopia, oculomotor paresis and optic atrophy. The duration varies from a few months to 15 or 20 years. The cerebrospinal fluid shows a raised protein content with reduced glucose and chlorides. There is a lymphocytosis as in tuberculous meningitis. The cryptococci may be present in abundance but may only be demonstrated by washing the deposit in saline and mounting in China ink to stain the particles. In periods of remission cryptococci may be present in the C.S.F. although cultures may remain negative.

Dermal cryptococcosis

This is usually associated with a systemic infection, but cases have been diagnosed without previous pulmonary infection. The skin lesions may be papules, pustules or subcutaneous abscesses which ulcerate. The ulcers may be solitary or multiple and may resemble carcinoma. Similar lesions may occur on the oral or nasal mucosa.

Involvement of the bones

Bone involvement occurs in 10% of reported cases. They are associated with pain and swelling of many months' duration and are osteolytic, often spreading to the skin. The cryptococci can be demonstrated only with difficulty in the glairy pus and biopsy material can be mistaken for Hodgkin's disease unless special stains are used to demonstrate the cryptococci.

Visceral spread

Infection may spread to any part of the body, where the granulomatous lesions bear a resemblance to carcinoma. Cryptococcal granuloma of the breast is a rare phenomenon in man. Endocarditis is a rare manifestation.

DIAGNOSIS

Isolation of the organism may be made on direct examination of fresh material stained with China ink and by culture on glucose agar or Sabouraud's medium at $37°C$ to distinguish it from non-pathogenic cryptococci. Pathogenic cryptococci can be tested by intracerebral, intraperitoneal or intravenous inoculation of a mouse.

TREATMENT

Amphotericin B has proved useful in some cases but not all patients recover and relapse is common. Treatment is with a total dose of over 2 grammes and using this dosage only 8 of 22 patients died and only 1 of 10 under 50 years of age (Furcolow 1963).

Seriously ill patients responded to intrathecal and intracisternal injection within a few weeks.

5-Fluorocytosine had a good effect on 3 patients who had all failed to respond to an initial course of amphotericin B (McGill *et al.* 1969). The dose used was 2–4 grammes daily for 7–40 weeks.

It is difficult to assess cure since cryptococci may be absent from the cerebrospinal fluid for long periods only to reappear at a later date.

Candidiasis

Synonyms

Moniliasis; thrush; *Candida* perionychia; *Candida* endocarditis; bronchomycosis; mycotic vulvovaginitis.

Definition

Candidiasis is an acute, chronic, superficial or disseminated mycosis caused by species of *Candida*.

AETIOLOGY

Candida albicans is the most frequent cause of any of the clinical types of the mycosis but *C. parapsilosis*, *C. guilliermondi*, *C. tropicalis* and *C. stellatoidea* may also be responsible.

Candida albicans grows on cornmeal as spherical macroconidia (chlamydospores), 8–12 μm in diameter, and characteristic spherical clusters of blastospores or yeasts. Fermentative reactions are useful in differentiating species of *Candida*.

TRANSMISSION

C. albicans is a frequent commensal in the alimentary canal and transmission is by direct inoculation on to the mucous surfaces of the mouth, vulva or intestines, from which systemic spread may occur rarely.

IMMUNOLOGY

Man is normally resistant to infection with *Candida*, which usually causes a local infection of the skin, nail, and mucous membranes, but where the immune response has been altered by the presence of lymphoma or leukaemia or suppressed by immunosuppressive drugs or steroids and where long courses of broad-spectrum antibiotic treatment have been given, systemic candidiasis occurs. *Candida* endocarditis is well recognized following cardiac catheterization and open-heart surgery. The antibody response depends on the depth and site of infection and is of little use in diagnosis.

Skin tests

Both immediate (Type 1) and delayed (Type 2) hypersensitivity reactions are found in 10–15% of the adult population and are probably related to early repeated contacts (Holti 1966). They are of little diagnostic significance.

Serum antibodies

These develop quite rapidly in children after birth, presumably because of commensal contact (Brody & Finch 1960).

Precipitin tests

These have been made especially with Mannan A and positive results have been obtained in healthy subjects as well as 72% of asthmatics with pulmonary infiltrations and eosinophilia (Pepys *et al.* 1967). Quantitative precipitin and agar gel diffusion tests using group specific cell wall polysaccharides have been used to separate Groups A and B of *C. albicans*.

Fluorescent antibody tests

These have been used to differentiate *Candida* species.

EPIDEMIOLOGY

Reservoir of infection

C. albicans causes candidiasis in monkeys, fowls, turkeys and pigeons and occurs as a commensal in the cat, dog, goat, hedgehog, rabbit and rat. It can survive in contaminated soil but is not known to have a natural habitat in inanimate nature.

The other species of *Candida* have a common saprophytic existence apart from the animal host.

Human infection

Oral candidiasis (thrush) is seen in the newborn and aged and in debilitated patients and is also associated with long continued therapy with broad-spectrum antibiotics. Intertriginous candidiasis and paronychia are seen in diabetic and obese persons and in those whose hands are frequently immersed in water for prolonged periods.

Vulvovaginitis occurs during pregnancy. Bronchopulmonary candidiasis is secondary to another disease, and endocarditis is associated with indwelling cardiac catheters.

Systemic candidiasis is an 'opportunist' infection associated with prolonged use of immunosuppressive drugs or the presence of lymphoma and leukaemic disorders.

Oral and intestinal candidiasis have been found as terminal infections in sprue in the tropics and at one time were thought to be the cause of the disease.

PATHOLOGY

In autopsy material *Candida* may be seen in superficial ulcers of the mucous membrane of the alimentary tract developing in the last stages of a terminal illness.

Systemic candidiasis

In this form the lesions caused are widespread, occurring as micro-abscesses in lungs, heart, kidney, brain and other organs. In candidiasis endocarditis the exuberant vegetations contain large numbers of hyphae and blastospores. Meningitis and intracranial candidiasis have been described (Miale 1943). The histological picture of terminal candidiasis is that of focal suppuration with the formation of small abscesses in which neutrophils abound.

Granulomatous form

Chronic granulomatous lesions occur in the mouth, skin and nails, causing leukoplakia-like lesions with ulceration and deforming scars. It starts in infancy or early childhood and is associated with debilitating conditions and nutritional deficiencies. It lasts until early adult life when death occurs from intercurrent disease.

Pulmonary candidiasis

This is a frequent terminal infection in pulmonary tuberculosis as an extension from the mouth and has not been recognized as a primary disease. Complete casts of the bronchial tree have been recorded in pulmonary candidiasis.

Alimentary candidiasis

Alimentary infection occurs as a local or general invasion of the alimentary mucosa followed by a *Candida* septicaemia as a terminal event in diabetics and others suffering from chronic cachexial conditions. Alimentary candidiasis provoked by antibiotic therapy may lead to systemic infection of various organs and sometimes embolism and infarction. The pathogenicity of these fungi in the deeper tissues is not great and if the alimentary infection is treated with nystatin spontaneous cure will occur (Mackinnon & Artagaveytia-Allende 1956).

CLINICAL FEATURES

Oral candidiasis (oral thrush)

The tongue, soft palate, buccal mucosa and other oral surfaces are characteristically covered with discrete or confluent patches of a cream-white to grey pseudomembrane composed of hyphae and yeasts of *C. albicans*, which may be deep and extensive enough to interfere with swallowing or breathing. Oral lesions may be associated with hypertrophy of the papillae of the tongue (black hairy tongue), and *C. albicans* grows freely in this environment although it is not the cause. When oral candidiasis extends to the angles of the mouth it may be a fortuitous invasion of the lesions of *perlèche*.

Cutaneous candidiasis

This is of particular importance in warm climates where the humid state of the skin especially in the intertriginous areas greatly conduces to the disease.

These cutaneous lesions generally resolve spontaneously with the removal to a cool climate or with the onset of the cool season, but recur with return to warm humid conditions. The forms of cutaneous candidiasis are intertriginous, generalized, paronychia, onychia, perianal and anogenital *perlèche*.

The intertriginous form occurs in the inguinal, genital, crural, gluteal, perianal, inframammary, axillary and interdigital clefts of the hands and feet.

The genitocrural infection is manifested at first by little papules or vesicles 1–2 mm in diameter, isolated or in groups. The papule is slightly raised, of a dull red colour with a scaly surface and surrounded by a narrow inflammatory zone. These initial lesions increase in size and coalesce to form large raised plaques and as these increase in size the central part becomes less scaly, is erythematous or violaceous in hue and still shows the crusts of dried vesicles and some excoriations. The marginal zone is active and covered with a thick layer of whitish sodden epithelium in which vesicles are common and ends abruptly in a prominent raised border surrounded by a zone of inflammation. Satellite lesions are common and in consequence the border often presents as a festooned outline. Although the appearance may be slightly modified by the chafing of opposed surfaces the general character is very typical of candidiasis, being unlike the picture of tinea cruris.

The interdigital type presents the same basic character and on the foot may be mistaken for tinea pedis.

The generalized form is found chiefly in infants associated with oral candidiasis or infection of the napkin area. It spreads to the main flexures and eventually may involve the entire skin in an erythemato-squamous vesicular and pustular eruption.

Among United States personnel in Japan, intertriginous candidiasis occurred more or less severely every summer owing to unsuitable uniform, although the local civilian population were free (Higdon 1956).

Paronychia (perionychia), onychia

This occurs in persons exposed occupationally to water, such as housewives and fruit packers. There is swelling, redness and pain at the base of the paronychium containing very little pus covered with an intact skin showing little scaling. The nail is brownish and sometimes shows striation.

Vulvovaginal candidiasis

Vulvovaginal infection consists of eczematoid lesions with slight erythema or with severe pustules, excoriations or even ulcers covered with a grey membrane composed of hyphae and yeasts of *C. albicans*.

Bronchocandidiasis

This is described as a chronic bronchitis characterized by cough, varying amounts of sputum, medium and coarse râles at the lung bases and X-ray appearances of peribronchial thickening or hazy linear fibrosis. It is difficult to evaluate *C. albicans* as the cause of this syndrome since it may be present in any chronic condition of the respiratory tract.

Pulmonary candidiasis

Pulmonary symptoms are characterized by low grade fever, cough with mucoid and sometimes blood-stained sputum, pleurisy and effusion. There may be patchy bronchopneumonia. Since *C. albicans* can be isolated from the sputum in almost any chronic bronchopulmonary disease, in most cases it can be disregarded as a causal agent.

DIAGNOSIS

Diagnosis is made by demonstration of the fungus. Direct examination of sputum, pus or scrapings is made in a drop of sodium hydroxide warmed gently and examined for the egg-shaped budding cells and hyphae of *Candida*. The yeast is Gram-positive in stained films. Culture is made on Sabouraud's modified agar with chloramphenicol and incubated at 30°C or room temperature.

TREATMENT

Nystatin is specific in the treatment of all forms of candidiasis. It can be administered orally in the treatment of deep forms of the infection or it can be given in conjunction with broad-spectrum antibiotics to counteract their effect.

Amphotericin B intravenously has also been used successfully in the treatment of severe forms of the infection.

Cutaneous candidiasis

A nystatin lotion or powder gives immediate relief and eventual cure in many cases. Nystatin lotion is prepared by suspending the antibiotic powder in 60 ml of a basic lotion of talc 6 grammes, zinc oxide 5 grammes, glycerine 6 ml, bentonite magna 12 ml and water to 60 ml, to give a concentration of 35 000 units of nystatin/ml. The lotion is applied thrice daily. It does not keep and should therefore be dispensed in small quantities and stored in the cold.

Sporotrichosis

Definition

Sporotrichosis is a chronic, subcutaneous, lymphatic mycosis which may remain localized for months but may become generalized involving bones, joints and other organs. Lesions may be granulomatous or may suppurate, ulcerate and drain.

AETIOLOGY

Sporotrichosis is caused by *Sporothrix schenckii*, also known as *S. beurmanni* and *Rhinocladium beurmanni*. *S. schenckii* is dimorphic. In tissues the yeast form appears as spherical budding cells which may reach a diameter of 10 μm or as cigar-shaped budding cells 1 × 3–10 μm. This form grows well on a high glucose medium at 37°C. In culture at room temperature (24°C) *S. schenckii* forms branching septate hyphae not exceeding 1–2 μm in diameter. Conidiophores bearing elliptical conidia 2–3 × 3–6 μm arise from the hyphae. At room temperature *S. schenckii* forms a moist colony with a wrinkled surface and newly isolated strains produce pigment, at first yellow, later becoming black.

Intraperitoneal inoculation into a male mouse causes orchitis within a week to 10 days.

TRANSMISSION

The infection is transmitted by direct inoculation into the skin or a pre-existing abrasion or cut, from an infected source.

IMMUNOLOGY

Skin sensitivity tests are of use in diagnosis of the common lymphatic variety and in the rare cases of disseminated disease complement fixation and agglutination tests may be of great value.

Skin test (sporotrichin test)

The specific capsular polysaccharide antigen of *S. schenckii* is most specific and a positive sporotrichin test is almost invariably a sign of infection with *S. schenckii*, either past or present, since positive reactions have been obtained in 6–24% of subjects in an endemic area compared with none of 55 in a non-endemic area (Wernsdorfer *et al.* 1963), and in 11–30% of healthy individuals the highest percentage being found in nursery gardeners (Schneidau *et al.* 1964). The sporotrichin skin test is especially useful in the differential diagnosis from cutaneous leishmaniasis.

Complement fixation and agglutination tests

The most specific antigens used in serological tests are prepared from yeast phase cells by autoclaving or grinding acetone treated cells. The precipitin test appeared most useful (Norden 1951) and has been used in the diagnosis of the disseminated disease.

Fluorescent antibody tests

These tests have proved useful in detecting *S. schenckii* in exudate from lesions and homologous *S. schenckii* fluorescein-labelled sera stained both yeast and mycelial phase cultures of 8 different strains and showed no cross-reactivity with heterologous species (Kaplan & Ivens 1960).

EPIDEMIOLOGY

Source of infection

S. schenckii is a saprophyte which grows in man's environment and causes disease after accidental inoculation. It occurs naturally on berberis, rose, poinsettia, sphagnum and salt marsh grass. It can grow on wood and causes 'bud rot' when inoculated into carnations. Infection is often related to minor punctures by rose or barbary thorns, splinters or even metal particles such as steel wool, which may have been contaminated by soil containing spores.

Animal reservoir

Sporotrichosis has been found in wild rats, dogs and horses and mules, in which it resembles epizootic lymphangitis, but the disease in lower animals does not constitute a reservoir of infection for man.

Occupation

Sporotrichosis occurs sporadically or in groups in many parts of the world and is particularly common in florists, horticulturists, and people who handle raw packing material. From 1941 to 1944 an epidemic of sporotrichosis involving 2825 cases occurred in 2 mine shafts on the Witwatersrand where conditions of temperature (26·1–28°C) and humidity (96–100%) were very favourable for the growth of *S. schenckii* on the sound but unpreserved mine timbers. The infection was associated with contamination of cutaneous abrasions common in the mine workers. In Uruguay Mackinnon (1948) found that the infection rate was related to seasonal conditions of temperature and rainfall comparable to the temperature and humidity recorded in the Transvaal mines.

PATHOLOGY

The infection starts as a primary lesion at the site of inoculation and extends along a superficial lymphatic vessel causing an ascending mycotic lymphangitis with development of secondary gummas along the course of the thickened vessel. These secondary gummas tend to break down and ulcerate but except from secondary bacterial infection there is generally an absence of secondary lymphadenopathy.

Histopathology

The basic histopathological lesion is a combination of a pyogenic and granulomatous reaction also seen in blastomycosis, coccidioidomycosis and chromoblastomycosis. Typically there are small nodules composed of histiocytes, some of which are epithelioid cells; in these small granulomas there is a central focus of neutrophils bordered by a rim of epithelioid cells. Langhans giant cells may be present. *S. schenckii* is difficult to demonstrate in skin lesions and those which are characterized by pseudo-epitheliomatous hyperplasia and a mixed pyogenic epithelioid cell granulomatous reaction in which neither fungi nor bacteria can be demonstrated should be suspected as sporotrichosis. In secondary and disseminated lesions the histological picture is the same.

The asteroid body consists of a central rounded or oval yeast-like somewhat basophilic structure 3–5 μm in diameter which is bordered by a radiate eosinophilic substance which forms a covering of approximately 10 μm thickness. The central yeast-like body reacts positively to fungus stains. Although asteroid bodies can be found in coccidioidomycosis and aspergillosis, if they are present in skin and secondary lesions they are presumptive evidence of sporotrichosis. *S. schenckii* may be more easily identified in lesions of susceptible animals and in visceral sporotrichosis by special fungus stains as oval, cigar-shaped or rounded bodies.

CLINICAL FEATURES

Localized lymphatic sporotrichosis

The commonest type of sporotrichosis follows the subcutaneous implantation of spores in a penetrating wound caused by a thorn or splinter. The incubation period is from 7 to 14 days but can be as long as 1 month, and very rarely 6 months.

The primary lesion is a cutaneous gumma, firm, elastic, painless and movable on the deeper tissues, measuring on the average about 1·5–2·0 cm. As the gumma enlarges its centre becomes necrotic and breaks down, becoming fluctuant, and the surface becomes dull red or violaceous in colour. A shallow ulcer with a little sinus may form at the apex and become crusted, but eventually the sinus enlarges, the summit breaks down and the contents of mucoid pus in which the fungus can be found by culture are discharged, leaving an indolent ulcer with overhanging violaceous walls and a non-sloughing granulomatous base from which a serosanguineous fluid exudes and forms a crust.

Lymphatic spread occurs along the lymphatics draining the area, which become indurated and cord-like; the lymph glands become swollen and eventually suppurate. The lesions may persist for years.

Disseminated sporotrichosis

Rarely there may be haematogenous spread from the primary lesion or from suppurating lymph glands. In some cases it seems possible that the infection could have had a respiratory origin.

Dissemination to the skin is manifested by numerous widespread skin lesions starting as nodules and developing into papules, pustules, ulcers and confluent areas of folliculitis. Occasionally there are lesions of the oral and nasal mucosa.

Dissemination to the visceral organs is rarely observed and is accompanied by fever. Pyleonephritis, orchitis, mastitis and pulmonary disease may all occur. Lesions of the bones are characterized by periostitis and osteomyelitis and of the joints by synovitis and destruction of cartilage.

DIAGNOSIS

The diagnosis by culture is made by sowing material from a gumma on glucose agar slants or Sabouraud's medium and incubating at room temperature (24°C). After 5–12 days the young colonies of characteristic appearance will be found.

The localized form must be distinguished from anthrax, tularaemia, cutaneous leishmaniasis, syphilis and tuberculosis; the disseminated form from other mycoses.

TREATMENT

Potassium iodide is specific in this disease, commencing with 600 mg to 1·0 gramme by mouth in 100 ml of milk or water thrice daily after food and increasing by about 300 mg/dose/day until a maximum of 3·0–3·3 grammes/dose is reached. This dosage should be maintained until clinical cure is achieved and continued in a diminishing scale for a further 4 weeks to insure against recurrence. In simple cases the treatment takes about 6–8 weeks but the response will depend on the state of the disease and the individual patient.

Histoplasmosis

Synonyms

Darling's disease; reticulo-endothelial cytomycosis.

Definition

Histoplasmosis is an intracellular mycosis of the reticulo-endothelial system involving lymphatic tissues, lung, liver, spleen, adrenals, kidneys, skin, central nervous system and other organs of the body. It may be asymptomatic, a benign acute or chronic pulmonary disease or widely disseminated and fatal.

AETIOLOGY

Histoplasma capsulatum is a dimorphic fungus which grows within cells of the reticulo-endothelial system (rarely in giant and polymorphonuclear cells) in the form of budding oval cells 2–3 × 3–4 μm. It grows readily on Sabouraud's medium at room temperature as a white to brown mould which reproduces by spherical smooth to spiny conidia 2–5 μm in diameter and by spherical macro-conidia 8–14 μm in diameter. A yeast-like phase can be obtained by sowing the mycelial form on to blood agar and by incubating at 37°C. The mycelial phase only occurs below 34°C.

Histoplasma duboisii (Van Breuseghem 1952) can be distinguished from the classical form by the large size of the intracellular form which measures 3–4 times the size of *H. capsulatum*. The oval cells are 6–12 μm in length and are readily cultivated at 26°C on glucose agar and maltose agar producing white cottony colonies.

Isolation from soil

Histoplasma may be isolated from soil by culture or by exposing animals in cages in suspected caves or by the intraperitoneal injection of soil into mice.

TRANSMISSION

Infection from human and animal cases does not occur.

Histoplasma capsulatum is found in soil and man is usually infected by inhalation of spores from the soil.

IMMUNOLOGY

Most primary infections with *Histoplasma* are asymptomatic or benign with rapid recovery and a lasting immunity to reinfection. Immunity is both cellular and humoral. Cellular immunity develops along with delayed hypersensitivity and humoral immunity is shown by the presence of serum antibodies. When delayed hypersensitivity is marked 'benign pulmonary histoplasmosis' results.

Where the immune process breaks down or fails to develop, widely dissemina-ted lesions result. Histoplasmosis is a common 'opportunist' infection.

Histoplasmin is a standardized preparation of a filtered culture autolysate of the mycelial form of *H. capsulatum* grown for several weeks in a chemically defined synthetic liquid medium at room temperature. The usual dilution is 1/1000. Both immediate (Type 1) and delayed (Type 4) reactions occur. 0·1 ml is injected intradermally and the reaction read at 12, 48 and 72 hours. The minimum positive reaction is an area of induration 5 mm in diameter. The skin test with histoplasmin is capable of producing serum antibodies, and cross-reactions with North American blastomycosis are very strong. Serial skin tests which show a change from negative to positive during an illness may be diagnostic but a positive skin test merely means past infection. Serological tests in regular diagnostic use are the intradermal, complement fixation and precipitin tests.

Intradermal test

The first test to become positive is the intradermal reaction to histoplasmin, which becomes positive within 2–20 days.

Complement fixation test

The antigens used are prepared in different ways either from the mycelial (histoplasmin) or yeast form. Tests should be performed with both types of antigen because some sera react with histoplasmin or with yeast cell antigen. Complement fixing antibodies are found in moderately severe and severe cases, about the end of the acute stage during the first 1–3 months. The antibody titre rises sharply and falls as steeply, although a low titre may persist for a time and is proportional to the degree of infection; antibodies may never appear, may appear only transiently or may persist for months. Transient cross-reactions occur with tuberculosis. A complement fixing titre of 1 in 8 with either histoplasmin or yeast phase antigen is generally considered as presumptive evidence of histoplasmosis, although not necessarily an active or present infection (Schubert & Wiggins 1963).

Precipitin test

Precipitin tests in agar gel using concentrated histoplasmin have been reported (Heiner 1958). Both specific (H) and non-specific (M) bands occur. M bands may be induced by histoplasmin skin testing but in the absence of a recent skin test the M band may be an early indication of disease (Kaufman 1966).

Latex agglutination test (Hill & Campbell 1962)

A commercial antigen has been used to coat latex particles and a titre of 1 in 32 or greater is significant and there were few false positives. The antibodies appear earlier but do not persist so long as complement fixing antibodies.

Fluorescent antibody methods have been used to differentiate between *H. capsulatum* and *H. duboisii* and fluorescent antibody inhibition tests have proved to be simple and effective in detecting yeast antibody and in differentiating from other serologically related mycotic infections (Kaufman & Kaplan 1963).

Fluorescent antibody tests on sera in combination with agar gel precipitation tests allow early recognition of the true positives among *H. capsulatum* reactive sera.

The serological response of *H. duboisii* is relatively weak in African histoplasmosis. The histoplasmin skin test may be negative even in proved cases.

EPIDEMIOLOGY AND GEOGRAPHICAL DISTRIBUTION

Histoplasmosis has been reported from 30 countries of the world and occurs in both temperate and tropical zones. It is chiefly a disease of the New World, particularly the United States. Sporadic cases and small groups of infection have been identified in the Old World—Australia, Austria, Belgium, Bulgaria, Great Britain, France, Germany, Holland, Spain, Turkey, India, Indonesia, Philippines, East Africa, South Africa and Portugal.

Reservoirs of infection

Soil. Histoplasma has been isolated from the soil of chicken houses, caves, hollow trees and barnyard soil. Growth of the fungus is most frequently associated with the decayed or composted manure of chickens, birds or bats.

Animals. In the United States *H. capsulatum* has been found to cause natural infection in the dog, cat, brown rat, mouse, spotted skunk and opossum. Chickens cannot maintain the infection, although they may harbour it for a few weeks. 14 species of bats have been found naturally infected in the Americas (Ajello *et al.* 1967). In Africa natural infection has been found in the baboon (Walker & Spooner 1960).

Endemicity

All age-groups are affected, with a maximum incidence in the second decade. Males are affected more than females.

Histoplasmosis is endemic in an enormous area in the Mississippi–Missouri–Ohio River valleys in a relatively mild and usually subclinical form. Histoplasmin skin testing has shown significant reactor rates in areas where histoplasmosis had not been expected. Histoplasmosis has a predominantly rural or village distribution and its occurrence is related to exposure to soils enriched by the faecal material of chickens, other birds and bats. Important urban sources of exposure have been shown by the isolation of *Histoplasma* from soil collected under trees used by starlings as roosting areas in cities.

Epidemics

Small epidemics of the benign pulmonary form of the disease occur in groups of persons infected through cleaning of chicken coops, pigeon lofts or disused silos. Others have been infected on visits to cellars or bat infested caves (cave disease). Outbreaks of histoplasmosis or cave disease have been reported in Venezuela, the Transvaal (Murray *et al.* 1957), Rhodesia (Dean 1957) and Tanganyika (Ajello *et al.* 1959), where the benign pulmonary form has attacked speleological expeditions.

PATHOLOGY

A primary lesion, histoplasmoma ('coin lesion'), occurs at the site of infection and is followed in the majority of cases by healing without any signs, causing a subclinical infection. Healing may occur with calcification, which may appear in later life on X-ray examination. If the infection is heavy the development of delayed hypersensitivity is accompanied by pulmonary signs (benign pulmonary histoplasmosis) or more rarely disseminated disease with lesions spread throughout the reticulo-endothelial system of the body.

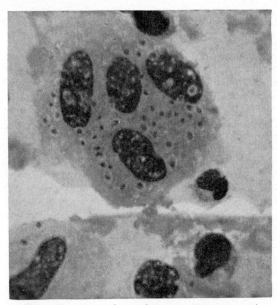

Fig. 201.—*Histoplasma capsulatum* from a smear preparation from a cutaneous lesion. (*Dr Alvarez Crespo, Guyaquil*)

The characteristic and diagnostic feature is the appearance of histoplasma cells. These are histiocytes containing the yeast form of the organism which appears as a small spheroid body measuring 1–5 μm in diameter averaging approximately 3 μm. In H. & E. sections it appears to have a rigid wall from which the protoplasm has been retracted by the fixative, giving the appearance of an unstained capsule (Fig. 201). Under low magnification the appearances closely resemble *Leishmania* and more superficially *Toxoplasma*, but they can be differentiated by PAS stain. They also have to be differentiated from other PAS-positive fungi: *Coccidioides immitis, Cryptococcus neoformans,* and *Blastomyces dermatitidis.* The characteristic cellular reaction is an epithelioid granuloma with or without Langhans giant cells.

The solitary pulmonary nodule or histoplasmoma of primary histoplasmosis is situated just beneath the pleura and there is fibrous thickening on the pleural surface and the centre is caseous. Healing occurs by fibrosis and later calcification. All the demonstrable histoplasma cells are usually within the caseous part.

In fatal disseminated histoplasmosis the reticulo-endothelial system is invaded by *Histoplasma,* and histoplasma cells multiply in great numbers eroding and replacing the normal tissue. Lesions may occur in any part of the body but chiefly the liver, spleen, adrenals, lymph glands, mucous membrane of the mouth, gastro-intestinal tract and bone marrow. Caseous necrosis develops, especially in the adrenals, but abscesses may occur anywhere in the body including the brain. Oropharyngeal lesions are not uncommon.

CLINICAL FEATURES

The disease occurs in an asymptomatic subclinical form, a benign pulmonary form which undergoes spontaneous cure and an uncommon grave disseminated form with a high mortality rate.

Pulmonary histoplasmosis

Benign pulmonary histoplasmosis resembles primary tuberculosis, is the form most commonly associated with 'epidemic' histoplasmosis, and develops as a result of delayed hypersensitivity. The incubation period is 9–14 days and in the acute stage the symptoms are those of a moderately severe pneumonitis with lassitude, headache, fever, pains in the limbs and joints, backache, coryza and non-productive cough. There may be high fever with rigors and a persistent dyspnoea. There may be patchy dullness suggesting virus pneumonia, and X-ray of the lungs shows widespread miliary nodules or localized groups of pea-sized nodules and a general increase in the bronchovascular shadows and enlarged hilar glands.

This acute stage lasts 1–3 weeks and is usually followed by complete recovery. All cases develop specific cutaneous hypersensitivity to histoplasmin in 4–8 weeks after the onset of symptoms, which persists, and complement fixing antibodies appear in the blood. Other forms of pulmonary histoplasmosis are a chronic infection with the development of fibrotic disease resembling phthisis, a mediastinal form resembling lymphosis and a diffuse interstitial form resembling miliary tuberculosis.

X-ray appearances show widespread diffuse 'fluffy' miliary mottling in the early stages, associated with hilar adenopathy, and many large areas of consolidation, either widely disseminated miliary lesions or a lung lesion with mediastinal glandular enlargement. Healing occurs with either miliary calcification or a calcified focus with calcified hilar glands.

Disseminated histoplasmosis

This is a rare form and appears only sporadically. Symptoms include continued fever, sweating, malaise, weakness and loss of weight. A syndrome may result, closely resembling kala-azar, with fever, leucopenia and anaemia often of a severe form with involvement of the blood-forming organs and haemorrhage. When the adrenals are involved symptoms of Addison's disease result. In infants the blood picture resembles that of 'aleukaemic leukaemia'.

Mucous membrane lesions are common and ulcerative lesions of the tongue, mouth and oropharynx may be the presenting signs of the infection.

Skin lesions may occur, sometimes papular and sometimes ulcerative.

DIAGNOSIS

The diagnosis of the benign pulmonary form can be made by serial histoplasmin skin tests, which show a conversion from negative to positive during illness. Complement fixing antibodies appear about the end of the acute stage and in some cases *Histoplasma* can be isolated from the urine.

In the disseminated form examination of sputum, urine, excised lymph glands, ulcer base, bone marrow or peripheral blood may show *Histoplasma*. Smears may be made and stained with Giemsa or Wright's stain. The fungus appears intracellularly within the macrophages or lying as an oval cell $2-3 \times 3-4$ μm with a large vacuole and a cup-shaped mass of red-stained protoplasm at the large end of the cell. The fungus may be isolated by culture on Emmons's modification of Sabouraud's medium (1% neopeptone, 2% glucose, 2% agar, pH $6\cdot5-7$); cultures should be incubated at or below $34°$C.

Animal inoculation

Material may be mixed with penicillin and streptomycin and inoculated intraperitoneally into a mouse which should be killed $2-4$ weeks after inoculation and cultures made from the liver and spleen.

TREATMENT

Amphotericin B is the drug of choice in treatment. It should be started in a low daily dosage of $0\cdot25$ mg/kg body weight increasing to a maximum daily dose of 1 mg/kg body weight. Total dosage need not be more than $2\cdot0$ grammes. When the adrenals are involved supporting treatment with cortisone is necessary. In histoplasmosis caused by *H. capsulatum* a favourable response has been observed in some patients but relapses are frequent. In 29 cases of active histoplasmosis treated with amphotericin B the total dosage varied between 600 mg and $2\cdot1$ grammes and lasted from $3-6$ weeks to $3-5$ months.

Of patients with severe histoplasmosis treated with amphotericin B 12 showed apparent recovery, 33 some improvement, 9 relapsed, 7 showed no change and 2 died (Furcolow 1963).

African histoplasmosis responds quickly and well to amphotericin B (Cockshott & Lucas 1964a).

Test of cure should include negative cultures and smears for *Histoplasma*, falling titres of complement fixing antibodies and arrest or remission of lesions.

AFRICAN HISTOPLASMOSIS, LARGE-CELL
HISTOPLASMOSIS (*Histoplasma duboisii*)

Histoplasma duboisii is found in tropical Africa, especially West Africa. It differs morphologically (page 700) and immunologically (page 701) from *H. capsulatum*.

The localized form of the disease may present as a solitary skin nodule or an isolated bone lesion but at the other extreme the disseminated form may involve the skin, subcutaneous tissues, lymph glands, bones, joints, lungs and abdominal viscera. A detailed classical description is given by Cockshott and Lucas (1964a).

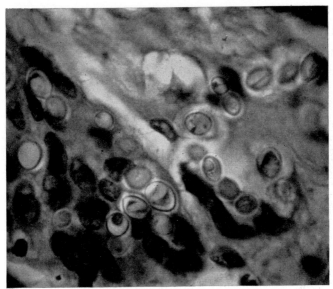

Fig. 202.—*Histoplasma duboisii* in a skin section × 2000 approx. (*W. St C. Symmers*)

Skin and subcutaneous tissues

The skin granulomas may present as nodular, ulcerative, circinate, eczematous or psoriasiform lesions with a well defined hyperpigmented halo surrounding them. In the disseminated form in the tissues these skin lesions are multiple and are continuously evolving.

Subcutaneous abscesses may arise from lesions in the underlying bone or independently. The abscesses present as firm, tender, hot swellings and the pus contains numerous yeast cells of *H. duboisii*.

Bone

The occurrence of bone lesions is an important feature. The bone lesions may be isolated or widespread in disseminated cases and are often asymptomatic and discovered only in the course of a radiological survey of the skeleton. When the abscess ruptures through the skin the resultant mass of granulation tissue may simulate a malignant neoplasm. Spontaneous fractures occasionally occur (Cockshott & Lucas 1964b).

Other lesions

Neurological complications may arise from compression of the spinal cord by lesions in the vertebrae. Lymphadenopathy is usually confined to the area of a local lesion, but is generalized in the disseminated form. Abdominal visceral lesions may be found in the liver, spleen, bladder and large bowel. The manifestations have included abdominal pain with jaundice (Cole *et al.* 1965). Systemic reaction with fever and rigors is often present in patients who have the disseminated form of the disease. Lungs are involved only rarely but cases have been recorded (Clark & Greenwood 1968) and miliary lesions have been found in the lungs in the disseminated disease.

Phycomycosis (Mucormycosis)

Definition

A group of mycoses caused by fungi belonging to the class Phycomyces.

AETIOLOGY

The phycomycoses include infection caused by species of *Absidia, Mucor, Rhizopus, Mortierella, Basiodobolus, Entomophthora* and *Hyphomyces destruens,* The commonest phycomycosis in the tropics is caused by *Basiodobolus* species. *Basiodobolus ranarum, B. meristosporus* and *B. haptosporus* (Dreschler 1956). Rhino-entomophthoromycosis (Clark 1968) is caused by *Entomophthora coronata.*

Most of the pathogenic phycomyces grow rapidly on neo-peptone agar and other media at 26–37°C.

SUBCUTANEOUS PHYCOMYCOSIS (*Basiodobolus* spp.)

The fungi which cause subcutaneous phycomycosis in man are numerous in the environment on the dung of herbivorous animals and decaying vegetation and fruit. *Basiodobolus ranarum* is present as a saprophyte in the intestinal canal of beetles, frogs, toads, and lizards.

Epidemiology

Subcutaneous phycomycosis has been described from Indonesia (Lie-Kan-Joe *et al.* 1956), Uganda (Jelliffe *et al.* 1961) and Nigeria. Males are attacked more frequently than females and it is predominantly a disease of childhood and adolescence.

Pathology

Basiodobolus species cause a granuloma with a chronic inflammatory reaction in the centre of which are found large degenerated poorly stained hyphae. Necrotizing eosinophilic debris surrounds the hyphae and the cellular reaction contains many eosinophils, neutrophils, fibroblasts and thick walled capillaries. Foreign body giant cells are common.

Clinical features

The infection begins as one spot of hard woody subcutaneous infiltration which spreads rapidly to involve extensive areas over the neck, arms and upper chest. The process involves subcutaneous tissue and muscle fascia. The infection usually heals spontaneously but deeper structures may be involved and visceral involvement has been reported (Ridley & Wise 1965). Sometimes some cheesy material may be squeezed out of the indurated areas.

Treatment

Potassium iodide has been used successfully in treatment. The drug should be administered commencing with 600 mg to 1·0 gramme by mouth in 100 ml of milk or water thrice daily and increasing by about 300 mg/dose until a maximum of 3·0–3·3 grammes/dose is reached.

Rhino-entomophthoromycosis (Clark 1968)

Aetiology

Entomophthora coronata occurs in soil and decaying vegetation and causes disease in insects.

Epidemiology

The disease occurs in adult males in the third and fourth decade of life living in lowland regions of tropical rain forest in Nigeria, India, Columbia and Brazil. Transmission is probably by the inhalation of spores.

Clinical features

The primary site of infection is in the nasal mucosa, and cases present with a nasal obstruction which eventually involves the paranasal sinuses, pharynx and subcutaneous muscles of the face in a chronic granulomatous swelling.

Protothecosis

A condition resembling 'mossy foot' has been described in a rice farmer in Sierra Leone from which *Prototheca sebgwema* was cultured both from the skin and a femoral gland (Davies & Wilkinson 1967).

Cercosporamycosis

Cercosporamycosis caused by *Cercospora apii* has been described in a single case from Indonesia (Lie-Kan-Joe *et al.* 1957). The patient was a boy with extensive indurated verrucous and ulcerated cutaneous and subcutaneous lesions of the face which later extended to other areas. The patient later died. The disease had started in early infancy. The fungus was easily seen in biopsy specimens as brown septate hyphae and was also cultured. Experimental infection of tomato plants gave rise to 'leaf spot disease'.

Rhinosporidiosis

Definition

A disease due to a yeast-like organism, *Rhinosporidium seeberi*, which infects the mucous membrane of the nose, producing nasal polypi and tumours on the cheek, conjunctiva, lacrimal sac, uvula, ear, glans penis and skin.

AETIOLOGY

Rhinosporidium seeberi is a spherical or oval non-motile organism which occurs in polypoid growths, usually lying between the connective-tissue cells. The earliest stages are about 6 μm in diameter, with a chitinous envelope, vacuolated cytoplasm and vesicular nucleus containing a karyosome (Fig. 203). When fully grown, the cyst, or sporangium, may measure 0·25–3 mm in diameter. In early stages the nucleus commences to divide by binary fission, until thousands are produced, of which the majority become daughter spores, though a considerable proportion remain unchanged. The fully formed sporangium (Fig. 203) finally bursts and discharges the spores, which are enclosed in chitinous envelopes; they

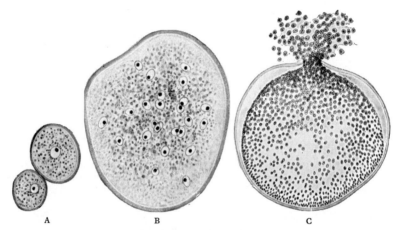

A   B   C

Fig. 203.—*Rhinosporidium seeberi*. (*After Ashworth. By permission of the Royal Society of Edinburgh*)

A, Trophic stages. × 400. B, Section of a stage with 64 nuclei, 24 of which lie in this section. × 400. C, Sporangium from which spores are being discharged, accompanied by mucoid substance, through a wide orifice. The peripheral spores lie in a fairly firm mucoid matrix. Stretching of the envelope, due to growth of the sporangium, has not only reduced its thickness, but has almost caused the disappearance of the thickened annulus round the pore. × 180.

then spread into the connective tissues via the lymph channels, and on reaching suitable spots the trophic stage at once begins and the cycle is repeated.

Attempts at cultivation proved partially successful in Ashworth's hands, and multiplication of the spores took place, but slowly, on Sabouraud's medium.

EPIDEMIOLOGY AND GEOGRAPHICAL DISTRIBUTION

Rhinosporidiosis is found most often in India and Ceylon, but has also been reported from Indonesia, Malaysia, Philippines, Iran, South Africa, Italy, England, Scotland, the southern United States, Mexico, Cuba, Argentina, Brazil, Paraguay and Ecuador. It is most often seen in children and young adults and in men more than women, but can also occur at any age. There are no racial differences in susceptibility. Infection is most often seen in labourers who are frequently exposed to water in streams and pools, and cases have occurred in groups of men diving to recover sand. This suggests that *R. seeberi* has a natural habitat in water, growing either as a saprophyte or as a parasite of fish or water insects. A closely related form, *R. equi*, has been found in the nasal cavities of horses and cattle and an organism closely resembling *R. seeberi* has been found in nasal polyps of two waterfowl in the Congo (Fain & Herin 1957).

PATHOLOGY

The most striking feature is the presence in the stroma of polyps of numerous sharply defined globular cysts varying in size from 10–200 μm in diameter. There is a chronic inflammatory reaction and occasionally micro-abscesses occur. Eosinophils are inconspicuous.

CLINICAL FEATURES

Friable, highly vascular, sessile and pedunculated polyps may appear on almost any mucosal surface, but only rarely on the skin. Extension can occur beyond the mucocutaneous border. The nose, nasopharynx and soft palate are most commonly affected, but the eye, lacrimal sac and to a less extent the larynx, penis and vagina may also be involved (Allen & Dave 1936).

Dissemination

Multiple pedunculated tumours on the nose and face, generally with secondary tumours on both feet, which ultimately became distributed over the whole body, have been described (Allen & Dave 1936). Haematogenous dissemination with rhinosporidial cells in the urine, peripheral blood and ascitic fluid has been described (Rajam 1955), and nodules on the palate and lower eyelid with visceral involvement of the lungs, liver, spleen, and skin (Agarwal *et al.* 1959).

DIAGNOSIS

The diagnosis is made by demonstrating the sporangia up to 350 μm in diameter in sections of excised tissue. Culture and animal inoculation are unsuccessful.

TREATMENT

Treatment is essentially surgical and consists in removing the polypi from the nares by a wire snare. Neostibosan was used by Allen and Dave (1936) but is not always effective.

REFERENCES

ABBOTT, P. (1956) *Trans. R. Soc. trop. Med. Hyg.*, **50**, 11.
ABERNETHY, R. S. & HEINER, D. C. (1961) *J. Lab. clin. Med.*, **57**, 604.
AGRAWAL, S., SHARMA, K. D. & SHRIVASTAN, J. B. (1959) *Archs Derm.*, **80**, 22.
ALLEN, F. R. W. K. & DAVE, M. (1936) *Indian med. Gaz.*, **71**, 276.
AJELLO, L. (1967) *Systemic Mycoses*. Ciba Foundation Symposium, p. 132. London: Churchill.
—— HOSTY, T. S. & PALMER, J. (1967) *Am. J. trop. Med. Hyg.*, **16**, 329.
—— MANSON-BAHR, P. E. C. & MOORE, J. C. (1959) *Am. J. trop. Med. Hyg.*, **9**, 623.
BAILEY, J. W., HUPPERT, M. & CHITJIAN, P. (1965) *Bact. Proc.*, **11**, 19.
BAKER, K. C. & KEMBERLING, S. R. (1960) *Archs Derm.*, **81**, 373.
BALOWS, A. (1963) *VII Int. Cong. Microbiol.*
BAXTER, M., MURRAY, I. G. & TAYLOR, J. J. (1966) *Sabouraudia*, **5**, 138.

BAYLET, J., CAMAIN, R., BEZES, H. & REY, M. (1961) *Bull. Soc. Path. éxot.*, **54**, 902.
——— ——— & SEGRETAIN, G. (1959) *Bull. Soc. Path. éxot.*, **52**, 448.
BIRKETT, D. P., WILSON, A. M. M. & JELLIFFE, D. B. (1964) *Br. med. J.*, **i**, 1669.
BOJALIL, L. F. & ZAMORA, A. (1963) *Proc. Soc. exp. Biol. Med.*, **113**, 40.
BOSWELL, W. L. (1959) *Am. J. Roentg.*, **81**, 224.
BRODY, J. I. & FINCH, S. L. (1960) *Blood*, **15**, 830.
BUCKLEY, H. R. & MURRAY, I. G. (1966) *Sabouraudia*, **5**, 78.
BUSEY, J. F. (1964) *Am. Rev. resp. Dis.*, **89**, 659.
CLERK, B. M. (1968) *Systemic Mycoses*, Ciba Foundation Symposium, pp. 179–197. London: Churchill.
——— & GREENWOOD, B. M. (1968) *J. trop. Med. Hyg.*, **71**, 4.
COCKSHOTT, W. P. & LUCAS, A. O. (1964a) *Q. Jl Med.*, **33**, 233.
——— ——— (1964b) *Br. J. Radiol.*, **37**, 653.
——— & RANKIN, A. M. (1960) *Lancet*, **ii**, 1112.
COLE, A. C., RIDLEY, D. S. & WOLFE, H. R. (1965) *J. trop. Med. Hyg.*, **68**, 92.
CONTI DIAZ, I. A., VIGNALE, R. & PENA DE PERIERA, M. E. (1966) *Revta urug. Patel. clin.*, **4**, 149.
CONVERSE, J. L. (1965) *Am. Rev. resp. Dis.*, **92**, 159.
COSTELLO, M. J., DE FEO, C. P. & LITTMAN, M. L. (1959) *Archs Derm.*, **79**, 184.
COURTOIS, G., DE LOOF, C., THYS, A. & VAN BREUSEGHEM, R. (1954) *Ann. Soc. belge Med. trop.*, **34**, 371.
DAVIES, R. R. & WILKINSON, J. L. (1967) *Ann. trop. Med. Parasit.*, **61**, 112.
DEAN, G. (1957) *Cent. Afr. J. Med.*, **3**, 79.
DE BRITO, T., RAPHAEL, A., FAVA NETTO, C. & SEMPAIO, S. DE A. P. (1961) *J. invest. Derm.*, **37**, 29.
DIAS, L. B., SEMPAIO, M. M. & SILVA, D. (1970) *Revta Inst. Med. trop. S. Paulo*, **12**, 8.
DONNAN, M. G. F. (1959) *J. Fac. Radiol.*, **10**, 17.
DRECHSLER, C. (1956) *Mycologia*, **48**, 655.
EMMONS, C. W. (1942) *Pub. Hlth Rep. Wash.*, **57**, 109.
——— (1955) *Am. J. Hyg.*, **62**, 227.
EVANS, E. E. (1950) *J. Immunol.*, **64**, 432.
FAIN, A. & HERIN, V. (1957) *Mycopath. Mycol. appl.*, **8**, 54.
FAVA NETTO, C. (1965) *Mycopathologia*, **26**, 349.
FIESE, M. J. (1962) *Coccidiomycosis*, p. 99. Springfield, Ill.: Charles C. Thomas.
FURCOLOW, M. D. (1963) *Med. Clins N. Am.*, **47**, 1119.
GORDON, M. A. & AL-DOORY, Y. (1965) *Fonsecaea J. Bact.*, **89**, 551.
——— & VEDDER, D. K. (1966) *J. Am. med. Ass.*, **197**, 961.
HEINER, D. C. (1958) *Pediatrics, Springfield*, **22**, 616.
HICKEY, B. B. (1956) *Trans. R. Soc. trop. Med. Hyg.*, **50**, 393.
HIGDON, R. S. (1956) *Archs Derm.*, **74**, 620.
HILL, G. B. & CAMPBELL, C. C. (1962) *Mycopathologia*, **18**, 169.
HOLTI, G. (1966) in *Symposium on Candida Infections* (ed. Winner, H. I. & Hueley, R.), p. 73. Edinburgh & London: Livingstone.
JELLIFFE, D. B., BURKITT, D. P., O'CONNOR, G. T. & BEAVER, P. C. (1961) *J. Pediat.*, **59**, 124.
KAPLAN, W. & CLIFFORD, M. K. (1964) *Am. Rev. resp. Dis.*, **89**, 651.
——— & IVENS, M. S. (1960) *J. invest. Derm.*, **35**, 51.
KASE, A. & MARSHALL, J. D. (1960) *Am. J. clin. Path.*, **34**, 52.
KAUFMAN, L. (1966) *Pub. Hlth Rep. Wash.*, **81**, 177.
——— & KAPLAN, W. (1963) *J. Bact.*, **85**, 986.
LEVINE, H. B. & KONG, YI-CHI-M. (1966) *J. Immunol.*, **37**, 297.
LIE-KAN-JOE, ENG, N. I. T., ROHAN, A. & VAN DER MERILEN, H. (1956) *Archs Derm.*, **74**, 378.
——— & SARTONO KERTOPATI (1957) *Archs Derm.*, **75**, 864.
LOPES, C. F., ALVARENGA, R. J., CISALPINO, E. O., MARTINELLI, B., SANTOS, P. V. & ARMAND, S. (1969) *Hospital, Rio de J.*, **75**, 1335.
——— & ARMAND, S. (1968) *Hospital, Rio de J.*, **73**, 1245.

LOPES, C. F., FURTADO, T. A., CISALPINO, F. & HERMETO, A. (1966) *Hospital, Rio de J.*, **70**, 285.
McGILL, P. E., SEQUEIRA, R., JINDANI, A., NGULI, E. T., FORRESTER, A. T. T. & FULTON, W. F. M. (1969) *E. Afr. med. J.*, **46**, 663.
MACKINNON, J. E. (1948) *Mycopathologia*, **4**, 367.
—— & ARTAGAVEYTIA-ALLENDE, R. C. (1956) *Trans. R. Soc. trop. Med. Hyg.*, **50**, 31.
MAHGOUB, E. (1969) *J. trop. Med. Hyg.*, **72**, 218.
MIALE, J. B. (1943) *Archs Path.*, **35**, 427.
MURRAY, I. G. (1966) *Trans. R. Soc. trop. Med. Hyg.*, **60**, 554.
—— & EL MOGHRABY, I. (1964) *Trans. R. Soc. trop. Med. Hyg.*, **58**, 557.
MURRAY, J. F., LURIE, H. I., KAYE, J., KOMINS, C., BOROK, R. & WAY, M. (1957) *Sth Afr. med. J.*, **31**, 245.
NORDEN, A. (1951) *Acta path. microbiol. scand.*, Suppl. 89.
PEPYS, J., FAUX, J. A., LONGBOTTOM, J. L., McCARTHY, D. S. & HARGREAVE, F. E. (1967) in *Clinical Aspects of Immunology* (ed. Gell, P. G. M. & Coombs, R. R. A.), 2nd ed., p. 108. Oxford: Blackwell Scientific.
POLLOCK, A. Q. & WARD, L. M. (1962) *Am. J. Med.*, **32**, 6.
POUNDEN, W. D. (1952) *Am. J. vet. Res.*, **13**, 121.
RAJAM, J. V. (1955) *Indian J. Surg.*, **17**, 269.
RESTREPO, M. A. (1966) *Sabouraudia*, **4**, 223.
RICHARDSON, H. B. jun., ANDERSON, J. A. & McKAY, R. M. (1967) *J. Pediat.*, **70**, 376.
RIDLEY, D. S. & WISE, M. (1965) *J. Path. Bact.*, **90**, 675.
SCARPA, C., NINI, G. & GERALDI, G. (1965) *Minerva derm.*, **40**, 413.
SCHNEIDAU, J. D., LAMAR, L. M. & HAUSTON, M. A. (1964) *J. Am. med. Ass.*, **118**, 371.
SCHUBERT, J. H. & WIGGINS, G. L. (1963) *Am. J. Hyg.*, **77**, 240.
SEELIGER, H. P. R. (1956) *J. invest. Derm.*, **26**, 81.
—— LACAZ, C. DA S., & ULSON, C. M. (1959) *VIth Int. Cong. trop. Med. Malar.*, **4**, 636.
SMITH, C. E., SAITO, M. T. & SIMONS, S. A. (1956) *J. Am. med. Ass.*, **160**, 546.
—— WHITING, E. G., BAKER, E. E., ROSENBERGER, H. G., BEARD, R. R. & SAITO, M. T. (1948) *Am. Rev. Tuberc.*, **57**, 330.
VAN BREUSEGHEM, R. (1952) *Bull. Acad. r. Méd. Belg.*, **23**, 686.
VOGEL, R. A., SELLERS, T. F. & WOODWARD, P. (1961) *J. Am. med. Ass.*, **178**, 921.
WALKER, J. & SPOONER, E. T. C. (1960) *J. Path. Bact.*, **80**, 346.
WERNSDORFER, R., PEREIRA, A. M., GONCALVES, A. P., LACAZ, C. DA S., FAVA NETTO, C. CASTRO, R. M. & DE BRITO, A. (1963) *Revta Inst. Méd. trop. S. Paulo*, **5**, 217.
WHITING, D. A. & CLOETE, G. N. P. (1968) *Sth Afr. med. J.*, **42**, 883.

SECTION IX

MISCELLANEOUS SKIN DISEASES

34. MISCELLANEOUS SKIN DISEASES

LEUCODERMA

LEUCODERMA or vitiligo is extremely common throughout the tropics, and is by no means confined to any particular race. Almost any part of the body may be affected. The atrophied, unpigmented patches of skin slowly enlarge peripherally, and may coalesce. Occasionally the whole body is affected, and a certain amount of symmetry may be observed; the hair of the affected parts may also become white (Fig. 204). The texture and glands of the skin remain normal. The aetiology of the disease is unknown.

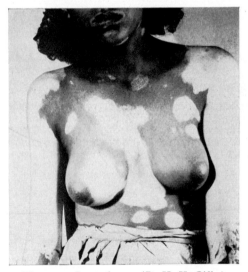

Fig. 204.—Leucoderma. (*Dr H. K. Giffen*)

Treatment

Bouchi oil injections have for many years been employed by the Calcutta School of Tropical Medicine. The oil is extracted from the seeds of *Psoralia comyfolia* and is also commonly used for external application. The dose is o·o5–o·1 ml intradermally at the margins of the patch and the number of injections varies according to its size. After 2–3 weeks the formation of pigment is noticed and gradually spreads. A second or even third series of injections may subsequently be given.

Psoralen obtained from the plant *Ammi majus* has been used; extracts of this plant were employed in Egypt as an ancient folk remedy. Psoralen has photosensitizing properties and this substance taken by mouth or applied topically will induce formation of pigment in some areas of vitiligo if administered before the skin is exposed to ultra-violet light. Pigmentary response is obtainable only in those areas in which some melanocytes remain, and the incidence of severe inflammatory reactions to the topical application of psoralens is high. Oral administration may cause nausea, diarrhoea and headache.

8-Methoxypsoralen (Meloxine) has been used by Lanceley *et al.* (1962) orally in doses varying from 2·5 mg in infants to 5–10 mg in older children, increasing gradually to a maximum of 30 mg. 2 hours after the dose the affected areas are exposed to the noonday sun for 5 minutes and exposure is increased by 1 minute each day after subsequent doses if the reaction is not excessive.

CHELOID (KELOID)

Hypertrophic scars are common enough in Europeans consequent upon surgical scars or burns, but some Europeans are predisposed to develop the extensive hyperplasia known as cheloid. Africans are especially liable, and in some tribes cheloidal scars on the back, thigh or chest constitute readily recognizable tribal marks. Similar fibrosis may occur in these people after a cautery, a healed syphilitic chancre, or even mosquito bites.

When fully developed, the growth is well defined; on a white skin it is pinkish or brownish, but it has a distinct red or chocolate tinge on a dark person. Growth takes place very slowly and, rarely, sarcomatous changes may supervene in the fibrous tissue. The growth may cause intense pain or a continuous ache when forming.

Treatment

The most efficacious method, according to Macleod, is by radium. A full strength radium plate is screened off by a silver sheet 1 mm in thickness. The exposure should last 18–30 hours. Less brilliant results are obtained by CO_2 snow, especially in early lesions. Electrolysis (3 m/amp.) is also useful, while occasionally X-rays are satisfactory.

Keloid ought not to be diagnosed as nodular leprosy, but the mistake has been made.

LYMPHOSTATIC VERRUCOSIS (MOSSY FOOT)

Definition

A chronic lymphoedema of the lower limbs with hypoplasia of the lymphatics, unconnected with filariasis.

Aetiology

The exact aetiology is uncertain but it is associated with hypoplasia of the lymphatics of the lower limbs. Repeated trauma and mild infections consequent upon the absence of shoes leads to a chronic inadequacy of lymphatic drainage and lymphoedema of the lower limbs appearing during the second decade of life.

Epidemiology and geographical distribution

Lymphostatic verrucosis is found in the tropics in widely separated areas such as Ecuador, West Africa (Manuwa 1935), Uganda (Loewenthal 1934) and

Kenya and Ethiopia (Cohen 1961). It is especially common at higher altitudes where Bancroftian filariasis is unknown and is found in both sexes during the second decade of life in people who do not normally wear shoes.

Pathology

Lymphangiography has shown that there is little spread of dye through the superficial lymph plexuses and that there is a marked hypoplasia of the main lymph channels below the knee, in contrast to filarial lymphoedema in which the lymph channels are dilated and the lymph flow retrograde (Cohen 1961). In developed cases the skin may be up to 2·5 cm thick and is firmly attached to the subcutaneous tissues and deep fascia. It is moist with lymph and not adherent to the underlying muscle. Microscopically there is a chronic fibrosis with giant cells (Loewenthal 1934).

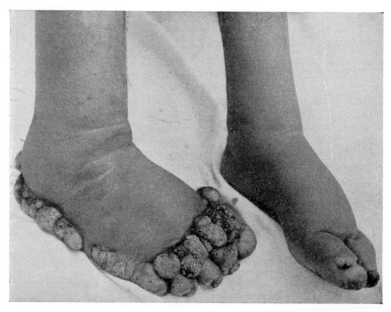

Fig. 205.—Lymphostatic verrucosis from Ecuador. (*Dr L. A. Leon, Quito*)

Clinical features

The onset is gradual during the second decade of life, with swelling of the dorsum of the foot gradually extending up to the knee. At first the swelling may be unilateral but later becomes bilateral. The oedema which pits at first later becomes firmer and does not pit as the skin thickens and 'moss' or verrucosis appears on the foot (Fig. 205) but never involves the sole. Folds of skin appear at the ankle and usually become infected. The condition is painless and slowly progressive until a gross elephantoid condition has developed.

Diagnosis

In the early stages the condition closely resembles idiopathic phlebitis and later filarial elephantiasis, from which it can be distinguished by the absence of filarial glandular enlargement and the absence of signs of filariasis elsewhere, especially in the penis, scrotum and vulva, which remain unaffected.

Treatment

The treatment is that of chronic lymphoedema. Infected areas should be cleaned up and firm bandaging applied, followed by the continual use of an elastic stocking. It is possible that the wearing of shoes from an early age may prevent the condition.

TROPICAL PHAGEDAENIC ULCER

This is defined by Loewenthal (1963) as 'an acute, specific, localized necrosis of skin and subcutaneous tissue endemic in, but not confined to, tropical regions. After the acute stage a chronic, non-specific ulcer may persist'. It is common in Africa, India ('Naga sore'), tropical America and elsewhere, and is one of the most disabling of diseases which, if neglected or badly treated, can give rise to serious effects.

Aetiology

The cause is disputed, but certain facts are established. It is commonly initiated by some trauma (which may be very slight), for instance a scratched mosquito bite (Thomson 1956), on the feet or legs, much less commonly on the arms. It is prevalent in people living on a poor diet, and rare in those eating plenty of animal protein, vitamins, fat and (possibly) calcium. It is therefore largely a disease of poverty, uncommon in the rich. It is largely a disease of agricultural communities, not of city dwellers. Fusiform bacilli and Vincent's spirochaetes (*Borrelia vincenti*) are found fairly constantly in the early stages (though not in the unbroken primary blebs); the same organisms are often present in the mouth, and in cancrum oris, and may be merely secondary invaders in tropical ulcer; they are anaerobic organisms probably growing in necrotic tissue, but only very doubtfully capable of invading normal tissue. Other organisms are also often found in the ulcers, including *Proteus*, *Pseudomonas*, staphylococci, haemolytic streptococci and diphtheroids, but these are contaminants, either accidental or resulting from treatment (Ngu 1967).

Clinically, however, the condition shows enough uniformity to suggest that some infective agent is involved, perhaps pathogenic only in suitable nutritional circumstances.

Epidemiology

Incidence is most usual at age 5–15 years (Ngu 1960). Outbreaks can occur in communities living in crowded conditions, subject to trauma and debility from disease, without medical care and on poor diets. For instance, tropical ulcer is notorious in refugees from war or famine, in prisoner-of-war camps, and in carriers such as the African Carrier Corps of the war of 1914–18, whose work was hard and whose diet consisted mainly of maize (Loewenthal 1963).

Apart from these extreme conditions, tropical ulcer is largely endemic and sporadic, and the existence of outbreaks does not necessarily imply actual transmission from one person to another, though there is some evidence that material from one sore can, if applied to another suitable person, initiate a typical sore in that person.

Clinical findings

The ulcer is usually solitary, but occasionally there may be more than one. It begins as a small bleb containing serosanguineous fluid, which breaks down within a day or so leaving a grey, foul-smelling slough. The ulcer spreads rapidly; it has a raised edge, and the surrounding tissues are oedematous. It is very painful. It spreads deeply as well as widely, with necrosis of skin and subcutaneous tissue, gangrene of muscles exposing tendons and penetrating to bone and causing periostitis, local necrosis and even osteomyelitis. Regional lymph nodes may be enlarged, though this is not very common and is probably due to secondary infection.

When seen at this stage the ulcer has often been treated by local herbalists, who may have used saliva or other possibly infectious material, to the detriment of the patient.

If the acute stage becomes modified, a more chronic phase supervenes, with firm sclerotic edges and a base of unhealthy pinkish granulation tissue. The surrounding skin is usually thin, atrophic and depigmented, and there is fibrosis in and around the ulcer. If healing takes place a scar is left which is fixed to deeper structures. This ulcer may be unable to heal without surgical intervention, and may go on to cause contractures and deformities or epithelioma.

Diagnosis

In the acute stage the ulcer has a typical appearance which is usually diagnostic, and the fusiform bacilli and Vincent's spirochaetes can usually be found, supporting (though not necessarily confirming) the diagnosis. In the chronic stage these organisms may not be present (and other types of ulcer may be contaminated with them). A biopsy is then helpful.

Tropical ulcer is to be differentiated from the late ulcerating granuloma of yaws; in this the serological tests for yaws are valuable, and also the X-ray appearances which in yaws show destructive lesions of the bone cortex, whereas in tropical ulcer they usually show periostitis with new bone formation (Ngu 1967). Malignant change may take place in bone. Tropical ulcer must also be distinguished from veld sore and buruli ulcer. Varicose ulcers may be contaminated by Vincent's spirochaetes and fusiform bacilli; the presence of varicose veins helps the diagnosis. Malignant melanoma may cause confusion but, when cleaned, the true nature of the pigmentation becomes apparent and can be confirmed by biopsy. Squamous cell carcinoma may develop, producing a rolled, everted edge, with destruction of the underlying bone demonstrable by X-ray, and possibly accompanied by enlarged lymph nodes. A biopsy should give the diagnosis.

Tetanus and gas gangrene are rare but possible complications requiring appropriate treatment. Chronic lymphoedema may result from constriction of lymphatics by scar tissue, and from chronic lymphangitis and lymphadenitis.

Treatment

Local. In the early stages the patient should if possible be admitted to hospital for complete rest to the affected limb. A swab should be taken for diagnosis and sensitivity tests on the bacteria isolated.

Old-fashioned antiseptics such as acriflavine should not be used; they damage the epithelium and therefore delay healing.

The ulcer should be dressed with gauze soaked in eusol or normal saline, changed several times in the day. If it is necrotic and dirty, however, hydrogen peroxide should be applied to it 3 times daily until bland dressings can be used. An alternative is a dressing of Sofratulle, a sterile paraffin gauze impregnated with 1% framycetin (Shrank 1965). Minor infections can be eliminated with antibiotic cream or 0·5% silver nitrate applications (changed every few hours) for a day or two. On this treatment pink, healthy granulations soon appear. Small ulcers do not need skin grafting, but large ulcers should be covered with split-skin grafts.

If the patient cannot stay in hospital, the ulcer should be treated with similar dressings, changed as before if possible, and when healthy granulations are seen, paraffin gauze dressings should be applied, under firm bandaging, and the whole limb may be encased in a plaster cast. This allows epithelium to grow (Ngu 1967). Antibiotics can be used locally, under a boot of Unna's paste. Care should be taken that antibiotics do not cause allergic sensitization.

For more chronic and intractable ulcers excision and skin grafting are needed and, in extreme cases, even amputation. For skin grafting the patient should be in hospital. It is essential to remove necrosed bone and tendon.

More heroic surgery, such as periarterial sympathectomy and ganglionectomy, has been used as an anti-ischaemic measure, but these involve surgical techniques beyond the scope of this book, as indeed does skin grafting.

If there is cancerous change it may be necessary to excise widely (or even to amputate) with block dissection of the regional lymph nodes.

General. In the acute stage penicillin, up to 1 mega unit, and strepto-mycin, up to 1 gramme, should be injected daily for 7–10 days (adult doses). If secondary invaders are resistant to these, other antibiotics are indicated. This general treatment relieves pain and diminishes smell very quickly.

If the patient cannot stay in hospital, long-acting penicillin can be given once each week, perhaps with a sulphonamide by mouth. An investigation with metronidazole has shown that in doses of 200 mg 3 times each day for 7 days it quickly reduces the size of the ulcers, compared with controls, and leads to healing in a shorter time. The ulcers were covered with dry dressings only. This treatment could be further explored (Lindner & Adeniyi-Jones 1968).

Prevention

In populations subject to tropical ulcer the general diet and standard of living probably need to be improved. In controlled communities such as plantation or mine workers (who are particularly subject to minor injuries in which tropical ulcer tends to start) this can be done centrally by the employers, and is done in many places. Otherwise, for uncontrolled populations it is a matter of raising the general standards, and altering some of the traditional patterns of diet. A generous amount of protein, especially animal protein, and fat (for instance red palm oil) would help.

The other great preventive principle is to report and seek proper treatment for abrasions of the skin of the legs and feet. Even small cuts and scratches should be attended to at once, cleaned with sterile water, perhaps treated with tincture of iodine and covered with a dressing. On mines and plantations this can be made a matter of discipline, so that every abrasion, however slight, is treated at the medical centre. This system has proved highly successful.

For the general population the hope is to induce patients to seek modern treatment rather than the often harmful treatments traditionally used by local herbalists.

VELD SORE (BARCOO ROT)

Veld sore is an ulcer, usually of the leg, often caused by *Corynebacterium diphtheriae*, and occurring in hot desert conditions. It was reported in British soldiers in the South African war and the two world wars, in the first of which

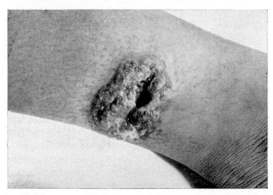

Fig. 206.—Veld sore on the leg, containing a growth of *Corynebacterium diphtheriae*. (*Dr H. K. Giffen*)

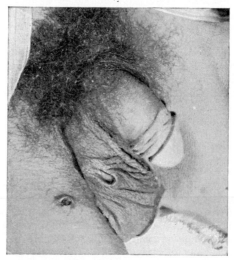

Fig. 207.—Veld sore. Primary lesions on the adductor aspect of the thigh and secondary contact sore on the scrotum. (*Captain Manton*)

Sir Philip Manson-Bahr saw it most often in men associated with horses and camels. In the war of 1939–45 veld sores and extra-faucial diphtheria were common in soldiers operating in North Africa. *C. diphtheriae mitis* was isolated from sores a number of times in this campaign (Prior 1970). Faucial diphtheria is by no means uncommon in hot countries, for instance in India and the Far East, throughout Africa and the Americas, and in 1964–65 the incidence reported in Iran was the highest in the world (Zaimiri 1970), and extra-faucial diphtheria is often reported in these areas. Transfer of *C. diphtheriae* from the throat to abraded skin is easy, and it is well known that carriers of the organism, themselves healthy, are not rare. For instance, a carrier rate of 7% was found in Ugandan children by Bezjak and Farsey (1970a). *C. diphtheriae* has also been isolated from small abrasions and even from normal skin in the hot, humid coastal areas of Colombia.

In other parts of the tropics respiratory diphtheria is rare or unknown, yet in these areas *C. diphtheriae mitis* is often found in skin lesions or ulcers, or even unabraded skin. This skin reservoir is probably important in the development of specific immunity (Bezjak & Farsey 1970b).

Clinical findings

The sore may start from diphtheritic infection of a scratch or other abrasion, commonly on the leg or arm, or even in skin irritated by the rubbing of clothing. The sores can be aggravated by sand, and serum oozing from them can be contaminated by *C. diphtheriae* from the throat of the patient himself, or of a contact (Walton 1970). The organism is less likely to be isolated from a chronic sore than from a sore in the acute stage.

The sore shows first as a vesicle full of straw-coloured fluid and is very painful. On bursting this leaves a shallow ulcer with a thin grey pellicle or chamois-leather slough, which may spread; the raw surface is exquisitely tender. After 2–3 weeks the ulcer becomes chronic. It is punched-out, circular, with undermined edges and thick margins. The base is covered with grey and scaly debris, beneath which there may be an adherent membrane. The edges become indurated and the thickened tissue has a cyanotic appearance. The ulcer may persist for many months. If healing takes place, a thin, paper-like scar is left.

The nervous system is likely to become involved, the first symptom being blurring of vision, numbness and coldness of the extremities. Paralysis of accommodation, and of the pharynx, with wrist drop and ankle drop, may follow, and there may be ataxia, loss of knee jerks, anaesthesia and incoordination. The initial local paresis is related to the site of the sore, which possibly indicates direct passage of toxin along the nerves to the central nervous system. General pareses usually appear in the second week; polyneuritis is usually delayed for 3 weeks or more.

Treatment

Once the diagnosis is established, diphtheria antitoxin (at least 20 000 units) should be injected subcutaneously or intramuscularly (with the usual precautions for serum injections), preferably near the sore or sores. These may also be dressed with antitoxin.

Penicillin is effective and should be given in full doses.

Prevention

Prevention, apart from the general adoption of active immunization in the population, involves the care of skin abrasions as in tropical phagedaenic ulcer.

REFERENCES

BEZJAK, V. & FARSEY, S. J. (1970a) *J. trop. Pediat.*, **16**, 12.
——— ——— (1970b) *Bull. W.H.O.*, **43**, 643.
COHEN, L. B. (1961) *E. Afr. med. J.*, **37**, 53.
LANCELEY, J. L., LANCELEY, E. S. & JELLIFFE, D. B. (1962) *J. Pediat.*, **60**, 572.

LINDNER, R. A. & ADENIYI-JONES, C. (1968) *Trans. R. Soc. trop. Med. Hyg.*, **62**, 712.
LOEWENTHAL, L. J. A. (1934) *Ann. trop. Med. Parasit.*, **28**, 47.
———— (1963) *Int. Rev. trop. Med.*, **2**, 267.
MANUWA, S. L. A. (1935) *Trans. R. Soc. trop. Med. Hyg.*, **29**, 289.
NGU, V. A. (1960) *W. Afr. med. J.*, **9**, 247.
———— (1967) *Br. med. J.*, **i**, 283.
PRIOR, A. (1970) *Lancet*, **i**, 1395.
SHRANK, A. B. (1965) *W. Afr. med. J.*, **14**, 215.
THOMSON, I. G. (1956) *Trans. R. Soc. trop. Med. Hyg.*, **50**, 485.
WALTON, H. C. M. (1970) *Lancet*, **i**, 1395.
ZAIMIRI, I. (1970) *Lancet*, **i**, 1112.

SECTION X

NEUROLOGICAL DISEASES

35. NEUROLOGICAL DISEASES

NEURASTHENIA IN THE TROPICS

It is probably true that expatriate residents in the tropics or in developing countries who suffer from disorders of the mind would do so if they lived in their own countries, but that certain environmental factors tend to exacerbate these conditions. Expatriate men have usually chosen to live abroad for economic reasons or for the adventure of seeing the world. To this extent they take the advantages and disadvantages willingly. This does not always hold with their wives, many of whom do not realize the conditions of life they are about to enter, and sooner or later begin to wish they were settled at home, particularly when children must be sent away to school. Domestic situations of this kind lead to friction and quarrels, not only within families, and sometimes to neurasthenia and psychosomatic ailments.

Other men and women adapt more easily, and make their lives and homes abroad, and they, like those who have been born and brought up abroad from childhood, tend to experience less mental stress than the people who long for the surroundings of their native countries.

There is evidence from laboratory studies and industrial experience that there are critical zones of temperature for unacclimatized and acclimatized man, above which most forms of work are unlikely to be performed effectively. For unacclimatized men this zone is about $18\cdot3°–21\cdot1°C$ effective temperature; for acclimatized men about $26\cdot7°C$, but there is a great range of variation (Pepler 1964). The detrimental effects of heat can be at least partly offset by an increase in effort to maintain a normal level of performance, either in physical or mental work, but this fact supports the view that heat reduces willingness to work rather than capacity for work (Pepler 1964).

These stresses, chiefly social but to some extent climatic, tend to increase the liability to those neurotic disorders which have been called tropical neurasthenia. The symptoms are widely varied, from a sense of persecution and ineffectual self-sacrifice, to withdrawal from ordinary social intercourse, or alternatively to extravagant behaviour requiring constant stimulation through convivial parties conducted on a scale which can lead to alcoholic excess and sexual promiscuity. There is probably more true alcoholism in such communities than in more settled conditions.

Psychosomatic illness is also common, needing psychological rather than physical treatment, of which perhaps the most important is a period of leave. Convinced Christians and members of other religions who sincerely observe their religious duties are probably happier than those who have no such support.

Actual disease undoubtedly influences the tendency to neurasthenia, especially perhaps the intestinal infections. The fear of amoebiasis can be very real, leading to the attention of the patient becoming riveted on his digestive system, and never happy unless reassured by repeated examinations. Attacks of non-specific diarrhoea, of bacillary dysentery and its sequelae or of sprue encourage hypochondria. Malaria is less important in this respect; most people profess to be able to recognize an attack, and to be able to deal with it. In the quinine days an attack of blackwater fever sometimes brought their confidence to an end. Hookworm infection is rarely severe enough to cause trouble in expatriate adults, but may do so in children. The fear of this and other helminthic infections, however, can add to general mental depression.

Mental illnesses in the indigenous inhabitants of tropical countries are important, and are receiving increasing study, but are beyond the scope of this book. Doctors practising in the tropics, however, are aware of the effect of the rapid change now occurring from the old, stable and emotionally satisfying tribal life, with its discipline and order, to the new, unstable and emotionally confusing urban and industrial life in which the criterion is not so much dignity and companionship as competition and antagonism. In such industrial communities there are immense opportunities for crime, violence and emotional disturbance on a large scale. 'Disease is now seen to be as much related to the social environment acting through the neuroendocrine system as it is to pathogens gaining entrance from outside' (Audy 1964). But the well known good humour and friendliness of many tropical peoples are factors of lasting value.

The indigenous peoples of tropical areas and developing countries have over the centuries evolved clear conceptions of human affairs governed in detail by supernatural agencies which are easily offended and which can be invoked for good or evil by practitioners of witchcraft. The prevention and cure of a multitude of diseases, though partly in the hands of herbalists skilled in traditional plant medicines, are partly in the hands of witch doctors who can influence these supernatural agencies to relax their hold on the victims of evil wishers. For a long time now, people brought up to accept these beliefs in supernatural agencies have been taught by Christian missionaries that their beliefs are false, but that belief in the Christian hierarchy of supernatural agencies is true. This change of attitude takes place with little difficulty in converts, but could cause confusion, and lead to mental instability in those who question the sources of belief, and this confusion may result in what we call neurasthenia.

Intellectual disturbance of this degree is therefore likely to impinge on medical practice. The intellectually advanced members of any community are by no means free from irrational fears for their own health, and psychosomatic troubles are to be expected among them. It is difficult, if not impossible, to prescribe any coherent regimen of treatment in these cases, but understanding of the underlying stresses may help.

KURU

Definition

A subacute cerebellar degenerative disease found in members of the Fore tribe in a small area of the Eastern Highlands of New Guinea.

Aetiology

Two possible factors have been suggested as the cause of kuru: one an infective agent such as a 'slow virus', similar to scrapie in sheep, and second a genetic susceptibility present in the affected persons.

Slow virus. The infective nature of kuru has been demonstrated in an experiment in which material from the brains of 8 patients who had died from kuru was inoculated into the brains of chimpanzees and produced a similar disease after a long incubation period (Gajdusek *et al.* 1966).

Genetic susceptibility. When first described kuru was found to affect children of either sex and young adult females and it was suggested (Gajdusek 1963) that a predisposition to kuru existed depending on a single gene dominant in females only and causing fatal disease in homozygotes of either sex and heterozygote females in adult life. More recent studies have suggested that genetic factors play no important role in the predisposition to kuru (Hornabrook & Moir 1970).

Transmission

Glasse (1963) first considered that the transmission of kuru was related to the practice of cannibalism formerly widespread in the Fore region but which has now died out. This concept has been studied in greater detail (Mathews *et al.* 1968) and it has been suggested that kuru is acquired from the consumption of the brains of victims and that the incubation period varies from 10 to 20 years.

Epidemiology and geographical distribution

Kuru is principally a disease of the Fore-speaking people and occurs in a strictly limited area South of Mount Michael in the Eastern Highlands of New Guinea (Zigas & Gajdusek 1957), which has not increased in size since 1957. Although confined mainly to the Fore people about 20% of kuru deaths each year have occurred in people of other linguistic groups (Hornabrook & Moir 1970), and the disease has also occurred in a few women who have entered the kuru area from outside.

Age and sex. When first described the disease affected chiefly children of either sex and young adult females. Adult males were only rarely affected but there has been a progressive rise each year since 1957 in the number of men who have died of kuru.

Incidence of the disease. When first described in 1957 kuru was common in the affected tribe when about 1% of the population were affected, reaching as high as 10% in some districts. Since 1957 there has been a rapid decline in mortality from the disease.

Relation to cannibalism. Cannibalism practised almost entirely by women and children was formerly common in the Fore area but was abandoned in the 1950s. If kuru is transmitted by cannibalism then the generation born since its cessation will not be affected and this observation has been borne out by the virtual disappearance of kuru among children in recent years.

Pathology

The cerebellum is primarily affected and there is a marked degeneration of the neurons in the cerebellar cortex, dentate nucleus, thalamus, corpus striatum, globus pallidus and focal areas in the cerebral cortex. The degenerative changes are most marked in the cerebellum particularly the vermis and its afferent and efferent connections. There is a slow progressive degeneration of the spino-cerebellar and lateral corticospinal tracts. The cytoplasm of the affected cell becomes basophilic and vacuolated and the Nissl substance is reduced. Astroglial and microglial proliferation occurs but neuronophagia is absent (Fowler & Robertson 1959). Occasionally there is some perivascular cuffing.

Clinical features

The incubation period is prolonged, up to 10–20 years after the consumption of infected material, and the onset is insidious with ataxia. As the ataxia progresses a destructive tremor appears, irregular but fine, involving head, trunk and limbs, which is exaggerated by excitement or fatigue and subsides during relaxation and sleep. Choreiform and wild athetotic movements occur when the patient tries to stand up. There are pronounced emotional changes and easily provoked inordinate laughter. Later there is a progressive dysarthria with convergent strabismus, flexed posture and Parkinsonism.

The course of the disease is invariably progressive, with death in from 3 months to 2 years, with an average of 6–9 months. In the terminal stages the patients, who are confined indoors, mute and doubly incontinent, die from starvation or intercurrent infection.

The rest of the nervous system is unaffected and the pyramidal tract is not involved. The cerebrospinal fluid is unchanged.

Treatment

There is no effective treatment.

LÂTAH

Lâtah, a word signifying 'nervous' or 'ticklish', is not uncommon in the people of Malaysia, Java and the neighbouring islands. It occurs more frequently in women, especially young women, than in men; children are seldom affected; it rarely appears before puberty and is especially common at the menopause.

A somewhat similar affliction is described among the Ainu people, usually in women, and is known as *imu*. This manifests as psychomotor attacks precipitated by some emotional shock. If a sufferer is startled, she may continue to echo everything that is said to her.

Lâtah persists for years. The main characteristics of this state are the same, though there is considerable variety in the intensity of the symptoms. The condition is incurable, shows no tendency to become worse, and does not terminate in insanity.

As the Malays say, an *orang lâtah* never becomes an *orang gila* (âmok). The subjects of 'lâtah' at first appear to differ in no way from their neighbours and relations, but on some sudden and striking impression, such as a loud sound, or in response to some overt suggestion by word or deed, they pass into a peculiar mental state in which they involuntarily utter certain sounds and execute certain movements. In other instances they will imitate words or movements, or yield to suggestions from others. During this hypnotic-like state, which may last for a few minutes or longer, the victim is at the mercy of his prompter and will unerringly follow any lead indicated. Although the manifestations of high degrees of lâtah may be followed by exhaustion, or even by swooning, as a rule nothing of the kind occurs. The infirmity is usually discovered by accident. Swettenham, for instance, used to relate that it was only necessary for anyone to attract the attention of these men by the simplest means, such as holding up a finger, or calling them by name in a pointed way, touching them, or looking them steadfastly in the face, in order to make them lose control of themselves and be willing to execute whatever was suggested by a sign. On one occasion, one of them, on being told that a roll of matting was his wife, embraced it with every sign of affection; but when the other lâtah subject, a policeman, was convinced that the same roll was his wife likewise, he too embraced it, and the two men fell to the ground struggling for the possession of the 'lady'.

Lâtah folk are favourite subjects for the practical joker, and in a few instances they very much object to being made a show of, and may become dangerous. Lâtah seems to be akin to certain emotional stresses which are common in all underdeveloped countries.

Abraham has seen the afflicted, if suddenly startled, fall down and imitate the gestures of anyone in sight; for instance, an old lady startled by a bicycle bell, will instantly imitate the pedalling of the cyclist till exhausted.

The most profound study of the pathodynamics of lâtah from the modern psychological aspects has been published by Yap (1952). From this it appears that lâtah reaction is related to 'sleep intoxication' and the so-called 'startled neurosis', and is to be differentiated from convulsive tics or 'primitive hysteria'. A special modifying of personality and the organization of fear in persons belonging to cultures of low technological level are suggested. He has drawn attention to the resemblance of lâtah to the 'jumpers' or 'shakers', a group of religious people, originating from the Methodist congregation of Wales during the time of the evangelist, Whitefield. They practised ritualistic jumping and shaking to the accompaniment of incoherent gutturals.

Unless unforeseen accidents occur, lâtah is not fatal. Gimlette and others have called attention to the medico-legal aspects of the disease. Fortunately, examples in which lâtah has been shown to play a part in crime are rare. Temperamentally, all the Malay races are very highly strung and nervous, although externally impassive, and there appears to be an hereditary tendency to the lâtah state in every Malay.

Young-dah-hte is a state closely related to lâtah. Mongolian races are predisposed. Heredity does not seem to play any part. It differs from lâtah in that the patient continuously remains in the imitative condition and is always liable to reactions.

Nat-win-de (Burma) is a religious dance with closed eyes and swinging movements. It is started by professionals and taken up by others.

There appears to be a somewhat similar affection among the Samoyedes which is known as 'ikota', and it is believed that the curious epidemics of religious ecstasy, which swept over Europe during the Middle Ages, were of similar origin.

Mirzachit is a hypnagogic intoxication seen in Siberia and has been compared to *Schlaftrunkenheit* and is practically the same as ikota.

Banga is a hysterical affliction in Congo women at puberty. The subject is convulsed and rushes about uttering wild cries.

ÂMOK

Âmok (or running âmok) is a term used somewhat loosely for a condition which, in the fully developed form, drives its victims to blind fury and to kill without reason.

Usually the 'âmok' runner (or âmoker) has a grievance upon which he allows himself to brood, and after a period of sullenness decides to kill the suspected person and at the same time to destroy as many other people as possible. He therefore arms himself, runs 'âmok', and buries his *kris*, when out to slay, in friend and foe alike, with the expectation of being killed in turn.

In other cases there may be premonitory signs in which a person mutters and has delusions. Quite suddenly he will run 'âmok' and after the attack may fall into a deep slumber and become comatose. The liability to 'âmok' attacks is greatest in the Malays, and their drugs, such as Indian hemp (*Cannabis indica*), are known to be potent predisposing causes of the attack. Van Loon found that in Java 'âmok' runners are often suffering from some infectious disease, and that the symptoms are hallucinations and confusion; such patients are impelled to flight and attack as reactions to imaginary dangers and the agony and terror caused thereby.

KORO

Koro occurs amongst the Macassars and the Buginese in Celebes, and is also well known among the Chinese as *Shook Jong*, originally described by Blonk in 1895. The term signifies 'shrivelling', and a feeling occurs at regular intervals of the penis retracting into the abdomen; if help is not forthcoming the patient dies. In his anxiety, the patient grasps the penis, and if unable to do so, obtains assistance from others. It may be days before the attack subsides, and the sufferer cannot bear to be left alone. If help be not to hand, he will actually tie the penis to his leg with string, anchor it by means of a pin or may even employ a double-bladed clasping instrument known as *li teng hok*, which is used by jewellers. This tendency is regarded as the 'Yin' principle, representing the female power, dominating the 'Yang' principle, which represents the male element. In order that a 'Yin' disease may be cured, a 'Yang' medicine must be employed. The sufferers are generally neurotics, and the anxiety arises out of sexual conflicts. Various pathological conditions, such as oedema of the lower abdomen, hernia, hydrocoele and elephantiasis of the scrotum, may evoke fear of an attack. An analogous state, characterized by diminution of the genital labia and shrinkage of the breasts, is known to occur in women.

Other neurological diseases are considered in Chapter 40.

REFERENCES

AUDY, J. R. (1964) *Public Health and Medical Sciences in the Pacific*. Hawaii: University of Hawaii Press.
FOWLER, M. & ROBERTSON, E. (1959) *Aust. Ann. Med.*, **8**, 16.
GAJDUSEK, D. C. (1963) *New Engl. J. Med.*, **268**, 475.
—— GIBBS, C. J. & ALPERS, M. (1966) *Nature, London*, **209**, 794.
GLASSE, R. M. (1963) *Cannibalism in the Kuru Region*. Papua and New Guinea Department of Public Health (Quoted by Glasse, R. M. (1967) *Trans. N.Y. Acad. Sci.*, **29**, 748).
HORNABROOK, R. W. & MOIR, D. J. (1970) *Lancet*, **ii**, 1175.
MATHEWS, J. D., GLASSE, R. M. & LINDEBAUM, S. (1968) *Lancet*, **ii**, 449.
PEPLER, R. D. (1964) in *Heat Stress and Heat Disorders* (ed. Leithead, C. S. & Lind, A. R.). London: Cassell.
YAP, P. M. (1952) *J. mental Sci.*, **98**, 515.
ZIGAS, V. & GAJDUSEK, D. C. (1957) *Med. J. Aust.*, **2**, 21.

SECTION XI

DISORDERS DUE TO THE ENVIRONMENT

36. DISORDERS DUE TO HEAT

BODY temperature fluctuates only slightly in healthy people so long as they are reasonably protected against extremes of environmental heat or cold, and consume suitable amounts of food and water. Body temperature depends upon:

1. Heat created by the metabolic processes of the body acting upon food and fluid ingested.
2. Physical activity which can quickly raise the metabolic rate, and therefore body temperature, but only moderately in health.
3. Heat absorbed by the body from the environment, which may be:
   a. Radiant heat from hot objects (e.g. in engine rooms).
   b. Convected heat from the air (e.g. in deserts).
   Conducted heat from actual contact with hot objects is rarely significant.
4. Heat lost from the body via:
   a. The lungs.
   b. The skin, partly by dissipation due to vasodilatation in the skin, which entails vasoconstriction of the splanchnic vessels, and partly (more important) through evaporation of sweat from the skin surface.

Evaporation of sweat is the main defence against heat stress, and sweat is apparently produced solely to provide water for evaporative cooling.

Sweat can be absorbed by the keratinaceous layers of the skin, which may swell and block the sweat ducts, reducing the amount of sweat and causing the condition of miliaria.

But the control of heat exchange is governed by complex physiological mechanisms, ultimately from a centre situated in the hypothalamus, which also controls water balance and vasomotor and humoral activities aimed at maintaining the temperature level. The heat-regulating centre comprises two distinct sub-centres, one for dissipation of heat (cutaneous vasodilatation and sweating) and one for heat conservation (cutaneous vasoconstriction and shivering). The mechanisms activating these centres are not precisely known (Leithead & Lind 1964).

In hot conditions the heat lost by evaporation of moisture from the lungs and from the surface of the body (as insensible perspiration or actual sweat) is greater than in cool conditions, but evaporation depends not only on external heat, but also on humidity. Skin exposed to hot dry wind remains dry because of the intense evaporation, though the actual production of sweat is very great; body temperature therefore is reduced in proportion. Skin covered from such wind remains wet because sweat is continually produced and evaporation is prevented. Skin exposed to even moderate heat in conditions of high humidity remains wet because evaporation is slow; body temperature is therefore less effectively reduced.

In all cases fluid is lost in sweat much more quickly in hot conditions than in cool, and therefore the secretion of urine is reduced unless the intake of fluid is increased. Fluid balance is therefore a primary factor in heat regulation. With fluid loss in sweat there is loss of salt, and salt depletion is another important factor in heat balance.

The hormone system is involved, and in dehydration, through excessive sweating, an anti-diuretic hormone is released from the pituitary. This hormone acts by reducing the output of urine through reabsorption of water in the renal tubules, and thus conserving body fluid. The production of aldosterone and possibly other adrenocortical substances is also increased, resulting in reduction of salt loss in sweat.

Acclimatization

There is evidence that people can become to some degree acclimatized to heat, so that body temperatures and pulse rates do not rise as high in experienced persons, whose sweating mechanism becomes more efficient (Edholm 1969), as in people unaccustomed to heat. But there is also evidence that, especially in older subjects, heavy work in the heat produces fatigue of the sweat glands during the work session, with consequent rise in body temperature and increased strain on the cardiovascular system.

HEAT STRESS AND HEAT STRAIN

Heat stress is defined as the total load of heat which must be dissipated if the body is to remain in heat balance. There are 5 components of 4 main features:

1. The metabolic rate of the subject, which varies with physical activity, body build and constitution.
2. Air temperature:
   a. Dry bulb.
   b. Wet bulb.
3. Air movement.
4. Radiant temperature (black globe reading).

Various indices based upon these factors have been devised, of which the Corrected Effective Temperature scale is perhaps the most well known. The details of these should be studied by doctors working in ships, mines and other places where heat stress is great; descriptions and references are available in the works of Leithead (1967), Leithead and Lind (1964) and Edholm (1969).

Heat strain is defined as the physiological or pathological displacement resulting from heat stress; it includes sweating, raised heart rate and body temperature, dehydration, syncope and other disorders discussed below (Leithead 1967). The important factors are sweat loss, heart rate, deep body temperature, acclimatization, age, body build, physical fitness and clothing. Increasing age (because of the cardiovascular strain) and obesity are detrimental. Some of these factors can easily be measured—the heart rate, for instance, indicates the demands imposed by work and heat load on the circulatory system (WHO 1969). A continuously rising rectal temperature can easily be measured, and is a serious danger signal. Intercurrent infectious disease adds to this risk. Sweating can be assessed clinically. A dry skin, indicating absence of sweating (except where sweat is evaporated at once in hot dry air), is easily noted and is a sign of serious heat effect in a person with a high pulse rate and rectal temperature. A sweat rate of 1 litre/hour in a desert environment may achieve thermal equilibrium even with heavy work, without rise in body temperature or cardio-vascular strain, but in a humid climate it could be accompanied by great strain if only 0·5 litre/hour evaporated and the rest was deposited on clothing, or dripped off the body.

The normal adult intake of water in food and drink, in a moderate climate, is about 2·5 litres daily; the loss of water is about 1·5 litres in urine and 1·0 litre in sweat, faeces and expired air. Similarly, the normal intake of sodium chloride is about 10 grammes, most of which is excreted in urine and a small amount in sweat. When a man is suddenly exposed to severe heat the salt content of sweat is initially high, up to 4 grammes/litre. But if severe sweating continues, maximal reabsorption of sodium and chloride from the renal tubules may be enough to maintain balance, and the salt content of the sweat may fall to as little as 1·0 gramme/litre. The speed at which this mechanism of salt conservation develops is important, and salt-depletion heat exhaustion is mostly observed in new-comers to heat.

When sweating is heavy—over 5 litres in 8 hours of work—however, the intake of salt, as well as that of water, should be increased.

HEAT DISORDERS

The pathological conditions resulting from failure to maintain heat balance are (Leithead & Lind 1964):

1. Disorders resulting from the processes of heat regulation:
   a. Circulatory instability:
      Heat syncope
   b. Water and electrolyte imbalance:
      Heat oedema
      Water-depletion heat exhaustion
      Salt-depletion heat exhaustion
      Heat cramps
   c. Skin changes:
      Prickly heat
      Anhidrotic heat exhaustion

2. Disorders resulting from failure of heat regulation:
   a. Heatstroke
   b. Heat hyperpyrexia

3. Disorders resulting from apathy, fatigue etc.:
   a. Chronic tropical fatigue
   b. Acute heat fatigue

The conditions in group 3 are discussed by Pepler (Leithead & Lind 1964) under the heading of psychological effects of heat, and may not be attributable solely to heat. They are referred to above (page 721). The various factors are shown in Fig. 208.

Heat syncope

This is a fainting attack due to collapse in vasomotor tone leading to cerebral anoxia, in the absence of water depletion or salt depletion. It is more common in hot humid conditions than in hot dry conditions.

The patient becomes pale, with slow pulse and slow, sighing breathing; consciousness is usually lost for a few minutes, but returns as the cerebral

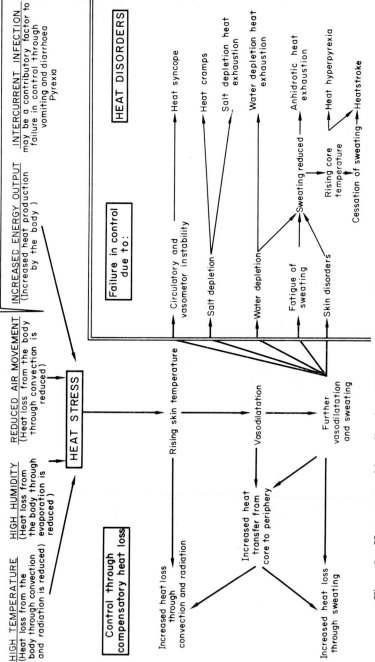

Fig. 208.—Heat stress and heat disorders. (*Wellcome Museum of Medical Science, after Leithead & Lind 1964*)

circulation is restored when the patient lies down. The patient may recover quickly, or may be shaken by the experience, and need a period of rest and quiet before complete recovery.

Other causes of loss of consciousness must be excluded; such an attack may be the prelude to more serious disorders due to heat. The patient should be taken to lie down in cool surroundings and given drinks if necessary.

Heat oedema

This affects the feet, and usually occurs within 10 days of first experience of hot climates; it disappears with acclimatization. The pathogenesis is uncertain. The swelling is usually slight, and is partially relieved by a night's rest. A short period of rest is usually enough to end the condition.

Water-depletion heat exhaustion

This is due to loss of fluid by sweating and insufficient intake of fluid to replace it; an accessory factor may be loss of fluid by vomiting or diarrhoea. The commonest factor is an inadequate supply of water to labourers or troops. It should be remembered that a man doing heavy work in severe heat (say $43°C$) can lose more than 1 litre of sweat/hour, and if working in the sun or in a boiler room, or if marching, for 8 hours a day, can lose up to 10 litres of sweat.

The patient becomes thirsty, and the secretion of urine is much reduced. The extracellular fluid is reduced, and water moves from the cells themselves into the extracellular fluid. If this process is severe, reabsorption of sodium from the renal tubules is increased, although the plasma sodium is already high, and this further induces water to move from the intracellular fluid to the extracellular fluid, including the plasma. Potassium excretion, however, continues. Eventually, in spite of these transfers of fluid, the amount of extracellular fluid becomes insufficient to maintain efficient circulation.

The thirsty patient's mouth is dry, and there is difficulty in swallowing. Fatigue and weakness follow, with a sense of foreboding, and even dulling of the mental capacity and judgement. In the late stage there may be paraesthesias, restlessness and hysteria, with giddiness and incoordination of limb movements, leading to delirium, coma and death. In extreme desert conditions death may occur in 12–48 hours.

Signs include increased pulse rate and temperature, and evidence of dehydration—the skin is inelastic, the cheeks hollow and the eyes sunken; breathing is fast, even leading to tetany, and there is cyanosis. As dehydration advances, sweating diminishes.

Diagnosis is important. Conscious patients complain of intense thirst, but irrational or comatose patients cannot do so. There is little urine and its specific gravity is high; unlike the urine in salt-depletion heat exhaustion, it contains measurable quantities of sodium chloride. The patient may be anuric.

It is obviously important to decide whether the heat exhaustion is due mainly to water depletion or to salt depletion (page 732), and the sodium content of plasma is significant in this respect. Sweat being hypotonic, more water is lost than salt, but if the patient has drunk some water without salt, more salt may have been lost than water. The distinguishing features of the two conditions are set out in Table 38 (from Leithead & Lind 1964).

Treatment of water-depletion heat exhaustion consists of rest in bed in cool surroundings, and high fluid intake, about 6–8 litres in the first 24 hours, and until the temperature is down and urinary excretion satisfactory. Heavily salted drinks are not indicated.

Unconscious patients may need intravenous fluid, and if there is a doubt whether such a patient is suffering from water depletion or salt depletion, isotonic saline should be given, 4 litres or more in the first 24 hours, and then according to progress. Otherwise the fluid of choice is 5% glucose solution. Plasma sodium should be watched if possible, and the output of urine observed. There is a risk of overloading the circulation with intravenous fluid.

Prevention of water-depletion heat exhaustion entails a plentiful supply of drinking water, or water flavoured with fruit juice, easily available for workers in the heat and for travellers, who should ensure adequate supplies for all journeys.

Table 38. Differential diagnosis of heat exhaustion

	Predominant salt depletion	Predominant water depletion
Duration of symptoms	3–5 days	Often much shorter
Thirst	Not prominent	Prominent
Fatigue	Prominent	Less prominent
Giddiness	Prominent	Less prominent
Muscle cramps	In most cases	Absent
Vomiting	In most cases	Usually absent
Thermal sweating	Probably unchanged	Diminished
Haemoconcentration	Early and marked	Slight until late
Urine chloride	Negligible amounts	Normal amounts
Urine concentration	Moderate	Pronounced
Plasma sodium	Below average	Above average
Mode of death	Oligaemic shock	High osmotic pressure; oligaemic shock; heatstroke

Salt-depletion heat exhaustion

The average daily diet of Europeans contains about 10 grammes of salt, and about as much is excreted daily, but in hot conditions sweating increases the loss of salt, even though sweat is hypotonic. This applies especially to newcomers.

The deficit of sodium is more important than the deficit in chloride. The extracellular fluid contains most of the sodium, and when sodium is lost in sweat the osmolarity of the extracellular fluid is reduced, and some of that fluid passes into the cells. Less water than usual is reabsorbed from the renal tubules, and there is therefore an increase in urine, with secondary depletion of water, and further reduction of extracellular fluid. In cases with marked symptoms plasma sodium and chloride are clearly reduced, and both are virtually absent from urine and sweat.

Plasma volume is reduced, and haemoconcentration therefore occurs, with high blood urea; this may be a factor in the tendency to nausea and vomiting.

The clinical features are fatigue, giddiness, anorexia, nausea, vomiting and muscle cramps. Fatigue is very marked—the patient is too desperately weary to give an account of his condition. Anorexia, diarrhoea and vomiting reduce the already inadequate intake of salt, establishing a vicious circle. Muscle cramps are common and very painful. Thirst is not a feature, but becomes prominent in progressive water depletion. The body temperature is usually normal, and the condition does not predispose to heatstroke.

The sodium chloride content of urine is negligible, and this, together with the other symptoms, helps in diagnosis. In the absence of laboratory facilities for estimating sodium and chloride the Fantus test on urine is simple and useful.

Fantus test for chlorides in urine (Leithead & Lind 1964). To 10 drops of clear centrifuged urine in a clean test-tube add one drop of 20% potassium chromate solution as an indicator. Then add 2·9% silver nitrate solution drop by drop, shaking well after each drop, until the colour changes from yellow to the brick red of silver chromate. This is the point at which the silver has combined with all the chloride, and is therefore available to combine with the chromate. The number of drops of the silver nitrate solution required to produce the end-point colour change is the concentration of chloride in the urine, expressed as grammes of sodium chloride/litre. If the colour change occurs with the first drop of silver nitrate it means that for practical purposes there is no chloride in the urine. The silver nitrate should be kept in a coloured bottle in the dark, and each reagent should be tested from time to time against distilled water. The normal NaCl value is 9 (3-15) g/litre of urine, and in the presence of the appropriate history and clinical features a level of 1-3 g/litre warrants a diagnosis of salt-depletion heat exhaustion.

Treatment involves rest in bed in cool conditions, and plenty of salt in the form of salted drinks. One teaspoonful of salt should be added to one pint of cool fruit drink (7 grammes/litre) and salty foods such as soup, beef tea and tomato juice should be encouraged, salt being added liberally to all appropriate food. The daily intake of salt in predisposing surroundings should be 20 grammes, and this should be weighed out each day; discipline is needed to ensure adequate intake.

For comatose patients isotonic saline may be given intravenously in doses of 2–4 litres during 12–24 hours. Pulse rates and blood pressures should be watched, and the volume, chloride content and specific gravity of the urine measured and recorded. The neck veins and lung bases must be examined for signs of overloading of the circulation, and cardiac failure.

Prevention entails the provision of salt for fluids and food, especially for people working in severe heat such as in engine rooms, and especially for people not acclimatized.

Heat cramps

These painful cramps are probably due to water intoxication or salt depletion, and occur in people who are sweating heavily and are at the same time drinking large amounts of unsalted fluids (Leithead & Lind 1964). The cramps may be mild or quite severe, with the affected muscles contracted into stony hard lumps. They usually last less than one minute, occasionally for 2 or 3, but they may recur every few minutes for several hours.

For severe cramps intravenous normal saline (0·5–1·0 litre) can be given, or even a small quantity of 5% (hypertonic) saline. This should be followed by liberal salt taken by mouth until the urine contains 2–3 grammes of chloride/litre.

Prevention entails the provision of salted drinks at the place of work; men differ in their need for extra salt.

Skin changes

Prickly heat (miliaria rubra). This common condition is due to prolonged wetting of the skin by sweat, and is found in those parts of the skin in which evaporation is poor, for instance where the skin is covered and chafed by clothing, and where there is friction. A high concentration of salt in sweat, possibly due to adrenocortical hypofunction or fatigue, may be a factor; bathing in sea water is thought to aggravate the condition (*Br. med. J.* 1964).

The essential lesion is obstruction of the sweat ducts by plugs of keratin debris, and distension of the ducts by retained sweat. There is round cell infiltration round the ducts. In skin persistently wet with sweat the epidermis tends to become oedematous and liable to infection; injury may also play a part.

The rash consists of many small red papules, going on to vesicles, on a mildly erythematous skin, chiefly in the bends of the elbows and knees, over the sternum, round the waist and in the axillae. In severe cases most of the trunk is involved, but not the palms or soles. The rash is accompanied by a prickling or tingling sensation which comes on in waves and which may be so irritating as to interfere seriously with sleep and therefore with general health. The rash may go on to pustule formation or eczema.

The best treatment is to remove the patient to a cooler climate. Otherwise the condition may be relieved by avoiding sweating, wearing light, airy, loose clothing or remaining as naked as possible, and by careful drying of the skin when wet by water or sweat.

Mildly astringent lotions, such as mercuric chloride (1 in 2000 in 95% alcohol), are useful. Another lotion (Wardle 1966) is:

Arachis oil	5%
Adeps lanae	2·2%
Lanette wax	6·7%
Salicylic acid	2·0%
Glycerin	6·7%
Tragacanth mucilage	25·0%
Water to	100·0%

Mercuric chloride or hexachlorophene can be added to this. Hexachlorophene soap, or a lotion or cream containing neomycin, helps to avoid infection.

Prickling can be relieved by a cool shower, thorough drying of the skin, and the application of calamine lotion or zinc oxide powder. Oral Phenergan relieves it.

For prevention, measures to avoid sweating are obviously desirable, and excessive use of soap (especially alkaline soap) is to be avoided. Hindson (1968) advises ascorbic acid, 15 mg/kg daily, for children subject to prickly heat.

Anhidrotic heat exhaustion. This affects people exposed for several months to heat, and is characterized by numerous discrete vesicles (miliaria profunda, mammillaria) in the skin, mainly of the trunk and proximal parts of the limbs, and by diminished or absent sweating (anhidrosis) in the area of the rash (Leithead & Lind 1964). It was described in troops in World War II, but not much since then.

The skin is relatively dry because there is obstruction to the delivery of sweat to the surface, caused by keratin plugs deep in the epidermis. The condition may evolve from prickly heat. The pathogenesis is disputed; there may be a factor of unexplained failure of the renal tubules to respond to antidiuretic hormone, and a defect in the secretion of aldosterone.

The patient is unduly fatigued, with headache and a feeling of uncomfortable warmth at first in the heat of the day, but later throughout the day but worst during exercise. The skin is dry, hot and tense (except the palms, which may sweat), and there is dizziness, nausea, tachycardia and hyperpnoea. Some patients pass more urine than usual because loss of fluid by sweating is reduced. The rectal temperature may be raised to 38·9°C.

The miliaria rash consists of discrete pale elevations like those of gooseflesh, and is present everywhere except on the palms and soles, perineum, groins and axillae.

Treatment involves cool surroundings. 10% salicylic acid in 70% alcohol may be applied to the anhidrotic area, followed after desquamation by inunction of lanolin cream.

Heatstroke and heat hyperpyrexia

In heatstroke the patient is usually unconscious, with or without convulsions, there is no sweating and the body temperature is very high. In heat hyperpyrexia the patient is conscious and may be sweating; the body temperature is not so high as in heatstroke.

The factors are heat, humidity, physical activity and lack of acclimatization. Except in industry these conditions are most common in infancy and in old age, when degenerative cardiovascular disease is a factor. In desert climates the failure of mothers to provide for their infants adequate fluid to compensate the great losses due to sweat is very important. In older people excessive food or alcohol is probably deleterious. Administration of atropine, for instance as a prelude to operation, can be dangerous by inhibiting sweating. Infections such as malaria and other fevers increase the risk of heatstroke.

The sweat mechanism may become fatigued, and anhidrotic heat exhaustion and severe water depletion (with some reduction of sweat) predispose to heatstroke, as does that rare condition in which sweat glands are defective or absent. Clothing is also a factor.

Pathology. The basic change is widespread cellular damage of vital organs, as a result of high body temperature (*Lancet* 1968).

At post mortem there may be cyanosis and ecchymoses. The meninges and brain are oedematous, with petechial haemorrhages (except in the cerebral cortex and hypothalamus). Haemorrhages are also common in serous cavities, the heart, kidneys, adrenals, liver and gastro-intestinal mucosa. The blood coagulation mechanism is affected, prothrombin and fibrinogen levels fall and platelet counts are below normal, probably as a result of liver damage. The organs are congested. The kidneys are damaged, with hyperaemia and petechial haemorrhages, and the urine is scanty and turbid, with protein and abundant casts. Intravascular clotting may lead to renal insufficiency (Haanen 1968). There may be acute renal failure. Liver damage is one of the most prominent features, with raised serum bilirubin, iron and SGOT, SGPT, lactic dehydrogenase (LDH) and creatine phosphokinase, and reduction in prothrombin and fibrinogen already mentioned. SGOT, SGPT and LDH are not raised in acute infections without heatstroke.

Polymorphonuclear leucocytosis (10 000–30 000) is usual in severe cases.

Clinical findings. The onset of heatstroke may be acute, relatively acute or insidious.

The acute onset is the most common, occurring without warning. The relatively acute onset is preceded by prodromal symptoms lasting minutes or hours. The insidious form is preceded by prodromal symptoms lasting several days, but this is not common.

The prodromal symptoms may include headache, confusion, disorientation, stupor, emotional outbursts, faintness, dizziness, anorexia, locomotor disturbances, excessive thirst and polyuria (*Lancet* 1968).

Typically, the patient is in coma, with a temperature of 40·6°C or more, and there may be involuntary movements closely resembling epilepsy, with tonic and clonic convulsions and incontinence of urine and faeces. It has often been said that the skin is hot and dry, and this may be so, but if the patient has been engaged in strenuous physical exercise in the heat, he may be sweating freely though suffering from heatstroke. This indicates that the thermo-regulatory mechanism has been overloaded, rather than that it has broken down (*Lancet* 1968).

The eyes are fixed and the pupils do not react to light; the conjunctiva is injected and the corneal reflex is lost. The face is cyanosed or blotched, and there may be petechiae on the head, neck and arms. Watery diarrhoea and vomiting (both with blood) are common and tend to a state of dehydration. Hyperpnoea is also common and may lead to tetany. The pulse is fast, and in severe cases the blood pressure is low (systolic below 90) indicating a state of shock, which is a bad sign; peripheral circulatory failure sometimes occurs. The myocardium may be damaged.

The patient may die before or during treatment, or the response to cooling may be only temporary, or may be complete. Delay of more than 4 hours in beginning active cooling, or ineffective cooling, may mean that the patient fails to respond, or if he does recover, he may have a residual disability such as paresis of a limb. Shock, jaundice, oliguria, pulmonary oedema and myo-cardial infarction are sometimes present, and there may be acute adrenal insufficiency.

In differential diagnosis the most important disease is *P. falciparum* malaria, for which appropriate treatment is urgently needed. Other fevers such as meningitis and arbovirus infections, and nervous affections such as tetanus and cerebral (pontine) haemorrhage, can lead to difficulty. It is important to examine the skull and surrounding parts for signs of injury—patients may have been aggressive, or have injured themselves during convulsions or at the onset of coma.

Treatment. The patient must be cooled efficiently and immediately, by a combination of convection and evaporation. He is placed on a slatted bed which exposes as much of his skin as possible to the air, and he is subjected to a fine spray of cold water in good air movement, by an electric fan if possible. The room should preferably be air-cooled, or made as cool as possible by other means. Alternatively the patient can be placed in a bath of water and ice, or cold water alone, and his body and limbs should be massaged vigorously to promote good circulation. However, these measures may cause vasoconstriction of the blood vessels of the skin, impeding heat loss, and the patient may struggle. It may be better to apply numerous ice-bags to the skin.

These measures can reduce body temperature to 38·9°C within 20–60 minutes, and it is extremely important to stop cooling at this temperature, otherwise it may fall to subnormal levels and shock may occur.

These facilities (ice and electric fans) should be available in hospitals where heatstroke is to be expected. If not available, the patient can be cooled by sponging in cold water, or by wrapping him in a wet sheet and fanning him. The room should not only be cool, but should be large, so that it does not become humid.

Cooling is effective, but drugs may be useful—for instance, chlorpromazine as a sedative. For shock oxygen is valuable if there is cyanosis or pulmonary oedema, and intravenous 5% dextrose in saline for water or salt depletion, or prolonged coma, though with care to avoid overloading the circulation. If the shock has a cardiac origin 1·0 mg of digoxin may be given intravenously. To avoid intra-vascular clotting Haanen (1968) advises the use of heparin; a subcutaneous dose of 7500 units every 6 hours has proved satisfactory (Weber & Blakeley 1969).

Pressor agents such as noradrenaline or metaraminol (Aramine) can be at least temporarily beneficial in hypotensive patients. These should not be given until the patient has been cooled, because they produce vasoconstriction which could interfere with heat loss.

If treatment is not given, heatstroke is fatal, and even in treated patients mortality is high (20–50%). In heat hyperpyrexia (in which the patient is conscious) treatment reduces mortality to about 5%.

Sequelae include persistent headache, difficulty in concentrating, personality changes and nerve damage of various kinds.

Prevention. Prevention of the ill-effects of heat entails, for doctors working in mines, ships and other places where the risk occurs, knowledge of the techniques for measuring the various environmental factors—heat, humidity and air movement to assess the Corrected Effective Temperature—and the factors relating to people at work or rest in those conditions. These techniques require more information than can be given here, and the reader is referred to Leithead and Lind (1964), WHO (1969) and other standard works on the physiology of people under heat stress. An essential is to have a prepared centre where effective cooling treatment can be given at once, without delay, to any patient in need.

REFERENCES

Br. med. J. (1964) Editorial, **ii**, 772.
EDHOLM, O. G. (1969) *J. R. Coll. Physns London*, **4**, 27.
HAANEN, C. (1968) *Lancet*, **ii**, 400.
HINDSON, T. C. (1968) *Lancet*, **i**, 1347.
Lancet (1968) Editorial, **ii**, 31.
LEITHEAD, C. S. (1967) *Trans. R. Soc. trop. Med. Hyg.*, **61**, 739.
—— & LIND, A. R. (1964) *Heat Stress and Heat Disorders*. London: Cassell.
WARDLE, E. N. (1966) *Br. med. J.*, **ii**, 221.
WEBER, M. B. & BLAKELY, J. A. (1969) *Lancet*, **i**, 1190.
WORLD HEALTH ORGANIZATION (1969) *Wld Hlth Org. tech. Rep. Ser.*, 412.

SECTION XII

NUTRITIONAL DISEASES

37. NUTRITIONAL DEFICIENCY SYNDROMES

Nutritional requirements in the tropics

THE caloric requirement for an adult man of 25 years for an 8-hour working day is estimated at 3200 calories/24 hours in the temperate countries. The effect of a hot climate on these requirements is not more than a 10–20% decrease at the most.

It has been estimated that some villagers consume only 2040 calories/day and are permanently hungry.

Pregnancy and breast feeding increase the caloric requirement and a baby during the first 6 months at the breast will require an extra 600 calories/day in the mother's food intake. Growing children require extra, so that pregnant women and nursing mothers, as well as growing children, are the most vulnerable to food deficiencies. This is shown by the average lower weight of children from underdeveloped countries as compared with well fed children from the temperate countries. Diets in the tropics are unbalanced as well as being deficient in calories. In the United Kingdom, of the 3200 calories daily intake, 88 grammes are protein of which 54 grammes are animal protein. In India of the 2040 calories daily intake 53 grammes are protein of which only 6 grammes are animal protein.

In addition to the calorie deficient unbalanced diet available to tropical people there is the added effect of the bacterial and parasitic infections which are so prevalent. Social and cultural customs and the breakdown of society from the impact of towns and industrial development have all played a major part in producing the nutritional deficiencies which are so common in many tropical areas.

NUTRITION AND INFECTION

The relationship between infection and nutrition is reviewed in detail by Scrimshaw *et al.* (1968). Infection may have an effect on the nutritional status, or the nutritional status may affect the resistance to infection of the individual.

Infection and nutritional status

Infection has its most serious effect in protein nutrition on the nitrogen balance. Intestinal infections may cause some decrease in absorption of nitrogen from the gastro-intestinal tract but the most important effect is from increased excretion of urinary nitrogen and diminished intake from anorexia (Scrimshaw *et al.* 1968). An outstanding feature of kwashiorkor is the frequency with which it is precipitated by an attack of acute diarrhoeal disease. The increased excretion of nitrogen and decreased intake of food associated with active tuberculosis is of considerable importance in regions where protein malnutrition is common. All virus diseases exert a detectable adverse effect on nitrogen balance, and measles of all the communicable diseases imposes an unusually severe nutritional stress. Morley (1962) believes that measles precipitates kwashiorkor in West Africa more frequently than any other infectious disease and measles is an important contributory cause of kwashiorkor in many tropical areas. Heavy *Ascaris* infection especially may divert protein from the host, since an adult worm contains a lot of protein. Any unusually heavy infection with an intestinal helminth can probably induce protein malnutrition in persons whose diet is otherwise adequate, and many observers believe that infection with helminths may precipitate kwashiorkor. The consequence of moderate and light helminthic infections is more debatable, and adequate epidemiological studies to determine their effect are not available.

Infection may have an effect on vitamin deficiencies. There is some evidence (Rodger 1957) that blindness caused by onchocerciasis is less common in areas where red palm oil, which is high in vitamin A content, is used.

Infectious diseases can precipitate clinical beri-beri in persons on a diet deficient in vitamin B_1.

Systemic infections are able to induce anaemia when folic acid is deficient and fish tapeworm may cause anaemia because of its high requirement of vitamin B_{12}.

Hookworm disease is responsible for iron deficiency anaemia, due to iron loss from blood passing through the worms' intestinal canal. Malaria often results in significant iron loss. Chronic infections of bacterial or viral origin produce an 'anaemia of infection' by interfering with iron binding capacity and red cell life span.

Heavy infections with *Giardia* or *Strongyloides* may interfere with fat absorption but unless the infection is heavy, intestinal helminths as a rule do not interfere with fat absorption.

Malarial infection is characterized by low levels of blood glucose and liver glycogen because of the requirements of the parasite.

Malnutrition and resistance to infection

When malnutrition weakens resistance to infection the effect is termed synergic; when malnutrition affects the infectious agent more than the host then it is termed antagonistic. Many observations have shown that tuberculosis is commoner in malnourished persons and that diarrhoeal diseases and upper respiratory illnesses occur more frequently and last longer than among well nourished children. There is some evidence, especially in Africa, that amoebic dysentery is more severe in persons who are on a deficient diet.

A variety of published evidence demonstrates conclusively that protein malnutrition has a profound effect on resistance to infection. Synergism is usual and antagonism is rare. From experimental studies on animals synergism is the characteristic reaction with bacteria, rickettsiae, intestinal protozoa and helminths. On the other hand antagonism is relatively common with viruses.

The results of studies support a general view that moderate to severe nutritional deficiencies increase the seriousness of infection in man.

NUTRITIONAL DEFICIENCY STATES

Certain well defined disturbances of nutrition occur most commonly in the tropics. These are:

1. Protein–calorie malnutrition: kwashiorkor and marasmus.
2. Vitamin A deficiency: xerophthalmia (see page 836).
3. Vitamin B_1 deficiency: beri-beri.

4. Vitamin B_2 deficiencies: pellagra and ariboflavinosis.
5. Nutritional neuropathies.

Certain other deficiencies are not nearly so common but can also occur: vitamin C deficiency (scurvy), vitamin D deficiency (rickets, osteomalacia) and iodine deficiency (endemic goitre).

PROTEIN-CALORIE MALNUTRITION (PCM)

The term protein–calorie malnutrition covers a number of syndromes which vary according to whether protein or calorie deficiency is the most prominent. The most typical in the advanced or severe stage are kwashiorkor and marasmus. Intermediate forms are not uncommon and mild and moderate forms almost universal among children in many tropical areas where they constitute one of the most serious health problems (Scrimshaw & Behar 1959; Trowell et al. 1954). Most indigenous children in the tropics pass through a stage of some degree of malnutrition, since comparison with European growth charts shows that the weight gain is much the same for the first 9 months but that from then on the charts show maximum retardation from the second to fourth years of age and do not catch up until after the fifth year.

KWASHIORKOR

Synonyms

Mehlnährschaden (Germany), obwosi (Uganda), diboba, m'buaki (Congo), culebulla (Mexico), bouffisure d'Annam (Indochina), depigmentation oedème syndrome, pellagroide beri-berico (Cuba).

History

Kwashiorkor is similar to Mehlnährschaden, a starch or flour dystrophy described by Czerny and Keller in Vienna in 1906. The first clinical description in the tropics was given in Kenya (Procter 1927; Gillan 1934). In Ghana Cicely Williams first gave it its distinctive name, kwashiorkor or 'deprived child', and described its pathology (Williams 1933).

Aetiology

Kwashiorkor is the result of a diet low in proteins but sufficient in calories for the needs of the child at the time of weaning and after. Kwashiorkor is a disease of artificially fed or weaned infants and is not usually found in adults. The onset of the disease may be triggered by loss of, or removal from, a parent or an attack of measles or infective diarrhoea (Figs 209, 210). Kwashiorkor has been seen in breast-fed babies who receive an excess of sugar and starches in addition to small amounts of breast milk (Davies 1955) and who are called 'sugar babies' in the West Indies (Jelliffe et al. 1954).

Pathophysiology

Practically every system of the body is affected by the upset in metabolism which follows on a general dysfunction of enzymes and many other vital functions.

Liver. A marked fatty change is always found in the acute stage. The fat appears first in the periportal area as small droplets, which coalesce to form large fat globules filling practically the whole cell. With adequate treatment the

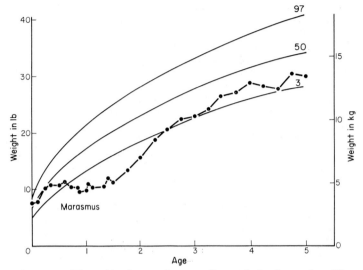

Fig. 209.—Effect of inadequate breast milk supply in the mother. The figures 97, 50 and 3 represent percentiles. (*Morley 1968*)

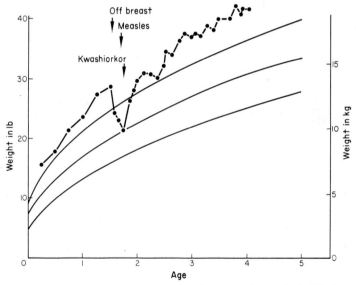

Fig. 210.—Effect of measles. Recovery after a stay in hospital. (*Morley 1968*)

fat disappears in the reverse order and the fatty changes are totally reversible. Although there is an increase in the number of lymphocytes and plasmacytes in the sinusoids during recovery the available evidence indicates that cirrhosis is not a late result (Umana & Tejada 1961).

Gastro-intestinal tract. There is a marked atrophy of the intestinal villi similar to that observed in primary malabsorption syndromes. Some degree of villous atrophy may be seen months after recovery.

Exocrine glands. There is considerable atrophy of the acini and hypofunction of the pancreas, shown by conspicuous loss of zymogen granules. Collapse of the reticulum, which has been interpreted as fibrosis, has been described (Trowell *et al.* 1954). There is marked atrophy of the parotid, submaxillary and lacrimal glands. Fatty degeneration of the cells of the convoluted tubules and hyalinization of the glomeruli in the kidneys have been observed. The atrophy and hyperkeratosis of the skin is similar histologically to the dermatosis of pellagra.

Thymus. A secondary thymic atrophy is characteristic of kwashiorkor, and there is some impairment of immune reactions of the cellular type (Watts 1969), but the ability to produce serum antibodies is not diminished.

Blood changes. Some degree of anaemia is always found in children with kwashiorkor, but this is usually mild to moderate; severe anaemia is due to other superimposed factors. Practically every type of anaemia has been described in kwashiorkor and it varies from region to region. The severe protein deficiency contributes to the deficiency of haemopoietic factors. When the anaemia is of the iron deficiency microcytic hypochromic type the response to iron therapy is inadequate until the protein deficiency has been corrected. A megaloblastic anaemia is also frequently found and is due to folic acid deficiency (Trowell & Simpkiss 1957).

Normocytic normochromic anaemia is also commonly observed and may be due simply to haemodilution. A dimorphic anaemia, in which there are microcytes and macrocytes circulating as two different red cell populations, is not rare.

Whatever type of anaemia is present this changes rapidly during treatment owing to a stimulation of the metabolism. A normocytic or macrocytic anaemia may be converted to a microcytic one when the iron stores become depleted. The serum iron and copper are low, but the total iron binding capacity is also low. Since adequate iron deposits may be demonstrated in the reticulo-endothelial cells of the liver and bone marrow this is probably due to the reduced level of protein carriers, transferrin and caeruloplasmin. The bone marrow is hypoplastic but is rapidly transformed by adequate treatment into a hyperplastic marrow with a peripheral reticulocystosis. Red cell hypoplasia responding to prednisone has occurred in some series of cases of kwashiorkor during treatment (Walt *et al.* 1962).

Water, electrolyte and circulatory changes. Oedema is a constant characteristic of kwashiorkor and is caused not only by hypoalbuminaemia but by other factors including hydrodynamic changes and altered water and electrolyte balance. The heart is small and atrophied; there is thinning and atrophy of the muscle fibres, which show degenerative changes (Smythe *et al.* 1962). There is no evidence of right heart failure but decreased cardiac output has been found, suggesting tissue anoxia as a factor in the production of oedema. There is increased fluid in all spaces (Smith 1960) and a decrease in osmolarity of the intravascular and intra- and extracellular compartments (Gordillo *et al.* 1957). Renal function tests show a decreased glomerular filtration rate, lowered renal plasma flow, decreased osmolar clearance, increased free water clearance and impaired renal response to a water load (Gordillo *et al.* 1960). Magnesium and phosphorus depletion have also been observed (Metcoff *et al.* 1960).

Carbohydrate metabolism. Hypoglycaemia is frequently observed and may be due to liver failure; it is one cause of death. Glucose absorption, and the handling of intravenous glucose and galactose loads is abnormal (Viteri *et al.*

1966). Enzymatic abnormalities of glucose oxidation have been described (Metcoff *et al.* 1960).

Lipid metabolism. An intestinal mucosal defect is responsible for marked reduction in the absorption of different fat fractions (Viteri *et al.* 1966), which persists for many weeks after clinical recovery. Intolerance to milk fats has been described (Dean & Swanne 1963). Abnormalities in lipid transport are probably related to a deficiency of protein carriers.

Protein and amino acid metabolism. There is a severe disturbance of protein metabolism in kwashiorkor. The serum proteins are invariably reduced. The serum albumin is low owing to decreased albumin synthesis (Picou & Waterlow 1962). The α_1 and α_2 globulins are relatively increased and the β globulin frequently decreased. The gammaglobulin is also high and the A/G ratio inverted. As a result of impaired hepatic circulation and altered serum proteins the flocculation and turbidity liver function tests are abnormal and there is a high bromsulphthalein retention in kwashiorkor. Nitrogen balance studies have shown that there is retention of a larger proportion of dietary protein than in normal children and there is increased recycling of body amino acids (Picou & Waterlow 1962).

Blood urea and urinary excretion of urea are low. Urinary creatinine is reduced but amino acid nitrogen, purine derivatives and protein and amino acid metabolites are high.

The serum activity of various enzymes, amylase, pseudocholinesterase and alkaline phosphatase, is constantly reduced but the levels of other enzymes associated with destruction of parenchymatous organs are raised.

Clinical features

The main clinical features of kwashiorkor are failure to grow, oedema, skin lesions, hair changes, diarrhoea and mental changes.

Failure to grow. Of all the measurements made which can foretell protein–calorie malnutrition weight records are the most valuable (Morley 1968). And the effect of removal of the child from the mother for social reasons and the results of an attack of measles are well shown in Figs 209 and 210 (page 741). In prolonged protein–calorie malnutrition the growth becomes stunted and the ossification of the bones is delayed (Fig. 213).

Oedema. Pitting oedema is of variable degree, from a slight pitting of the legs to a generalized oedema in which the child is blown up, with massive swelling of the eyelids which block the eyes (Fig. 211). The oedema may be deceptive and the child looks fat and plump so that when recovery begins and the oedema is lost he changes into a wizened little oaf with sunken cheeks, pot-belly and spindly legs.

Skin lesions. Skin lesions, which may be slight or absent, are very characteristic of kwashiorkor (Fig. 212). The skin always shows some degree of atrophy but the typical dermatosis is seen with varying frequency. It starts as large areas of erythema resembling second degree burns, which become progressively dry, hyperkeratotic and hyperpigmented. In other cases the lesions start as small areas of hyperkeratosis and hyperpigmentation which grow and become confluent. The epidermis peels off, leaving a depigmented, often tender and reddish oozing surface known as 'crazy pavement', 'alligator' or 'mosaic' skin. The dermatosis affects mainly the pressure areas and is not, like the dermatosis of pellagra, limited to areas exposed to sunlight. It first appears in the napkin areas or lower legs, spreading to the thighs, elbows and flexures of the knee and groin. Linear flexural fissures extending into the subcutaneous tissues may be seen around the pinna of the ear and back of the knee. In severer cases the dermatosis is well marked over the legs and in milder cases over the lumbar region. There is a tendency for the skin to break down, giving rise to deep necrotic ulcers of the skin, and gangrene of the limbs may ensue.

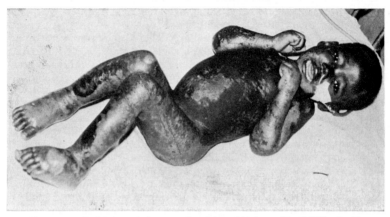

Fig. 211.—Oedema and dermatosis of kwashiorkor. (*Dr Jelliffe & Dr Barber*)

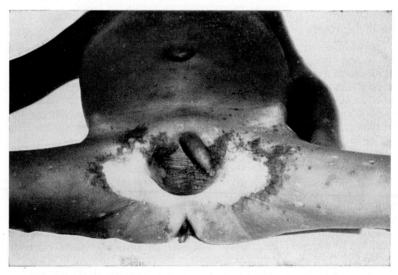

Fig. 212.—Kwashiorkor in a Fijian male child aged 2, showing characteristic dermatosis, depigmentation and hyperpigmentation. (*P. E. C. Manson-Bahr*)

Hair changes (achromotrichia). Hair changes are almost a constant feature, but are variable. The hair becomes dry and thin, loses its normal sheen and can easily be pulled out. Hair grown during periods of malnutrition loses its colour; black hair becomes brown or reddish yellow or even white, and periods of depigmented growth alternating with periods of more pigmented growth are responsible for the 'flag sign' (signale la bandera) (Pena Chavarria *et al.* 1948). Similar but less marked changes may be seen in the eyelashes and nails.

Diarrhoea. Diarrhoea is almost always present. The stools are fatty, soft, semi-fluid and offensive and the steatorrhoea may be so pronounced as to resemble the stools of malabsorption syndromes. Undigested food is frequently present. Vomiting is frequent, especially if the child is forced to eat more than the small amount of food he will accept.

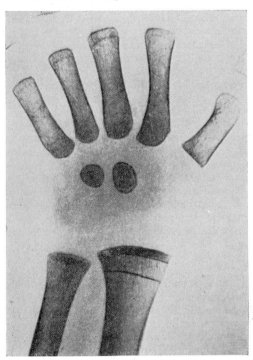

Fig. 213.—X-ray of the wrist in severe kwashiorkor, showing the transverse line across the radius and the thin bone texture of the metacarpals. (*Jones & Dean 1956*)

Mental changes. The kwashiorkor child is dull, apathetic and miserable. He rarely screams or cries but gives rise to a low and miserable whimper and resists examination. He never fights or screams. There is a great falling off in expression and comprehension (Geber & Dean 1956). A syndrome resembling encephalitis has been described with coarse tremors, postural abnormalities, exaggerated tendon reflexes and myoclonus, which are transient features and disappear with treatment (Kahn & Falcke 1956). Transient EEG abnormalities have been reported (Nelson & Dean 1959). Brain weights of children dying of malnutrition are significantly lower than in control non-malnourished children (Brown 1965). EEG and histological evidence of brain damage has been found in protein deficient animals (Platt *et al.* 1964) but there is as yet no evidence that these findings are applicable to the progress of children recovering from protein–calorie malnutrition.

Cardiovascular changes. Since the heart is small and atrophied patho-logically, some disturbance of cardiovascular function is to be expected. The heart is small on X-ray and there is a low cardiac output. The extremities are frequently cold and cyanotic and the blood pressure is low with a small pulse pressure. The low serum potassium and magnesium affect the myocardial excitability and the heart is extremely sensitive to digitalis. During recovery there may be marked cardiovascular changes with an increase in heart diameter with gallop rhythm, and cardiac failure may occur after blood or plasma infusions (Smythe *et al.* 1962).

Electrocardiogram. The ECG shows non-specific changes, dwarfing of all complexes and abnormally short or long P–R interval and flat or inverted T waves over the left praecordium. During recovery bizarre S–T and T patterns have been noted, often with asymmetrical peaking of the T wave (Smythe *et al.* 1962).

Hormonal changes. No constant hormonal changes have been found in kwashiorkor.

Associated nutritional deficiencies. Associated vitamin deficiencies are frequently seen but are not constant and vary from one region to another. Vitamin A deficiency is favoured since its absorption, transport and utilization are impaired in kwashiorkor (Arroyave *et al.* 1959), and there is a high frequency of severe ocular lesions due to vitamin A deficiency in children with protein-calorie malnutrition in areas where vitamin A deficiency is endemic (Oomen 1954). Vitamin E deficiency is often the cause of anaemia in kwashiorkor in Nigeria (Marvin & Audu 1964). Associated infections are common. Bronchitis and bronchopneumonia occur and a patient with kwashiorkor may die suddenly of respiratory failure due to bronchopneumonia without having shown fever or dyspnoea.

Treatment

Treatment is based fundamentally upon the administration of a diet high in protein of good biological value and containing sufficient calories. Dehydration and electrolyte imbalance must be corrected and since there is usually a severe potassium deficiency potassium must be given. Since the cardiac reserve is diminished intravenous fluids must be given cautiously. The basis of treatment is skim milk powder (50 grammes) which can be used with calcium caseinate (50 grammes), sugar (20 grammes) and cotton seed oil (30 grammes) in water to 1 litre. The milk powder is made to a paste with cold water, hot water is added and brought to the boil and the whole is blended and made up to 1 litre (Dean & Skinner 1957). A total intake of 3–5 grammes/kg body weight of protein of high biological value should be maintained and the total calorie intake should be about 120–140 Cal./kg body weight/day. Small frequent feeds are necessary from the start. Specific supplements are needed only if there is a particular deficiency, such as vitamin A, which should be given intramuscularly. Potassium chloride 1 gramme daily is also recommended and rapid improvement in the ECG and in the child is achieved by adding magnesium. Blood transfusion may be needed; iron should be given in the case of iron deficiency anaemia and folic acid for megaloblastic anaemia. The weight curve and consistency of the stools form important guides and weight may be lost at first because of loss of oedema. In some infants diarrhoea may develop owing to carbohydrate intolerance, especially of lactose (Dean 1956). Lactose-free material made from groundnuts 150 grammes, wheat flour 50 grammes, maize flour 100 grammes, cotton seed oil 25 grammes and sugar 75 grammes made into biscuit has been used successfully.

Recovery takes place in 2 stages (Brock *et al.* 1955). During the first stage the oedema disappears and the major biochemical and physiological alterations return to normal values. This stage lasts 2–3 weeks and weight is lost. During the second stage the child recovers the weight lost and reaches the normal weight for his height. This takes 2–3 months.

Prevention

Prevention depends on educating the mothers to avoid artificial feeding in the absence of the correct knowledge of how to handle it, and in adopting satisfactory weaning habits using local products containing available protein.

Incaparina prepared by the Institute of Central America and Panama is an economic, easily cooked mixture of ground maize, whole ground sorghum, cotton seed flour, yeast and calcium carbonate, enriched with vitamin A, and is a protein supplement widely used in Central America to prevent the development of protein-calorie malnutrition.

MARASMUS

The commonest form of marasmus in the tropics is of primary origin and is the result of starvation in small children.

Aetiology

Children are fed a diet which is adequate qualitatively but is grossly deficient in calories to fill the requirements of the rapidly growing child. Calories are the limiting factor and the child lives on its own tissues. The picture develops in infants fed on mother's milk, which is deficient in amount in malnourished mothers, or fed by prolonged breast feeding, with inadequate supplementation or inadequate artificial feeding with over-diluted cow's milk or starchy gruels. Social changes and urbanization are forcing mothers to wean early, and the adoption of artificial feeding brings infective diarrhoea, with marasmus as the result.

Pathophysiology

There is marked atrophy of all the organs and tissues. There is no anaemia unless a superimposed cause is present. Intestinal absorptive mechanisms are adequate (Thompson & Trowell 1952). The duodenal enzymes are normal in marasmus, in contrast to kwashiorkor (Vegelhyi 1948).

Serum proteins are normal and serum enzymes like amylase and pseudo-cholinesterase are not affected (Waterlow 1959).

Clinical features

Marasmus is more frequent in infants than older children because they are growing more rapidly and are more likely to be subject to the marasmus-producing type of diet. With restriction of food intake growth almost ceases and the infant utilizes the subcutaneous fat and then the muscles. The infant is hungry and cries continuously. There may be constipation because of the diminished food intake. Infectious diseases act as precipitating and aggravating factors. The child is extremely emaciated; the muscles are atrophic. The skin is thin, flaccid and wrinkled. The hair is not altered. The mind is alert, but the typical face of the marasmic child looks like that of a very little old man. Often there is added dehydration from infective vomiting and diarrhoea.

Treatment

Practically all cases will recover with adequate dietary treatment unless severe complications, such as dehydration, electrolyte imbalance or infection, are present. The diet should be complete and balanced and be adequate for the apparent biological age and higher in calories than would be required for a normal child. 200 cal./kg body weight daily are needed (Jelliffe 1970). Progress must be followed by regular weighing.

ENDEMIC GOITRE

Aetiology (Stanbury & Ramalingaswami 1964)

The immediate cause of endemic goitre is failure of the thyroid gland to obtain a supply of iodine sufficient to maintain its normal structure and function. This failure may be brought about by an environmental deficiency of iodine or by factors (goitrogens) which impose an abnormal demand on the thyroid or interfere metabolically with the utilization of iodine by the thyroid (Scrimshaw 1958).

Thiocyanate compounds and fluoride interfere with the ability of the gland to trap iodine from the circulation, and thiouracil prevents the production of protein-bound iodine. Antimony and cobalt also interfere with hormone production.

Studies in the Andes, Venezuela, Holland, India, Thailand, New Guinea and the Congo have shown results consistent with the iodine deficiency hypothesis.

Geographical distribution

Endemic goitre is widely scattered throughout the world. It is classically associated with mountain ranges such as the Andes, Himalayas, and Alps. It is however found in some parts of the tropics—Congo, India, Indonesia, New Guinea and other areas.

Clinical features and diagnosis

Large goitres are easy to recognize. Moderate degrees of thyroid enlargement are diagnosed on goitre surveys and are graded by inspection, palpation and measurement of the neck. The presence of thyroid enlargement in a significant number of persons living in an area is sufficiently strong evidence for the diagnosis of endemic goitre. In areas of endemicity serum protein bound iodine levels are low and the uptake of ^{131}I is an indication of the degree of iodine deficiency and may reveal the presence of unsuspected goitrogenic factors.

Where the iodine deficiency is severe and prolonged, hypothyroidism may occur and cretins become common. Usually the thyroids are euthyroid. There is no evidence that endemic goitre predisposes to carcinoma (Stanbury & Vickery 1962).

Treatment

Iodine should be administered as a solution of potassium iodide in water. The solution is 30 mg potassium iodide made up to 20 ml distilled water and administered as 4–6 drops daily in a glass of water. Results will be observed in 4–6 weeks.

Advanced goitres may have to be treated by surgical excision.

Prevention

The most practical method of goitre control is by the use of iodized salt. 100 μg of iodine added to the diet daily are sufficient to prevent the development of goitre. In New Guinea a single injection of 4 ml of iodized oil containing 2·15 grammes of iodine corrected iodine deficiency for 4–5 years and visible goitres regressed in size (Buttfield & Hetzel 1967).

FAMINE OEDEMA

True famine oedema is due to a deficiency of protein in adults. It occurs during war and other social disturbances and was common in Central Europe during the First World War. Famine oedema was common in Japanese prison camps during the Second World War and was confused with beri-beri. The 'hungeroedem' of the Dutch was synonymous with the wet beri-beri of the British medical staff.

The condition is due to a lack of fat and protein in the diet. The primary effect is a reduction in the serum protein below 4–5 grammes/100 ml. A generalized oedema develops without albuminuria or evidence of heart failure or peripheral neuritis. The serum albumin is greatly reduced. Recovery takes place when the patients are placed on a diet containing sufficient protein of high biological value. Many of the cases of so-called adult kwashiorkor are in reality famine oedema. Epidemic dropsy caused by the consumption of contaminated cotton seed or mustard oil can also produce a similar picture.

REFERENCES

ARROYAVE, G., VITERI, F., BEHAR, M. & SCRIMSHAW, N. S. (1959) *Am. J. clin. Nutr.*, **9**, 186.

BROCK, J. F., HANSEN, J. D. L., HOWE, E. E., PRETORIOUS, P. J., PAVEL, J. G. A. & HENDRICKSE, R. G. (1955) *Lancet*, **ii**, 355.

BROWN, R. E. (1965) *E. Afr. med. J.*, **42**, 584.

BUTTFIELD, I. & HETZEL, B. S. (1967) *Bull. Wld Hlth Org.*, **36**, 243.

DAVIES, J. N. P. (1955) *E. Afr. med. J.*, **32**, 283.

DEAN, R. F. A. (1956) *Bull. Wld Hlth Org.*, **14**, 798.

———— & SKINNER, M. (1957) *J. trop. Pediat.*, **2**, 215.

———— & SWANNE, J. (1963) *J. trop. Pediat.*, **8**, 97.

GEBER, M. & DEAN, R. F. A. (1956) *Courrier*, **6**, 3.

GILLAN, R. W. (1934) *E. Afr. med. J.*, **11**, 88.

GORDILLO, P. G., SOTO, R. A., METCOFF, J., LOPEZ, M. E. & GARCIA, A. L. (1957) *Pediatrics, Springfield*, **20**, 303.

JELLIFFE, D. B. (1970) *Diseases of Children in the Tropics and Subtropics*, 2nd ed. London: Arnold.

———— BRAS, G. & STUART, K. L. (1954) *W. Indian med. J.*, **3**, 43.

KAHN, E. & FALCKE, H. C. (1956) *J. Pediat.*, **49**, 37.

MARVIN, H. N. & AUDU, I. S. (1964) *W. Afr. med. J.*, **13**, 3.

METCOFF, J., FRENK, S., ANTONOWICZ, I., GORDILLO, P. G. & LOPEZ, M. E. (1960) *Pediatrics, Springfield*, **26**, 960.

MORLEY, D. C. (1962) *Am. J. Dis. Childh.*, **103**, 230.

———— (1968) *Trans. R. Soc. trop. Med. Hyg.*, **62**, 200.

NELSON, G. K. & DEAN, R. F. A. (1959) *Bull. Wld Hlth Org.*, **21**, 779.

OOMEN, H. A. P. C. (1954) *Br. J. Nutr.*, **8**, 307.

PENA CHAVARRIA, A., SAENZ HERRERA, C. & CORDERO, C. E. (1948) *Revta med. Costa Rica*, **6**, 170.

PICOU, D. & WATERLOW, J. C. (1962) *Clin. Sci.*, **22, 459.**

PLATT, B. S., HEARD, C. R. C. & STEWART, R. J. C. (1964) 'Experimental protein deficiency' in *Mammalian Protein Metabolism* (ed. Munro, H. N. & Allison, J. B.). New York: Academic Press.

PROCTER, R. A. W. (1927) *Kenya med. J.*, **3**, 284.

RODGER, F. C. (1957) *Trans. ophthal. Soc. U.K.*, **77**, 267.

SCRIMSHAW, N. S. (1958) *Fedn Proc. Fedn Am. Socs exp. Biol.*, **17**, 57.

—— & BEHAR, M. (1959) *Fedn Proc. Fedn Am. Socs exp. Biol.*, **18**, 82.

—— TAYLOR, C. E. & GORDON, J. E. (1968) *Wld Hlth Org., Monograph*, 57.

SMITH, R. (1960) *Clin. Sci.*, **19**, 275.

SMYTHE, P. M., SWANEPOEL, A. & CAMPBELL, J. A. H. (1962) *Br. med. J.*, **i**, 67.

STANBURY, J. B. & RAMALINGASWAMI, V. (1964) *Nutrition*, **1**, 373.

—— & VICKERY, A. L. (1962) *Indian J. Path. Bact.*, **5**, 1.

THOMSON, M. D. & TROWELL, H. C. (1952) *Lancet*, **i**, 1031.

TROWELL, H. C., DAVIS, J. N. P. & DEAN, R. F. A. (1954) *Kwashiorkor.* London: Arnold.

—— & SIMPKISS, M. J. (1957) *Lancet*, **ii**, 265.

UMANA, C. R. & TEJADA, V. C. (1961) *Revta clin. Méd. Guatemala.*

VEGELHYI, P. (1948) *Acta chir. belge*, **2**, 347.

VITERI, F. E., ARROYAVE, C. & BEHAR, M. (1966) *7th Int. Congr. Nutr.*, **12**, 170, 46.

WALT, F., TAYLOR, J. E. D., MAGILL, F. B. & NESTADT, A. (1962) *Br. med. J.*, **i**, 73.

WATERLOW, J. C. (1959) *Fedn Proc. Fedn Am. Socs exp. Biol.*, **18**, 113.

WATTS, T. (1969) *J. trop. Pediat.*, **15**, 155.

WILLIAMS, C. D. (1933) *Archs Dis. Childh.*, **8**, 423.

38. MALABSORPTION IN THE TROPICS

THE malabsorption syndrome is characterized by the passage of fatty stools (steatorrhoea), loss of weight and the occurrence of various signs and symptoms attributable to specific nutritional deficiencies.

Physiology of absorption

The intestinal villi are elevations 0·1–0·25 mm long and number 10/mm^2 of mucosal substance. They are normally finger-like and in a state of continuous movement stimulated by a hormone, villikinin. The villi are lined with columnar cells or enterocytes (Booth 1970) which have a well defined brush border composed of microvilli and a well marked structure visible on electron microscopy. They play a fundamental part in intestinal absorption by means of various enzymes formed in the cell. Glucose, xylose, iron, water-soluble vitamins and divalent cations are absorbed in the jejunum. Fat, protein and certain fat-soluble vitamins are absorbed to a certain extent proximally, but complete absorption takes place in the ileum, which also absorbs vitamin B$_{12}$ (Booth 1965). Fat is ingested as the triglyceride in emulsion in the lumen of the small intestine and the emulsifying system is dependent on a triple combination of fatty acid, bile salt and monoglyceride.

Intestinal absorption in tropical peoples

In tropical countries there is a widespread incidence of subclinical jejunal abnormalities (Baker *et al.* 1962; Banwell *et al.* 1964; Lindenbaum *et al.* 1966) and tests of intestinal absorption are abnormal when judged by Western standards. Xylose malabsorption has been found to vary between 5 and 40% in different regions (Mathan & Baker 1968). In the tropics primary malabsorption is usually caused by tropical sprue, and gluten-induced enteropathy (coeliac disease, idiopathic steatorrhoea) is uncommon.

Light infections with intestinal parasites do not usually cause malabsorption, but heavy infections with *Strongyloides* (page 272), *Giardia* (page 187) and hookworm (page 258) can all cause a well marked malabsorption syndrome. Malabsorption of many substances occurs in protein–calorie malnutrition in the advanced case (see Kwashiorkor, page 745). Other causes of malabsorption in the tropics are intestinal tuberculosis and pancreatic disease (see Pancreatic Calcification, page 10).

TROPICAL SPRUE

Synonyms

Tropical diarrhoea; aphthae tropicae; psilosis; Ceylon sore mouth.

Geographical distribution (Fig. 214)

Tropical sprue is found in South China, the Philippines, Vietnam, Japan, Indonesia, Malaysia, Ceylon, India, Burma and Mauritius, and a few cases have come from Fiji. In the Western hemisphere it occurs in the West Indies, Puerto Rico, Southern United States (formerly), Central America and Guyana; also Queensland. Isolated cases have been recorded from Iraq, Egypt, Israel,

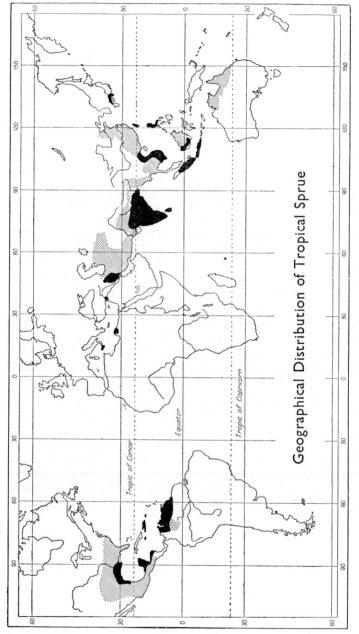

Fig. 214.—Geographical distribution of tropical sprue.

Jordan, North Africa and Russian Turkestan. It is very doubtful if sprue ever occurs in West, East or Central Africa. During the 1939–45 war a few cases were seen in British soldiers from the Mediterranean—Malta, Southern Italy and Gibraltar.

Aetiology and pathogenesis

The features of tropical sprue are caused essentially by impaired absorption of all nutrients, including fat, protein, carbohydrate, vitamins, minerals and even water. Abnormal losses of nutrients in the faeces, often associated with inadequate dietary intake, result in steatorrhoea, loss of weight and the development of anaemia, hypoproteinaemia, hypokalaemia and tetany as well as

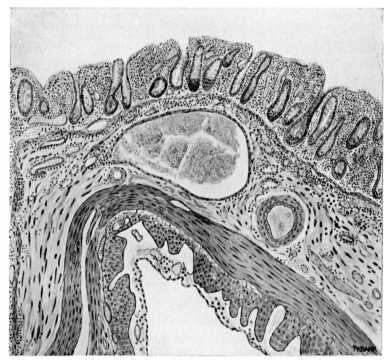

Fig. 215.—Section of the ileum in tropical sprue, showing shrinking, deformity of the villi and round cell infiltration of the mucosa. (*P. H. Manson-Bahr*)

deficiency states, including deficiency of minerals and vitamins. The pathogenesis of this malabsorption is now considered to be due to a defect in the intestinal mucosa accompanied by bacterial contamination of the small intestine (Banwell & Gorbach 1969).

Intestinal mucosal defect. The chief lesions in tropical sprue are to be found in the villi of the jejunum and ileum. Originally these changes were described at autopsy (Bahr 1915) and have been confirmed by laparotomy and by jejunal biopsy (Shiner 1956). Under a binocular microscope the villi may look like fingers or leaves, or there may be ridges or convolutions. A flat mucosa found in other malabsorptive conditions is rare in tropical sprue. Microscopically the villi are broadened and fused together. The epithelial cells (enterocytes) stain poorly and are reduced to low columnar or cuboidal types. The cells are vacuolated with a well defined brush border; goblet cells are numerous, the fundi of Lieberkuhn's follicles distended and the interstitial tissues infiltrated with round and plasma cells. The microvilli of the enterocytes are grossly abnormal on electron microscopy.

Similar changes may be found in apparently normal subjects in tropical areas who show no clinical signs of malabsorption (O'Brien & England 1966), and

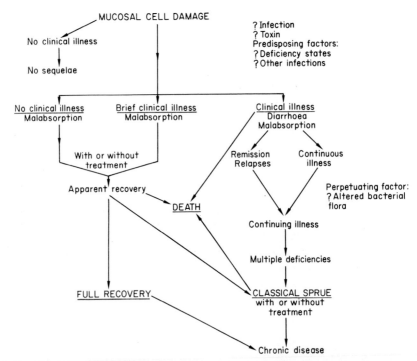

Fig. 216.—Schematic representation of the natural history of tropical sprue. (*After Baker 1967*)

may also develop in expatriates after a period of residence there (Lindenbaum *et al.* 1966). These changes may be reversed rapidly with folate and vitamin B_{12} therapy but may persist after antibiotics have restored vitamin B_{12} and fat absorption to normal. The initiating agent is still unknown, though in some instances at least it may be an infective agent, possibly a virus (Baker 1967); alternatively it could be some 'toxic' factor, possibly caused by the excessive splitting of bile acids by the contaminating bacteria.

Bacterial contamination

Certain features of sprue suggest that it is associated with an abnormal intestinal flora. The condition often follows an attack of acute gastro-enteritis and epidemic tropical sprue occurred in Burma in World War II (Leishman

1945), prisoner-of-war camps (Stefanini 1948) and villages in South India (Mathan & Baker 1968). Intestinal bacteriology and absorption are altered after gastro-enteritis and the subsequent development of sprue may be determined by the micro-organisms responsible and the susceptibility of the mucosa to injury and its ability to recover. An abnormal intestinal flora may interfere with vitamin B_{12} absorption by binding the vitamin, as occurs in the 'blind-loop' syndrome. The rapid initial improvement of vitamin B_{12} absorption in half the cases of sprue after antibiotics suggests that this is so. In the other half of the cases the lack of improvement with antibiotics could be due to insensitive bacteria (Baker & Mathan 1967).

Fat absorption is interfered with by a different mechanism. Small intestinal bacterial overgrowth interferes with fat absorption by splitting the bile acids so that the concentration of conjugated bile acids is reduced below the critical level necessary to emulsify fats. In addition ineffective ileal resorption of conjugated bile salts, due to ileal lesions, reduces the bile salt pool further in the small intestine. In this way tropical sprue resembles the 'distal' blind-loop syndrome, as is seen in Crohn's disease and ileal stricture.

Dietary factors

Dietary factors have been suggested as being causal in the tropical sprue syndrome, by its occurrence in areas where unsaturated fats predominate in the diet, and its absence from the predominantly maize-eating areas of Africa, where saturated fats are in use.

Aetiology of nutritional deficiencies. Malabsorption of fat, folic acid, vitamin B_{12} and other nutrients is responsible for much of the nutritional deficiencies, but loss of nutrients from the gut may also be important. Dehydration, hyponatraemia and hypokalaemia are extremely common in the more severe cases of sprue (Black 1946). Excessive loss of albumin via the intestine (protein-losing enteropathy) occurs in a proportion of cases (Vaish et al. 1965) and folic acid may also be lost in a similar manner (Baker & Mathan 1967).

Epidemiology

Tropical sprue occurs both endemically and epidemically. Sprue is endemic throughout India, South-east Asia and the Far East, including Northern Australia, as well as the tropical and subtropical areas of South and Central America.

Atmospheric temperature has no influence, for sprue originates at high altitudes in Ceylon and the Himalayas.

Epidemic sprue is present today in many parts of India where 13 epidemics have been recorded (Baker 1967). In World War II sprue behaved in Burma like an epidemic disease (Leishman 1945), with an incubation period and a seasonal incidence, and a large epidemic occurred in India in 1960–1 (Baker et al. 1962). The disease has disappeared in the last 20 years from many of its old haunts. In Singapore and Ceylon it has disappeared since the introduction of deep refrigeration. Both sexes are affected but children are rarely attacked. All races may be attacked and the indigenous inhabitants of the East are commonly affected.

In East India the sprue season lasts from March to September with a peak incidence in June, coinciding with the fly season. In epidemics the disease starts in a village with a few cases and then spreads through the community over the next 3–4 years with a clustering in space and time and a concentration in some houses, others being unaffected. There used to be residences in Bombay and Ceylon which were notorious for the incidence of sprue and were known as 'sprue houses'. The disease is apt to occur in one or more members of a family. In one study in India an 'incubation period' of 5–6 days was suggested (Baker 1967).

Clinical features

Symptoms. The onset is usually gradual in persons who are in an endemic area. The disease may appear for the first time some time after returning to a temperate climate after residence in an endemic area. Diarrhoea is the commonest symptom and is prominent in the majority of cases, although occasionally there is sprue without diarrhoea, and only pale copious but solid stools.

The diarrhoea, especially in the early stages, may be intermittent, being present for several weeks then remitting, only to return at a later stage. Repeated remissions and relapses continue for months or years. In other cases the diarrhoea may persist throughout the course of the disease with little or no remission.

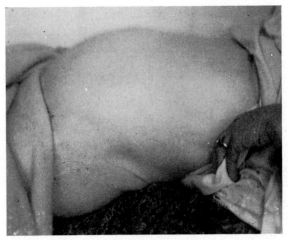

Fig. 217.—Sprue abdomen, showing intense meteorism in a Sinhalese. (*P. H. Manson-Bahr*)

The stools in established cases are pale, fermenting, acid and foul-smelling and may contain a large amount of fat and float in water. Often the stools are not noted to be especially abnormal. Dyspepsia caused by carbohydrate malabsorption is troublesome, with feelings of weight, oppression and gaseous distension after eating. The abdomen may feel like a drum and borborygmi roll through the bowel (Fig. 217).

Anorexia, nausea and vomiting are often prominent in the early stages but may persist or appear at any stage.

Loss of energy and lassitude are important symptoms and may be marked. Mental and physical fatigue and emotional irritability are common and may overshadow the other symptoms and end in a depressive state. Loss of weight is invariable and considerable and may lead to emaciation in a chronic case.

Sore tongue and mouth occur in 50% of cases, and usually follow the diarrhoea, but may at first be the only symptom, to be followed later by the other symptoms of sprue. The only manifestation of the glossitis may be a change in or loss of taste. Cramps in the hands and legs, the result of hyponatraemia, may be particularly distressing.

Signs. Glossitis and stomatitis are the result of vitamin B_2 deficiency and the mouth lesions though painful are very superficial and vary in intensity from day to day. During an exacerbation the tongue looks red and angry; superficial erosions, patches of congestion and perhaps minute vesicles appear on its surface, particularly about the edges and tip. The sides of the tongue have the appearance of being fissured. The filiform papillae cannot be made out although here and there the fungiform papillae stand out pink and swollen (Plate V). Patches of superficial erosion, sometimes covered with an aphthous looking pellicle, may be seen on the fraenum, the inside of the lips, cheeks and occasionally the palate. The pharynx and uvula may become raw and sore. Loss of weight and wasting are evident in advanced cases with emaciation.

Clinical pathology

Steatorrhoea, the result of malabsorption of fat, is found in 95% of patients. The stools of sprue are characterized by their light colour and excessive size and they may be 5 or 6 times the normal amount. They are pale and frothy and although bile pigments are present they contain excess fat; microscopic examination frequently shows fat globules. Normally neutral fats in the faeces are in the proportion of 1 to 2 to fatty acids; in pancreatic disease this ratio is reversed to as high as 15 to 1, while in sprue more splitting of fat takes place and the proportion of neutral fats to fatty acids is more even, 1 to 3 or 1 to 5. In fat balance tests, in which the patient is given a fixed diet of 50 grammes daily for several days, sprue patients do not retain the normal amount of fat (90% of the ingested fat), the figure being less than 85%. With an intake of 50 grammes of fat daily the steatorrhoea ranges between 6 and 25 grammes of fat a day and an excretion of more than 10 grammes a day establishes the presence of steatorrhoea.

Anaemia is almost invariable in fully developed sprue, and is more prominent in sprue in the Western hemisphere. Deficiencies of iron, vitamin B_{12} and folic acid play a part either alone or in combination. The serum folate falls rapidly and FIGLU (formiminoglutamic acid) appears in the urine after 20 grammes of histidine. The vitamin B_{12} falls and the absorption of radioactive vitamin B_{12} given with intrinsic factor is decreased.

There is a progressive fall in haemoglobin, and the marrow, which is normoblastic in the early stages, shows some degree of megaloblastosis after 2 months and frank megaloblastic change after 4 months (O'Brien 1967). The blood picture of a fully developed case of tropical sprue is a megaloblastic macrocytic (cells varying from 7·8 to 8 μm) anaemia with a normal white cell count or leucopenia associated with a relative lymphocytosis. Blood crises may occur and are characterized by a rapid fall in haemoglobin and red cells.

An associated iron deficiency is often found in women and in cases of sprue in India where iron deficiency is common. The serum iron is low and the total iron binding capacity is high. In a group of Indian patients the serum iron was half that of a control group and stainable iron was never found in the marrow even in the presence of gross megaloblastic change (Baker 1967).

Subacute combined degeneration of the cord may occur and mild neuritic signs are common; occasionally a peripheral neuropathy resembling beri-beri develops which responds to thiamine.

Carbohydrate malabsorption is responsible for a flat glucose tolerance curve and low D-xylose absorption.

Electrolyte and salt malabsorption may cause sodium deficiency in advanced cases of sprue with low blood pressure, signs of peripheral circulatory failure and the oedema which occasionally occurs in sprue and which is due in part to salt depletion.

Calcium deficiency can cause tetany and a positive Trousseau's sign, although osteoporosis is not found in tropical sprue.

Low serum potassium causes flaccidity of the muscles, reduced tendon reflexes and electrocardiographic changes with occasional arrhythmia.

Hypoproteinaemia causes muscle wasting and occasionally generalized oedema with a low serum albumin.

Table 39. The clinical pathology of sprue

	Normal	Sprue
Serum		
Albumin	4·0–5 2 grammes/100 ml	Diminished
Carotene	0·06–0·4 mg/100 ml	Diminished
Calcium	7·0–10·5 mg/100 ml	Diminished
Cholesterol	150–250 mg/100 ml	Diminished
Potassium	3·5–4·7 mEq/litre	Diminished
Magnesium	1·7–2·0 mEq/litre	Diminished
Folate	3·5–8·5 ng/ml*	Diminished
Vitamin B_{12}	150–850 pg/ml*	Diminished
Iron	50 μg/100 ml	Sometimes diminished
Total iron binding capacity	Less than 300–400 μg/100 ml	Sometimes increased
Tolerance tests		
D-Xylose (25 grammes orally)	Urinary excretion 4–5 grammes or greater in 5 hours	Diminished (normal in pancreatic deficiency)
Glucose (100 grammes orally)	35 mg rise in fasting plasma level	'Flat curve'
Vitamin A (0·22 grammes/ kg of oily solution containing 60 000 units/ gramme (2 mg β carotene))	Rise of at least 50 May units in 3–8 hours	Diminished
Stool fat		
Chemical determination (100 grammes/day)	5 grammes/day	Increased
[131]I Triolene (3-day collection)	Up to 4%	Increased
[131]I oleic acid (3-day collection)	Up to 4%	Increased

*For symbols n and p see p. xiii.

Vitamin deficiency

Vitamin A deficiency is shown by the skin, which is dry, often with marked follicular hyperkeratosis. A high incidence of xerosis of the conjunctivae is related to a poor vitamin A intake of the population. Vitamin B deficiency is responsible for the glossitis and cheilosis, and angular stomatitis seen in 20% of cases of acute sprue. Vitamin C deficiency can produce scorbutic phenomena; petechial haemorrhages, noticeable on the thighs and legs, formerly occurred in patients fed on milk and disappeared on the administration of adequate amounts of vitamin C. Small subcutaneous haemorrhages are common in atrophic cases of sprue. Amino acid excretion in the urine of sprue patients is decreased (Satwekar & Radhakrishnan 1965). Porphyrinuria can occur as in pellagra.

Evidence of disordered pituitary–adrenal function as shown by a low blood pressure, delayed water excretion and low output of 17 keto and ketogenic steroids in the urine is common. The basic lesion is a functional depression of pituitary in the unstimulated state and the pathogenesis is obscure (Baker *et al.* 1967).

Sprue in women

Amenorrhea and menstrual disturbances are extremely frequent in women with advanced sprue. Symptoms of sprue become exacerbated during pregnancy. There may be premature labour with death of the fetus or the infant may be born with various deformities—spina bifida and incomplete ossification of the calvarium, suggesting deficiencies of vitamins A, B and D.

Course of the disease

The disease often appears to be self-limiting, but in some villages in India up to one-third of those affected died (Baker 1967). Expatriates may recover spontaneously after return to a temperate climate but once the disease has been present for a year or more it is persistent. Intestinal atrophy consequent on sprue may ensue and the patient's absorptive mechanisms are permanently impaired. Slight irregularities in the quality or amount of food, chill, fatigue and other trifling causes suffice to bring on dyspepsia accompanied by flatulence and diarrhoea. These cases may linger on for years. Usually they improve during the summer in temperate climates, getting worse during the winter and spring or during cold weather. Ultimately these patients die from general atrophy, diarrhoea or some intercurrent disease.

Radiological changes

The radiological changes are those of a deficiency or malabsorption pattern.

The mucosal folds of the small intestine are reduced in number and are irregular in width and spacing with thick transverse barring seen on X-ray. Peristalsis is disordered and in advanced cases the mucosal folds may be entirely absent (Patterson *et al.* 1965).

Diagnosis

The diagnosis of tropical sprue is made by finding evidence of malabsorption as shown by steatorrhoea, reduced D-xylose and carotene absorption and diminished serum folate and vitamin B_{12} (Table 39). Confirmation of the condition of the small intestine can be obtained by intestinal biopsy.

Other causes of malabsorption to be distinguished are coeliac disease and idiopathic steatorrhoea which are caused by gluten intolerance and, unlike sprue, respond to a gluten-free diet. Lactose intolerance responds to a milk-free diet. Intestinal parasitism, giardiasis and strongyloidiasis are diagnosed by stool examination or duodenal aspiration. In chronic pancreatitis neutral fats predominate in the stool and the diastatic index of the urine is increased. Intestinal tuberculosis and lymphosarcoma of the mesenteric glands will show signs elsewhere. Whipple's disease, intestinal lipodystrophy, can be distinguished by biopsy and gastrojejuno-colic fistula and blind-loop syndrome by radiology. Other causes of megaloblastic anaemia may cause difficulty, especially where anaemia is the prominent feature of sprue. Signs of malabsorption are not found in nutritional megaloblastic or pernicious anaemia.

Pellagra may be distinguished by the characteristic rash and absence of malabsorption.

Treatment

The object of treatment is to correct the bacterial contamination of the bowel and restore the deficiencies caused by malabsorption. This is done by the administration of broad-spectrum antibiotics, vitamins, proteins and electrolytes.

Antibiotics. Tetracycline 2 grammes daily for 2–3 weeks will improve the vitamin B_{12} absorption and reduce the steatorrhoea to normal in 5 days in about half the cases (Baker & Mathan 1967). Folic acid is specific in many cases, and should be commenced directly the diagnosis has been established. It is given in doses of 10 mg 3 times daily for 10 days, followed by 10 mg twice daily for 10 days, and then 5 mg once daily as a maintenance dose for the duration of stay in an endemic area. Vitamin B_{12} should be given in conjunction with the folic acid to prevent the onset of cord changes and should be given intramuscularly once weekly in doses of 1 mg.

The progress of the case will be measured by the degree of steatorrhoea, the glossitis, haemoglobin level, body weight and intestinal absorptive capacity as measured by the D-xylose and carotene tests. If there is evidence of other vitamin deficiencies these should be corrected by the appropriate vitamin. Electrolyte abnormalities should be corrected and calcium administered as calcium gluconate intravenously if tetany is present.

In severe cases of anaemia blood transfusion may be necessary.

Diet. No special diet is necessary any longer. If there is hypoproteinaemia then a high-protein diet should be given.

Results of treatment are variable. Most cases improve rapidly on antibiotics and folic acid. In South India half of the patients treated with antibiotics alone for 2–3 weeks showed some improvement in steatorrhoea, but in only one-fifth did the fat excretion return to normal (Baker & Mathan 1969).

Long-term antibiotic treatment for a number of months has produced some improvement in intestinal function. Vitamin B_{12} and folic acid have the greatest effect on the anaemia, but folic acid alone has arrested the diarrhoea in some cases, and produced considerable improvement in alimentary function. In other cases little or no effect is noted. In cases of sprue of long duration permanent damage may be suffered by the absorptive apparatus and atrophic changes in the small bowel may persist into old age. These individuals show permanent signs of malabsorption and develop diarrhoea if careful attention is not paid to their diet.

Convalescence. In many cases of sprue, the intestinal defect persists although the symptoms of malabsorption have disappeared. If possible, sprue patients ought not to return to the tropics if they are aged over 50. Young adults usually recover completely. If they do return to a hot climate a maintenance dose of 5 mg of folic acid daily is recommended.

REFERENCES

BAHR, P. H. (1915) *A Report on Sprue in Ceylon*. London: Cambridge University Press.
BAKER, S. J. (1967) in *Tropical Medicine Conference* (ed. Walters, J. H.). London: Pitman Medical.
────── & MATHAN, V. I. (1967) quoted by Baker (1967).
────── ────── & JOSEPH, I. (1962) *2nd Wld Congr. Gastroent.*, 4.
BANWELL, J. G. & GORBACH, S. L. (1969) *Gut*, **10**, 328.
────── HUTT, M. S. R. & TUNNICLIFFE, R. (1964) *E. Afr. med. J.*, **41**, 46.

BLACK, D. A. K. (1946) *Lancet*, **ii**, 671.
BOOTH, C. C. (1965) in *Symposium on Advanced Medicine* (ed. Compston, N.). London: Pitman Medical.
——— (1970) *Br. med. J.*, **ii**, 725.
LEISHMAN, A. W. D. (1945) *Lancet*, **ii**, 813.
LINDENBAUM, J., KENT, I. H. & SPRINZ, H. (1966) *Br. med. J.*, **ii**, 1157.
MATHAN, V. I. & BAKER, S. J. (1968) *Am. J. clin. Nutr.*, **21**, 1077.
O'BRIEN, W. (1967) in *Tropical Medical Conference* (ed. Walters, J. H.). London: Pitman Medical.
——— & ENGLAND, N. W. J. (1966) *Br. med. J.*, **ii**, 1157.
PATERSON, D. E., DAVID, R. & BAKER, S. J. (1965) *Br. J. Radiol.*, **38**, 181.
SATWEKAR, K. & RADHAKRISHNAN, A. N. (1965) *Clinica chim. Acta*, **12**, 394.
SHINER, M. (1956) *Lancet*, **i**, 17.
STEFANINI, M. (1948) *Medicine, Baltimore*, **27**, 379.
VAISH, S. K., IGNATIUS, M. & BAKER, S. J. (1965) *Q. Jl Med.*, **34**, 15.

Scurvy

Aetiology

SCURVY is caused by a deficiency of vitamin C (ascorbic acid), which is present in all living tissues; fresh fruits and plants are the best source and the intake largely depends on the consumption of fresh vegetables. Vitamin C is destroyed by heat, especially prolonged cooking in the presence of alkalis. Foods which are steamed and cooked rapidly retain much of their vitamin C. The recommended allowance of vitamin C is 30 mg daily for infants, 40–50 mg for children and 70 mg for adults. Scurvy is not common in the tropics since vitamin C is abundant in tropical and subtropical areas. Cases can occur in infants who are fed on dried cereals and boiled milk. Epidemics are apt to occur in labourers who are fed on dried cereals and preserved foods and soldiers who are living in desert areas on dry rations.

Vitamin C deficiency causes increased permeability of the capillary endothelium, and a haemorrhagic diathesis.

Symptoms and signs

The onset of scurvy is insidious, with loss of weight, progressive weakness and stiffness in the leg muscles. Haematomas forming in the leg muscles may be the first sign. The acute symptoms are often brought on by hard physical exertion. The gums soon become affected, with swelling and sponginess of the alveolar margin, and fungating masses project beyond the teeth, which loosen and fall out.

Subcutaneous petechiae form on the limbs and trunk producing scorbutic purpura.

In infantile scurvy the epiphyses of the long bones separate owing to haemorrhage and a 'scurvy rosary' forms along the costochondral junctions.

Diagnosis

The capillary permeability test of Hess is performed using a sphygmomanometer to occlude the venous return of the arm, when petechiae will appear in scorbutic cases.

Vitamin C deficiency can also be diagnosed by the vitamin C saturation test, which is performed by saturating the body with ascorbic acid and measuring the excretion in the urine. If any ascorbic acid is retained then there is a deficiency of vitamin C.

Treatment and prevention

Scurvy is easily treated by the administration of 200–500 mg daily of ascorbic acid. Fresh orange juice and other fresh fruits are also curative.

Scurvy is prevented by the administration of 30 mg of ascorbic acid daily when fresh foods are not obtainable.

Rickets

Since rickets is prevented and cured by vitamin D it is rare in most tropical and subtropical countries, where the action of sunlight on the skin produces adequate vitamin D.

In certain circumstances, however, rickets may occur among children in both tropical and subtropical zones. The sunlight may be cut off by high buildings in Asia (Jelliffe 1955), the San Blas Indians of Panama protect their children from the sun because of the high incidence of albinism (Jelliffe & Jelliffe 1961) and in Guatemala some cases have been found in sunny rural areas where the toddlers are kept in the houses because the mothers have to go out to work.

Rickets in the tropics is no different from classical rickets. The typical bossing of the skull must be distinguished from that of sickle cell disease and other chronic haemolytic anaemias and from infantile scurvy and congenital syphilis.

Osteomalacia

Primary osteomalacia due to inadequate amounts of calcium or vitamin D in the diet is endemic in wide areas of northern India, where it occurs in 'purdah' women, and in northern China. The custom of keeping women in seclusion (purdah) prevents the action of sunlight on the skin to produce vitamin D. Osteomalacia occurs chiefly in women and may be more severe in each succeeding pregnancy owing to the demands made by the fetus and by the mammary glands on the calcium reserves of the mother. The bones, especially the pelvic girdle, ribs and femora, become soft, painful and deformed. Deformation of the pelvis may be so severe as to necessitate Caesarean section. Symptoms recur with each succeeding pregnancy but tend to clear up after lactation is completed. The serum calcium is low (6–7 mg/100 ml) and tetany is a common complication. The bones of the fetus show no signs of rickets.

Treatment

Administration of calcium salts alone does not relieve the condition but the administration of cod liver oil or vitamin D cures or prevents the disease and restores the normal serum calcium level.

Beri-beri

Synonyms

Kakke; barbiers; polyneuritis endemica.

AETIOLOGY

Beri-beri is caused by a deficiency of vitamin B_1 (aneurine, thiamine) in the diet. It was noted that fowls or pigeons fed exclusively on paddi or unhusked rice throve, whereas those fed on a diet exclusively of polished rice developed peripheral neuritis (polyneuritis colombarum and gallinarum). Recovery took place after injection of an extract of the germ centre of rice grains. Fraser and Stanton showed in classical experiments that the antineuritic element was located in the pericarp of the rice grain in the aleurone layer and were further able to show in experiments on 24 life prisoners that beri-beri was non-communicable and that it could be produced in man solely by diet.

Acting on these findings the governments of Singapore and Malaya forbade the use of polished rice in jails, mental institutions, schools and hospitals with the result that beri-beri almost vanished as a disease. The same results followed the banning of polished rice in Indonesia, the Philippines, Burma and the Japanese Navy so that beri-beri is now rarely seen as a primary nutritional deficiency in the Far East.

HISTORY AND GEOGRAPHICAL DISTRIBUTION

Until recently beri-beri was common in tropical and subtropical areas and was formerly the scourge of mines and plantations in Malaysia, China, Indonesia and other parts of the Far East, wherever rice was the staple diet, and was the cause of an enormous mortality and morbidity. It was common among workers in the tropics on such major engineering projects as the Panama Canal and Congo Railway. Outbreaks have occurred in institutions such as mental homes in Ireland, the U.S.A. and France and in fishermen in Newfoundland, the North American coast and Iceland. Beri-beri was formerly a major problem in the Japanese Navy and was almost universal in prisoner-of-war and internment camps in the Far East in World War II.

Ship beri-beri

Beri-beri was formerly prevalent in the crews of ships on the high seas. From 1894 to 1920 the disease was common in the crews of Swedish and Norwegian ships and yet was comparatively rare in British ships. The explanation was that during these years bread baked from white flour or a mixture of wheat and rye was used in the Scandinavian ships, so that the crew's diet was inadequate in vitamins.

PATHOPHYSIOLOGY

Vitamin B_1 is found in the tissues in the phosphorylated form as diphospho-thiamine which acts as a coenzyme for the metabolism of carbohydrate in the Krebs citric acid cycle and plays a part in the oxidative breakdown of pyruvic acid. Since the brain and all nervous tissue and heart muscle use glucose in large amounts as a primary source of energy, carbohydrate metabolism is especially deranged in these tissues in vitamin B_1 deficiency. Pyruvic acid accumulates in the blood and central nervous system and is excreted in excess in the urine.

Vitamin B_1 is widely distributed in raw foodstuffs, the richest sources being whole cereals and especially rice, in which it is found in the pericarp in the aleurone layer and in the embryo of the grain (Fig. 218). The rice grain in its natural condition is enclosed in a husk. In 'husking' the husk is removed but the pericarp is retained; this is unpolished rice. In milling and 'polishing' both the embryo and pericarp are removed and the grains are polished by rubbing with talc between sheepskins (Fig. 219). This is known as polished or white rice. Vitamin B_1 is also found in yeast which is an exceptionally potent source and can be used as a dietary supplement. Vitamin B_1 is a colourless water-soluble crystalline substance melting at 248–250°C and in dry conditions is stable at 100°C for 24 hours. The rate of destruction is increased by the presence of water and alkali but ordinary cooking in the absence of soda does not destroy the vitamin; it is, however, destroyed by pressure cooking and autoclaving when yeast and liver are subjected to heat and pressure. The larger part of vitamin B_1 is stored in the liver, kidneys and muscles and it is abundant in the normal heart. Vitamin B_1 is excreted in the urine in which the kidney concentrates it from the plasma, but only a small part of the vitamin given by the mouth is excreted, the rest being destroyed in the body. It is also excreted in the milk but not in the faeces. An excretion of less than 12·1 I.U./day in the urine is evidence

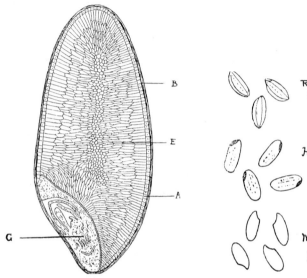

Fig. 218.—Diagram of a longitudinal section through a grain of wheat, showing (A) the aleurone layer of cells forming the outermost layer of the endosperm, removed with the pericarp during milling; (B) the pericarp forming the branny envelope; (E) parenchymous cells of the endosperm; (G) the embryo or germ. (*Reproduced from 'Report on the Value of Bread made from Different Varieties of Wheat' by J. M. Hamill, by permission of H.M. Stationery Office*)

Fig. 219.—The various stages in the milling of the rice grain. 1, The rice grain in its natural condition enclosed in the husk or enclosing glumes. 2, After removal of the husk, but retaining the pericarp or 'silver-skin' and the embryo. 3, After milling and polishing. Both 'silver-skin' and embryo are removed when the grains are polished by rubbing with talc between sheepskins. (*After Chick & Hume*)

of vitamin B_1 deficiency. The International Unit is the antineuritic activity of 3 μg of pure vitamin B_1. The minimum daily requirement of an adult of 70 kg on 3000 cal./day would be 300 I.U. or 1 mg, but 500–700 I.U. (1·75–2·3 mg) is desirable. A larger amount is required where metabolic rates are increased in pregnancy, lactation, infancy and childhood and there is a high incidence of beri-beri among pregnant women and mothers. Hard physical work also increases the requirements; thus beri-beri is more prevalent among stokers than sailors. Since the metabolic rate rises during fever there is an association of beri-beri with malaria and other pyrexias.

Secondary (alcoholic) beri-beri

Alcoholic cardiomyopathy causes a low output type of heart failure, has a complicated aetiology and is not due to beri-beri (Brigden & Robinson 1964).

True alcoholic beri-beri is a form of oedematous heart disease with high output failure occurring in certain severe alcoholics, which responds rapidly to vitamin B_1. It is not common in the West, but has been described as 'palm-wine tappers' heart' in Gambia (Walters & Smith 1952) which develops in palm tappers whose work is arduous and involves the climbing of many palm trees and the consumption of the fermenting sap.

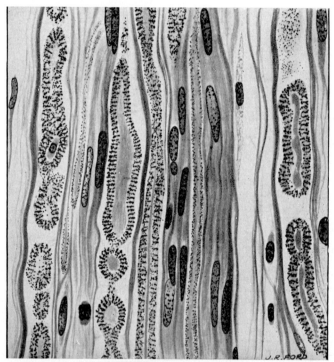

Fig. 220.—Longitudinal section of the external popliteal nerve in beri-beri. One medullated nerve fibre in the centre is practically intact; the others show typical fragmentation of the myelin sheath, with swelling of the remains of the nerve fibre. (*From a preparation by Dr A. C. Stevenson*)

Drug-induced beri-beri has been reported from East Africa from the use of nitrofurazone in the treatment of trypanosomiasis which interferes with pyruvate metabolism.

PATHOLOGY

As a result of the breakdown of carbohydrate metabolism those systems of the body which utilize glucose most rapidly are affected. These are the central nervous system, peripheral nerves and cardiac muscle. Degenerative nerve changes may be detected in the nerve centres, neurons (Fig. 220), in the anterior and posterior horn cells and sympathetic ganglia. The vagus is involved with degenerative changes in its nucleus in the floor of the fourth ventricle.

Microscopically the nerve trunks show changes from a slight medullary degeneration to complete destruction of the nerve (Wallerian degeneration). Regenerative processes can occur side by side with the degenerative. Some fibres of the vagus and sympathetic nerves escape and the bronchial and oesophageal twigs are usually unaffected. In Wernicke's encephalopathy foci of congestion and haemorrhage are scattered symmetrically in the grey matter of the brain stem and hypothalamic regions. The mamillary bodies are nearly always affected. The lesions show specific selectivity for the vegetative centres, being most severe in the lateral horns and Clarke's nuclei at the thoracic level. There are also numerous perivascular haemorrhages and widespread degenerative changes throughout the brain. In the heart the primary lesion is a loss of contractibility of the heart muscle due to water retention. Microscopic examination of the heart muscle shows intracellular oedema, sarcolysis and hydropic degeneration probably due primarily to an excess of lactic acid brought about by defective oxygenation (Wenckebach 1928). These changes cause 'beri-beri heart' the essential features of which are a hyperkinetic circulation, peripheral vasodilatation, enlargement of the right side of the heart and dilatation of the pulmonary artery with an increased circulation time, causing a high output failure (Weiss & Wilkins 1937).

The cause of the hyperkinetic circulation is not exactly clear. It may be a compensatory mechanism which is brought into play to counteract tissue anoxia, which is simulated by a failure of carbohydrate metabolism, or the vasodilatation in the muscles may be responsible by causing an arteriovenous shunt.

The post mortem appearances are those of severe right heart failure. The right side of the heart is dilated, especially the right auricle, the walls of which may be paper thin. There is gross congestion of the venous return and right auricle and ventricle. There are serious effusions into the pleural and peritoneal cavities and cellular tissues. There is oedema of the lungs and severe central congestion of the liver with 'nutmegging'.

SYMPTOMS AND SIGNS

Beri-beri assumes varying clinical forms according to the extent and degree of cardiac involvement. There are two main forms of the disease; paraplegic or 'dry' beri-beri, and oedematous or 'wet' beri-beri. In all its forms beri-beri is the same disease and a mixture of the two forms is usual.

The period of development of beri-beri in man after being placed on a vitamin B_1 deficient diet was determined by Fraser and Stanton as between 80 and 90 days. The onset is usually insidious but may occasionally be ushered in by acute symptoms, ending fatally within a few hours without any symptoms referable to the central nervous system.

Paraplegic or dry beri-beri

The signs and symptoms are those of a peripheral neuropathy of a mixed motor and sensory type. There is a gradual onset of weakness of the lower limbs followed by ataxia; there may be paraesthesiae with burning and tingling in the limbs.

Motor signs. A flaccid weakness with wasting develops at first in the muscles of the lower limbs. The extensors of the foot and toes are involved with foot and toe drop and the gastrocnemii become weak and wasted. This weakness gradually spreads up to involve the extensors of the legs and later the extensors and flexors of the thigh. At this stage the patient is not able to rise from the squatting position with his hands held above his head. This is the 'jongck' or 'squatting test'. The upper limbs are eventually affected with weakness and wasting of the thenar, hypothenar, plantar and arm muscles, which may show fibrillary twitchings. There may be marked wrist drop (Fig. 221). There is a loss of the deep reflexes. The knee jerks, ankle jerks and arm reflexes are all lost. The fibres of the affected muscles show myoedema and contract painfully when struck by the patellar hammer. Electrical reactions show the reaction of degeneration.

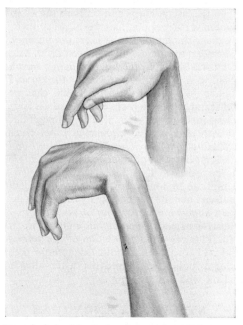

Fig. 221.—Paraplegic beri-beri, showing wasting of the extensor muscles and wrist drop.

Sensory changes. Sensory changes are marked. There is a sensory neuropathy of the peripheral type with glove and stocking anaesthesia spreading up from the feet over the tibiae to the thighs. A similar loss of sensation spreads up from the tips of the fingers. There is loss of sensation to pain, light touch and heat and cold, and deep sensibility elicited by compression of the Achilles tendon is lost.

A severe ataxia develops owing to the marked loss of postural sensation and the patient is unable to button his jacket or pick up a pin. The gait becomes ataxic and he walks with a high stepping gait on a broad base, requiring the use of a stick (Fig. 222). The cranial nerves are not involved and there are no tremors. The bladder and rectal sphincters are not involved until the terminal stages.

Cardiac or wet beri-beri

Cardiac beri-beri is a high output right heart failure in which the circulation time is increased.

Oedema. The reis generalized oedema of the arms, legs, hands and trunk and

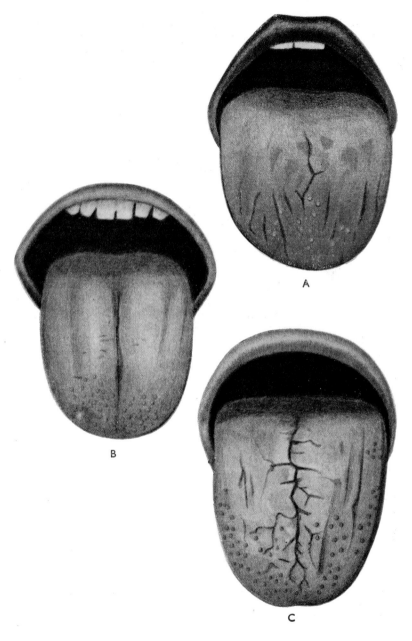

PLATE V

Prepellagrous and sprue tongues.

A, Avitaminosis B_2 tongue, showing angular stomatitis. B, Acute stage of sprue with typical aphtha. C, Chronic sprue tongue. (*P. Manson-Bahr*)

[*To face p. 768.*

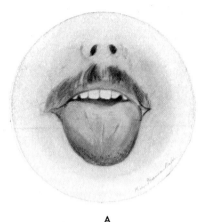

A

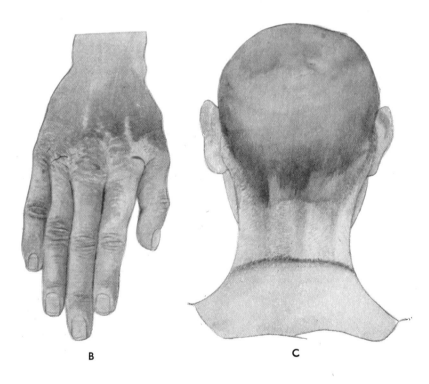

B   C

PLATE VI

Pellagra.

A, Characteristic inflamed tongue of acute pellagra, with angular stomatitis. B, Early pellagrous rash, with cellular infiltration and pigmentation. C, Typical pellagrous rash over the occiput and mastoid processes, with formation of a 'rosary' round the neck. (*The late Dr J. I. Enright*)

the face is puffy (Fig. 223). The urine is scanty, of high specific gravity and contains no albumin.

Circulatory changes. The extremities are warm, the pulse rapid with a raised pulse pressure and low diastolic pressure. 'Pistol shot' sounds may be heard over the larger arteries and occasionally heart block may occur. The jugular venous pressure is greatly raised with a marked venous pulse in the neck due to tricuspid incompetence. The heart is enlarged to the right and the heart sounds are evenly spread, causing a tic-tac rhythm with reduplication of the second heart sound. A loud pansystolic murmur is heard over the whole of the praecordium including the tricuspid area. Paralysis of the recurrent laryngeal nerve by a

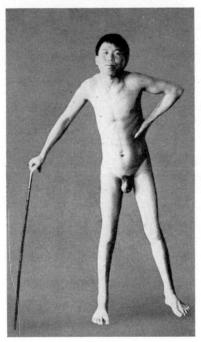

Fig. 222.—Ataxic or paraplegic beri-beri, showing the characteristic attitude.

grossly distended auricle has been recorded. The liver is enlarged and tender and may pulsate. There is usually a single or double hydrothorax and ascites.

Radiography of the heart shows a typical globular enlargement affecting the right and left ventricles. Pericardial effusion is rare at this stage. The electrocardiogram shows distinct changes of low voltage, inverted or flattened T waves in all leads, a decreased P–R interval and a prolongation of the Q–T interval. Changes of right ventricular strain are also found.

Progress

Most patients die from paralysis and right heart failure complicated and aggravated by oedema of the lungs, diaphragmatic paralysis, hydrothorax or hydropericardium. Sudden cardiac failure is common (Shôshin of the Japanese).

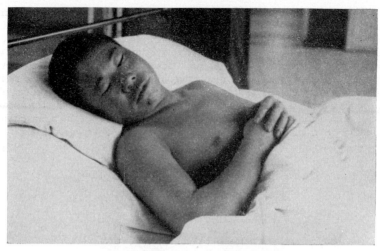

Fig. 223.—Wet or oedematous cardiac beri-beri. (*Philip Manson-Bahr*)

INFANTILE BERI-BERI

Infantile beri-beri occurs in breast-fed infants of vitamin B_1 deficient mothers, especially if they are taking a high carbohydrate diet. It can also occur in artificially fed infants if the feed is deficient in vitamin B_1 or the carbohydrate level is too high.

Aetiology

It is probable that vitamin B_1 deficiency is not the only cause of infantile beri-beri (Fehily 1944) and that some of the features are caused by certain toxic products in the breast milk. It is considered that breakdown products from the incomplete metabolism of carbohydrate, especially methyl glyoxal (Sato 1964), are toxic to the infant.

Clinical features

Characteristically the onset is during the second and third months of life especially the ninth, tenth and eleventh weeks (Bray 1928). The baby is rather fat and flabby. The onset is with restlessness, attacks of crying, oliguria and a little puffiness of the body. This may be followed by vomiting of the milk (Fig. 224).

Cardiorespiratory phase. This is the most dramatic and rapidly fatal form of the disease. There is a fairly sudden onset of peripheral and central circulatory failure. The lungs become moist, the heart enlarges with a tic-tac rhythm and the pulse becomes rapid and thready. There is venous engorgement of the neck veins with tender enlargement of the liver. Oedema collects and the child may die in 36–41 hours from cardiorespiratory failure.

Chronic phase. This occurs in slightly older infants .There is anorexia, loss of weight and constipation. Dysphonia and aphonia, ascribed to a paralysis of the left recurrent laryngeal nerve from pressure of the left auricle, are common and give rise to a characteristic cry. There is oedema and oliguria. Paralysis of muscles and loss of tendon reflexes are found (polyneuritic phase).

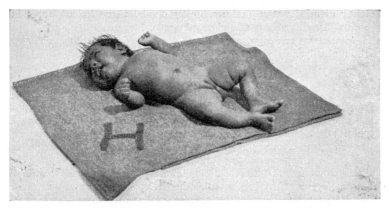

Fig. 224.—Nauruan child in convulsions of infantile beri-beri. Note the general anasarca. (Dr G. W. Bray)

Laboratory diagnosis

The thiamine concentration in the milk can be estimated (Simpson & Chow 1956). The critical level may be about 6–7 μg/100 ml.

WERNICKE'S ENCEPHALOPATHY

The combination of ataxia, clouding of consciousness and ophthalmoplegia was described by Wernicke in 1881. Subsequently this syndrome was associated with chronic alcoholism. From 1933 onwards its connection with vitamin B_1 deficiency was suspected and a similar condition was described in a nutritional disease of silver foxes in America. Outbreaks of this disease occurred in prisoner-of-war camps in the Far East in World War II and have been described by De Wardener & Lennox (1947) and Spillane (1947). Diagnosis was established at autopsy by demonstration of haemorrhages in the mamillary bodies (see Pathology, page 767). The cause of the syndrome was established as vitamin B_1 deficiency by the rapidity with which it responded to injections of vitamin B_1. Predisposing causes were dysentery, diarrhoea, failure to adapt to a rice diet and febrile conditions such as sepsis and malaria.

Symptoms and signs

In 90% of cases of the B_1 deficiency type other forms of beri-beri are associated. There are signs of severe disturbance of the mid-brain with oculomotor signs and cranial nerve lesions, with general clouding of the consciousness. The first symptom is persisting anorexia, followed by cranial nerve lesions.

General signs. These include clouding of consciousness, insomnia, disorientation and semi-coma.

Oculomotor signs and symptoms. Wavering of the visual fields on looking to the side, diplopia, and photophobia occur. Horizontal nystagmus is the earliest sign. In a quarter of the cases there is an external rectus palsy, sometimes with complete disconjugate wandering of the eyes. There are loss of visual acuity, ptosis and retinal haemorrhages.

Other cranial nerve lesions. Other cranial nerve lesions occur in the trigeminal, facial, auditory and glossopharyngeal nerves.

The symptoms and signs are relieved promptly by injections of vitamin B_1 50–100 mg daily.

DIAGNOSIS

Dry beri-beri must be distinguished from alcoholic peripheral neuropathy in which there are associated tremors and mental changes including Korsakoff's psychosis; from tabes dorsalis, in which there are Argyll–Robertson pupils and posterior column changes; from arsenical neuritis, in which there are pigmentation of the skin, hyperkeratosis of the palms and soles of the feet; from chronic lead poisoning, in which there is a blue line on the gums and the neuropathy is purely motor; from lathyrism, in which there is a pyramidal lesion with spasticity of the legs, increased tendon reflexes and extensor plantar responses; from triorthocresyl phosphate (ginger or jake) paralysis in which there is a pure motor flaccid paralysis; from other nutritional neuropathies such as burning feet and combined degeneration of the cord when both posterior columns and the pyramidal tracts are involved. In the rapidly ascending paralysis of the Guillain–Barré syndrome the cerebrospinal fluid shows a raised protein content. Wet beri-beri must be distinguished from other causes of right heart failure with a high cardiac output: anaemic heart failure, hookworm disease and also chronic nephritis. In famine oedema and epidemic dropsy signs of peripheral neuropathy are absent.

Laboratory tests. The pyruvic acid level of the blood is raised and is of diagnostic value. In acute beri-beri the level of pyruvic acid is about 2 mg/100 ml and in untreated chronic beri-beri about 1·5 mg/100 ml. After aneurine injection the level falls to about 0·5 mg/100 ml.

Meyers test. There is an increase in the audible sounds in the antecubital fossa after the subcutaneous injection of adrenaline.

Volhard's diuresis test. In a normal fasting person after drinking 1 litre of water, all the fluid is excreted in 4 hours. In beri-beri there is water retention, which disappears after treatment with aneurine.

Acute cardiac beri-beri will respond dramatically within a few hours to the intravenous injection of 50–100 mg of vitamin B_1.

TREATMENT

Wet beri-beri

The specific treatment of beri-beri is with thiamine. Crystalline preparations are available—Benerva and Betavel. Benerva is issued as tablets of 3, 10, 25, 50, 100 and 300 mg and ampoules of 25 and 100 mg; Betavel is issued as tablets of 50 mg and in ampoules of 100 mg as an injection. Dramatic effects are observed in acute cardiac cases when large doses are given intravenously (Hawes 1938). Immediate intravenous injections of 50 mg of aneurine should be repeated 2–3 times in the 24 hours until serial X-rays show that the heart has been reduced to a normal size. In moribund patients the injection has been made straight into the jugular vein. In severe cases venesection taking 250–300 ml of blood from the arm is of great value. In the ordinary case the patient should be confined to bed and given a high-protein diet with restriction of salt and fluids and the addition of aneurine to the diet in the form of tablets or by intramuscular injection.

Dry beri-beri

The treatment with injections of thiamine will relieve the pain and subjective dysthesiae. The signs of peripheral neuropathy take some time to disappear but results are disappointing in some parts of the world where the patients will inevitably relapse when they return home and resume a diet of polished rice.

Infantile beri-beri

After an injection of thiamine improvement will be noted in a few hours; sometimes it is dramatic. In acutely ill children 25 mg of thiamine should be injected intravenously and a further 25 mg given intramuscularly once or twice a day until the symptoms have subsided, when an oral dose of 10 mg should be given daily for several weeks. The child should be removed from the breast and given artificial feeds for 24 hours while the mother is given thiamine. The breast milk must be drawn off and discarded so that after 24 hours she is ready to feed her baby again.

PREVENTION

Beri-beri can be eradicated by the prohibition of the use of polished rice. This has been attempted in some countries but to legislate against the use of white rice in countries where rice is the staple food leads to the appearance of a black market in polished rice. Unpolished (red) rice and parboiled rice, in which the vitamin is retained, are good foods. Beri-beri can also be prevented by using mixed diets containing other sources of thiamine, such as pulses, ground nuts, whole wheat, vegetables, fruit and milk.

Health education and the development of methods of milling rice in which the germ is not removed have led to the disappearance of beri-beri from most eastern communities.

Pellagra

The name pellagra is derived from the Italian, *pelle* (skin) *agra* (rough).

AETIOLOGY

Pellagra is a syndrome caused by a deficiency of a variety of specific factors, with nicotinic acid (nicotinamide, niacin) as the most important. The amino acid tryptophan is a precursor of nicotinic acid in man, so that a diet with a high tryptophan but low nicotinic acid content is not pellagrogenic.

The richest source of nicotinic acid is liver, kidney and yeast, and important sources are whole-meal flour and green vegetables. Of staple foods maize contains the least available nicotinic acid, possibly because a large proportion of the nicotinic acid is in a bound form which can be liberated by alkaline hydrolysis and is achieved by the treatment of maize with lime practised in Central America. The daily need of nicotinic acid is about 10–15 mg but can be replaced by excess dietary tryptophan. Nicotinic acid is found in the tissues as a nucleotide, diphosphopyridine nucleotide (DPN) usually called coenzyme I, formed by the combination of adenine ribose phosphate and nicotinamide. There is also a corresponding coenzyme II, triphosphopyridine nucleotide.

Coenzymes I and II are the coenzymes responsible for the oxidative enzyme dehydrogenases and act as intermediate carriers for the hydrogen released from various substrates by the dehydrogenase enzymes. The enzymes containing nicotinamide are concerned with many of the important energy producing reactions of metabolism. Nicotinic acid deficiency leads to metabolic disturbances in many tissues and the nervous system is seriously involved.

Pellagra and maize

Pellagra appeared soon after the introduction of maize to Europe and advanced with the extension of maize cultivation. Epidemics of pellagra occur among maize (or sorghum) eaters. Pellagra is also found in non-maize-eating countries, such as India, Cuba and Brazil. In Central America, where maize is the staple, pellagra is rare. This may be due to the treatment of the maize with lime which releases more tryptophan or to the consumption of coffee, which is rich in niacin (Bressani et al. 1961). The cause of pellagra is more complicated than a simple deficiency and is due to the disturbance of a delicate chemical balance between certain toxins present in relatively large amounts in maize and some essential dietary factors, of which nicotinic acid and tryptophan are the most important. Leucine, for instance, which is plentiful in sorghum, affects the metabolism of tryptophan and nicotinic acid in man. Analogues of nicotinic acid can produce pellagra-like effects in animals, but it is not certain whether these are the poisonous substances present in maize. The problem of pellagra is one of biochemical imbalances.

Secondary pellagra is due to non-absorption of the necessary vitamins by a non-functioning intestinal mucosa. It also occurs after prolonged treatment with large doses of isoniazid which replaces the nicotinic acid in the oxidative reduction coenzyme DPN.

GEOGRAPHICAL DISTRIBUTION AND EPIDEMIOLOGY

Pellagra has been reported from most parts of the world, especially from countries where maize is consumed as a staple. Since World War II pellagra has vanished from most of its former range and is now found only occasionally in some tropical areas, or after social disturbances.

Seasonal incidence

In Europe pellagra used to appear during the spring and autumn quarters, being most severe in the spring. In Egypt the incidence was similar. In Malawi, south of the equator, pellagra was prevalent during August, September and October, the southern spring. In the northern U.S.A. the disease exhibited the usual double incidence, the spring outbreak occurring during May and June and the autumnal in September and October. In the deep south the disease used to appear as early as January. This definite seasonal periodicity indicates that climatic factors have an important though indirect effect and it is likely that exposure to sunlight which exacerbates all the manifestations of pellagra is responsible.

Sex

Both sexes are liable to the disease, but in different places the disease exhibits a different predilection for one or other sex in accordance with the occupation and habits of the people. In the U.S.A. it was more prevalent in women of child-bearing age because of the debilitating effects of menstruation, pregnancy and lactation. Old people living alone are especially liable, owing to their monotonous diet.

Age

Pellagra is a disease of middle age, the majority of cases occurring between 20 and 50. 'Infantile pellagra' is now known to be due to protein–calorie malnutrition and is not a pellagrous condition.

Occupation

Pellagra is most prevalent amongst field labourers doing hard manual work. It is very prevalent among the prison population and in mental institutions and breaks out when the inhabitants are suddenly exposed to hard physical labour.

Diet

The dietary factor is all-important. In the southern U.S.A. pellagra was common when the main diet was molasses and corn (maize). With improved social and economic conditions and the development of supermarkets pellagra preventing foods, such as milk and eggs, became more freely available and pellagra has vanished from the community. Pellagra is a disease of poverty, backwardness and subsistence agriculture in large populations of plantation labour.

PATHOLOGY

There is an increased excretion of coproporphyrin in the urine in pellagra which has been regarded either as indicating faulty metabolism or abnormal absorption. It occurs especially in alcoholic pellagra but Beckh et al. (1937) have shown that the amount of coproporphyrin in the urine is inversely proportional to the nicotinic acid intake. Since the oral gastro-intestinal and neurological manifestations of pellagra can be evoked by exposure to sunlight it has been suggested that there is an abnormal porphyrin metabolism in pellagra. There is great emaciation of the body. The viscera show fatty degeneration and a characteristic deep pigmentation. The intestinal walls and villi, the liver and the spleen are atrophied. The suprarenal capsules may be atrophied and the cortex black; the medulla may be the seat of haemorrhages. The heart shows brown atrophy.

Central nervous system (Spillane 1947)

In the brain the main alterations are found in the Betz cells of the motor cortex and to a less extent in the Purkinje cells, the periventricular cell groups and the nuclei of cranial motor nerves. Chromatolysis, poor staining of nuclei and nucleoli and an increase of intracellular pigment are the most constant findings. The frontal lobes are most affected but the basal ganglia may show some degree of change. There is some endothelial thickening and hyaline degeneration of the walls of capillary blood vessels. In advanced cases there may be some gliosis.

The spinal cord shows a more or less symmetrical degeneration of the dorsal columns in the form of scattered demyelinization. The spinocerebellar and pyramidal tracts are involved to a lesser extent. The cells of Clarke's column show chromatolysis and pigmentary degeneration, the column of Goll being most affected. Myelin degeneration of the peripheral nerves of some degree is common. The myelin sheaths become irregular from swelling and atrophy and may present a honeycombed appearance.

CLINICAL FEATURES

The cardinal signs of pellagra constitute the well known diagnostic triad, 'diarrhoea, dermatitis and dementia'.

Prepellagrous state

The initial symptoms are composed of vague psychological digestive disturbances which recur with repeated exacerbations and periods of quiescence for years without the appearance of skin eruptions. The patient appears pale, has a peculiar lifeless staring look with dilated pupils and complains of non-specific symptoms, giddiness and vague but often severe pains in the back and joints. The complexion is muddy with bluish leaden-coloured sclerae. The character changes, becoming irritable and at the same time stupid and morose. Since the

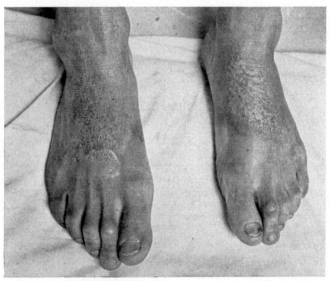

Fig. 225.—Pellagra rash on the feet. The dorsa of the feet had been exposed to the sun in the area between the turned-up trousers and the uppers of the shoes. (*Dr A. D. Bigland*)

earliest signs are difficult to define a great many people who suffer from chronic ill health in an endemic pellagra area may really be in the prepellagrous state.

Other early vitamin B deficiencies may be associated with the prepellagrous state: angular stomatitis (Plate V), an atrophic condition of the lips (*perlêche*) and cheilosis (page 781) are associated with ariboflavinosis.

The disease may not advance beyond this point but may progress to the fully developed syndrome.

Gastro-intestinal symptoms and signs

The gums become swollen and bleed easily (alpine scurvy). The tongue may be scarlet, raw and fissured and the lingual papillae atrophied. A characteristic symptom is pyrosis or a burning sensation in the oesophagus causing dysphagia. The appetite is variable. There is tenderness in the epigastrium and over the lower abdomen. There may be constipation but diarrhoea is common and the stools are often pale and fermenting, resembling those of sprue.

Skin lesions

The skin lesions appear on sites exposed to the sun and pressure. At first an erythema not unlike a severe sunburn is observed on the parts of the body which are as a rule unclothed and exposed to the sun (Plate VI). The eruption is symmetrical and characteristic. It appears suddenly first on the back of the hands and feet, then on the forearms, legs, chest, neck, face and sometimes on the scrotum and female genitalia, anus and other regions subject to mechanical pressure and irritation. The patches of erythema are irregular in outline and intensity. Very characteristic is a symmetrical eruption behind the mastoid process or a ring and collar round the neck (Casal's necklace, Plate VI). The affected area is swollen and tense and is the seat of burning or itching sensations, which become acute on exposure to the sun. The congestion disappears completely but temporarily on pressure. Petechiae are common on the affected parts; blebs with clear opaque or blood-stained contents of feebly alkaline reaction may form. The eruption usually lasts about a fortnight and is followed by hyperkeratosis and desquamation, which leaves the skin rough, thickened and permanently stained a light sepia. This is specially marked on the backs of the hands and on the elbows, thus constituting recognizable evidence of pellagra. There may be malar or supraorbital pigmentation. Hyperkeratosis may follow and involve the whole body. Linear haemorrhagic strips of purpura may occur after exposure to the sun and after trauma caused by increased permeability of the blood vessels (Simons 1946), and was observed in prisoners in Indonesia.

Pellagra differs in coloured races and erythema becomes a blackish or purplish patch on black skin. In olive-skinned races these appear sepia.

After the eruption has subsided atrophic patches of skin remain in the interdigital clefts and these, combined with wasting, produce the appearance of 'washerwoman's fingers'. The hands become aged and the nails atrophic and brittle.

Nervous system

The brain, cord and peripheral nervous system may all be involved.

Central nervous system. The time of appearance of mental symptoms is subject to the widest variations. They may be present from the start or occur during convalescence. The patient suffers from obstinate insomnia but occasionally from sleepiness. In general there is anxiety neurosis with dep essive features and depression is common. Psychosensory disturbances are common with intolerance of bright light, colours and noises and the patient becomes fidgety, quarrelsome and irritable. General deterioration of mental and physical health may antedate continued manifestations of disease or acute mania and confusion may herald the end.

Encephalopathy and nicotinic acid deficiency. Acute encephalopathic states associated with a deficiency of nicotinic acid are accompanied by an acute metabolic disturbance of a reversible nature (Spillane 1947). Certain stuporose and psychotic states in malnourished individuals have been found to respond in a significant manner to nicotinic acid. A certain clinical picture has been described of clouding of consciousness, cogwheel rigidity of the extremities and uncontrollable gasping and sucking reflexes. This syndrome has been observed in association with pellagra, alcoholism, polyneuritis, Wernicke's encephalopathy and scurvy. No response was obtained with thiamine, but after 1000 mg of nicotinic acid daily in divided doses parenterally, recovery occurred between the third and fifth days of treatment (Jolliffe *et al.* 1941). Stupor, delirium and acute psychotic symptoms are sometimes seen in association with a mild pellagrous rash and may respond dramatically to intravenous nicotinic acid.

Psychosis and pellagra. Pellagra may not only cause insanity but may result from it. It has been estimated that from 4 to 10% of patients with pellagra become permanently insane and in the U.S.A. pellagrins used to be numerous in the lunatic asylums. Not only may pellagra lead to insanity but those insane from other causes used to be very liable to pellagra. Goldberger and Wheeler (1920) found that in certain mental institutions in the U.S.A. the number of mentally insane developing pellagra was a constant proportion of the total. In a review of pellagra in asylums in England it was found that at the time of onset pellagrins had been resident from 6 months to several years. The type of psychosis is a most profound melancholia with suicidal tendencies preceded by restlessness and insomnia; it may closely resemble general paralysis of the insane. The mental aberration may be characterized by profound dementia, hallucinations and catatonia.

Spinal cord and peripheral nerve disturbances. Disturbance of the spinal cord or peripheral nerves may precede, accompany or follow the cutaneous, oral and alimentary lesions of pellagra. In the early stages of pellagra the neurological manifestations are commonly those of a psychoneurotic kind but later peripheral neuropathy or paraplegia of the ataxic or spastic type or a combination of both may develop. Cord changes are commoner than those of a neuropathy. Tremors and rigidity, possibly of extrapyramidal origin, may occur. Burning, tingling and aching feet suggest neuropathy; exaggerated knee jerks and extensor plantar responses suggest a pyramidal lesion and ataxic paraplegia is not uncommon in the late stages of pellagra. The cranial nerves may be involved and eighth nerve deafness, retrobulbar neuritis and central scotomas have all been recorded.

The variable incidence of these neurological complications in different pellagrous communities and the fact that they sometimes appear after recovery from pellagra and are resistant to treatment with nicotinic acid suggests that they are caused by associated vitamin B deficiencies and are not features of pure pellagra. They are considered more fully in nutritional neuropathies (page 783).

Associated vitamin B deficiencies

Ariboflavinosis with angular stomatitis and cheilosis may occur in the early stages of pellagra. Burning feet is a common symptom in pellagra and is probably associated with pantothenic acid deficiency.

Ocular changes

The eyes may be affected with oedema of the conjunctiva, corneal dystrophy and lens opacities of three types—powder-like, multiple irregular and tongue-like opacities extending from the peripheral zone towards the centre of the lens.

Progress

The symptoms may abate 2–3 months after onset and although the affected skin areas remain dark and rough the disease appears to be arrested. Next spring, however, if the diet is the same, it recurs in a more severe form. The eruption assumes a darker colour and the depression of spirits deepens into melancholia which may have maniacal interludes with a peculiar tendency to suicide. The general feeling of weakness increases, the patient loses weight and is unable to work and his gait becomes uncertain and of the spastic paraplegic type. The tongue is tremulous. The pains in the back become very acute and there may be lightning pains, cramps, twitching, tremors and even epileptiform convulsions of the cortical type. Diarrhoea becomes troublesome. The duration of pellagra is extremely variable: it may last only 2 or 3 years but usually extends to 10–15 or more.

SECONDARY PELLAGRA

Pellagra due to voluntary restriction of diet has been recognized for several years; slimming, ketogenic and faddist diets have all been responsible. It is stated that hyperthyroidism predisposes to pellagra.

Surgical pellagra

Pellagra may follow upon surgical operations on the gastro-intestinal tract, such as partial colectomy, total or partial gastrectomy. It may also be associated with some organic lesion in the gastro-intestinal tract, such as oesophageal stricture, carcinoma of the stomach, pyloric ulcer, pyloric stenosis, carcinoma of the ileum, stricture of the rectum, rectal polyposis, Crohn's disease, chronic intestinal amoebiasis and malabsorption syndromes such as coeliac disease and sprue. Failure of biosynthesis of vitamins is the probable cause in these cases.

Alcoholic pellagra

Alcoholic pellagra occurs especially in America in those who drink methyl alcohol; it is possible that chronic gastritis interferes with the production of intrinsic factor and the absorption of nicotinic acid.

Drug-induced pellagra

Isoniazid, which is used in the treatment of tuberculosis, may cause pellagra when administered in doses of more than 300 mg daily by displacing nicotinic acid in the oxidative reduction coenzyme DPN. In these cases extra nicotinic acid must be given along with the isoniazid. Sulphonamides are also capable of interfering with the action of nicotinic acid and may cause pellagrous rashes.

DIAGNOSIS

In acute pellagra the blood nicotinic acid has been found to be 0·31 mg/100 ml and to rise on treatment to 0·55 mg/100 ml. A combination of localized erythema of seasonal recurrence with neurological, particularly mental, disturbance in a person coming from an endemic pellagrous area is not likely to be confused with any other disease.

The rash may be mistaken for acrodynia, erythema multiforme, dermatitis venenata, lupus erythematosus or eczema solare. The combination of mental and neurological signs must be distinguished from hysteria, cerebrovascular syphilis, G.P.I., ergotism, lathyrism and other nutritional neuropathies. 'Pink disease' in children may also be mistaken for pellagra as the distribution of the skin lesions is similar.

TREATMENT

The most important part of the treatment of pellagra is to provide an ample and balanced diet and most pellagrins will improve as rapidly on a good hospital diet as on any other treatment. There is evidence that rapidly increasing the intake of one vitamin may precipitate imbalance and produce deficiency in another. A high-calorie diet is necessary—3000–4000 calories with good supplies of fresh meat, liver, milk, eggs and in addition a source of the vitamin B complex, such as yeast 25–50 grammes daily.

Nicotinic acid

Nicotinic acid should be given in doses of 50 mg 3 times a day for 10–14 days and double this quantity in severe cases. There is usually a reaction with tingling and warmth over the malar regions and neck. Overdosage may cause tingling and numbness of the tongue and lower jaw.

In acute mania or encephalopathy associated with pellagra intravenous nicotinic acid in large doses (1000 mg daily in divided doses) may cause a dramatic recovery. The spinal symptoms of pellagra are largely resistant to treatment, and nicotinic acid has not been of much use in chronic psychotic pellagrins (Sydenstricker *et al.* 1938).

Maize and sorghum, both associated with pellagra, contain large amounts of leucine, which affects the metabolism of tryptophan and nicotinic acid. Isoleucine counteracts this metabolic effect, and Krishnaswamy and Gopalan (1971) have treated pellagrous patients (sorghum eaters) with 5 grammes of isoleucine daily, curing them in about 15 days. Controls kept on the sorghum diet without isoleucine did not improve.

Riboflavine

Since ariboflavinosis frequently accompanies pellagra treatment should be reinforced with riboflavine 1–3 mg daily.

Parenterovite

Parenterovite is a multivitamin preparation which is of great use in the treatment of pellagra.

PREVENTION

Pellagra may be prevented by a change in the economic and social conditions that cause it. In institutions and prisons the diet must not be confined to maize meal but must include fresh fruit and vegetables and foods containing vitamin B. Hard physical work must be avoided when the diet is not of a good mixed nature.

ARIBOFLAVINOSIS

Aetiology

Riboflavine (vitamin B_2) is found in tissues as a dinucleotide, flavinadenine dinucleotide (FADN) or flavine, which occupies a key position in reactions leading to the oxidation of hydrogen to water. The main sources are meat, milk and wholemeal flour. Riboflavine is destroyed on exposure to light, and signs of riboflavine deficiency occur when the daily intake is 0·2–0·3 mg/1000 cal. A daily intake of 0·35–0·5 mg/1000 cal. is adequate. An average daily intake of 2 mg of riboflavine is considered adequate for an adult.

Signs

Sore red lips (cheilosis), a marked increase in the vertical fissuring of the lips (*perlêche*), a sodden fissured condition at the angles of the mouth (angular stomatitis) and a purplish raw tongue covered with granular enlarged papillae are among the most constant signs of ariboflavinosis (Bicknell & Prescott 1953). Other signs are facial lesions consisting of seborrheic excrescences (dyssebacia), varying in length up to 1 mm and sparsely scattered over the face (Fig. 226). The mouths of the sebaceous glands are plugged with inspissated sebum giving the skin a roughened appearance which, when it occurs on the shoulders, arms and legs, is known as follicular hyperkeratosis, phrynoderma, or toad's skin. This may, however, be a manifestation of vitamin A deficiency, and not caused by ariboflavinosis. Scrotal dermatitis, an eczematous condition of the scrotum

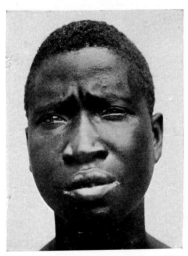

Fig. 226.—Avitaminosis B_2 in a West African Negro, showing the characteristic facies of ariboflavinosis. (*Dr D. Fitzgerald Moore*)

is due to ariboflavinosis. Ariboflavinosis frequently complicates other deficiency syndromes such as pellagra and protein–calorie malnutrition and was frequently associated with the deficiency syndromes occurring in prisoner-of-war camps in the Far East in World War II.

Treatment

Ariboflavinosis is quickly cured by the administration of 2–5 mg of riboflavine daily. Measures designed to improve the diet in a general manner and an increased diet of legumes, roots and animal proteins will prevent any deficiency.

REFERENCES

BECKH, W., ELLINGER, P. & SPEIS, T. D. (1937) *Lister Inst. prev. Med. coll. Pap.*, **33**, 4.
BICKNELL, F. & PRESCOTT, T. (1953) *The Vitamins in Medicine*, 3rd ed. London: Heinemann.
BRAY, G. W. (1928) *Trans. R. Soc. trop. Med. Hyg.*, **22**, 9.
BRIGDEN, R. W. & ROBINSON, J. (1964) *Br. med. J.*, **ii**, 1238.

DE WARDENER, H. E. & LENNOX, B. (1947) *Lancet*, **i**, 11.

FEHILY, L. (1944) *Br. med. J.*, **ii**, 591.

GOLDBERGER, J. & WHEELER, G. A. (1920) *Archs intern. Med.*, **25**, 451.

HAWES, R. B. (1938) *Trans. R. Soc. trop. Med. Hyg.*, **31**, 474.

JELLIFFE, D. B. (1955) *Monograph Ser. W.H.O.*, 29.

——— & JELLIFFE, E. F. P. (1961) *J. Pediat.*, **59**, 271.

JOLLIFFE, N., WORTIS, H. & FEIN, H. D. (1941) *Archs Neurol. Psychiat.*, **46**, 569.

KRISHNASWAMY, K. & GOPALAN, C. (1971) *Lancet*, **ii**, 1167.

SATO, A. (1964) *Tokuku J. exp. Med.*, **83**, 103.

SIMONS, R. D. G. P. (1946) *Ned. Tijdschr. Geneesk.*, **90**, 351.

SIMPSON, I. A. & CHOW, A. J. (1956) *J. trop. Pediat.*, **2**, 3.

SPILLANE, J. D. (1947) *Nutritional Disorders of the Nervous System*. Edinburgh: Livingstone.

SYDENSTRICKER, V. P., SCHMIDT, H. L., FULTON, M. C., NEWS, J. S. & GEESLIN, L. E. (1938) *Sth med. J., Nashville*, **31**, 1155.

WALTERS, J. H. & SMITH, D. A. (1952) *W. Afr. med. J.*, **1**, 21.

WEISS, S. & WILKINS, R. W. (1937) *Ann. intern. Med.*, **2**, 104.

WENKEBACH, K. A. (1928) *Lancet*, **2**, 265.

40. NUTRITIONAL NEUROPATHIES

THIS group of disorders includes a variety of syndromes which fall into three main categories (Cruickshank 1969):

The vitamin deficiencies

Vitamin B_1 : Dry beri-beri, Wernicke's encephalopathy.
Vitamin B_6 : Pyridoxine deficiency induced by drugs.
Vitamin B_{12}: Subacute combined degeneration of the cord in pernicious anaemia.
Pantothenic acid deficiency (burning feet syndrome).

The toxic neuropathies

Lathyrism.
Other lateral sclerosis syndromes.

A wide range of neuropathies of uncertain aetiology

These occur either individually or in combination and include retrobulbar neuropathy, eighth nerve deafness and cord syndromes which may be purely motor, purely sensory or a mixture of both.

VITAMIN DEFICIENCIES

Vitamin B_1 deficiencies have been discussed on page 763.

Pyridoxine

Pyridoxine and its derivatives and their phosphates (the vitamin B_6 group) act as coenzymes for many of the metabolic reactions of amino acids including the transamination reactions. Pyridoxine deficiency may occur in patients undergoing treatment with isoniazid for tuberculosis. The symptoms of pyridoxine deficiency under these circumstances are pains in the soles of the feet which can be cured by adding 10 mg pyridoxine daily to the dose of isoniazid.

Burning feet syndrome

Synonyms. Chachaleh (Buchanan 1932; Somalia); barasheh; kalerichal; Gopalan syndrome (Gopalan 1946); dysaesthetic phenomenon (Spillane 1947), pyralgia; melalgia; happy feet.

Definition. A disorder in which 'burning feet' has been the only or outstanding complaint, probably due to a deficiency of pantothenic acid.

Aetiology. Pantothenic acid occurs in nearly all foodstuffs, being especially rich in liver, kidneys and yeast. The bran of cereals is a good source. It is concerned as a dinucleotide referred to as coenzyme A with reactions involving the active form of organic acids. Volunteers in whom pantothenic acid deficiency was induced by an antagonist, omega-methyl pantothenic acid, developed burning pains in the feet which rapidly improved on the addition of pantothenic acid to the diet (Cruickshank 1960).

Geographical distribution. Before World War II 'burning feet' was common in Malaya (Dugdale 1928), Somalia (Buchanan 1932), India (Gopalan 1946) and West Africa. It was common among prisoners-of-war in the Far East during World War II and in German prisoners-of-war in the Middle East (Spillane 1947).

Symptoms and signs. The symptoms commence slowly, taking some months to develop, with a deep aching in the soles of the feet spreading to the toes and instep, until eventually the whole of both feet is involved with the most acute 'pins and needles'. The pain is worse at night so that the legs are kept outside the blankets. The condition progresses with excruciating pain shooting up and down the feet and calves. The palms of the hands are only rarely involved. There is no erythromelalgia. Signs of peripheral neuropathy are minimal with some analgesia to pin prick and light touch of stocking distribution and diminution of the knee and ankle jerks. Most of the advanced cases exhibit signs of associated deficiencies with retrobulbar neuritis, eighth nerve palsy and ariboflavinosis.

Treatment. The condition responds well to the administration of yeast and other products rich in vitamin B as well as to pantothenic acid.

TOXIC NEUROPATHIES

Pathophysiology of toxic and nutritional neuropathies

An intact nervous system depends upon a series of intricate biochemical reactions. A variety of factors operating at different levels can produce selective damage to the most susceptible tissues. Those parts of the nervous system which carry the heaviest metabolic load are the upper motor neuron, first sensory neuron for proprioception and the optic and auditory nerves. The aetiological agent varies and may be a vitamin deficiency, a toxin or a combination of the two. Some of the toxins responsible are thought to be organic complexes in which cyanide is bound.

Chronic cyanide intoxication

A variety of compounds basically of the nitrite configuration which contain the cyanide radicle have been isolated from the *Lathyrus* family of legumes which have produced mesenchymal damage in rats. The cycad nut which is consumed by the Chamorros in Guam contains a substance with a cyanide radicle which is thought to be an aminonitrile. Cyanide radicles are found in quantity in cassava and certain of the yam family, but are normally removed by cooking. These roots form a major part of the diet in Africa and the West Indies.

Lathyrism

Definition. A neurological disease in which changes take place in the lateral columns of the spinal cord, characterized by ataxic spastic paraplegia and caused by a toxic agent in the pea *Lathyrus sativus*.

Aetiology. The disease occurs in Ethiopia, Algeria and India in the districts in which vetches, 'khashari', *Lathyrus sativus* and allied species are the staple food. There are two varieties of vetch, one larger called 'lakh' or 'teova', the other smaller called 'takhori' or 'teovi'. Cyanide-containing compounds have been isolated from the lathyrus family. *Lathyrus sativus* is more drought resistant and as the percentage of *Lathyrus* consumed rises during droughts so the incidence of paraplegia increases, especially among active young males.

Pathology. The lateral columns of the spinal cord are chiefly affected by a demyelinating process although associated posterior column changes have been described (Buzzard & Greenfield 1921).

Signs and symptoms. The disease is very chronic. There is gradual onset of a spastic paraplegia which causes a typical 'scissors gait' (Fig. 227). Incontinence of urine and impotence are common and early symptoms. Ataxia due to posterior column changes is less marked but is found in advanced cases.

Treatment. It is claimed that cases rapidly improve on dietetic and vitamin treatment.

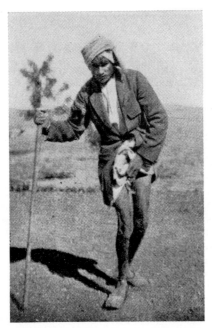

Fig. 227.—Scissors gait due to adductor spasm in lathyrism. (*Reproduced from McCombie & Young* (1927) *Indian J. med. Res.*, **15**, 453)

Amyotrophic lateral sclerosis syndrome

A hereditary form of paralysis has been known to occur on Guam for many years which was reported as amyotrophic lateral sclerosis after World War II (Koerner 1952). In nearly 10% of the population of Chamorros on the island a syndrome occurs which closely resembles amyotrophic lateral sclerosis. It is familial and accounts for 10% of all deaths among adults. The disease shows the same high incidence in Guamanians who have emigrated to other islands. There is no essential difference between the clinical and histological features of the Guamanian and sporadic cases of amyotrophic lateral sclerosis observed elsewhere in the world, except that other tissue abnormalities are found in association with the condition on Guam. A cycad nut, which contains a nitrile compound, is extensively consumed on Guam. It is possible that a toxic factor acting against a strong familial background is responsible for this disease (Kurland 1962).

Parkinsonian dementia complex (Kurland 1962)

A progressive and fatal neurological disease also occurs on Guam which accounts for the death of 7% of Chamorros. It is familial and closely related to the amyotrophic lateral sclerosis syndrome. The mean age of onset is 50; males outnumber females by 3 to 1 and death occurs after 3–5 years. There is progressive mental degeneration with Parkinsonism. Pathologically there is cortical and pallidal atrophy and depigmentation of the substantia nigra, with widespread ganglion cell degeneration without inflammatory changes. These changes are widespread throughout the frontal and temporal lobes and the substantia nigra and tegmenta of the brain stem.

NEUROPATHIES OF UNCERTAIN AETIOLOGY

This group includes retrobulbar neuropathy, cord syndromes with the pyramidal tracts affected alone or in combination with the posterior columns and eighth nerve disturbances.

These syndromes have been described from many parts of the tropical world—Malaya (Landor & Pallister 1935), Central Africa (Stannus 1936), Ceylon (Nichols 1933), Jamaica (central neuritis; Scott 1918; Cruickshank et al. 1960), Nigeria (Money 1960) and in World War II prisoners-of-war (Spillane 1947).

Aetiology

No evidence of vitamin B_{12} deficiency has been found, but recent research in Nigeria (Monekosso 1968) has shown foci of endemic neuropathy in areas where cassava is consumed as a farina called 'gari'. The cassava is inadequately peeled and the cyanide is not removed. The close relationship between vitamin B_{12} and cyanide, which has already been described, may be responsible for these neuropathic syndromes.

Pathology

There are widespread patches of demyelination with a peripheral distribution affecting chiefly the posterior and lateral columns. There is perivascular inflammation involving the vessels of the pia arachnoid and spreading into the cord via the penetrating vessels.

Clinical manifestations

The presenting features of these syndromes vary in different areas. Severe posterior column damage, retrobulbar neuropathy and eighth nerve deafness are the commonest presenting features. Pyramidal tract damage is rare and the burning feet syndrome is intermediate in occurrence. There is a striking difference between the cases described from Africa, where there is a low incidence of pyramidal tract damage, and Jamaica, where the incidence is very high (Cruickshank 1969).

Treatment

In any one case it may not be possible to find out whether a toxic substance (cyanide) or a vitamin deficiency is the major factor. The diet should be a good mixed one and possible cyanide-containing staples must be avoided. Large doses of vitamin B_{12} (0·1 mg daily for 12–14 days), vitamin B_1, pantothenic acid and pyridoxine should all be administered. Response to treatment is poor and not much improvement can be expected in advanced cases.

REFERENCES

BUCHANAN, J. C. R. (1932) *Trans. R. Soc. trop. Med. Hyg.*, **25**, 383.

BUZZARD, E. F. & GREENFIELD, J. G. (1921) *Pathology of the Nervous System.* London: Constable.

CRUICKSHANK, E. K. (1960) *Control of Malnutrition in Man.* American Public Health Association.

────── (1969) in *Neurological Disorders in the Tropics* (ed. Williams, D.). London: Butterworths.

DUGDALE, J. N. (1928) *Malay med. J.*, **3**, 74.

GOPALAN, C. (1946) *Indian med. Gaz.*, **81**, 22.

KOERNER, D. R. (1952) *Ann. intern. Med.*, **37**, 1204.

KURLAND, L. T. (1962) quoted by Cruickshank (1969).

LANDOR, J. V. & PALLISTER, R. A. (1935) *Trans. R. Soc. trop. Med. Hyg.*, **29**, 121.

MONEKOSSO, G. L. (1968) *Abbottempo*, **3**, 6.

MONEY, G. L. (1960) *W. Afr. med. J.*, **9**, 3.

NICHOLS, L. (1933) *Indian med. Gaz.*, **68**, 681.

SCOTT, H. H. (1918) *Ann. trop. Med. Parasit.*, **12**, 109.

SPILLANE, J. D. (1947) *Nutritional Disorders of the Nervous System.* Edinburgh: Livingstone.

STANNUS, H. S. (1936) *Trop. Dis. Bull.*, **33**, 729.

SECTION XIII

POISONS

41. CHIGGERS, MITES AND ANIMAL POISONS

THE CHIGGER OR SANDFLEA

This insect, formerly confined to the tropical parts of America (30° N. to 30° S.) and to the West Indies, appeared on the West Coast of Africa for the first time about the year 1872. Since that date it has spread all over the tropical parts of that continent, and even to some of the adjacent islands—Madagascar, for example. As a cause of suffering, invaliding and indirectly of death from secondary infections, it is an insect of some importance. It is now extremely prevalent on the East Coast of Africa, whence it has been introduced into India.

The chigger (*Tunga penetrans*) is not unlike the common flea either in appearance or, with one exception, in habit. It is somewhat smaller (1 mm), the head being proportionately larger and the abdomen deeper than in the flea. It is red or reddish brown. Like the flea, its favourite haunt is dry, sandy soil, the dust and ashes in badly kept huts, the stables of cattle, poultry pens, and the like. It greedily attacks all warm-blooded animals, including birds and man.

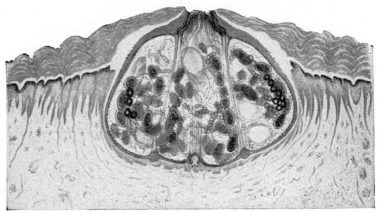

Fig. 228.—Section of a female chigger in the stratum lucidum of the skin. (*Fülleborn*)

Until impregnated, the female, like the male, is free, feeding intermittently as opportunity offers. As soon as she becomes impregnated she burrows diagonally into the skin of the first warm-blooded animal she encounters where, being well nourished by the blood, she proceeds to ovulation. By the end of this process her abdomen, in consequence of the growth of the eggs it contains, has attained the size of a small pea (Fig. 228). As seen in Fig. 228, the chigger within the

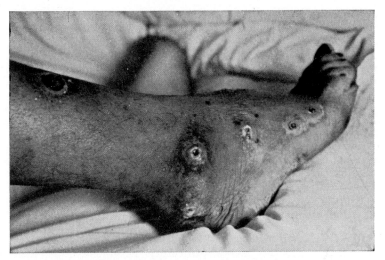

Fig. 229.—Septic lesions of the foot caused by chiggers.

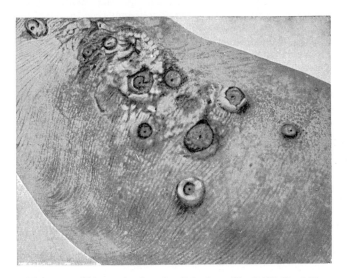

Fig. 230.—Chiggers in the sole of the foot. (*Dr C. W. Daniels*)

epidermis enters the stratum lucidum, which it invades and pushes before it. (See also Appendix III.)

The chigger is not a good jumper and therefore she seldom attacks the skin of the leg *above* the dorsum of the foot.

The soles (Fig. 230), the skin between the toes, and that at the roots of the nails are favourite situations. Other parts of the body are by no means exempt; the scrotum, the penis, the skin around the anus, the thighs and even the hands and face are often attacked. Usually only 1 or 2 chiggers are found at a time;

occasionally they are present in hundreds, the little pits left after their extraction, or expulsion, being sometimes so closely set that parts of the surface may look like a honeycomb.

During her gestation the chigger causes a considerable amount of irritation. In consequence of this, pus may form around her distended abdomen, which now raises the inflamed integument into a pea-like elevation. After the eggs are laid (according to some, before this process) the superjacent skin ulcerates, and the chigger is expelled, leaving a small sore which may be infected by some pathogenic micro-organism, such as the organisms causing phagedaena or tetanus, with grave consequences (Fig. 229).

Ulceration is common, and may follow removal of the chigger or natural extrusion of the egg-sac. The ulcer commences as a tiny pit and, as it extends, the sloping edge may develop into a septic ulcer. It remains more or less circular in outline, except under the nail or nail margin, where the outline is more irregular and a pocket of pus forms underneath it. Chronic absorption of pus may lead to thrombophlebitis.

Treatment

In chigger regions the houses, particularly the ground floors, must be frequently swept and accumulations of dust and debris prevented. The housing of cattle, pigs and poultry demands the same precautions. The floors should often be sprinkled with carbolic water, pyrethrum powder, DDT or similar insecticide, and walking bare-footed must be avoided. A daily bath must be taken, and any chiggers that may have fastened themselves on the skin at once removed. They may be killed by pricking them with a needle, or by the application of chloroform, turpentine, mercurial ointment or similar means, after which they are expelled by ulceration. The best treatment, however, is not to wait for ulceration, but to enlarge the orifice of entrance with a sharp, clean needle and neatly to enucleate the insect entire. Some women, from long practice, are experts at this little operation. The part must be dressed antiseptically and protected until healed. A daily inspection of the feet, especially under the nails, is advisable. Should any black dot be discovered, the chigger should be removed at once.

Prophylaxis

If avoidable, camps should not be formed in chigger-infested spots or in the neighbourhood of existing villages. The camping-ground should be swept or, if necessary, fired; the floors of huts and tents may be sprayed with DDT and naphthalene. Balfour recommended that the feet be rubbed thoroughly with a mixture consisting of 5 drops of Lysol, or liq. cresol. sap., in 28 grammes of soft paraffin. Special attention should be paid to the interdigital clefts. Pigs should not be kept in the vicinity of dwelling-houses, as these animals are severely attacked by chiggers.

ACARINE DERMATOSIS

Several forms of mites inhabiting sugar, grain or copra may live as temporary parasites on the skin of man, and set up an intense irritation not unlike that produced by scabies. One of the most familiar of these is 'grocer's itch', set up by mites of the genus *Glyciphagus*, which are common in raw sugar and cause an erythematous rash. Among the copra workers in Ceylon and the Pacific islands a similar skin affection is due to *Tyroglyphus*. 'Grain itch', an urticarial and papular eruption of the exposed parts of the body, is caused by *Pediculoides ventricosus* (Fig. 231) in those who handle grain, cotton seeds or beans. These mites give rise to a severe pruritus. Preventive treatment consists in the application of 5% betanaphthol ointment, and dilute phenol solution to kill the mites. Preparations of gamma benzene hexachloride may be used.

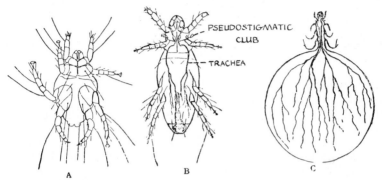

Fig. 231.—*Pediculoides ventricosus.* A, Male. B, Adult female. C, Pregnant female with brood sac. (*After Alcock*) × 80.

NUNEZ ANDRADE'S DISEASE

A parasitic dermatitis resulting from the bites of the larvae of *Neoschöngastia nunezi* is found in Brazil. Molluscoid lesions are accompanied by pruritus. This insect, 0·33–0·45 mm in length, is a common parasite of fowls and produces petechiae of the skin resembling spots of ground brick.

Haematosiphoniasis in Mexico is due to bites of *Haematosiphon inodora*— locally known as *chinche de los gallos* (chicken bug), an insect 5 × 3 mm, which is greenish-red in colour. It produces a polymorphous dermatitis with pustules, scabs and linear scars.

DERMATOSES AND DERMATITIS DUE TO BUTTERFLIES, MOTHS, BEETLES AND CATERPILLARS

Leger, Mougels and Bozé have described urticaria, conjunctivitis and facial oedema due to contact with a saturniid moth, *Hylesia urticans*, in French Guiana. In Celebes similar lesions are evoked by another, *Scirpophaga innotata*. The dorsal sides of the wings of this moth are covered with a greyish-white powder which is the irritating agent.

Le Gac and colleagues describe a similar dermatitis due to a moth, *Anaphe renata*. The imago and the larvae are clothed with detachable irritating hairs. Africans as well as Europeans are affected in Equatorial Africa. Similar moths occur also in Ghana. In Brazil flannel moths (*Megalopygidae*) are well known.

In Texas the 'puss caterpillar', *Megalopyge opercularis*, produces thousands of cases of dermatitis in children, necessitating the closing of schools.

In Japan it was reported in 1955 that the poisonous moth *Euproctis slava* had affected 300 000 people, two-thirds of them in Nagoya.

Caterpillar dermatitis is common in the northern parts of Kenya; in Israel every year it is prevalent in the months of February and May, caused by the hairs of *Thaumatopoea pinivora*. In Israel *T. wilkinsoni* also appears to be implicated (Ziprkowski *et al.* 1959).

The nests of moths appear in pine trees and have become more numerous as the result of afforestation. Skin irritation and conjunctivitis last 2–8 days. Only the hairs of the caterpillar contain the irritant. Epidemics of urticaria have been described in troops in New Guinea and others have been recorded in N. Australia due to a moth, *Ochrogaster contraria*. Some developed urticaria within a few minutes. Caterpillar urticaria is common in the Panama Canal Zone due to *Megalopygida lanata* which produces rapidly developing eosinophilia (8–22%), numbness and vesication. It is pale yellow, 5 cm long by 1·5 cm. The body is covered with long black hairs.

Beetle dermatitis

Canthariasis is due to beetles of the family *Meloidae* which contain a cytotoxic principle, cantharidin, which, when applied to the skin, produces vesicular dermatitis. The Staphylinidae (rove beetles) embrace forms with vesiculating properties. They occur in Java, tropical S. and E. Africa and in S. America.

Two species of *Sessinea* (coconut beetles) cause burning pains at the point of contact, followed by large blisters.

Earle has described 'fuetazo dermatitis' in those engaged in oil exploration on the coast of Ecuador. This is caused by a blackish-green beetle (*Paederus ornaticornis*), 1 cm in length. 'Fuetazo' is said to be Spanish for whiplash.

A variety of lesions are caused by contact with the secretions of this insect, the most common of which is a papulo-vesicular rash.

BEE AND WASP STINGS

The stings of hymenoptera of the tropics resemble those of temperate climates, but can be more severe. Stinging bees, *Apis indica* and *A. florea*, the small bee, as well as the giant Indian bee, *Apis dorsata*, may attack in swarms in temples and caves, and may cause death. In N. Africa the species is *A. mellifica addisoni*. The antidote is injection of adrenaline. Sensitization may ensue leading to anaphylaxis which may be fatal. A parasitic wasp in Tokyo is *Scleroderma nipponensis* of which the female is ant-like and wingless. In one incident 340 people were attacked, showing reddish swellings and injuries leading to suppuration and lymphangitis.

Massive anaphylaxis causes muscular paralysis and suggests a curare-like action at synapses of muscle end plates. Hymenoptera venoms contain histamine, acetylcholine and enzymes. 5-Hydroxytryptamine is a constituent of wasp venom which is distinctly more active than that of the honey bee.

There is often a history of allergy in patients who react badly to stings, and symptoms may include shock, vomiting, cyanosis, diarrhoea and abdominal cramps, dyspnoea and laryngeal stridor—tracheostomy may even be needed. Besides adrenaline, oral antihistamines are valuable, and in acute cases steroids may be used. Stings should be scraped, as forceps may express further venom from the sac attached to the sting.

Marshall (1957) finds that toxic reactions resemble those of rattlesnake poisoning with haemolytic and neurotoxic effects. Allergic shock develops quickly, in the course of 20–30 minutes. In bees hypersensitivity is believed to be due to water-soluble protein derived from its body. Wasps, being scavengers, may introduce bacteria with their stings.

POISONOUS SNAKES

For a full discussion of poisonous snakes, see Bucherl *et al.* (1968) and Russell (1965).

Snakes form a sub-order of the reptiles and have definite characters. The quadrate bone is articulated to the skull, but there is no tympanic cavity. The brain capsule is osseous and the mandibles are united mesially by a highly elastic ligament. The limb girdles are absent or reduced to mere vestiges. A peculiar feature is that there are no movable eyelids, but the eyes are covered with a transparent disc, which is shed with the rest of the epidermis. The tongue is deeply bifid and is retractile into a basal sheath; but is protrusible when the mouth is closed through a notch in the rostral shield (Fig. 232). As in the lizards, the anal cleft is transverse.

Characters used for identification and classification

Osteological and dental characters are employed to determine families and genera, and it is therefore necessary to understand the various types of ophidian

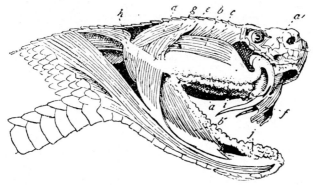

Fig. 232.—Poison apparatus, venom gland and muscles of the rattlesnake (lateral view). (*After Duvernoy*)

a, Venom gland. *a'*, Venom duct. *b*, Anterior temporal muscle. *b'*, Mandibular portion of the same. *c*, Posterior temporal muscle. *d*, Digastricus muscle. *e*, Posterior ligament of gland. *f*, Sheath of fang. *g*, Middle temporal muscle. *h*, External pterygoid muscle. *i*, Maxillary salivary gland. *j*, Mandibular salivary gland.

skulls and the different arrangement of fangs and solid teeth. For generic and specific distinctions the form and number of the epidermal shields and scales are of great importance.

The arrangement of the scales on the head is shown in Fig. 233, and that of the prefrontal and preocular scales varies in different species and genera. In the crotalidae, or pit vipers, there is a sensory uveal pit situated between the eye and the nostril. Viperine snakes can generally be distinguished from the colubrinae by their smaller size, the angular shape of the head, and the sharp stumpy tail. The maxillae are vertically erectile, with enormously enlarged tubular fangs situated anteriorly (Fig. 234).

The more important poisonous snakes

The poisonous snakes are distributed among the following families and subfamilies:

(a) *Viperidae,* or true vipers, found only in the Old World.

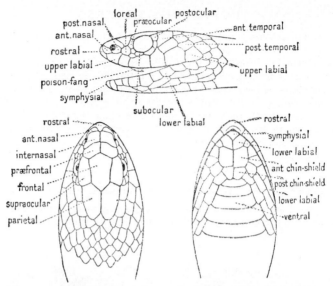

Fig. 233.—Head shields of *Causus rhombeatus*. (*After Boulenger*)

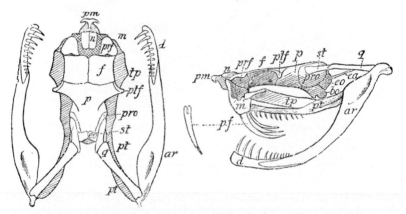

Fig. 234.—Skull of *Trimeresurus gramineus*, upper view and side view.
(*After Boulenger*)

ar, Articular, *bo*, Basioccipital. *ca*, Columella auris. *d*, Dentary. *eo*, Exoccipital. *f*, Frontal.
m, Maxillary, *n*, Nasal. *p*, Parietal. *pf*, Poison fang. *pm*, Praemaxillary. *prf*, Praefrontal.
pro, Prootic. *pt*, Pterygoid. *ptf*, Postfrontal. *q*, Quadrate. *st*, Supratemporal. *tp*, Transpalatine.

(*b*) *Crotalidae*, or pit vipers, found in the New World and in Asia.

(*c*) *Elapidae*, represented by coral snakes and cobras, found in all continents
except Europe.

(*d*) *Colubridae*, to which nearly two-thirds of the known species of snakes
belong, but in which the only poisonous varieties are some of the rear-
fanged reptiles seldom found outside Africa.

(*e*) *Hydrophinae*, or sea snakes, which can be dangerous, especially to
fishermen in Malaysia.

The Americas

Two families, the Crotalidae and the Elapidae, are present in U.S.A. The pit vipers (Crotalidae) are abundant and the presence of 35 species and sub-species has been established, including the true rattlesnakes, the pigmy rattlers and the 'massasauga' of the genus *Sistrurus*, the 'copperhead' (*Ancistrodon contortrix*) and the 'water mocassin' (*A. piscivorus*). The family Elapidae is represented by coral snakes. Poisonous snakes are more abundant in South and Central America than in Northern America. In the two former, the majority of fatalities are caused by members of the Crotalidae, especially the tropical rattlesnake (*Crotalus terrificus*) and the members of the genus *Bothrops* (*B. atrox* or *fer-de-lance, B. jararaca, B. schlegeli*) and the bushmaster (*Lachesis muta*).

In Brazil the number of annual snakebite deaths is about 2000 (a death rate of 4 per 100 000).

The large majority of deaths occur from the bite of *C. terrificus, Bothrops jararaca, B. jararacussu* and *B. alternata*.

In Trinidad, Tobago and West Indies, the most poisonous species is *B. atrox* (*fer-de-lance*). The coral snake (*Micrurus corallinus*) is also found.

Asia

All families containing venomous snakes are represented from West Pakistan to Malaysia. The region includes countries with the highest snakebite death rates in the world.

The vast majority of deaths are caused by Viperidae (true vipers) and the Elapidae (cobras and kraits).

In Burma an average of 2000 deaths from snakebite are registered every year. The mortality is highest there, where the annual snakebite death rate is about 15·4 per 100 000 population.

The majority of deaths are caused by Russell's viper or 'daboia' (*Vipera russelli*).

Cobras and kraits (*Bungarus*) account for the large proportion of the snakebite mortality. In Ceylon the death rate is 4·2 per 100 000. Russell's viper (*Vipera russelli*), the cobra (*Naja naja*) and the Indian krait (*Bungarus caeruleus*) are the most dangerous. The Malayan pit viper is *Ancistrodon rhodostoma*.

India and Pakistan. In India, before partition, the recorded snake-bite deaths were from 10 000 to 15 000 a year. The later annual death rate from snakebite is 5·4 per 100 000 population. The largest numbers of deaths are reported from Bengal, Uttar Pradesh, Madras, Bombay and Bihar. The area of highest snake-bite mortality is in W. Bengal in the Delta of the Ganges, in certain districts, Dinajpur, Nadia, Murshi-dabad and Midnapore.

Cobra (*Naja naja, N. hannah* or 'hamadryad'), krait (*Bungarus caeruleus, B. fasciatus*), Russell's viper or 'daboia', and *Echis carinatus* are the commonest terrestrial poisonous snakes in India and Pakistan. There are a few other species of poisonous snakes, such as the green pit viper (*Trimeresurus gramineus*), the coral snake (*Calliophis*) and the Himalayan pit viper, *Ancistrodon*, which seldom inflict fatal bites.

In Thailand (Siam) deaths from snakebite total 1·3 per 100 000. The large majority occur from the bites of the cobras (*Naja naja* and *N. hannah*), kraits (*Bungarus caeruleus, B. fasciatus*), coral snakes, *Calliophis, Doliophis* and Russell's viper.

Australia

There are over 70 poisonous snakes. The most aggressive is the tiger snake (*Notechis scutatus*), which is responsible for a high percentage of the deaths. The 'taipan' (*Oxyuranus scutellaris*) and the 'death adder' (*Acanthopis antarcticus*) are specially active and dangerous in the sandy areas. The brown snake (*Demansia textilis*) and the Australian black snake (*Pseudechis porphyriacus*) are widely distributed.

In Papua and New Guinea the venomous snakes are Elapidae—the taipan (*Oxyuranus scutellatus canni*), the death adder (*Acanthopis antarcticus rugosus*), and the Papuan black snake (*Pseudechis papuanus*).

In Japan the 'mamushi' (*Ancistrodon blomhoffi*) is the most common poisonous snake.

Africa

It is estimated that the annual snakebite deaths average 800 which gives the death rate of 0·4 per 100 000. There are no poisonous snakes in Mauritius, Seychelles, Madagascar and Comoro Islands.

The following are the most dangerous:

Viperidae: *Bitis* (*arietans, gabonica, nasicornis*), *Echis carinatus*, *Causus rhombeatus* or 'night adder'. Elapidae: *Naja* (*nigricollis, melanoleuca, haje*), *Dendraspis* or 'black mamba' (*angusticeps, jamesoni, viridis*), *Dispholidus typus* or 'boomslang', the ringhals or spitting cobra (*Sepedon haemachates*).

Europe

The only poisonous snakes found in Europe and in N. Asia belong to the family Viperidae. Of this family the common viper or adder (*Vipera berus*) is most extensively distributed, and is the only poisonous species in the British Isles. The asp (*V. aspis*) is found in S. France, S. Italy, Yugoslavia, the Apennines and Pyrenees.

The long-nosed viper (*V. ammodytes*) occurs in Austria, Yugoslavia (Bosnia) and other Balkan countries. *V. renardi* is found in the Crimea and parts of E. Russia extending into Central Asia.

It is estimated that 50 deaths occur annually due to bites of vipers in Europe.

Poison apparatus and venom

The poison apparatus consists of a pair of venom-secreting glands connected by ducts to the poison fangs in the maxillae; they are analogous to the parotid glands in mammals. These glands, situated in the temporal regions, are operated during the act of biting, when they are squeezed by the contraction of the temporal muscle, the venom being expelled by means of the grooved or tubular fangs (Fig. 232). In the African 'spitting cobras' the venom, which contains an active haemolytic and anticoagulant factor, is ejected with great force into the face of the enemy.

In striking, the snake throws itself forward with great violence. On the whole vipers strike with greater velocity than colubrines. Most strike with the jaws closed, but as the head approaches the victim, the mandibles are depressed by rapid contraction of the digastric and other muscles and simultaneously the fangs are elevated and rotated forward. The fangs of colubrines are grooved and shorter than those of vipers. Closure of the jaw is brought about by the simultaneous contraction of the temporal muscles which strongly elevate the mandible (Fig. 235). In vipers, expulsion of the venom is instantaneous, and independent of fixation of the lower jaw. Immediately after the insertion of the fangs and accompanying discharge of venom, contraction of the retractor muscles drags the elevated fangs downwards and backwards through the tissues. Impression of the fangs and the pterygopalatine indentations may be made in Kerr's impression compound of dental wax, and by this method it has been found that the distance between the fang punctures affords a fair index to the venom yield. Death may follow inoculation from a single fang. Snakes, especially the poisonous species, are nocturnal or semi-nocturnal, and are generally believed to bite most commonly at night; it has been shown, however, that the cobra bites as frequently by day as by night.

The lethal dose of venom varies within wide limits when tested on different species of animals. The numbers of certainly lethal doses for sheep, in the average yields of various snakes, were found by Fairley to be: 118 for the Australian tiger snake (*Notechis scutatus*), 31·7 for the cobra, 2·2 for Russell's

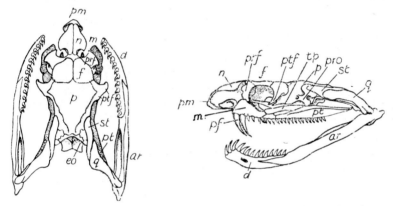

Fig. 235.—Skull of *Naja naja*, upper view and side view. (*After Boulenger*)
ar, Articular. *d*, Dentary. *eo*, Exoccipital. *f*, Frontal. *m*, Maxillary. *n*, Nasal. *p*, Parietal. *pf*, Poison fang. *pm*, Praemaxillary. *prf*, Praefrontal. *pro*, Prootic. *pt*, Pterygoid. *ptf*, Postfrontal. *q*, Quadrate. *st*, Supratemporal. *tp*, Transpalatine.

viper, 84·7 for the Australian death-adder (*Acanthopis antarcticus*), 8·9 for the copperhead (*Denisonia superba*), and 1·5 for the black snake (*Pseudechis porphyriacus*).

The *venom*, a clear, amber-coloured fluid, is composed of modified proteins. It is of 3 kinds; that of the Viperidae (vipers) acts principally upon the vascular system, but that of the Colubridae and Elapidae, i.e. cobras, acts upon the nervous system and brings about respiratory paralysis; that of Hydrophinae (sea snakes) is myotoxic and causes muscle necrosis. The complexity of venoms is determined by physical methods, such as electrophoresis, cross-neutralization tests with different venoms and anti-sera. Antisera for one venom can neutralize venoms of other snakes belonging to the same family. There is more than one proteolytic enzyme in cobra venom and also a haemolytic ferment and a phospholipase. A venom, in general, consists of a mixture of several individual proteins which constitute 90–92% of its dry weight. Elapid venom contains a highly potent neurotoxin, cobra venom a haemolysin. A cardiotoxin has also recently been isolated. The presence of an acetylcholine as a hydrolysing enzyme has been proved by Iyengar.

Hyaluronidase, as a spreading factor, is present in most venoms and is surprisingly high in that of the common krait (*Bungarus caeruleus*).

Viper venom contains two factors, a haemorrhagic vasculotoxic factor and a procoagulant defibrinating factor. A fibrinogen-consuming substance has been isolated from Malayan viper venom and has been used commercially as an anticoagulant, Arvin (Esnoub & Tullah 1967).

Russell's viper bites are characterized by haemorrhagic, haemolytic and nephrotoxic features. More recently neurotoxic features have also been described (Visuvaratnam *et al.* 1970).

The toxin of the venom of the tropical rattlesnake (*Crotalus t. terrificus*) contains crotamine which produces paralysis in experimental animals. It is composed of a proteolytic enzyme which clots fibrinogen and a neurotoxin which corresponds to crototoxin.

Naja nigricollis in Rhodesia and S. Africa is one of the spitting cobras and can eject venom as far as 2 m and can aim at the eye of its victims. It causes extremely painful conjunctivitis which subsides only after several days. The eye should be washed out with milk alone or in a solution of potassium permanganate and a few drops of antivenene instilled into it.

SYMPTOMS OF SNAKEBITE IN MAN

The physiological action and symptoms produced by snake venoms can be classified into three groups, related to the Elapidae (cobras), vipers, and seasnakes.

Cobras

In cobra bite (Fig. 236) (*Naja naja*) there is severe pain and the part becomes inflamed and oedematous. Early signs are slight ptosis, nasal voice, and paralysis of the extrinsic muscles of the eyes, with nausea, vomiting, salivation, and paralysis of tongue and larynx. There may be haematuria or melaena. Soon the

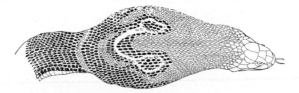

Fig. 236.—The cobra (*Naja naja*).

respiratory centre becomes involved and respiration ceases entirely. Should the patient survive the paralysis, recovery is rapid. The pupil is contracted throughout. The king cobra, or hamadryad, is the most formidable and aggressive of all the cobras.

Reid (1964) in Malaysia, however, points out that the dogma that cobra bites are usually neurotoxic is incorrect; the main clinical feature is local necrosis. In half the 47 verified cases of bite by *Naja naja* the effect was negligible, 20 developed local necrosis, and systemic neurotoxic poisoning developed in only 6, of whom 2 died. Pain, swelling, and local necrosis were usual, and systemic poisoning showed as drowsiness, difficulty in opening eyes and mouth, in speaking and swallowing, and general weakness; there was proteinuria. Specific antivenom (minimum dose 100 ml intravenously) is the most important treatment, to be given only after systemic poisoning becomes evident (paresis and apathy), but it does not prevent local necrosis.

The bite of the krait (*Bungarus fasciatus*, Fig. 237) is extremely dangerous, especially in Northern India; the symptoms are similar to those produced by the cobra. *Dendraspis viridis*, a very agile and aggressive species, is regarded as the most dangerous of African snakes.

The symptoms caused by the bite of the Australian Elapidae may not be very severe, but constitutional effects appear with great rapidity—sometimes in as short a period as 15 minutes. A feeling of faintness and irresistible desire to sleep are soon followed by paresis of both legs, vomiting and cardiac paralysis. The pupil is widely dilated and insensitive to light. Should the patient survive the coma, recovery is complete and no sequelae occur.

Vipers

For the type of lesion produced by the viperines, that of Russell's viper, the daboia (*Vipera russelli*, Fig. 238) may be taken as an example. This species can be extremely deadly. The symptoms produced depend upon the amount of

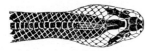

Fig. 237.—The krait (*Bungarus fasciatus*).

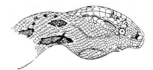

Fig. 238.—The daboia (*Vipera russelli*).

venom injected. In 30% of cases there is no envenomation. In another 30% there are only local signs, while in the remaining 40% some systemic envenomation occurs.

The local signs are severe pain at the site of the bite with blood-stained discharge and ecchymoses around the site of the punctures. Later there may be extensive sloughing of the tissues followed by scarring.

The general signs of systemic envenomation are those of a defibrination syndrome with non-clotting blood, haematuria, melaena, haemoptysis and

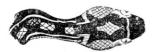

Fig. 239.—The phoorsa (*Echis carinatus*).

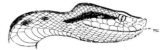

Fig. 240.—The rattlesnake (*Trimeresurus lanceolatus*).

bleeding from mucous membranes and into the skin. Renal failure is found in a proportion of cases with falling urinary output and anuria.

The bite of *Echis carinatus* (Fig. 239) is less dangerous than that of the daboia, but is in many ways similar in its effects.

The bites of the rattlesnakes—*Trimeresurus* and *Crotalus* (Figs 240, 241)—are remarkable for the local disturbance they produce. Constitutional paralytic symptoms come on quickly, usually in less than fifteen minutes. Should the patient recover, swelling and discoloration extend up the limb and trunk, and general symptoms of blood-poisoning with pyrexia, restlessness and delirium set in. The wound suppurates freely and may become haemorrhagic, or even gangrenous. The South American *Crotalus terrificus*, though a viper, has neurotoxic venom.

The symptoms produced by the bite of the European vipers resemble those of *Crotalus*, but are very much milder.

The mortality from snakebite, even of the most venomous varieties, is not so great as is popularly supposed. That it is not more is probably due to the fact that the reptile is seldom able to inject a full dose of venom. If given a fair chance, the cobra is able to inject the equivalent of twenty lethal doses at a time.

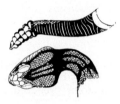

Fig. 241.—The rattlesnake (*Crotalus terrificus*). The tail with its rattle is shown above.

Sea snakes

Sea snakes inhabit the shores of the Indian and Pacific oceans, ranging from the Persian Gulf to S. Japan, the coast of tropical Australia and the S. Pacific Isles.

These snakes can be identified by their flat, rudder-like tails. *Water* snakes, which are also common along these shores, are harmless and have round tapering tails.

The commonest sea snake is *Enhydrina schistosa* which is 0·9–1·2 m long and 2·5–5 cm thick and recognizable by a deep cleft in its chin. Some species of *Hydrophis* grow to the length of 2·7 m, but are relatively slender, with small heads.

Members of the genus *Astiotia* are mostly massive, being up to 10 cm thick.

Pelamis platurus has the widest distribution and is recorded off the west coast of tropical America and the shores of S.E. Africa. The genus *Laticauda* is amphibious.

All sea snakes are able to secrete a highly toxic venom, which is myotoxic, through small fixed fangs. Sea snake bite is mainly an occupational hazard to fishermen and rarely affects bathers. Significant envenomation is only found in about one-third of cases and such bites give rise to little *local* pain and inflammation.

Sea snake venom is myotoxic but also causes renal tubular necrosis and hepatic parenchymal necrosis. Symptoms develop within 30–60 minutes and if there is no muscle pain or stiffness within 1 hour of being bitten then no further symptoms will develop. The symptoms are due to muscle damage, with pain, stiffness and immobilization of certain muscle groups, the jaw (trismus), eye and tongue muscles being commonly affected, causing ophthalmoplegia and dysphagia. Myoglobinuria develops about 3–6 hours after evenomation and impaired renal function may persist for some weeks. Permanent muscle damage does not occur. Hyperkalaemia is a feature and death can occur from respiratory failure, acute renal failure or hyperkalaemic cardiac arrest (Reid 1959). A double strength antivenom against *E. schistosa* has been prepared at the Commonwealth Laboratories, Melbourne, see Treatment, page 802 (Reid 1961).

Victims are usually fishermen. Bathers and paddlers in shallow water do not usually see the offending snake.

CLINICAL NOTES ON SNAKEBITE

By Dr H. A. Reid, M.D., F.R.C.P. (Ed.), F.R.A.C.P, D.T.M. & H., Liverpool School of Tropical Medicine, formerly Director of the Snake and Venom Research Institute, Penang

Diagnosis

In India it is generally fairly easy to diagnose that snake bite has occurred, and it is not difficult to distinguish between krait and cobra bites. Krait bites are much rarer than cobra bites, and if the victim survives more than a few hours there will, in cobra bite, be local swelling followed in a day or two by necrosis (if the victim is one of the 50% in whom venom was actually injected). The distinction in India is somewhat academic, since the same antivenom will be given whether for cobra or krait bite; ptosis is the predominant systemic sign indicating antivenom.

The most useful early sign of systemic viperine poisoning is blood-tinged spit, often seen only if the victim is asked to cough hard. Non-clotting blood is also a most valuable sign, but may not develop until several hours after the bite in moderate systemic poisoning.

Poisoning	Elapid	Sea snake	Viper
1. Nil	50%	75%	30%
2. Local only	Cobra: Swelling then necrosis 35% Other Elapids: no local effects usually	None	Swelling 30% (Necrosis 10%)
3. Systemic (with or without local effect)	15% *Neurotoxic* Ptosis then glosso-pharyngeal then respiratory and general paresis	25% *Myotoxic* Muscle movement pains. Paresis. Myoglobinuria. Hyperkalaemia	40% *Haemotoxic* Haemoptysis. Other bleeding symptoms. Shock. Non-clotting blood

First-aid treatment of snakebite

First-aid treatment of snakebite is defined as the 'measures taken by the victim or associates prior to receiving medical treatment'. Unfortunately it is often confused, especially by doctors, with medical treatment. Recommendations for first-aid treatment should be short, simple, practicable and more beneficial than harmful. Although it might be theoretically desirable to vary recommendations according to the country, the type of victim (or associates), the species of snake, the time after the bite, the site of the bite and so on, in practice such variations would make the recommendations impossibly confusing. Measures such as immediate amputation if a toe or finger is bitten, though fully effective in preventing poisoning, are impracticable. Other measures such as incision and suction have been shown to be beneficial in laboratory experiments, but in practice are more harmful than helpful because of the danger of introducing infection.

The short and sensible answer is 'Leave the bite alone and go to the nearest hospital as quickly as possible'. Unfortunately, most people feel they must 'do something'. Accordingly the following compromise recommendations have been evolved in the light of some years of clinical work dealing with snakebite:

1. The common symptom in human snakebite is *fright and fear of rapid death*. But the danger of poisonous snakebite in human victims has been greatly exaggerated: one-half of the people bitten by poisonous snakes such as cobras, vipers and sea snakes develop no significant poisoning (because little or no venom is injected). Serious poisoning is rare in man and death is *highly exceptional*—particularly if adequate medical treatment is received within a few hours of the bite.

2. Wipe the site of the bite and then cover with a handkerchief or cloth. *Do not incise* the bite as this does more harm than good (for example it often introduces infection).

3. Apply a firm (but *not* tight) ligature above the bite—use cloth, handkerchief or grass.

4. Go to the nearest hospital. Bring the snake if available (kill it by one or two sharp blows on the neck: lift by the tail).

Medical treatment of snakebite

Land snake bite. 1. *If there is no local swelling 2 or more hours after the bite* (which means that in viper and cobra bites, poisoning has *not* occurred: swelling does not occur in over one-third of bites) give vitamin B complex, 1·0 ml, intramuscularly as a placebo to reassure the patient.

2. *If there are no systemic signs* do not give antivenom (it does not *prevent* local poisoning). Give vitamin B complex as before (as a placebo). Observe for 6 hours for systemic signs.

3. *If systemic signs occur, antivenom is indicated.*
Systemic signs of Elapid poisoning (usually cobra): Ptosis, glossopharyngeal palsy, paresis of the neck, trunk and limbs.

(a) *With local swelling* (necrosis follows)—cobra. Give cobra or polyvalent antivenom with cobra fraction, 100 ml (10 ampoules) by intravenous drip (see below); repeat in 1–2 hours if there is no clinical improvement.

(b) *Without local swelling*—in Africa—mamba (therefore give mamba antivenom); in Asia—krait (therefore give krait antivenom or polyvalent antivenom with krait fraction). Dosage as for cobra.

Systemic signs of Viper poisoning: Sputum blood-stained (ask the patient to cough hard and then spit into a dish); later the blood will not clot (leave 1 ml of blood in a test-tube for 20 minutes, and then inspect it for clotting). Give viper or polyvalent antivenom, 50 ml by intravenous drip for an average case; but for more severe cases with shock give 100 ml.

Sea snake bite. 1. Note that *local pain excludes sea snake bite*. Absence of general muscle pains on movement, 1 or more hours after the bite, *excludes significant poisoning* (there is no poisoning in two-thirds of sea snake bites). Give the placebo intramuscularly, as above.

2. *Systemic signs of sea snake poisoning.* General muscle aches and pains on movement, starting ½–1 hour after the bite; passive movement of the limbs or trunk by the doctor is painful; myoglobinuria occurs 3–6 hours after the bite, the urine is dusky yellow, then red-brown, and is positive for protein. Give 2–3 ampoules of sea snake antivenom by intravenous drip; in severe cases with ptosis, external ophthalmoplegia, or slow reaction of the pupil to light, give 4–5 ampoules.

Administration of antivenom

Note that only a minority of patients need antivenom. Clinical trials show that specific antivenom is successful in severe poisoning even if it is not given until several hours after the bite. Therefore *wait for clear clinical evidence of systemic poisoning before giving antivenom* (but signs of systemic poisoning *must be looked for carefully*).

First inject 0·2 ml subcutaneously to test for sensitivity to the serum (0·02 ml in subjects who give a positive history of allergy). If anaphylactic reactions occur, attempt desensitization with graded doses. If this is unsuccessful, abandon antivenom.

Intravenous drip should initially be slow (40 drops/minute), as reactions may occur despite negative sensitivity tests. These can usually be controlled by intramuscular adrenaline (1·0 ml of a 1 in 1000 solution). The speed of the drip should then be slowly increased to 150 drops/minute, to complete administration in 30–50 minutes.

Children require doses of antivenom similar to those needed by adults.

General medical treatment

Release any tourniquet which has been applied. Leave the bite alone (interference often causes bacterial infection). If the lower limb has been bitten, rest the patient in bed. If the upper limb has been bitten, rest it in a sling.

If local necrosis develops give prophylactic tetanus antitoxin. *If respiratory failure develops* in Elapid or sea snake poisoning (shown by *confusion, stupor, rapid shallow breathing, rise in pulse rate and blood pressure*) perform *tracheostomy.* Artificial respiration may also be needed, by manual compression of a rebreathing bag and carbon dioxide absorber from an anaesthetic machine. Intragastric drip feeds may be needed until glossopharyngeal palsy resolves.

(See page 804 for list of institutes making antivenoms for snakebite in various continents.)

Other measures. Cortisone has been used by some other workers with some success in the treatment of bites of the Malayan pit viper (*Ancistrodon rhodostoma*). Cortisone is given orally in 25 mg tablets. During the first 24 hours it is given 4-hourly and during the next equal period, 6-hourly. Steroid therapy should usually be reserved for the treatment of reactions to antivenom.

Surgical treatment may be required for the late results of infected snake bites and the deep gangrenous conditions which may follow them.

ANTIVENOMS

Antisera are produced in various areas of the tropics and subtropics to neutralize the venoms of the locally important venomous snakes. Some of these antisera are specific so that a precise identification has to be made, but there are also polyvalent antisera available which are effective, for example, against the venom of the locally occurring crotalidae and elapidae. Certain venoms have a medicinal use. Russell's viper venom has for some time been used to promote local clotting, and more recently Arvin, a fraction of the venom of the Malayan pit viper, has been used as a defibrinating anticoagulant.

Institutes making antivenoms for snake bite in Europe, Africa, America and Asia (Russell & Lauritzen 1966)

EUROPE

Serotherapeutisches
Institut Wien,
Triesterstrasse 50,
Wien,
Austria.

Institut Pasteur,
36 Rue du Docteur Roux,
Paris 15,
France.

Behringwerke AG,
Postfach 167,
355 Marburg,
Germany.

Swiss Serum and Vaccine Institute,
3001 Berne,
P.O. Box 2707,
Switzerland.

Istituto Sieroterapico e
Vaccinogeno 'Sclavo',
Via Fiorentine 1,
Siena,
Italy.

Tashkent Institute,
c/o Ministry of Health,
Moscow,
U.S.S.R.

Institute for Immunology,
Rockefellerova 2,
Zagreb,
Yugoslavia.

AFRICA

Institut Pasteur d'Algérie,
Rue Docteur Laveran,
Alger,
Algeria.

FitzSimmon's Snake Park,
P.O. Box 1,
Snell Parade,
Durban, Natal,
Republic of South Africa.

CAPS,
P.O. Box 2279
Salisbury,
Rhodesia.

South African Institute
for Medical Research,
P.O. Box 1038,
Johannesburg,
Republic of South Africa.

ASIA

Central Research Institute,
Kasauli, R.I.,
Punjab,
India.

Perusahaan Negara Bio Farma,
9 Djalan Pasteur,
Bandung,
Indonesia.

Institute d'Etat des Serums et
Vaccins Razi,
P.O. Box 656,
Teheran,
Iran.

Haffkine Institute,
Parel,
Bombay 12,
India.

Laboratory of Chemotherapy and
Serum Therapy,
Kumamoto City,
Kyushi,
Japan.

The Takeda Pharmaceutical Co.,
Osaka,
Japan.

ASIA—*continued*

Rogoff Institute,
Beilinson Hospital,
Tel-Aviv University,
Tel-Aviv,
Israel.

Taiwan Serum Vaccine Laboratory,
130 Fuh-lin Road,
Shih-Ling,
Taipei,
Taiwan.

Institute for Infectious Diseases,
University of Tokyo,
Tokyo,
Japan.

Queen Saovabha Memorial Institute,
Rama 4 Road,
Bangkok,
Thailand.

Pasteur Institute,
Nha Trang,
Vietnam.

Serum and Vaccine Laboratories,
Alabang,
Muntinlupa,
Rizal,
Philippine Republic.

AUSTRALIA

Commonwealth Serum Laboratories,
Poplar Road,
Parkville,
Melbourne,
Victoria,
Australia.

NORTH AMERICA

Wyeth Laboratories,
Box 8299,
Philadelphia,
Pennsylvania,
U.S.A.

Laboratory 'MYN' S.A.,
Ave Coyoacan 1717,
Mexico 12,
D.F.,
Mexico.

Instituto Nacional de Higiene,
Czda,
M. Escobedo No. 20,
Mexico 13,
D.F.,
Mexico.

SOUTH AMERICA

Instituto Nacional de Microbiologia,
Vélez Sarsfield 563,
Buenos Aires,
Argentina.

Instituto Butantan,
Caixa Postal 65,
São Paulo,
Brazil.

Instituto Pinheiros,
Productos Therapeuticos,
Caixa Postal 951,
São Paulo,
Brazil.

Instituto Nacional de Salud,
Calle 57,
Numero 8–35,
Bogotà,
D.E.,
Colombia.

Laboratorio Behrens,
Ave Principal de Chapellin,
Apartado 62,
Caracas,
Venezuela.

VENOMOUS LIZARDS

All lizards are absolutely non-poisonous, with the exception of a single genus, easily recognized, inhabiting Mexico and Arizona. *Heloderma* consists of 2 species, *H. suspectum*, and *H. horridum*, both heavy, stout lizards, yellow or shrimp-pink in colour, with black bead-like scales. They are desert dwellers, and store fat in their swollen tails to tide them over periods of famine. Popularly known as the 'Gila monsters', they were first discovered near the village of Gila.

The poison apparatus is in the lower jaw, where venom-secreting submaxillary glands are connected by ducts with grooved teeth. Symptoms of poisoning start with paralysis. A large dose produces dyspnoea and convulsions. Post mortem examinations on experimental animals show a greatly dilated heart and venous congestion of the internal organs. Changes in the spinal cord ganglion cells have also been observed.

VENOMOUS MARINE ANIMALS

For details of venomous marine animals, see Cleland and Southcott (1965), Halstead (1965) and Russell (1965).

Poisonous fishes

Poisonous fishes exist in most tropical waters, especially among the coral reefs of the Pacific and Indian Oceans. Their venom may be conveyed to man either through the bite or by stings. In one case the poison is secreted by certain epithelial glands within the mouth; in the other, by poison glands connected

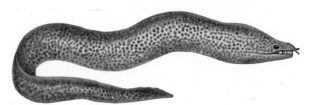

Fig. 242.—*Muraena moronga.* (*After Calmette*)

with barbs in the dorsal fin. The former comprise more than 100 species of the genus *Muraena*, all of which possess powerful teeth capable of inflicting bites (Fig. 242). The poison secreted by the glands courses down the hollow teeth. The effect of the venom on man is neurocardiac. In some, the poison finds its way to the exterior only when the barbs are broken, and produces severe inflammation in the wound and, it may be, tetanic symptoms. *Synanceja*, a spinous genus, is widely distributed throughout the Indian and Pacific Oceans and is one of the Scorpaenidae (scorpion fish); *S. verrucosa* is the most toxic. The poison apparatus is connected with the dorsal fin. *Plotosus anguillaris*, known as 'machoira' in Mauritius, has a similarly wide distribution, while *Saccobranchus fossilis*, in the waters of India and Ceylon, produces much the same symptoms.

Stingrays are common. The tropical species is *Aetobatis narinari*. The venom is secreted by the glandular epithelium sheath of caudal sting. Death may ensue. Treatment is effected by washing out the wound, which may be extensive, with water. Heat is the most effective treatment for the pain. The affected part must be immersed in water as hot as the patient can stand and removed as soon as the pain goes, to be recommenced as often as is necessary (Russell 1965). The integumentary sheath of the sting should be removed if found, and debridement and suture may be needed. Antitetanus agents should be given.

Over 40 species of *Scorpaena* are found in tropical waters. Their integument is provided with numerous spines, the stings of which may excite convulsions and even cause death. The symptoms usually evoked are pain extending up the limbs, profuse sweating, pallor, dyspnoea and tachycardia. There is often also a morbilliform or scarlatiniform rash. Pain can be mitigated by infiltration of 2% procaine and 1 in 1000 solution of adrenaline.

In South American waters, several species of *Thalassophryne* have dorsal spines containing a central poison-duct connecting with glands. Species of *Trachinus* (weeverfish), in northern waters as well as in the Mediterranean, have 2 sets of poison barbs situated on the operculum as well as on the dorsal fin. The venom has a general action on the heart, besides causing severe pain and mydriasis.

Toadfish stings are caused by *Batrachus grunniens* in W. Indies tropical waters and by *Thalassophryne dowi* on the Pacific Coast of Panama.

Stonefish (*Synanceja trachynis*) in the coral reefs of the waters of New Guinea and the Indian and Pacific Oceans possess dorsal spines which inject a toxin into the feet of people who tread on them, causing intense pain, local oedema and necrosis, with severe shock. Phleps (1960) found that injection of 0·5–1 ml of a solution of emetine hydrochloride (60 mg in 1 ml) into each puncture, within one hour of the sting, was most effective; an antivenom has been prepared, which can be given at the same time.

The sting of the lionfish (*Pterois volitans*) may be followed by cardiovascular collapse; treatment with adrenaline may be necessary.

Poisoning from ingestion of poisonous fishes. Cases of fish poisoning arising from eating the flesh of fishes containing some intrinsic toxin occur more commonly in the tropics than in more temperate countries. In many instances these fish may be eaten with safety, except at certain seasons of the year; in others the poisonous qualities are acquired only after feeding or living in certain localities.

The barracuda (*Sphyraena barracuda*), a pike-like fish, is eaten widely throughout the South Atlantic; it is the large examples, especially those that are spawning, which are apt to be poisonous, and the symptoms are mainly gastrointestinal, with paraesthesia. Local people regard as poisonous fishes which show a whitish, watery fluid when cut up, or a black, purplish discoloration at the base of the teeth.

Ciguatera poisoning results from eating fish of many different kinds, which inhabit seas between latitudes 35° N. and 34° S., especially in the Pacific and the West Indies; the fish most commonly implicated are snappers, groupers, pompano or jack, barracuda, moray eels, and surgeon fishes. Some are toxic at all times while in others the flesh is only toxic at certain seasons when the small fish feed on dinoflagellates and blue green algae and are in turn ingested by larger fish.

Symptoms include abdominal pain, diarrhoea and vomiting, but the toxin also exerts a profound neurotoxic effect in some cases, with paraesthesia, incoordination, hypotension, muscular weakness or paralysis; it may be fatal. Recovery is often slow. Treatment with neostigmine methylsulphate 0·5 mg intramuscularly every hour, with or without Tensilon (edrophonium chloride) 2 mg every 2–3 minutes for 10–15 minutes, may have some effect. Intravenous fluid with hydrocortisone 100 mg during the first hour and 50 mg an hour for the next 2 hours, may also be helpful. Neostigmine bromide, 15 mg by mouth every 2 hours, may be substituted for the methylsulphate as the patient improves.

There are various sprats (*Clupidae*) in tropical waters which acquire poisonous properties; among them is *C. longiceps*, a sardine found in Ceylon waters, which occasionally may produce collapse and even death.

Puffer fish poisoning. Many species of the widespread genus *Tetrodon* are poisonous, such as the 'death fish' of Hawaii, *T. hispidus*, and other species in Korea and Japan, where it is a special hazard. The poison, tetrodotoxin, is contained in ovaries and eggs and causes gastro-intestinal and nervous symptoms, sometimes culminating in syncope or coma.

The flesh of certain large fishes normally constituting excellent food, such as the king-fish (*Scomberomorus cavalla*), may occasionally exhibit toxic properties.

In all forms of fish poisoning the most effective *treatment* is to evacuate the poison by washing out the stomach and administering purgatives. Other symptoms must be treated on general lines with stimulants, hot-water bottles, and injections of morphine, if necessary, to alleviate pain.

Poisonous shellfish

In the South Pacific Islands fatal cases of poisoning may be due to bites of certain shellfish of the genus *Conus*, all of which are adorned with brightly coloured shells. Six at least are known: *Conus tulipa*, *C. marmoreus*, *C. striatus*, *C. geographus*, *C. textilis* and *C. aulicus*. They are provided with a long tubular proboscis which can be protruded beyond the shell, and opening into it is a sac containing two rows of hollow teeth. The poison is not delivered directly from the poison gland, but probably on to the wounded surface. The symptoms are acute pain, swelling, numbness and spreading paralysis. There may be early drowsiness, dysphagia, deepening into coma and death. When bitten in this manner, the Polynesians make small incisions round the bite to cause blood to flow freely. Fatalities have been reported in North Australia and Polynesia.

Of the bivalves, mussels produce paralytic shellfish poisoning—*Mytilus edulis* and congeners. Toxicity is due to dinoflagellates (*Gonyaulax catenella*) in their bodies.

In Japan shellfish poisoning is due to *Venerupis semidecussata*. The toxic principle is venerupin which causes acute yellow and red atrophy of the liver.

Murex poisoning

Murex brandaris and *M. trunculus* occur mostly on the Syrian coast. The active principle is murexine, a choline derivative allied to adrenaline, which produces paralysis of the central nervous system.

Annelida (segmented worms)

The stinging sea-mouse (*Chloeia flava*) is a polychaete which causes lesions in sea-bathers due to its poisonous calcareous spicules, and is known as the bristleworm. Other species are *C. viridis* in West Indies, *Eurythoe complanta* in Australia and *Hermodice carunculata* in tropical E. America and Gulf of Mexico.

Poisonous corals (Anthozoa) and sea anemones

Coral dermatitis results from cuts in the skin which cause indolent lesions from contact with the anthozoa. The surrounding skin becomes red, oedematous and itchy.

Sea-anemones of the genus *Hellenopolypus* and *Aktinion* give rise by contact to sponge-fishers' or 'Skevos-Zervos' disease, itching and vesication, pustulation, nausea and vomiting being produced. The toxin acts like cantharides, and the lesions are due to urticating cells in the tentacles. Washing with vinegar and the application of olive oil is the best treatment.

Poisonous Echinoidea, sea urchins

In the West Indies, especially Barbados, spiny sea urchins cause septic lesions on hands and feet from punctures by the spines. The poisonous species are *Tripneustes esculentus, Diadema antillarum, Centrechinus antillarum* and *Athenosoma varium* in Australian waters, which also have poisonous ovaries and eggs, when symptoms resembling fish allergy are produced. *Diamina setosum* occurs off the African coast to Australia, South Sea islands and Japan: *Paracentrotus lividus* in the Azores, Africa and Mediterranean: *Toxopneustes pileolus* in Malaysia and Japan: *Sphaerechinus granulosus* in Mediterranean and E. Atlantic. The venom is injected by globiferous pedicellariae which have blades with a venom gland attached.

Jelly-fish poisoning

Medusae of the genus *Obelia* contain in their ectoderm numerous clear ovoid bodies, the stinging capsules or nematocysts, which serve as weapons of offence. The whole apparatus is developed in an interstitial cell (cnidoblast) which, as it approaches maturity, migrates towards the surface and at one point is elongated by a delicate process—the cnidocil or trigger hair. When this is touched the cnidoblast undergoes a sudden contraction and causes an eversion of the thread, at the base of which are minute barbs, which are poisonous and produce a numbing effect. The stings produce a painful local swelling and a disagreeable urticaria, and, in susceptible individuals, shock and collapse.

Cyanea is common off the Queensland coast and produces stings in bathers; it resembles 'a mop hiding under a dinner plate', measuring 25 cm across.

The Portuguese man-of-war (*Physalia*) or *agua viva* is provided with a characteristic stinging apparatus. From the underside of the float there hang filamentous tentacles (gastrozooids, dactylozooids and branching blastostyles), some of which are long and retractile and contain batteries of stinging capsules which produce severe dermatitis and irritation in the skin of those who come into contact with them. Extract of the tentacles contains 5-hydroxytryptamine, a potent causer of pain and a releaser of histamine. It is a vasodilator, and is found in wasp venom, and in the stinging hairs of nettles. Antihistamine cream is curative.

The sea wasp (*Chironex fleckeri*) has caused at least 50 deaths off the East Coast of Australia from cardiorespiratory failure (Keen 1970). Contact with the tentacles can also result in acute local pain and inflammation often with permanent scarring.

Gymnothorax poisoning is caused by several species, in the Red Sea, Indian Ocean and tropical Pacific. *G. javanicus* is found as above; *G. meleagris, G. pictus* and *G. petelli* range to the sea of Japan.

Twenty minutes after ingestion there is numbness, laryngeal spasm and aphonia. Mortality is about 10%. Paraldehyde is the best drug to control the convulsions.

SCORPIONS AND SPIDERS (ARACHNIDA)

Scorpions

Scorpions are very common in the tropics, and their stings are very painful and cause a considerable amount of inconvenience, though they are not exactly dangerous, except to young children, in whom, in addition to local symptoms, muscular cramps, profuse perspiration, pyrexia, vomiting and convulsions may be produced. Deaths have been reported from North and South Africa, the West Indies, Mexico, Korea and Manchuria. In Trinidad, glycosuria, hyperglycaemia, pancreatitis and even pancreatic cysts, are described as sequelae to scorpion stings. In general the symptoms are lacrimation, salivation and sphincter relaxation.

In Southern Europe and North Africa black scorpions, *Euscorpius italicus* and *Buthus maurus*, in Mexico the 'durango' (*Centrurus*), in Brazil *Tityus serrulatus* and *T. bahiensis*, in Manchuria *Buthus martensi*, are dreaded (Fig. 243). In South

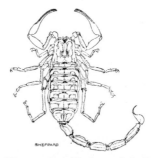

Fig. 243.—The scorpion (*Buthus* sp.), half natural size.

Africa the genera are *Hodogenes*, *Opisthophthalmus* and *Parabuthus*. In Algeria and N. Sahara the most formidable species are *Androctonus australis*, *Buthus occitanus*, *Buthacus arenicola* and *A. amoreuxi*.

Paired poison glands are situated in the last or postanal segment of the tail which is jointed and very flexible, so that it can be curved forwards over the body when the scorpion is striking. The venom which it ejects is in many respects like that of the cobra, but far less toxic.

The toxins in amorphous and crystalline form are isolated by grinding up dried poison glands with quartz sand, extracting with normal saline, clarifying by aluminium sulphate and precipitating by acetone. The venom is obtained by electrical excitation of the distal coils of the tail.

In South Africa, Grasset and colleagues have found neuromotor symptoms to follow intravenous injections of toxins of the three main genera. Neuro-toxins and haemorrhagins have been isolated from the genus *Parabuthus*. The venom of *Centruroides sculpturatus* caused hypertension, respiratory failure and skeletal stimulation in anaesthetized animals because pressor substances were released from the adrenal (Patterson 1960).

In Trinidad, Poon-King (1963) records myocarditis as a sequel of sting by the scorpion *Tityus trinitalis*; there is disturbance of the electrocardiogram with inversion of the T-wave, and acute pancreatitis following scorpion bite has been described in Trinidad by Bartholomew (1970). The sting of a scorpion, *Buthus tamulus*, has caused a defibrination syndrome in Ceylon (Sita Devi 1970).

In the treatment of scorpion sting in children, it may be necessary to incise and thoroughly wash out the sting with a strong solution of potassium permanganate. Dyce Sharp, from experiences mostly in his own person, advocated immediate injection of procaine hydrochloride and adrenaline in the vicinity of the sting. For the severe intoxications of children, an efficient antitoxin is prepared. The venom extracted from dried stings and venom glands by normal saline is toxic to horse, goat, and most laboratory animals. The antitoxin has been prepared from horses by subcutaneous injection of graduated doses of venom. In doses of 5 ml it exerts both prophylactic and curative action. Sergent states that severe symptoms disappear very rapidly after serum injection which when administered early enough and in sufficiently large doses saves many lives. Mortality is less than 3·1% in all treated cases.

Spiders

Nearly all spiders (*Araneae*) possess poison glands, the venom of which is injurious to insects, but few are dangerous to man. Certain of the genus *Latrodectus* are poisonous. In New Zealand one, *L. hasselti*, is known as the 'katipo', Maori term for 'night-stinger'. In Southern Europe, *L. tredecimguttatus*, the 'malmignatte' (Fig. 244); in Israel, Jordan and N. Africa, *L. lugubris* and *L. revivensis*, in North and South America, *L. mactans*, *L. curacaviensis*, and *L. geometricus* are credited with toxic properties.

L. mactans is known in California as the 'black widow spider'; the adult female is glossy black with crimson hourglass markings on the abdomen; in Turkestan *L. tredecimguttatus* is the 'karakurt spider'; in Australia, *Atrax robustus* is the 'funnelweb spider' and in South Africa *L. indistinctus* is known as the 'kroppie spider' or 'button spider'.

The toxin of the poison glands has been shown to be a powerful haemolysin, causing inflammation and oedema at the site of injection, together with numbness of the part and, it may be, urticarial rash. Most observers describe intense nerve pain, which is said to be due to stimulation of the myoneural junctions by the venom. The venom of *L. tredecimguttatus* contains a neurotropic toxin which acts centrally and peripherally. Rigidity and spasm of most of the muscles supervene, especially those of the abdomen, which becomes 'board-like', simulating appendicitis. Sloughing of the skin in the neighbourhood of the bite may occur.

Fatal cases of the bite of *Atrax robustus*, the funnelweb spider, have been described from Australia. Deaths from respiratory failure occur mostly during November and March. The venom of the male spider is more toxic than that of the female. No haemotoxic effects have been described (Wiener 1957).

In Brazil, the species are *Lycosa raptora* and *Ctenus nigriventer;* the venoms posses a proteolytic action similar to that of hyaluronidase.

Treatment consists in washing out the wound with a solution of potassium permanganate (1 in 4000).

Intravenous injections of calcium gluconate (10 ml of a 10% solution) are said to relieve the pain and decrease the muscular spasm. In South Africa a serum which neutralizes the venom of *L. indistinctus* has been prepared by Finlayson, and similar methods have been used in the Argentine and Russia against local species of *Latrodectus*. Allen advocates 9 mg D-tubocurarine chloride solution given intravenously for relief of pain. It causes immediate relaxation. Corticotrophin is effective in black widow spider poisoning, and subcutaneous atropine has been successful. When infection occurs penicillin is indicated. An antivenom is available in Mexico.

In Peru a pruning spider, *Mastophora gasteracanthoides*, which lives in the leaves of vines, and is identified by its ash-grey colour and large globular abdomen with two prominent tubercles, produces, according to Escomel, the same symptoms as *Latrodectus*, and sometimes haematuria.

The 'tarantula' spider, *Lycosa tarentula* (Fig. 245), occurs in Southern Europe. Mysterious properties have been attributed to its bite; apparently in some specially susceptible people oedema of the eyelids and pyrexia are apt to result, and gave rise to hysterical manifestations known in the Middle Ages as 'tarantism'. The tarantulas of tropical countries are bird-eating spiders of the family Mygalidae. They are trap-door spiders, terrestrial in their habits, with prominent projecting mandibles which give them a terrifying appearance. The North African species, *Chaetopelma olivacea*, is feared by Arabs, and its bite is said to give rise to acute inflammation.

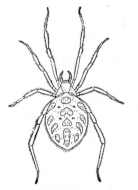

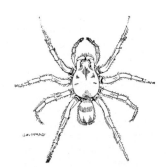

Fig. 244.—*Latrodectus tredecimgutt-atus*, twice natural size. (*After Hirst*)

Fig. 245.—The tarantula spider (*Lycosa tarentula*), half natural size.

Brown spiders (*Loxosceles*) are found in Chile, California, Arizona, Israel and elsewhere. They are distinguished by a violin or fiddle shaped marking on the dorsal side of the carapace. The species which have caused symptoms in man are *Loxosceles laeta* in Chile ('Arana de los rincones'), *Loxosceles unicolor* and *L. arizonica* in California and Arizona and *Loxosceles rufescens* in Israel. These spiders attack mostly at night while the victims, mostly women, are sleeping. The bite is on the face and causes local necrosis followed by ulceration and sometimes scarring from tissue destruction. In about 10% of cases in Chile there is systemic envenomation with haemoglobinuria and haemolytic anaemia. In treatment the local application of fibrinolysin and antihistamines is of value while in systemic envenomation corticosteroids and blood transfusion are used (Schenone 1959).

CENTIPEDES (MYRIAPODA)

The Chilopoda, to which the poisonous genus *Scolopendra* belongs, are widely distributed in the tropics. They are large creatures, and possess a poison apparatus at the base of the first pair of appendages, which are modified to form jaws. The tropical species, *Scolopendra morsitans*, reaches a large size, up to 15 cm; the venom causes both local and general symptoms. The site of the bite becomes inflamed and the starting-point of lymphangitis; dizziness, headache and vomiting may ensue.

Treatment consists in bathing the part with a strong solution of ammonia, 1 in 5 or 1 in 10. It may be necessary to give hypodermic injections of morphine to allay pain.

MILLIPEDES

Some species of millipede cause vesicular dermatitis.

ACARIASIS

There is some evidence of a close association of the acarine mite, *Dermatophagoides pteronyssinus* and asthma (*Lancet* 1968). The mites become airborne during bed-making and are present in house dust, and there is a possibility that allergic lung disease of different kinds may be caused by exposure to mites and their products.

A case of pulmonary acariasis has been described by Kijima (1963) in which a resected segment of lung showed large quantities of black-brown pigment granules free and taken up by histiocytes, the product of a *Tyroglyphus* mite which was found in the sputum.

TICK PARALYSIS

For details see Editorial (*Br. med. J.* 1969) and Stanbury and Huyck (1945).

Tick paralysis is a rapid progressive flaccid paralysis which follows tick bite and is probably caused by a neurotoxin in the tick saliva. The pathogenesis is obscure, but a conductance block in the motor fibres, interference with the monosynaptic pathways, a depolarizing block at the neuromuscular junction or a muscle lesion have all been suggested.

Tick paralysis has been reported from the North-west states of America and Canada, Australia, South Africa, Somaliland and South-eastern Europe. A similar disease has been recognized among sheep in South Africa and sheep and cattle in Canada. The ticks responsible are *Dermacentor andersoni* and *D. variabilis* in America, *Ixodes holocyclus* and *I. ricinus* in Australia, *I. pilosus*, *Haemaphysalis cinnabarina* and *Rhipicephalus simus* in South Africa. Children are more frequently and more severely affected than adults, and girls more than boys, possibly because of ticks concealed by their long hair.

The patient becomes restless 5 or 6 days after the attachment of the tick, and there is numbness and tingling of the extremities, lips, throat or face, which is followed within a day or two by an ascending flaccid paralysis of the Landry type; affecting arms and legs, sometimes with loss of sphincter control. The reflexes are absent. There are no sensory changes. Pain, nausea, vomiting and dizziness are rare. Signs of bulbar involvement may appear rapidly, with dysphagia, dysarthria and respiratory distress. Local skin changes and morbilliform rashes have been reported. The condition, which must be differentiated from poliomyelitis, may be fatal from respiratory paralysis. Complete recovery follows removal of the tick, and although recovery may take more than a week it has occurred in 48 hours.

The tick must be removed completely, as the salivary glands are the source of the toxin. A protective serum has been used in dogs and tried successfully in several human cases. Travellers to tick-infested areas should be warned to look for ticks at the end of the day, and to pay particular attention to children.

REFERENCES

BARTHOLOMEW, C. (1970) *Br. med. J.*, **i**, 666.

BUCHERL, W., BUCKLEY, E. E. & DEUIOFEU, V. (1968) *Venomous Animals and Their Venoms, Vol. I, Venomous Vertebrates.* New York & London: Academic.

CLELAND, J. B. & SOUTHCOTT, R. V. (1965) *Injuries to Man from Marine Invertebrates in the Australian Region.* Special Report Series 12. Canberra: National Medical Research Council.

EDITORIAL (1969) *Br. med. J.*, **iii**, 314.

ESNOUB, M. P. & TULLAH, G. W. (1967) *Br. J. Haemat.*, **13**, 581.

HALSTEAD, B. W. (1965) *Poisonous and Venomous Marine Animals of the World, Vol. I, Invertebrates.* Washington: U.S.A. Government Printing Office.

KEEN, T. E. B. (1970) *Med. J. Aust.*, **1**, 266.

KIJIMA, S. (1963) *Br. med. J.*, **i**, 451.

Lancet (1968) Editorial, **i**, 1295.

MARSHALL, J. K. (1957) *Practitioner*, **178**, 712.

PATTERSON, R. A. (1960) *Am. J. trop. Med. Hyg.*, **9**, 410.

PHELPS, D. R. (1960) *Med. J. Aust.*, **1**, 293.

POON-KING, T. (1963) *Br. med. J.*, **i**, 374.

REID, H. A. (1959) *Practitioner*, **183**, 530.

―― (1961) *Lancet*, **ii**, 299.

―― (1964) *Br. med. J.*, **ii**, 540.

SCHENONE, H. (1959) *Bol. chil. Parasit.*, **14**, 7.

RUSSELL, F. E. (1965) *Adv. mar. Biol.*, **3**, 255.

――& LAURITZEN, L. (1966) *Trans. R. Soc. trop. Med. Hyg.*, **60**, 797.

SITA DEVI, C. (1970) *Br. med. J.*,

STANBURY, J. B. & HUYCK, J. M. (1945) *Medicine, Baltimore*, **24**, 219.

VISUVARATNAM, M., VINAYAGAMOORTHY, C. & BALAKRISHNAN, S. (1970) *J. trop. Med. Hyg.*, **73**, 9.

WIENER, S. (1957) *Med. J. Aust.*, **2**, 377.

ZIPRKOWSKI, L., HOFSHI, E. & TAHORI, A. S. (1959) *Harefuah*, **56**, 141.

42. PLANT POISONS

FOR a full discussion of poisonous plants, see Watt and Breyer Brandwijk (1962), North (1963) and Kingsbury (1964).

ALLERGIC AND TOXIC DERMATITIS

Pyrethrum dermatitis

Pyrethrum dermatitis has been noted in Kenya, and is caused by the leaves and flowers of *Chrysanthemum cinerariaefolium*, which grows at altitudes of 150–2100 m and flowers throughout the year. The content of pyrethrins and cinerins is 1–2%. Absorption is facilitated by constant sweating, and exposure to sunlight greatly exacerbates the lesions. Some persons on contact exhibit merely a local dermatitis; others show a widespread allergy. Itching commences at the corner of the eyes, and is followed by lacrimation, an irritating vesicular rash, peeling of the skin, and formation of painful fissures.

Poison ivy dermatitis (dermatitis venenata)

Many tropical plants cause dermatitis which may assume an erythematous, vesicular or urticarial form. Intimate contact with the plant or its leaves is

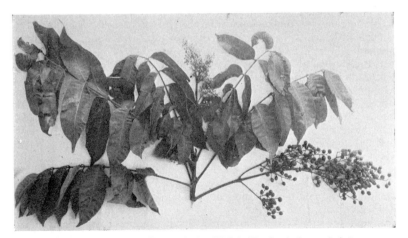

Fig. 246.—Poison ivy (*Rhus juglandifolia*). (*Dr L. A. Leon, Quito*)

necessary. Poison ivy (*Rhus toxicodendron* and *R. juglandifolia*) (Fig. 246), poison sumac (*R. vernix*), poison wood (*Metopium toxiferum*) in North Eastern and Southern United States cause intense dermatitis. Repeated attacks do not produce immunity. The venom is toxicodendrol. Treatment consists of washing the skin with soap and water; alcoholic or oily solutions must be avoided. Clothes must be decontaminated by immersion in 1% calcium hypochlorite for twenty minutes.

Other forms of dermatitis

Several other plants and flowers may cause severe allergic dermatitis, such as *Cypripedium* (lady's slippers), *Euphorbia*, primroses, lilies and vanilla beans; sometimes also mangoes and, in Japan, lacquer made from *Rhus vernicifera*.

Seaweed dermatitis has been reported from Hawaii, and appears to be due to contact with a blue-green filamentous alga tentatively identified as *Lyngbya majuscula*, which produces an erythematous and vesicular rash in persons bathing in the sea off windward beaches. The condition is a reaction to a toxin, and is not allergic in origin. It subsides quickly on local treatment.

Iroko dermatitis. Idiosyncrasy to wood dust is not uncommon. Iroko is a trade name for *Chlorophora excelsa*, a tree of East and West tropical Africa, and known as African teak. The dust produces the usual signs of allergy, with skin irritation, oedema of face, blepharospasm, acute coryza and pharyngitis. Other woods, such as satin wood, teak and mahogany, also produce allergy in susceptible persons. Obeche, or Wa-Wa (*Triplochiton scleroxylon*), a soft wood, produces similar symptoms.

VEGETABLE POISONS

Poisons used for criminal purposes

The inorganic poison most generally used by tropical races is arsenic in some form, cleverly intermingled, as a rule, with flour, inserted into the grains of maize or millet, or introduced into sweets, as in Egypt; in Malaysia, powdered croton seeds or datura are used. The actions of poisons are usually well known.

In Brazil, common poisons are derived from *Paullinia pinnata*, which contains an alkaloid, timboin, and from the fruit of *Thevetia ahonai*, the active principle of which is thevetosin; both of these cause vomiting and respiratory failure.

In Indonesia a poison extracted from the roots of *Milletia sericea* produces debility, headache, diarrhoea, collapse and death.

In the Pacific Islands poison is derived from the fruit of *Barringtonia speciosa*.

In India a large number of vegetable poisons are in use. In the Madras and Bombay States an extract is obtained from the roots of *Nerium odorum*, the white oleander, which contains two glycosides exerting a specific action on the heart. Similar substances, urechitin and urechitoxin, from *Urechites suberecta*, exert a cumulative action, and therefore sudden death may be produced without arousing suspicion of poisoning.

The juice of an *Asclepias* (or milkweed) is used in India as an infanticide; the symptoms are vomiting, salivation and cramps. The roots of various species of aconite (*Aconitum ferox*, etc.) are used for the same purpose; death takes place rapidly—in 3–6 hours, as a rule. Several species of Apocynaceae, such as *Cerbera odollam* and *Thevetia neriifolia*, the sap and seeds of which contain a glycoside, *thevetin*, are very deadly, death from cardiac failure taking place in twelve to fifteen hours. In Southern India, Burma, and Ceylon a decoction of the fruit of *Gloriosa superba*, one of the Liliaceae, allied to squill, is employed for criminal and suicidal purposes. The active principle, superbin, causes gastro-intestinal irritation and cardiac failure within 4 hours. The commonest poison in India and Ceylon is datura, one of the Solanaceae, of which there are several species. The seeds, mixed with food or drink, produce a state of extreme mental exaltation, followed by coma; the active principles are atropine, hyoscyamine, and scopolamine.

In Africa the leaves of *Hyoscyamus fahezlez*, containing *hyoscyamine* and *scopolamine*, as active principles, are used by Tuaregs of the Sahara. On the West Coast of Africa, a decoction of a cactus, colloquially known as 'oro', produces blisters in the mouth, vomiting and gastro-intestinal irritation, collapse and death. In China, opium is the suicidal poison most frequently used, especially by women.

Curare, the potent arrow poison of S. American Indians, was known to Sir Walter Raleigh in 1595. The material was obtained from the giant vines of the Amazon and Orinoco, called 'bushropes' by explorers, which include *Chondodendron tomentosum* which is the main source of curare. Curare poisons by causing paralysis of the muscles as shown by Claude Bernard in 1857. It has a molecular structure similar to that of acetylcholine. As a result of this molecular similarity the 'receptors' in the muscle, upon which acetylcholine acts, cannot distinguish between them and in this physiological manner relaxation of the muscle is produced. It has now revolutionized anaesthesia; the active principle is D-tubocurarine chloride. Synthetic forms of curare have been discovered and are being widely used.

In the Congo almost all the poisons used on arrow-heads contain cardiotoxic glycosides derived from species of *Strophanthus*, particularly k-strophanthin and ouabain; many contain haemolytic saponins and organic bases.

Atriplicism

A combination of cutaneous and nervous symptoms in China is caused by eating leaves of *Atriplex littoralis*. The earliest symptoms consist of itching of the hands, followed by oedema, and often by bullae; the finger-tips may become gangrenous, cutaneous haemorrhages may occur and the face and eyelids become cyanotic and oedematous. In many aspects it resembles Raynaud's disease and erythromelalgia. Yu Ky described a syndrome after eating the leaves of *Atriplex serrata*, or *Chenopodium hybridum*, in which the symptoms and signs are similar, and it is thought that the skin lesions can be ascribed to light-sensitive dermatosis.

Ackee poisoning (vomiting sickness of Jamaica)

An acute and fatal condition, locally termed 'the vomiting sickness', has been known for many years in Jamaica. It is found principally in rural districts in circumscribed epidemics. The causation and nature were neither apprehended nor understood, although several Commissions had attempted to elucidate them. To Sir Harold Scott belongs the merit of clearing up this mystery, and of indicating simple and practical methods of prevention, which have saved the lives of many children. It is estimated that since 1886 over 5000 lives have been lost in Jamaica from this cause.

Aetiology. Scott showed, on what must be regarded as convincing evidence —clinical, seasonal, epidemiological, and experimental—that vomiting sickness is the result of poisoning by a fruit, much used by Negroes in Jamaica, called ackee, the fruit of *Blighia sapida* (Fig. 247), a tree very common in the island. A similar species is found on the West Coast of Africa, where it is known as Irsin. When mature and in good condition, this fruit is wholesome enough; if gathered, before it is quite ripe and before it has opened while on the tree, or if gathered from an injured branch, or opened after falling to the ground, it is poisonous. The poisonous element in the immature and unsound fruit appears to be soluble in water, for 'pot water' in which the ackees have been cooked is much more toxic than cooked fruit. The poison is precipitated by alcohol. Jordan and

Burrows showed that the toxic principle is also contained in the seeds and in the arilli of the ackee which have not yet 'opened'.

Cicely Williams (1954) has stated that this disease is not caused only by ackee, but by other herbs used for 'bush teas'. Recently other observers, such as Hill (1952), have raised doubts of the very existence of vomiting sickness as a separate entity. Stuart *et al.* (1955) found extreme hypoglycaemia (blood sugar levels as low as 22 mg/100 ml) in children with this illness. They laid the foundations for its logical treatment by prompt and large doses of glucose. Biopsy and necropsy showed fatty changes in the liver with almost complete absence of glycogen. The course of the disease suggested a temporary enzyme block, inhibiting gluconeogenesis for which the name of *acute toxic hypoglycaemia* is proposed. The ackee, when studied by Hassall and Reyle (1955), was found to contain in its seeds two polypeptides—hypoglycin A and B—which produced fatal hypoglycaemia in laboratory animals. This study may be important to the fuller understanding of carbohydrate metabolism in diabetes mellitus.

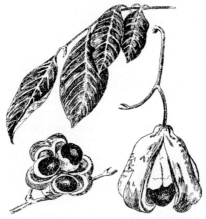

Fig. 247.—Ackee fruit (*Blighia sapida*), quarter natural size. (*After Byam & Archibald*)

Vomiting sickness is confined to the West India Islands, practically to Jamaica, and occurs principally in the cooler months, from November to April.

Symptoms. A previously healthy child suddenly complains of abdominal discomfort, vomits several times, recovers, and perhaps falls asleep. Three or 4 hours later, vomiting—now of a cerebral type—returns. Within a few minutes, convulsions and coma supervene, and death follows, on an average, about 12 hours from the initial vomiting, though it may take place in $1\frac{1}{2}$ hours. The case mortality amounts to 80–90%. In those who recover, convalescence is complete in 24 hours.

During the attack the temperature is normal or subnormal, rarely rising to 38·3°C; the pulse rate is 90 to 100; the respirations are 26–30, sometimes, as death approaches, of Cheyne–Stokes type. The pupils are slightly dilated and, until near the end, react to light. Except during the convulsive seizures, there is no muscular rigidity. Post mortem examination reveals hyperaemia of viscera with a tendency to minute intestinal haemorrhages, together with marked fatty changes, especially in the liver and kidneys, and sometimes in the pancreas and heart muscles.

introduction of the latex into the conjunctival sac. Severe dermatitis brought about by handling dried wood powder is thought to be allergic.

If the fruit is eaten, as it may be by ignorant visitors, children or insane people, vesiculation of the buccal mucous membrane with diarrhoea and blood and mucus stools may ensue. Fatal poisoning may result.

Manchineel juice on the skin should be washed off with sea water. Blisters should be kept aseptic, and, if extensive, should be treated like a second degree burn. When the fruit has been eaten, emesis should be induced.

Alcoholism and drug habits

Alcohol poisoning. This occurs in varying degrees among nearly all tropical races, and in symptoms and course does not differ materially from alcoholism in other parts of the world. Rum (65–72% of alcohol), obtained from the fermentation of molasses, is used in the West Indies and South America; arrack (50–60% alcohol) is manufactured in India, China and Java from fermented rice or from palm sap; while a slightly fermented drink, toddy, is obtained from sweet sap of various palms, and is drunk in India, Ceylon and West Africa. In South America a potent alcoholic drink is made from the fermented juice of *Agave americana*, and is known as 'pulque'.

Opium poisoning. The opium habit, either eating or smoking—the symptoms of which are too well known to require description—is common throughout the tropics. Opium poisoning is also a favourite form of suicide, especially among women.

Cannabis indica. Indian hemp, or hasheesh, grows in India, Iran and Arabia, and is a variety of the common hemp, *Cannabis sativa*. The leaves are powdered down, and either chewed or smoked in a preparation known as bhang; an extract of the flowers is known as ganja. Both these preparations cause great nervous excitement and, if persistently used, often lead to permanent insanity, the main features of which are hallucinations and illusions. Hasheesh, in various preparations, often with the addition of extracts of various Solanaceae, such as datura and nux vomica, is habitually taken daily by millions of the inhabitants of Africa and Asia. The most stringent government regulations have been framed to suppress trade in this drug.

Kava or yangona. The powdered root of one of the Piperaceae, prepared to form a beverage, is drunk on festive occasions throughout Polynesia. Formerly the root was masticated by specially selected girls in the preparation of the drink, a practice which was then a prolific source of tuberculosis. Overindulgence in kava induces a state of hyperexcitement, with loss of power in the legs. Chronic intoxication produces debility, with coarse roughened skin.

Betel. Chewing betel, the leaves of *Piper betel*, together with lime and areca nut (*Areca catechu*), is a common practice in India and Ceylon, and generally throughout the East. The mouth, lips and teeth are stained a bright red colour. It produces a flushing of the face, and has mild stimulant and possibly anthelmintic properties. In Central Africa the nuts of the kola tree (*Sterculia* sp.) are chewed habitually, and act, like betel, as a stimulant, without, it is said, producing any detrimental effects.

Cocaine. Erythroxylon coca is widely used in India and in parts of South America as a stimulant and intoxicant. The leaves, first dried in the sun, are chewed with lime or, as in India, with betel. This drug produces a loss of sensation in tongue and lips, the pulse is accelerated and there ensues a period of hilarity and exaltation. The drug addict soon becomes emaciated and cachectic.

Mushroom poisoning

There are many poisonous species of mushroom, particularly the genus *Amanita* in Southern Europe and U.S.A., more especially *A. phalloides*, the 'death cap'. These mushrooms cannot be distinguished by their taste and are said to possess an agreeable flavour. They can be recognized by persistence of a portion of the veil encircling the stem a little below the cup. *A. muscaria* contains an alkaloid, *muscarine*, which is allied to pilocarpine. Atropine constitutes an efficient antidote.

Flax darnel (*Lolium linicolum* or *L. temulentum*) poisoning

Brinton (1946) has described recurrent epidemics of food poisoning in the local population of Aden due to Ethiopian wheat containing this poisonous weed, known in local Arabic as Miscara ('tipsy'). Each weed seed is covered by a mould known as temuline. Within a quarter of an hour the patient becomes dizzy, with headache, slurred speech and generalized tremors and staggering gait. Sometimes there is diarrhoea, nausea and abdominal pain. Stupor and coma supervene and last for about 10 hours. This state is known as 'lolism' and is common in Ethiopia.

Catha edulis or miraa poisoning

Miraa is a local name (muiragi, khat, cafta) of a tree, *C. edulis*, about 6 m in height, indigenous to Africa. The leaves or twigs may be chewed or infused to make 'bushman's tea', or may even be smoked, when they induce a happy mellow sense of friendliness. Cases of mental disturbance in addicts have been described. *C. edulis* contains 3 alkaloids, cathine, cathinine and cathidine. Except that it is not an analgesic the action resembles that of cocaine.

Epidemic dropsy (argemone oil poisoning)

Epidemic dropsy somewhat resembles beri-beri. Clinically, it is characterized by dropsy associated with cardiac symptoms, but without paralysis or anaesthesia.

History and geographical distribution. This condition was first noted in Calcutta in 1877; it has since occurred there sporadically, but vanishes in the hot season. In Mauritius, in 1879, it affected one-tenth of the coolies, of whom a large number died. An epidemic broke out in Fiji in 1926 and was limited to Asians; no native Fijians were affected. In Purulia (Nagpur, India) there have been epidemics at intervals since 1913, the worst being in 1934 when over 2000 were attacked. Meaker (1950) has described an outbreak in coloured labourers in N.W. Cape District of South Africa.

Aetiology. In spite of the apparently wide distribution of this disease, most of the information comes from India, where this form of poisoning is especially seen in the Hindus, particularly in females. Children under puberty are less liable than adults; sucklings are seldom affected. The weak and the robust are equally susceptible. It has been remarked that very few are of the poorer class, nearly all coming from the middle and upper classes.

The outbreak in Fiji in 1926 was attributed to mustard oil used in the preparation of curries, and later, Banerji and Ghosh in Bengal came to the same conclusion. The Mexican poppy, *Argemone mexicana*, is a common weed in India as well as in Australia, where it has been mixed with wheat and fed to fowls. In them it produces changes in the comb, paralysis of legs and oedema of wattles and subcutaneous tissues reminiscent of epidemic dropsy in man. Bhattacharjee was the first to bring forward evidence that oil from the seeds of this poppy was responsible for toxic manifestations in man. Later, Pasricha showed that the toxicity of contaminated mustard oil could be eliminated by heating to 240°C for 15 minutes. Lal and his colleagues found that the seeds of *A. mexicana* (Sialkanta, in Hindu) are present in many stocks of mustard seed in India, used in the preparation of katakar oil for cooking. Sanguinerine is believed to be the toxic principle of argemone oil. In animal experiments it has been found to cause capillary dilatation and interferes with oxidation of pyruvic acid. Cullinan *et al.* (1946) described an outbreak among African troops in Madagascar which, however, appeared to be due to fungus-infected rice.

The aetiology now appears clear. Argemone oil, under experimental conditions, produces symptoms indistinguishable from those of 'epidemic dropsy'. It can be detected by a simple colour test, on adding nitric acid to contaminated mustard oil. Sarkar did not consider that this is sufficiently delicate, but stated that argemone oil, when heated with ferric chloride, in the presence of strong hydrochloric acid and ethyl alcohol, gives an orange-red precipitate. Two ml of the oil to be tested are taken in a test-tube, 2 ml of concentrated hydrochloric acid are added, mixed and heated in water-bath at 33·3°–35° C for 2 minutes. Then 0·8 ml of ethyl alcohol is added, the mixture shaken thoroughly and kept in a water-bath for 1 minute. Two ml of ferric chloride solution are then run in, the contents mixed thoroughly by shaking, and the whole heated in a water-bath for another 10 minutes.

Pathology. De described as characteristic extensive vascular dilatation in the deeper layers of the skin. The heart muscle shows no degenerative changes, but there is thinning of the muscle walls, and muscle fibres are separated by dilated capillaries. Shanks also found capillary dilatation wherever the vessels are least supported, and this is most obvious in fatty tissues, whether subcutaneous, subpericardial or subperitoneal. Similar changes are seen in the lungs, in the cervix uteri, in the ovaries and in the intestines. The liver usually presents a 'nutmeg' appearance (Shaha). The chief changes occur in the blood vessels, which are dilated and surrounded by proliferating endothelial cells.

For effects on the eye, see Chapter 44.

Chatterjee and Halder found that in an average case the total erythrocyte count is about 3·8 millions, while the haemoglobin is reduced to 11 grammes/100 ml. The lymphocyte percentage is raised and there is usually considerable eosinophilia. The reticulocytes are not increased as a rule.

Symptoms. Dropsy is almost invariably present. It usually appears first in the legs, and in some instances is confined to them; in others it involves the entire body. Occasionally, it is very persistent, recurring during convalescence. Fever also is very constant; sometimes it precedes, sometimes it accompanies, sometimes it follows the dropsy. It is rarely high, ranging usually from 37·2° to 38·9°C. Diarrhoea and vomiting generally ushered in the disease in the Mauritius epidemic. In Calcutta these symptoms were not so frequent, although by no means rare, occurring at both earlier and later stages. The total duration is about 6 weeks. An outbreak in the employees of the E. Indian railway was reported in 1945. There were 476 cases. The largest proportion were oedematous and a considerable number had diarrhoea and pyrexia. Oedema of feet and legs lasted for 2 weeks. There was patchy pigmentation over nose, malar bones and shins. Tachycardia was common and mortality 4·4%.

Peripheral neuritis is absent and the knee jerk is not abolished, but usually distressing aching of muscles, bones and joints is prominent. An exanthem, erythematous on the face, rubeolar on the trunk and limbs, was frequently seen in Mauritius, less so in Calcutta. It appeared about a week after the oedema and lasted from 10 to 12 days. On the skin, vascular naevi often appear and may bleed profusely, while telangiectases are common. The eruptions have been described as nodular, resembling sarcoids in some epidemics, while lesions on the mucous membranes have been noted. They do not inconvenience the patient, but may bleed uncontrollably. Ecchymotic patches consist, not of haemorrhage, but of telangiectases. Three to 6 weeks after the first symptoms, nodular excrescences are seen; there may be 100 or more; they may be sessile or pedunculated, varying in size from a pea to a lemon, and they bleed readily (Fig. 249).

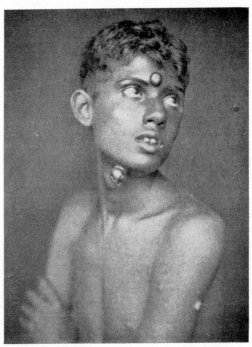

Fig. 249.—Nodular lesions (sarcoids) in epidemic dropsy. (*After De & Chatterjee*)

Disturbances of the heart and circulation are prominent in nearly all the cases. The pulse is weak, rapid and irregular, the blood-pressure low; cardiac bruits are often noted. Breathlessness on exertion occurred in all cases, severe orthopnoea in many. Signs of pleural and pericardial effusion, of oedema of the lungs, of pneumonia, and of cardiac dilatation are common. Hawes stated that the lung signs are characteristic and resemble a bronchial spasm with defective aeration. Anaemia is usually marked, and so are wasting and prostration. The urine is not albuminous, but of low specific gravity and greatly increased in amount. Concurrent primary glaucoma is not uncommon.

It may be necessary to differentiate epidemic dropsy from the war oedema as observed in Central Europe and Egypt during the 1914–18 and 1939–45 wars. The latter occurred in a population undergoing dietetic restrictions, and was characterized by great emaciation and a high degree of anaemia. Experiments with rats fed on diets deficient in proteins and salts produce a condition not unlike nutritional oedema. From oedematous beri-beri epidemic dropsy is differentiated by pyrexia, the peculiar erythematous rash, and persistence of the deep reflexes. A history of family outbreaks following the use of mustard oil suggests epidemic dropsy. Not all batches of oil are contaminated with argemone oil.

Treatment is based upon the facts that:

1. The adulterant argemone oil is the primary cause.
2. It is a cumulative poison.
3. It causes capillary dilatation and permeability.
4. The serum albumin and calcium are reduced, and serum globulin is increased.
5. Carbohydrate metabolism is checked at the pyruvic acid stage.
6. Myocardial damage is set up.

Antihistaminic drugs, such as Phenergan, benefit, though no rise in blood histamine has been demonstrated. Restoration of damaged capillaries by vitamins C and E and by hesperidin or rutin extracts of citrus fruits, protection of the liver by a diet rich in protein and fat with glucose and insulin (10 units twice daily) is indicated. The calcium deficiency is restored by 10% calcium Sandoz intravenously.

REFERENCES

BRINTON, D. (1946) *Proc. R. Soc. Med.*, **39**, 173.
CULLINAN, E. R., KEKWICK, A., WATTS, A. S. & TITMAN, W. L. (1946) *Q. Jl Med.*, **15**, 91.
EKPECHI, O. L. (1967) *Br. J. Nutr.*, **21.**, 537.
HASSALL, C. H. & REYLE, K. (1955) *W. Indian med. J.*, **4**, 83.
HILL, K. R. (1952) *W. Indian med. J.*, **3**, 243.
KINGSBURY, J. M. (1964) *Poisonous Plants of the United States and Canada*. Cornell, N.J.: Prentiss Hall.
MEAKER, R. E. (1950) *Sth Afr. med. J.*, **24**, 331.
NORTH, P. (1963) *Poisonous Plants and Fungi*. London: Blandford.
STUART, K. L., JELLIFFE, D. B. & HILL, K. R. (1955) *J. trop. Pediat.*, **1**, 69.
WATT, J. M. & BREYER BRANDWIJK, M. G. (1962) *Medicinal and Poisonous Plants of Southern and Eastern Africa*. Edinburgh: Livingstone.
WILLIAMS, C. D. (1964) *Report on Vomiting Sickness in Jamaica*. Kingston: Government Printer.

SECTION XIV

LEECHES

43. LEECHES AND LEECH INFESTATION

LEECHES which attack man belong to:

Phylum	Annelida
Class	Hiridinea
Order	Gnathobdellida
Family	Hirudinidae

Gnathobdellid leeches are invertebrates, having a smooth cuticle, a mouth lacking a proboscis but with 3 jaws, 2 suckers (one surrounding the mouth, the other at the posterior end) and powerful muscles, circular and longitudinal. When unfed they are usually about 2·5 cm long and 5 mm thick; some are bigger. When full of blood they are dark bloated objects.

The muscular jaws are covered with chitin, and produce a characteristic triradiate wound in the skin of the victim. The mouth leads to a pharynx, with salivary glands which secrete the anticoagulant hirudin, a crop in which ingested blood can be stored, a stomach, intestine, rectum and an anal pore near the posterior sucker. The excretory system consists of 17 pairs of nephridia. There is a vascular system and a nervous system.

Leeches are hermaphrodites, each one possessing testes and ovaries, the spermatozoa of one individual being deposited during copulation on the cuticle (to migrate through the tissues to reach the ovary) or into the vagina, of the other member of the copulating pair. Some leeches deposit egg masses on objects submerged in water, others form a cocoon to be deposited in water or mud, from which the young hatch and attach themselves to water plants. Others carry their young until they are able to suck.

Leeches live by sucking the blood of other animals—frogs, turtles, molluscs and land vertebrates such as cattle, horses and man. Aquatic leeches haunt water; land leeches live in the vegetation of tropical rain forests. Both will attack man, but the land leeches are more notorious in this—they tend to breed and live near springs, streams and wells frequented by cattle, horses, man and other vertebrates.

The species noted for attacks on man include *Haemadipsa zelanica*, *H. sylvestris*, *H. picta*, *Phytobdella catenifera* and *Dinobdella ferox*. This last deposits its eggs on water plants, whence the young offspring invade the mouths or nostrils of animals drinking the water, and can pass to the deeper respiratory passages or the oesophagus.

LAND LEECHES

The punctures made in the skin by these are painless, and remain open and bleeding after the leech has gone; healing is slow. Leeches take much more blood than they need, and if they remain attached, or are numerous, they can take so much that the patient becomes seriously anaemic and may even die from loss of blood.

Treatment

Leeches which attach themselves to the skin must be induced to detach, but they must not be simply pulled off because they may then leave behind their jaws, which could become the starting point of phagedaenic ulceration. Drops of strong salt solution, alcohol or strong vinegar applied round the mouth, or heat from a lighted match applied to the body, will cause the leech to release its hold. The wound can then be treated with a styptic and an antiseptic.

Prevention

People in countries where these leeches are common (particularly South-east Asia, the Pacific Islands, the Indian sub-continent and South America) should, when travelling in infested country, wear boots and trousers thick enough to prevent access by the leeches (from vegetation) to the skin. Additional and effective protection is afforded if the garments or the skin are treated with repellents such as dimethyl or dibutyl phthalate, Rutgers 612, or indalone. Dibutyl phthalate lasts longer on clothing than dimethyl phthalate, and if applied about once every 2 weeks at the rate of 28 ml per set of garments, or about 4 ml/ 30 cm^2, is a good repellent. On the skin these are effective for only 3–5 hours, or less if sweating is excessive. Dimethyl phthalate should not be used on rayon garments.

AQUATIC LEECHES

Internal leech infestation is less common than external attack on the skin, but it does occur, and can be very dangerous. Aquatic leeches can enter the mouth or nostrils of man if he approaches his face to water, to drink or wash, and they can also attack the conjunctiva, the vulva and vagina and the male urethra in persons bathing in infested water. Leeches of the species *Limnatis nilotica* and *L. maculosa* are among those which can be dangerous in this way. *L. nilotica* is very large, haunting quiet waters and ponds.

Having entered the mouth or nostrils the leech can quickly pass to the naso-pharynx, epiglottis or oesophagus, and even to the trachea and bronchi. When it attaches itself to the mucous membrane it secretes its anticoagulant and engorges. The natural result is bleeding, according to the site of attachment— epistaxis, haemoptysis or haematemesis—which may lead to severe anaemia. A leech in the nares may also give prolonged headache; if in the larynx there is a cough with bloody discharge, hoarseness, dyspnoea, pain and even suffocation; if in the epiglottis region there is likely to be difficulty in swallowing. Infestation of these parts by leeches may be one cause of 'halzoun' (marrara), more often attributed to *Fasciola hepatica*, or more certainly to nymphs of *Linguatula serrata* (Schacher et al. 1969 (Appendix III)).

Treatment

In treating leech infestation of the upper respiratory passages an attempt should be made to see the leech. If it is in the posterior pharynx, larynx, trachea or bronchi, the patient should be placed in the Trendelenburg position so that the leech cannot fall back and block the lower passages. If it is in the nares or upper pharynx it can be treated with a cocaine preparation and extracted with forceps or a hooked probe, but it is difficult to grasp. If lower down, the use of cocaine is not advised; a pair of long hooked forceps can be introduced through a laryngoscope, and the leech pulled out gently, but tracheostomy may be necessary. If in the oesophagus the leech should be seen through an oesophagoscope, and can be treated with cocaine; it will then fall into the stomach where the gastric juice will render it harmless. For a leech in the genito-urinary apparatus irrigation with strong salt solution is useful.

Prevention

To avoid attack by aquatic leeches it is important to wear appropriate clothing and to use repellents when in contact with water in the affected parts of the world, and to drink only water which has been filtered or at least strained through fine gauze, and preferably (for this and other reasons) boiled.

Since leeches take in large amounts of blood, sometimes necessarily containing blood parasites, Marsden and Pettit (1969) thought that the medicinal leech, *Hirudo medicinalis*, might be used in the xenodiagnosis of Chagas's disease, but their experiments showed that although *Trypanosoma cruzi* can survive in a recognizable form for 72 hours in the gut of the leech, there was no indication that this would be a useful method of xenodiagnosis.

REFERENCES

MARSDEN, P. D. & PETTITT, L. E. (1969) *Trans. R. Soc. trop. Med. Hyg.*, **63,** 413.
SCHACHER, J. F., SAAB, S., GERMANOS, R. & BOUSTANY, N. (1969) *Trans. R. Soc., trop. Med. Hyg.*, **63,** 854.

SECTION XV

OPHTHALMOLOGY IN THE TROPICS

44. OPHTHALMOLOGY IN THE TROPICS
By A. McKie Reid, *M.C.*, *T.D.*, *O. St. J.*, F.R.C.S., D.O.M.S.

GENERAL CONSIDERATIONS

It is irrational to think or speak of tropical ophthalmology as we speak of a foreign language in a country remote from our own and without a single root common to our native tongue, for congenital abnormalities, new growth, simple or malignant, traumas, inflammation acute or chronic, cyst formation and infections and infestations in the eye, as elsewhere in the body, follow the same basic pathological processes in all parts of the world. Conditions of life in the tropics may, it is true, modify these processes and there are, of course, many diseases affecting the eye which originate exclusively in tropical countries.

We should agree, therefore, with the semantics of E. J. Somerset, who writes of 'ophthalmology in the tropics' rather than of 'tropical ophthalmology'.

Nevertheless, the importance of ophthalmology in the tropics and the high incidence of diseases of the eye with their accompanying suffering, blindness and economic loss, both to the individual and to the community, cannot be too strongly emphasized.

Socio-economic factors

Poverty and malnutrition, particularly protein deficiency; housing and sanitary conditions; ignorance and lack of education; indifferent personal hygiene often associated with a poor water-supply; the havoc wrought by unqualified and unskilled practitioners using unscientific methods of treatment, such as couching for cataract with an acacia thorn—all play their part. A peculiar and interesting factor is that which comes into play, in primitive and isolated communities, by inbreeding. Examples of this are the high incidence of retinitis pigmentosa in Tristan da Cunha, albinism in Brandywine in Maryland and hereditary microphthalmia in Alabama (Gillespie & Covelli 1963) and among the Nanticokes in Delaware. In the Pingelap Atoll in the Eastern Caroline Islands, 4–10% of the 900 inhabitants are blind from birth, manifesting nystagmus, night blindness, colour blindness and eventually cataract. The cause is attributed to a typhoon about 1780 which reduced the male population to 9. As well as inbreeding a dietetic factor may be responsible for precipitating the disease in children who are genetically susceptible. In these conditions recessive disorders are favoured where the population is rural and immobile, where there is a high degree of consanguinity and where large families are the rule.

Psychological factors

Psychological factors such as apathy and fatalism, superstitious beliefs and suspicion of outside help and treatment are found predominantly in deprived people. These attitudes are not, however, confined to torrid countries, for even in an advanced country such as we believe our own to be, we find patients who through hope, fear, apathy or sheer stupidity allow blindness to overtake them and who, in the present decade, use carrot poultices and cold tea or urine as eye lotions.

Climatic conditions prevalent in the tropics, such as glare, heat, humidity and dust, are other adverse factors.

Bacteria, fungi, parasites and insects, if not all specific, are abundant in the tropics and productive of much eye trouble.

Many of these factors will be discussed where they are pertinent; but two factors, glare and malnutrition, may appropriately be dealt with forthwith.

Glare and the use of sunglasses

Nature has made reasonably adequate provision for regulating the amount of light entering the eye—eyelashes to screen the light from above or reflected from below, the orbicularis to 'screw up' the eye, the active pupil and the uveoretinal pigment. The Eskimos make use of slotted strips of bone or wood to cut out snow-reflected light, but many races and individuals survive, without adventitious aid, the fiercest rays of the sun. Spectacles are, however, worn to indicate that the wearer is 'literate' for why should they be worn if he is unable to read? The wearing of sunglasses has become a social custom for some people, as much as a practical necessity. Many people wear dark glasses to see without being seen, or to add a fictitious glamour or mystery to an otherwise unconvincing physiognomy. Neither the softly shaded lighting of a restaurant or hotel lounge nor the light out of doors on dull days menaces even the most photophobic eyes, yet no other optical product is manufactured, distributed in such enormous quantities and worn so indiscriminately and capriciously.

A High Court judge (Mr Justice Philamore) in giving judgement against a driver recently said: 'I do not suppose her ability to keep a proper look-out was enhanced by wearing dark glasses. It seems an extraordinary thing to do when driving a car by night.'

Sunglasses were probably worn before spectacles were invented to correct errors of refraction. The emerald through which Nero watched the flames was in the nature of a sunglass, and tourmaline lenses with their polarizing quality were used by the Chinese. The ophthalmic surgeon is often asked for advice by those living or contemplating living in countries where the sun is more evident than in northern climes. A brief review of the physiological principles involved may help to explain the conditions under which the use of tinted lenses is expedient.

Visible light consists of electromagnetic vibrations of wavelengths between the values of 4000 and 7600 Ångstrom units. Below 4000, ultraviolet radiations, and above 7600, infrared radiations replace the visible spectrum. Prolonged exposure to infrared rays may produce lens changes, as in glassblower's cataract, and exposure to excessive ultraviolet radiation may produce a variety of effects such as solar photophthalmia or snow blindness, in which photophobia, lacrimation, ciliary neuralgia, blepharospasm, oedema of the eyelids and even corneal ulceration may occur. Industrial photophthalmia occurs in occupations where sources of light rich in short waves are used, such as in arc-welding and oxyacetylene burning or where short-circuiting of high-tension currents is likely to occur. Exposure to these wavelengths may cause oedema of the macula, followed by pigment proliferation and a central scotoma. Similar changes follow sun-gazing or watching an eclipse. Hence possibly some cases of unexplained amblyopia.

Indications for the wearing of tinted or sunglasses are:

a. Clinical. Many surgeons advise the wearing of smoked or tinted glasses after cataract extraction as the retina cannot immediately tolerate the increased intensity of light following the removal of the opaque cataract.

In keratitis, iritis and acute inflammatory conditions of the posterior segment bright light may cause photophobia and headache.

In some myopes in whom the pupil is habitually dilated, in blond people who lack uveal pigment and especially in albinos and cases of aniridia the wearing of dark glasses is justifiable. Many people wear dark glasses to disguise the wearing of strong spectacle lenses.

b. Occupational. Oxyacetylene and arc-welders must wear ultraviolet lenses, with side-pieces as a safeguard against flashes from the side; in addition, in many such occupations, a protective tinted screen is also used.

Dark adaptation: night-fighters and night-pilots, who may depend on visual control rather than on instrumental control, and night-drivers and dark-room workers such as radiographers can achieve maximum dark adaptation before starting on their duty by wearing dark glasses for a period, with a minimum of 15 minutes, which varies with the individual and his age.

c. Casual and recreational. In sun-bathing, especially if reading or sewing in sunlight, in motoring on glaring roads or facing the sun low in the horizon, in boating in small boats on bright days, and in skiing on snow glistening with sunlight, the wearing of protectively tinted lenses is justified. People from northern climes holiday-making in the south may, with reason, wear dark glasses when outside.

Types of sunglasses. Although glass is normally employed, the use of plastic filters is increasing. These have the advantage of lightness and are not so easily broken. The most popular types of filter are those without optical correction, and are worn by persons with normal visual acuity or as 'clip-on' lenses attached to the clear glass spectacles worn to correct an error of refraction.

The essential qualities of the lens are that visible radiation in all wavelengths is transmitted evenly; that ultraviolet and infrared rays are largely absorbed and that the lens should be ground or moulded in such a way as to prevent distortion of vision which, if not actually harmful, is irksome; and that the tint should not be deeper than necessary. For motoring and country sports an absorption of 50% of visible radiation is permissible, while for aquatic sports and for snowy terrain from 50 to 75% may be absorbed with advantage.

The actual colour of the lens is of minor importance; brownish, greenish and bluish-grey are in common use. Although the transmitted colour of surroundings is obvious on first using the lenses, the ocular perception registers colours normally and colour-confusion has not been recorded. In cases of colour-blindness or defective colour vision, tinted glasses will not remedy the defect.

In cases where corrective lenses are habitually worn, these may be dispensed in coloured glass, but where there is considerable variation in thickness in different parts of the lens, as in high myopia where the optical centre of the spectacle lens is very thin and in high hypermetropia where the centre is thick, the absorption varies in different parts of the lens. To overcome this, instead of glass-dyed lenses, a composite lens has been designed with a transparent carrier layer covered by a thin tinted layer of even thickness or, more recently, coated lenses in which the lens is smoked in a vacuum and absorbs an even layer of pigment.

To sum up, indiscriminate use of sunglasses is to be deprecated. They should not, unless clinically necessary, be worn indoors or in conditions of artificial illumination, or out-of-doors unless the condition of glare warrants their use. They are rarely necessary, though often worn, by persons in whom the ocular pigment is heavy, as it is in dark-skinned races. Finally, discretion should be exercised in allowing their use by troops on active service, unless on special duties such as driving or snow-trekking, for if they are habitually worn, and are then lost or broken, the result can be incapacitating.

Solar retinopathy—a warning!

The phenomenon of an eclipse of the sun has in some parts of the world a religious significance and, indeed, wherever it can be observed, the spectacle attracts well merited curiosity.

In scanning the sky for aircraft, an adventitious hazard is a direct glimpse of the sun; mentally disturbed patients are recorded as having sustained retinal injury by sun-gazing.

An increasing number of cases of eclipse blindness are on record and recently a young woman, a patient of the writer, had to abandon a university career because of this.

The sudden intense glare of the sun at the end of the eclipse may unexpectedly throw a ray into the unprotected eye. This may cause an actual burnt-out hole in the macular area with loss of central vision and a positive scotoma. Minute haemorrhages, oedema and detachment of the retina are other sequelae. The ultimate prognosis varies with the severity of the lesion and with the length of time taken for the scotoma to subside.

Smoked glass or sunglasses, however dark, or exposed camera film do *not* offer adequate protection. Specially made gelatin filters confer some degree of safety but they should be authoritatively made by makers of repute.

Indirect observation of the image projected on to a white, grey or black screen through a pinhole, on the principle of a pinhole camera, is the only safe method for an amateur observer.

Socrates advised looking at a solar eclipse by watching its reflection in still water, a procedure unsafe enough in cloudy Britain but fraught with danger in the translucent atmosphere of Greece.

The Ministry of Health (1968) suggests a filter of density 4·5 which does not transmit more than one part in 30 000 of the total strength of solar radiation.

It is possible that some cases of unexplained amblyopia are due to solar retinopathy.

NUTRITION AND THE EYE

Deficiency disease, apart from sheer starvation or deprivation of food of any kind, implies disease caused by deficiency, ingestion of food below minimal requirements, defective utilization in the body of food substances or the absence in the food of protein, vitamins and amino acids and other essential chemicals.

Nowhere in the body is the impact of deprivation more in evidence than in the eye and in the visual sense.

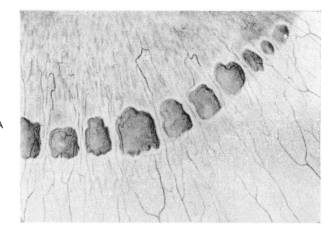

A

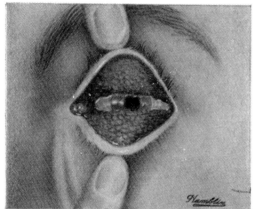

B

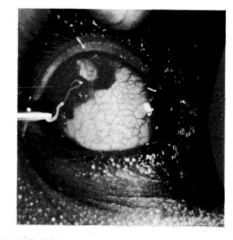

C

PLATE VII

Eye conditions in the tropics.

A, Herbert's pits in trachoma. B, Advanced trachoma. C, Extraction of *Loa loa* from the eye.

[*To face p. 832.*

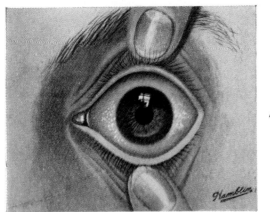

A

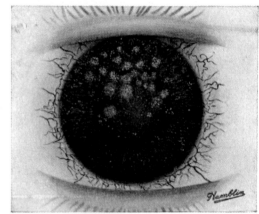

B

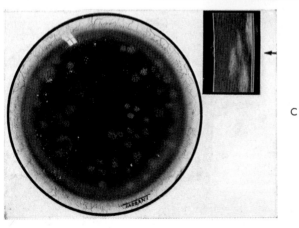

C

PLATE VIII

Eye conditions in the tropics.

A, Xerophthalmia. B, Leprosy of the cornea. C, Onchocerciasis.

Metabolism of the eye

The nutrition of most of the organs and tissues of the body is subserved directly by the blood stream, the haemoglobin of which carries oxygen to and extracts carbon dioxide from the tissues, while the plasma directly conveys nutrient metabolites. The mature eye differs from other organs and tissues in that its optical media—the cornea, aqueous, lens and vitreous—must of necessity be transparent. They are, therefore, avascular and devoid of blood vessels and direct blood supply. These transparent media are not inert, for in them occur metabolic processes which concern growth, maintenance and, particularly in the cornea, repair. The cornea is surrounded at its circumference by the blood capillaries of the limbus and both its surfaces are bathed by circulating fluids, the anterior by lacrimal secretion and the posterior by the aqueous. These fluids contain glucose, which is the main metabolic fuel of the cornea. Some of the glucose is built up into glycogen in high concentration in the epithelium. Glycolysis or the breakdown of glucose into lactic acid, the end-product of aerobic and anaerobic metabolism, is mediated by enzymes and co-enzymes which are in the main derived from vitamins. The lens also derives all material for growth and maintenance from its circumambient aqueous and vitreous humours. Much of its metabolism is dependent upon the reactions of enzymes of vitamin derivation. Other substances, amino acids and traces of mineral elements, also play an important part.

Historical review

From time to time during the past hundred years attention has been drawn to the effect of malnutrition upon the eyes of specific groups of people under specific conditions.

Hubbenet, the chief medical officer of the Russian Army in the Crimea (1860), recorded the occurrence in soldiers and in prisoners-of-war of xerosis of the conjunctiva, loss of lustre of the cornea and night blindness.

Bitot (1863) described what are now known as Bitot's spots in children in a foundling institution in Bordeaux. Simeon Snell (1876) reported on the occurrence of night blindness and xerosis in children in Sheffield and pointed out the beneficial effect of cod-liver oil in these patients. The people of Sheffield called these patches of conjunctival xerosis 'fish scales' and McLaren (1963) pointed out that in 3 countries where the condition is still common—Indonesia, Thailand and East Pakistan—the vernacular name has the same connotation.

Eijkman (1897) investigated nutritional ophthalmia which occurred among the officers of the Japanese Navy, while ratings escaped. He found that the staple diet before the mast was unhulled barley while the officers fed upon the more sophisticated diet of polished rice.

In Denmark during the war in 1917 all fresh butter was exported to Germany and margarine was substituted for home consumption. Children suffered from xerophthalmia and keratomalacia until butter, and margarine reinforced with vitamins, was added to their ration (Ehlers 1969).

In Vienna after the First World War many cases of keratitis were ascribed to tubercular infection, although no organism was isolated. Later reflection attributed these cases of xerophthalmia to protein and vitamin deficiency. In the Second World War prisoners-of-war in the Far East suffered from Wernicke's encephalopathy and 6% of them exhibited a greater or lesser degree of retrobulbar neuritis.

Atkinson (1955) reported xerophthalmia in Texas among the share-croppers who subsisted on a diet of over-milled corn-bread, and Thomson (1956) found acute corneal ulceration in Northern Nigeria, which he ascribed, in the thorn-scrub country, to the absence of that rich source of carotene, the oil-palm *Elaeis guineensis* Jacq.

The writer recollects the case of a young wife and mother who, in 1946 in England, manifested ocular signs of deficiency—night blindness, xerophthalmia and corneal ulceration—because she had diverted her balanced ration of butter and other fats to her working husband and young children. Under intensive hyperalimentation she made a good recovery apart from some residual corneal scarring.

Distribution of malnutrition

At the present time the manifestations of deficiency disease are to be found mainly in underdeveloped countries. Protein deficiency arises where production

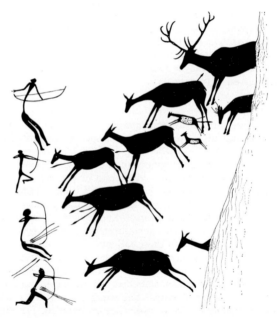

Fig. 250.—The search for protein, a cave painting from Castellón de la Plana. (*Ars Hispaniae*)

of cattle is inadequate, for instance because of disease, such as trypanosome infection. In Africa, between the southern limits of the Sahara down to latitude 20° S., 'nagana', the disease in animals caused by trypanosome infection, reduces the cattle-carrying capacity of the country by more than 50%. Wild animals and some breeds of cattle arrive at an understanding with the trypanosome risk to which they are exposed, so as to be able to absorb it, not without being infected, but without clinical manifestation. If the mechanism were understood, we should be in possession of a tool which could, beyond any other available, enlarge the production of available animal protein in the tropics (Lumsden 1969).

Rinderpest and East Coast fever are other factors in this part of the world. In India, religious restriction limits the amount of meat available as food and in other parts of the world, Latin America and Asia, meat is simply too dear.

Contributory factors

Mankind through the ages has progressively acquired knowledge of improved methods of cultivation and animal breeding but, *pari passu*, adverse factors have arisen. Soil erosion, a disease of civilization, has been caused by destructive methods of agriculture, such as the neglect of contour-ploughing, deforestation in which trees have been ruthlessly felled to supply fuel and building-timber, the ravages of undisciplined herds of goats which devour every burgeoning blade of herbage and eat the bark off trees, the use of animal manure as fuel instead of as fertilizer and the improvident utilization of water supply. An uncontrolled birth rate has increased competition for the relatively reduced amount of protein. The late Jawaharlal Nehru dared to say: 'We should be a far more advanced nation if our population were half what it is'.

Family customs and behaviour play their part. In West Africa the last-born child is carried strapped to the mother's back near to the source of nutriment until its successor arrives. It is then precipitately weaned and placed on a fully farinaceous diet of cassava, kenki or rice without milk or protein or any source of carotene. When meat, chicken or goat is eaten, the father has his fill, the mother next and the children in order of age. Only rarely does the weanling find a meat-bone to pick.

In other countries potentially milk-yielding animals—cows, buffaloes, camels, sheep and goats—are kept as stock animals and not milked. In places where fish is available the vitamin-rich liver is regarded as offal and thrown to the dogs. In the green humid tropics, where leafy green vegetation abounds, it is often overlooked as a food rich in vitamins, proteins and minerals.

In some parts of the world, infants suffering from ocular complications perish from general disease or from intercurrent infections without being admitted to hospital. The mortality may be high, but it reduces the social consequence of blindness, reduces the statistical impact of destructive eye disease and contributes to neglect of this problem.

Vitamin factors

The study of nutritional disease in man is a complex problem for, whereas in experimental animals isolated deficiencies can be inflicted, it is unusual for single deficiencies to occur clinically in man. In their sources and metabolism vitamins and accessory food factors are closely associated, but signs ascribable to one factor may dominate the picture. When so many factors are involved, even when a disease is proved to be well localized geographically, it cannot necessarily be concluded that one factor alone is incriminated.

With the reservations noted in the preceding paragraph there are, nevertheless, certain derangements of the eye associated with specific food deficiencies.

Vitamin A. Vitamin A, derived from carotene, occurs in milk products, carrots (hence the name), turnips, leafy vegetables, egg yolk and the livers of salmon, cod and halibut, and of seals and polar bears which eat these fish. This vitamin is mobilized by enzyme action to maintain a constant level in the plasma with a reserve in the liver. It is found in rhodopsin, the visual purple of the rod cells, and it is essential for dark adaptation. Night blindness is thus a symptom of deficiency. In retinitis pigmentosa a persistently low level in the blood has been described, so that this disease may be a hereditary deficiency disease due to faulty metabolism. Uyemura (1928) described small white spots in the fundus in severe hypovitaminosis A which disappeared under cod-liver oil therapy, and fundus changes, resembling retinitis punctata albescens, which responded to vitamin A treatment, were described by Teng-Khoen-Hing (1959). Bitot's spots are triangular areas of roughened epithelium covered with a foamy crust. They certainly occur in undernourished children, but their specific association with vitamin A deficiency is not universally agreed. These 'spots' respond rapidly to treatment with zinc sulphate 0·5% drops.

Xerophthalmia and keratomalacia. A low level of serum vitamin A affects the anterior segment of the eye. The conjunctiva becomes dry, wrinkled and opaque. The changes result from keratinization of the epithelial cells and are most marked in the interpalpebral fissure. A more advanced stage of the deficiency

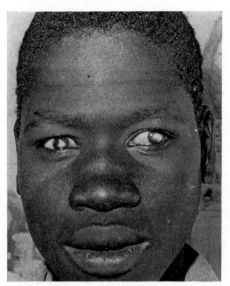

Fig. 251.—Keratomalacia in a Matabele boy of 14 years. (*Reproduced by permission of the Central African Journal of Medicine*)

leads to involvement of the cornea. In addition to the dull dry epithelium, there is infiltration of the stroma, and the cornea assumes a blue-grey appearance. There is little or no neovascularization. As the morbid process advances loss of substance occurs, the cornea becomes soft and excavation or ulceration occur, particularly in the central part. In advanced cases perforation follows with prolapse of the iris, which may become adherent to the cornea—the condition of leucoma adherens. Loss of vitreous, extrusion of the lens, hypopyon, endophthalmitis and total destruction of the eye often complete the picture. In the earlier stages the condition is described as xerophthalmia; when the whole cornea is involved it is called keratomalacia. When the tissue of the cornea melts away into a cloudy, gelatinous, yellowish mass, the descriptive term colliquative necrosis is applied (McLaren 1963). Affections limited to the conjunctiva may persist for months, but keratomalacia is a matter of days—and of life or death. Xerophthalmia, with its sequelae, is a major cause of blindness in children throughout the world. The percentage of malnourished children who show specific eye signs varies from country to country; from Indonesia incidences of 50-70% are regularly reported. Observers also suggest that for every survivor there is one child who dies; even after surviving the actual affection the chances of subsequent survival are worse than for his age partner (Ooman *et al.* 1964).

It is estimated that in the world there are 80 000 new cases per annum; in Indonesia 200 cases per million; in North Vietnam, with a population of 4 million, 280 children were admitted to one hospital in 1953. In Jordan, where accurate records are kept, there was recently an annual incidence of 238 cases in a population of 2 million. According to a recent estimate in rural Matabeleland, with a population of 800 000, there were 250 new cases in 1966. Infectious diseases, particularly measles, seem to push border-line cases into acute vitamin A deficiency and many patients with general diseases escape observation until too late. A World Health Organization bulletin, in a trenchant paragraph, states that 'the parents may not have their attention drawn to the seriousness of this condition until the corneae are dissolving away behind the closed eyes of their infant.'

Vitamins B_1, B_2. The germ-cells of cereals, milk, eggs, yeast, beef and leguminous vegetables are rich in these vitamins. Vitamin B_1 is thiamine or aneurine and B_2 is riboflavine. Absence of B_1 is responsible for beri-beri, in which the ocular symptoms are a dry burning conjunctivitis, keratitis and optic neuritis progressing to optic atrophy. Wernicke's encephalopathy with its nystagmus and external rectus palsy, together with cerebral symptoms, is attributable to thiamine deficiency. Vitamin B_2 deficiency or ariboflavinosis is manifested by vascular arcades at the limbus with vascular invasion of the cornea.

Vitamin PP or nicotinic acid. Deficiency of this vitamin together with B_1 and B_2 is considered to be a causative factor in pellagra. Exposure to sunlight causes hyperpigmentation of the skin and this is manifested in the eyelids, the lid margins and the conjunctiva in pellagra. The bulbar conjunctiva is chemosed, with linear erosions, particularly on the temporal side. In the cornea there are deeply placed ovoid opacities. In the lens, powder-like opacities and peripheral tongue-shaped opacities are found. In the affected subject, normal sunlight causes retinal hyperpigmentation and appearances at the macula similar to a burn, with hyperaemia and loss of the foveal reflex. These central changes result in a reduction of visual acuity (Mathur 1969).

Vitamin B_{12} or cyanocobalamin. This is poorly absorbed in Addisonian anaemia, in which disease retinal haemorrhages may appear.

Vitamin C or ascorbic acid. This vitamin is found in many fruits, particularly citrus fruits, and in milk products. The classical lesion is scurvy and this tendency may result in marginal blepharitis. In this complaint, which is distressing alike to the sufferer and to the beholder, the patient often admits to an adherence to a starchy diet and an avoidance of fruit and green vegetables.

Ocular lesions in scurvy are rare. The typical lesions are haemorrhages in the eyelids, conjunctiva, subconjunctival and episcleral tissues and, infrequently, in the iris and retina. Intracranial haemorrhages may cause ptosis and external ophthalmoplegia. Conjunctival lesions in volunteers who were subjected to ascorbic acid deprivation disappeared rapidly during repletion with ascorbic acid.

Vitamin D or calciferol. This is found in fish liver, eggs, milk and the hull of grains. The predominant deficiency manifestation is rickets. In experimental animals, deprivation has caused cataract. Zonular cataract and the cataract of tetany may be associated with a deficiency of this vitamin.

Vitamin K or naphthaquinone. Without this factor prothrombin disappears and clotting is inhibited. It is not absorbed from the gut unless the bile salts are present; thus retinal haemorrhages in diabetes when the liver is involved may be connected with defective absorption of this vitamin.

In conclusion, we may reflect that the traveller, lay or medical, is often dismayed at encountering, in the highways and byways of the East and in other parts of the world, so many sightless, light-searching eyes and empty sockets.

A generation ago, and unfortunately even in these days in many places, much of this blindness was attributed to trauma, ophthalmia neonatorum, trachoma or, in specific regions, onchocerciasis. Although these still take a heavy toll of sight, in many cases we are becoming increasingly aware of the true aetiology of much of this blindness—sheer starvation—and of its prevention.

The Chinese have an adage: 'Give a man a fish and you feed him for a day; teach him to fish and you feed him for life.'

EXAMINATION OF THE EYE

Examination of the eye not only implies the investigation of an isolated organ but may call for the examination of the patient as a whole because of the impact of general diseases upon the eye. The examination of the eye itself should be carried out in accordance with a definite routine, otherwise the attention may be directed to an obvious sign or symptom while something else equally important is overlooked.

The clinical examination may be divided into subjective and objective examinations.

SUBJECTIVE EXAMINATION

The subjective examination comprises the testing of the function of each eye separately and, in the case of squint, diplopia and muscle imbalance, of the two eyes together. The functions to be tested are visual acuity, field of vision, colour vision, light sense and binocular and stereoscopic vision.

Visual acuity

In testing for distance vision the subject is required to read letters or identify symbols on a test-type chart placed at 6 m distance. Snellen's test type consists of letters, but for illiterates Landolt's ring-test or the 'E' test is used. The size of the letter or symbol diminishes from above downwards. The uppermost is of such a size that it can be read or identified by the normal eye at 60 m and the letters or symbols lower down are such as can be read at 36, 24, 18, 12, 6, 5 and 4 m. The visual acuity is then expressed as an apparent fraction. The symbol 6/18, for example, implies that the subject reads at 6 m the line which should be read at 18 m if distance vision is normal.

Near vision is tested by test-types for near vision on which are printed types of various sizes. The smallest type which can be read is the visual acuity for near vision.

The field of vision

The field of vision represents the limits of peripheral vision while the eye remains fixed upon a central spot. This test can be carried out by a perimeter.

Where this instrument is not available, the confrontation test can provide useful information. The subject sits facing the examiner and with one eye covered he fixes his gaze upon the opposite eye of the examiner whose other eye is closed. The examiner's hand or a bright object is brought in from the periphery and the subject's field is tested against that of the examiner.

Limitations or defects in the field of vision may indicate diseases of the eye itself, such as glaucoma and pigmentary degeneration; of the optic nerve, such as optic atrophy and retrobulbar neuritis associated with multiple sclerosis and toxic amblyopia; or of the central nervous system, such as pituitary enlargement, cerebral tumours and intracranial vascular lesions.

Colour vision

This can be examined in many ways. The standard methods are (a) the Board of Trade lantern in which light is shone through an aperture in which screens of coloured glass are placed, or (b) the Ishihara colour charts. The matching of skeins of different coloured wool or coloured beads is used in testing children and illiterate patients.

Light sense

The light sense is the power of perceiving gradations in the intensity of illumination. The adjustment of the eye in passing from bright light to partial darkness, or vice versa, is known as adaptation. This factor is essential in deciding upon the suitability of candidates for such tasks as night-flying and night-driving. Adaptation varies with individuals. It decreases with age and is reduced in glaucoma and in vitamin A deficiency. Accurate estimation is a laboratory rather than a clinic room procedure.

Medical officers in remote places, who are not ophthalmic specialists, may be called upon to report upon the visual acuity of candidates for public services and should be familiar with the testing of visual acuity. Colour vision is important in commerce and industry. A case is recalled in which a representative of a textile firm who was colour-blind ordered from abroad large quantities of material of the wrong colour, with unfortunate results.

OBJECTIVE EXAMINATION

In the first place the patient should face a good even light such as a north-facing window or artificial light. The eyes are examined in relation to each other. In this way many anomalies may be demonstrated, such as facial asymmetry, unilateral swelling of the eyelids and surroundings of the eyes as in the case of a lacrimal abscess, unilateral exophthalmos, unilateral ptosis, squint and differences in iris pigmentation or heterochromia iridis.

Further examination of each eye proceeds in a routine order.

The conjunctiva

The palpebral conjunctiva lines the eyelids. The lower eyelid is pulled down to expose the deep surface of the lid and the lower fornix; then the upper eyelid is everted. This exposes the tarsal conjunctiva which covers the tarsal plate.

The eye is then rotated downwards to display the folds of the upper fornix.

The bulbar conjunctiva, the white of the eye, can be examined by causing the eye to be rotated fully in every direction.

The cornea

Gross changes can be seen with the naked eye, but wounds and pathological conditions of the cornea, although serious, are often so minute that intense oblique illumination from a focused lens or torch, and examination by a loupe lens or corneal magnifier, is essential. A slit-lamp, if available, will be used in the routine examination of any suspected corneal lesions.

The anterior chamber

After an injury or acute inflammation of the eye blood may lie in the angle of the anterior chamber; this is known as hyphaema. In iridocyclitis pus may be found in a similar situation; this is known as hypopyon. These conditions and larger foreign bodies can be seen with the naked eye. Magnification is required to detect the presence of inflammatory cells or of keratic precipitates (KP) adhering to the posterior surface of the cornea. Gonioscopy, or examination of the angle of the anterior chamber, such as is required in the investigation of glaucoma, is a specialist procedure.

The iris and pupil

A routine procedure will become instinctive with practice. The diameter of the pupil, its regularity, that is, whether it is circular or scalloped, the equality of the pupils of the two eyes and their reaction to light and accommodation and consensuality are all noted. The colour of the iris, the clearness of its pattern or whether it is muddy-looking, the presence of new vessels where none should be seen and presence of nodules or cysts, or of an adhesion of the iris to the cornea or to the lens (called anterior and posterior synechia respectively) are all of importance in the diagnosis of, for instance, leprosy of the iris and of other types of iritis.

The lens

The lens can be examined with a loupe or slit-lamp but full examination requires dilatation of the pupil with a mydriatic such as homatropine. The main departure from the normal is cataract, a condition to which reference will be made later (page 865). Dislocation of the lens may be found as a congenital lesion, as in Marfan's disease, or as a result of an injury.

The vitreous

The examination of the vitreous usually requires a dilated pupil. The vitreous is avascular and there is no true inflammation in such a structure, but haemorrhage from the retina may spill into the vitreous, or it may be invaded by new vessels arising from the retina. Any departure from normal interferes with the transparency of this medium, with resultant lowering of the visual acuity.

The fundus

An examination of the background of the eye requires the use of an ophthalmoscope. Here again a systematic search is essential and the more often normal fundi are examined, the less likely are departures from normal to be missed.

The disc is examined first. In colour it may be pale, suggesting atrophy, or hyperaemic; the margin may be blurred and the disc swollen, suggesting increased intracranial tension; it may be cupped or excavated, suggesting glaucoma. The macula in the direct line of the visual axis should then be examined.

Irregular pigmentation and haemorrhage may be noted, and here it may be mentioned that in 23% of patients over the age of 70 registered as blind in the United Kingdom blindness is due to senile macular degeneration.

The vessels must then be examined for changes in calibre, tortuosity, sheathing and other anomalies and then every quadrant of the retina right up to the periphery must be explored with the circle of light from the ophthalmoscope. Haemorrhages, exudates, pigmentation, tears, detachments and tumours may thus be found. The amazing variety of pictures to be seen cannot be described here but it may fairly be said that the clinical examination of a patient suffering from any disease, apart from local lesions, is incomplete without an ophthalmoscopic examination.

DISEASES OF THE CONJUNCTIVA
CONJUNCTIVITIS

Conjunctivitis, in one form or another, is one of the commonest conditions which occurs in the practice of ophthalmology in any country. The forms it assumes range from a simple catarrhal conjunctivitis to acute blinding ophthalmia neonatorum and chronic sight-destroying trachoma.

Signs and symptoms

Conjunctivitis in the absence of complications is not painful. Discomfort and a feeling of dryness or grittiness are common complaints and watering or running of the eye is often experienced. The sticking together of the eyelids on waking is a complaint frequently made. Photophobia is rarely present unless the cornea or iris is involved. In simple conjunctivitis there is no interference with vision though flecks of mucous secretion may cause transient blurring.

In the normal eye, the bulbar conjunctiva is white with a few branching blood vessels in the actual membrane. The palpebral conjunctiva which lines the eyelids is a smooth, regularly pink coloured, glistening, mucous membrane. Departure from these criteria is shown by increased vascularity or by irregularities of the smooth surface.

Increased vascularity may be generalized, the 'blood-shot' eye, or localized, when the conjunctiva is red in a particular region as in phlyctenular or angular conjunctivitis or in the dark red patch of a subconjunctival haemorrhage. Irregularities of the surface are seen in conditions such as the swelling or chemosis of a chemical burn or vernal catarrh, the follicles in the lower fornix in follicular conjunctivitis and the granules on the tarsal conjunctiva in trachoma.

Aetiology

The causes may be divided into four groups:

a. Infection with micro-organisms through contact with fingers or towels or with infected dust or dirt.

b. Allergic, as in hay-fever.

c. Febrile conditions, such as the common cold and the exanthemas such as measles and scarlatina, smallpox and typhus; in the first stage of Weil's disease in which there is intense congestion.

d. Traumatic, direct injury by foreign bodies, irritant or corrosive fluids and substances and by exposure to heat or ultraviolet light.

In the first three groups the conjunctivitis is usually bilateral with the exception of epidemic keratoconjunctivitis. In unilateral conjunctivitis a localized trauma or possibly a foreign body is suggested.

Dipyridilium compounds, such as Paraquat and Diquat, used as herbicides and defoliants, sprayed into the eyes may produce destruction of conjunctival and corneal epithelium. The onset of symptoms may be delayed, and, as in the case of lime burns, the chemical may be bound to the tissues. In the presence of a surface-active agent, irrigation is relatively ineffective and treatment difficult. Snake venom from the spitting cobra, *Naja nigricollis*, may cause a painful conjunctivitis with chemosis. Irrigation of the eye with a bland lotion such as normal saline and the instillation of anaesthetic drops such as amethocaine or 1% cocaine relieve the symptoms. If the cornea is involved atropine should be instilled. The condition usually clears up without sequelae, but defective vision may remain as a result of the scarring of the cornea.

Common forms of conjunctivitis

Phlyctenular conjunctivitis. This disease occurs predominantly in undernourished children and is often associated with tonsil and adenoid infection, otorrhoea and cervical and hilar adenitis. Although the tubercle bacillus cannot be isolated from the conjunctiva the disease is caused by an allergic endogenous protein, usually tuberculoprotein. The actual phlycten appears as a small (3 mm) yellow swelling in the conjunctiva, surrounded by a localized leash of blood vessels. The phlycten may occur on the cornea, where it breaks down to cause a corneal ulcer. When the ulcer heals an irregular semi-opaque scar remains. If the scar is in the central area of the cornea, vision may be affected.

Treatment. Investigation of the nasopharyngeal condition and X-ray of the hilar region are followed by specific treatment if tuberculous infection is verified, by hyperalimentation associated with vitamin therapy and by the topical application of steroid drugs.

Vernal or spring catarrh. This is also an allergic reaction, but to exogenous allergens. The topical application of steroids as in the case of phlyctenular keratoconjunctivitis has revolutionized the treatment of this disease.

Follicular conjunctivitis. This is characterized by rows of follicles of seed-pearl size, particularly in the lower fornix. The condition occurs in children, often as a sequel of one of the exanthemas. Improvement in the general condition is followed by recovery. Follicular enlargement is also found in adenoviral and acute bacterial infections and also in association with molluscum contagiosum of the skin near the eyes.

Angular conjunctivitis. In this disease the conjunctival infection is localized near the canthi, and a foamy secretion lodges in the canthi. The neighbouring skin is red and excoriated or eczematous. This condition is found mostly in older subjects. The specific organism involved is a saprophyte, the diplobacillus of Morax-Axenfeld.

Although sometimes intractable, the condition often responds to zinc sulphate applied as a lotion or as drops, in a strength of 0·125% (30 mg to 28·5 ml of water or saline).

Mucopurulent conjunctivitis. This is a general infection but petechial subconjunctival haemorrhages are often seen and the discharge is a straw-coloured fluid in which float flakes or strands of mucus, described as 'junket floating in whey'. This condition occurs mainly as the result of infection with the Koch-Weeks bacillus, and is often epidemic among small boys in boarding-schools who make use of each others' towels and sponges. The disease rapidly responds to treatment by irrigation with normal saline or 1 in 10 000 solution of mercury perchloride, or by painting the conjunctiva with a 2% aqueous solution of mercurochrome. Penicillin or other antibiotics are indicated if bacteriological sensitivity tests are made. Labelled towel-hooks and disciplined hygiene will prevent a recurrence in schools or families.

The Koch-Weeks bacillus has been found in Samoan and Fijian conjunctivitis and in Egyptian epidemic conjunctivitis.

In addition to these diseases, many other types of conjunctivitis occur—diphtheritic, rosacea associated with acne rosacea, Parinaud's, which is allied to, if not identical with, oculoglandular tularaemia, and tuberculous conjunctivitis.

Differential diagnosis

Apart from the characteristics of different types of conjunctivitis, disease of other ocular tissues must be excluded. The behaviour of the vascular tree often indicates the nature of the lesion, as, for instance, the circumcorneal injection in iritis.

Episcleritis. In this condition there is a localized, somewhat elevated, deep red, circular area of congested vessels. If the conjunctiva is gently moved over the area the faint conjunctival vessels move with the membrane, but the deeper, congested episcleral vessels remain fixed.

Keratitis. In its various forms keratitis is accompanied by ciliary injection. Superficial vessels from the conjunctiva may ramify over the surface of the cornea as in phlyctenular or rosacea disease, in contrast with the brushes of parallel vessels which invade the deeper layers of the cornea in interstitial keratitis. When corneal ulceration has occurred staining with fluorescein will indicate the extent of the ulcer.

Herpes simplex is one of the commonest infective causes of corneal damage. The eye is red and painful and may resemble an acute conjunctivitis but it is usually unilateral, whereas conjunctivitis, with the exception of epidemic keratoconjunctivitis, is bilateral. Staining with fluorescein reveals the typical branched pattern. Steroids should not be used as they cause destructive spreading of the ulcer. 5-Iodo-2-deoxyuridine (IDU) is often an effective line of treatment.

Iritis. The conjunctival redness is confined to a circle of fine injected vessels which surround the cornea, the so-called ciliary injection or ciliary blush. These vessels are branches of the anterior ciliary vessels which pierce the sclera to reach the ciliary region about 4 mm outside the limbus. Other signs of iritis are seen such as vascularity of the iris, keratic precipitates and synechiae.

Glaucoma. In acute and subacute glaucoma the conjunctiva is intensely congested; the cornea is hazy and other signs of glaucoma are present.

Treatment in general

Simple conjunctivitis will respond in many cases to lavage with a saline solution or with the following lotion:

Chlorbutol	60 mg
Sodium chloride	800 mg
Cherry-laurel water	1·3 ml
Elder-flower or distilled water to	30 ml

A portion of the lotion is diluted with warm water and the eye bathed with an eye-cup or a pledget of cotton-wool. The dilution renders the saline isotonic with the conjunctiva. This washes away irritant exudates and dilutes the infection. Antibiotics and sulphonamides may be called for in severe cases. Cortisone may occasionally be used, with circumspection. It is not bactericidal and it may be actually harmful if the corneal epithelium is involved. Mercurochrome in a 2% solution used as drops or painted on the conjunctiva is a harmless and valuable agent. Silver preparations are not in favour; some are actually dangerous and others tend to produce argyrosis or permanent staining of the conjunctiva.

Lime burns. Inactivation of the lime by the chelating agent trisodium ethylenediamine tetraacetate, applied as drops, mitigates the severity of conjunctival and corneal damage.

Conjunctivitis, in general, has been sketched, but a discussion of three types of conjunctival infection is of paramount importance in considering ophthalmology in the tropics. These are ophthalmia neonatorum, epidemic keratoconjunctivitis (EKC) and trachoma, and will be discussed in this section. Two other diseases, leprosy and onchocerciasis which may cause blindness, although they are not primarily eye diseases, are discussed here because of their great importance as public health and socio-economic problems.

OPHTHALMIA NEONATORUM

Ophthalmia neonatorum is the most important bacterial conjunctivitis at the present time in the Western world. It occurs throughout the world and in underdeveloped countries is surpassed in numbers only by such diseases as nutritional keratoconjunctivitis and trachoma.

Definition

Under the Public Health (Ophthalmia Neonatorum) Regulations 1926, ophthalmia neonatorum is defined as 'a purulent discharge from the eye of an infant commencing within 21 days from the date of its birth'. Any discharge, even if only watery, must be suspect, for an infant does not usually begin to secrete tears until 7–10 days after birth. The disease is notifiable in the United Kingdom.

Incidence

In a study of causes of blindness in England prior to 1948, 10% of children in the age-group 0–4 and 12% in the age-group 15–19 were blind through ophthalmia neonatorum. Improvements in notification and treatment have reduced these figures to less than 2·0% but in many countries the figures are still very high.

Micro-organisms

The organisms which have been found are many and often there is a mixture. The *Staphylococcus* is by far the most common and the TRIC agent and the gonococcus are next in order of frequency. For many years the Gram-negative *Neisseria gonorrhoeae* held first place, but antenatal screening has reduced its ascendency so that, today, many nurses working in the maternity hospital of a large industrial city with a mixed population have never seen a baby suffering from this specific infection. Treatment is often, rightly, begun on clinical grounds before the nature of the organism is confirmed by laboratory investigation.

A non-bacterial form of ophthalmia neonatorum was recognized in 1884 by Kroner, and in 1909 inclusion bodies similar to those of trachoma were found in the conjunctiva in these cases. The term inclusion blennorrhoea was applied by Lindner (1909). Later work confirmed the resemblance or near identity of the occlusion bodies and the name TRIC, an acronym for trachoma-inclusion conjunctivitis, was applied to this agent.

Neonatal TRIC infection resembles gonoccoccal ophthalmia also in its train of transmission—male urethritis→maternal cervicitis→neonatal conjunctivitis (see Trachoma, page 847).

Infection

At birth the eyes are tightly closed but during the passage of the head down the infected birth canal infected discharge is smeared on the outside of the eyelids. The most dangerous type of confinement is a protracted labour with a face presentation. Immediately after birth infection may be introduced by wiping the eyes carelessly so that discharge on the outside of the eyelids is introduced into the conjunctival sac; or by bathing the new-born baby in such a way that infected material from the body is washed into the eyes. Later, the eyes may be infected by soiled dressings or linen, or by contaminated fingers.

The defences of the new-born are poor in that there are no tears, there is no subconjunctival lymphoid barrier layer and the eyes are kept almost constantly closed.

Clinical course

The incubation period is from a few hours to 3 days. Both eyes are usually involved. The conjunctival discharge is initially serous and blood-stained and, if untreated, rapidly becomes frankly purulent. The lids are red, swollen and glazed and tightly closed so that they can only be opened with difficulty. The bulbar conjunctiva is chemosed so that there is a circumcorneal depression or gutter. The cornea may become involved and a greyish area of infiltration appears which breaks down to form an ulcer, central, marginal or circumferential. The ulcer may perforate and the iris become prolapsed. In more severe cases the lens and other contents of the eye may be extruded. The end result may range from a localized opacity to a dense leucoma involving the whole cornea, or an anterior staphyloma, in which the softened cornea yields to form a prominent bulge. Sight may be impaired or completely and irrevocably lost, so that the first glimpse of light seen by the child is the last.

Treatment

Prophylactic. Pre-natal examination and treatment of the mother if infection is present.

Hygienic. Precaution in dealing with the new-born at birth and after.

Therapeutic. Immediately a discharge from the eyes, however slight, is noticed, the baby is wrapped in a towel imprisoning the arms: the head is held firmly and the eyelids are wiped. The lids are gently opened and great care must be taken that discharge under pressure behind the lids does not spurt in the eyes of the medical or nursing attendant. Penicillin drops in a strength of 5000 units/ml are instilled between the lids at the rate of 1 drop every minute for 5 minutes; 1 drop every 5 minutes for half an hour; 1 drop every half hour for 2 hours; and then hourly for 24 hours. Penicillin by injection is indicated where ophthalmic trained staff are not available. Sulphonamide therapy may be used in conjunction with penicillin, or independently; sulphadiazine or sulphamerazine are crushed in milk and given by mouth, 0·5 gramme initially and 0·25 gramme every 8 hours. Irrigation is sometimes indicated. The conjunctival sac is irrigated from a drop-bottle with 2·5% sodium bicarbonate at intervals of 3 hours. If the cornea begins to show greyish patches, atropine is instilled. Silver salts are no longer used either prophylactically or therapeutically; prophylactic instillation of drops of any kind into the eyes of a new-born baby is no longer a routine duty of the midwife. The modern practice is that all suspected cases should be referred for medical opinion.

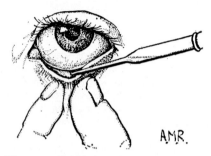

Fig. 252.—Instillation of drops into the eye.

EPIDEMIC KERATOCONJUNCTIVITIS

Epidemic keratoconjunctivitis (EKC) is a specific eye disease which occurs in endemic form in India and the Far East particularly in summer and autumn and in epidemic form in the U.S.A. and elsewhere.

The organism is a small epitheliotropic virus, a member of the adenoidal-pharyngeal-conjunctival (APC) virus group. In Taiwan 252 patients were investigated and adenovirus type 8 was isolated in 72% of these and type 4 in 13%. Other types were found in single cases. The clinical severity was similar irrespective of type. The virus is air-borne and is favoured by dust and wind. Humid coastal climates likewise favour the disease.

Signs and symptoms

The earliest sign is that of a mild conjunctivitis with injection of the vessels, accompanied by irritation of the eye. When the upper lid is everted small follicles are seen in the loose conjunctiva but rarely in the tarsal area. The bulbar conjunctiva is chemosed. An early watery discharge may become purulent in untreated cases owing to secondary infection.

The cornea shows subepithelial infiltrates which break down to form superficial punctate ulcers which stain with fluorescein. Petechial haemorrhages are seen in some cases. The pre-auricular gland is enlarged and tender. This is one of the few types of infective conjunctivitis in which in most cases only one eye is infected. Somerset gives a ratio of 7 to 1 in favour of uniocularity.

Some patients exhibit pharyngeal symptoms. Severe, untreated or late-treated cases may develop keratitis profunda, disciform keratitis, swelling of the nerve head and retinal haemorrhages.

Treatment

Irrigation with normal saline and the instillation of atropine drops, 1%, to full dilatation of the pupil, is usually effective within a week. Cortisone is contra-indicated as it delays the repair of the cornea and may precipitate the perforation of a corneal ulcer.

KERATITIS NUMMULARIS

This is an acute keratoconjunctivitis characterized by coin-shaped opacities deep in Bowman's membrane. It occurs in paddy-field workers in Indonesia. Stellwag (1889) reported a similar condition in central Europe. The cause may be a virus related to the virus of EKC.

TRACHOMA

Trachoma ($\tau\rho\alpha\chi\acute{\upsilon}s$, rough) is a communicable keratoconjunctivitis usually of chronic evolution, characterized in its developed stage by a granular appearance particularly of the conjunctiva of the upper tarsus, by vascularization and subepithelial infiltration of the cornea and resolving by cicatrization of and distortion of the conjunctiva and opacification of the cornea. Untreated patients suffer from gross visual disability and blindness.

Social history

The history of trachoma is as old as written human history and embraces at least five millenia. No disease of the eye, or indeed no disease of any kind, has caused more suffering, blindness and personal and national economic loss.

Trachoma was endemic in China in the twenty-seventh century B.C.; it was endemic in Egypt in the twentieth and nineteenth centuries B.C., and the Ebers papyrus of Thebes dated 1500 B.C. gives a clinical account of the disease. Hippocrates in the fifth century B.C. ascribed the cause of trachoma to a corrupt humour emanating from the brain. Celsus described scarification and cautery with copper salts in the treatment of trachoma in A.D. 14. Dioscorides in A.D. 60 named it 'trachys' for its rough feel; and Galen in A.D. 160 described the four stages of the disease. Epilation forceps were found in Tutankhamen's tomb and instruments recovered from excavations in the Roman dominions (Fig. 253) were used in the treatment of the disease. Armies and travellers spread it; the Crusaders brought it, with leprosy and the donkey, to Europe and later the Spanish conquerors took it across the Atlantic. Muslim armies carried it far into Asia. Soldiers returning from the Napoleonic campaigns in Egypt in 1798 brought the infection from its putative original habitat in the Middle East to France and England where it was known as 'Egyptian' or 'military' ophthalmia.

From papers in the Public Record Office it appears that the two regiments having the largest number of casualties from ophthalmia were the 20th Foot (later the Lancashire Fusiliers) and the 24th Foot (later the South Wales Borderers). In the regimental hospital in Malta on 18 December 1801, of the 24th Foot there were 32 soldiers blind in 1 eye and 66 blind in both eyes. Vetch (1807) states that between August 1805 and August 1806, in the 54th Foot, which had returned to England, 636 cases of ophthalmia, including relapses, were admitted to hospital. Of these 50 were dismissed with the loss of both eyes and 40 with that of 1 eye.

The librarian at the Ministry of Defence (1969) stated that although the army suffered many casualties, the numbers were not as great as those quoted in some text-books.

The question arises as to whether all these were cases of trachoma. The acute epidemicity and the clinical descriptions of many of the cases suggest that there was some confusion between trachoma and purulent, possibly gonococcal, ophthalmia. After all, at that time bacteriological examination did not exist. Moorfields Eye Hospital in London was founded to deal with the Egyptian ophthalmia.

Trachoma was endemic in Ireland in the middle of the nineteenth century, and later schools for children suffering from ophthalmia were opened at Hanwell in 1889, at Chigwell and in the Portobello Road in 1897 and in other places. About the turn of this century, Eastern Europeans on their way in to the New World brought fresh waves of infection. Shipping companies suffered heavy penalties if they landed infected immigrants into Canada or the United States. There is, at the present time, a potential danger of renewed spread in England by immigrants from countries where trachoma is endemic. In 1969

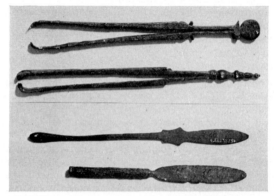

Fig. 253.—Epilation forceps and conjunctival forceps from the second century A.D., of the Gallo-Roman oculist Gaius Firmius Severus, found in a tomb in Rheims. (*By permission of the Wellcome Museum of Medical Science*)

attention was directed to the rising incidence of trachoma in the West Midlands (Howells 1969). Most of the patients were immigrants from the Jullunder district in the Punjab where, according to a recent survey, 80% of the population are infected.

Aetiology

Although, as has been shown, trachoma is not confined to the tropics, it is more common in those areas than elsewhere. In underprivileged parts of the world where protein food is in short supply and malnutrition is the common lot of millions of people, where housing conditions are squalid and overcrowded, where domestic sanitation is noticeable by its absence and where there is an inadequate supply of water, the disease is endemic. Dust, dirt and flies are ever-present factors. Contagion and infection and reinfection by direct or indirect contact cannot be controlled. Under such conditions the disease is contracted in the first few years of life in the home, in the alleys and in the schools. Adults living under similar conditions, such as soldiers in armies on campaign, are just as vulnerable.

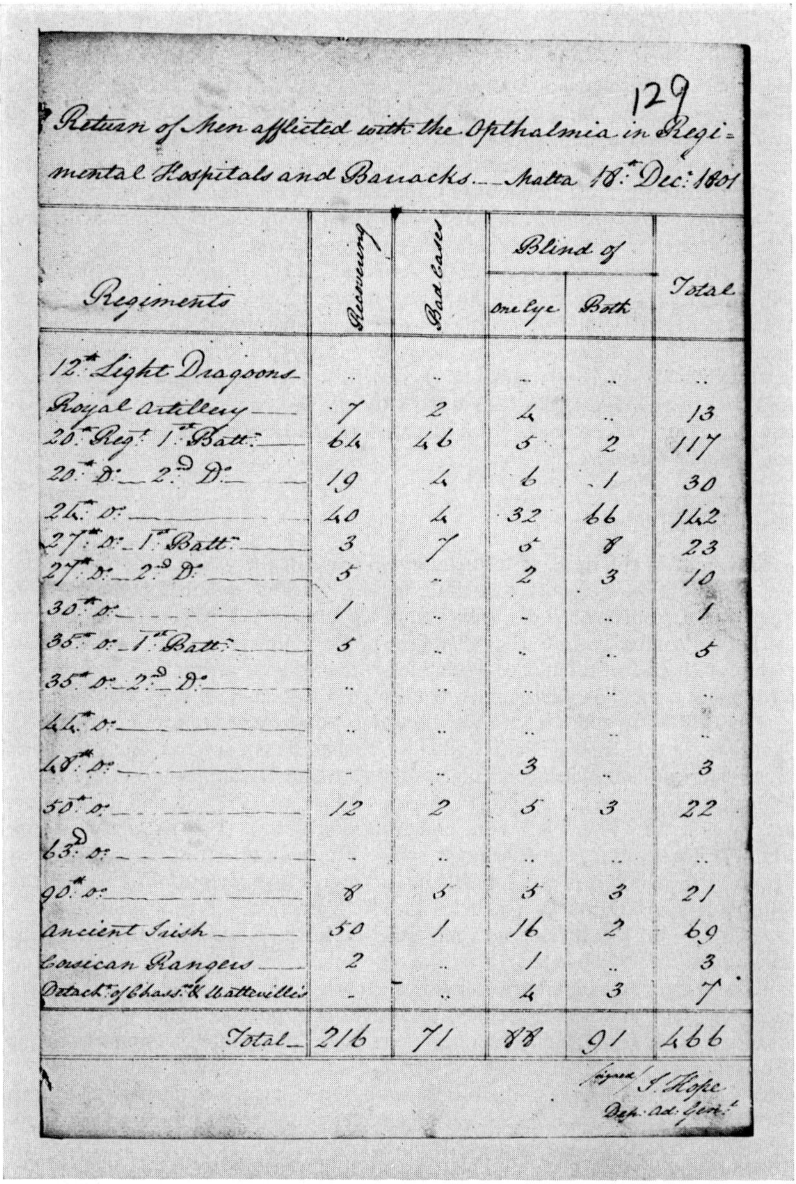

| Regiments | Recovering | Bad Cases | Blind of | | Total |
			one Eye	Both	
12.th Light Dragoons	..	..	..	..	..
Royal artillery	7	2	4	..	13
26.th Reg.t 1.st Batt.n	64	46	5	2	117
20.th D.o 2.d D.o	19	4	6	1	30
24.th D.o	40	4	32	66	142
27.th D.o 1.st Batt.n	3	7	5	8	23
27.th D.o 2.d D.o	5	..	2	3	10
30.th D.o	1	..	..	..	1
35.th D.o 1.st Batt.n	5	..	..	..	5
35.th D.o 2.d D.o	..	..	..	..	..
44.th D.o	..	..	..	..	..
48.th D.o			3	..	3
50.th D.o	12	2	5	3	22
63.d D.o			..	..	
90.th D.o	8	5	5	3	21
ancient Irish	50	1	16	2	69
Corsican Rangers	2	..	1	..	3
Detach.t of Chas.tk & Watteville's	..	..	4	3	7
Total	216	71	88	91	466

Return of Men afflicted with the Opthalmia in Regimental Hospitals and Barracks. Malta 18.th Dec.r 1801

129

Sign.d J Hope
Dep. ad Gen.l

Fig. 254.—Papers from the Public Record Office, London, showing the incidence of ophthalmia in regiments returning from Egypt in 1801. (*By permission of the Public Record Office*)

Many theories have, in the past, been advanced and rejected regarding the specific aetiological factor. Halberstaedter and von Prowazek (1907) described, originally in the orang-utang, granular inclusion bodies in the cytoplasm of epithelial cells in scrapings of infected conjunctiva. They stained with Giemsa and were called inclusion bodies. Lindner (1909) described inclusion blenorrhoea, now called inclusion conjunctivitis, and found similar bodies; and Bedson (1952) isolated similar bodies in psittacosis and lymphogranuloma venereum. T'ang (1957) cultivated a virus and from 1958 onwards Collier and Sona produced typical trachoma by inoculation with the virus; and from the lesions the virus was again isolated. The virus of inclusion conjunctivitis was isolated from the conjunctiva and from the genital tract.

The viruses are interrelated and the acronym TRIC virus (trachoma-inclusion conjunctivitis) is widely used; however, it has not been universally accepted. A view held, particularly by some French trachomatologists, is that, while the agents cannot be differentiated in laboratory tests, they produce manifestations as clinically distinct as trachoma and inclusion conjunctivitis. The dualists hold that the convenience of the unicist theory should not lead to its exclusive and premature acceptance. Such discussion is healthy and stimulating. *Tot homines quot sententiae!*

Distribution

Trachoma is the most widespread eye disease in the world. WHO estimates that 500 million persons, one-sixth of the world's population, suffer from trachoma. In Europe the disease, even in the present century, is endemic in all the Balkan countries. In Serbia 3% of the population were affected 20 years ago. Although there are still areas of endemicity, an energetic campaign decentralized throughout the country has almost eradicated the disease. In Bulgaria, trachoma is responsible for 9·8% of cases of blindness; and there are areas in Southern Spain where the disease is still endemic. Trachoma is prevalent in the Eastern Mediterranean countries, particularly Lebanon and Jordan. South of the Mediterranean the countries in North Africa—Morocco, Tunisia and Egypt—are heavily affected. There is a high endemic rate, with a peak incidence in pre-school children, in Sudan (Majucuk 1966). Throughout Africa there is scarcely a country in which it is not a problem. An interesting exception is Liberia; this country is surrounded by countries in which trachoma is rife, but Liberia is covered by rain forest, dust and fine sand do not pervade the atmosphere and trachoma is almost absent.

To Asia again—trachoma is endemic in Arabia, Iran and other Arab countries. In India, trachoma with associated bacterial infections is a major public health problem and is responsible for a high percentage of blindness. An examination of migrants from Kurali in the Punjab to British Columbia revealed that 20% carried the active disease and a further 40% showed signs of inactive trachoma. Statistics relating to China are not available, but in Singapore, where socio-economic conditions are high with abundant water and an efficient medical service, of the relatively few persons suffering from trachoma, 77% had migrated from China. Trachoma is prevalent in Indonesia, in the Pacific Archipelago and in Japan. Trachoma has been recognized in Australia since the latter part of the eighteenth century and was at one time the predominant form of eye disease (Hansman 1969). A reservoir continues to exist among Aborigines but white inhabitants are now rarely affected. The disease began to disappear before the introduction of sulphonamides and antibiotics. The decline was probably due to improvement in hygiene. In New Zealand statutory notification is enforced.

Trachoma will thus be seen to have encircled the globe.

Sex incidence

There is in general a higher prevalence of active trachoma in women than in men. This difference occurs in early life and seems to increase with age.

Sex difference is not due to host sensitivity, but to environmental and behavioural factors. In many countries the girl baby receives less care than the boy; a young girl of 5 is often in charge of younger brothers and sisters, whereas a boy never undertakes this duty. The youngest child is carried on its mother's back until the next child is born when the displaced child, carrying with it bacterial and TRIC infection, is given into the care of and into intimate contact with its elder sister.

Signs and symptoms

In endemic areas many children are infected but manifest no symptoms and only a minimum of signs. The disease of this mild type recovers spontaneously. Faint horizontal scars on the tarsal conjunctiva and ghost vessels, the remains of pannus invading the upper part of the cornea and found only with the corneal loupe or the slit-lamp, are the only indications of a healed infection. Secondary bacterial infection is a potent factor in potentiating the trachoma agent.

The evolution of this disease is conveniently differentiated into 4 stages:

Stage I: In this early stage lacrimation and slight oedema of the eyelid may occur. The conjunctiva of the upper eyelid shows tufts of dilated capillaries and the formation of epithelial papillae. These follicles may be 2–3 mm in size and give the conjunctiva a granular appearance. The lower eyelid and the bulbar conjunctiva are not involved at this stage. With the slit-lamp fine epithelial infiltrates may be seen at the margin of the cornea. The TRIC virus is found in epithelial scrapings. This stage may persist for many months.

Stage II: Blood vessels, prolongations of the terminal vascular arcades, invade the cornea at its upper limbus, continuing as non-anastomosing brushes of fine vessels at whose tips there is a grey infiltrate between the epithelium and Bowman's membrane. The infiltrate later penetrates the substantia propria. This combination of new vessels and infiltrate, known as pannus, spreads from the periphery to involve the whole cornea. The cornea is covered with, as it were, granulation tissues with consequent impairment of sight. Ulceration may occur and, when these ulcers become epithelialized, facets are left which cause distortion of vision. The infiltration may cause softening of the cornea, with ectasia and rupture. This stage may last from 6 months to a year or more in untreated patients. The virus is recoverable throughout.

Stage III: In this stage, for trachoma is a self-limiting disease, linear cicatrization begins in the tarsal conjunctiva and in the sub-tarsal groove. Ruptured follicles are replaced by star-shaped white cicatrices forming a mosaic pattern. When active cicatrization has ceased the conjunctiva becomes smooth, white and avascular. The conjunctiva of the lower eyelid and the fornices may be covered with a bluish haze, giving it a skimmed-milk appearance.

In the cornea also the follicles rupture or cicatrize. The craters of the ruptured follicles become lined with clear epithelium and produce at the limbus a series of lacunae called Herbert's pits.

In the cornea, the invading vessels retrogress and infiltration is absorbed. Remnants of the vessels can always be seen with the loupe or slit-lamp and a diffuse haze pervades the cornea. If a major disaster, such as ectasia or rupture, has not involved the cornea, useful economic sight is often regained at this stage and persists.

Virus invasion at this stage is less intense and is difficult to demonstrate.

The affected eye may remain in this state for many years.

Stage IV: At this stage the follicles have been replaced by scar tissue and active morbidity in the cornea has ceased. No virus is to be found. The active disease is now burnt out. The leading role is now assumed by an inexorable and progressive cicatrization of the scar tissue already present. The upper eyelid becomes grossly deformed due to buckling of the tarsal plate and the margin of the eyelid is turned in towards the cornea, the condition of entropion. The lash-bearing area of the eyelid is distorted, and irregular, secondary lines of eyelashes appear, thrusting out in all directions, the condition of trichiasis. Entropion–trichiasis (Fig. 255) is essentially an adult complication. The already damaged cornea is now excoriated by the continual impact of the inturned eyelashes and once more becomes vascularized and ulcerated. It loses its sensitivity and is laid open to further damage by particles of dust and sand.

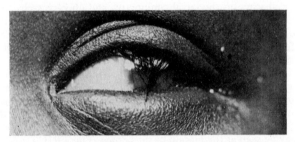

Fig. 255.—Trichiasis–entropion in trachoma. (*Reproduced by permission of Dr S. C. I. Sowa and the Editor of the British Journal of Ophthalmology*)

Cicatrization of the fornices leads to their obliteration and to the cutting-off of lacrimal secretion. The condition of xerosis is established and cornea and conjunctiva are covered with a skin-like membrane. In long-standing cases, as the result of the blocking of lymphatics by scar tissue, the eyelid becomes swollen and heavy; this, combined with involvement of the levator muscle, causes trachoma ptosis—the drooping 'bedroom eyes of the Orient'.

Field studies

The changes from stage to stage are a continuum and borderline cases present problems of clinical judgement. The World Health Organization has suggested that in order to attain reasonable uniformity in the results of field studies, cases between Stages I and II should be categorized as Stage II; between II and III as Stage III and between III and IV as Stage IV. The comparison of results in different fields is more accurate if patients are examined independently by two observers who compare their observations and arrive at an agreed classification. The questions to be asked in a field study are:

a. Is a given case trachomatous?
b. In which stage is the case to be placed?
c. What is the degree of disablement?

Diagnosis

In field studies where laboratory investigation is not available, two of the following signs must be present to establish a positive diagnosis:
Folliculosis.
Linear scarring of the tarsal conjunctiva of the upper eyelid.
Active keratitis.
Pannus in the upper third of the cornea.

Laboratory investigations include:
a. Examination of conjunctival scrapings for Halberstaedter–Prowazek inclusion bodies which stain with Giemsa or iodine.
b. Inoculation of scrapings into chick embryos, followed by virological investigations.
c. Examination of conjunctival flora by culture.
d. The finding by the immunofluorescence test of antibodies to trachoma in conjunctival secretion (McComb & Nichols 1969).

Differential diagnosis. In trachoma the maximum conjunctival involvement is in the upper eyelid; and the maximum pannus in the upper third, whereas in inclusion conjunctivitis the maximum involvement is in the conjunctiva of the lower eyelid. Pannus, keratitis and scarring are absent. In ariboflavinosis the vascular invasion of the cornea is to be found in any sector and not markedly in the upper third. Epidemic keratoconjunctivitis has no pannus or lid involvement. Fluorescein staining demonstrates the punctate ulcers on the cornea, just as in dendritic keratitis fluorescein marks the branching ulcer.

In vernal catarrh eosinophilia is present in conjunctival scrapings; there is often a fibrinous membrane on the conjunctiva and a ring of circumcorneal oedema. Follicular conjunctivitis shows regular rows of seed-pearl-like follicles 1 mm in size in the lower fornix. There is no pannus. Tarsal follicles are found in adenoviral and acute bacterial infections and in association with molluscum contagiosum. Immunofluorescent tests of conjunctival scrapings are valuable in countries in which trachoma is endemic.

Treatment

General considerations. It has been emphasized that trachoma is endemic and flourishes in favourable environmental conditions, natural or man-made. A trachoma map would include most of the desert and semi-desert parts of the world, especially where the dust particles are fine.

In relation to some of the factors favouring the persistence of trachoma, Gilkes (1962) quoted the opinion of two eminent authorities: 'An increase in living standards of 1% results in a fall of the trachoma incidence of 10%', and 'A water-tap in every village and a bottle of the simplest eye-drops in every dwelling would end trachoma in our generation'. As people move from water-scarce areas to a piped water supply transmission of the disease in the home will tend to move into low levels and schools will remain the most important loci of infection. Marshall (1968) relates that in a school in Naha water is plentiful and cleansing of hands and faces is enforced. Children have their own towels, but 12 children have been seen to wipe their faces with one towel. It is ironic that transmission occurs in places where water is scarce, and in other places transmission may take place because it is plentiful. It is not, however, only in developing countries that the communal towel is used, for the present writer recalls that in an expensive preparatory school in England 'pink-eye' was endemic until it was observed that small boys, returning from games, used not their own towels but grabbed the first towel to hand. Discipline, not drugs, controlled their infection.

The association of trachoma with low socio-economic and sanitary levels, and its tendency to disappear as a serious public health problem when living conditions improve, are potent factors which must be taken into account at the same time as the individual treatment of the patient.

Vaccines. The prolonged course of the natural disease has been thought to be due to the failure of the causative agent to stimulate antibody formation. The successful cultivation of the trachoma agent in 1957 encouraged the hope that this would soon be followed by the development of a vaccine for the effective control or prevention of the disease. The cultivation of the agent did, in fact, open up a new era in trachoma research and much of the progress which has been made has come from studies aimed at the development of a vaccine. A 5-year study supported by statistical analysis on the use of a live trachoma vaccine in northern Transvaal confirmed that no clear-cut benefit was obtained in severe trachoma, though encouraging results had been obtained in mild trachoma (Scott & Kerrich 1971).

Methods of treatment

Many forms of mechanical treatment have been given a trial over the centuries. Expression of the follicles by the finger-nail or by special intruments has been used since remote times and is still occasionally applied. Massage and brossage, in which tufts of raw wool, the skin of a fish or other excoriants were used to rub down exuberant follicles, is obsolete. Xysis still has its adherents. The follicles are curetted and the conjunctiva is then massaged or injected with one of the following chemical—oxycyanide of mercury, phenol, copper sulphate or boric acid. Successful results have been claimed.

Physical treatment includes such methods as cauterization with the actual or the electric cautery and diathermy. Beta-ray radio-active strontium 90 applied with a surface applicator, it has been claimed, causes the follicles to melt away; cryogenic application with CO_2 snow or the cryogenic applicator induces cicatrization and is less severe than diathermy (Vancea & Vancea 1968).

Biological treatment. The subconjunctival injection of milk, blood, placental extract and other proteins has produced no clear results. Corticosteroids, although useful in certain complications, precipitate the occurrence of herpes simplex, and should not be used as a routine measure.

Sulphonamides and antibiotics. Treatment to-day is essentially based on the use of sulphonamides and of antibiotics. The action of sulphonamides and antibiotics on trachoma has been attributed, in part, to their action upon the associated bacterial flora. This may play a part important in itself and is thus an additional indication for their use. The knowledge of the mechanism of these drugs and of the structure and metabolism of the trachoma agent justifies the belief that the effect of these drugs on the disease is in a great part caused by specific action on the agent. Both an inhibitory effect on the agent in the laboratory and a beneficial effect clinically have been observed.

Sulphanilamide. Sulphanilamide (*p*-aminobenzene sulphonamide), the basic compound of all sulphonamides, is a structural analogue of *p*-aminobenzoic acid which is required by micro-organisms for the synthesis of folic acid, an essential metabolite. Sulphonamides thus act as microbial inhibitors by interfering with folic acid metabolism.

Antibiotics. The chemical structures of the most commonly used reflect their mode of action. The penicillins are peptides and interfere with cell-wall synthesis and membrane function. Aminoglycosides (streptomycin, neomycin) interfere with protein synthesis by causing misreading of the genetic information supplied by mRNA (Davies 1965). Tetracyclines act by binding the aminoacyl tRNA to the ribosome mRNA complex and thus provoke the formation of aberrant ribosome subunits. Macrolides, which include erythromycin and carbomycin, inhibit protein synthesis by acting on the peptide bond-forming step at the ribosomal level.

Choice of drug. Particularly with the sulphonamides there are different characteristics with regard to solubility, absorption and excretion, and therefore with different indications for their use. Sulphadiazine is characterized by a high concentration in the tissues, and by its potency, rapid absorption and relatively slow excretion. Sulphamethoxypyridazine and sulphadimethoxine are long-acting and characterized by rapid absorption, pronounced plasma-binding and poor tissue diffusion, thus obviating the need for frequent administration. Sulphonamides in solution, as ointments or by systemic administration, provided they are well tolerated, give better results than other drugs. Systemic administration by mouth is recommended in a dosage of 40–50 mg/kg body-weight, or approximately 2·5 grammes daily for 10–15 days. Supervision is essential, with attention to the blood-picture and renal function. Diuresis is important. A combination of local with systemic treatment may give the best results.

Tetracycline (Achromycin) and oxytetracycline (Terramycin) are the antibiotics which have been most extensively used and give the best results. They are given by local application as solutions, suspensions or ointments at 1–3%, 2 or 3 times a day over periods of at least several weeks. Erythromycin and rifampicin (Rifamycin) have also given favourable results.

Association of drugs. The efficacy of treatment in general is often increased by a combination of oral sulphonamides with local antibiotics. Particularly in the early stages, local treatment with ointments and drops may be effective, but when the conjunctiva is thickened with deep crypt formation systemic administration is indicated in conjunction with local treatment.

Side-effects. It should be borne in mind that even the most effective preparations are not free from side-effects and that this sometimes limits their application in large-scale campaigns.

In communities with a low educational level, as is the case where trachoma is highly prevalent, indiscriminate use may present an added health hazard. This, particularly in the case of sulphonamides, reflects the experience accumulated in the use of these drugs in the treatment of so many diseases. Because of the risk of complications following sulphonamide treatment in the U.S.A. package inserts contain a warning; in Hungary and Czechoslovakia the use of sulphamethoxypyridazine is restricted; in Western Australia, in 1961, oral sulphonamides were forbidden in the treatment of trachoma (Tarrizzo & Nataf 1970).

It is important to recognize that, whatever method of treatment is used, the trachoma organism can sometimes be recovered from clinically quiescent patients. Such patients are therefore potential sources of infection until they are cleared by negative laboratory results.

Pannus, which persists even after the tarsal conjunctiva is clear, may respond to subconjunctival injections, under local anaesthesia, of 0·75 ml of normal saline.

Surgical treatment. Only the treatment of complications of trachoma will be reviewed here and no attempt will be made to discuss the problem of other ophthalmic conditions which may occur in trachoma patients. The main indications are thickening and deformity of the tarsal plate, which is a frequent cause of corneal ulceration even when there is no trichiasis, blepharophimosis, in which the palpebral aperture is contracted, trichiasis–entropion, a condition in which the tarsal conjunctiva contracts and brings the inturned eyelashes into contact with the cornea, and symblepharon.

Simple tarsectomy. The skin of the upper eyelid is incised and the anterior surface of the tarsus is exposed. The irregular thickened portion is excised. Sufficient tarsal plate should remain to give shape and firmness to the upper eyelid.

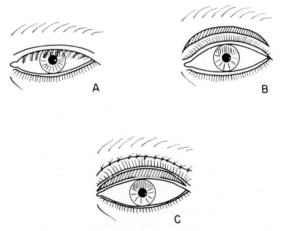

Fig. 256.—The Jasche–Arlt operation. A, Trichiasis–entropion before operation, with pannus in the upper third of the cornea. B, The margin of the upper eyelid is split and a lanceolate strip of skin is removed. C, The strip of skin is transplanted between the lash-bearing area and the conjunctival edge of the eyelid.

Canthoplasty for blepharophimosis consists essentially in a surgical prolongation of the outer angle of the eyelids.

Trichiasis–entropion is the most important complication of trachoma. Many operations have been devised to deal with this deformity. Two of these, the Hotz–Anagnostakis and the Jasche–Arlt will be described.

Hotz–Anagnostakis operation. The upper lid is everted and a linear incision made along the middle two-thirds of the conjunctiva in the tarsal groove. This cuts through the cicatricial tissue and mobilizes the lid margin. A skin incision is then made along the whole width of the lid 3 mm above the lid margin. The orbicularis muscle is incised and the tarsal plate exposed. A wedge-shaped gutter is cut out of the tarsal plate. Sutures are inserted into the upper lip of the gutter and brought out through the lower lip of the skin incision. When they are tightened the gutter is closed and the margin of the eyelid, mobilized by the conjunctival incision, is relatively everted, withdrawing the lashes from the cornea. The sutures are strapped to the eyebrow. No skin sutures are required.

Jasche–Arlt operation (Fig. 256). The lid margin is split along the grey line posterior to the lash-follicles to a depth of 4 mm. A lanceolate strip of skin is then removed from the upper eyelid 3 mm from the lid margin and 4 mm wide at its centre. The margins of the incision are sutured, bringing the lash-bearing area away from the eye. The strip of skin is then placed on the bare area at the lid margin and sutured into position.

This operation is indicated where the Hotz–Anagnostakis operation does not give enough clearance.

Operation for symblepharon. In advanced cases the fornices are obliterated and the lids are adherent to the globe. To relieve this condition the eyelid is dissected off the globe to the depth of the normal fornix. The mucous membrane of the lower lip is infiltrated tensely with lignocaine, and a thin layer stripped off as in Thiersch skin-grafting technique. The sheet of mucous membrane is attached by one edge to the lower fornix, smoothly stretched over the eyelid and sutured to the lid margin. Another sheet of mucous membrane is attached by the same sutures to the fornix and brought over the denuded surface of the globe and sutured into position. A similar procedure is used for the upper fornix.

The cornea in these cases is usually covered with an opaque membrane resembling skin. This membrane is dissected off at a later operation; a lamellar graft is applied and, subsequently, a penetrating graft.

The obliteration of the tear-ducts by cicatrization may result in a completely dry conjunctival sac. Artificial tears, in the form of drops, cannot cope with this absolute dryness. Stensen's duct is mobilized by submucous dissection under the mucosa of the cheek along to the parotid gland. It is then transplanted in a tunnel under the mucosa and cheek muscles until the orifice of the duct can be brought out into the lower fornix. Here it is sutured into position. The salivary secretion thus moistens the conjunctival sac. Hypersecretion can be controlled by X-ray of the parotid gland.

This treatment is practised in the Filatov Institute at Odessa with some degree of success.

Other complications and sequelae. Canaliculitis with stricture formation and dacryocystitis are other complications which call for operation only if they do not respond to conservative treatment.

Irrigation with alpha-chymotrypsin has been used in the treatment of involvement of the lacrimal passages.

LEPROSY

There are at least 12 million people suffering from leprosy in the world; estimated numbers vary up to 15 or 16 million.

Ocular involvement

There is a great variation in the incidence of ocular involvement. Some observers consider that the ocular tissues are eventually involved in all long-standing cases of the disease; others assess the incidence at between 5 and 10% of all cases, whereas in Bengal, it is stated that 25% of patients suffering from both the tuberculoid and the lepromatous types of the disease develop ocular complications. In West Africa, on the other hand, ocular complications are uncommon.

These differences are due to variations in the type and severity of the disease in different countries, and also to difficulty in the early recognition of the disease in the eye. Unless the eyes are examined by an expert, preferably

by microscopy or at least with a loupe and focal illumination, the earliest signs
may be missed.

Pathology

The clinical and pathological features of the polar and intermediate types are
described elsewhere in this volume, but as ocular involvement varies according
to the type of this disease it may be recalled that in the tuberculoid type, epithelioid cells, lymphocytes and Langhans-type giant cells are found in cutaneous
nerve twigs. The relatively frequent invasion of the facial and trigeminal nerves
results in ocular involvement. In the lepromatous type, *Mycobacterium leprae*
are found in the cytoplasm of the Schwann cells which ensheath sensory nerves.
The dermis is severely attacked and hair-follicles and sweat and sebaceous
glands are destroyed. The third method of attack is by participation of ocular
tissues in the reactive phase which is a generalized allergic reaction.

Ocular manifestations

Eyelids and eyebrows. Madarosis, or loss of hair of the eyebrows and especially
of the outer third of the eyelashes, is characteristic. Tylosis is the name applied
to the swollen, rolled appearance of the lid margin.

Conjunctiva and episclera. The conjunctiva is not directly invaded but infective conjunctivitis often complicates the leprous eye.

Cornea. The cornea is involved in two ways: by paralysis of the facial nerve,
and by invasion by *Mycobacterium leprae.*

Lagophthalmos or imperfect closure of the eyelids due to paralysis of the
seventh nerve, combined with swollen and stiff upper eyelids and overaction of
the levator muscle, causes a wide-open eye and staring look which startles the
observer. The paralysed lower eyelid falls away from the eye in a state of paralytic ectropion. The punctum is everted, and this leads to epiphora. The partially
uncovered cornea becomes dry; keratitis and ulceration may occur, and hypopyon, perforation, endophthalmitis or secondary glaucoma may bring about
the destruction of the eye.

In leprotic keratitis the *Mycobacterium* may be found in corneal scrapings.
The corneal nerves enter the cornea radially. Beading and thickening of the
nerves can be observed especially in the upper quadrants. Granulomatous
infiltrations in the corneal stroma accompany the nerve involvement. They
appear as discrete cloudy opacities. At the same time, superficial punctate
keratitis occurs as chalky-white grains in the epithelium and subepithelial
layers. Pannus now makes its appearance equally around the limbus, unlike
that of trachoma which is more dense in the upper third of the limbus.

When infiltration is advanced the cornea becomes opaque and thickened—
hyperplastic keratitis.

Episclera and sclera. The organism may infiltrate the episcleral tissues in
the same way as it invades the skin and produces raised nodules, gelatinous and
yellowish in colour, hard to the touch and near the limbus. They first appear in
the upper temporal quadrant but may eventually surround the limbus and simulate the bulbar type of spring catarrh. They are 3–4 mm in diameter and are
surrounded by slight hyperaemia. They are extremely chronic and show no
change for years. In some cases an active reaction takes place with increased
redness, swelling, pain and irritation. The adjacent cornea may develop an
opaque interstitial keratitis.

The iris. The onset of iritis is insidious and in its early stages challenges clinical diagnosis. The invasion is chronic but is nevertheless inexorably progressive; it is one of the most serious of the ocular complications and may, of itself, lead to blindness. In the early stages posterior synechiae may become evident when the pupil is dilated with homatropine. There are the usual signs of iritis—blurring of vision, lacrimation, photophobia, a ciliary blush and keratic precipitates. Eventually, after an acute phase, exudates are deposited on the anterior capsule of the lens and the vision is seriously impaired. In 30% of patients nodules are found on the iris itself or on the synechiae. They present the appearance of seed-pearls less than 1 mm in diameter. There is little or no surrounding reaction, whereas in syphilis the nodules produce a local reaction and vascularity of the iris.

In tuberculoid leprosy the nodules are larger and less discrete or clearcut in appearance. They may disappear spontaneously, leaving only a minute area of iris atrophy or retro-illumination. In a heavy infection with apparently low resistance a leproma may develop in the anterior chamber, emerging from the angle. Secondary glaucoma due to closure of the pupil and blocking of the angle may develop and in long-standing cases the lens becomes cataractous.

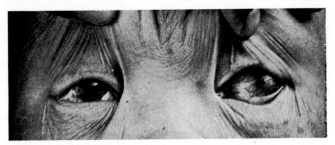

Fig. 257.—Leprosy, showing keratitis, loss of eyebrows and iridiocyclitis. (*Wellcome Museum of Medical Science*)

Posterior segment. Involvement of the choroid and retina is rarely seen, probably because the iris is involved earlier and observation of the fundus is difficult. When the fundus can be examined, two types of lesion may be seen— refractile deposits at the periphery and, behind the equator, discrete yellowish nodules similar to iris 'pearls'.

Diagnosis

The chalky appearance of superficial punctate keratitis and the iris pearls are pathognomonic of leprosy. In every case of iritis slit-lamp or loupe examination is essential. Lagophthalmos is not pathognomonic but should lead to a search for other signs of the disease.

Treatment

The general treatment of leprosy is not in the province of the ophthalmologist but general treatment alone will not suffice to combat ocular infection.

The treatment of iritis, *pari passu* with general treatment, is essentially the prevention of synechiae and it is of paramount importance that the pupils should be kept dilated with atropine. Synechiae may be broken down with mydricaine injected subconjunctivally. Cortisone may be injected at the same time and cortisone drops tend to inhibit the formation of synechiae. In the acute stage of iritis hot steaming, or an electric eye-warmer, often brings relief from pain. Dark glasses may be advisable where photophobia is present.

Sulphone, especially in the treatment of erythema nodosom leprosum, may liberate substances which bring about an allergic response in the eye, manifested by keratitis, iris lepromas, plastic iridocyclitis and secondary glaucoma. For treatment of secondary glaucoma corticosteroids, Diamox and possibly paracentesis should be considered.

Surgical treatment. In lagophthalmos, where the cornea is exposed and ulceration is imminent, lateral tarsorrhaphy is indicated. Where the orbicularis is completely paralysed, a nylon suture may be inserted along the margins of both lids in a purse-string fashion as described by Axenfeld. The temporalis sling operation is effective in severe cases. Two strips of temporalis fascia are inserted into tunnels near the margins of the upper and lower eyelids and united at the median tarsal ligament. Voluntary closure of the lids synchronizing with that of the other eye is brought about. This operation is described in detail by Somerset (1962).

The Kuhnt–Dimmer operation is effective in tightening the flaccid lower eyelid and is recommended by the writer for seventh nerve paralysis from other causes.

For cosmetic purposes a grafting operation may be carried out to replace the denuded area of eyebrow. A superficial strip of scalp from behind the ear, suitably shaped, is effective donor materal.

Operations on the globe. When the pupil is occluded an optical iridectomy may be performed to make an artificial pupil. This operation is only undertaken in the later stages of the disease when the iris is avascular, otherwise the new pupil becomes blocked immediately with haemorrhage.

Iridectomy is also indicated in the secondary glaucoma which may supervene upon a completely blocked pupil.

Operations other than iridectomy may be performed for glaucoma and the extraction of a cataractous lens may be carried out. Such operations are best performed when general treatment has reduced the virulence of the disease and when the cornea and iris in particular are in a quiescent state.

Posterior synechiae may complicate the removal of the lens, and for this reason and also because the corneal incision may excite a reaction or a recurrence of iritis, a preliminary iridectomy is advocated by some surgeons. A disadvantage of this procedure is that the patient may not return for the definitive operation.

Recently, a patient of the writer, a European who contracted leprosy in South-east Asia, developed bilateral leprous iritis and eventually cataract. After a bilateral cataract extraction in which he recovered 6/6 visual acuity in each eye his criterion of success was that he played golf better than ever.

ONCHOCERCIASIS

History

In 1893, Leuckart discovered *Onchocerca volvulus* in a cyst sent to him from the Gold Coast (Ghana) and, later, cutaneous lesions were attributed to this worm, but it was not until 1915 that Robles in Guatemala discovered the connection between the occurrence of onchocercal nodules and the existence of serious ocular symptoms which were described by Pacheco-Luna. In 1931, Torroella, under slit-lamp examination, saw the microfilaria of *O. volvulus* in the anterior chamber. Onchocerciasis appeared to be a cutaneous disease in

Africa and a blinding disease in Central America, until, in 1931, Hissette established that, if looked for, ocular lesions similar to those observed in America could be demonstrated in onchocerciasis patients in Africa; and in 1935 Bryant confirmed the onchocercal cause of ocular lesions by conjunctival snips and the presence of microfilariae in aspirated aqueous humour.

Distribution

The endemic zones are situated in Central America and in tropical Africa. The connection between these zones may well have been the importation of infected Africans as slave labour in Central America by the Spaniards in the sixteenth century. It is estimated (Choyce 1964) that in Central America 2000 and in Africa 50 000 people are totally blind as the result of this disease; in some regions 2 out of every 3 blind persons are blind through onchocercal lesions of the eye. There is a remarkable difference in the situation of the ocular lesions in these two great endemic areas, for whereas in Africa anterior and posterior segment lesions occur, in Central America optic atrophy and choroido-retinitis are rare and onchocercal iritis is the main cause of blindness. The distribution of nodules on the body is a significant factor. Eye lesions are common when nodules are found on the head but relatively infrequent when the nodules are confined to the lower part of the body.

Ocular manifestations

Lesions of the anterior segment, conjunctiva and cornea. A simple conjunctivitis occurs in response to the local presence or local death of the micro-filariae. The patient complains of irritation, lacrimation and photophobia, and on examination of the cornea superficial punctate keratitis is found. By slit-lamp examination microfilariae are seen in the substantia propria near Bowman's membrane close to the limbus, particularly in the temporal region. They are immobile and probably dead and in a few weeks the outline becomes blurred and 'cracked-ice' or 'snow-flake' opacities are seen. They may resolve and disappear or become converted ito 'nummular' opacities, disc-shaped and with a clearcut margin. In long-standing and intense infections a sclerosing keratitis may develop, starting at the lower limbus and extending upwards to involve the pupillary area. This opacity is pigmented and sparsely vascularized with new vessels. If trachoma is present the upper part of the limbus also may be invaded by new vessels. When secondary glaucoma supervenes corneal oedema appears with, as an end result, epithelial degeneration and calcification.

Anterior chamber. In the anterior chamber microfilariae may be seen with the slit-lamp and, rarely, hypopyon may complicate severe iritis.

Iris. Iritis with secondary glaucoma is a major cause of blindness. The classical signs of acute or chronic iridocyclitis occur, with ciliary injection, flare and keratic precipitates. Pigment is deposited on the anterior capsule of the lens and the iris becomes bound down by posterior synechiae. The iris may display patches of atrophy. Progressive loss of vision takes place as the pupil becomes occluded, and secondary glaucoma may supervene. (See Plate VIII.)

Lesions of the posterior segment. In 1931, when Hissette published his classic paper, he described the choroidoretinal lesions associated with onchocerciasis. The statistical relationship between anterior and posterior lesions cannot be accurately stated for there are many cases in which posterior lesions cannot be seen because of corneal opacities and occlusion of the pupil.

Papillitis is seen in early cases. There is never gross swelling of the nerve head and it probably never exceeds 2–3 dioptres. Consecutive optic atrophy may follow the papillitis. Microfilariae have been demonstrated in the optic nerve of an excised eye.

Choroidal exudate. This is an early sign and usually confined to the macular area. The exudate appears as a fine grey or white mottling and is rarely accompanied by an overlying vitreous haze.

Retinal pigmentation. The first sign produced by disturbance of the retinal pigment layer is a tigroid or mottled appearance of the fundus. The retinal changes begin at the periphery and spread towards the disc. Familiarity with the normal African fundus, particularly in the elderly, is essential as a criterion. There is at this stage no diminution of the visual acuity unless there is involvement of the cornea or of the iris. At a later stage, dense masses of heaped-up pigment are seen and pigment surrounds the margins of areas of choroidal atrophy.

Choroidal atrophy. This begins as a clearly circumscribed area. Later it may include the disc and macula and in advanced cases large areas of the fundus. At first the bright red vessels of the choroid are seen as a tangled skein but later the colour changes to orange or yellow and in advanced stages the vessels are sclerosed and obliterated and the white sclera shows through.

Retinal vascular sclerosis. The vessels are attenuated and sheathed as they leave the disc.

Optic atrophy. As in other choroidoretinal degenerative processes, such as disseminated choroiditis and primary pigmentary degeneration, a secondary optic atrophy develops. The disc margins are well defined, in contradistinction to the optic atrophy consecutive to papillitis, in which the margins and the lamina cribrosa are obscured by neuroglial tissue.

Conditions of the fundus similar to those described can occur in many diseases and genetically determined degenerations, in patients in whom there is no evidence of onchocerciasis and in regions where there is no endemic onchocerciasis. By the same token, many onchocercal patients may present intercurrent fundus lesions. There is now, however, general agreement that fundus lesions occur which are specifically onchocercal in origin though not necessarily specific in their appearance.

The incidence of fundus lesions increases with the intensity of infection in the community. Choroidoretinal lesions, as might be expected in an endemic area, occur in several members of the same family, but an equal incidence has been found among males who are blood relations and among their wives who are not related by blood.

Vitamin deficiency, particularly of the B complex, seems to potentiate the severity of the fundus lesions.

Diagnostic criteria

1. Residence in an endemic area.
2. Prodromal skin irritation and rash.
3. Eosinophilia.
4. Finding of microfilariae in skin and conjunctival snips.
5. Demonstration of microfilariae in the cornea and anterior chamber.

Treatment

Treatment comes under two headings:

1. Treatment of the patient by removal of nodules and drugs.
2. Local treatment of affected eyes.

General treatment is dealt with elsewhere (see page 233).

Conjunctivitis. Whether specific or intercurrent, conjunctivitis is dealt with by lotions to wash away surface organisms and by the wide range of sulphonamides and antibiotics which are available. Mercurochrome in a 2% aqueous solution is valuable as drops or for painting the conjunctiva. It not only inhibits the organisms, but also dries up the florid oedematous conjunctiva. Cortisone should not be used if there is any question of superficial corneal erosion or ulceration.

Iritis is treated as any other non-specific iritis by mydriatics, such as atropine or phenylephrine, in an attempt to keep the pupil dilated and so prevent synechiae involving the central area of the pupil. Mydricaine injected subconjunctivally is of value in this respect and cortisone may be injected with mydricaine to limit the inflammatory exudate. In cases where photophobia is troublesome, dark glasses are indicated, but not otherwise.

Glaucoma may call for operative treatment such as iridectomy to relieve the tension. If senile or complicated cataract develops, and the disease is under control, a cataract operation may be performed.

Whether the blindness attributable to onchocerciasis is referable to lesions of the anterior or of the posterior segment, or both, the disease is of considerable social importance and the majority of workers agree that wherever it is endemic effective control measures are necessary and urgent.

OCULAR FOREIGN BODIES

In our early biological studies we learned that a minute extraneous fragment of matter inside the shell of an oyster can become the nucleus of a pearl of great price; and so a minute foreign body lying on the outside of the eyeball or, more so, if it penetrates into the eye, can cause discomfort disproportionate to its size, and complications which may lead to the loss of vision or loss of the eye itself.

Site

Extraocular. A foreign body may lie loose in the conjunctival sac moving here and there with the movement of the eye; it may lie on the surface of the conjunctiva or may lodge in the subtarsal groove, the shallow sulcus on the conjunctival surface of the upper lid above the sharp margin of the lid. This can be seen only when the lid is everted. A foreign body may lie on the surface of the cornea or become embedded in the corneal epithelium.

Such cases account for 34% of all new cases in the casualty department of an eye hospital in an industrial city.

Intraocular. A foreign body or missile may penetrate the coats of the eye by perforating the cornea or the sclera. Having entered the eye it may be enmeshed in the iris, become buried in the lens, float loosely in the vitreous or lodge in the choroidoretinal tissues in the fundus. An intraocular foreign body is often described in a case-sheet as an 'IOFB'.

Incidence

The most common accident in ophthalmology is that of a foreign body on the surface of the eye. In domestic life ashes, coal dust, cigarette-ash (and this occurs frequently in babies' eyes), eyelashes, scraps of ceiling plaster and fragments of textile material are often found. In industry, flakes from tools and grindstones, dust from loose cargo, debris from building operations and iron and rust in boiler-making and scaling are hourly incidents. As casual accidents, dust from cinder-paved sites, street and road dust in dry and windy weather, sparks from engines add their quota and, in the tropics, myiasis which is dealt with in a separate section. Ocular foreign bodies associated with warfare are, optimistically, omitted.

Diagnosis

The history is that of the rapid onset of an irritable or painful eye, with lacrimation. Acute conjunctivitis is rarely unilateral and in every such case the presence of a foreign body must be suspected.

If the eye is painful, a local anaesthetic, such as 1% amethocaine, will aid inspection. The lower fornix is easily seen; in the cornea a foreign body can be seen against the dark pupil. Then the upper lid must be everted. This is more easily done by requesting the patient to look down, then by grasping the margin of the lid between the finger and thumb and turning the lid inside out as it were, just as if turning up the edge of a cuff. Thus the whole conjunctival sac can be explored.

Removal of a foreign body

A loose foreign body can be washed out and a foreign body lightly embedded in the cornea can be wiped off with a pledget of cotton wool rolled up into a stiff pencil. If the foreign body is embedded deeply, the eye is anaesthetized with cocaine or amethocaine, the patient is placed with the head on a couch or head-rest and the eyelids are retracted with a speculum or an assistant's fingers. The point of a foreign body needle—a minute spear-like knife—is placed at the edge of the foreign body and the fragment is prised out. The old-fashioned spud with its rounded end makes an unnecessary furrow in the tissue. A drop of sulphacetamide or Chloromycetin (chloramphenicol) is instilled and, if there is circumcorneal injection, betokening ciliary irritation, atropine 1% is instilled. The eye is covered with a pad and it is advisable to request the patient to return the following day for inspection. A legal point may be scored against a doctor who does not give this advice. Cortisone should not be used as it may retard the healing of the ulcer. The foreign body, stuck to a piece of sticky tape, should be retained and attached to the record card.

Complications

A traumatic ulcer on the cornea may become infected, particularly if there is a blocked tear-duct, and a hypopyon ulcer may develop, sometimes followed by secondary glaucoma or endophthalmitis. Admission to hospital is essential if the ulcer does not heal rapidly.

Intraocular foreign bodies

The treatment of a penetrating injury is beyond the scope of casualty department surgery. X-ray examination and admission to hospital are essential in these cases.

OTHER EYE CONDITIONS ARRANGED ALPHABETICALLY

Many conditions of the eye have been dealt with in the preceding sections but there are many others in which the ocular condition is either primary or complicates a general disease.

An aetiological or pathological classification would merely recapitulate the general classification observed in the book. It is thought, therefore, that an alphabetical classification of eye diseases which have not already been considered and of the ocular complications of general diseases, will be convenient and, it is hoped, acceptable.

Angiostrongylus cantonensis INFECTION

This parasite, the lung-worm of rats, has been found in man in the meninges and in the cerebrospinal fluid. In Thailand, an adult male worm was removed from the anterior chamber of the eye. In the case described, the presenting symptoms were clouding of the vision, pain and lacrimation. Iritis and keratic precipitates followed and a small, white, thread-like filament with both ends buried in the iris was observed. The worm, 13 mm in length, was removed through a corneal incision (Kobchai 1962; Rendtorff *et al.* 1962).

BRUCELLOSIS

Brucellosis in man has been clearly recognized for 35 years. It is the major zoonosis in the United Kingdom and it is a disease of diverse presentation and protean symptomatology. It may present as an undulant fever but eye symptoms may first draw attention to the disease.

In the early stages pain in the eyes, especially on side-to-side movement, is the presenting symptom. This symptom, due to tenonitis, is often associated with a generalized headache, anorexia and malaise. Catarrhal conjunctivitis is present in the febrile phases.

Plastic iridocyclitis is a relatively early complication and may give rise to secondary glaucoma.

Involvement of the central nervous system may lead to papilloedema, optic neuritis and optic atrophy with loss of sight.

External ophthalmoplegia due to involvement of the sixth cranial nerve is not uncommon.

The most troublesome and refractory complication is detachment of the retina. This is an unlocalized, irregular and often shallow detachment, caused by retroretinal exudate.

Treatment

Iridocyclitis is treated primarily with mydriatics to prevent the formation of synechiae. Pain in the acute stage may be relieved with hot steaming or an electric eye-pad. Secondary glaucoma may require paracentesis. When detachment of the retina occurs, retroretinal exudate may absorb spontaneously. Operation, whether diathermy, retinal resection or light coagulation, must, of course, be resorted to in many cases, but the prognosis should be guarded as recurrence happens time and again.

In all patients general treatment of this disease is essential. The disease affects dairy workers but the general public is at risk in that Britain is among the diminishing number of countries in which the disease has not been eradicated. A wider awareness of ocular complications could stimulate legislation.

Eradication areas have now been designated in Britain.

CATARACT

Aetiology

In a highly organized and well documented community the obtaining of statistics presents little difficulty; and it is known that of the 10 000 persons

registered as blind in 1959 in the United Kingdom, cataract was responsible for 22%. It is accepted that senile cataract occurs more frequently and
matures at an earlier age in tropical countries than in comparatively sunless
latitudes, although accurate figures are not obtainable. In considering the
relative frequency, three factors at least must be considered: (a) ultraviolet
radiation, (b) nutrition, and (c) genetic influences.

Ultraviolet radiation. Senile cataract usually starts in the lower sector of the
lens where incident sunlight falls more directly. It is thought that the continual
absorption of ultraviolet light over a long period may bring about a denaturation
of the lens proteins and subsequent opacification.

Nutrition. Animal experimentation has demonstrated that lack of a specific
vitamin, with the possible exception of riboflavine, does not appear to affect the
lens. The examples of experimental cataract caused by dietary deficiency are
concerned with protein or amino acid deficiency and it is this type of deficiency
which is prominent in the undernourished inhabitants of tropical countries.

Genetic influences. Parents and children and brothers and sisters often display
a tendency to the development of senile cataract; where the incidence of
cataract is already high, this factor would tend to become more prominent.

Diagnosis

Cataract may be congenital, traumatic or associated with metabolic diseases
such as diabetes, tetany and galactosaemia, but the type with which we are
concerned is senile cataract. From time to time patients are referred as suffering
from cataract when in reality the opacity is in the cornea—though both conditions
may be found in the same eye.

The history and the age of the patient are helpful data, but essential to the
diagnosis is the adroit projection of a narrow pencil of light from an electric
torch into the eye. The pupil may need to be dilated. That the opacity is in the
lens is then beyond doubt.

Treatment

Where vision is affected to the point where the patient is unable to carry out
his normal work, operation is indicated. When one eye only is cataractous,
operation may be delayed until deterioration begins in the hitherto useful eye.

If, in this better eye, the lens opacity increases rapidly, operation on the
worse eye should be advised before bilateral blindness supervenes. The
management of every case will depend upon individual conditions. Advanced
age, provided the patient is otherwise fit for operation, is not a contra-indication.
The burden of years may be lightened, even in the very aged, by a successful
operation.

The operation for cataract may be extracapsular or intracapsular. Intracapsular extraction, in which the lens is removed with its capsule intact, is the
more generally indicated. The patient is subjected to one operation only,
whereas in the extracapsular operation the capsule may require a subsequent
capsulotomy for which the patient may never return from his distant village.
Moreover, there is likelihood of an inflammatory reaction following the
extracapsular procedure. A cataract operation should be performed only
by a trained operator and, if possible, in a hospital where trained nursing is
available.

Finally, no medical treatment, as yet, has been found effective in the treatment of cataract.

CHOLERA

An early ocular sign in this disease is a bluish discoloration of the skin of the eyelids. The general dehydration which characterizes the disease causes the lacrimal secretion to dry up and the eyeballs to sink into the orbits. When the patient is unconscious the eyelids are kept half open, the condition of coma vigil. The exposed, dry cornea quickly ulcerates and massive sloughing of the cornea and sclera may take place. If this disastrous termination is avoided the healed ulcer often leaves a characteristic scar in the lower part of the cornea. The retinal arteries are narrow and dark and the blood-column in the veins may be broken.

Cataract may develop rapidly in the stage of collapse. This may be due to changes in the osmotic pressure of the body fluids or to loss of nutrients in the circumambient media of the lens. In lesser degrees the opacity of the lens is reversible.

Treatment

In the stage of coma vigil the cornea is kept moist with liquid paraffin or with methyl cellulose 1% solution. Artificial tears (gelatin 0·3 gramme, chlorbutol 0·3 gramme, Locke's solution 30 ml) serve the same purpose. The exposed cornea is protected against dust and infection by a tulle gras eye pad or by a Buller's shield. If the cornea becomes ulcerated, atropine and antibiotics are indicated. Cortisone is contra-indicated in corneal ulceration.

Cataract may be avoided by vigorous measures to control general dehydration. If cataract develops and the patient survives, an extraction of the lens may be carried out after convalescence.

COCCIDIOIDOMYCOSIS

This generalized infection has not hitherto been held responsible for much eye involvement, but clinical reports and necropsy findings have increasingly shown that the choroid and optic nerves may be involved, possibly from vegetating endocarditis; at least one case is recorded in which the eye was enucleated and revealed endophthalmitis and abounding spherules.

The present writer saw many patients suffering from the disease in the hot, dry and dusty San Joaquin valley and also in laboratory workers in Los Angeles, who had become infected during their work, but he saw no ocular lesions. A routine examination of the fundus, even in the absence of ocular symptoms, might show that ocular involvement is not such a rarity.

Treatment of the eye condition is that of the general disease with amphotericin B. If there is overt uveitis, atropine and local corticosteroids are indicated (Olavarria & Fajardo 1971).

DRACONTIASIS

The filaria *Dracunculus medinensis* (guinea-worm) is usually found in the lower limbs but occasionally the female travels upwards to the head of the human host and may be found in the eyelid, where it causes intense oedema in the soft tissue, or in the conjunctiva. The worm has been known to penetrate the eyeball resulting in loss of the eye.

Treatment

Whereas surgical excision is a recognized line of treatment when the worm is in the leg, the tortuosity of its body makes surgical extraction from the orbit difficult and dangerous.

A West African method of treatment observed by the writer is to await the appearance of the head through the ruptured blister and then to apply a drop of the juice from a macerated, fresh tobacco leaf to the head of the worm. The body then begins to appear and is carefully rolled around a match-stick. Each day this process is repeated until the whole worm is extruded. Traditional methods are not always to be decried! The treatment is with niridazole (Ambilhar) or diethylcarbamazine (see page 244).

DYSENTERY

Amoebic dysentery

Conjunctivitis and iritis have been ascribed to this disease but the association is probably adventitious. Papilloedema may occur as in other intracranial space-occupying lesions when an amoebic cerebral abscess develops, but this complication is very rare.

Bacillary dysentery

Conjunctival congestion occurs during the acute febrile stage of the disease. Iridocyclitis, associated with polyarthritis, may occur within four weeks of the onset of the intestinal symptoms. Other causes of iritis such as Reiter's disease, Behçet's syndrome, etc., must be excluded. The routine treatment of iritis is indicated, with the promotion of mydriasis by atropine and hot steaming to allay the pain.

FILARIAL INFECTIONS OTHER THAN ONCHOCERCIASIS

Two other nematodes are of importance to the ophthalmologist, *Wuchereria bancrofti* and *Loa loa.*

Filariasis due to *Wuchereria bancrofti* is found in the tropics of every continent and occasionally in sub-tropical countries such as Southern Spain. Although the disease is common, the eye is rarely involved. The adult worm has been found in the anterior chamber and in this situation, although it moves about like an eel in a tank, curiously enough there is little local reaction. Atropine is said to cause the death of the worm. The dead adult worm, unlike the living nematode, may excite in the eye a reaction characterized by severe iridocyclitis, keratitis and secondary glaucoma. The worm has been observed in the vitreous chamber, apparently causing no trouble. It can be removed from the anterior chamber, under a local anaesthesia, by a keratome incision at the limbus. The rush of aqueous washes out the worm, or its removal may be assisted by forceps.

Setaria found in the anterior chamber of horses in Southern India can be removed in the same way.

Unlike those of *Onchocerca* the microfilariae of *Wuchereria* do not affect the eye.

Tropical eosinophilia

In this syndrome, of which infection by *Wuchereria bancrofti* may be one of the causes, a severe iridocyclitis and posterior uveitis may supervene. The usual treatment of iritis is carried out but the condition may not subside without specific general treatment.

Loiasis

This disease is due to infection by *Loa loa* and is endemic in West and Central Africa and in Southern Sudan. The worm, about 30–70 mm in length, may be seen under the bulbar or palpebral conjunctiva, or moving immediately under the skin of the eyelid. In the conjunctiva the parasite causes irritation and congestion and sometimes actual pain. Calabar swelling (Fig. 258), the allergic response to filarial toxins, may occur in the eyelid causing a tense swelling with inability, while it persists, to open the eyelid.

Treatment. Apart from general treatment the worm can sometimes be removed from the eye. A local anaesthetic, amethocaine or cocaine 1 %, is rapidly instilled

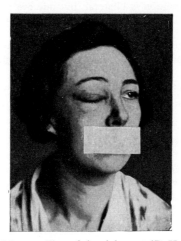

Fig. 258.—Calabar swelling of the right eye. (*P. H. Manson-Bahr*)

into the conjunctival sac. The worm is gripped through the conjunctiva by forceps. The conjunctiva is incised and the worm is gripped by another pair of forceps and withdrawn.

Although modern chemotherapy may render this procedure unnecessary there is some satisfaction in removing an uninvited guest.

Tapeworm

The parasite has been dealt with elsewhere (see page 337) in this book, but it might be appropriate to mention here that it has been suggested that optic atrophy may result from the treatment.

The female of the plant *Hagenia abyssinica*, called 'kosso' in Ethiopia, is widely used as a tapeworm remedy. The active principle kosotoxin is said to be similar to filicic acid, the anthelmintic agent in filix mas.

General poisoning even with fatal results may follow overdosage especially in hypersensitive patients.

A recent paper reports (Rokos 1969) the occurrence of primary optic atrophy in 12 patients as a further complication. The optic atrophy is associated with peripheral or total loss of the visual fields and is usually bilateral.

High dosage of vitamins B_1 and B_{12} is suggested empirically by way of treatment.

GLAUCOMA IN EPIDEMIC DROPSY

Maynard (1909) described the association of glaucoma with epidemic dropsy in Calcutta. The condition became known as Bengal glaucoma.

Signs and symptoms

The presenting symptom is the subjective appearance of halos around lights. In long-standing cases the field of vision becomes contracted; untreated patients eventually lose their sight.

The general symptoms of epidemic dropsy may not necessarily accompany the glaucoma. The condition is bilateral, but one eye may be worse than the other. Pain is unusual even when the tension is consistently high and the discs show cupping.

The diagnosis is particularly indicated when the symptoms occur in different age-groups in one family, or in people indulging in communal feeding over a long period.

The effects of this disease are increased where the basic diet is carbohydrate, such as rice.

Aetiology

The dropsy and its concomitant glaucoma is considered to be due to contamination of mustard-oil used in cooking with the seeds of the common prickly poppy, *Argemone mexicana*. The possible toxic factor is the isoquinoline alkaloid, sanguinerine, which is found in the seeds of *A. mexicana*. Animal experiments have demonstrated that the injection or ingestion of this substance may increase intraocular pressure.

Treatment

The treatment of the general disease and the elimination of suspected cooking-oil are paramount. Locally, the increased intraocular tension does not respond well to the usual miotics.

Diamox and other carbonic anhydrase inhibitors are useful in many cases but others may require a tension reducing operation. Even in cases which appear to have settled down, periodical examination is important as recurrence after apparent recovery is not uncommon.

HAEMOGLOBINS RETINOPATHY

The haemoglobinopathies (page 26) are a group of haemolytic diseases caused by the presence of abnormal haemoglobin in the blood stream. Haemoglobin A is the adult type of haemoglobin and haemoglobin F is the fetal type, usually replaced by A by the age of 12. Abnormal types—haemoglobin S, differing from haemoglobin A by the substitution of a valine molecule for a glutamic molecule, or haemoglobin C, in which a lysine molecule replaces the glutamic molecule—may replace haemoglobin F in the first month of life.

The haemoglobin gene follows a Mendelian model in the determination of the appearance of either haemoglobin A or an abnormal type.

Haemoglobin C and S occur primarily in Negroes and in some Mediterranean people. Approximately 10% of American Negroes possess an abnormal haemoglobin.

Haemoglobin S under certain conditions, associated with changing oxygen saturation, has the ability to change the shape and viscosity of blood cells. These characteristics bestow the name of sickle cell anaemia and bring about thrombosis, ischaemia and infection of tissues and their sequelae.

The pathological changes in the eye run the whole gamut of vascular pathology. Conjunctival capillary stasis can be seen in over 80% of patients. In the interior of the eye the following manifestations have been noted: dilated and tortuous retinal veins, sheathed and occluded arterioles and venules, choroidoretinal scars, vitreous and retinal haemorrhages, retinal exudates and refractile bodies, presumably cholesterol deposits, retinal vasoproliferation with micro-aneurysms, glial proliferation, vitreous haemorrhages and retinal detachment, papilloedema and angeoid streaks and occlusion of the central retinal artery or vein (Kerney 1967).

The retinopathy in sickle cell disease is related to and is similar to the retinopathies seen in diabetes mellitus, venous occlusion, Eales's disease and advanced hypertension.

HISTOPLASMOSIS

The characteristic ophthalmological complications are disseminated areas of choroiditis. These are yellowish-white, one-tenth of a disc-diameter in size and unpigmented. Macular involvement may simulate central serous retinopathy or cause haemorrhages with organized mildly pigmented scars indistinguishable from the Junius–Kuhnt form of macular degeneration. Serous exudates may result in disciform detachment. The choroiditis may also exhibit a circumpapillary pattern (Schlaegel 1968).

Diagnosis is made by the clinical picture confirmed by a positive histoplasmin skin-test. Histoplasmin and brucellergin are two examples of skin-test antigens used in ophthalmology to elicit a positive serological response.

KERATOMYCOSIS

Keratomycosis or mycotic keratitis (Fig. 259)—corneal infection with fungi—was recognized by Leber as early as 1879, but only in recent years has it assumed the proportions of a major ophthalmological problem. It is significant that fungus infections of the cornea have become increasingly common following the widespread use of local applications of antibiotics and corticosteroids. Experimentally, corticosteroids facilitate corneal infection by fungi, and, clinically, in cases of keratomycosis nearly 75% of the patients have undergone local steroid treatment.

The condition presents as a superficial ulcer in the central third of the cornea. The margins are irregular but well defined and delineated by a yellowish-grey, subepithelial infiltration. The base of the ulcer is heaped up and has a dry, crumbly, grey appearance. Hypopyon is common. The ulcer seldom perforates but when bacterial infection supervenes a violent reaction occurs with deepening of the ulcer, which may lead to perforation and endophthalmitis. The intraocular tension may be raised.

Organisms

Thirty different fungi have been isolated from the eye. *Aspergillus* spp. have been observed most commonly, but *Nocardia* spp., *Candida albicans*, *Blasto-myces dermatitidis*, *Penicillium* spp. and *Sporothrix schenckii* are all relatively common.

Diagnosis

Fungus infection should be suspected in chronic hypopyon ulcers which are resistant to routine treatment and where a fungus is found on examination. Material for culture is taken with a platinum loop and inoculated on Sabouraud's glucose medium, MacConkey's agar or blood agar.

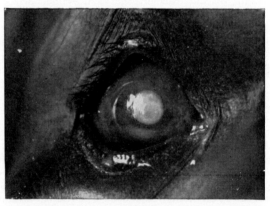

Fig. 259.—Mycotic keratitis. (*British Journal of Ophthalmology*)

Treatment

Full mydriasis with atropine 1 or 2% drops or ointment is essential. Intractable cases may respond to curettage of the ulcer and iodine cautery. A solution of iodine 7% and potassium iodide 5% in alcohol is applied directly to the anaesthetized cornea which is dried with filter paper.

Nystatin (Mycostatin, 1 tablet = 500 000 units) by mouth has been used with benefit. Secondary infection may be controlled with mercurochrome 2% aqueous solution or with sulphacetamide. What is certain is that corticosteroids alone or combined with antibiotics should be used with caution, lest perforation may be precipitated. Raised tension is treated with Diamox or repeated para-centesis. Therapeutic keratoplasty has been advocated.

LEISHMANIASIS

Kala-azar, oriental sore and espundia are three distinct clinical conditions caused by *Leishmania* spp.

Kala-azar. Ocular manifestations are relatively rare. Retinal haemorrhages may be seen and are secondary to the anaemia. Thrombosis of the central vein has been recorded.

Nodules may be found on the eyelids. The palpebral conjunctiva is not involved but small nodules may occur in the episclera near the limbus and may extend on to the cornea with resulting opacification and neovascularization. A chronic iritis accompanies corneal involvement. The early symptoms are lacrimation and irritation, with photophobia when the disease spreads to the cornea and an increasing loss of vision as the opacities spread from the periphery to the centre of the cornea. Treatment of the general disease brings about regression of the ocular trouble. Atropine and dark glasses to relieve the photophobia are indicated when the cornea and iris are implicated.

Oriental sore. There is no specific ocular lesion attributable to this disease but the lesion may be seen on the upper or lower eyelid.

Espundia. Destructive ulceration starting in the skin/mucosa junction of the nose or in the skin of the face may spread to destroy the eyelids. General treatment is indicated, to be followed by plastic operative procedures when the disease is controlled.

Linguatula serrata INFECTION

In man this pentastomid is found in the gastro-intestinal tract and in the lung, but rarely in the eye. When it does occur in the eye the presenting symptoms are pain and blurred vision followed by acute iritis with secondary glaucoma, due to the growth of the parasite within the eye. The nymph form of the parasite, $4 \cdot 5 \times 1 \cdot 5$ mm, lies in the anterior chamber enclosed in a fine translucent capsule. Peristaltic movements may be detected. Treatment is by removal through a simple corneal incision (Rendtorff *et al.* 1962).

LYMPHOMA OF THE ORBIT (BURKITT'S TUMOUR)

Ex Africa semper aliquid novi (Pliny)

A highly malignant tumour syndrome affecting children in tropical Africa has, within recent years, received considerable attention (Burkitt 1962).

The distribution map of this tumour is from approximately 15°N. to 20°S. of the equator where the average minimum temperature does not drop below 15·6°C and the rainfall is over 50 mm a year. The fact that the tumour distribution is dependent on climatic factors suggests a vector-borne virus as the responsible agent. The EB virus, which almost certainly causes infectious mononucleosis, is at least associated with Burkitt's tumour (Stoker 1970). New Guinea is the main area outside Africa where this tumour has been recognized.

It is not a tumour of Africans but a tumour of children in Africa, of 'place' not 'race'. The tumour presents in children between the ages of 2 and 14, with a peak incidence at the age of 5. It may arise in the maxilla or mandible, in the testis, spine, femur or arm or present as an abdominal mass.

Ocular manifestations

This tumour is the commonest cause of unilateral exophthalmos in young children in the endemic areas (Fig. 260). An analysis of the diagnosis of proptosis due to orbital neoplasms in a series of 60 Ugandan children revealed that 28 were due to Burkitt's lymphoma. The next in frequency was chloroma (Templeton 1971). Oedema of the eyelids is an early sign followed by marked

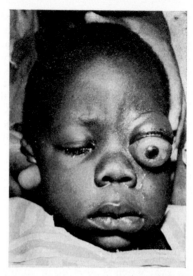

Fig. 260.—A tumour involving the orbit and presenting with proptosis in a boy aged 2 years. (Dr D. Burkitt)

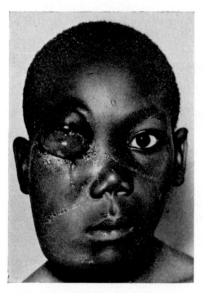

Fig. 261.—Lymphoma of the orbit.
(Dr D. W. Ellis-Jones)

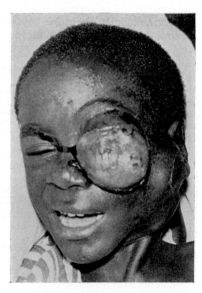

Fig. 262.—Retinoblastoma.
(Dr D. W. Ellis-Jones)

chemosis. These cases are thus often first seen in the eye department. Proliferation of the tumour within the orbit results in exophthalmos and displacement of the eye, which may be thrust almost out of the skull. The globe itself is not invaded until the later stages and this distinguishes it from advanced retinoblastoma (Figs 261, 262).

Treatment

Radiotherapy has not proved to be successful. Nitrogen mustard gave immediate results but in many cases induced neurotoxicity followed by recurrence
and death (Clifford 1966). The long-term results of pteroylglutamic acid
were disappointing.

At the present time trial is being given to a combination of Endoxana (cyclophosphamide) and ortho-melphalan given intravenously with cytosine arobino-
sine and methotrexate administered intrathecally. The mortality of patients
under this treatment has been reduced to 30% as opposed to the certain mortality of untreated patients or patients treated by other methods (Bisley 1970).

Burkitt's tumour, although described comparatively recently, may not in
fact be a new disease. The clinical appearance of advanced untreated retinoblastoma may resemble that of Burkitt's tumour presenting in the orbit.

In earlier days before expert pathological examination was available patients
may have been diagnosed as suffering from retinoblastoma when they were in
fact victims of ocular lymphoma.

MALARIA

Ocular involvement

In general, true malarial involvement of the ocular tissues is rare and many of
the complications attributed to malaria are incidental.

In the acute stage, as in many febrile conditions, the conjunctiva becomes
hyperaemic and this congestion may lead to petechial, or larger, conjunctival
haemorrhages. In this phase of the disease infection with the virus of herpes
simplex may occur. The resulting dendritic ulcer, the outline of which can be
demonstrated by staining with fluorescein, occurs in 5% or less of patients with
otherwise healthy eyes.

Transient amaurosis may follow the comatose state and may persist with
signs, eventually, of optic neuritis.

In the fundus, capillary obstruction, brought about by leucocytic or parasitic
emboli, may cause small peripheral or larger central haemorrhages. When the
latter are absorbed permanent pigmentary macular changes may result.

In the hazy margin of an inflamed disc, a peculiar chestnut greyish coloration,
due to the deposition of pigmented leucocytes, is considered to be pathognomic
of malarial papillitis. This was described by Sulzer (1890) as papillary melanosis
(mélanose de la papille).

In chronic or cachectic patients, who suffer from anaemia, more severe
haemorrhages may cause widespread retinal disorganization.

These vascular complications recall to the mind that the original author of
this volume said: 'What one sees in the peripheral circulation is only a reflection
of the drama occurring in the internal circulation.'

Blepharitis, xerosis, pigmentation of the cornea, iridocyclitis and choroiditis
have been attributed to the main disease. Ocular palsies involving the third,
fourth and sixth cranial nerves, paralysis of accommodation and even an
Argyll–Robertson pupil have been reported. In view of the experience of later
years, the view may be accepted that the association of at least some of these
conditions with malaria is fortuitous.

Treatment

The initial conjunctivitis may be relieved by a saline lotion or by cold water
pads. Dendritic keratitis must be treated energetically by cauterization with

phenol or by the instillation into the conjunctival sac of IDU (5-iodo-2 deoxy-uridine) an anti-viral drug which resembles thymidine. Antibiotics are ineffectual.

Iritis, whether attributable or intercurrent, is treated with atropine. Other ocular conditions respond, or otherwise, to the general treatment.

Complications of treatment. *Quinine.* The standard treatment for 300 years, quinine seems for a time to have lost its ascendency as a prophylactic or therapeutic drug. In some parts of South-east Asia and in South America some strains of *P. falciparum* have developed chloroquine resistance. In primary infections of *P. falciparum* malaria, delay in effective treatment may endanger the life of the patient. Many authorities are now advising that, in severe cases of *P. falciparum* malaria, parenteral quinine should be given initially. Quinine may thus be restored to the therapeutic front line and quinine amblyopia and blackwater fever may be encountered again. Quinine amblyopia is due to a hypersensitivity to the drug, and even small doses may bring on this condition in idiosyncratic people. The onset is sudden. The loss of vision may be absolute, with no perception of light. The pupils are dilated and react sluggishly, if at all. The fundi show marked constriction of the retinal arteries; there is pallor of the disc and a cherry red spot at the macula, such as is seen in occlusion of the central artery. Vision may return in a few hours but may take days or weeks. A woman, seen by the writer, took 30 grains as an abortifacient and although she retained her fetus she regained perception of light only. When recovery occurs the fields of vision may be greatly contracted almost to tubular vision. If the case is seen at an early stage a retrobulbar injection of tolazoline hydrochloride may bring about vasodilatation.

Chloroquine. Chloroquine and hydroxychloroquine are responsible in sensitive subjects for a variety of ocular side-effects.

Loss of sensitivity of the cornea is an early symptom, associated with blurring of vision and the appearance of halos. Later, white granules appear in the epithelium which may become aggregated into curved lines below the centre of the cornea. Posterior subcapsular lens opacities develop later.

The gravest changes are in the fundus. The macula develops a mottled appearance and pigment granules appear. A 'doughnut' picture develops with a central dark area, a clear zone and then a ring of pigment. Narrowing of the vessels and peripheral pigmentation may follow.

The visual acuity should be noted before the start of, and at regular intervals throughout, the course of this treatment. Treatment should be discontinued if the visual acuity falls, and particularly if macular pigmentation becomes evident.

Mepacrine was widely used in the Second World War in West Africa as a prophylactic. It stained the skin and conjunctiva a deep yellow, a cosmetic effect resented particularly by the nursing sisters, to save whose faces and to keep the peace physicians found it expedient to use, prophylactically, the dwindling stocks of quinine with, fortunately, successful social and medicinal results.

To the lately arrived medical officer unfamiliar with the drug the pigmentation sometimes suggested the icterus of hepatitis, and in another field of war wily patients, reluctant to return to jungle warfare, deliberately used mepacrine to stain the conjunctiva in the hope of postponing their return to the fighting line.

MEASLES

A Parsee proverb runs: 'Smallpox will make your child blind, measles will send him to his grave.' The mortality of measles is not in dispute but in some parts of the world measles is a significant cause of blindness.

It is not the purpose of this article to give the geographical distribution of the disease, nor the general clinical features or treatment, but the following references suggest the prevalence and severity of ocular involvement. In the Luapula Province of Zambia in 1966, the overall figure of uniocular blindness in children between the ages of 6 and 14 was 9·48 per 1000. Measles, smallpox and chickenpox, in that order, were responsible for 68% of all cases. Blindness due to measles in this province is particularly in evidence in the river and lake-side areas.

In Upper Volta, measles is stated to be a significant cause of blindness.

In West Africa, measles led to damage or destruction of one or both eyes in 31 of 2164 patients (1·4%). In Rhodesia, the combination of measles and vitamin A deficiency is believed to be the main cause of blindness in children.

In contrast, in England and Wales in the first two weeks of January 1970, 8268 cases of measles were notified. There were no deaths and no cases of blindness were recorded.

Ocular involvement

The presenting sign is an oculonasal catarrh with profuse conjunctival watery discharge which, because of secondary infection, becomes mucopurulent. There is profound photophobia. The condition is invariably bilateral. Superficial keratitis punctata is found in many cases and the lesions can be demonstrated by fluorescein staining. If treatment is timely and energetic, this condition may resolve in 3–4 days. In other patients, where heavy bacterial infection and malnutrition are accompanying factors, ulceration and perforation of the cornea may occur, with prolapse of the iris and leucoma adherens in the lower half of the cornea.

Other complications are iritis, choroidoretinitis, retinal oedema and optic neuritis. Occlusion of the central artery has been reported. Endophthalmitis and panophthalmitis may lead to rapid and complete destruction of the eye. Perforating keratomalacia, in which a part or the whole of the cornea sloughs off, may occur in cases of gross nutritional deficiency.

Treatment

Gentle bathing with tepid normal saline, or with 2.5% sodium bicarbonate lotion if the eyelids are crusted and sticky, is sufficient in the early stage.

If the secretion shows signs of becoming purulent, before a bacteriological examination has verified the organism, the painting of the palpebral conjunctiva with 2% aqueous mercurochrome tends to control the discharge; or mercuro-chrome drops of the same strength may be used.

If a specific pyogenic organism is found specific antibiotics, drops or ointment may be used.

Atropine 1% drops are indicated if the corneae become hazy, or if superficial keratitis or discrete ulceration can be demonstrated. Atropine is also indicated at any stage if iritis is seen.

Corticosteroids should NOT be used at any stage of the disease: their use may precipitate the perforation of an ulcer which might otherwise resolve.

In undernourished children, large doses of vitamin A are indicated, but this comes under general treatment of the disease rather than the specific eye treatment.

MYIASIS

Myiasis is the condition produced by the invasion of the tissues by maggots, the larvae of flies. The fly may deposit ova or the actual larvae in wounds or in the natural openings of the body.

Ocular myiasis

The larvae may be found in swellings with sinuses in any part of the eyelids (Fig. 263). They may be deposited in the conjunctival sac and are found particularly in the upper fornix. Occasionally they burrow under the conjunctiva and rarely through the sclera into the interior of the eye-ball. The symptoms range from those of catarrhal conjunctivitis to violent iridocyclitis. In debilitated patients and in neglected children larvae may penetrate deep into the orbital tissues, so that the eye and orbit are converted into a mass of inflammatory tissue.

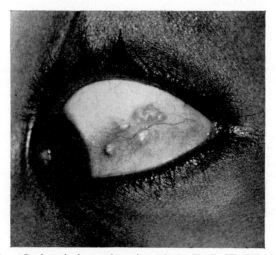

Fig. 263.—Conjunctival granuloma in myiasis. (*Dr D. W. Ellis-Jones*)

Diagnosis

This depends upon finding and identifying the maggots. Flies of many different families are involved (see Appendix III).

Treatment

If the eye is involved in myiasis the upper eyelid must be everted and the upper fornix examined. Larvae, if seen, are then picked off with forceps and any sinus which is present should be explored under local anaesthesia. Mercurochrome 2% aqueous solution as drops or antibiotics are used to control secondary infection. When the larvae are intraocular attempts at removal may be made but the prognosis as regards vision is unfavourable.

Conjunctival granuloma

Although no actual larvae have been identified, this condition may possibly be a form of myiasis. These granulomas, each 3–4 mm in size, appear often in groups of 6 or more under the bulbar conjunctiva, particularly on the temporal side. They may disappear spontaneously in 4–5 weeks but occasionally they ulcerate.

The microscopic appearance shows fibroblastic response surrounding a necrotic area in the centre of which is a small lumen suggesting the burrow of a larva or other parasite, but no parasite has as yet been identified. In Uganda they are known as Ower Hennessey granulomas.

In the treatment of this condition the conjunctiva is kept clear of secondary infection by sulphonamide drops or ointment. Excision of the tumour is rarely called for. When ulceration occurs the sinus may be treated with mercurochrome 2% aqueous solution.

ONYALAI

This disease, which is identical with essential thrombocytopenia, is described on page 19, but is mentioned in this section because one of the presenting signs in the sudden onset of the disease is suffusion of the conjunctiva. Later subconjunctival haemorrhages occur. Retinal and intraocular haemorrhages have not been described.

PARAGONIMIASIS

The distribution, aetiology and pathology are dealt with on page 327.

In the endemic areas 0·8% of patients suffering from the pulmonary form of the disease develop cerebral complications variously manifested in Jacksonian epilepsy, plegias, aphasia, arachnoiditis, abscesses and granulomas. The larvae have been thought to travel along the tissues surrounding the jugular vein towards the brain (Oh 1968).

Ocular complications

Homonymous hemianopia, papilloedema and impaired visual acuity are the main signs. Defects in the field of vision, constriction and hemianopia, are explained by involvement of the temporoparietal and occipital lobes. Papilloedema is explained by space-occupying granulomas or abscesses which cause an increase in intracranial pressure. In the Foster–Kennedy syndrome a granuloma or abscess exerts direct pressure on one optic nerve causing optic atrophy while the same lesion produces generalized increased intracranial pressure and papilloedema in the contralateral eye.

Pathological and pneumo-encephalographic evidence has shown that basal arachnoiditis, which is common in the cerebral type of the disease, is also a cause of optic atrophy and a major cause of impaired vision.

Ophthalmological examination is an important factor in the diagnosis of this disease.

Armillifer (Porocephalus) armillatus INFECTION

A. armillatus is a member of a small group of blood-sucking arthropods of the class Pentastomida. The adult form is a parasite found in the lungs and trachea of the West African royal python. Larval forms (Fig. 264) are found in the lion and other quadrupeds. Infestation of the eye is rare. It has been found in the human eye lying in the subconjunctival plane (Figs 265, 266), and in the

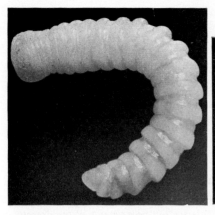

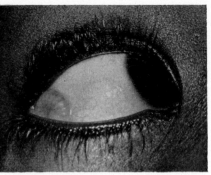

Fig. 264.—*Armillifer armillatus* larva. (*Dr. D. Ellis-Jones; British Journal of Ophthalmology*)

Fig. 265.—Subconjunctival porocephalus. (*Dr. D. Ellis-Jones; British Journal of Ophthalmology*)

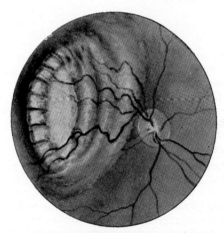

Fig. 266.—Intraocular porocephalus. Drawn by A. Mckie Reid. (*British Journal of Ophthalmology*)

choroidoretinal space where it produced a detachment of the retina. From the former situation it can without difficulty be removed by operation (Reid & Jones 1962).

PTERYGIUM

Pterygium ($\pi\tau\acute{\epsilon}\rho\upsilon\xi$, a wing) is an arrow-head fold of bulbar conjunctiva which creeps over and becomes attached to the neighbouring cornea. It consists of connective tissue containing elastic fibres and is continuous with the subconjunctival tissue. It invades the cornea as deeply as Bowman's membrane, which undergoes degeneration.

Pterygia are found particularly in hot, dry climates where there is much dust and aridity. The condition is prevalent in Southern India. Heredity may be a factor but this view should be accepted with caution as similar environmental and climatic conditions obtain in successive generations. Pterygia occur from time to time adventitiously in patients who live sheltered lives in temperate climates.

Signs and symptoms

The pinkish-yellow apex shows up clearly on the cornea against the background of the dark iris and advice is often sought for cosmetic reasons. The apex tends to progress towards the centre of the cornea and when it reaches the pupillary area vision is interfered with (Fig. 267).

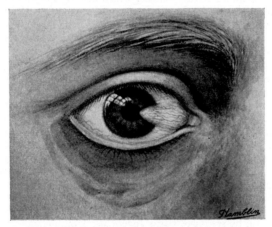

Fig. 267.—Pterygium.

Treatment

If the pterygium has shown no signs of advancing it may well be left alone but if the apex is seen to be travelling towards the centre of the cornea surgical treatment is advisable before vision is menaced.

Simple excision. The apex is carefully sliced off the cornea. Delicate handling is essential as the cornea has been perforated in this procedure. The new tissue is then dissected off the underlying sclera and the whole mass cut away with scissors. The conjunctiva is then undercut and sutured to cover the gap. The recurrence rate is high, up to 25%, in this method.

Transplantation. The apex is dissected off the cornea and the scleral attachment released. The apex is then transfixed with a suture and brought down under the conjunctiva towards the lower fornix where it is anchored with a suture. The bed of the pterygium may be gently touched with a diathermy applicator or with phenol and the conjunctival gap is repaired. This method may leave an unsightly swelling at the site of transplantation.

McGavic's technique. The apex is sliced away from the cornea as described above. Horizontal incisions are made along the upper and lower borders of the pterygium as far as the canthus. The subconjunctival fibrous tissue is dissected off the overlying conjunctiva and removed. The conjunctiva is then replaced and the edges are replaced. A small area at the apex of the conjunctival flap is excised leaving a bare area of sclera. This prevents the granulating free edge of conjunctiva from becoming adherent to the cornea at the limbus. The free edges of the conjunctiva along the gap may be sutured to the episcleral tissue (McGavic 1949).

Pseudo-pterygium is an attachment of a fold of conjunctiva to the raw floor of a corneal ulcer near the limbus. When the acute phase has passed the fold may be dissected off. Recurrence is unlikely.

RHINOSPORIDIOSIS

A general description of this disease, which is due to a yeast-like organism, *Rhinosporidium seeberi*, is given in another part of this volume (page 707). Ocular lesions come next in frequency to those in the nose and nasopharynx. In 93 cases of oculosporidiasis reported in India since 1900 the lesions occurred in the lacrimal sac, conjunctiva, eyelid, sclera and canaliculus in that order of frequency. Scleral involvement has been recorded in 2 patients. As thinning of the sclera carries with it the threat of rupture and loss of the eye, a lesion involving this tissue calls for careful consideration.

In one case the scleral involvement was described as a staphyloma and in the more recent case (Lambda *et al.* 1970) as scleral ectasia. In this patient a conjunctival polyp 10 mm in diameter was associated with a cystic swelling in the ectatic sclera. Treatment in the second case consisted in the wide excision of the conjunctival polyp, aspiration of the scleral cyst and the grafting of preserved homologous sclera over the scleral defect. Fascia lata, as used in scleral staphylomas from other causes and in scleromalacia perforans, would probably serve the same purpose should preserved homologous sclera not be available.

There is a tendency for ocular lesions as well as lesions elsewhere to recur, owing to invasion by spores of tissue spaces and lymph channels.

RUBELLA

The finding of lamellar cataract in infants who have been exposed to the influence of maternal rubella during the first sixteen weeks of pregnancy is well recognized. Fundus lesions have been established as occurring in congenital rubella in the United States, in South America and in Europe (Stark 1966; Kresky & Nauheim 1967).

The typical appearance is the aggregation of dust-like pigment particles, interspersed with larger dots, concentrated at the posterior pole. The pigment does not assume bone-spicule formation. The condition may be unilateral or bilateral and does not interfere with visual acuity, dark adaptation or peripheral vision.

Associated lesions may be deafness, ataxia, diplegia, mental defects, heart lesions and metaplasia of the teeth.

The significance of the observation of the fundus lesion is the ability to establish the aetiology of other congenital malformations in the absence of a definite history of rubella.

Prophylactic vaccine therapy gives promise of limiting the ravages of this disease.

In the meantime, the devastating effects of rubella lend truth to the observation that 'the best birthday present to an as-yet-unmarried daughter may well be an attack of rubella'.

SCHISTOSOMIASIS AND THE KATAYAMA SYNDROME

Ocular manifestations

In the invasive stage urticaria and oedema of the face and eyelids may be observed. The conjunctiva is occasionally invaded and pinkish-yellow, soft, painless tumours may be seen in the palpebral conjunctiva of the upper eyelid and in the fornix.

Microscopic examination shows schistosome ova surrounded by endothelial cells, lymphocytes, plasma cells, eosinophils and giant cells. The adult worm has been found in a dilated vein near the caruncle.

In the later stages, intracranial involvement may occur with granulomatous swellings of the meninges and of the cerebral cortex. Ova have been demonstrated in these swellings.

Visual disturbances up to total blindness may result from involvement of the optic tract and the visual cortex.

Treatment

When granulomas are found in the conjunctiva surgical excision is indicated (Sparrow 1966).

SMALLPOX

In some parts of the subcontinent of India and in Algeria smallpox is held to be responsible for a quarter of all cases of blindness. About the fifth day catarrhal conjunctivitis occurs with subconjunctival haemorrhages in the haemorrhagic type. Pustules resembling early stage phlyctenules are comparatively rare but may be found on the bulbar or palpebral conjunctiva or on the caruncle. When they occur at the limbus corneal ulceration follows and secondary infection leads to hypopyon. The corneal ulcer may perforate, leading to endophthalmitis and phthisis bulbi. The other eye may be involved in sympathetic ophthalmitis. Even in less severe cases the deep corneal ulceration leaves a dense white leucoma.

On the eighth day, when secondary fever returns, the lids become tensely swollen and closed and the eye is difficult to examine. Seroplastic iritis with ring synechiae may develop unobserved and thus be untreated. If the eye, and the patient, recovers, small depigmented atrophic scars—vitiligo iridis, in which the stroma is thin or absent—may be left in the iris.

Retinal haemorrhages and optic neuritis may also occur, and encephalomyelitis may lead to ocular motor palsies particularly of the sixth nerve.

Ulcerative lesions on the lid margins may result in madarosis and trichiasis; and cicatrical contraction to phimosis and symblepharon. Acute dacryocystitis may complicate the condition.

Treatment

Even when, or particularly when, the eyelids are greatly swollen and difficult to examine they should be opened with lid hooks. If the cornea is involved or iritis is apparent atropine is essential and mercurochrome 2% or antibiotics should be instilled to combat secondary infection.

SPARGANOSIS

Invasion of the orbital tissues by sparganum, the plerocercoid form of *Diphyllobothrium mansoni*, is a condition well recognized in the Far East, and one case of ocular infection has been described in a woman in Uganda (Jones 1962). The mode of infection in China is ascribed to the custom of applying a raw split frog as local treatment to an inflamed eye, although this method did not appear to apply in the case of the Uganda patient.

Symptoms

Pain, redness of the eye, oedema of the eyelids, ptosis and lacrimation are the presenting symptoms (Fig. 268). The worm has been found in a cystic swelling lying under the bulbar conjunctiva near the caruncle, with a second worm in a flattened, yellow plaque, high up in the superior fornix, having the appearance of a nodule of fat.

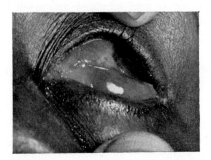

Fig. 268.—Sparganosis. A cyst containing *Sparganum mansoni* under a bulbar conjunctiva.

Treatment

The general treatment is by intravenous neoarsphenamine 0·3–0·45 gramme repeated after 4–5 days.

Surgical treatment consists in removal of the cyst or swelling with the worm; but it has been suggested that simple incision with removal of the worm, leaving the sac in situ, is quicker and appears to cause no local reaction.

THELAZIASIS

Thelazia callipaeda (*Filaria circumlocaris*, *F. lacrimalis*) or the oriental eye-worm is a nematode which inhabits the conjunctival and lacrimal sacs of man and dogs, and of cats in California. It is also found in India, Burma and China.

The female is 7 mm long and the male somewhat smaller.

Symptoms

Conjunctival irritation and pain, lacrimation, ectropion and partial facial paralysis are the symptoms.

In Australia, another nematode *F. habronema* is responsible for the condition of 'blue eye' or 'bung eye'.

The vector is a fly.

The lesion presents as a granulomatous tumour and the treatment is by excision.

TOXOCARIASIS

Visceral larva migrans (Wiseman & Woodruff 1967) is the term applied to the clinical syndrome which occurs in children as the result of the invasion of the tissues by the larva of a nematode which is normally parasitic in lower animals.

The ascarids of the dog and cat, *Toxocara canis* and *T. cati*, are responsible for ocular lesions which have within the last decade been shown to be attributable to the parasites.

In the past, some ocular lesions now known to have been caused by *Toxocara* have been diagnosed variously as organized haemorrhages or exudates, as Coats's disease, or as choroiditis or retinoblastoma. Because the last-named has been diagnosed, eyes have been removed.

Aetiology

Toxocara is common throughout the world in dogs and cats, and especially in puppies and kittens. Some recorded figures are 82·8% of 100 dogs in Calcutta, 61% of cats in Wales, 13·5% of dogs in Marseilles and 21% at Battersea Dogs' Home. The chances of an infant coming in contact with an infected animal are considerable, for children fondle domestic pets and crawl on floors and in yards and gardens which may be fouled with ova excreted by infected animals. Children addicted to the habit of pica are particularly susceptible.

Clinical signs and symptoms

Infection in early infancy is characterized by a wide pattern of constitutional symptoms, such as recurrent febrile attacks, anaemia, upper respiratory infections, pneumonitis and hepatomegaly. When laparotomy is performed minute granulomas may be found on the surfaces of the liver.

In the early stage of this disease eye symptoms are not present, but after an apparently latent period ocular lesions present themselves in older children or in adolescents or later. A low-grade iridocyclitis with posterior synechiae formation may progress to chronic endophthalmitis, detachment of the retina or secondary glaucoma. A case has been reported in which the infestation presented as acute uveitis with hypopyon. An anterior retinal mass developed and the eye was enucleated as it was thought to be a retinoblastoma (Smith & Green 1971).

The retinal lesion presents as a solitary granuloma one disc-diameter in size at or near the macula. It is raised above the level of the retina and may mimic a retinoblastoma. When the acute phase has subsided, if the media are clear the lesion may be seen as a clear-cut circumscribed area of retinal degeneration. Many of the lesions formerly ascribed to tuberculosis or to one of the exanthemata are now known to be larval granulomata. If the lesion is central, central vision is reduced or lost and strabismus due to macular damage is the presenting symptom.

Diagnosis

No clinical investigation can give unequivocal affirmation. X-ray examination displays an absence of calcification which is present in some retinoblastomas. Eosinophilia of up to 12% is suggestive. An intradermal test with an antigen prepared from dead larvae and a *Toxocara* fluorescent test on the serum are aids to diagnosis. The number of larvae required to produce a serious pathological condition in the eye is less than is required to implicate the liver or respiratory tract. Hence antigenic stimulus may be too weak to yield detectable antibody. Liver biopsy may support a diagnosis.

Treatment

No drug is effective against the migrating larvae of *Toxocara*. Diethylcarbamazine 2 mg/kg body weight thrice daily may shorten the acute phase.

Prevention is the main line of defence, with a realization by parents and others of the potential danger to small children playing with animals known to be affected. Domestic animals with worm infection may be treated with piperazine phosphate but this drug is ineffective against larvae.

The dog may be 'man's best friend' but the puppy is not always a good friend to the children of man.

TOXOPLASMOSIS

The aetiology, description of the organism and an account of the general disease is given on page 148.

The eye may be involved in three ways: (*a*) by congenital infection; (*b*) by the reactivation of congenital lesions; and (*c*) by acquired infection.

Clinical manifestations

Anterior uveitis. Toxoplasmosis is an uncommon cause of pure anterior uveitis, but a severe and intractable form may accompany toxoplasmic choroidoretinitis. There is no pathognomonic feature in iridocyclitis from this cause.

Choroidoretinitis. The typical picture is an acute choroidoretinitis occurring in a male or female between 11 and 40 years of age. The lesion may present at the margin of an old scar of an earlier or congenital infection. In the acute stage a browny red swelling up to 6 disc diameters in size appears in the region of the macula, the disc and the larger vessels. The inflammation is focal and surrounding areas of the retina are normal. There may be a slight overlying haze in the vitreous. In the quiescent stage the lesion presents as a sharply demarcated area of choroidoretinal atrophy with masses of black pigment aggregated on the lip and in the floor of the crater. The nerve head may show some degree of pallor. The vitreous is clear.

Strabismus and lowered visual acuity occur when the macula is involved and a central scotoma can be demonstrated.

Diagnosis

The place of toxoplasmosis in the aetiology of intraocular infection is undoubted but its relative significance is in dispute. The descriptions of earlier studies resemble the older descriptions of ocular tuberculosis, and investigation has often failed to substantiate the clinical diagnosis.

The main points in diagnosis are: (*a*) a history of hunting and handling wild game; (*b*) occupations such as meat-handling and animal farming; and (*c*) the habit of eating raw meat.

The methylene blue dye test and the complement fixation test provide evidence. One author states that juxtapapillary choroidoretinitis is usually toxoplasmic (Perkins 1961).

Treatment

When the history and clinical appearance are suggestive of an acute phase of the disease the prognosis is said to be better if treatment is instituted before the results of laboratory tests are available.

Systemic corticosteroid therapy, combined with sulphadimidine and pyrimethamine, has been successful in controlling acute infections. The last-named drug must be given with caution as it may bring about a severe anaemia.

TROPICAL TYPHUS

Tsutsugamushi, Japanese river fever or scrub typhus is due to infection by *Rickettsia orientalis* of which the vector is a mite, for example *Leptotrombidium deliense*.

Ocular manifestations

In the initial stages, hyperaemia of the conjunctiva occurs, sometimes associated with haemorrhages. Bilateral uveitis frequently occurs, followed by a hazy vitreous, engorgement of the retinal vessels and swelling of the nerve-head.

The eye symptoms are often overlooked because of the severity of the general condition. Local treatment consists in energetic treatment of the iritis to prevent the formation of synechiae. General treatment is dealt with elsewhere.

Rocky Mountain spotted fever. When the typhus condition prevails, there is intense photophobia and headache and, if consciousness is retained, there may be a complaint of impaired vision.

TRYPANOSOMIASIS (AFRICAN)

Ocular manifestations

Urticarial swellings of the eyelids occur soon after infection. They often appear as baggy, fluid swellings overhanging the cheek-bone, and the preauricular gland may be enlarged.

Interstitial keratitis with neovascularization of the cornea occurs later and may be associated with iridocyclitis. In Africa and other places where onchocerciasis is found, the two infections may co-exist and the latter may be the cause of the corneal trouble. External ophthalmoplegia, ptosis, papilloedema and optic atrophy are later manifestations of involvement of the central nervous system.

Treatment

Keratitis and iridocyclitis call for mydriasis with atropine. Tryparsamide, when it is used in the general treatment of the disease where the central nervous system is involved, may cause optic neuritis and an irreversible optic atrophy. During the course of such treatment it is important to test the visual acuity and to make an ophthalmoscopic examination regularly and often.

Lowering of the visual acuity or pallor of the discs would call for immediate cessation of this line of treatment.

TRYPANOSOMIASIS (SOUTH AMERICAN), CHAGAS'S DISEASE

After an incubation period of two weeks, a primary lesion, the chagoma, develops in the skin and frequently on the eyelids. In endemic areas, oedema of the eyelids of one eye, known as Romaña's sign, is of diagnostic significance (Fig. 269). The conjunctiva may be the port of entry. Dacryocystitis is a further complication.

Intraocular manifestations have not been described.

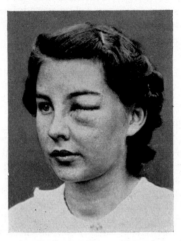

Fig. 269.—Unilateral palpebral oedema (Romaña's sign) in Chagas's disease. (*Dr S. B. Pessôa, Sâo Paulo*)

TULARAEMIA

In 1889, Parinaud described an infective conjunctivitis of animal origin, usually uniocular. Clinically, granules appear on the tarsal and bulbar conjunctiva and there is a muco-fibrinous discharge which never becomes purulent. Associated with the conjunctival involvement the pre-auricular and parotid glands become enlarged and tender. The cornea is not involved. The syndrome described by Parinaud is now recognized to be oculoglandular tularaemia. A somewhat similar condition occurs in ocular lymphogranuloma venereum, but in this condition keratitis, uveitis and optic neuritis may complicate the disease. The intradermal Frei test, positive in the latter disease, differentiates the aetiology of the two diseases.

YAWS, GANGOSA, GOUNDOU

Involvement of the eye has not been described in the primary stage. In the widely distributed lesions of the secondary stage the eyebrows and eyelids are often affected and ulcerated granulomas or soft papillomas occur on the skin of the eyelids. Granulomas are not found on the conjunctiva but there may be an associated catarrhal conjunctivitis in the secretion of which *Treponema pertenue* may be found. Interstitial keratitis and iritis have been recorded.

Gangosa is regarded as a sequel of yaws. In this condition a destructive ulcerative rhinopharyngitis may spread through the nose to involve the eyelids and lead to cicatricial ectropion with exposure and consequent ulceration of the cornea (Fig. 270).

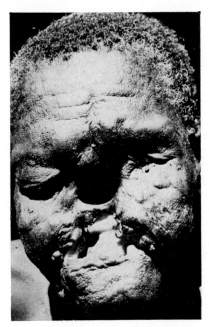

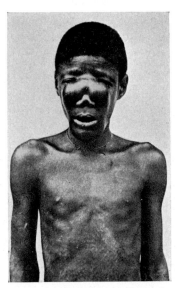

Fig. 270.—Extensive gangosa in a woman aged 40. Serum Kahn + + + +. (*Dr C. J. Hackett, by permission of the Wellcome Museum of Medical Science*)

Fig. 271.—Goundou obstructing vision, from the Ivory Coast. (*London School of Hygiene and Tropical Medicine*)

Goundou is a symmetrical hyperostosis beginning in the nasal processes of the superior maxillae. The paranasal swellings increase to the size of an orange or larger, encroach upon the orbits, interfere with the fields of vision, displace the globes and may in extreme cases press upon and destroy the eyes (Fig. 271).

YELLOW FEVER

In the early stages there is hyperaemia of the face and conjunctiva. The eyes are bright red, watery and brilliant and have been described as having a 'ferrety' look. The lids are swollen and photophobia is evident. Later the conjunctiva becomes icteric and effusions of blood appear.

Many patients complain of a frontal headache which is fixed, intense and persistent and which they attribute to the eyes.

REFERENCES

ATKINSON, R. L. (1965) *J. Nutr.*, **55,** 387.
BEDSON, S. P. (1952) *Irish J. med Sci.*, **332,** 385.
BISLEY, C. G. (1970) Personal communication.
BITOT, C. (1863) *Gaz. med. Paris*, **1,** 435.
BURKITT, D. (1962) *Ann. R. Coll. Surg. Edin.*, **30,** 211.
———(1966) *J. R. Coll. Surg. Edin.*, **11,** 170.
CHOYCE, D. P. (1964) *Trans. R. Soc. trop. Med. Hyg.*, **58,** 11.
CLIFFORD, P. P. (1966) *E. Afr. med. J.*, **7,** 43, 179.

COLLIER, L. H. & SONA, J. (1958) *Lancet*, **i**, 993.
DAVIES, J. (1965) *Antimicrob. Agents Chemother.*, **1945**, 1001.
EHLERS, H. (1969) Personal communication.
EIJKMAN, R. L. (1897) *Virchows Arch. Path. Anat. Physiol.*, **148**, 523.
GILKES, M. J. (1962) *Chem. ther. Rev.*, **4**, 176.
GILLESPIE, F. D. & COVELLI, B. (1963) *Am. J. Ophthal.*, **55**, 1263.
HALBERSTAEDTER, L. & VON PROWAZEK, S. (1907) *Dt. med. Wachr.*, **33**, 1285.
HANSMAN, D. (1969) *Med. J. Aust.*, **1**, 151.
HOWELLS, J. G. (1969) *Br. med. J.*, **ii**, 813.
HISSETTE, J. (1932) *Ann. Soc. belge Med. trop.*, **12**, 433.
HUBBENET, M. (1860) *Annls Oculist.*, **2**, 293.
JONES, D. W. E. (1963) *Br. J. Ophthal.*, **47**, 169.
KERNEY, W. F. (1967) *Clin. int. Ophthal.*, **7**.
KOBCHAI, P. (1962) *Am. J. trop. Med. Hyg.*, **11**, 759.
KRESKY, B. & NAUHEIM, J. (1967) *Am. J. Dis. Childh.*, **113**, 305.
LAMBDA, P. A., SHUKLA, K. N. & GANAPATHY, N. (1970) *Br. J. Ophthal.*, **54**, 565.
LINDNER, K. (1909) *Wien klin. Wschr.*, **22**, 1555.
LUMSDEN, W. H. R. (1909) *Sandoz J. med. Sci.*, **9**, 35.
McCOMB, D. E. & NICHOLS, R. L. (1969) *Am. J. Epidemiol.*, **90**, 278.
McGAVIC, J. S. (1949) *Archs Ophthal.*, **42**, 726.
McLAREN, D. S. (1963) *Malnutrition and the Eye*, p. 162, New York: Academic.
MAJČUK, J. F. (1966) *Bull. Wld. Hlth. Org.*, **35**, 262.
MARSHALL, C. L. (1968) *Archs envir. Hlth.*, **17**, 215.
MATHUR, S. P. (1969) *Br. J. Ophthal.*, **53**, 350.
MAYNARD, F. P. (1909) *Indian med. Gaz.*, **44**, 373.
MINISTRY OF HEALTH (1968) *Br. med. J.*, **iii**, 633.
OH, S. J. (1968) *Trop. geogr. Med.*, **20**, 13.
OLAVARRIA, R. & FAJARDO, L. F. (1971) *Archs Path.*, **92**, 191.
PERKINS, E. S. (1961) *Uveitis and Toxoplasmosis.* London: Churchill.
REID, A., McK. & JONES, D. E. W. (1963) *Br. J. Ophthal.*, **17**, 169.
RENDTORFF, R. C., DEWEESE, M. W. & MURRAH, W. (1962) *Am. J. trop. med. Hyg.*, **7**, 62.
ROKOS, L. (1969) *Ethiop. med. J.*, **7**, 11.
SCHLAEGEL, T. F. (1968) *Trans. Am. Acad. Ophthal. Otolar.*, **72**, 355.
SCOTT, J. G. & KERRICH, J. E. (1971) *Br. J. Ophthal.*, **55**, 189.
SMITH, P. H. & GREEN, C. H. (1971) *Br. J. Ophthal.*, **55**, 317.
SNELL, S. (1876) *Trans. Ophthal. Soc. U.K.*, **1**, 270.
SOMERSET, E. J. (1962) *Opthalmology in the Tropics.* London: Baillière, Tindall & Cassell.
SPARROW, C. H. (1966) *Cent. Afr. J. Med.*, **12**, 55.
STARK, G. G. (1966) *Archs Dis. Childh.*, **41**, 420.
STELLWAG, K. VON L. (1889) *Wien klin. Wschr.*, **31**, 614.
STOKER, M. (1970) *Br. med. J.*, **iii**, 536.
SULZER, D. E. (1890) *Arch. Ophthal. Paris*, **10**, 193.
T'ANG, C. H. (1957) *Chin. med. J.*, **75**, 445.
TARRIZZO, M. L. & NATAF, R. (1970) *Révue int. Trachome*, **46**, 7.
TEMPLETON, A. C. (1971) *Br. J. Ophthal.*, **55**, 254.
THOMSON, I. G. (1956) *J. trop. Med. Hyg.*, **59**, 155.
UYEMURA, M. (1928) *Klin. Mbt. Augenheik.*, **81**, 186.
VANCEA, P. & VANCEA, P. P. (1968) *Révue int. Trachome*, **45**, 155.
VETCH, J. (1807) *An Account of the Ophthalmia which has appeared in England since the Return of the British Army from Egypt.* London: Longman.
WISEMAN, R. S. & WOODRUFF, A. W. (1967) *Trans. R. Soc. trop. Med. Hyg.*, **61**, 827.

SECTION XVI

DRUGS

45. DRUGS

By P. H. REES, M.B., M.R.C.P., M.R.C.P.(Ed.), D.C.M.T.

Dosages

DOSAGES given are for the average 70 kg adult. Care should be taken to reduce the dose for children and small adults on a weight for weight basis. This is particularly so with the more toxic preparations, but is relatively unimportant with those drugs that are not absorbed (e.g. bephenium). It is rarely necessary and often unsafe (e.g. niridazole) to increase the dose for heavier individuals.

Some drugs are included for their historic interest, and if they are but little used now, their dosages are not given. Dosages of newer drugs are also omitted where regimens are not yet established. Drugs are classified as follows:

1. *Heavy metals*
   Antimony, trivalent and pentavalent
   Arsenic, trivalent and pentavalent
   Bismuth
   Heavy metal antagonists

2. *Plant derivatives and related drugs*
   Berberine sulphate
   Emetine, dehydroemetine and E.B.I.
   Glaucarubin
   Kousso
   Male fern
   Pelletierine tannate
   Quinine

3. *Dyes and dye derivatives*

   Aminoquinolines—chloroquine and primaquine
   Clofazimine (B663)
   Dithiazanine iodide
   Rosanilines
   Lucanthone
   Hycanthone

   Methylene blue
   Mepacrine
   Pyrvinium pamoate
   Stilbazium iodide
   Sulphobromphthalein sodium
   Suramin

4. *Folate inhibitors and related drugs*

   Sulphonamides
   Para-aminosalicylic acid (PAS)
   Sulphones

   Pyrimethamine
   Proguanil
   Trimethoprim

5. *Miscellaneous anti-protozoal compounds*

Clefamide	Metronidazole
Diloxanide furoate	Pentamidine
Diminazene aceturate	Hydroxystilbamidine isethionate
Iodinated quinolines	

6. *Miscellaneous anthelmintics*

Amphotalide	Hexylresorcinol
Bephenium hydroxynapthoate	Niclosamide
Bithionol	Niridazole
Dichlorophen	Tetramisole hydrochloride
Furapromidium	Thiabendazole

7. *Semicarbazones and related drugs*

Thiacetazone	Isoniazid
Methisazone	Nitrofurazone

8. *Chlorinated hydrocarbons*

Carbon tetrachloride	Tetrachloroethylene
Hexachloroparaxylene	

9. *Piperazine and related drugs*

Piperazine	Diethylcarbamazine

10. *Antibiotics and antifungal agents*

Amphotericin B	Nystatin
Chloramphenicol	Paromomycin
5-Fluorocytosine	Fumagillin
Griseofulvin	Puromycin
Neomycin	Penicillins
Gentamycin	Rifamycins
Kanamycin	Streptomycin
Novobiocin	Tetracyclines

11. *Topical applications including parasiticides and repellents*

Benzyl benzoate	Dimethyl phthalate
Chlorbutol	Gamma benzene hexachloride
Chrysarobin	5-Iododeoxyuridine
Crotamiton	Methoxsalen
Desitin	Metriphonate
Dicophane (DDT)	Pellidol
Dibutyl phthalate	Zinc undecenoate
Diethyl toluamide	

12. *Immunizing and related preparations*

Antivenoms, see page 804	Measles
Anthrax	Pertussis
BCG	Plague
Botulism	Poliomyelitis
Cholera	Rabies
Diphtheria	Smallpox
Gas gangrene	Tetanus
Hepatitis	Typhoid
Influenza	Typhus
Leptospira	Yellow fever

1. HEAVY METALS

ANTIMONY

Organic compounds of trivalent antimony are more toxic to both host and parasite than pentavalent compounds. Trivalent compounds are used for the treatment of schistosomiasis, whereas pentavalent compounds are used for leishmaniasis.

Trivalent antimony

Several compounds are available. In general, toxicity and efficacy are related to the total weight of antimony given. *S. haematobium* is the most susceptible to treatment, and *S. mansoni* and *S. japonicum* progressively less so. Phosphofructokinase, an enzyme essential to schistosome glycolysis, is inhibited by antimony compounds. There is a hepatic shift of the adult worms and the production of eggs is disturbed.

Trivalent antimonials have also been used in trypanosomiasis, leishmaniasis, filariasis, lymphogranuloma venereum, granuloma inguinale, mycosis fungoides and lepra reactions. Oral preparations have been used as emetics and as reflex expectorants.

Antimony is excreted slowly, mainly in the urine.

Toxicity. The important toxic effects are on the heart and liver. Sudden death may occur at any stage in treatment.

Immediate symptoms of toxicity include cough, chest pain, pain in the arms, vomiting, abdominal colic, faintness and collapse which may be fatal but may be reversed by an injection of 1/1000 adrenaline. Those preparations that are given intravenously should be given slowly through a fine needle. Local leakage may cause great pain because of tissue damage. An anaphylactoid reaction may occur after the sixth or seventh intravenous injection, with an urticarial rash, husky voice and collapse. Delayed reactions may occur during the course of treatment or later and include a multiplicity of symptoms, such as nausea, vomiting, anorexia, diarrhoea, pains in muscles and joints, arthritis, pneumonia, headache, fatigue, pruritus, back pain, excessive salivation, dizziness, a metallic taste in the mouth, skin rashes, constipation, fever, herpetic lesions and conjunctival injection. ECG changes with prolonged QT interval, and ST segment and T-wave changes are almost invariable, reverting to normal within about 6 weeks, but a fall in blood pressure or bradycardia necessitates discontinuation of treatment. Cardiovascular collapse or fatal arrhythmia may occur at any time. Haemolytic anaemia, sulphaemoglobinuria, retrobulbar neuritis and encephalopathy have been reported with some preparations. A rise in liver enzymes is common. Liver damage with hepatic failure and death is especially likely to occur in those with pre-existing liver disease.

Contra-indications. Liver, heart, renal and lung disease.

Route. Slow intravenous injection is required for most preparations but some (TWSb and stibophen) are given intramuscularly. Oral administration for schistosomiasis is not satisfactory because of the local emetic action and uncertain absorption.

Dose. The number of injections and the length of the course varies with preparations. In general a total dose of 0·5 gramme of trivalent antimony is given.

Preparations of trivalent antimony. *Antimony lithium thiomalate* (*Anthiolimine, Anthiomaline*). Available as a 6% solution for intramuscular injection, equivalent to 10 mg of antimony/ml. Given over a period of 30 day on alternate days to a total of 40–60 ml.

Antimony potassium tartrate (tartar emetic, potassium antimonyl tartrate). The sodium salt of antimony tartrate is usually preferred, thus avoiding the intravenous administration of potassium ions.

Antimony sodium tartrate (sodium antimonyl tartrate) contains 38% of trivalent antimony, and is given as a 2% solution by slow intravenous injection. An initial dose of 30 mg is increased on alternate days to a maximum dose of 150 mg and continued until a total of 2 grammes has been given.

Sodium antimony tartrate   TWSb/6 (antimony sodium dimercaptosuccinate)

Antimony sodium thioglycollate.

Sodium antimonyl gluconate (Triostam) contains approximately 36% of trivalent antimony. 190 mg are given intravenously daily for 6 days.

Stibocaptate (Astiban, antimony dimercaptosuccinate, Friedheim's TWSb) a combination form of trivalent antimony and a dimercaprol derivative analogous to melarsoprol (Mel B), it contains 25–26% of trivalent antimony. 500 mg are given on alternate days, twice weekly or weekly by intramuscular injection to a total of 2·5 grammes.

Stibophen (Fouadin, Fantorin, Neoantimosan, Repodral) contains approximately 16% of trivalent antimony. A 6·3% solution contains 8·5 mg of trivalent antimony/ml. Given intramuscularly, an initial dose of 2 ml is increased to a maximum of 5 ml and continued to a total course of 40–80 ml over a period of 2–4 weeks.

Pentavalent antimony

This is used in the treatment of visceral, cutaneous, and mucocutaneous leishmaniasis, and has been used in schistosomiasis. Toxic effects are similar to but less frequent and less severe than with trivalent antimony.

Preparations

Ethyl stibamine (Neostibosan)

Sodium stibogluconate (Sodium antimony gluconate, Pentostam) contains 30–34% of pentavalent antimony. There are solutions of differing strengths. A solution containing 10% pentavalent antimony is given intramuscularly or intravenously. The adult dose is 6 ml daily (2 grammes sodium antimony gluconate, 600 mg antimony). For children aged 8–14 the dose is 4 ml, and 2 ml for children under 5. A full course for most forms of leishmaniasis is 30 daily injections, totalling 18 grammes of antimony. The course may be repeated after 1 or 2 weeks.

Ethyl stibamine (Neostibosan, Neostam) is given intravenously. The dose is 100 mg on the first day, 200 mg the second and 300 mg on the third day and daily thereafter for 8 injections.

Urea stibamine (Stiburea) is a compound of urea with stibamine and should not be exposed to the air. The dose is 100-200 mg intravenously on alternate days for about 1 month for adults. Total dosage for adults is 3 grammes and for infants 650 mg.

Meglumine antimoniate (Glucantime) is given intramuscularly. The dose is 60-100 mg/kg daily in a course of 12-15 injections, which may be repeated after 15 days.

$$CH_2OH \qquad\qquad CH_2OH$$
$$| \qquad\qquad\qquad |$$
$$CHOH \qquad\qquad CHOH$$
$$| \qquad\qquad\qquad |$$
$$CHO \diagdown \quad OH \qquad ONa \diagup CHO$$
$$| \qquad \diagdown | \qquad | \diagup \qquad |$$
$$CHO-Sb-O-Sb-CHO$$
$$| \qquad \diagup \qquad\qquad \diagdown \qquad |$$
$$CHO \diagup \qquad\qquad\qquad \diagdown CHO$$
$$| \qquad\qquad\qquad\qquad |$$
$$COO.Na \qquad\qquad COO.Na$$

Sodium stibogluconate

ARSENIC

Trivalent arsenicals are more potent and more toxic than pentavalent arsenicals. Pentavalent arsenic owes its activity to its conversion to trivalent arsenic *in vivo*, and its relative non-toxicity to its ability to penetrate parasite cells more readily than host cells.

The main use of arsenicals is in the treatment of African trypanosomiasis. Sulphydryl enzyme systems of the trypanosomes are blocked. Arsenicals have also been used in spirochaetal infections (syphilis, yaws, relapsing fever, ratbite fever, Vincent's angina), anthrax, protozoal diseases (malaria, amoebiasis, trichomoniasis) and in helminthic infections (pulmonary tropical eosinophilia, filariasis (effective against adult worms—macrofilaricidal), schistosomiasis and threadworm infection).

Toxicity

In general the more toxic preparations have been discarded, and arsenicals themselves have been displaced as elective therapy in situations where less toxic drugs are available.

Immediate reactions include anaphylactoid arsenical shock, especially with tryparsamide. The face is flushed, with oedema of the tongue and eyelids, a burning taste in the mouth, nausea, vomiting, dyspnoea, cyanosis, precordial distress, sweating and coma. Herxheimer reactions may occur with fever and exacerbation of symptoms secondary to the effect on the trypanosomes.

Delayed toxicity includes rashes (particularly exfoliative dermatitis), nephritis, acute yellow atrophy of the liver, blood dyscrasias, peripheral neuritis, optic neuritis and encephalopathy.

Sudden death may occur at any stage of treatment. The dose varies with the preparation, but small initial dosages should be used especially in debilitated patients. Arsenic is excreted slowly in the urine and faeces. It persists in certain tissues for long periods and may remain in a hair throughout its life.

Preparations

Trivalent arsenic. *Arsphenamine.* Ehrlich's original 'therapia magna sterilisans' for relapsing fever. Replaced by less toxic neoarsphenamine.

Melarsen oxide. Replaced by less toxic melarsoprol.

Melarsonyl potassium (Mel W). Similar to melarsoprol, though water-soluble, and so can be given intramuscularly, but probably more toxic and less effective. It is a macrofilaricidal drug, but is too toxic for general use in filariasis.

Melarsoprol (Mel B). A combination of melarsen oxide and dimercaprol (BAL). It is effective in Rhodesian and Gambian trypanosomiasis, on blood forms as well as those in the nervous system, and on trypanosomes resistant

Mel B (melarsoprol)

to other arsenicals. It is given by slow intravenous injection as a 3·6% solution in propylene glycol to a maximum daily dose of 5 ml (180 mg) and to a total dose of 30–40 ml over a period of 3 weeks.

Neoarsphenamine (NAB). Still sometimes used for pulmonary tropical eosinophilia. It is given intravenously in doses of 150–600 mg weekly for 8–10 weeks.

Sulpharsphenamine. Less effective than neoarsphenamine; the dose is 100–600 mg subcutaneously or intramuscularly.

Pentavalent arsenic. *Tryparsamide (Tryparsone, Novatoxyl).* Effective in African trypanosomiasis with central nervous system involvement. A drug effective on blood parasites (e.g. suramin) should be given concurrently. A freshly prepared 20% solution of tryparsamide is given in an initial dose of 1 gramme, followed weekly by 9–10 doses of 2 grammes.

Tryparsamide

Carbarsone introduced by Ehrlich has been used for non-invasive amoebiasis— now superseded.

BISMUTH

Intramuscular injections of bismuth salts played an important part in the control of yaws in the pre-antibiotic era of this century. Combined with arsenic, the oral preparation of bismuth glycollylarsanilate (glycobiarsol, Milibis) has been used in the treatment of amoebiasis.

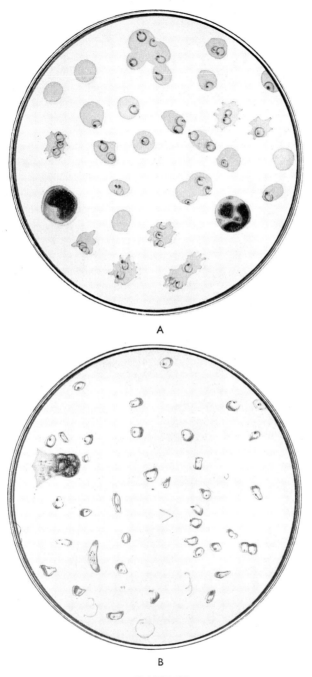

A

B

PLATE IX

The blood picture of subtertian malaria.

A, Blood film from a fatal case of subtertian malaria, showing heavy 'ring' infection. Giemsa. B, Thick blood film preparation of subtertian rings and crescent to show appearances after dehaemoglobinization. × 1000. Leishman. (*From a preparation by Dr H. Seidelin*)

[*To face p. 896.

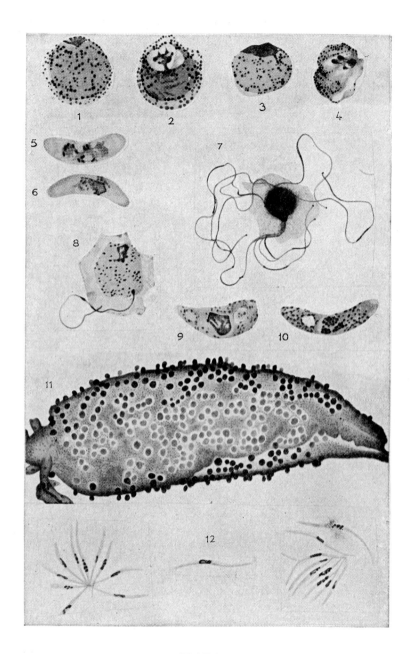

PLATE X

Malaria parasites.

1, *P. vivax* macrogametocyte. 2, *P. vivax* microgametocyte. 3, *P. malariae* macrogameto-cyte. 4, *P. malariae* microgametocyte. 5, *P. falciparum* microgametocyte. 6, *P. falciparum* macrogametocyte. 7, *P. vivax* exflagellating microgametocyte. 8, *P. vivax* fertilization of macrogametocyte. 9, 10, *P. vivax* oökinetes. 11, *P. vivax*. Midgut of an *Anopheles* showing mature oöcysts. 12, *P. vivax* sporozoites. All parasites stained with leishman and the midgut with Weigert's haematoxylin. (*From an original painting by B. Jobling; reproduced by kind permission of the authors and publishers from Shute & Maryon 1966*)

HEAVY METAL ANTAGONISTS

Dimercaprol (BAL). Used in the treatment of poisoning with organic antimonials and arsenicals.

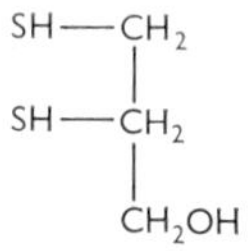

$$SH\!-\!CH_2$$
$$SH\!-\!CH_2$$
$$CH_2OH$$

Dimercaprol (B.A.L.)

Side-effects are common but the drug is not cumulative. A course of intramuscular injections is given at intervals of not less than 4 hours. The dose
ranges from 1 to 3 mg/kg repeated every 6 hours for 3 days, and thereafter
twice daily until recovery.

Sodium calcium edetate is given intravenously in lead poisoning.

D-*Penicillamine hydrochloride* is administered orally in Wilson's disease, lead
poisoning and haemosiderosis.

Desferrioxamine mesylate is given orally or by injection for acute or chronic
iron intoxication.

2. PLANT DERIVATIVES AND RELATED DRUGS

BERBERINE SULPHATE

An alkaloid present in various species of *Berberis* and other plants. Used
orally as a bitter, and by local injection for oriental sore (cutaneous leishmaniasis).

EMETINE

An alkaloid present in the roots of the South American plant *Cephaelis
ipecacuanha*. The crude preparation (ipecacuanha, Brasil root) was introduced
into Europe in the seventeenth century for the treatment of dysentery, though

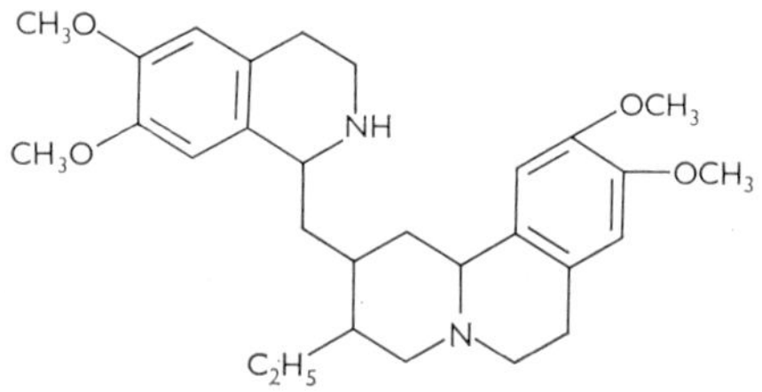

Emetine

the specific action of emetine against *Entamoeba histolytica* was not appreciated
until 1912. It has a direct amoebicidal action and parenteral emetine affords
rapid symptomatic and clinical improvement in amoebic involvement of the
liver, amoebic dysentery, amoeboma, and other forms of invasive amoebiasis.

When given by injection it does not affect *E. histolytica* in the intestinal lumen. However, the oral preparation, emetine and bismuth iodide, is a most effective luminal amoebicide. Emetine injected locally relieves the pain of scorpion stings. It has been used for its emetic and expectorant properties, and has an antibacterial action which has been utilized in the treatment of septic conditions.

Toxicity

Emetine is a protoplasmic poison. Damage to the heart is the most important side-effect. Full dosage of emetine almost invariably produces changes in the electrocardiogram. Flattening or inversion of T-waves and a prolonged QT interval are the main features. Reversion to normal may take several weeks. Tachycardia, which may be marked on the least exertion, hypotension, arrhythmias and precordial pain resembling a coronary thrombosis may occur. In deaths from emetine a degenerative myocarditis may be found. Weakness with muscle pain indicates myositis, and both this and cardiac toxicity are aggravated by the hypokalaemia that may complicate invasive amoebiasis. Nerve involvement with motor and sensory loss is probably very rare. Pain due to local necrosis may occur at the site of injection. Other side-effects include nausea, vomiting, diarrhoea, depression, liver and renal damage and striation of the nails. Therefore emetine should only be given to patients on full bed-rest under constant supervision. Should signs of toxicity occur, especially in the cardiovascular system, treatment must be discontinued. The synthetic preparation dehydroemetine is weight for weight probably less toxic. The oral preparation EBI is less toxic, but as some of the emetine is absorbed it is dangerous if given during or immediately after parenteral emetine. Emetine is slowly excreted, mainly by the kidneys, over a period of weeks, so that there is a risk of cumulative toxicity.

Contra-indications

Heart, liver and renal disease and pregnancy. Care should be taken to reduce the dose on a weight for weight basis in children and in adults who are debilitated and have lost weight.

Route

Emetine is given subcutaneously or intramuscularly but never intravenously.

Dosage

A maximum daily dose of 60 mg is given. In amoebic dysentery 3 daily injections may suffice, but in other forms of invasive amoebiasis the injections should be continued for a maximum of 10 days.

Preparations

Emetine hydrochloride injection. A sterile solution in water containing 60 mg/ml is the usual preparation but different concentrations are available.

Dehydroemetine hydrochloride is more rapidly excreted than emetine. Indications and cautions for use are similar to those of emetine. It has also been used in the treatment of schistosomiasis and cutaneous leishmaniasis.

The injection is available in 2 ml ampoules (Mebadin) containing 30 mg/ml. There are tablets of dehydroemetine resinate containing 20 mg of the base, and of dehydroemetine and bismuth iodide.

Emetine and bismuth iodide tablets. Tablets of 60 mg.

Dehydroemetine

GLAUCARUBIN

A preparation from the South American plant *Simaruba glauca*. Formerly used in the treatment of intestinal amoebiasis.

KOUSSO

Prepared from the flowers of *Brayera anthelmintica*. It has been used for the expulsion of tape worms, particularly *Taenia saginata*. It has structural similarities to filicin, the active principle of male fern.

MALE FERN

Prepared from the rhizome, frond bases and apical bud of *Dryopteris filix-mas*. It is effective in the expulsion of tape worms, its action probably depending on the paralysis of smooth muscle by filicin. The paralysed worm is unable to maintain its position against peristalsis.

Toxic effects

Rare in therapeutic dosage, but absorption and subsequent toxicity is increased by the presence of fat in the intestine. Nausea, vomiting, diarrhoea and headache may occur. Rarely neurological lesions with visual disturbances, permanent blindness, coma and convulsions, hyperbilirubinaemia, and respiratory, cardiac and renal failure may occur.

Administration

Preliminary starvation and purgation for 1 or preferably 2 days is necessary. The drug (3–8 ml of male fern extract) is best given as a draught or an emulsion with suitable flavouring. A purgative follows (magnesium sulphate), which will not only result in the rapid expulsion of the worm, but will also expel the drug and minimize the risk of absorption of filicin and subsequent development of side-effects. A search is made for the head so that a cure can be confirmed.

Preparations

Male fern extracts (aspidium oleoresin, filix mas), a thick greenish brown liquid containing 21–23% of filicin.

Male fern extract capsules of 1 ml.

Male fern extract draught. 3·6 grammes of male fern extract in 45 ml of water with acacia.

PELLETIERINE TANNATE

Prepared from the bark of *Punica granatum*. Previously used in the expulsion of tapeworms.

QUININE

An alkaloid prepared from the bark of various species of cinchona tree. It was introduced to Europe from South America in 1633. There are many other alkaloids in cinchona bark, one of which is quinidine, the D-isomer of quinine. The main use of quinine at present is in the treatment of *P. falciparum* infections resistant to 4-aminoquinolines. Quinine has been widely used as a prophylactic and for the treatment of acute attacks of all forms of malaria. It is a schizontocide, acting on early ring forms (trophozoites) with a rapid therapeutic response.

$$CH(OH)—CH—\ N\ —CH_2$$
$$CH_3O.$$
$$CH_2$$
$$CH_2$$
$$CH_2—CH—CH\ CH::CH_2$$

Quinine

The growth of the trophozoites is arrested, the cytoplasm may become clumped with loss of the vacuole, and there may be disintegration of the nuclear chromatin. Such changes may be observed within hours of administering the drug. Damaged parasites may persist in the peripheral blood for 24–48 hours. Quinine is also gametocytocidal in the benign malarias. Its precise mode of action is uncertain but it may interfere with lysosome function or with nucleic acid synthesis.

Quinine is also used as a bitter. It is an analgesic and an antipyretic, and has a quinidine-like action on the heart. It increases the refractory period of skeletal muscle and depresses the excitability of the motor end-plate and thus is useful in the management of myotonia.

Toxicity

This is related to dose, 8 grammes usually being fatal, but some individuals show intolerance, so that side-effects may occur at very low dosage. The combination of tinnitus, headache, nausea and visual disturbances is known as cinchonism and may also occur with salicylates and cincophen. It is irritant, so that gastric discomfort may follow oral administration, sterile abscesses intramuscular injection and venous thrombosis intravenous injection. Peripheral vasodilatation occurs and may be useful in the treatment of night cramps. Unwanted cardiovascular effects include a fall in blood pressure and ventricular arrhythmias. It has an oxytocic action. However, the effect is not marked until late in pregnancy, so that it is a poor abortifacient in early pregnancy. Toxic effects on the fetus include blindness and deafness. In subjects with a glucose-6-phosphate dehydrogenase deficiency a haemolytic episode may be provoked. Hypersensitivity reactions may occur. Quinine bound to platelets may be antigenic, and the subsequent production of platelet antibodies may lead to thrombocytopenia. Similarly, massive haemolysis may occur, especially in *P. falciparum* infections (blackwater fever) and in pregnancy. Agranulocytosis, anaphylactic shock, rashes and fever are further hypersensitivity reactions.

Administration

The oral route is satisfactory as it is rapidly absorbed. Excretion is rapid, mainly in the urine, so that frequent dosage is required. In comatose or vomiting patients it may be given intravenously.

Dosage

In *P. falciparum* infections resistant to chloroquine, 600 mg every 8 hours for 14 days.

Preparations

Quinine bisulphate. Tablets of 300 mg.
Quinine dihydrochloride. Injection, usual strength, 300 mg/ml which must be diluted at least 10 times in water for injection, and given by very slow intravenous injection.
Quinine hydrochloride. Tablets of 300 mg.
Quinine sulphate. Tablets of 300 mg.

3. DYES AND DYE DERIVATIVES

Some dye derivatives with particular actions, such as the sulphonamides (anti-folate), will be described in other sections.

AMINOQUINOLINES

Chloroquine

A 4-aminoquinoline, chloroquine, has the quinoline nucleus in common with quinine and the side chain in common with mepacrine. Developed in the 1930s, as a result of the intensive investigation into dyes and dye derivatives, it was not widely available until after the Second World War.

Quinoline

Choroquine

Its main use is in malaria. It is a schizontocide, acting on the early ring forms. Growth is arrested, the cytoplasm becomes ragged, and pigment granules are clumped. Damaged parasites may sometimes persist in the peripheral blood for 48 hours or more. Gametocytes may also be damaged but may remain viable. The precise action is unknown, but it may be due to lysosome damage or to interference with nucleic acid synthesis.

Chloroquine effects a radical cure in *P. falciparum* infections, but is only suppressive in the benign malarias (*P. vivax*, *P. ovale* and *P. malariae*). Some strains of *P. falciparum* (Far East, especially Vietnam, and South America, especially Brazil) are resistant to chloroquine. Cross-resistance occurs with mepacrine and amodiaquine.

Chloroquine is also used in hepatic amoebiasis, in lung and liver fluke infections, and in taeniasis and giardiasis. It has an anti-inflammatory action that has been used in lepra reactions, collagen diseases, sarcoidosis, urticaria and light-sensitive eruptions.

Toxicity. In malarial dosage side-effects are few, though deaths in children from cardiorespiratory collapse have been recorded after a few tablets (0·075–2 grammes) and from intravenous administration.

In adults headache, visual disturbances, nausea, vomiting and pruritus may occur, especially if chloroquine is used for long-term prophylaxis. In the large dosages that are used for its anti-inflammatory effect, side-effects are more frequent. Difficulty in accommodation, diplopia, bleaching of the hair, changes in the electrocardiogram (T-wave depression), skin rashes and weight loss occur.

Chloroquine is particularly deposited in melanin-containing tissues, and persists for many months. A retinopathy with a mottled appearance around the macula may be followed by pigmentary clumping with visual defects which may be permanent. Chloroquine is also deposited in the iris and in the cornea, in the latter causing opacities which usually resolve on cessation of treatment. A myopathy may occur which usually is proximal. Psychotic behaviour, agranulocytosis, thrombocytopenia and a blue-black pigmentation of the palatal mucosa and of the subungual tissues may occur.

Dosage. Chloroquine is rapidly absorbed, so that parenteral administration is unnecessary unless the patient is vomiting or comatose. Tissues, especially the liver, spleen, kidneys and eyes, are avid for the drug so that a loading dose is required. It is partially metabolized and excreted over a period of weeks or months in the urine.

Dosage. Various salts of chloroquine, the products of acids with the base chloroquine, are available so that the dosage is described in terms of the weight of chloroquine base rather than of the chloroquine salt.

Malaria. For treatment of acute attack 600 mg of the base at once, followed by 300 mg 6 hours later and 300 mg daily for 2 days or more. Suppressive 300 mg weekly.

Cerebral malaria. Children: Intramuscular injection in a dose of 5 mg of the base/kg repeated in 6 hours if necessary to a total of 25 mg/kg in 4 days. *For a warning on toxicity see page 74.* Adults: 200 mg of the base well diluted by very slow intravenous injection, or 200 mg intramuscularly, to a maximum of 900 mg in 24 hours.

Preparations. *Chloroquine phosphate.* Injection, usual strength 40 mg of chloroquine base/ml.

Chloroquine phosphate. Tablets (Aralen, Avloclor, Resochin) of 250 mg containing approximately 150 mg of chloroquine base.

Chloroquine sulphate. Injection, usual strength 40 mg of chloroquine base/ml.

Chloroquine sulphate. Tablets (Nivaquine) containing approximately 150 mg of chloroquine base.

Other 4-aminoquinolines. Uses and toxic effects similar to chloroquine.

Amodiaquine hydrochloride (Camoquin)
Amopyroquine hydrochloride (Propoquin)
Hydroxychloroquine sulphate (Plaquenil)

Primaquine

The least toxic of many 8-aminoquinolines. It is used for the radical cure of benign malarias (*P. vivax, P. ovale, P. malariae*) as it is effective against the exo-erythrocytic cycle of these parasites. It also has a weak schizontocidal action, a marked gametocytocidal action and some action against the pre-erythrocytic cycle of all species. It is rapidly absorbed.

Primaquine

Toxicity. In the recommended dosage side-effects are unusual, but with higher dosage side-effects become increasingly severe. Abdominal pain, methaemoglobinaemia and haemolytic anaemia occur. In patients with a deficiency of the enzyme glucose-6-phosphate dehydrogenase, a haemolytic crisis may be precipitated.

Dosage. In the radical cure of benign malarias 7·5 mg of the base twice daily for 14 days. It is too weak a schizontocide for treating the acute attack, which should be controlled by the concurrent or previous administration of a powerful schizontocide such as a 4-aminoquinoline.

Preparations. *Primaquine phosphate.* Tablets containing 7·5 mg of primaquine base. American tablets may contain 15 mg of primaquine base.

Other 8-aminoquinolines. Pamaquin (Plasmoquine), Pentaquin, Quinocide.

CLOFAZIMINE (B663)

An orange-red dye which has been used in the treatment of acid-fast infections. More useful in leprosy than in tuberculosis, it is one of the few drugs that appear to have some effect in Buruli ulcer (*Mycobacterium ulcerans*). It also has some anti-inflammatory action.

Dose

100–400 mg daily (but see Leprosy, page 440).

Preparation

B663 (*Lamprene*). Capsules of 100 mg.

DITHIAZANINE IODIDE (TELMID)

A blue cyanine dye formerly used in the treatment of strongyloidiasis. Administered orally, the drug is little absorbed by the healthy intestine. The stools are stained blue. However, the drug may be absorbed, particularly in severe strongyloidiasis. Side-effects are then common and fatalities have occurred, post mortem revealing generalized blue discoloration of the viscera. The drug has been withdrawn.

ROSANILINES

Gentian violet (methylrosaniline chloride). A violet dye that has a bactericidal and an anthelmintic action. It has been used in strongyloidiasis and threadworm infections.

Pararosaniline and rosaniline hydrochlorides. Bactericidal and fungicidal, the main constituents of Castellani's paint.

Pararosaniline pamoate and its active fraction, tris (p-aminophenyl) carbonium pamoate, are under trial for the mass treatment of schistosomiasis, particularly *S. japonicum* infection.

LUCANTHONE

A yellow dye. An oral schistosomicide, but side-effects, particularly vomiting, have limited its use. The skin is stained yellow.

Lucanthone

Dose

0·5–1·0 gramme twice daily for 3 days.

Preparation

Lucanthone tablets (Nilodin). Tablets containing 250 mg of lucanthone hydrochloride. Miracil D and American preparations contain 200 mg of the hydrochloride.

HYCANTHONE

A derivative of lucanthone. Initial trials suggest that the drug is more effective than lucanthone in schistosomiasis. It may be especially useful in *S. mansoni* infections. Nausea, vomiting and anorexia are common and appear to be related to dosage. Transient elevation of liver enzymes may occur and deaths have resulted from acute liver failure. Induration may occur at the injection site, and the urine may be stained yellow. It is contra-indicated in active liver disease, pregnancy, and any severe coexisting illness.

Dose (see page 314)

3 mg/kg by single intramuscular injection to a maximum of 200 mg. An alternative is 1·5 mg/kg to a maximum of 100 mg on 2 occasions 7 days apart.

Hycanthone

Preparation

Hycanthone methanesulphonate (*Etrenol*). Ampoules containing 200 mg of the base. Water for injection, 2 ml, is added immediately prior to the injection. Tablets are also available.

METHYLENE BLUE

This blue dye was shown to have some antimalarial activity by Ehrlich and Gutman in 1891. The extensive research into the chemotherapeutic properties of dyes and dye derivatives stems from this finding.

Methylene blue

MEPACRINE (ATEBRIN)

A yellow dye introduced for malaria therapy in the 1930s. Of great importance in the Second World War, it is now largely superseded. The side-chain is identical with that of chloroquine.

Mepacrine

Acridine

Its action in malaria is similar to that of chloroquine and quinine. It is also used in tapeworm infections and giardiasis, and has anti-inflammatory properties similar to those of chloroquine.

Toxicity

The skin and urine are stained yellow. Dizziness, headache, nausea, vomiting and mental changes may occur. Skin rashes occur and deaths have been reported from exfoliative dermatitis and also from hepatitis. Toxicity is increased if an 8-aminoquinoline is administered concurrently.

Dosage

Malaria. Suppresive, 100 mg daily. Curative, 900 mg on the first day, 600 mg on the second day and 300 mg daily for 5 days, in divided doses.
Tapeworm. 1 gramme by duodenal tube.
Giardiasis. 100 mg thrice daily for 1 week.

Preparation

Mepacrine hydrochloride (Quinacrine). 100 mg tablets.

PYRVINIUM PAMOATE

A bright red dye used in the treatment of threadworm infections. The stools are stained bright red. Toxic effects include nausea, vomiting and diarrhoea, and it should be used with caution in the presence of renal or hepatic disease.

Dose

5 mg of pyrvinium base/kg body weight as a single dose.

Preparations

Pyrvinium pamoate. Tablets containing 50 mg of pyrvinium base.
Pyrvinium pamoate oral suspension (Viprynium mixture, Vanquin) containing 1% of pyrvinium base.

STILBAZIUM IODIDE

Stilbazium iodide (monopar), a red dye, is said to be one of the few drugs effective in trichuriasis, also effective in ascariasis and enterobiasis. Not generally available.

SULPHOBROMPHTHALEIN SODIUM (BROMSULPHALEIN SODIUM)

A dye used in the assessment of liver function. After intravenous injection it is rapidly excreted in the bile by the healthy liver. 45 minutes after injection (5 mg/kg) the blood should contain less than 7% of the injection.

SURAMIN (BAYER 205; MORANYL)

A derivative of the trypan dyes, introduced in the 1920s for the treatment of African trypanosomiasis. It is also used in the treatment of onchocerciasis. Its mode of action in trypanosomiasis is unknown. It does not reach the cerebrospinal fluid so is of no value when the central nervous system is involved, though a single injection may usefully precede a course of Mel B in such cases. In onchocerciasis suramin's main action is on the adult worms (macrofilaricidal).

Toxicity

Immediate reactions include nausea and anaphylactic shock; 24 hours later photophobia and peripheral neuritis may occur. Albuminuria is a common late effect. Agranulocytosis and haemolytic anaemia are rare. The drug should be given under close medical supervision. If albuminuria is marked or casts appear, it should be stopped.

Route and dosage

It is given by slow intravenous injection. Only freshly prepared solutions should be used. The initial dose in trypanosomiasis is 0·5–1·0 gramme. There-after it is given weekly to a total dose of 7·0 grammes.

Preparation

Suramin injection (Antrypol). A sterile powder to be dissolved in water for injection immediately before use.

4. FOLATE INHIBITORS AND RELATED DRUGS

Differences in folate metabolism in man, protozoa and bacteria have led to the development of antiprotozoal and antibacterial antifolate drugs with limited human toxicity. The drugs act mainly by substrate inhibition, having structural similarities either to para-aminobenzoic acid (PABA) or to folic acid.

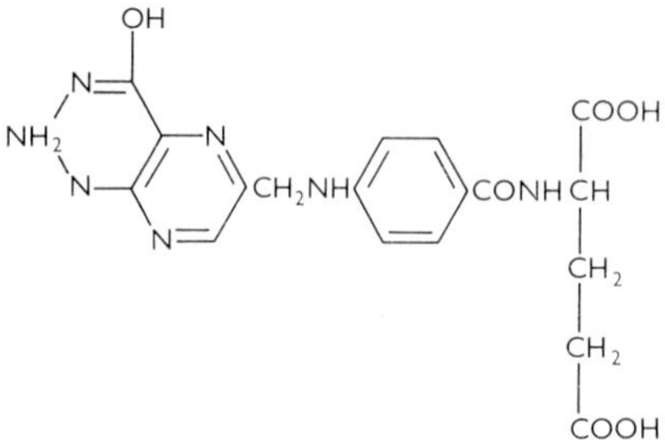

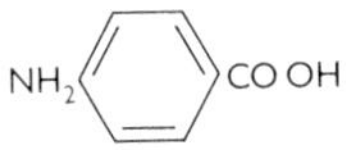

PABA (Para-aminobenzoic acid)

Folic acid

Pteridine + PABA

Block 1

Folic acid

Dihydrofolic acid

Dihydrofolate reductase → ← Block 2

Tetrahydrofolic acid

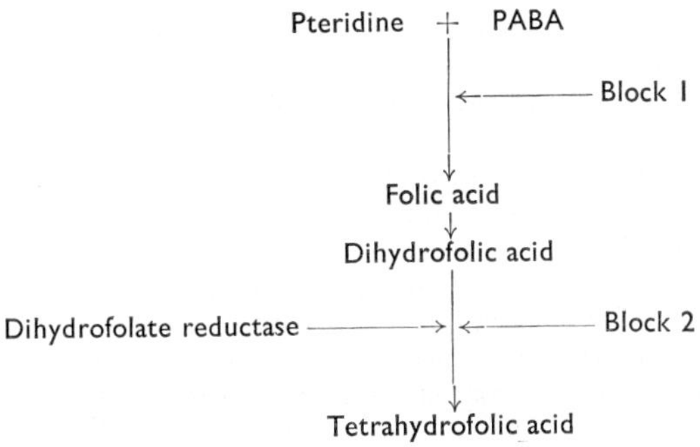

Block 1 is unimportant to human cells for they are permeable to preformed folic acid. Drugs acting at this point include sulphonamides, and probably also sulphones and para-aminosalicylic acid (see page 909).

Block 2. Dihydrofolate reductases vary from order to order so that a drug may have a more marked effect in bacteria or protozoa than in man. Drugs acting at this point include pyrimethamine and proguanil (mainly protozoa especially plasmodium species), trimethoprim (bacteria and protozoa) and methotrexate (man).

SULPHONAMIDES

Domagk (1935) demonstrated the chemotherapeutic value of these drugs, which were developed from the azo dyes. Their mode of action is to block the synthesis of folic acid. They are bacteriostatic, but may be bactericidal when used in combination with dihydrofolate reductase inhibitors, and in such combinations have an antiprotozoal effect which has been used in malaria and toxoplasmosis. It has recently been suggested that high blood levels of sulphonamides may have a lethal effect on feeding mosquitoes.

$$NH_2 \diagdown\diagup SO_2NH\,(R)$$

Sulphonamides

Toxic effects

In general, the slowly excreted protein-bound sulphonamides are more likely to cause severe toxic effects. The poorly soluble sulphonamides have been largely superseded because of the risk of crystalluria and renal damage. General side-effects include nausea, vomiting, anorexia, fever, meth- and sulphaemo-globinaemia, goitre, hypothyroidism, vertigo, tinnitus and ataxia. Skin rashes, of which the Stevens–Johnson syndrome, a severe form of erythema multiforme, is the most dangerous, acute haemolytic anaemia, agranulocytosis, thrombocytopenia and hepatitis may also occur.

Preparations

Group 1. Well absorbed, relatively soluble, rapidly excreted—the drugs of choice for routine use.

Sulphadimidine. Tablets of 0·5 gramme; 0·5–1·5 gramme 6 hourly. Injection 1 gramme in 3 ml intramuscularly or intravenously.

Sulphadiazine. Tablets of 0·5 gramme; may be more effective than sulphadimidine in meningococcal meningitis.

Sulphasalazine (Salazopyrin). A compound of salicylic acid and sulphapyridine used in ulcerative colitis 0·5–1·5 grammes 6 hourly.

Group 2. Poorly absorbed, previously used for bacilliary dysentery, but now largely replaced by Group 1 drugs: phthalylsulphathiazole, succinylsulphathiazole, sulphaguanidine.

Group 3. Medium- to long-acting, bound to protein.

Sulfalene. Used in combination with trimethoprim.

Sulphormethoxine (Fanasil)

Sulphamethoxazole. Used in combination with trimethoprim (Septrin, Bactrim) (see page 912).

Sulphalene

Sulphamethoxypyridazine (Lederkyn)
Sulphaphenazole (Orisulf, Orisul)

PARA-AMINOSALICYLIC ACID (PAS)

A weakly tuberculostatic drug, of little value by itself, but useful in the prevention of the development of resistant organisms when combined with other antituberculous drugs. Structurally similar to para-aminobenzoic acid, its mode of action may be comparable to that of the sulphonamides. Side-effects resemble those of aspirin, and include anorexia, nausea, vomiting, diarrhoea, gastric haemorrhage and a possible association with peptic ulceration. Hypersensitivity may occur with fever, joint symptoms and skin rashes.

PAS (Para-aminosalicylic acid)

Leucopenia, agranulocytosis, lymphocytosis, thrombocytopenia, liver damage, pancreatitis and nephritis may also occur. The prothrombin time is often prolonged, and a number of patients develop a goitre and sometimes evidence of hypothyroidism.

The drug is well absorbed, and is rapidly excreted by the kidneys. It should be used with caution in renal disease.

Dose

Dose is 6–12 grammes in single or divided doses daily, in conjunction with at least one other antituberculous drug.

Preparation

Sodium aminosalicylate. Cachets of 1·5 grammes. Many other preparations are available, particularly combined with isoniazid.

SULPHONES

Derivatives of diaminodiphenylsulphone (DDS, dapsone). Their main use is in the treatment of leprosy, but they have also been used in combination with dihydrofolate reductase inhibitors in the treatment and prophylaxis of malaria. Many of the sulphones are metabolized to DDS *in vivo*. DDS is the most widely used preparation.

Sulphones

DDS (Dapsone)

Toxic effects

Reactional leprosy may be precipitated and this is the most important unwanted effect in the management of that disease. Other effects include fever, malaise, lymphadenopathy, skin rashes, anaemia, methaemoglobinaemia, depression, psychoses and hepatitis.

Dose

In leprosy 5–200 mg weekly in single or divided doses.

Preparations

Diaminodiphenylsulphone (Dapsone, DDS). Tablets of 5 and 100 mg.
Diethyl dithiolisophthalate (Ditophal). A yellow viscous liquid with an odour of garlic. By inunction.
Sodium sulfoxone. No longer marketed.
Thiambutosine (Ciba 1906). Not a sulphone but a useful alternative in the management of leprosy. Tablets of 500 mg.

PYRIMETHAMINE

Pyrimethamine has structural similarities to folic acid, and acts by substrate inhibition, blocking the enzyme dihydrofolate reductase. The effect is most marked in malaria but is also useful in toxoplasmosis. In large doses an antifolate effect can be demonstrated in man with the production of a macrocytic anaemia. Pyrimethamine has been used in the treatment of polycythaemia vera. Its action in malaria is on the dividing schizonts and it has little action on the ring forms, so that its action is too slow for use in the acute attack.

Pyrimethamine

It has an action on the pre-erythrocytic stage of *P. falciparum* so that it is a causal prophylactic of *P. falciparum*. It is a suppressive prophylactic of the benign malarias. Some strains of *P. falciparum* are resistant to pyrimethamine, and in these there is a cross-resistance to proguanil. However, pyrimethamine has been used in combination with other drugs in the treatment of chloroquine-resistant malaria. Pyrimethamine inactivates gametocytes so that they do not mature in the mosquito.

Toxic effects

These are rare in suppressive doses. The prolonged course used in treating toxoplasmosis may cause a macrocytic anaemia. Massive doses cause vomiting, collapse, convulsions and death.

Dose

Malaria prophylaxis. 25–50 mg weekly continued for 2–4 weeks after leaving the malarial zone.

Toxoplasmosis. 25–50 mg daily for 3–6 weeks, concurrently with a sulphonamide.

Polycythaemia vera. The dose required to maintain a normal haemoglobin varies from patient to patient. Thrombocytopenia and leucopenia may occur.

Preparation

Pyrimethamine (Daraprim). Tablets of 25 mg. Also an elixir.

Pyrimethamine is also available in combination with chloroquine sulphate (Daraclor), dapsone (Maloprim) and sulphadoxine (Fansidar).

PROGUANIL

Developed from research into pyrimidine derivatives, it is much used for malarial prophylaxis. Probably with little antiplasmodial activity itself, it is metabolized in the body to cycloguanil, a triazine derivative. Cycloguanil

Proguanil   Cycloguanil

has structural similarities with pyrimethamine and likewise is probably an inhibitor of dihydrofolate reductase in plasmodia. Like pyrimethamine its action is on the dividing schizonts, it is a causal prophylactic of *P. falciparum* malaria and a suppressive prophylactic of the benign malarias, and it inactivates gametocytes. Cross-resistance exists with pyrimethamine-resistant strains of *P. falciparum.* However, the metabolite, cycloguanil, is much more rapidly excreted than is pyrimethamine, so that daily administration is required. Proguanil is singularly free from toxic effects and appears to exert no anti-folate activity in man. Loss of appetite, nausea, vomiting and diarrhoea may occur, perhaps owing to inhibition of gastric secretion. Large doses may cause haematuria.

Dose

Malaria prophylaxis: 100 mg or more daily continued for 4 weeks after leaving the malarial zone.

Preparations

Proguanil hydrochloride (Paludrine). Tablets of 25, 100 and 300 mg.

Chloroproguanil hydrochloride (Lapudrine). Slowly excreted. Prophylactic dose 20 mg weekly.

Cycloguanil pamoate (Camolar). The pamoate of the active metabolite of proguanil. It is excreted slowly so that a single intramuscular injection of 5 mg/kg may protect against malaria for 3 to 6 months. It is used in the treatment of leishmaniasis.

TRIMETHOPRIM

Trimethoprim has a structural similarity to folates and thus acts as a spurious substrate for dihydrofolate reductase. The subsequent inhibition of tetra-hydrofolic acid production is most marked in bacteria and plasmodia but is minimal in man in the therapeutic dose range. It exhibits synergism with sulphonamides so that whereas individually at a given concentration the drugs are feebly bacteriostatic, together they are bactericidal.

Trimethoprim

Combinations of trimethoprim and sulphonamides are used for their broad-spectrum bactericidal properties. It has also been shown that they are effective in malaria, and of possible use in chloroquine-resistant *P. falciparum* infections.

Preparations

Trimethoprim (80 mg) and sulphamethoxazole (400 mg) tablets (Septrin, Bactrim). Bactericidal dose 2 tablets 6-hourly for 1–2 weeks.

Trimethoprim has been used with sulphalene in the treatment of malaria. A single administration of trimethoprim 10 mg/kg and sulphalene 20 mg/kg to a maximum of trimethoprim 0·5 gramme and sulphalene 1·0 gramme has been found effective.

5. MISCELLANEOUS ANTI-PROTAZOAL COMPOUNDS

CLEFAMIDE (MEBINOL)

A luminal amoebicide, in 250 mg tablets.

DILOXANIDE FUROATE

An effective luminal amoebicide, curing some 90% of *Entamoeba histolytica* cyst passers. It is used as a supplement to other drugs in invasive amoebiasis to ensure that the parasite is eradicated from the bowel lumen. It is free from serious side-effects, but flatulence may occur.

Dose

The dose is 500 mg orally 3 times daily for 10 days.

Preparation

Diloxanide furoate (Furamide). Tablets of 500 mg.

DIMINAZENE ACETURATE (BERENIL)

Widely used in veterinary medicine for the treatment of trypanosomiasis, babesiasis and bacterial infections. Has been used for human trypanosomiasis in a dose of 2 mg/kg intramuscularly each day for 7 days.

IODINATED QUINOLINES

These drugs are used in the treatment of amoebic cyst passers, and to a lesser extent in amoebic dysentery. Toxic effects include diarrhoea, nausea and vomiting, pruritus ani, iodism, goitre and liver damage.

Preparations

There are a large number of preparations available, with much variation in presentation. Chiniofon (Iodoquinoline); Clioquinol (Iodochlorohydroxy-quinoline, Enterovioform); Di-iodohydroxyquinoline (Diodoquin, Embequin).

METRONIDAZOLE

Introduced for the treatment of trichomoniasis, metronidazole has been found to be valuable in all forms of amoebiasis. It may be as effective as emetine in hepatic amoebiasis and in amoebic dysentery, and is relatively non-toxic. It is also a luminal amoebicide. It is effective in giardiasis. It has been used in alcoholism, the taste for alcohol being diminished, but if alcohol is taken concurrently a confusional state may occur. It is well absorbed after oral administration. Side-effects include nausea, vomiting, rashes and mental changes. The urine becomes dark in some patients. There may be a fall in the leucocyte count, but agranulocytosis has not been reported.

Dose

In trichomoniasis and giardiasis 200–400 mg 3 times daily for 5–10 days. *E. histolytica* cyst passers 400–800 mg 3 times daily for 5–10 days. Invasive amoebiasis 400–800 mg 3 times daily for 5–10 days.

Preparation

Metronidazole (Flagyl). Tablets of 200 mg (U.K.); American tablets of 250 mg.

PENTAMIDINE

A diamidine used as a second line drug in the treatment of African trypanoso-miasis and visceral leishmaniasis. It is not effective in trypanosomiasis if the central nervous system is involved. It is excreted very slowly, and single injections are used to give long-term prophylaxis in trypanosomiasis. The precise mode of action is unknown but it has been suggested that the glucose metabolism of the trypanosome may be disturbed. An alternative explanation is that the lysosomal enzymes may be affected. Rapid intravenous injection may cause hypotension. Other toxic effects include hypoglycaemia and pain at the site of intramuscular injection. The development of a temporary diabetic state after a course of pentamidine has also been noted.

Dose

By intramuscular injection. Treatment of African trypanosomiasis 10 injections of 4 mg/kg over a period of 10–20 days. Prophylaxis of African trypanosomiasis, a single injection of 4 mg/kg may protect for up to 6 months. Treatment of visceral leishmaniasis, a course similar to that used in African trypanosomiasis.

Preparations

Pentamidine injection (Lomidine). An ampoule, the contents of which should be dissolved in water for injection immediately before use.

HYDROXYSTILBAMIDINE ISETHIONATE

Hydroxystilbamidine isethionate is allied to pentamidine and is used in the treatment of antimony-resistant kala-azar. and some deep mycoses. There is a fall in blood pressure after intravenous injection, and this must be counteracted by the simultaneous administration of an antihistaminic such as mepyramine maleate (Anthisan) 50–100 mg twice daily.

Dose

250 mg daily by slow intravenous injection for 10 days, repeated after 7 days. The total number of courses for an adult in most forms of kala-azar is 3, a total of 7·5 grammes of the drug.

6. MISCELLANEOUS ANTHELMINTICS

AMPHOTALIDE (SCHISTOMIDE)

Oral, non-antimonial drug previously used for the treatment of schistosomiasis.

BEPHENIUM HYDROXYNAPHTHOATE

This drug was developed after investigation of the anthelmintic properties of quaternary ammonium compounds. It is used in the treatment of hookworm infections. It is thought to be more effective against *A. duodenale* than against

Bephenium

N. americanus. It also has some action against roundworms and *Trichostrongylus.* Absorption is negligible, so that toxic effects are limited to the gastro-intestinal tract and include nausea, vomiting and diarrhoea.

Dose

5 grammes (2·5 grammes of base) as a single dose or daily for 3 days (see page 260).

Preparation

Bephenium granules (Alcopar). Sachets containing 5 grammes of bephenium hydroxynaphthoate.

BITHIONOL

This drug has bactericidal properties but has also been shown to be useful in fluke infections including paragonimiasis and fascioliasis. Toxic effects include gastric irritation with nausea, vomiting and diarrhoea, urticarial skin rashes and transient albuminuria.

Dose

30–50 mg/kg (orally) on alternate days for 3–4 weeks.

Preparation

Bithionol (2,2' thiobis; 4,6-dichlorophenol; Actamer, Bitin).

DICHLOROPHEN

This drug is much used in veterinary medicine, but it has also been used in

Dichlorophen

the treatment of tapeworm infections in man. The worms are killed and part digested, so that it is impossible to identify the scolex and confirm the cure immediately. It may be used in *Taenia saginata* infections, but is contra-indicated in *T. solium,* because of the risk of auto-infection and subsequent cysticercosis. Toxic effects include nausea, vomiting, diarrhoea, urticaria, lassitude and jaundice. Rarely, fatalities have followed large doses.

Dose

6 grammes (orally) daily for 2 days.

Preparation

Dichlorophen. Tablets of 500 mg.

FURAPROMIDIUM (F 30066)

Oral, non-antimonial drug used in *S. japonicum* and *Clonorchis* infections.

Dose

50–80 mg/kg daily in divided doses for 10–15 days.

HEXYLRESORCINOL

Hexylresorcinol has anthelmintic, antiseptic and spermicidal properties. As an anthelmintic it has been largely superseded, but hexylresorcinol enemas may yet be the most effective treatment for severe trichuriasis.

NICLOSAMIDE

This drug, widely employed as a molluscicide (Bayluscide), is effective in tapeworm infections, the worms being excreted in a partially digested or unrecognizable form. The drug is not absorbed and does not appear to irritate the gastro-intestinal tract so that side-effects are minimal. There is no need for preliminary starvation or purgation. It is contra-indicated in *T. solium* infections.

Niclosamide

Dose

1 gramme, chewed and washed down with water, followed 1 hour later by 1 gramme.

Preparation

Niclosamide (*Yomesan*). 0·5 gramme tablets.

NIRIDAZOLE

Useful in the treatment of schistosomiasis, it is also effective in amoebiasis and in guinea-worm infections. High cure rates are obtained in *S. haematobium* infections but in *S. mansoni* infections results are less good, and side-effects are more frequent, particularly in the presence of portal hypertension. The drug has also been reported to be effective in *S. japonicum* infections. The mode of action in schistosomiasis is uncertain but may be related to an inhibitory action on the enzyme glucose-6-phosphate dehydrogenase of the adult worm. Niridazole is well absorbed and is metabolized rapidly by the liver so that it is necessary to give the drug twice daily. The metabolites are excreted in the urine, giving it the colour of Coca-Cola. The most important toxic effects are on the central nervous system and include changes in mood, confusional states and convulsions. Other side-effects include nausea, vomiting, anorexia, headache, drowsiness, urticarial rashes, a temporary haemolytic anaemia in subjects with glucose-6-phosphate dehydrogenase deficiency, tachycardia and ECG changes with flattening or inversion of T-waves. In animals spermatogenesis may be inhibited, but this has not been confirmed in man. It should not be used concurrently with isoniazid, and with caution in those with liver, heart, renal or neurological diseases.

Dose

25 mg/kg (by mouth) in divided doses daily to a maximum of 1·5 grammes daily for 5–10 days.

Preparation

Niridazole (*Ambilhar*). 500 and 100 mg tablets.

TETRAMISOLE HYDROCHLORIDE

A veterinary anthelmintic that has recently been shown to be as effective as piperazine in the treatment of human *Ascaris* infection, and may be of use in hookworm infections. It acts by interfering with the carbohydrate metabolism of nematodes and inhibiting the production of succinate dehydrogenase; this produces complete muscular paralysis of the worms. Dose 2·5 mg/kg in a single dose. Side-effects are few: nausea, vomiting, abdominal pain, dizziness.

Tetramisole

Preparations

Laevo-tetramisole (*Levamisole, Ketrax*). The L-isomer and active form. 40 mg tablets.

THIABENDAZOLE

A broad-spectrum anthelmintic which is particularly useful in the treatment of strongyloidiasis and creeping eruption. It also has some effect on hookworm, *Ascaris*, and *Enterobius*. It is possible that it has some value in trichinosis, but it has little effect in trichuriasis. Toxic effects include dizziness, anorexia, nausea and vomiting, pruritus, skin rashes, headache, drowsiness and a fall in blood pressure.

Dose

25 mg/kg (by mouth) twice daily for 2 days.

Preparations

Thiabendazole (*Mintezol*). 500 mg tablets, also available as an emulsion.

7. SEMICARBAZONES AND RELATED DRUGS
THIACETAZONE

This drug is used in the treatment of tuberculosis, particularly in combination with isoniazid where economic considerations are paramount. It is also of some use in leprosy.

Toxic effects include nausea, vomiting, anorexia, headache, vertigo, blurred vision, urticaria and dermatitis, fever, anaemia, agranulocytosis, Stevens–Johnson syndrome and liver damage.

Preparations

Thiazina. Tablets containing thiacetazone and isoniazid. Varying combinations are available, including tablets of thiacetazone 150 mg and isoniazid 300 mg, and thiacetazone 75 mg and isoniazid 150 mg.

Thiacetazone (TBI, Thioparamizone). Tablets of 25 mg, 50 mg and 75 mg.

METHISAZONE

A thiosemicarbazone used in the prophylaxis of smallpox. It is effective only if taken early in the incubation period. It has also been used in the treatment of eczema vaccinatum and vaccinia gangrenosum.

Toxic effects

These include nausea, vomiting, diarrhoea and fluid retention. These effects may be aggravated by alcohol.

Dose

3 grammes (by mouth) twice daily.

Preparations

Methisazone (Marboran). A chewable capsule of 1·5 grammes.

ISONIAZID

This most effective and inexpensive tuberculostatic drug was developed as an intermediate product in the synthesis of the thiosemicarbazone of iso-nicotinaldehyde, which it was hoped would have useful antituberculous properties itself.

Toxic effects

Not perhaps as frequent as with other antituberculous agents. Peripheral neuritis may occur but can be prevented by the concurrent administration of pyridoxine. Changes in mood may occur, and this observation led to the development of iproniazid and other monoamine oxidase inhibitors for the treatment of depression. Isoniazid is not a monoamine oxidase inhibitor itself.

Nausea, headache, anorexia, dry mouth, ataxia, drowsiness, tinnitus, fever, liver damage, skin rashes, pellagra, hesitancy and agranulocytosis may occur, but rarely unless high dosages are used. Some individuals have an inherited disposition governed by a recessive gene to inactivate isoniazid slowly.

Dose

200–300 mg (by mouth) daily.

Preparations

Isoniazid. Tablets of 50 and 100 mg. A syrup and an injectable form are also available, as are many preparations combined with either para-aminosalicylic acid or thiacetazone.

NITROFURAZONE

Related to the urinary antiseptic nitrofurantoin (Furadantin), this drug, besides similar antibacterial properties has some value in the management of trypanosomiasis. It is not a first line drug, but may be used in infections showing resistance to the usual trypanocidal drugs.

Toxic effects

Nausea, vomiting, headache, arthralgia, peripheral neuritis and haemolytic anaemia in subjects with a glucose-6-phosphate dehydrogenase deficiency have been reported.

Preparation

Nitrofurazone. Tablets containing 100 mg of nitrofurazone. (Furacin is a 0·2% ointment or solution).

8. CHLORINATED HYDROCARBONS

CARBON TETRACHLORIDE

Carbon tetrachloride (CCl_4) previously used for the treatment of hookworm, roundworm and tapeworm, is now replaced by less toxic drugs.

HEXACHLOROPARAXYLENE (HEXACHLOROPARAXYLOL, CHLOXYLE, HETOL)

Shown to be effective in the treatment of fluke infections including clonorchiasis, fascioliasis and paragonimiasis. Although little toxicity has been reported in man, renal damage has occurred in dogs. Only available in certain parts of the world (Far East), not generally available in Europe, America and Africa. Dose 50–70 mg/kg daily in divided doses (morning and evening after food) for 5 days (see also page 327).

Hexachloroparaxylene

TETRACHLOROETHYLENE (TCE)

Effective against hookworm, probably by causing a reversible paralysis.

Tetrachloroethylene

There is disagreement as to whether it is more effective in *A. duodenale* or *N. americanus* infections. In either case the worm load is likely to be reduced by half by a standard course of treatment.

Toxic effects

It has a central action in some respects similar to that of chloroform ($CHCl_3$) but with proper administration little is absorbed or inhaled. However, headache, faintness, giddiness and loss of consciousness may occur. Local effects include nausea, vomiting, and abdominal pain. The drug is hepatotoxic. It should not be administered to ill patients, particularly those with liver diseases. Its administration should be preceded by a low fat diet as its absorption is enhanced by fat. It may precipitate intestinal obstruction in patients with coexisting *Ascaris* infections.

Dosage

2–3 ml of tetrachloroethylene. Side-effects are frequent with higher dosage.

Preparations

Tetrachloroethylene draught. 3 ml of tetrachloroethylene in 45 ml of flavoured water.
Tetrachloroethylene capsules. 1 ml.

9. PIPERAZINE AND RELATED DRUGS

PIPERAZINE

Piperazine was originally introduced for the treatment of gout as it is a good solvent of uric acid *in vitro*, but clinically it was found to be ineffective. It is now used for the treatment of roundworm and threadworm infections. Piperazine paralyses roundworms, probably by acetylcholine blockade. The worms, no longer able to maintain their position in the gut, are expelled by peristalsis.

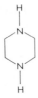

Piperazine

Toxicity

It is a safe drug, but excessive dosage in small children may cause vertigo, muscular incoordination and other neurological effects. Nausea, vomiting, diarrhoea and urticaria may occur. Rapidly absorbed, it is mainly excreted in the urine, so that piperazine should not be given in renal disease.

Dosage

Ascariasis. 3–6 grammes daily for 1–2 days.
Enterobiasis. 2 grammes daily for 1 week, or as for ascariasis.

Preparations

Piperazine adipate (Entacyl). Tablets of 300 mg of piperazine adipate equivalent to 250 mg piperazine hydrate. Entacyl suspension contains 300 mg in 2 ml.

Piperazine citrate (Antepar elixir). The elixir containing equivalent of 750 mg of piperazine hydrate in 5 ml.

Piperazine hydrate

Piperazine phosphate (Antepar). Tablets containing 520 mg of piperazine phosphate equivalent to 500 mg of piperazine hydrate.

Pripsen. A 10 gramme dose contains piperazine phosphate (4 grammes) and standard senna.

DIETHYLCARBAMAZINE

A derivative of piperazine. It is used in the treatment of filariasis and is more active against microfilariae (microfilaricidal) than against adult worms (macrofilaricidal). Its macrofilaricidal effect is most marked in *Loa loa* infections. It is usually effective in pulmonary tropical eosinophilia. Its action on microfilariae is probably to sensitize them, making them more susceptible to phagocytosis.

Diethylcarbamazine

Toxic effects

These are slight, but release of foreign protein following the death of microfilariae may lead to allergic reactions. This is especially so in onchocerciasis, and the subsequent skin reaction forms the basis of the Mazzotti test. Severe systemic reactions have been reported in heavy *Loa loa* infections. Reactions may be controlled by antihistamines or steroids.

Dosage

Filariasis. Initially 50 mg daily increased to a top dose of 150–450 mg in 3 divided doses daily for 3 weeks.

Pulmonary tropical eosinophilia. 150 mg 3 times daily for 5–10 days.

Preparation

Diethylcarbamazine (Banocide, Hetrazan, Ethodryl). 50 mg tablets of diethylcarbamazine citrate.

10. ANTIBIOTICS AND ANTIFUNGAL AGENTS

General texts deal fully with this group, so that only a selection of drugs particularly useful in tropical medicine will be mentioned.

AMPHOTERICIN B

A toxic antibiotic produced by the growth of *Streptomyces nodosus,* and used in the treatment of systemic fungal infections. Given intravenously, it may cause thrombophlebitis. Systemic side-effects are invariable. A fever during the course of the infusion is common. Nausea, vomiting, anorexia, malaise, bone-marrow depression, renal damage, hypokalaemia and visual disturbance are frequent. Deaths have been reported.

Dose

Initially 0·1 mg/kg daily by slow intravenous infusion, well diluted in 0·5–1 litre 5% dextrose in water, given over 6 hours. The dose may be increased slowly to a maximum of 0·25 mg/kg and the total dosage should not be more than 2 grammes. The blood urea must be estimated regularly, and if it is elevated the drug should be withheld until it has returned to normal, when the dose which was tolerated before the renal damage may be continued. No further increase in dosage must be made. Side-effects such as rigors and fever should be controlled with small doses of steroids.

CHLORAMPHENICOL

A broad-spectrum bacteriostatic antibiotic. Toxicity limits its use to the treatment of typhoid and *Haemophilus* meningitis.

Dose

In typhoid 500 mg 6-hourly for 7–14 days (see page 540).

Preparations

Chloramphenicol (*Chloromycetin*). Capsules of 250 mg. Parenteral preparations are also available.

5-FLUOROCYTOSINE

An antimetabolite of cytosine in fungi but not in man. It shows promise in the treatment of systemic fungal infections such as cryptococcosis. Side-effects are less common than with amphotericin B. Serum transaminases may be elevated and pancytopenia has been reported. It is excreted in the urine.

Dose

2–4 grammes by mouth daily for 6 weeks or more (see page 692).

GRISEOFULVIN

An antifungal substance produced by the growth of *Penicillium griseofulvum*. It is effective in the treatment of fungal infections of the skin, nails and hair. Tinea imbricata is readily cured by griseofulvin. It has no apparent effect on systemic fungal infections. Side-effects are generally mild. However, allergic reactions and anaphylaxis may occur and there may be cross-sensitivity with penicillin. Leucopenia, lupus erythematosus, proteinuria, mental changes, oestrogenic activity and changes in porphyrin metabolism have been described.

Dose

0·5–1 gramme (by mouth) daily in divided doses. The duration of the treatment varies. Fungal infections of the nails may require prolonged treatment over several months.

Preparation

   Griseofulvin. Capsules and tablets of 125 mg and 250 mg.

NEOMYCIN

Produced by the growth of *Streptomyces fradiae*. Generally too toxic to use systemically. Is not absorbed and is used in the suppression of nitrogen-producing gut flora in hepatic failure. Topical preparations are used in the treatment of infected skin disorders.

Preparations

   Neomycin. Tablets of 500 mg.
   Neomycin ointment. 1%.

GENTAMYCIN

Like neomycin, an aminoglycoside, poorly absorbed, broad-spectrum antibiotic, but less toxic, though eighth nerve damage occurs. Given intramuscularly, it is mainly excreted in the urine.

KANAMYCIN

Also similar to neomycin. Parenteral use leads to the eighth nerve and renal damage. Of some value in tuberculosis resistant to first line drugs.

NOVOBIOCIN

A well absorbed, broad-spectrum antibiotic, now obsolete as side-effects are very frequent.

NYSTATIN

Used in the local treatment of moniliasis. Produced by the growth of *Streptomyces noursei*. It is poorly absorbed and parenteral preparations are too irritant to be practicable in the treatment of systemic mycoses.

Preparations

   Nystatin. Tablets of 500 000 units, pessaries, ointments, ear-drops, eye-drops, oral suspension and paints.

PAROMOMYCIN

An antibiotic produced by the growth of *Streptomyces rimosus*. Used in the treatment of both amoebic and bacillary dysentery, and in non-invasive amoebiasis (carrier state). It has recently been shown to be useful in *Taenia saginata* and *Hymenolepis nana* infections. It is not absorbed, so that toxic effects with oral preparations are restricted to irritation of the gastro-intestinal tract. However, parenteral administration may give rise to side-effects similar to those of streptomycin.

Dose

1–2 grammes daily in divided doses for 5–7 days.

Preparation

Paromomycin (Humatin). Capsules containing paromomycin sulphate 250 mg.

FUMAGILLIN

An antiprotozoal antibiotic and luminal amoebicide, now withdrawn.

PUROMYCIN

An antiprotozoal antibiotic, experimentally valuable against *T. cruzi*, but toxic.

PENICILLINS

Pencillins vary in their routes of administration, duration of action, resistance to staphylococcal penicillinase and spectrum of activity.

1. Standard penicillins

Derivatives of benzyl penicillin. Bactericidal and the penicillins of choice against sensitive Gram-positive cocci and bacilli and Gram-negative cocci. Short-acting parenteral preparations are the most effective. Toxic effects are common to all penicillins, hypersensitivity reactions being the most important.

Oral. *Phenoxymethyl penicillin (Penicillin V).* Resistant to gastric acid. Usual dose 250 mg every 6 hours.

Parenteral. The duration of action of these penicillins depends on the rate of release of benzyl penicillin from the injection site.

Benzyl penicillin. Crystalline penicillin G. Short-acting—4–12 hours. Dose 0·5–2 mega units 2–12-hourly by intramuscular or intravenous injection.

Procaine penicillin. Medium-acting—12–24 hours. Dose 0·3–0·9 mega units daily by intramuscular injection.

Penicillin aluminium monostearate (PAM). A medium-acting penicillin previously used for the out-patient treatment of yaws.

Benethamine penicillin. Medium/long-acting penicillin. Effective blood levels for 3–4 days following a single intramuscular injection. Dose 0·3–0·6 mega units.

Benzathine penicillin. Long-acting penicillin. Effective blood levels for 1–2 weeks following a single intramuscular injection. Dose 1–3 mega units.

2. Broad-spectrum penicillins

Active against many Gram-negative bacilli as well as other penicillin sensitive organisms.

Ampicillin (Penbritin). Available as capsules of 250 mg, as tablets of 125 mg, as a syrup and as an intravenous injection. Dose 1–6 grammes daily in divided doses. At the lower dose range the drug may be only bacteriostatic, but it may be bactericidal at the higher range.

Cephalosporins (Cephaloridine, Cephalothin). Related to penicillin, they are poorly absorbed, broad-spectrum antibiotics with some resistance to penicillinase. There is cross-allergy with penicillins. They are given by intramuscular injection.

3. Penicillinase-resistant penicillins

Cloxacillin (*Orbenin*). Available as capsules of 250 mg and as an injection. Dose 1·5–3 grammes daily in divided doses.

Erythromycin is not a penicillin but is effective against penicillin-resistant staphylococci, but resistance rapidly develops. It is toxic to the liver. *Triacetyloleandomycin* is similar.

RIFAMYCINS

A group of antibiotics derived from *Streptomyces mediterranei*. They appear to be useful against infections with acid-fast bacilli (tuberculosis, leprosy, and Buruli ulcer). Rifampicin, a semi-synthetic derivative, shows particular promise. It is probably bactericidal against both *Myco. tuberculosis* and *Myco. leprae*. Its mode of action is by inhibition of bacterial RNA synthesis.

STREPTOMYCIN

A broad-spectrum bactericidal drug, which, because of the rapid development of resistant organisms, is mainly reserved for the treatment of tuberculosis; it is effective in plague. However, the combination of streptomycin and another bactericidal drug, such as penicillin, forms a useful combination in urgent situations when tuberculosis can be excluded. Side-effects are well known. In particular the drug is toxic to sensory nerve endings in the inner ear. Vestibular function is disturbed before auditory. The drug crosses the placenta and may damage the fetal ear. It is not absorbed, so may only be given parenterally.

Dose

In tuberculosis 0·5–1·0 gramme daily by intramuscular injection. There is now a tendency to reduce both the frequency and the duration of the course of injections.

Preparation

Streptomycin injection. A solution in water for injection.

TETRACYCLINES

Bacteriostatic broad-spectrum antibiotics. There are several preparations with little advantage over one another. Tetracycline itself is usually the least expensive.

Toxic effects

The more severe toxic effects include hepatic and renal damage and a general bleeding tendency. These effects are especially likely to be seen in pregnancy, in renal or hepatic disease or if the drug is given intravenously. Degradation products of outdated tetracycline may be nephrotoxic. Tetracyclines are deposited in growing bones and teeth. Teeth may be discoloured and there may be enamel hypoplasia. As tetracycline crosses the placenta, the dental damage that may result is a further reason for not giving the drug during pregnancy. Dental damage may also occur if tetracycline is given during the first 8 years of life.

Dose

By mouth 250–500 mg every 6 hours. By injection 0·5–1·0 gramme in divided doses daily, but in severe infections a total daily dose of 2 grammes may be used but not exceeded.

Preparations

There are a large number of preparations available. Parenteral preparations are usually for either intramuscular or intravenous use, and may only be given by the indicated parenteral route.

11. TOPICAL APPLICATIONS INCLUDING PARASITICIDES AND REPELLENTS

BENZYL BENZOATE

Effective in scabies as it is lethal to *Sarcoptes scabiei*. It is not so useful in pediculosis. It may cause skin eruptions, particularly in eczematous individuals.

Application

The patient is first scrubbed with soft soap. Immediately after drying benzyl benzoate is applied to the whole body below the neck. It is sometimes necessary to repeat the application.

Preparation

Benzyl benzoate application (*Ascabiol*). Benzyl benzoate 25% w/v with emulsifying wax and water.

CHLORBUTOL

This is antibacterial, antifungal and possibly antipruritic. It is used in many dusting powders, and also as a preservative for injections and eye drops. It is related to chloral hydrate, and has sedative and anti-emetic actions.

CHRYSAROBIN

A parasiticide, but stains brown-violet, and is toxic if absorbed. Now largely superseded.

CROTAMITON

Used in the treatment of scabies; also as an antipruritic.

Preparation

Crotamiton (*Eurax*). Available as a cream or lotion containing 10% crotamiton.

DESITIN

A powder, ointment or ointment spray containing cod liver oil and zinc oxide.

DICOPHANE (DDT)

An insecticide which may be used to eradicate fleas and lice. Acute toxic signs include vomiting, diarrhoea, paraesthesiae, giddiness, tremors, anxiety and liver, bone marrow and renal damage.

DDT

Preparations

Dicophane. Available as an application and as a dusting powder.

DIBUTYL PHTHALATE

An insect repellent and mite repellent. Rubbed into clothes it may give protection for 2 weeks.

DIETHYL TOLUAMIDE

An insect repellent. May be applied direct to skin but the eyes and mouth must be avoided.

Preparation

Diethyl toluamide solution (Mylol). Available as 50 and 75% solutions in alcohol, and as a cream, a liquid and in pressurized containers.

DIMETHYL PHTHALATE

An insect, mite and tick repellent. Should be applied away from the eyes and mouth, and should not be allowed to come into contact with plastics and other synthetic materials.

Preparation

Dimethyl phthalate cream (Sketofax)

GAMMA BENZENE HEXACHLORIDE

Used to eradicate lice and scabies. Toxic effects are similar to those of dicophane.

Preparation

Gamma benzene hexachloride (Lorexane). Available as a cream, dusting powder and application.

5-IODODEOXYURIDINE

An antimetabolite which disrupts DNA synthesis and thus prevents the replication of certain viruses. A 0·1% solution instilled into the conjunctival sac every 1–2 hours may control the keratitis of herpes simplex or vaccinia.

METHOXSALEN

This induces hypersensitivity to ultraviolet light. The subsequent stimulation of melanin pigments may be useful in idiopathic vitiligo, though not in secondary leucoderma. Side-effects including nausea and depression are common. It is toxic to the liver and may cause dermatitis.

Dose

20 mg daily by mouth followed 2 hours later by exposure of vitiliginous area to ultraviolet light for 5 minutes increasing to 30 minutes. Alternatively a 1% lotion may be applied locally once a week and followed by a 1 minute exposure to ultraviolet light. Treatment may need to be continued for months.

Preparations

Methoxsalen (*Xanthotoxin, Meloxine, Meladinine, Methoxa-dome*). 10 mg tablets.
Methoxsalen. 1% lotion.

METRIFONATE (DIPTEREX, TRICHLORPHON, NEGUVON)

An organophosphorus insecticide, *o,o*-dimethylhydroxy-2,2,2-trochlorethyl-phosphonate, it acts by inhibiting cholinesterase. It is effective against some intestinal nematodes when given by mouth, and also against *S. haematobium* and *S. mansoni*, presumably by cholinesterase inhibition and subsequent paralysis of the worms.

$$\begin{array}{c} CCl_3 \\ | \\ CHOH \\ | \\ (CH_3O)_2\ P{=}O \end{array}$$

Trichlorphon:

Toxic effects

When concentrated it is very toxic if inhaled, swallowed or spilled on the skin. There may be a fall in plasma and red cell cholinesterase after administration. Gastro-intestinal disturbances, abdominal pain, nausea and vomiting are common. Solutions must be freshly prepared.

Antidote. The enzyme reactivator pralidoxime iodide (2-PAM). Atropine gives symptomatic relief.

Dose

7·4 mg/kg in very dilute solutions may be given by mouth after food once every 14 or 28 days for 3 doses, or 15 mg/kg repeated once after 24 hours, or 5 mg/kg daily for 12 days, or 10 mg/kg daily for 6 days. It has been used as a cream for local application to creeping eruption.

PELLIDOL

Diacetylaminoazotoluene, a red powder related to scarlet red. It is used as a dusting powder or ointment to promote the healing of wounds, burns and ulcers.

ZINC UNDECENOATE

A topical fungicide, frequently combined with undecenoic acid. Available as a dusting powder, spray or ointment (Mycota, Tineafax).

12. IMMUNIZING AND RELATED PREPARATIONS

These fall into 2 main groups, the globulin preparations or antisera which convey short-lived passive immunity, and the antigenic preparations, or vaccines, which provoke active immunity. Foreign protein reactions, including anaphylaxis and serum sickness, are especially likely to occur with antisera, and partially for this reason and partially because of the uncertainty of their action and the development of more effective treatment, in particular antibiotics, many of the antisera included here are becoming obsolete. The problem of anaphylaxis and serum sickness is not mentioned with individual preparations, but it should be constantly borne in mind in making a decision whether or not to use a particular antiserum.

Many preparations of multiple vaccines are available. Their availability varies from area to area and they have not been mentioned. Individual program-mes for multiple vaccination vary considerably with the area and the expected exposure and have not been dealt with. In general live vaccines should not be given concurrently, and the greater the interval between the administration of different live vaccines the better the immune response and the fewer the side-effects.

For vaccination schedules see page 4.

Antivenoms are discussed on page 804.

ANTHRAX

Sclavo's ass serum has been replaced by antibiotics in the treatment of this disease. For workers at risk a vaccine is available.

Anthrax vaccine. 0·4 ml by intramuscular injection repeated at 6 weeks and 6 months, and subsequently annually.

BCG

A suspension of living attenuated tubercle bacilli, which gives protection against tuberculosis and perhaps also against leprosy. An ulcer may develop at the site of the vaccination. Other side-effects include eczema, lupus vulgaris, keloid formation, regional adenitis, fatal BCG infection (especially in individuals with hypogamma-globulinaemia or lymphopenia) and osteitis.

Bacillus Calmette–Guérin vaccine (BCG vaccine). 0·1 ml by intradermal injection.

BOTULISM

A globulin preparation (antitoxin) capable of neutralizing the toxins of *Clostridium botulinum* is available. Its value is uncertain.

Botulinum antitoxin. Polyvalent 10 000 to 50 000 units by intramuscular (prophylactic) or intravenous (therapeutic) injection, repeated as necessary.

CHOLERA

A suspension of killed cholera vibrios of Inaba and Ogawa strains which gives a short-lived immunity, is available. An El Tor vibrio vaccine is also available.

Local swelling and redness may occur, as may fever, headache, malaise and anaphylactic shock.

Cholera vaccine. 0·5 ml by subcutaneous injection followed by 1 ml in 2–4 weeks, and thereafter at intervals of 6 months, if necessary.

DIPHTHERIA

A toxoid is available for active immunization, and an antitoxin for passive immunization and treatment.

A local reaction is common after administration of the toxoid. A general reaction may occur. Neurological complications are very rare.

Diphtheria vaccine. Various preparations are available.

Diphtheria antitoxin. Prophylactic, 500–2000 units by subcutaneous or intramuscular injection. Therapeutic, 10 000–100 000 units by intramuscular or intravenous injection.

GAS GANGRENE

A number of specific and polyvalent globulin preparations (antitoxins) are available for neutralizing the toxins of the various species of clostridia that cause gas gangrene. Their value is uncertain.

Mixed Gas Gangrene antitoxin contains antitoxins to the toxins of *Clostridium oedematiens, Cl. septicum,* and *Cl. welchii.* Prophylactic, 25 000 units intramuscularly; therapeutic, not less than 75 000 units intravenously.

HEPATITIS

Human normal immunoglobulin may give passive protection against infective hepatitis for 6 months, and also against measles and rubella.

Human normal immunoglobulin. Preparations and dosage vary.

INFLUENZA

Various vaccines are available. Their status is not yet established.

LEPTOSPIRA

A globulin (antiserum) preparation against strains of *Leptospira icterohaemorrhagiae* is available. Its value is uncertain.

MEASLES

A live attenuated and an inactivated vaccine are available. For immediate prophylaxis human normal immunoglobulin may be given. Side-effects from the live vaccine, which is generally preferred to the inactive vaccine, are frequent, a mild measles-like illness developing around the sixth day. Rarely high fever, delirium, convulsions, cerebellar ataxia and other neurological complications occur. Thrombocytopenic purpura has been recorded.

Measles vaccine (live attenuated). 0·5 ml subcutaneously, to be given immediately after preparation.

PERTUSSIS

A suspension of killed *Bordetella pertussis* for active immunity is available. Severe reactions may occur.

Pertussis vaccine. 0·5 ml by subcutaneous injection repeated at 4–8 weeks.

PLAGUE

A suspension of killed *Pasteurella pestis* is commonly used. Its value is uncertain (see page 460).

Plague vaccine. 0·5 ml subcutaneously, followed by 1 ml subcutaneously 1–3 weeks later.

POLIOMYELITIS

A live attenuated and a killed vaccine are available. Side-effects from either vaccine are rare, but neurological complications have been reported with both. Paralytic poliomyelitis is a very rare complication of the live vaccine.

Poliomyelitis vaccine (inactivated), Salk. 1 ml subcutaneously repeated at 6 weeks and 9 months.

Poliomyelitis vaccine (oral), Sabin. Contains live attenuated virus. Types 1, 2 and 3. Dose is 3 drops by mouth, repeated at 6 weeks and 6 months.

RABIES

Inactivated vaccines and antisera are available for the pre- and post-exposure prophylaxis of rabies in man. Live attenuated vaccines are restricted to animal use. Of the inactivated vaccines, those prepared from duck embryo cultures are now generally preferred to those prepared from brain tissue cultures (Semple) as the risk of encephalitis is reduced, though allergy to egg protein may rarely cause a severe reaction. Local reactions at the site of injection are not uncommon.

Rabies antiserum. 2000 units by intramuscular injection as soon as possible after exposure, but not more than 48 hours, to be followed by a course of a rabies vaccine.

Rabies vaccines. Semple type or Duck embryo vaccine (DEV). Pre- and post-exposure regimens will vary with preparations and the type of exposure (see page 406).

SMALLPOX

The vaccine contains the living virus of vaccinia. Dangerous reactions are more likely after a primary vaccination than re-vaccination, and include encephalomyelitis, vaccinia necrosa and eczema vaccinatum. Less severe are generalized vaccinia, auto-inoculation vaccinia and sensitivity rashes. Other side-effects include thrombocytopenic purpura, myocarditis, nephrotic syndrome, transplacental infection, abortion and local reactions including bacterial infection and keloid formation.

Smallpox vaccine. About 0·2 ml applied to the skin by scarification or pressure inoculation.

TETANUS

A vaccine containing modified tetanus toxin (toxoid) and an antiserum containing an antitoxin are available. Important side-effects to the toxoid are rare although severe sensitivity reactions and peripheral neuropathy have been recorded.

Tetanus vaccine (tetanus toxoid). Dose varies with the preparation, and is repeated in 6 weeks and 6 months and subsequently at intervals of from 5 to 10 years.

Tetanus antitoxin. Therapeutic, 3000 I.U. locally and 10 000 I.U. or more by intramuscular or intravenous injection. Prophylactic, 1500 I.U. by subcutaneous injection.

TYPHOID

An inactivated suspension of *Salmonella typhi*, usually combined with *S. paratyphi* A and B. Preparations vary widely in their useful antigenic properties. The paratyphoid vaccines are of unproved efficacy and of the typhoid vaccines the acetone-killed, phenolized vaccine may be better than the heat-killed, phenolized vaccine. Local reactions occur in about 75% and general reactions, with headache, fever, malaise, nausea and diarrhoea, are common. Rare complications may include nephropathy, arthritis, urticaria and encephalitis.

Typhoid/paratyphoid A and B vaccine (TAB). By subcutaneous or intradermal injection. The dose varies with different preparations and is repeated in 6 weeks.

TYPHUS

A suspension of inactivated rickettsiae of epidemic and murine typhus (*R. prowazeki* and *R. mooseri*). Protection may last about 6 months.

Typhus vaccine. 0·25–1·0 ml subcutaneously, repeated in 10–20 days.

Live attenuated vaccine. E strain. Protection lasts 5 years. Febrile reactions are common.

YELLOW FEVER

The preferred vaccine is a suspension of chick embryo tissue infected with living 17D strain yellow fever virus. A single injection, after a period of 10 days, confers immunity for at least 10 years. Reactions are rare but the chicken protein may cause allergic reactions and encephalitis may occur, especially in infants. Side-effects are more common with other preparations, such as mouse brain tissue cultures.

Yellow fever vaccine. Not less than 1000 mouse LD_{50} doses by subcutaneous injection.

For detailed information on vaccines the reader should consult:

CANNON, D. A. (1969) *Trans. R. Soc. trop. Med. Hyg.*, **63**, 867.

APPENDIX I

MEDICAL PROTOZOOLOGY

MALARIA PARASITES*

PHYLUM: PROTOZOA Goldfuss, 1818

SUBPHYLUM: SPOROZOA Leuckart, 1870

CLASS: TELOSPOREA Schaudinn, 1900

SUBCLASS: COCCIDIOMORPHA (COCCIDIA) Doflein, 1901

ORDER: COCCIDIIDA Labbé, 1899

SUBORDER: HAEMOSPORIDIIDEA Doflein, 1916

FAMILY: PLASMODIIDAE Mesnil, 1903

GENUS: *Plasmodium* Marchiafava & Celli, 1885

SUBGENERA (of those affecting man): *Plasmodium, Laverania*

The genus *Plasmodium* includes the malaria parasites of man and animals (including birds). The species affecting man are:

Quartan group

P. (*Plasmodium*) *malariae* (Grassi & Feletti, 1892)
P. (P.) *inui* (Halberstädter & von Prowazek, 1907)
P. (P.) *brasilianum* (Gonder & von Berenberg-Gossler, 1908)
P. (P.) *shortti* Bray, 1963

Benign tertian group

P. (P.) *vivax* (Grassi & Feletti, 1890)
P. (P.) *cynomolgi* Mayer, 1907
P. (P.) *cynomolgi bastianellii* Garnham, 1959

Malignant tertian group

P. (*Laverania*) *falciparum* (Welch, 1897)

Ovale group

P. (P.) *ovale* Stephens, 1922
P. (P.) *simium* Fonseca, 1951

Knowlesi group

P. (P.) *knowlesi* Sinton & Mulligan, 1932

Of these, *P. malariae*, *P. vivax*, *P. falciparum* and *P. ovale* are the most common and important. The others are primarily parasites of monkeys or apes, affecting man only incidentally, and not seriously. *P. malariae* can exist in a man-mosquito-man cycle, but in parts of Africa there is evidence that a reservoir exists in chimpanzees, the parasite apparently passing backwards and forwards between these animals and man.

---

*The information in the section on the malaria parasites has been revised, largely by reference to the authoritative descriptions contained in Professor Garnham's standard work (1966). This most comprehensive book contains references to the information collated from the work of vast numbers of scientists over the years, and of the distinguished author himself.

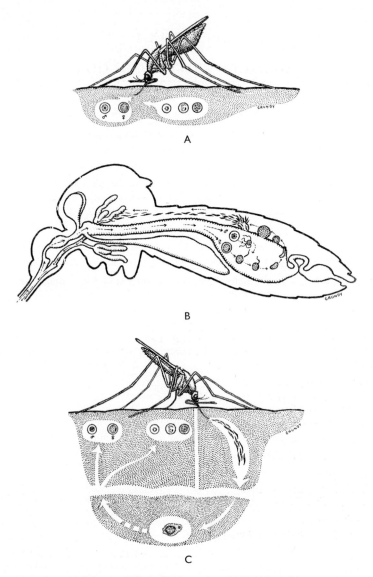

Fig. 272.—The malaria cycle. (*J. Hull Grundy*)

A, The female *Anopheles*, in feeding on a person with malaria, takes in blood containing the male and female gametocytes. B, The male and female gametocytes fuse in the stomach of the mosquito to become a single fertile egg-like body, which develops in the stomach wall producing a large number of sporozoites, which make their way to the salivary glands. This cycle lasts 7 days or more. C, When, after the development of the sporozoites, the infected mosquito again feeds on man, she discharges sporozoites in the human tissues. These may be detected in the blood for not more than half an hour after the mosquito has bitten. Thereafter they develop in the cells of the liver, and the malaria parasites to which they give rise may be found in the blood 6–9 days after the bite of the infected mosquito. The clinical attack of malaria usually begins within a day or two of their appearance in the blood. Exceptionally, in *P.vivax* infections, this process of development may be delayed for several weeks or months. (The sizes of the mosquitoes and parasites are not in proportion.)

The life cycles of these parasites have features in common. They are all carried from man to man or from animals to man by mosquitoes of the genus *Anopheles*, unlike the bird malaria parasites, which are carried by *Culex, Aedes* and other species. Some rodent malaria parasites are also carried by *Anopheles* (e.g. *P. berghei* and *P. vinckei*).

LIFE CYCLE OF THE MALARIA PARASITES OF MAN

The life cycle, taking the sporozoite as the starting point, comprises several well defined stages.

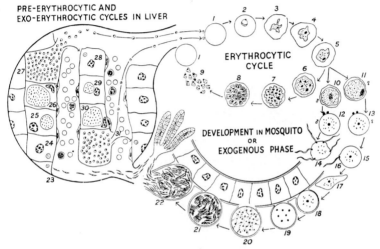

Fig. 273.—Schema of the complete life cycle of the mammalian malaria parasite based on *P. vivax* and *P. cynomolgi. (After Shortt & Garnham)*

1, Normal red cells. 2–5, Red cells containing young parasites (trophozoites). 6–8, Erythrocytic schizogony. 9, Liberation of erythrocytic merozoites into the blood. 10, 11, Development of male and female gametocytes in the circulating blood. 12, Mature male gametocyte extruding polar bodies. 13, Mature female gametocyte extruding polar bodies. 14, Exflagellation of male gametocyte producing male gametes (microgametes) in the stomach of the mosquito. 15, Female gamete, or macrogamete, being fertilized by the male to become a zygote. 16, Male gamete or microgamete. 17, Oökinete, or travelling vermicule, formed by elongation of zygote, about to penetrate the epithelial lining of the mosquito's stomach. 18–21, Oöcysts developing on the outer wall of the mosquito's stomach. 22, Mature oöcysts rupturing and liberating sporozoites, which enter the salivary glands. 23, Sporozoite from the salivary gland of the mosquito entering the liver cell of man. 24–26, Development of pre-erythrocytic schizont or cryptozoite in liver cells. 27, Pre-erythrocytic schizont liberating pre-erythrocytic merozoites (cryptomerozoites) which enter red cells, to commence the erythrocytic cycle, or to enter fresh liver cells to repeat the cryptozoic development, or exoerythrocytic schizogony. 28–30, Stages of exoerythrocytic schizogony ending in a second generation of merozoites (metacrypto-merozoites). 31, Rupture of exoerythrocytic cryptozoic schizont of any later generation to maintain cryptozoic cycle in the liver, or to produce relapse by restarting the erythrocytic cycle by metacryptomerozoites.

The *sporozoites* inoculated by the infected *Anopheles* enter the blood stream, but cannot be found in it after about half an hour. Parasites reappear in the blood 6–9 days later, but in an altered form, having undergone profound developmental changes. Some sporozoites enter the parenchyma cells of the liver, and there divide and multiply to form the first *exoerythrocytic (pre-erythrocytic) schizonts*, each developing within a liver cell, and bounded by a limiting membrane. Multiplication takes place by division of the nucleus of the original sporozoite, and continues until there are hundreds or thousands of separate nucleated parasites in each schizont. These eventually burst the limiting membrane and are shed into the circulation as free individual *merozoites*, some

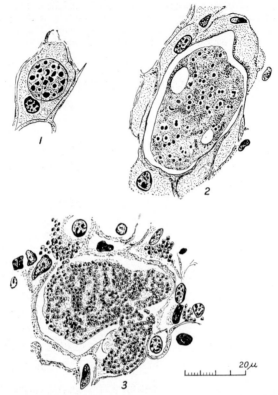

Fig. 274.—Pre-erythrocytic cycle of malaria parasites. (*After Shortt & Garnham*)

1, Pre-erythrocytic (cryptozoic) schizont of *P. cynomolgi* in a liver cell on the fifth day. 2, Pre-erythrocytic (cryptozoic) schizont of *P. vivax* in a liver cell on the seventh day, showing a form with 2 vacuoles. 3, A more advanced stage of the pre-erythrocytic schizont of *P. vivax*, showing the formation and release of pre-erythrocytic merozoites (crypto-merozoites.)

Table 40. Tissue phase of human malaria

Species	Duration of primary e-e schizogony (days)	Size of mature schizont (μm, approx)	Number of merozoites	Size of mero-zoites (μm)	Special features	Second-ary e-e schiz-ogony
P. vivax	8	45	over 10 000	1·2	Vacuoles	Present
P. ovale	9	70	15 000	1·8	Large nuclei	Present
P. malariae	12–16 (?)	45	?	?	Enlarged host cell nucleus	Probable
P. falciparum	5½	60	40 000	0·7	Small nuclei, cytomeres	Improbable

Reproduced from WHO (1963).

smaller (*micromerozoites*) and some rather larger (*macromerozoites*). These first generation merozoites are collectively known as *cryptozoites;* later generations as *phanerozoites.*
The micromerozoites find their way into the peripheral blood, and can be detected
there by subinoculation of the blood into a susceptible person.

The macromerozoites, on the other hand, in *P. vivax*, and probably in *P. ovale* and
P. malariae, are now assumed to reinvade the parenchyma cells of the liver, to go
through that part of the cycle again, to produce in a few days another batch of merozoites from the second (and succeeding) generations of exoerythrocytic schizonts.

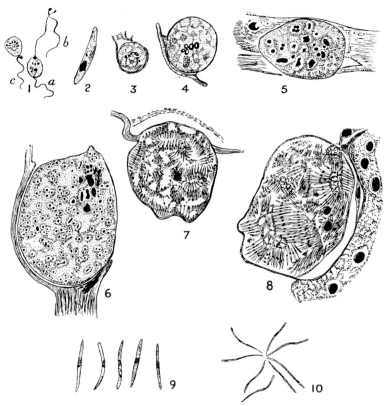

Fig. 275.—Stages in the development of *P. falciparum* in *Anopheles.*
×2000. (*After Wenyon*)

1a, Exflagellation of male gametocyte of *P. vivax*. 1b, Free flagellum (male gamete).
1c, Fertilization of female gamete. 2, Oökinete. 3, Encysted zygote in the stomach wall.
4-6, Oöcysts showing reticulated cytoplasm. 7, Section of oöcyst showing sporozoite
forming outgrowths from cytoplasmic reticulum. 8, Section of oöcyst into mature sporozoites. 9, Sporozoites from the salivary gland. 10, Sporozoites of *P. ovale*.

These in turn produce merozoites, some of which are shed into the peripheral blood,
and others apparently turn again to invade liver cells and repeat the whole process. In
the case of *P. falciparum* this reinvasion of liver cells does not occur, and the only
exoerythrocytic schizonts are those of the first, pre-erythrocytic generation. This is an
important distinction.

The result of the reinvasions, in the case of the first 3 species above, is that
periodically, every week or more, and in the absence of treatment, new waves of
parasites are released into the blood, and initiate recurrences of fever. The recurrences

may be separated by short or long periods of time, and in these intervals the liver cycle is presumably continuing.

In *P. falciparum* the repetition of the liver phase does not occur after the first schizonts have matured, and therefore recurrences of the type met in the other species do not take place, though recrudescences due to persistence of the blood phase do occur and cause renewed bouts of fever for up to 1–2 years after first infection in persons in whom that infection is not completely eradicated. Thus, though *P. falciparum* is much more dangerous than the other three species, partly (probably) because it multiplies much more prolifically than them, it is more easily cured by the drugs we now possess—except where drug resistance has appeared. *P. falciparum* is not repeatedly locked away inside liver cells where 4-aminoquinolines do not reach it.

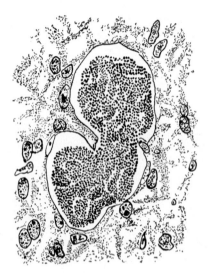

Fig. 276.—Pre-erythrocytic schizont of *P. falciparum* in the human liver on the sixth day.

The micromerozoites are shed into the peripheral blood, in enormous numbers, from the bursting liver phases, and their function is to invade the red cells, particularly the young red cells, the reticulocytes. They enter these cells, though how they penetrate the cell envelopes is not clear; the envelopes are apparently intact after the merozoites have entered. Some *P. falciparum* parasites seem to adhere to the outsides of red cells; these are known as *appliqué* forms. Once within the red cells, the parasites appear first as *ring forms*, each with a nucleus and cytoplasm surrounding a vacuole. This is the *trophozoite*, which feeds on the haemoglobin of the cell, and enlarges to assume an amoeboid form which may occupy the greater part of the red cell. It does not completely metabolize the haemoglobin, however, and a residue is left. This constitutes the *malarial pigment (haemozoin)* which appears as follows:

P. vivax: Numerous fine, yellowish brown, golden dust-like particles.
P. ovale: Numerous blackish brown particles.
P. malariae: Numerous coarse and dark brown particles.
P. falciparum: 1, 2 or at most 3 solid blocks of black pigment (an important diagnostic feature).

When the red cell finally disrupts because the parasites burst out of it (see below) the pigment is shed into the blood, and is taken up largely by cells of the reticuloendothelial system. It can be seen in those cells in the internal organs, and is strong evidence of previous malarial infection, though similar pigment is seen in the liver in intestinal schistosomiasis.

It has repeatedly been noticed that infection by *P. falciparum* is less intense in children who carry sickle-cell haemoglobin (HbS) or other abnormal haemoglobins (e.g. HbC), than it is in carriers of normal adult Hb. The explanation may be that these abnormal haemoglobins do not effectively supply the nutrients needed by the parasites, but another explanation may be that the circulation, being slowed down in the capillaries, favours the sickling process of the red cells, which collapse, and in which, therefore, the parasites die.

The micromerozoites which invade the red cells grow in size for some hours, and then begin to divide (*schizogony*), the nuclei splitting into daughter nuclei and forming the 'rosettes' characteristic of the *erythrocytic schizont* (or segmenter). Each daughter nucleus attracts its portion of the cytoplasm, and eventually, in about 48 hours (*P. vivax* and *P. ovale*) or 72 hours (*P. malariae*), the daughter parasites (*merozoites*) burst out of the red cells, to invade other red cells and start this phase of the life cycle all over again. In *P. falciparum* the periodicity is about 48 hours but is not so regular as in the other species. Moreover, although the dividing forms (*schizonts*, segmenters or rosettes) of *P. vivax*, *P. ovale* and *P. malariae* can be seen in the peripheral blood, in *P. falciparum* they are mostly present in the blood spaces of the internal organs; indeed, if they are found in the peripheral blood, this is a sign that the infection has become dangerous to life, and is an indication for immediate and urgent treatment, especially in primary infections in non-immune persons.

The numbers of merozoites formed in red cells are:

P. vivax	8–24 (usually 12–18)
P. ovale	6–12 (usually 8)
P. malariae	6–12 (usually 8–10)
P. falciparum	8–32 (usually 8–18)

Although most of the merozoites from the exoerythrocytic schizonts invade red cells, to initiate the asexual cycle as described above, some develop quite differently, into male and female sexual forms (*gametocytes*). The mechanism which determines which merozoites become asexual trophozoites and which become sexual forms is not clear, but the sexual forms appear in the blood, each within a red cell, at a predetermined date.

The gametocytes, male (*microgametocytes*) and female (*macrogametocytes*) do not divide in the human or animal body. Their next stage of development takes place in the stomach of *Anopheles*.

Gametocytes of *P. vivax* (and probably of *P. ovale* and *P. malariae*) can originate not only from merozoites of exoerythrocytic schizonts, but also from merozoites of asexual erythrocytic schizonts, in successive waves. Gametocytes can appear 3 days after the beginning of parasitaemia following heavy sporozoite infection, and about 5 days after infection by inoculation of blood forms which do not lead to exoerythrocytic schizogony. It has usually been thought that gametocytes take twice as long as schizonts to reach maturity, becoming fully grown in 4 days, and circulating in the blood for some time, reaching maximum numbers about 4–6 days after the peak density of asexual parasites.

Hawking *et al.* (1968), however, have produced evidence which strongly suggests that gametocytes of *P. knowlesi*, *P. cynomolgi* (in monkeys) and *P. cathemerium* (in canaries) do not follow this pattern. They take a few hours longer than their asexual cycles to develop to the stage of infectivity for mosquitoes, remaining mature for only a few (5–12) hours, and then quickly degenerate and disappear, to be followed by new gametocytes from each schizogony. This probably applies to all plasmodia which show a synchronous asexual cycle, except perhaps to *P. falciparum*, in which gametocytes take 9–12 days to develop. This biological feature is assumed to be a mechanism which produces short-lived mature gametocytes in the blood to coincide with the biting habits of vector mosquitoes. Further investigation will probably clarify this matter.

The gametocytes of *P. falciparum* when fully developed are crescentic bodies,

longer than the diameter of the red cells in which they grow, with the result that the
red cell membrane is stretched to accommodate this length. The name *falciparum*
reflects this shape; it is derived from the Latin *falx*, a sickle or crescent, and *parere*, to
bring forth.

In the other 3 species the gametocytes are round bodies which almost fill the red
cells in which they grow; they cannot easily be differentiated from trophozoites. The
pigment is scattered through the cytoplasm.

Gametocytes can persist in the blood after asexual forms have disappeared as a
result of treatment (in *P. falciparum* apparently as a result of a small but constant
supply from internal organs). They are not affected by the antibodies which are active
against the asexual forms.

When a thick drop of freshly drawn blood containing mature gametocytes is placed
in a moist atmosphere, a remarkable change which takes place in the male gametocyte

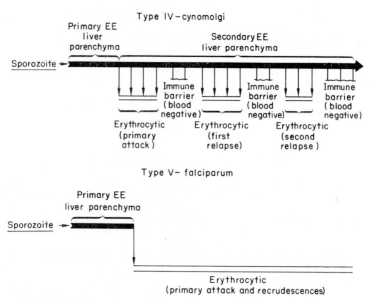

Fig. 277.—Types of exoerythrocytic schizogony. A, *P. cynomolgi*. B,
P. falciparum. (*After World Health Organization 1963*)

can be seen. The parasite sheds its erythrocyte envelope, and throws out several
slender, active *flagella*, each containing nuclear material from the original nucleus.
These flagella lash about vigorously, detaching themselves from the cell body, to swim
free in the plasma. The process of *exflagellation* takes about 10–12 minutes. The
function of these male elements is to fertilize female cells, after the fashion of spermatozoa in other forms of life.

Exflagellation can be achieved as follows (Shute & Maryon 1966): A layer of filter
paper is accurately cut to fit the bottom of a Petri dish, and another to fit the lid. These
papers are then saturated with hot water, completely but without excess. A triangular
piece of glass rod or tube is then placed in the dish, which is immediately closed, and
kept for 1 hour. The operator then makes a thick film of blood on a slide, breathes on
it, and at once places it on the glass rod and replaces the lid. Exflagellation at a temperature of 25°C is complete in 15 minutes for *P. vivax* and *P. ovale* and in 15–30
minutes for *P. falciparum*.

The process of exflagellation and fertilization can take place in the stomach of any biting insect, but only in certain species of *Anopheles* can the parasites infecting man develop further. When a susceptible *Anopheles* takes in mature gametocytes at a blood meal, the male elements go through this process of exflagellation, the flagella moving vigorously in the fluid stomach contents. They are now known as *gametes*.

The female gametocyte has in the meantime freed itself from the erythrocyte membrane, and is also known now as a *gamete*. If a flagellum (male gamete) now meets a female gamete, it enters it, thus fertilizing it, to form a *zygote*. This now elongates, becoming a *travelling vermicule* (*oökinete*) which is able to penetrate one of the epithelial cells lining the mosquito stomach. This done, the oökinete begins to develop, the fertilized nuclear material and the cytoplasm divide and subdivide continuously, forming a cyst (*oöcyst*) which grows and can be seen lying under the elastic membrane on the outer surface of the mosquito stomach if this is removed and examined. Mature oöcysts may number scores or hundreds in a single mosquito. Besides dividing forms, they contain pigment (Fig. 278).

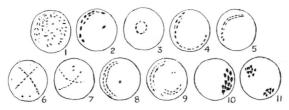

Fig. 278.—Typical arrangement of pigment granules in 3–4 day oöcysts. (*After Shute*)

1, Benign tertian with golden brown pigment. 2–5, Subtertian with black pigment. 6–9, Ovale tertian with dark brown pigment. 10, 11, Quartan with coarse black pigment.

Division of the oöcyst contents continues until it is filled with masses of slender, pointed and nucleated individual forms known as *sporozoites*, about 9 μm in length. These finally burst out of the limiting membrane, flooding the body cavity and even the limbs of the mosquito. Masses of them find their way into the cells of the salivary glands of the mosquito, and thence into the saliva itself, which is injected into the next host on which the mosquito feeds.

Recent work on the electron microscopic examination of sporozoites at high magnifications has shown that their structure is complex. The outer coat is thick, giving a degree of rigidity. At the anterior end there is an organelle which probably produces a proteolytic enzyme to assist penetration of the tissues of the host. Fibrils probably have a locomotory function and mitochondria provide a source of energy. There is a micropyle which may be the point of exit for infective material (Garnham 1966).

Ross's 'black spores'

Sometimes the development of oöcysts is halted, with the formation of these 'black spores' (which are not true spores). They are banana-shaped bodies, dark brown or black, within the thickened oöcyst wall and occasionally in the thoracic muscles near the salivary glands; they are, presumably, chitinized sporozoites. The mechanism of their formation is obscure; it may be the result of unfavourable environmental or biological conditions, and the deposition of dark material by some unknown biological action. Another view is that they are the result of the secretion of chitin around tracheoles or foreign bodies.

SUMMARY OF THE LIFE CYCLE OF MALARIA PARASITES

1. *Sporozoites* in the saliva of infected mosquitoes are injected into man, and enter liver cells where they develop into *exoerythrocytic schizonts* (first generation, *pre-erythrocytic*).

2. These produce *merozoites* (of which the first generation are *cryptozoites*). These:

   a. Enter the circulation (*micromerozoites*), or

   b. Re-enter liver cells (*macromerozoites*).

3. All *exoerythrocyte* generations occurring after parasitaemia becomes possible are known as *phanerozoites*.

4. In the circulation micromerozoites enter red cells to form:

   a. Asexual *trophozoites*, becoming *schizonts* which divide by *schizogony* to form new merozoites which again enter red cells, and

   b. Sexual forms, male (*microgametocytes*) and female (*macrogametocytes*).

5. In the mosquito stomach male gametocytes become *gametes* and produce *flagella* which fertilize female *gametes*, forming *zygotes*, which become motile *oökinetes*.

6. The oökinetes invade the mosquito stomach cells, producing *oöcysts* containing large numbers of *sporozoites* (*sporogony*).

7. Sporozoites enter the salivary glands, to be inoculated into man at subsequent mosquito feeds.

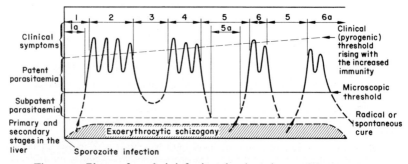

Fig. 279.—Phases of a malaria infection, showing relapses of the recurrent and recrudescent type. *(WHO 1963)*

1, Incubation period. 1a, Prepatent period. 2, Primary attack composed of paroxysms. 3, Latent period (clinical latency). 4, Recrudescence (short-term relapse). 5, Latent period. 5a, Parasitic latency. 6, Clinical recurrence (long-term relapse) followed by parasitic recurrence. 6a, Parasitic relapse.

The terms *relapse, recrudescence* and *recurrence* are commonly used, and need definition.

A *relapse* is a renewed manifestation of clinical symptoms, or parasitaemia, of a malarial infection, and comprises 2 types—*recrudescence* and *recurrence*.

A *recrudescence* is a renewed manifestation due to an increase in the surviving population of erythrocytic forms; blood infection persists.

A *recurrence* (or true relapse) is a renewed manifestation due to multiplication of the parasites in the blood from a secondary exoerythrocytic source; there is no erythrocytic schizogony in the latent period (Garnham 1966).

Malaria may be induced by means other than the bites of infected *Anopheles:*

1. Congenital malaria has been observed, but very rarely, the parasites presumably having crossed the placenta.

2. By the inoculation of infected blood, as in transfusion of inadequately stored infected blood, in malaria therapy for syphilis, or accidentally in drug addicts through the use of unsterilized syringes passed from one person to another. (Hepatitis and septicaemia are other common hazards of this practice.)

In such cases sporozoites are not involved, and therefore the liver stages do not occur; true relapses are not possible, though recrudescences from persisting parasites in the blood are possible. Malaria induced in these ways is easily curable by schizontocidal drugs.

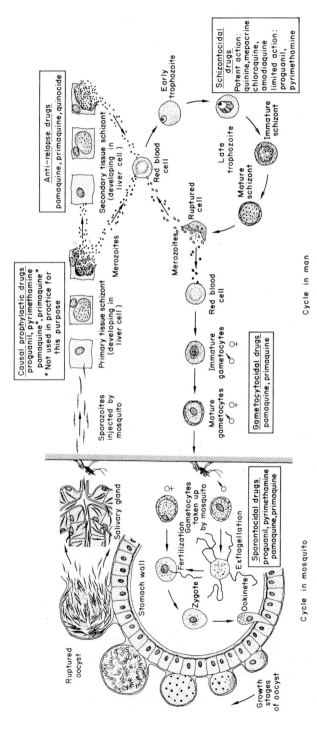

Fig. 280.—Action of antimalarial drugs in relation to the life cycle of malaria parasites. (*After Alvarado & Bruce-Chwatt 1962*)

FEATURES OF THE VARIOUS PARASITES OF MAN

Trophozoites

P. vivax. The first stage is the ring stage, when a vacuole forms, surrounded by a loop of thin cytoplasm, and a small round nucleus, sometimes in the loop. The ring enlarges within a few hours, and the cytoplasm becomes amoeboid, throwing out pseudopodia in rapid movements which justify the name *vivax.* Minute grains of light brown pigment appear in the cytoplasm.

The red cell enlarges and becomes pale, the whole cell developing the tiny spots known as Schüffner's dots, which stain red with Romanowsky stains at a suitably alkaline pH.

At about 24 hours the parasite occupies most of the red cell, the vacuole disappears, and the cytoplasm becomes more dense. At about 36 hours a proportion of the parasitized red cells retreat into the blood spaces of the internal organs (though not so many as in *P. falciparum*). The nucleus divides and subdivides until, typically, there are 16 daughter nuclei (though the number varies), each attracting a portion of cytoplasm. This is the rosette stage. The pigment granules agglomerate and at maturity consist of a very few dark brown collections, though not so well coalesced or so big as in *P. falciparum.*

The red cell is now enlarged to about 10 μm in diameter, is always heavily stippled and may be distorted; it ruptures to set free the merozoites and pigment. The pigment is taken up by phagocytes or by cells of the reticulo-endothelial system. The merozoites measure about 1·5 μm; they have no pigment.

Although the process of schizogony is never absolutely regular, maximum segmentation usually takes place in the afternoon.

In a mixed infection with *P. falciparum* the parasitaemia by *P. vivax* is likely to be inhibited because *P. falciparum* is dominant, overshadowing *P. vivax*, which may be missed. When the activity of *P. falciparum* subsides, *P. vivax* multiplies without hindrance, and can be seen.

The asexual cycle in the blood is repeated until a peak occurs about 2 weeks after the first patency. Parasites then become fewer until there is a recrudescence in about a month. Recrudescences are repeated a few times until a condition of latency occurs as immunity is established, when merozoites from the liver stages are taken up by phagocytes before they can do any harm. Immunity, which is stimulated by merozoites, then declines until, after a period, a relapse takes place.

P. ovale. The development of this species in red cells resembles that of *P. vivax*; its periodicity is rather more than tertian, the merozoites taking 49–50 hours to grow to mature schizonts. The red cells show dots which are less numerous than Schüffner's dots of *P. vivax*, and have a violet tinge; they have been named James's dots. The cells become slightly enlarged, with weakening of the cell envelope, so that in thin films the cells (which are globular and stick to the slide) are distorted by the process of spreading, and are seen as oval bodies with ragged or fimbriated edges. In humid conditions when films dry slowly this character may not be seen, but it is an important indication of a change in the physical state of the red cells.

P. ovale often shows prolonged latency of months before the first attack, and relapses tend to occur after intervals of about 3 months.

P. malariae. The asexual forms may be very scanty in the blood, even when the patient is experiencing definite attacks of fever every 72 hours. Trophozoites are seen in mature red cells, unlike the other species which favour reticulocytes, but cells harbouring very young rings have not been recorded. The trophozoites live longer in the red cells than the other species. They are less amoeboid than *P. vivax*, and band forms are characteristic, reaching from side to side of the cells. This appearance may be an artefact, the parasite being distorted by the process of spreading thin films—band forms do not occur in thick drops. The pigment is dark brown or black, and tends to collect on one edge of the band, and a linear nucleus is seen on the other edge.

The nucleus begins to divide after 48 hours, and the rosette form is mature at 72 hours, usually giving 8 merozoites, occasionally up to 12 but no more. The schizont usually ruptures in the morning or early afternoon.

P. malariae does not cause the red cell to enlarge, but after prolonged staining it produces characteristic (Ziemann) stippling with fine red-staining dots. This is difficult to demonstrate, and is more important by its absence than by its presence, since in a well stained film, parasites with undotted erythrocytes are almost certainly *P. malariae*.

P. falciparum is vicious; it attacks both young and mature red cells, which then show a brassy coloration. The rings are small (1·2 μm) and hair-like, with thin cytoplasm, a prominent nucleus and a vacuole. The nucleus may be double. Appliqué forms are common, as is multiple infection of red cells. The trophozoites are very variable in shape and size. Except in pernicious attacks, however, only the ring forms and gametocytes are usually seen in routine examination in the peripheral blood, the developing stages and schizonts usually hiding in the blood spaces of internal organs— spleen, bone marrow, placenta, brain and others. This has long been recognized as a feature of this infection. Schizonts, however, can often be found very scantily in the peripheral blood after careful critical scrutiny—in 2% of light infections to 26–60% of heavy infections. They tend to be found in non-immune or susceptible persons in whom there has been fever for several days before administration of antimalarial drugs.

At 24 hours the parasite is a thick ring and the vacuole begins to disappear; at this time the retreat to the internal organs begins, and consequently fewer may be seen in the peripheral blood.

The red cell begins to show 6–12 marks known as Maurer's clefts, which may be the result of loss of substance from the surface of the cell as a result of the attack by the parasite, and these show as red blotches if stained with a Romanowsky stain at pH 7·2–7·4, rather longer than usual. The red cell is now darker, and purplish, with a red edging.

In the internal organs the nucleus of the schizont begins to divide, and the pigment collects into a dark brown or black mass. The number of merozoites produced varies from 8 to 32, but these extremes are rare. The periodicity is tertian, at about 48 hours.

Of peripheral red cells 25% or more may be infected, and at this intensity a patient in his first attack, without acquired immunity (or passive from the mother in young infants) usually dies. Peak density is commonly reached in 10–14 days from the beginning of parasitaemia, after which the numbers quickly decline. In untreated cases recrudescences can be expected once or twice a month for 6–9 months, occasionally considerably longer.

Gametocytes (crescents) are never seen in the peripheral blood until about the tenth day of parasitaemia.

Gametocytes

P. vivax. Mature gametocytes appear about the third day of an attack, and immediately after a relapse. They are compact spherical bodies without vacuoles and with denser cytoplasm round a central nucleus. The red cells are enlarged and show Schüffner's dots. The fully grown gametocyte occupies most of the red cell, measuring 10–11 μm. The female stains bright blue with Romanowsky stains; the male is more grey. The male nucleus is larger than the female, and stains more pink. In each the pigment is in the form of fine granules (coarser in the male) throughout the cytoplasm. The male gametocyte is smaller than the female.

The gametocytes take 4 days to mature, reaching their peak density 4–6 days after the peak of asexual forms. There are more females than males. Exceptionally, red cells may contain 2 gametocytes, or a gametocyte and a schizont.

P. ovale. The gametocytes first appear, fully grown, on the fifth day of parasitaemia, becoming more numerous until in 3 weeks there are enough to infect mosquitoes effectively.

They resemble solid asexual forms, but the scanty pigment is coarser and darker. They fill the red cells, measuring about 9 μm. Stained gametocytes have a lilac colour, less vivid in the males.

P. malariae. The gametocytes do not usually appear until late, about 5–23 days after the asexual forms. They are at peak density about 6 days after the peak of asexual forms, and then they diminish. In endemic areas they are found only in young children. The male has a large nucleus which stains pink, the cytoplasm being greenish-grey owing to fine black pigment granules. The parasite fills the red cell, which is not enlarged. The female is difficult to identify because it resembles the large uninucleate asexual form. It is spherical, about 7 μm, with a central nucleus and fine pigment granules. The cytoplasm stains deep blue.

P. falciparum. Elongated gametocytes are numerous in the peripheral blood of young children (maximum at 9 months to 2 years of age) in endemic areas and after primary attacks, reaching 14 600/mm³; they are rare in older children and adults. Young children are therefore the effective sources of mosquito infection.

The gametocytes appear in the peripheral blood in a wave, fully grown, 8–11 days after the asexual forms, rising to a peak and slowly falling until at about 3 weeks they have usually disappeared, though some may be found for several months. They are not numerous after the parasitaemia of recrudescence, presumably because those of the first attack have provoked some immunity. If the first attack is aborted by quinine or sulphamethazine, gametocytes appear 10–14 days later in enormous numbers.

The gametocytes are characteristically crescentic, but may be spindle-, diamond-, oat-, or cigar-shaped, containing a few grains of pigment concentrated round the nucleus; the pigment does not clump as in the schizonts.

Occasionally certain inclusions known as Garnham bodies have been found in red cells harbouring developing gametocytes. These are thick filaments, loops or bars, staining deep red with Romanowsky stains. Their origin is uncertain.

Gametocytes of *P. falciparum* are not destroyed by the schizontocidal drugs, whereas gametocytes of *P. vivax* and probably also of *P. ovale* and *P. malariae* are destroyed by them.

INFECTION OF ANIMALS BY THE MALARIA PARASITES OF MAN

P. vivax

The chimpanzee is partially susceptible to sporozoites, which produce exoerythrocytic schizonts pursuing a normal course, though blood infection is submicroscopic. If the spleen is removed the animal is much more vulnerable and parasitaemia is heavy, with the production of infective gametocytes, and recrudescences. *Aotus* monkeys are very susceptible, but rhesus monkeys are totally immune.

P. ovale

The chimpanzee has been infected with sporozoites, to the stage of exoerythrocytic schizogony, but not further unless the spleen is removed, when the animal becomes completely susceptible, showing heavy parasitaemia, schizonts and gametocytes.

P. malariae

This is the only human parasite which occurs for certain in animals. In the chimpanzee it has repeatedly been found in nature in West Africa, though the incidence is low. It could conceivably be a natural source of infection for man. In the chimpanzee infection is light unless the spleen is removed, after which it flares up, with recrudescences and the production of gametocytes (Bray 1965).

P. falciparum

Blood containing trophozoites has been shown to be infective to newborn mice and splenectomized gibbons, and the gibbons have been infected by the bites of *A. balabacensis*. *Aotus* monkeys are susceptible, and young howler monkeys (*Alouatta palliata*) have also been infected by the injection of enormous numbers of blood forms. In the chimpanzee, sporozoites develop to exoerythrocytic schizonts, and merozoites invade red cells, but do not develop further unless the spleen is removed, when schizonts and gametocytes appear.

PARASITES OF ANIMALS CAPABLE OF INFECTING MAN

Apart from *P. malariae* of chimpanzees, several other malaria parasites of primates can infect man.

Benign tertian type

P. cynomolgi is a tertian parasite of *Macaca irus*, *M. nemestrina*, *Presbytis* spp. and other monkeys of the Far East. It is capable of infecting a large variety of *Anopheles*, and man is slightly susceptible to infection by sporozoites, though parasitaemia is light. Nevertheless, the clinical response may be quite severe, and infections can last for some weeks.

P. cynomolgi bastianellii is a tertian parasite of *M. irus* in the Far East, transmitted by several species of *Anopheles*. Man has several times been infected accidentally in the laboratory when working with infected mosquitoes, and although parasitaemia is low, the clinical response with fever, enlargement of the spleen and liver and production of gametocytes, is quite severe. In experimental work the red cells of Negroes are resistant whereas whites are susceptible; the red cells of New World monkeys are resistant, but liver stages have been found.

Ovale type

P. simium is a tertian parasite of *ovale* type, infecting *Alouatta fusca* in southern Brazil and, experimentally, *Saimiri sciureus* and *Callithrix jacchus*. Man has been infected in nature, and can be infected by the bites of infected *A. cruzii*.

Quartan type

P. brasilianum is a parasite of South American monkeys of the genera *Cacajao*, *Alouatta*, *Ateles*, *Cebus*, *Saimiri* and *Lagothrix*. It can be transmitted to man by the bite of infected *A. freeborni*, producing slight parasitaemia and quartan fever with splenomegaly.

P. inui is normally a parasite of *Macaca irus* (formerly known as *M. inuus*, hence the name), *M. nemestrina*, *M. mulatta* and other monkeys. In the Far East it is transmitted by *A. stephensi* and can experimentally infect other *Anopheles*. Man can be infected experimentally by the blood forms, but parasitaemia and febrile reaction are slight.

P. shortti is a parasite of *M. radiata* and *M. sinica* of S. India and Ceylon, probably transmitted by *A. stephensi*. Man has been infected experimentally with sporozoites, but the infection was mild (Coatney *et al.* 1966).

Knowlesi type

P. knowlesi is a quotidian (24-hour periodicity) parasite of *M. irus*, *M. nemestrina* and *Presbytis melalophos* in the Far East, in which it produces a low level of parasitaemia, though it is much more severe and fatal in *M. mulatta*. It is transmitted by *A. hackeri*, and experimentally by several other species. Man is susceptible to inoculation of blood forms, which produce clinical effects varying from mild to severe; it has been used for malaria therapy of advanced syphilis. Chin *et al.* (1965) reported probable infection of man by mosquitoes in nature, but this has not been proved experimentally. *P. knowlesi* has been extensively used in studies on pathology and immunity in monkeys.

MALARIA PARASITES OF RODENTS AND BIRDS

The malaria parasites of rodents—*P. berghei*, *P. berghei yoelii*, *P. vinckei*—have been much used in the study of parasites and their effects on vertebrate hosts. Man is not susceptible to them, and they are therefore not described here. The same is true of the parasites of birds—*P. gallinaceum*, *P. relictum*, *P. cathemerium*, *P. circumflexum* and others.

Biologists who wish to study these parasites, or to use them for research, are referred to the comprehensive book by Garnham (1966).

STAINING MALARIA PARASITES

The techniques briefly noted here are taken largely from a detailed paper by Shute (1966); readers are advised to consult the original.

Clean slides and neutral distilled water are essential for good results. Distilled water is usually too acid, and if possible the pH should be tested. If this is not possible, a test can be made by adding a few drops of haematoxylin stain to 5 ml of water in a test-tube; if the solution remains reddish pink after shaking, the water is acid, and alkali (a few drops of saturated lithium carbonate or other alkali solution, after filtration) should be added—about 5 drops of alkali to 5 litres of distilled water is about right. Buffer salts are better:

Potassium dihydrogen phosphate, KH_2PO_4	0·7 gramme
Disodium hydrogen phosphate, Na_2HPO_4 (anhydrous)	1·0 gramme
Distilled water	1000 ml

Or buffer tablets (G. Gurr, London) may be used. The pH (normally 7·2) should be tested, and necessary adjustments made. The solution keeps well for many months if well stoppered.

Thin films, Giemsa stain

Fix with 1–2 drops methanol; allow to evaporate. Make a 5% solution of the stain in the prepared distilled water, mix thoroughly and cover the film; leave for 20–30 minutes. Wash with distilled water from an aspirator.

Thin films, Leishman stain

With the slide on a level bench add 7–8 drops of stain. Leave for 20 seconds, *not more*, then add 12–15 drops of distilled water (pH 7·2). Mix thoroughly without spilling the stain; leave for 20 minutes and then wash off with distilled water from an aspirator.

Thick drops, Giemsa stain

The drops should be not too thick, about 10–15 leucocytes/field. They should be quite dry, having been protected against flies, which eat the blood. The slide should be placed in a plastic or glass staining jar, and the 5% stain (see above) should be gently poured on until the slide is submerged. Leave staining for 20 minutes, and then gently run in distilled water at one end, from an aspirator, to wash off the stain. This stain diluted with distilled water stains the envelopes of erythrocytes; to overcome this, dilution with normal saline is advocated; it dissolves the envelopes and leaves a clear background. Good results are claimed if the thick drop if first lysed with 3 drops of 0·5 or 1% saponin solution for about 5 sec (with gentle agitation); this is then drained off and the preparation is stained with Wright or Wright-Giemsa. The saponin does not appear to lyse the parasites, and there is less background debris (Umlas & Fallon 1971).

To prepare Leishman stain

Into a clean, dry and securely stoppered polythene jar or hard glass flask, place about 50 large glass beads, 200 ml methanol (analar) and 0·3 gramme of Leishman crystals. Stopper tightly and shake vigorously for a few minutes. Repeat the shaking at least 6 times at frequent intervals. The stain is ready in 24 hours.

Field's stain

Two solutions are used:

Solution A

Methylene blue (medicinal)	0·8 gramme
Azur 1	0·5 gramme
Disodium hydrogen phosphate (anhydrous)	5·0 grammes
Potassium dihydrogen phosphate	6·25 grammes
Distilled water	500·0 ml

Solution B

Eosin	1·0 gramme
Disodium hydrogen phosphate (anhydrous)	5·0 grammes
Potassium dihydrogen phosphate	6·25 grammes
Distilled water	500·0 ml

Dissolve the phosphate salts and then add the stain. Leave for 24 hours and then filter.

If the anhydrous salt is not available, sodium phosphate cryst. B.P. ($Na_2HPO_4.12$ H_2O), 12·6 grammes, can be used.

In surveys of an infected population (preferably children) there may be heavy infections of 1000 parasites/mm³ of blood. These can usually be found by examining a few fields of a thick film, but lighter infections of 100/mm³ or less may be missed on such cursory examination.

The World Health Organization (1963) suggests that the standard time for examination of a thick blood film should be 5 minutes, during which the average microscopist can examine 100 fields, representing 0·1–0·2 mm³ of blood. A thin film containing the same amount of blood will take 10–20 times as long to examine.

STAINING POST MORTEM AND BIOPSY MATERIAL
(Shute & Maryon 1966)

Post mortem material should be examined as soon as possible after death, because malaria parasites become unrecognizable within a few hours. Smears are better than sections because the parasites stain better, and smears can be made more quickly.

Brain

A small portion no bigger than a pin-head is squashed between two dry slides, which are then dragged over each other, under pressure, to give 2 thin smears. When quite dry they are fixed for 5–10 minutes in methyl alcohol, and stained with Geimsa (7 ml) in distilled water (100 ml) at pH 7–7·2 for 30 minutes, then flushed with distilled water and dried. They are then soaked for 5 minutes in normal saline to remove most of the methylene blue from the tissue cells, and washed with distilled water to remove all salt particles. In brain material the capillaries are well preserved. If a post mortem cannot be conducted, material withdrawn in a large hollow needle inserted beneath the eyelid and through the orbital plate into the brain is satisfactory; suction is applied.

Spleen and other organs

A small piece of pulpy material from the spleen is broken down in a few drops of saline, and thin films are prepared from this, fixed in methyl alcohol and stained with Giemsa. Material from the heart, liver, kidney and bone marrow can be treated in the same way.

CULTIVATION OF *P. falciparum* IN VITRO

About 10–20 ml of blood containing numerous rings of fairly large size (early rings do not grow well) are placed in a sterile test-tube and either defibrinated or prevented from clotting by the addition of heparin or sequestrene. The blood can be defibrinated with a thick wire passed through the cotton plug of the tube, and having a loop at the lower end. The wire is rapidly rotated and then withdrawn with the clot, after which the tube is plugged. 0·2 ml of a 50% sterile solution of dextrose is added and mixed thoroughly. The tube is incubated upright at 37°C.

The erythrocytes quickly become sedimented below the buffy coat, and the parasites grow in the erythrocytes immediately below the buffy coat. The tube must not be tilted when the upper erythrocytes are withdrawn by capillary pipette (with a little of the serum) for staining as thin films after incubation for various intervals up to 36–48 hours. Segmenting forms are usually most common after cultivation for 24–36 hours.

More complicated media have been developed. The techniques are elaborate; for information see Garnham (1966).

TEST FOR SENSITIVITY OF *P. falciparum* TO CHLOROQUINE

In this test 1 ml of blood, defibrinated with glass beads, is incubated for 24 hours at 37°C with glucose and chloroquine at various concentrations. Control blood is incubated with glucose only. Nuclear division is assessed in thick blood films stained with Giemsa and the controls are compared with the specimens exposed to various concentrations of chloroquine (Rieckmann *et al.* 1968).

FAMILY: BABESIIDAE (PIROPLASMS)
GENUS: *Babesia*

Members of this genus are parasites of cattle, dogs and other animals. They are pear-shaped bodies which invade and divide in red blood cells, and can be mistaken for malaria parasites when they appear in man, which has occurred very occasionally in persons whose spleens had been removed and who therefore had a defective immune mechanism. The parasites are transmitted by ticks. They have some immunological affinity with malaria parasites of animals. They cause piroplasmosis in animals and redwater in cattle, and a fever in man. Quinuronium sulphate (Babesan, Pirevan) is used in the treatment of animals with this infection. Chloroquine has been used in 1 human case, apparently with success.

COCCIDIA

ORDER: COCCIDIA
FAMILY: EIMERIIDAE

Coccidia are intracellular protozoa with a life cycle consisting of alternation of generations—an asexual cycle (*schizogony*), alternating with a sexual cycle (*sporogony*). A single zygote encysted as an oöcyst produces secondary cysts (*sporocysts*), which give rise to a number of sporozoites. The life history of a typical coccidium (*Eimeria*), which causes disease of the rabbit liver, closely resembles that of the malaria parasite. This led Pfeiffer in 1892 to predict, with some accuracy, the probable malaria cycle in the mosquito. The sporozoites, liberated from the sporocyst, penetrate epithelial cells where they develop into schizonts, characterized by a vesicular nucleus and karyosome. The *nucleus* divides by repeated fission till a number of daughter-nuclei are produced and the schizont divides into as many merozoites. When the cell bursts, *merozoites* are set free and, entering other cells, develop either into *schizonts* or *gametocytes*, male or female.

The male gametocyte develops by mitosis of the nucleus, forming *microgametes*, which are small, slender bodies. When the host cell bursts, these microgametes are liberated and enter the female cell (*macrogamete*). The fertilized cell (*zygote*) secretes a tough membrane and becomes an *oöcyst*.

The nucleus of the penetrating microgamete then fuses with the female nucleus (*synkarion*). The zygote breaks up into 4 *sporoblasts*, which, when enclosed by a tough envelope, are known as *sporocysts*, and within this the protoplasm divides into 2 *sporozoites*. In order to develop further, the oöcyst has to pass out in the faeces and be swallowed by a new host, whereupon the tough membranes dissolve and *sporozoites* are liberated.

Eimeria stiedae is a common parasite of the rabbit. A somewhat similar coccidium has been reported in the human liver, and named *E. gubleri* (Guiart 1922). The first cases of hepatic coccidiosis in man were described by Gubler in 1858 and by Virchow in 1860; three more were reported by Dobell in 1919. This parasite has a special affinity for hepatic tissue. The cysts are ellipsoid, measuring 46 × 34 μm. Woodcock and Wenyon originally discovered coccidial cysts (*Isospora*) in human faeces in 1915. Dobell (1919) described cysts of the genus *Eimeria* as occasionally occurring in man.

INTESTINAL COCCIDIA
GENUS: *Isospora*
Isospora hominis (Rivolta, 1898) Dobell, 1919 (Fig. 281)

Synonym: *I. belli*. (All authorities are not agreed that this synonym is correct. Hoare considers that *I. hominis* and *I. belli* are distinct; the former probably a parasite of the dog, the latter of man.) The oöcysts are found in the faeces and have been seen in fluid from duodenal intubation.

Though undoubtedly a parasite of the epithelium of the small intestine, possibly the duodenum, this coccidium is not seriously pathogenic, though it may be the cause of a debilitating diarrhoea, in which the stools contain pus cells and Charcot-Leyden

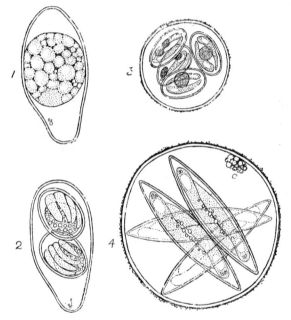

Fig. 281.—Oöcysts of Coccidia found in human faeces. × 1000 (*After Dobell*)

1, *Isospora hominis*, undeveloped cyst. 2, *Isospora hominis*, fully developed spores. 3, *Eimeria clupearum*, fully developed oöcyst and spores. 4, *Eimeria sardinae*, fully developed oöcyst and spores.

crystals, as shown by Connal in a technician who swallowed material containing ripe oöcysts of *I. belli*. In addition there were cysts in the faeces and associated eosinophilia. Nevertheless, the schizogonic cycle of development in the intestine is not yet known. The oöcysts are elongated, with tapering extremities; they vary in length from 18 to 33 μm and in breadth from 12·5 to 16 μm. The oöcyst wall is clear and colourless; the contained *zygote* is usually unsegmented, but occasionally segmentation into sporoblasts has been observed. Further development takes place in the faeces: two ovoid sporoblasts become enclosed in sporocysts measuring 14 × 7–9 μm. In each eventually 4 sporozoites are produced. At least 2 species of *Isospora* infect man, one corresponding to *I. belli* (Wenyon) and the other to *I. hominis* (Rivolta) as follows:

I. belli may be passed at all stages of development, immature forms mature in up to 5 days. Oöcyst 30 × 12 μm: sporocyst 11 × 9 μm. Usually no oöcystic residual body; sporocystic residual body finely granular with limiting membrane, compact and centrally placed between 4 sporozoites. The sporocysts are relatively larger than those of *I. hominis*.

I. hominis is usually passed fully developed. Oöcyst wall is usually absent. Sporocysts may be single or coupled in pairs, each being 15 × 10 μm. Sporocystic residual body of coarse loosely aggregated granules appearing polar in position, separate from the 4 sporozoites.

A single case of infection with *I. rivolta* has been reported and there is a possibility that *I. hominis* and *I. bigemina* are of the same species.

I. natalensis. This species resembles *I. rivolta* in its cystic stage. The cyst measures 30 × 24 × 21 μm and the sporocysts occupy an equatorial position and measure 17 × 12 μm. They contain an irregular residue of loose, coarse granules.

For clinical features see page 152.

Cysts of the genus *Eimeria* have been seen in faeces, but they are not really parasitic in man, but are passed through the intestine after eating fish infected with *E. clupearum* or *E. sardinae* (Fig. 281).

ORDER: EUCOCCIDIA
SUBORDER: EIMERIINA
GENUS: Toxoplasma (Nicolle & Manceaux, 1908)

Life history

Toxoplasma gondii is a coccidian parasite belonging to the Sporozoa. There is an asexual cycle of schizogony which takes place in an intermediate host (any mammal including man) and a sexual cycle of gametogony which takes place in the intestinal

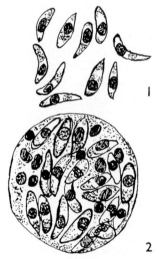

Fig. 282.—Types of spore of *Toxoplasma gondii*. (*After Carini & Mariel*).
1, Various forms. 2, Groups of spores resulting from schizogony.

epithelium of the definitive host, the cat, which is infected by eating uncooked flesh, e.g. of rodents or pigs. Trophozoites (toxoplasms) undergo schizogony and form merozoites intracellularly in many tissues; as the immune response of the host develops they form into schizonts (pseudocysts) containing up to 100 organisms. One schizogonic cycle or more occurs in the intestinal epithelial cells before merozoites are released; these develop into macro- and microgametocytes which form oöcysts from which sporozoites are released in the faeces and which are infective to the intermediate hosts.

Morphology

In man only 2 phases have been observed: the trophozoites or proliferative forms and the cysts (oöcysts and schizonts). Trophozoites are typically curved or crescent-shaped measuring 4–6 μm in length 2–3 μm breadth with one end more rounded. When stained with Giemsa the cytoplasm stains blue and the nucleus is a red or purple irregular mass occupying one-fifth or one-quarter of the cell and eccentric in position. The ultra-structure as shown by electron microscopy reveals the organism to be a sporozoan. There is a distinct membrane and a clump of densely staining material.

A *micropyle* 100 nm thick is found in the centre of the organism. Inside the organism there are peripheral fibrils (toxonemes) terminating at the polar ring. The anterior tip is provided with a strong *conoid* or truncated cone in which are the anterior parts of the paired *organelles* which are the secreting *mitochondria*. The *oöcyst* (cystic form) reaches the size of 100 μm in diameter and contains thousands of undeveloped *Toxoplasma*, each enclosed in a large red pellicle 6 μm in width. The *schizont* (pseudocyst) contains fewer (up to 100) *Toxoplasma* and represents schizogony in every type of parenchymal cell.

For details of pathology and treatment see page 148.

CLASS: ZOOMASTIGOPHOREA
ORDER: PROTOMASTIGIDA
FAMILY: TRYPANOSOMATIDAE Doflein, 1901

The Trypanosomatidae are haemoflagellates that live in the tissues of their hosts. The family is divided into six genera:

1. *Leptomonas*, which have an amastigote (*Leishmania*) and promastigote (*Leptomonas*) stage and are found only in invertebrates.

2. *Crithidia*, which have an amastigote, promastigote and epimastigote (*Crithidia*) stage and occur only in invertebrates.

3. *Herpetomonas*, which have an amastigote, promastigote, epimastigote, and trypomastigote (*Trypanosoma*) stage and occur only in invertebrates.

4. *Leishmania*, which like the genus *Leptomonas* have an amastigote and promastigote stage but have both vertebrate and invertebrate hosts.

5. *Phytomonas*, which have an amastigote and promastigote stage but have both an invertebrate and plant host.

6. *Trypanosoma*, which have an amastigote, promastigote, epimastigote and trypomastigote stage and have both an invertebrate and invertebrate host. They are classified as Salivaria (anterior station development) and Stercoraria (posterior station development). A sphaeromastigote stage, rounded with a flagellum, has been described.

Two genera can cause human disease:

1. *Trypanosoma*. The *T. brucei* group produces *trypomastigotes* in the blood of the mammalian host and *epimastigotes* in the invertebrate host. *Sphaeromastigote* forms have been seen completely blocking some of the capillaries in the choroid plexus of rats infected with *T. br. rhodesiense*. The *T. cruzi* group has trypomastigotes in the gut of the insect host and in the blood of man, amastigotes intracellularly in the mammalian host and epimastigotes in the midgut of the insect host.

2. *Leishmania*, which produce amastigotes intracellularly in the mammalian host and promastigotes in the midgut and proboscis of the insect vector.

GENUS: *Trypanosoma* Gruby, 1843

Trypanosomes are trypomastigotes, which are minute, actively motile, flattened, fusiform protozoa (Fig. 284). The body is slender, sloping to a fine point anteriorly,

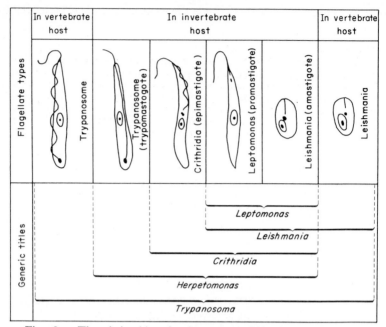

Fig. 283.—The relationships of various genera of blood and tissue flagellates and the morphology of the various developmental forms and species. (*After Wenyon*)

while the posterior may be pointed or blunt. In general shape it resembles a curved flattened blade.

Ultrastructure

The trypomastigote of the *T. brucei* group has a compact proteinaceous surface coat which, it has been suggested, contains the trypanosome's variant antigen.

The *nucleus* is centrally situated and contains a central *karyosome*, a distinct membrane and Feulgen-positive submembranous granules.

The *kinetoplast*, which is usually placed posterior to the nucleus, sometimes in close proximity, is disc-shaped, about 1 μm in size, consisting of a spherical or rod-shaped parabasal body of variable size connected anteriorly by one or more delicate fibrils with a small basic granule, the *blepharoplast*. The kinetoplast may be absent (akinetoplastic stage) especially in trypanosomes transmitted mechanically. The *axoneme*,

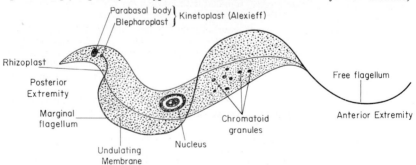

Fig. 284.—Schema of *Trypanosoma*. (*After Dobell*)

which is the striated sheathed axial filament of the flagellum, arises from the blepharo-plast and passes forward along the margin of the undulating membrane, terminating sometimes at the anterior end but more usually continuing forward as the *flagellum* which is composed of cross-striated parallel fibrils united to form a cable enclosed in a protoplasmic sheath. Granules and refractile cytoplasmic inclusions occur in the blood forms of certain trypomastigotes and some of these are *volutin* granules, the number and appearance of which may be connected with the antigenic response of the parasite to the resistance of the host, while others may be produced by drugs such as antrycide, dimidium and stilbamidine. The granules are composed of RNA and protein and those caused by chemotherapy contain the drug responsible for their production and this actually inhibits the growth of the cell. Trypaflavine dyes and prothidium induce akinetoplasia by inhibition of DNA synthesis in the kinetoplast.

Multiplication takes place by binary fission. The blepharoplast and kinetoplast divide first, followed by mitosis of the nucleus and formation of a new flagellum and membrane. The body then divides longitudinally in an anteroposterior direction.

If all the individual trypomastigote forms possess a free flagellum, then the species is monomorphic, e.g. *T. cruzi*. If some individuals do and some do not the species is polymorphic, e.g. *T. brucei*.

Metabolism

Respiration of the various species depends upon different enzyme systems. The blood forms of the *T. evansi* and *T. brucei* groups are not inhibited by cyanide, owing perhaps to the possession of a dehydrogenase system, while the *T. lewisi* group is strongly inhibited owing to the presence of a respiratory enzyme system dependent upon heavy metals. Trypomastigote respiratory metabolism is profoundly different from the epimastigote, the change being initiated in the short blood stream form.

Carbohydrate metabolism. Trypomastigotes cannot store carbohydrates and are dependent for sources of energy upon supplies from the host. The blood forms of the African trypanosomes have a high rate of sugar consumption, while *T. cruzi* consumes practically none at all. Cultural forms require less sugar. Glucose is the chief source of energy but fructose and mannose may also be used. Of the disaccharides, maltose and sucrose are utilized more than lactose. A number of glyocolytic enzymes have been identified and phosphorylation demonstrated. In *T. rhodesiense* the end-products of fermentation are pyruvic, lactic, formic, acetic and succinic acids, ethyl alcohol and glycerol.

The arsenical drugs block the early stages of carbohydrate metabolism in the African trypanosomes but have no effect on *T. cruzi*, since this consumes little sugar. Since the diamidines lower blood sugar this may interfere with the carbohydrate metabolism of the parasites.

Protein metabolism. Cultural stages can derive energy from protein but it is doubtful whether the blood forms of the African trypanosomes can break down protein.

Viability

T. br. rhodesiense and *T. br. gambiense* have remained viable for 8 months in citrated blood at $-79°C$ but only for 1–3 days at -20 to $-40°C$ and in 10% glycerol for 7 days at $-20°C$ and 14 days at $-40°C$. Blood, or culture or fly forms can be preserved for long periods at $-80°C$ (Cunningham *et al.* 1963).

Cultivation

Trypomastigotes can be cultured in non-cellular media, tissue culture and chick embryo. *T. br. gambiense* can be cultured in Weinman's medium and *T. cruzi* grows readily on media to which blood has been added, such as NNN medium.

NNN medium (Novy, MacNeal and Nicolle's medium). The formula is as follows:

Agar	14 grammes
Sodium chloride	6 grammes
Distilled water	900 ml

Mix and bring to the boiling point then distribute in tubes and sterilize in the auto-clave. The tubed medium is melted and cooled to 48°C and to each tube one-third of its volume of defibrinated rabbit blood is added. This is mixed well with the medium by rotating the tube, after which the tubes are slanted and allowed to cool. Water of condensation is allowed to form and it is in this water in which growth occurs.

Weinman's medium. The medium consists of NaCl 8 grammes and distilled water to make up 900 ml. Citrated human plasma and human haemoglobin (1 part of blood with 3 parts of distilled water) 20 ml. The NaCl solution is autoclaved, the haemo-globin mixture added and the medium adjusted to pH 7·4–7·5. It is dispensed in rubber-stoppered test-tubes and incubated at 26–28°C.

Separation from blood. Trypanosomes can be separated from large quantities of blood by concentration methods described on page 99. Trypanosomes of the *T. brucei* group can also be separated from blood by virtue of the fact that they bear a smaller negative charge than the erythrocytes. The technique involves blood diluted with phosphate buffered glucose saline at pH 8, which is layered on to the surface of an anion exchange column (DEAE-cellulose) and then added continuously to maintain a sharp descending front of erythrocytes. The trypanosomes are eluted with buffered saline, but the erythrocytes remain adsorbed. The trypanosomes are motile and in-fective. *T. cruzi* is not separated by this method (Lanham 1968).

Transmission

With the exception of *T. equiperdum*, which passes from horse to horse during coitus, trypanosomes are transmitted by bloodsucking invertebrates, usually insects, but in fish and turtles by leeches.

In *T. evansi* this transmission is mechanical and the bloodsucking fly, after feeding, bites an uninfected host within a short interval, in this manner inoculating directly those trypanosomes which adhere to the proboscis.

In most cases, however, transmission is effected by a development cycle (cyclical development) in the fly so that after an infective feed a definite intrinsic period is passed through before the fly is capable of conveying the disease. The infective stage is then known as a *metacyclic trypanosome*. The trypanosomes are classified according to which of two types of cyclical development takes place:

a. Salivaria (anterior station). Development commences in the stomach of the fly, trypanosomes spreading forward to the proboscis and salivary glands or solely confined to the proboscis. This group contains the *T. brucei* trypanosomes.

b. Stercoraria (posterior station). Development commences in the stomach and trypano-somes pass backwards to the hindgut. This group contains the *T. cruzi* trypanosomes. In the *Salivaria* metacyclic trypanosomes are inoculated during the act of biting, whilst in the *Stercoraria* they escape in the faeces of the insect and infect their host through the mucous membrane or the puncture made by the insect in the skin.

Life cycle of Salivaria

The pathogenic trypanosomes of Africa are transmitted by species of tsetse fly, *Glossina*, in which three subspecies developing in the anterior station are known to occur: *T. br. gambiense (Glossina palpalis, G. tachinoides), T. br. rhodesiense (G. morsitans, G. pallidipes, G. swynnertoni, G. fuscipes)* and *T. br. brucei (G. morsitans).* The ingested trypomastigotes start to develop in the stomach where long slender individuals are evolved. In the stomach an important function is subserved by the *peritrophic membrane.* This is a soft cylindrical membrane extending from the pro-ventriculus to the hindgut, where it is patent and is in reality a cylindrical tube sus-pended in the intestine. It is derived from an annular ridge or ring of gland cells in the proventriculus which secretes a viscous fluid which immediately solidifies as it is pushed progressively backwards, reaching the hindgut 2–4 days after the young fly has emerged from the pupa. The ingested blood does not, therefore, come into contact with the gut wall, but osmosis takes place through the peritrophic membrane and the trypomastigotes cannot penetrate it. Up to the fourth day the trypomastigotes actually within the lumen can migrate and pass round the open end and escape to pass forward

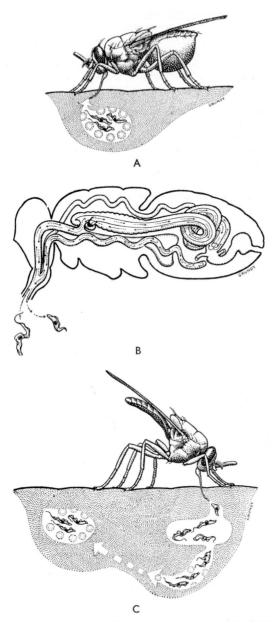

Fig. 285.—The trypanosomiasis cycle. (*By permission of J. Hull Grundy*)

A, The tsetse fly, male or female, takes up the blood of the sick person, which contains trypomastigotes. B, The trypomastigotes enter the gut of the tsetse fly and there develop and increase in numbers by a process of division. The trypomastigotes travel along the gut to the end of a lining membrane, and then double back between it and the gut wall, passing into the proboscis and from there into the salivary glands. C, From the salivary glands the trypomastigotes are injected into animals or man at subsequent feeds. The whole cycle in the tsetse fly occupies about 20 days. The sizes of the parasites and tsetse flies are not in proportion.

outside it to the proventriculus. They then find themselves in a cul-de-sac and penetrate the membrane at a point where it is still fluid. They then pass to the oesophagus and proboscis, to the end of the hypopharynx, and double back again to the salivary glands, which are slender coiled tubes lying in the abdomen. The salivary ducts lead through the thorax to the head where they unite to form a common duct leading to the hypopharynx. There the trypomastigotes become epimastigotes, attaching themselves to the salivary ducts for 2–5 days before becoming metacyclic trypomastigotes. The critical period is just after emergence from the pupa, since if the young fly does not take an infective blood meal within 4 days after emergence then it cannot become infected, since the peritrophic membrane has developed as far as the hindgut and the trypanosomes cannot penetrate it.

The whole cycle occupies some 20 days. The fly is not infective until this stage is reached, but thereafter remains so for life (about 8 months). *T. br. rhodesiense* trypomastigotes migrate from the ectoperitrophic space to the anterior station and can find their way through the membrane even at the front of the proventriculus (Fig. 284).

The infectivity of *T. br. gambiense* for *Glossina* is slight, less than 10% under experimental conditions, and in nature less than 1% are found infected. Strains of *T. br. gambiense* vary in infectivity and this property appears to become lost in long-standing infections. In laboratory strains long absence from the natural vector is a factor. Polymorphism is also lost and only long slender forms may be encountered.

Mechanical transmission. *T. br. gambiense* can survive on the proboscis of *Glossina* for varying periods, can be injected mechanically and direct transmission can occur, especially when there is interrupted feeding. It has been shown in Malawi that *Musca spectandra* feeding on exuded blood can ingest trypomastigotes and pass them out via the faeces into abrasions of the skin.

Life cycle of Stercoraria

T. cruzi is transmitted by reduviid bugs (*Panstrongylus, Triatoma, Rhodnius*) in which posterior development takes place.

The cycle of development may occur in the larva, nymph or adult and always takes place in the bug's intestinal tract.

Typical trypomastigote forms which are ingested by the insect become short epimastigotes which multiply to produce long epimastigotes in the posterior portion of the midgut. In from 8 to 10 days small trypomastigote forms develop from the epimastigotes and appear in the rectum. These metacyclic trypomastigotes are passed in the faeces (posterior station) and are infective to man and animals when rubbed into the puncture wound made by the insect or into an abrasion of the skin. The time required for bug faeces to become infective for all 5 larval stages and adults of *R. prolixus* is 7 days at 20°C and 3 days at 25°C (Phillips 1960).

Insect vectors. Although the major vectors are *Panstrongylus* (*Triatoma*) *megistus* and *Rhodnius prolixus* (see page 108) a large number of reduviid bugs have been found capable of transmitting *T. cruzi*. In Mexico no fewer than 15 species have been found naturally infected. Among these are: *Triatoma phyllosoma, T. pallidipennis, T. rubida, T. barberi, T. dimidiata, T. picturata, T. longipes, Rhodnius prolixus* and *Dipetalogaster maximus*. Other species in Brazil are *Panstrongylus megistus*; in N. Argentine, Chile and Uruguay, *T. infestans, T. sordida, T. vitticeps, T. dimidiata* var. *maculipennis*; in Venezuala *Rhodnius prolixus* and *Eratyrus cuspidatus*. Other species are *Eutriatoma maculata, E. nigromaculata, E. oswaldoi, E. patagonica, E. rubrovaria, E. sordida, Panstrongylus geniculatus, Psammolestes arthuri, P. coreodes, Rhodnius brumpti, R. domesticus, R. pallescens, R. pictipes, Parabelminus carioca, Triatoma brasiliensis, T. carrioni, T. capitis, T. chagasi, T. cruzi, T. geniculata, T. hegneri, T. maculipennis, T. platensis, T. protracta, T. rosenbuschi, T. sanguisuga, T. spinolai*.

A species common in California (*Triatoma protracta*), extending as far north as Salt Lake City, harbours a trypanosome resembling *T.cruzi*, though the human disease is unknown there, while, under experimental conditions, other members of the *Triatoma* genus in the United States can be easily infected, as well as cosmopolitan species, *T. rubrofasciata* and *T. dimidiata* (Ecuador). In Arizona it is *Eutriatoma uhleri;* in New Mexico *E. protracta woodi;* and in Texas *T. gerstaekeri*. It is probable that all species of *Panstrongylus* and *Triatoma* are susceptible to infection. Under laboratory conditions Brumpt has observed development in bugs, *Cimex hemipterus* (*rotundatus*), *C. lectularius, C. boueti, C. hirudinis,* and in ticks, *Ornithodorus moubata* and *O. savignyi,* but *O. hermsi* is resistant.

Trypanosoma brucei

The trypanosomes which infect man in Africa belong to the *T. brucei* group. There are 3 members of this species which are biological races and are morphologically indistinguishable:

1. *T. brucei brucei* is non-infective for man but highly infective for cattle and game.
2. *T. brucei rhodesiense* is well adapted to game and cattle but poorly adapted to man.
3. *T. brucei gambiense* is well adapted to man and has not been found naturally in any animal, although it will infect pigs.

Differentiation of *T. brucei* **group.** Various methods have been used for the differentiation of the *T. brucei* group: pathogenicity to laboratory animals, resistance to tryparsamide and infectivity for man.

T. brucei brucei is the most pathogenic for laboratory animals and causes a severe, rapidly fatal infection in white rats. It is resistant to tryparsamide and fails to infect man.

T. brucei rhodesiense is highly pathogenic to laboratory animals and commonly produces posterior nucleated forms in the rat. It is resistant to tryparsamide and can infect man.

T. brucei gambiense is the least pathogenic to laboratory animals, in which only a few posterior nucleated forms are produced. It is sensitive to tryparsamide and can infect man.

Blood infection incubation test (B.I.I.T.). Since human serum has a lethal effect on *T. br. brucei,* but not on *T. br. rhodesiense,* a test has been devised in which human serum is mixed with the strain of trypanosome under test and incubated for 5 hours at 37°C. The effect of the procedure on the strain's infectivity to rats is observed, since the infectivity of *T. br. rhodesiense* will not be affected by the procedure.

Occult phase (Ormerod & Venkatesan 1971). An occult phase of *T. brucei* has been described in the choroid plexus of rats, where amastigote and sphaeromastigote (amastigote with flagellum) forms develop out of reach of humoral antibodies and form the source of relapse strains of trypomastigotes which invade the blood stream. Swelling of the choroid plexus may be the cause of headache in the early stages of human trypanosomiasis.

Trypanosoma brucei gambiense

Morphology. In the blood *T. br. gambiense* occurs in 3 forms—a long slender trypomastigote form having a flagellum, a short broad one without a flagellum and an intermediate one (polymorphic).

In fresh blood the trypomastigotes may be seen as colourless spindle-shaped bodies moving rapidly among the red blood corpuscles. In preparations with Giemsa or Wright's stain *T. br. gambiense* measures 14–33 μm in length and 1·5–3·5 μm in breadth. In the blood of man the long trypomastigote form is predominant. The cytoplasm is granular and may be vacuolated. It stains a pale blue and contains dark blue volutin granules. Centrally located is the nucleus which stains reddish or reddish purple and in specimens stained with haematoxylin a definite nuclear membrane and large central karyosome may be distinguished. In most preparations the kinetoplast appears as a dark red dot and distinction cannot be made between the blepharoplast and parabasal body. The red staining flagellum arises from the blepharoplast and runs along the edge of the undulating membrane and becomes a free flagellum at the anterior end of the body.

PLATE XI

Malaria parasites

1, Early trophozoite of *P. vivax*.

2, Half-grown trophozoite of *P. vivax*.

3, *P. vivax* macrogametocyte with a schizont in the same erythrocyte.

4, Early trophozoite of *P. malariae*.

5, Later trophozoite of *P. malariae*.

6, Band form of *P. malariae*.

7, Mature schizont (rosette) of *P. malariae*.

8, Early trophozoite of *P. falciparum*.

9, Early trophozoite of *P. falciparum*, showing double chromatin dots or double infection.

10, Large trophozoite of *P. falciparum*.

11, Advanced schizont of *P. falciparum*.

12, Early trophozoite of *P. ovale*.

13, Half grown trophozoite of *P. ovale*.

14, Schizont of *P. ovale*.

15, Mature schizont of *P. ovale*.

16, Host stippling in *P. vivax*. Schüffner's dots.

17, Host stippling in *P. malariae*. Ziemann's stippling.

18, Host stippling in *P. falciparum*. Maurer's spots.

19, Host stippling in *P. ovale*. James's stippling.

Parasites 10 and 18 are rarely seen in the primary or subsequent acute attack, but are common in asymptomatic cases, at least in tropical Africa. All parasites stained with Leishman. (*From an original painting by B. Jobling; reproduced by permission of the authors and publishers from Shute & Maryon 1966.*)

PLATE XII

Intestinal Protozoa (stained Weigert's iodine)

First row: *Entamoeba histolytica*

1. Precystic form. Note diffuse iodine-staining substance.
2. Immature cyst with two nuclei and chromatoid rods.
3. Mature cyst with four nuclei, iodine vacuoles and chromatoid rods.
4. Quadrinucleated cyst of the minuta form.

Second row: *Entamoeba coli*

1. Active vegetative form with vacuoles and ingested food material.
2. Precystic form.
3. Immature cyst with two nuclei and vacuole.
4. Mature cyst with eight nuclei.

Third row: *Endolimax nana*

1. Active vegetative form with one nucleus and protoplasmic granules.
2. Mature cyst with four characteristic nuclei and iodine-staining substance.
   Iodamoeba bütschlii
3. Active vegetative form with one nucleus and iodine-staining vacuoles.
4. Mature cyst with one nucleus and iodine-staining vacuole.

Fourth row: *Giardia intestinalis*

1. Active form with sucking disc.
2. Active form (side view).
3. Cyst with four recently divided nuclei.
4. Four-nucleated cyst (end-on view).

Fifth row: *Trichomonas hominis*

1. Active form with undulating membrane.

   Chilomastix mesnili
2. Active form with peristome and contained flagellum.
3. Pear-shaped cyst of above with nucleus and peristome.
4, 5, 6. Various forms of *Blastocystis hominis*.

Trypanosoma brucei rhodesiense

This is indistinguishable from *T. br. gambiense* in human blood, the same 3 forms occurring. In the rat posterior nucleated forms are produced but, although commoner in *T. br. rhodesiense*, these are also found with some strains of *T. br. gambiense*. In the posterior nucleated forms a change occurs in the nucleus which assumes a position close to the kinetoplast or posterior to it. The proportion of posterior nucleated forms which are shorter than normal may be 50% in some laboratory animals (Fig. 286).

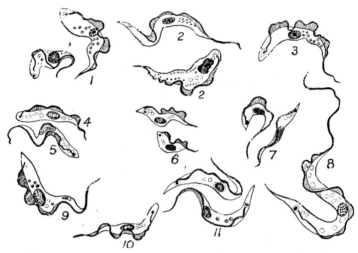

Fig. 286.—Various trypansosomes of man and animals. × 1300. (*After Wenyon*)

1, *T. br. gambiense*. 2, *T. br. rhodesiense*. 3, *T. evansi*. 4, 5, *T. uniforme, T. vivax*. 6, *T. congolense*. 7, *T. cruzi*. 8, *T. theileri*. 9, *T. equinum*. 10, *T. equiperdum*. 11, *T. lewisi*.

Reservoir hosts. Several antelopes probably harbour *T. br. rhodesiense* under natural conditions and a strain of this trypanosome has been transmitted to man, which had been passed through various animals for 10 years by *Glossina morsitans*. In nature *T. br. rhodesiense* has been isolated from a wild bushbuck (*Tragelaphus scriptus*) and from domestic cattle in Kenya.

Trypanosoma cruzi (Chagas, 1909)

Synonyms. *Schizotrypanum cruzi* (Chagas 1909), *Trypanosoma escomeli* (Yorke 1920), *Trypansoma triatomae* (Kofold & McCulloch 1916).

Morphology. *Trypanosoma cruzi* is a monomorphic trypanosome having two phases in its life cycle. In the mammalian host it occurs in the blood in a *trypomastigote* form and in reticuloendothelial and other tissue cells in an *amastigote* form. When it is about to escape from the tissue cell after multiplication it occurs in *promastigote* and *epimastigote* forms.

While in the insect host it occurs in *amastigote, epimastigote*, and *trypomastigote* form (Fig. 287).

Trypomastigote. In the blood of man *T. cruzi* occurs in trypomastigote form measuring 20 μm in length. Two forms are found in the blood, a long slender and a short broad form. Both forms have a central nucleus and the posterior end is pointed and contains a large kinetoplast consisting of a dot-like blepharoplast and a large oval parabasal body. The root of the flagellum, the axoneme, arises from the blepharoplast and extends along the edge of a narrow undulating membrane. In stained films the trypomastigote assumes a characteristic C-shape. With the electron microscope it can be seen that the kinetoplast is represented by a spherical vacuole containing a dispersed osmiophilic mass, while the basal granule (blepharoplast) of the flagellar axoneme lies at the anterior margin of the vacuole enclosing the kinetoplast. Within the cytoplasm of the trypomastigote there is a group of about 11 striae lying between the nucleus and the kinetoplast which is likened to the parabasal body of other protozoa and the Golgi apparatus in metazoal forms. It is absent from the amastigote forms.

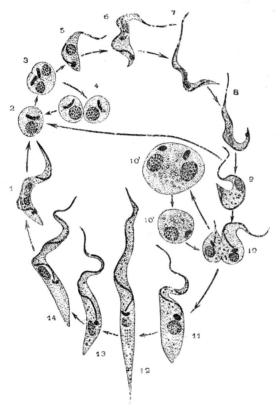

Fig. 287.—Evolutionary cycle of *T. cruzi*. Stages 2–9 occur in man or other vertebrate; stages 9–14 in *Panstrongylus, Triatoma* or *Cimex*. × 1500. (*After Brumpt*)

1, Metacyclic trypanosome infecting vertebrate. 2–4, Schizogony in organs. 5–9, Trans-formation to adult trypanosome (9). 10, Crithidial form about to divide in small intes-tine. 10′. *Leishmania* forms frequent in the proventriculus. 11–14, Progressive trans-formation of crithidia forms into metacyclic trypanosomes (1) in the hindgut.

The trypomastigote does not divide in the blood stream but multiplies only in reticuloendothelial cells as amastigote, promastigote or epimastigote forms.

Amastigote. The undulating membrane and flagellum disappear after entry into the cell, and the organism divides by fission producing amastigote forms which even-tually fill and destroy the cell. The amastigote forms (Fig. 287) with Giemsa stain are round or ovoidal in shape measuring from 1·5 to 4 μm in diameter. Each has a large nucleus, ruby red in colour, and a rod-like or spherical kinetoplast stained a deep violet or almost black. In tissue histiocytes and especially in the reticuloendothelial cells the amastigote form behaves like *L. donovani*, from which it is almost indistin-guishable as an intracellular parasite.

Other forms. The amastigote forms collect in the invaded cell within a cyst-like cavity and are liberated with destruction of the cells as amastigote, promastigote, epimastigote or trypomastigote forms but only trypomastigotes are found in the peripheral blood.

Electron microscopy has shown that a rounded form with a flagellum, a *sphaeromastigote*, develops into epimastigote and trypomastigote forms. The variation in shape and size of the kinetoplast during the cycle of development depends on how much DNA is present and whether the DNA loops are arranged in a single layer (amastigote forms) or in 3-4 layers (trypomastigote form).

In the transmitting insect both epimastigote and trypomastigote forms occur similar to those of other trypanosomes. Short and long epimastigote forms with the kinetoplast at the anterior end and a central nucleus; intermediate forms with the kinetoplast at various levels of the body; and metacyclic trypomastigote forms with the kinetoplast at the posterior end, a well developed undulating membrane and flagellum all occur.

Metabolism. *T. cruzi* has a high lipid content and contains 25% cholesterol. The presence of RNA and DNA has been confirmed.

Cultural characteristics. *T. cruzi* is cultured easily on NNN. The forms in culture are the same as in the transmitting insect. In tissue cultures on chick embryo luxuriant growth takes place in fibroblasts, histiocytes, macrophages, epithelial cells and cells of the nervous system. The trypomastigote forms are transformed into intracellular amastigotes followed by epimastigote and trypomastigote stages.

Reservoir hosts. The epidemiological situation in various countries of South America is controlled by several factors. In some the prevalence of Chagas's disease depends entirely on the introduction of *T. cruzi* from wild animal reservoirs, whereas in others it is purely endemic and independent of them. The multiplicity of the vicarious hosts of *T. cruzi* certainly indicates that the organism would spread to many countries, if other conditions remained favourable. These reduviid bugs are so easily infected that 100% become so at all stages of their existence and, moreover, remain so for the whole of their lives.

T. cruzi has been found in cats, dogs and pigs, but under wilder conditions it occurs mainly in several species of armadillo (Edentata), *Euphractus vellerosus* (the long-haired armadillo), *Dasypus novemcinctus* (the Peba armadillo), *D. novemcinctus fenestratus, Euphractus sexcinctus* (the 6-banded armadillo), *Cabassous unicinctus* (the broad-banded armadillo), *Chaetopractus vellerosus, C. pannosus, C. villosus cautinus, C. crassicauda* and *C. paranalis*; in *Zoedypus pichiy* (the little armadillo), *Tolypeutes matacos* and the tayra (*Tayra barbara*) in Brazil, all of which constitute the main reservoir hosts in country districts (Garnham).

Under experimental conditions all laboratory animals can be infected. In infected animals transuterine infection can take place and a similar process takes place in man. Other mammals include:

Canidae	*Pseudolopex culpaeus* (Colpeo Fox), *P. andinus, Pseudocyon gracilis.*
Chiroptera	*Histiotus caephotis, H. montanus, Myotis nigricans, M. dinellii, M. levis, Carollia perspicillata, Antibeus jamaicensis, Desmodus rotundus marinus* (Panama), *Darias albiventer, Talirida macrotis, Glossophagosoncina leachi, Carollia perspicillata azteca, Phyllostomus hastatus, Vroderma bilobatum* (Panama).
Mustelidae	*Grisonella huronax, G. ratellina* (Chilian grison).
Rodentia	*Octagon degus* (Chilean bush rat), *Dasyprocta aguti* (golden agouti), *Neotoma fuscipes* (woodrat, California). *N. albigula* (New Mexico, Arizona).
Marsupialia	*Didelphis azarae, D. paraguayensis, D. marsupialis mesoamericana* (California) (opossums), *Lutreolina crassicauda paranalis, Marmosa cinera* (ashy opossum), *M. metachirus nudicaudatus* (rat-tailed opposum).

Anteaters   *Tamandua tetradactyli kriegi.*

Sciuridae   *Leptosciurus argentinus* (Argentine squirrel).

Monkeys   *Saimiri sciureus* (Saimiri).

The Australian phalanger or opossum, *Trichosurus vulpecula*, is very susceptible.

Trypansoma rangeli (Tejera, 1920)

This species occurs in Guatemala, Uruguay, Colombia and Venezuela.

Morphology. In the blood stream of man and reservoir hosts *T. rangeli* exhibits a typical trypomastigote form but is much more elongated (31 μm) than *T. cruzi* (Fig. 288). The relatively ovoid nucleus is situated in front of the equatorial plane and the minute round blepharoplast lies at the posterior terminus of the undulating membrane an appreciable distance in front of the posterior end of the organism. No amastigote forms have ever been found. Epimastigote forms are found in the intestinal contents of bugs.

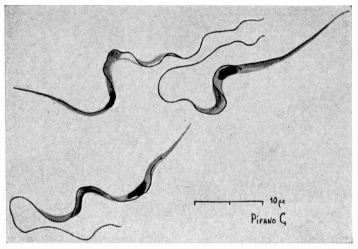

Fig. 288.—*T. rangeli.* Forms in culture from the peripheral blood. (*After Pifano & Mayer*)

Cultural characteristics. *T. rangeli* is easily cultured on the same media as *T. cruzi* but can also be grown in a liquid medium containing frozen sheep brain added to brain and heart infusion, in which *T. cruzi* will not grow.

Life cycle. Unlike *T. cruzi* trypomastigote forms exhibit longitudinal binary division in the mammalian host's blood.

In the insect host *T. rangeli* is not discharged in the metacyclic trypomastigote stage in the faeces of the bug, but rather in the salivary secretions after a period of migration from the midgut through the haemolymph to the salivary glands so that infection of the mammalian host results from the puncture of the bug's proboscis into the skin.

Reservoir hosts. This parasite has been demonstrated in the blood of man, cebus monkey and dog. In man it is considered to be non-pathogenic but may be found in association with *T. cruzi.*

Trypanosoma ariarii

Hoare and other authorities consider that this trypanosome is identical with *T. rangeli*

Trypanosoma lewisi (Kent, 1879)

This is a common parasite of the rat and is present in considerable numbers in the blood stream (Fig. 286) at the height of the infection. It was once recorded in large numbers in the blood of a Sikh child in Malaysia, but this is now thought to have been *T. conorhini*. It is, however, non-pathogenic to the rat. Individual trypanosomes vary considerably in size and appearance during the multiplication phase, but in the chronic stage average about 24 μm. The *nucleus* is situated at a point slightly anterior to the centre of the body.

    T. lewisi develops in *Ceratophyllus fasciatus, Xenopsylla cheopis*, and other fleas. Trypanosomes enter the epithelial cells of the stomach, where they become spherical and grow. The *nucleus* divides repeatedly and young trypanosomes are formed by multiple division. These pass into the hindgut, and after 2 days become crithidial forms. Eventually they escape as small metacyclic trypanosomes in the excreta. They are then ingested by the rat, which either licks up the flea faeces or devours the insect. Trypanosomes appear in the blood stream after an incubation period of 6 days.

GENUS: *Leishmania*

Species belonging to this genus have an *amastigote* stage in the mammalian host and a *promastigote* stage in the insect (sandfly) host (Fig. 289).

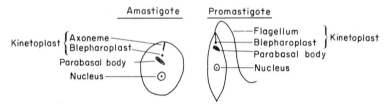

Fig. 289.—Amastigote and promastigote forms of *Leishmania*.

Species of *Leishmania* (For details see pages 120, 134, 139).

Morphology

    In all stages of development *L. tropica, L. brasiliensis* and *L. donovani* are indistinguishable from each other.

    Amastigote. In man and the mammalian hosts the amastigote appears as an ovoid or rounded body measuring about 2–3 μm in length and living intracellularly in monocytes, polymorphonuclear leucocytes or endothelial cells. In preparations stained with Giemsa or Wright stain the cytoplasm is pale blue and there is a limiting membrane. Within the cytoplasm is a relatively large *nucleus* which stains red and a *kinetoplast* which consists of a deep red or violet rod-like body, the *parabasal body*, and a dot-like *blepharoplast*. A delicate thread connects the two organelles near the parabasal body and an *axoneme* arises from the blepharoplast and extends to the anterior tip. Elongated so-called 'torpedo forms' may be observed, having pointed or rounded ends with the nucleus and kinetoplast closely associated.

    Multiplication. Multiplication is by binary fission, and is initiated in the kinetoplast, which elongates. The blepharoplast and parabasal body each divide into two portions. The nucleus elongates and divides mitotically. After division of the blepharoplast a new axoneme or flagellar root is formed by the daughter blepharoplast which is not attached to the old axoneme. The cytoplasm divides, and two individuals are produced. Dividing forms may be seen in spleen smears.

    Ultrastructure. The organism is surrounded by a double membrane below which is a row of 130–200 hollow fibrils. The *flagellum* arises from the blepharoplast containing 9 peripheral double fibrils ending on a plate from which the axoneme begins.

The blepharoplast lies on the margin of a well developed *flagellar vacuole* which may be the source of soluble antigens. The *kinetoplast* is a complex body and appears as an electron dense granular band with a distinct and regular fibrillar pattern lying inside a large body with a double membrane and having all the characteristics of mitochondria.

Change to promastigote form. At 26°C the amastigote grows and the anterior end, through which the flagellum will emerge, broadens. The flagellar vacuole increases in size and the first signs of a flagellum are seen. At first it consists of a short stumpy protrusion and when it has grown to about 1 μm in length it begins to move and rotate the organism. The flagellar protuberance becomes attenuated and the flagellum attains full size. Full length is attained 4–4½ hours after the first signs of appearance of the flagellum, by which time the body has assumed full promastigote form. The development of the flagellum is affected and inhibited by immune serum. This characteristic forms the basis of Adler's test (Adler *et al.* 1966), in which the development of promastigotes is inhibited in Locke serum agar by homologous serum and aflagellar forms appear massed together in clumps. Normal development of promastigotes takes place in the heterologous serum. With this test *L. donovani*, *L. tropica* and *L. braziliensis* can be distinguished from each other.

Promastigote. The *promastigote* forms which are found in cultures on NNN medium and in the digestive tract of the sandfly host are identical. Promastigotes have a single free flagellum arising from the kinetoplast at the anterior end and possess marked motility. The average length is 15–20 μm and the breadth 1·5–3·5 μm; the flagellum measures 15–28 μm. Short broad forms and rounded forms 4–5 μm in diameter with a long flagellum may be seen in old cultures in which they exhibit a tendency to agglomerate in clusters or rosettes with their flagella centrally directed. Volutin granules may be seen in both amastigote and promastigote forms.

Cultural characteristics

When introduced into NNN medium the amastigote transforms into the promastigote stage when incubated at 22–25°C. A small amount of material is inoculated into the water of condensation and growth appears in anything from 2–3 to 20 days. A small amount of penicillin and streptomycin should be added to prevent secondary contamination. The thermal death point of amastigotes is 40°C within 15–30 minutes. Amastigotes grow well in tissue culture with a base of human amniotic cells in medium 199. Cultures remain infected for up to 60 days at 33°C. Macrophages have been successfully infected in tissue cultures with promastigotes at 37°C.

Promastigotes may be stored for years at −79°C in 10% glycerol. The amastigotes may also be stored in homogenized splenic tissue in 10% glycerol at −79°C. The technique used is that of Cunningham *et al.* (1963).

Animal inoculation

All species of hamster are very susceptible to inoculation and the parasites multiply in the golden hamster (*Cricetus auratus*) in geometrical progression until death of the animal in about 6 months. The golden hamster is the most useful laboratory animal for isolation of the parasite.

Differentiation of *Leishmania*

The leishmaniae which infect man cannot be differentiated from each other morphologically. In culture strains may differ in the rate at which they grow. In animals the behaviour of the three species depends more on the route of inoculation than on the species. Serological methods have proved disappointing, although Adler's test can distinguish the three main species.

Xenodiagnosis

Material from human blood or spleen, or homogenized spleen or skin from wild animals is inoculated intraperitoneally into hamsters which are examined after 6 months for leishmanial infection. This is a very sensitive method of isolation of *Leishmania* from material.

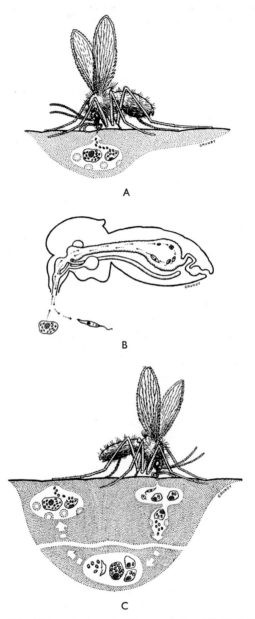

Fig. 290.—The leishmaniasis cycle. (*By permission of J. Hull Grundy*)

A, The sandfly takes up amastigote (round forms) when it bites a man or dog suffering from leishmaniasis. B, The amastigotes develop and increase in numbers by a process of division in the stomach of the sandfly. They become elongated and move forward to the pharynx, where they multiply so greatly that they block the passage. C, The sandfly then injects the elongated promastigotes into man or dogs, when it subsequently attempts to feed. The whole cycle in the sandfly takes about 10 days. The sandflies and parasites are not in proportion.

Material likely to be infected should be homogenized in normal saline or Locke's solution and incubated with small amounts of penicillin and streptomycin overnight at 4°C before inoculation into the hamster.

Life history in the sandfly

The cycle of development can be divided into two stages after the first and second blood meals. First the parasites enlarge and undergo binary fission, and promastigotes form on the second day. On the third day they become elongated and active in the midgut while the short forms remain attached to the gut wall. On the fourth day they occur in masses near the proventriculus (blocked sandfly) and the fly is ready to lay eggs when ready for the second blood meal. Transmission takes place so that when the sandfly next attempts to feed, the promastigotes are discharged from the buccal cavity and inoculated into the site of the bite (Fig. 290).

Susceptible animals

Animals found naturally infected are described in Chapter 7. Other animals susceptible to inoculation are the mouse, Mongolian gerbil (jird), cotton rat, Australian opossum (*Trichosurus vulpecula* and *Pseudochirus laviginosus*), American marsupials (*Didelphis marsupialis* and *Metachirus nudicaudatus*) and chinchilla. There is a spectrum of susceptibility varying from almost complete resistance in the rat and guinea-pig, through tolerance in the mouse, to complete susceptibility with death in the hamster, cotton rat and chinchilla (Stauber 1958).

Lizard leishmaniae

Nine species of *Leishmania* have been described from lizards and chameleons as species of *Leptomonas*.

They are important because the promastigotes, though morphologically distinct, may resemble human *Leishmania* when found in sandflies being examined for human infections. No lizard leishmaniae have been recorded from America or Australia.

L. adleri is infective for lizards of diverse genera. The infection is cryptic and can only be demonstrated by culturing heart blood. Transient infections which are cryptic

Table 41. Lizard *Leishmania*

Leishmania species	Lizard host	Geographical location
L. adleri	Latastia longicauda revoili	Kenya
L. agamae	Agama stellio	Tiberias, Israel
L. ceramodactyli	Ceramodactylus dorias	Baghdad
L. chamaeleonis	Chamaeleon vulgaris	Egypt, Israel
	C. ellioti	Uganda
	C. pardalis	
	C. ousteli	
	C. verrugosus	Madagascar
	C. lateralis	
	C. brevicornis	
L. gymnodactyli	Gymnodactylus caspiae	
	Agama sanguinolenta	U.S.S.R.
	Pharinocephalus heliodactylus	
	P. myctaceus	
L. hemidactyli	Hemidactylus gleadovii	India
L. henrici	Lizards of genus Anolis	Martinique
L. tarentolae	Tarentola mauritanica	N. Africa, Sicily
L. zmeevi	Unnamed species of lizards	Karakorum desert

have been demonstrated in the hamster and in the skin of white mice. Transient skin nodules in which amastigotes were demonstrated up to 5 days after inoculation have been produced by the inoculation of promastigote forms into the skin of man.

PARASITES OF UNCERTAIN ORIGIN
GENUS: *Pneumocystis*

Pneumocystis carinii Delanoë & Delanoë, 1912, is probably a protozoon, and has been found in dogs, guinea-pigs, mice, rats, rabbits, foxes, goats, sheep and man. The mode of transmission is unknown.

Morphology

The parasites appear as round, ovoid or cup-shaped cysts measuring 3·5–12 μm in diameter in smears from infected animals. Each cyst contains 8 corpuscles, averaging 1 μm in diameter, which may be pear-shaped, crescentic or amoeboid. Cysts and corpuscles are readily stained by Giemsa and are positive by the periodic acid Schiff technique.

Ultrastructure (Arean 1971)

The elementary corpuscles or trophozoites appear as thin-walled structures with a wall or pellicle enclosing a nuclear mass, a mitochondrion, round endoplasmic reticulum, round bodies and vacuoles. The larger trophozoites evolve into thick-walled structures or cysts. Within these develop 8 nuclear masses, surrounded by a membrane, together with a mitochondrion, membrane-bound vacuoles and round bodies. The fully developed thick-walled cyst contains 4–8 trophozoites anchored to the inner surface on the cystic wall by electron-dense stalks.

For details of pathology and treatment see page 153.

SUBCLASS: SARCOSPORIDIA
GENUS: *Sarcocystis*

Sarcocystis is a parasite of striped or cardiac muscle, mainly of herbivorous animals, but *S. lindemanni* has occasionally been found in man, in the tongue, larynx, diaphragm, chest, abdomen or extremities. It would probably be found more often if the muscles were examined microscopically more frequently.

The fully developed organism consists of an elongated fusiform body (Miescher's tube), varying in length from microscopic proportions to 5 mm, lying among muscle fibres. There is a surrounding membrane which encloses hundreds of round or crescentic trophozoites (Rainey's corpuscles) measuring 4–4·8 × 0·8–1·2 μm.

The cysts develop in muscle cells, without inflammatory reaction, though the cells are destroyed. The cysts may rupture, and the trophozoites may infect other muscle cells or invade the blood stream. Rupture stimulates an inflammatory reaction to remove the cyst remnants and damaged muscle, and scar tissue is left—it has been reported in heart muscle. A toxin (sarcocystin) is produced, which may provoke a general allergic state resembling periarteritis nodosa, and which appears to have a selective action on the spinal cord, causing temporary paralysis of the hind limbs in experimental animals. Similar effects have been reported in veterinary literature.

Infection in man may be symptomless, the diagnosis being made at autopsy, or on biopsy material. The Sabin-Feldman test for *Toxoplasma* is sometimes positive, but cannot distinguish between toxoplasmosis and *Sarcocystis* infection. Fulton and Voller (1964), however, found a high titre by immunofluorescence in the serum of a patient with *Sarcocystis* infection who was negative for *Toxoplasma*.

Localized muscular swelling lasting 2-4 days, often accompanied by slight fever, bronchospasm and eosinophilia, has been found associated with *S. lindemanni*, and Mandour (1965) reported a case in a patient who had lived in The Far East and who had intermittent painless swellings of the muscles of arms and legs, with progressive weakness of those muscles and paraesthesia of hands and feet. There was eosinophilia of 40%. Muscle biopsies showed the parasite and scar tissue, and X-ray showed faint shadows in the leg muscles, presumably cysts.

There is no intermediate host, and the infection is acquired by eating undercooked infected meat, or by oral contamination with faecal material, after which the organisms penetrate the intestinal epithelium.

THE SPIROCHAETES

Though formerly regarded as protozoa, the spirochaetes are more closely related to bacteria.

The 4 genera which relate to tropical medicine are:

Borrelia of relapsing fever.
Treponema of syphilis, yaws and pinta.
Leptospira of leptospirosis.
Spirillum of rat bite fever.

Members of the true genus *Spirochaeta* are not pathogenic, but the common name spirochaete is used loosely, on historical grounds, to cover the pathogenic genera.

Spirochaetes are motile, spiral organisms which move by flexion, rotation and translation from one place to another. *Borrelia*, *Treponema* and *Leptospira* have axial filaments, but probably no flagella. They multiply by transverse fission.

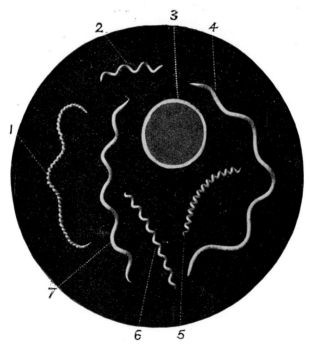

Fig. 291.—Different forms of spirochaetes. ×3500. (*After Dobell. By permission of the Wellcome Bureau of Scientific Research*)

1, *Leptospira ictohaemorrhagiae* (Inada & Ido) Noguchi, one cause of spirochaetal jaundice. 2, *Spirochaeta eurygirata* Werner, commonly found in human faeces, in both health and disease (e.g. dysentery). 3, Human red blood corpuscle on the same scale. 4, *Borrelia recurrentis* Leber (*Borrelia obermeiri* Cohn) occurs in the blood in relapsing fever. 5, *Spirochaeta pallida* (Schaudinn) Vuillemin (*Treponema pallidum* Schaudinn). Syphilis. 6, *Spirochaeta gracile* Levaditi & Stanesco. Found on external genitalia in health and in various diseased conditions. 7, *Spirochaeta refringens* Schaudinn (emend.) occurs in syphilitic lesions on the external genitalia.

The different species (or strains) of the tick-borne *Borrelia* (*B. duttoni, B. latychevi, B. persica, B. hispanica, B. parkeri, B. hermsi* and *B. venezuelensis*) are indistinguishable except serologically. *B. recurrentis* of louse-borne relapsing fever is also distinguished only by antigenic structure. In general they are about 10–16 μm long, with 5–10 loose spiral waves. They can easily be stained with ordinary dyes. They can be cultivated on the chorio-allantoic membrane of the developing chick embryo, but not satisfactorily in vitro. They can infect monkeys, rats and mice, but not rabbits or guinea-pigs.

B. vincentii is found in association with fusiform bacilli in the throats of patients with Vincent's angina, in which (as in tropical phagedaenic ulcer) it may be a secondary invader. It can be cultivated in vitro.

Treponema pallidum of syphilis, *T. pertenue* of yaws and *T. carateum* of pinta are slender, delicate organisms which can be stained by Giemsa, Ziehl-Neelsen, silver impregnation and other special methods, or can be recognized by dark ground techniques. Their length is about 6–14 μm and they have numerous primary spirals of about 1 μm. Treponemes can infect monkeys, rabbits and hamsters experimentally.

The genus *Leptospira* comprises 2 complexes, *L. interrogans* which includes the 15 serogroups affecting man (subdivided into over 119 serotypes), which are pathogenic, and *L. biflexa* whose members are not pathogenic for man. These serogroups and serotypes are not regarded as species; they are distinguishable serologically. The leptospires are delicate organisms about 6–12 μm long, having closely wound spirals of about 0·5 μm. When active, they can worm their way through Berkefeld candles, but when motionless they are held back, lying passively athwart the interstices. Pure cultures of the living leptospires can be obtained by such filtration. Leptospires can be stained with Giemsa or silver impregnation. They can be cultivated in vitro in various media containing serum. Guinea-pigs, hamsters and young chicks can be infected, but white mice and albino rats should not be used unless they are known to be free from leptospirosis; they are often naturally infected.

Spirillum minus (*S. morsus-muris*) of rat bite fever is short (2–5 μm) and rather thick, with few spirals but with terminal flagella. It is readily stained with aniline dyes, and it has been cultivated, but successive transfers have not been successful.

INTESTINAL AMOEBAE

CLASS: RHIZOPODA
FAMILY: ENTAMOEBIDAE
GENUS: *Entamoeba*

Entamoeba hystolytica Schaudinn, 1903

Entamoeba histolytica is a protozoan which normally lives and multiplies in the contents of the large intestine of man, but which can, in conditions which are not clear, invade the tissues, and in this pathogenic form can spread to the liver, brain, lungs, skin and other organs. The pathogenic forms can infect certain animals, especially kittens.

E. histolytica is closely related to *E. hartmanni*, which is considerably smaller and is never pathogenic.

There are several well defined stages or forms: *Trophozoites*, the vegetative, motile, dividing forms, which live either as commensals feeding on intestinal contents, or as pathogenic tissue-invading forms, ingesting erythrocytes, leucocytes and tissue debris, and producing necrosis in the bowel wall, liver etc.

The commensal trophozoites are rather smaller than the pathogenic forms, and are therefore sometimes referred to as 'minuta' forms, but they are bigger than *E. hartmanni*. The dimensions are given in Table 42.

The trophozoites (size 10–40 μm) have a characteristic nucleus (2·8–4·5 μm), a small central karyosome and peripheral chromatin in the form of fine granules (Fig. 292). The cytoplasm has 2 zones—outer with clear ectoplasm, and inner with granular endoplasm, enclosing food vacuoles which, in pathogenic strains, usually contain ingested erythrocytes.

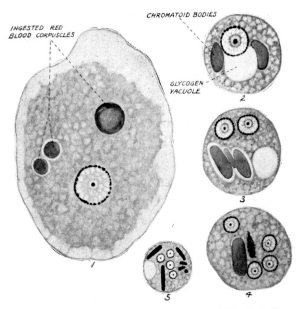

Fig. 292.—*Entamoeba histolytica.* ×2500. (*After Dobell*)

1, Active amoeboid form with ingested red blood corpuscles. 2, Uninucleate cyst. 3, Binucleate cyst. 4, Quadrinucleate cyst. 5, Quadrinucleate cyst, dwarf race, 6·6 μm in diameter. Note the distinct central karyosome in the nucleus.

Trophozoites multiply by binary fission. In wet preparations they move sluggishly by suddenly thrusting out pseudopodia from the ectoplasm, into which the other contents of the cell flow. This has been described as like a slug moving at express speed.

Table 42. Differential characters of the Entamoebae of the *E. histolytica* complex

		E. histolytica forms	
	E. hartmanni	Minuta	Large haematophagous
Trophozoite			
Body	3·0–10·5 μm	10·0–20·0 μm	20·0–40·0 μm
Nucleus	1·5– 3·2 μm	2·8–4·5 μm	
Cyst			
Body	3·8– 8·0 μm	9·5–17·5 μm	Absent (cysts produced only by minuta forms)
Nuclei			
1	1·8– 3·0 μm	4·0– 5·5 μm	
2	1·3– 2·0 μm	2·0– 3·2 μm	
4	0·7– 1·7 μm	1·4– 2·6 μm	
Glycogen	Small vacuoles	One large vacuole	

Cysts

The trophozoites inhabit the crypts of the caecum and the first part of the colon, where they feed on mucus and its contents and probably live in symbiosis with intestinal bacteria. As they pass down the colon, and the faecal material becomes drier, the conditions are less favourable, and the trophozoites protect themselves by encysting, though what factors actually influence encystment are uncertain—one element seems to be the right bacterial flora. The cysts are quiescent and resist various environmental conditions which would be fatal to trophozoites. In this process the trophozoites discharge undigested food and condense into a spherical mass (the *pre-cystic stage*), with a tough wall and still a single nucleus. They may contain a mass of glycogen and chromatoid bodies which stain black with iron–haematoxylin.

The next stage is the development of the fully formed cyst. In the fresh state this has a greenish, refractile appearance. At 9·5–17·5 μm this is smaller than the trophozoite, and more compact. The nucleus divides by mitosis to produce 2, then 4 nuclei,

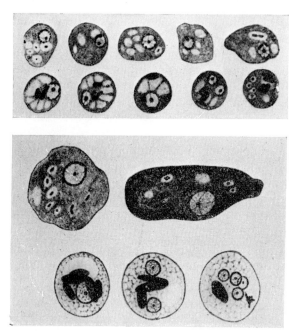

Fig. 293.—Entamoebae of the *E. histolytica* complex. ×1500. (*After Hoare*)

Above: E. hartmanni trophozoites (top) and cysts (bottom). *Below:* Typical *E. histolytica* trophozoites (top) and cysts (bottom).

which have the same characteristics as the nucleus of the trophozoite, though they become smaller. Each nucleus has a central karyosome and peripheral chromatin granules, as in the trophozoite.

The cyst wall is relatively tough, and within it there are one or more chromatoid bodies—oval bars staining black with iron–haematoxylin—and in the early stages glycogen staining golden brown with iodine. The glycogen gradually disappears, presumably being metabolized, and the chromatoid bodies become less conspicuous.

Cysts are usually found without trophozoites in the faeces of infected persons not suffering from actual disease, but in such persons trophozoites can be demonstrated after a purgative has been given. Cysts are never found in liver abscesses or lesions of other organs; only the haematophagous trophozoites are found in such lesions.

Cysts are the only infective forms. They are passed in faeces and can resist external environmental conditions which are not too extreme—for instance they can remain viable in an ice box at 4–8°C for several days, in cool faeces for 12 days or more, in cool water for several weeks. They can withstand passage through the intestines of filth flies, and viable cysts and even trophozoites have been recovered from the vomit and faeces of flies. Cysts can pass through cockroaches and remain viable. They are sensitive, however, to desiccation and to temperatures above 50°C and below −5°C. They can resist 1 in 2500 mercury bichloride, 5% HCl or 0·5% formalin for 30 minutes, and 1 in 500 potassium permanganate for 24–48 hours. They are killed by 1 in 20 cresol in 15 minutes, by 1% phenol in 30 minutes and by 5% acetic acid at 30°C in 15 minutes. They have considerable resistance to chlorine, but can be killed in drinking water by superchlorination and by iodine. Recorded experiments vary in the figures given for superchlorination. A *residual* of 2–3 p.p.m. of chlorine kills over 99% of cysts in 20–30 minutes, but this is influenced by the organic content of the water. If the organic content is high, for instance through faecal contamination, the required concentration of chlorine is also high. Dechlorination is necessary in this process. Ozone at 0·5–1·0 p.p.m. kills over 99% of cysts within 5 minutes, but ozone dissipates quickly and leaves no effective residual. Cysts pass through Mark 0 micro-straining metal fabric (aperture 23 μm) (Upton 1969). This is sometimes used as part of a treatment process for domestic water supplies. In relation to cysts coagulation and sand filtration are needed as well as chlorination.

When trophozoites are swallowed, they are destroyed in the acid contents of the stomach; cysts are not, and can therefore pass into the alkaline small intestine where excystation takes place with the release of 4 growing and multiplying trophozoites from each quadrinucleate cyst, to complete the cycle. Excystation can also be induced in vitro in conditions resembling those of the intestinal contents. In man, however, it occurs after a cyst is swallowed, but not, apparently, in the large intestines. In this cycle there is normally no invasion of the intestinal wall, no ulceration, and no spread beyond the intestinal lumen. The trophozoites and cysts in this cycle, though belonging to the large race (as distinct from *E. hartmanni*) may apparently be non-pathogenic (and world-wide) or pathogenic (mostly in hot countries). Yet the potentially pathogenic race can apparently live as non-pathogenic, commensal inhabitants of the intestinal lumen without invading the tissues, until some influence, at present obscure, causes the trophozoites to invade the intestinal mucosa and deeper tissues. These now pathogenic and invasive trophozoites destroy tissue, ingest red blood cells and tissue debris and, perhaps because of improved nutrition, become generally much larger than the commensal trophozoites. In faeces, active amoebae containing ingested red blood cells can confidently be diagnosed as *E. histolytica*.

The non-pathogenic entamoebae are sometimes called 'minuta' forms because, though belonging to the large race, they are smaller than the pathogenic invasive forms. But they are not *E. hartmanni*, which is also non-pathogenic and even smaller, forming cysts with 4 nuclei, and which never invades the tissues (see page 158).

The aggressive pathogenic trophozoites which invade tissues do not give rise to cysts. They pass out in the faeces and, because they do not possess the defensive properties of cysts, they are a dead end in the chain of reproduction. Cysts are formed only by the commensal trophozoites (Hoare 1957).

The virulent race is potentially pathogenic, and in certain circumstances (as has been stated) can invade the tissues, causing disease. The mechanism by which pathogenic *E. histolytica* gains entry into the tissues is not clearly understood. It can hydrolyse casein, fibrin, haemoglobin and the epithelium of guinea-pig gut. It has tryptic and peptic activity, and most pathogenic strains contain hyaluronidase and other enzymes. Trophozoites of various strains (pathogenic and non-pathogenic) are cytotoxic to leucocytes of some animals. Yet all these facts are not enough to explain invasiveness. These invasive entamoebae, causing disease, feed on erythrocytes both in the tissues and when they escape into the lumen of the bowel, and because they are in a better state of nutrition they increase in size to 20–40 μm. These large trophozoites (sometimes described as *magna* forms) multiply and are passed out in the faeces, where they can be recognized by their morphology, movements and the presence of ingested erythrocytes.

E. histolytica can be cultivated in vitro, and several media have been described, the most well known of which is that devised by Boeck and Drbohlav, composed of egg beaten up in Locke solution and inspissated as a slope, autoclaved, and then covered to a depth of 1 cm with sterile Locke solution and inactivated human serum (or 1% crystallized egg albumin) in equal parts. An essential addition to all media is a culture of enteric bacteria (organism 't') or *Klebsiella*, or *Trypanosoma cruzi*, as well as starch or rice flour.

It has also been grown in cultures of chick embryo tissue.

Table 43. Aetiology of amoebiasis

Hypotheses	Unicistic 1913	Dualistic 1925	Neodualistic 1957
Non-pathogenic amoebiasis	*E. histolytica* SMALL RACE LARGE RACE: Commensal phase ('minuta' form)	*E. hartmanni* *E. dispar*	*E. hartmanni* *E. histolytica* Avirulent large race
Pathogenic amoebiases			?
			Virulent large race:
Subclinical		*E. dysenteriae*	Dormant in lumen of gut
Clinical	Virulent (tissue) phase ('magna' form)		Invading gut wall

After Hoare (1961).

Recognition of *E. histolytica*

A small portion of fresh faeces should be emulsified in saline on a *warm* slide, and covered with a coverslip. The emulsion should not contain solid particles which could prevent the coverslip from lying flat, and it should allow light to pass through it easily; newsprint should be readable through it. Trophozoites of *E. histolytica* can be recognized by their pseudopodial movements, their ectoplasm and granular endoplasm, and (in pathogenic forms) by ingested erythrocytes; the nuclei are characteristic. Cysts have a greenish translucency and a 'ground glass' appearance.

An emulsion of this kind can be stained with iodine (one part in 2 parts of potassium iodide, water 100), a drop of this solution being placed on the faecal emulsion and then covered. The nuclei, glycogen granules and refractive chromatoid bodies can then be seen.

An emulsion can also be stained with eosin (0·5%), which stains the background pink, against which viable cysts stand out as clear unstained bodies. A cyst which takes the eosin stain is regarded as non-viable, a fact which is made use of in tests of disinfectants for chemical closets.

Emulsions can also be stained with haematoxylin, but the techniques are more elaborate than those described above. The haematoxylin specimens keep well if they are fixed before being stained.

The Merthiolate–iodine–formaldehyde (MIF) fixative stain consists of 250 ml distilled water, 200 ml tincture of Merthiolate (1 in 1000), 25 ml formaldehyde and 5 ml glycerol, to which 10–15 parts of fresh Lugol's 5% iodine in 10% potassium iodide in distilled water are added. This may be used for direct smears or for preserving

Table 44. Differential characters of the common intestinal amoeba

Entamoeba coli	Entamoeba histolytica	Endolimax nana
Size: 10–40 μm. Morphology: No distinction between endo- and ectoplasm	10–40 μm. Granular endoplasm; clear ectoplasm	6–12 μm. Granular and rather vacuolated cytoplasm
Ingests bacteria, other protozoa, etc.	May ingest red cells, tissue cells, etc.	Ingests bacteria and food granules
Nucleus distinct in fresh specimens. Coarse chromatin granules on nuclear membrane. Eccentric karyosome surrounded by coarse ring	Nucleus inconspicuous in fresh specimens. Fine chromatin granules on nuclear membrane. Central karyosome surrounded by delicate ring	Clear nuclear membrane and massive, irregular karyosome
Sluggish movement with granular pseudopodia	Active movement with clear, blunt pseudopodia	Sluggish movement with clear pseudopodia
Multiplication: By binary fission in faeces. Encystment and formation of spherical cysts. 10–30 μm in diameter, with 1, 2, 4, or 8 nuclei	By binary fission. Encystment and formation of spherical cysts, 9·5–17·5 μm in diameter, with 1, 2 or 4 nuclei	By binary fission in faeces. Encystment and formation of nucleated oval cysts 8–10 μm in length by 4–5 μm in breadth, with 1, 2, or 4 nuclei
Chromatoid bodies typically not present in the mature cyst	Chromatoid bodies especially present in the mature cyst	Chromatoid bodies not present in the cyst

faeces. For preservation 0·15 ml of Lugol solution is placed in a tube, followed by 2·35 ml of the MIF solution, and 0·25 gramme of faeces is added and thoroughly mixed. The parasites are well preserved.

Entamoeba moshkovskii (Tshalaia, 1941)

This species resembles *E. histolytica* in both trophozoite and cystic stages and has been recovered from sewage in Moscow, U.S.A., England and Brazil. Attempts to infect laboratory animals have been unsuccessful. *E. invadens*, a parasite of snakes, is also morphologically identical with *E. histolytica*.

Entamoeba coli (Grassi, 1879)

Unlike *E. histolytica*, this amoeba does not invade tissues; it is therefore a non-pathogenic species and a harmless commensal in the intestinal tract of man. A similar amoeba is found in monkeys and rats.

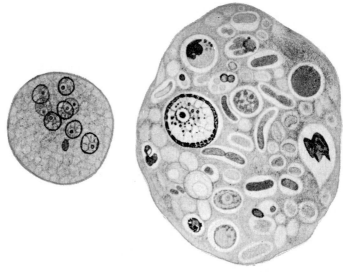

Fig. 294.—*Entamoeba coli.* ×2500. (*After Dobell*)

1, Cyst with 8 nuclei. 2, Active amoeboid stage with ingested food material. Note the characteristic nucleus with eccentric karyosome.

E. coli is a very common parasite in the tropics and wherever sanitation is primitive it is probable that no individual escapes infection. On the average, *E. coli* is larger than *E. histolytica*, but varies greatly. The active vegetative stage measures from 10 to 40 μm, but is usually 20–30 μm in diameter. It normally lives in the large intestine, does not invade tissues, but develops in intestinal contents, where it ingests bacteria, yeasts and other material. *E. coli* can be differentiated from *E. histolytica* by means of the fluorescent antibody technique.

Generally speaking, movements are much more sluggish than those of *E. histolytica*, and the individuals are less active. The organism does not move across the slide, but remains stationary. The ectoplasm is not clearly defined but is represented by a superficial clearer area merging into the endoplasm. This is extensively vacuolated, and food vacuoles contain bacteria, yeasts or even cysts of other protozoa, such as *E. histolytica*, *Giardia* and *Isospora*. Red blood corpuscles or tissue elements are not ingested. In general, *E. coli* is faintly grey, contrasting with the greenish tint and higher refractive index of *E. histolytica*. Sometimes individuals show various fissures or rectangular vacuoles representing degenerative changes.

The *nucleus*, compared with that of *E. histolytica*, is larger, coarser and more easily visible in the living organism (Fig. 294). The chromatin granules on the nuclear membrane are relatively coarse, and there are others on the linin network. The karyosome, larger than that of *E. histolytica*, is usually eccentric in position, surrounded by a clear area intersected by linin network with chromatin granules. These nuclear characteristics are best seen in fresh specimens but are obscured in degenerate individuals. *E. coli* reproduces by binary fission.

Precystic forms

Before encystment the amoebae undergo reduction in size, with the result that precystic forms are especially difficult to distinguish from those of *E. histolytica*, but are usually larger. Precystic forms are probably formed by division of larger individuals.

Cysts

The cyst wall is secreted round a spherical precystic amoeba. Individual cysts vary greatly in size, from 10 to 30 μm. Like *E. histolytica*, *E. coli* is a composite species consisting of a number of races distinguished by the dimensions of the cysts.

The cyst is at first uninucleate, the nucleus having the same characteristics as that of the active form. It divides repeatedly by mitosis, the nuclei progressively diminishing in size as their number increases. The quadrinucleate stage is passed through very rapidly and is therefore rarely seen. The mature cyst typically contains 8 nuclei. Immature binucleate and quadrinucleate cysts are occasionally seen, even supernucleate cysts with 16 nuclei. The binucleate cyst frequently contains a large quantity of glycogen, which replaces almost the entire cytoplasm, but this usually disappears before the quadrinucleate stage is reached.

Chromatoid bodies are usually not present, but, when they are, they appear as small granular, spicular or rod-like bodies, more especially in the binucleate stage. In the mature octonucleate form they may occasionally be seen as pointed threads or splinters, thus differing from the stouter bodies with blunted ends common in *E. histolytica*. When hatching, an octonucleate amoeba escapes from the cyst and gives rise to eight uninucleate amoebulae.

The life history of *E. coli* resembles that of *E. histolytica*, except that the vegetative forms inhabit only the faeces. This protozoan may be cultivated, but with difficulty, on the same media as are employed for *E. histolytica*. It is not affected by emetine. Cysts of *E. coli* can withstand drying while those of *E. histolytica* cannot. The cyst wall consists of two layers—a thick inner and a flexible outer wall measuring 1·0 μm in diameter.

Incidence

E. coli is common in man in temperate zones as well as in the tropics, and found in about 15% of normal people. It is most readily seen in dysenteric cases with diarrhoea. Some monkeys harbour a parasite closely resembling it.

Entamoeba polecki (Von Prowazek, 1912)

An intestinal amoeba of the frog and rhesus monkey has been reported from man in California. The trophozoite resembles *E. coli* in viscosity and movements.·

Entamoeba gingivalis (Gros, 1949) (Fig. 295)

This amoeba is of interest, not only for its occurrence in the mouth, but also because it was the first to be discovered in man. The claim that it might prove to be the cause of pyorrhoea alveolaris has been disproved. This species has been found in pulmonary suppuration by bronchoscopy. The importance of this lies in its differentiation from *E. histolytica*. *E. gingivalis* may be found in the sputum where it can be mistaken for *E. histolytica* from a pulmonary abscess.

E. gingivalis is a small species with great variations in size, from 10 to 25 μm depending on its metabolic activity. As in *E. histolytica*, endoplasm and ectoplasm are sharply differentiated. The cytoplasm is occupied by food vacuoles, and peculiar inclusions of a greenish refractile appearance of undetermined nature, which may be the remains of salivary corpuscles or polymorphonuclear cells; there are also numbers of ingested bacteria.

The *nucleus* is similar to that of *E. coli*. It is 2·5–3 μm, spherical and vesicular but slightly smaller in proportion to the rest of the organism than in *E. histolytica* or *E. coli*. The nuclear membrane is a definite structure, and is lined with peripheral chromatic granules.

E. gingivalis probably reproduces by binary fission, although all intermediary stages have not been studied and it is probable also that it does not form cysts.

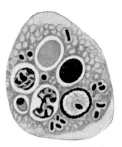
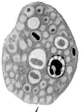

Fig. 295.—*Entamoeba
gingivalis* in the active
amoeboid form, with
eccentric nucleus and
ingested bodies. ×2500.
(*After Dobell*)

Fig. 296.—*Endolimax nana*. ×2500.
(*After Dobell*)

1, Active amoeboid form. 2, Quadrinucleate
mature cyst.

Endolimax nana (Wenyon & O'Connor, 1917) (Fig. 296)

This is a non-pathogenic species commonly inhabiting the intestinal tract of man (mainly of the large and to a lesser extent of the small intestine), especially in the tropics, and it is of importance because the spherical quadrinucleate cysts resemble those of the small race of *E. histolytica*; moreover, it is found in 33% of dysenteric or diarrhoeic faeces, and is often very abundant indeed.

E. nana is a small species, 6–12 μm in diameter; it has a characteristic vesicular *nucleus* with a large irregularly shaped karyosome. It ingests food granules and bacteria, but not red blood corpuscles or cells. Its movements are sluggish, but it may become quite active on a warm stage.

The *cysts* (Fig. 296) are of approximately the same size and appearance as the active form. When fully mature they have characteristic nuclei and contain a few refractile granules, but are devoid of vacuoles or chromatoid bodies. Sometimes they contain glycogen, especially the binucleate forms. In shape they vary from that of a typical oval to a sphere. Small individuals measure 6 μm in diameter. Occasionally, they contain small filamentous rods or granules.

E. nana is certainly non-pathogenic and is not amenable to emetine. This species has been successfully cultured on serum and egg media.

Iodamoeba bütschlii (Von Prowazek, 1912) (Fig. 297)

Synonym: *Endolimax williamsi*

Cysts of this species have long been known in man as 'iodine', or 'I.' cysts, and similar organisms are found in the faeces of monkeys and pigs.

I. bütschlii is small, intermediate in size between *E. coli* and *E. nana*, measuring from 9–20 μm in diameter, though smaller individuals, 5 μm in size, may occur. In form and habit it resembles small specimens of *E. coli*. The cytoplasm contains food vacuoles with bacteria and other food particles. There is no marked differentiation of ecto- and endoplasm. The movements are sluggish, like those of *E. coli*.

The *nucleus*, which is often indistinguishable in specimens containing many food granules, is large, being in diameter one-quarter to one-fifth of the whole organism. There is a large conspicuous karyosome which has a diameter of one-third to one-half of the nucleus.

The *cysts* are uninucleate, frequently irregular in outline, measuring 7–15 μm in diameter. There is a distinct cyst wall and inside the cyst is a rounded refractile body with a number of small *volutin* granules. There is usually a large and dense glycogen mass which shows up clearly in iodine solution, and sometimes even two or three separated masses may be observed within the same cyst.

The cyst nucleus, eccentrically placed, is comparatively large, 2–3 μm in diameter, whilst the karyosome, which is centrally placed in the nuclei of the precystic stage, gradually passes, during encystment, to the periphery, showing up as a large compact mass in close contact with the nuclear membrane.

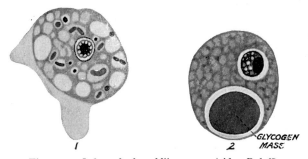

Fig. 297.—*Iodamoeba bütschlii*. × 2500. (*After Dobell*)

1, Active amoeboid form with ingested micro-organisms. 2, Mature cyst (iodine cyst) containing a large iodine-staining glycogen mass.

It is remarkable that very large numbers of cysts may be present in the faeces without any evidence of free forms. The mature uninucleate cysts, save for the disappearance of the contained glycogen, do not undergo any further changes outside the human body.

It is estimated that *I. bütschlii* occurs in 5% of human faeces, most commonly in the tropics, and is found, not infrequently, in association with *E. histolytica*. Both the active forms as well as the cysts are amenable to emetine and emetine and bismuth iodide. This amoeba has been cultivated on egg medium and Locke's solution.

Pathogenicity

A generalized amoebiasis thought to be due to *I. bütschlii* in a Japanese prisoner of war was described by Derrick (1948). This differed from any known infection of *E. histolytica* by the extent and bizarre nature of the lesions. These were ulceration of the stomach, small intestine and colon. Metastatic foci were present in the brain, both lungs, gastric and mesenteric lymph glands, but not in the liver. In most of the lesions the amoebae occurred in enormous numbers. In all tissues they had the same morphology and varied from 3 to 12 × 9 μm, on an average that of a leucocyte in sections. It is conceivable that a set of circumstances arose when the host's resistance was much reduced which caused the amoebae to invade the tissues—that there was a primary infection of the intestinal tract from which the amoebae spread to other organs. The invasion of vessels, arterioles, venules and lymphatics readily explains the widespread metastases. It was suggested that primarily there was a heavy infection of the faeces with *I. bütschlii* (but see page 980).

A second case has now been reported by Kernohan *et al.* (1960) in a six-year-old child from Tucson, Arizona, who had bruised the right parieto-occipital region in a fall. A granuloma was found, with cystic spaces filled with gelatinous matter in which amoebae were found, resembling *I. bütschlii*, but the forms in the brain were slightly larger than those in the faeces. It is now thought that these two cases were caused by *Naegleria*.

Dientamoeba fragilis (Jepps & Dobell, 1918) (Fig. 298)

This is a small species which may measure 3·5–12 μm, but its usual size is 8–9 μm; it inhabits the large intestine of man and has also been found in monkeys (macaques in the Philippines). It is very actively motile, throwing out pseudopodia which are lobed and indented. Each amoeba is typically binucleate. The spherical *nucleus*, measuring 0·8–2·3 μm, contains 6 chromatin granules. The 2 nuclei are connected by a thread (*centrodesmose*). In fresh preparations the amoeba rapidly degenerates and vacuoles form. It lives exclusively on bacteria and small micro-organisms, and is apparently amenable to emetine. No cystic stage is known.

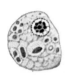 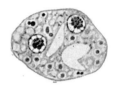

Fig. 298.—Uninucleate and binucleate forms of *Dientamoeba fragilis.* ×2500. (*After Dobell*)

Dobell has brought forward evidence that this amoeba is closely related to the flagellate *Histomonas meleagridis* (the parasite of 'blackhead of turkeys') which normally lives as a flagellate in the caecum, but can invade the liver, where it assumes the amoeboid form.

Burrows and Swerdlow (1956) have recorded an abnormally high association between the incidence of *D. fragilis* and that of *Enterobius vermicularis*. Of 22 appendices harbouring *D. fragilis*, 12 were also infected with the pinworm. The association is supported to some extent by the supposed passage of *Histomonas meleagridis* of turkeys through the nematode, *Heterakis*.

Parasitism. Most human amoebae are liable to be parasitized by a fungus *Sphaerita*— consisting of a small spherical mass of coccus-like bodies, which are refractile and occur within vacuoles of the cytoplasm.

FREE-LIVING AMOEBAE

GENUS: *Naegleria*

These free-living amoebae have been shown to cause primary amoebic meningoencephalitis (see page 185).

Morphology

Living amoebae in wet smears of cerebrospinal fluid (Carter 1968). The amoebae are slug-shaped, with 1 broad and 1 pointed extremity and are actively motile at 21°C. Movement is directional and quite brisk. Temporarily rounded forms, with diameters varying between 6 and 15 μm, may be found. A hyaline ectoplasmic layer is well differentiated from a finely granular endoplasm containing up to 6 small clear vacuoles. The nucleus is distinctive, with a centrally located nucleolus. A few organisms undergo a transient flagellate transformation, which is a free-living form of the parasite.

Morphology in sections. When stained with haematoxylin and eosin the amoebae have a diameter between 6 and 9 μm, and may be as large as 12 μm. There is a very fine haematoxophilic cell membrane, usually giving rise to a circular, occasionally oval, outline, which may be irregular. The cytoplasm has distinctive outer and inner zones, the outer packed with coarse magenta-stained granules and clear vacuoles, amorphous eosinophilic fragments and occasional red blood cells and granules of polymorpho-nuclear lymphocytes. The inner zone, up to half the diameter, consists of 4-6 vacuoles surrounding the nucleus, which is usually single, eccentrically situated and measures up to 2 μm in diameter. The nucleus contains a centrally located nucleolus 1 μm in diameter.

Culture

The amoebae may be cultured in a proteose peptone glucose medium (PPG) (Band 1959) and the cultures, inoculated intranasally in to mice, cause fatal meningo-encephalitis within 5 days.

INTESTINAL FLAGELLATES

ORDER: POLYMASTIGIDA
FAMILY: MONADIDAE
GENUS: *Enteromonas*

Enteromonas hominis (Da Fonseca, 1915) (Fig. 299)

Synonym: *Tricercomonas intestinalis* (Wenyon & O'Connor, 1917).
This is a minute but very active pyriform flagellate, measuring 4–10 × 3–6 μm. The posterior end is attenuated to a fine point.

The *nucleus* is single and vesicular, and 3 flagella of equal length arise from a blepharoplast. A fourth flagellum runs down the margin of the body to the posterior extremity and ends in a terminal lash. The combined movements of all these produce a sort of 'hovering effect' when in full action.

The *cysts* are small, oval, with a distinct cyst wall, resemble fungus spores, and contain iodophilic refractile bodies. This flagellate can be cultivated with comparative ease on Locke-egg medium. There is no evidence of pathogenicity.

FAMILY: EMBADOMONADIDAE
GENUS: *Embadomonas*

Embadomonas intestinalis (Wenyon & O'Connor, 1917) (Fig. 299)

A small but active flagellate, oval, 4–9 × 3–4 μm, which inhabits the intestinal tract. There are 2 flagella: the anterior longer and thinner; the posterior projecting from a laterally-situated mouth (cytostome), at the anterior extremity, supported by a ridge. The flagella act independently and thereby impart a peculiar jerky movement to the organism. The general shape is ovoid, with blunt anterior and pointed posterior extremities. The cytoplasm is vacuolated, containing ingested bacilli.

Cysts are pear-shaped, 4·5–6 μm in length, and appear structureless in the unstained state, but in iodine solution the *nucleus* can be discerned. This flagellate has been cultivated on egg medium. As in other members of this group, there is no evidence of pathogenicity.

FAMILY: CHILOMASTIGIDAE
GENUS: *Chilomastix*

Chilomastix mesnili (Wenyon, 1910)

Synonym: *Tetramitus mesnili* (Fig. 299).
This flagellate resembles *Trichomonas hominis* in general shape and size and occurs in the large intestine. There are 3 long flagella, but no undulating membrane or

axostyle. There is a large mouth (cytostome), which occupies two-thirds of the body length, and contains a flagellum arising from a granule situated anteriorly to the spherical nucleus. The posterior extremity is attenuated. The cytoplasm contains numerous vacuoles and bacteria which form the main food supply. Division takes place by longitudinal fission. Individual organisms vary very much in length, but measure on an average 14 μm in length by 5–6 μm in breadth.

In freshly-passed faeces, *Chilomastix* moves with active, jerky movements which distinguish it from the more deliberate rotatory action of *Trichomonas*.

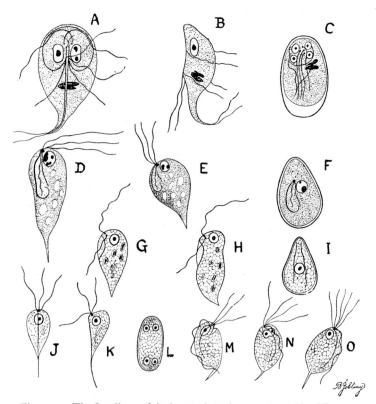

Fig. 299.—The flagellates of the human intestine. × 2000. (*After Wenyon*)

A–C, *Giardia intestinalis*, free and encysted forms. D–F, *Chilomastix mesnili*, free and encysted forms. G–I, *Embadomonas intestinalis*, free and encysted forms. J–L, *Tricercomonas intestinalis*, free and encysted forms. M–O, *Trichomonas hominis*, forms with 3, 4 and 5 flagella.

Cysts

'Lemon-shaped' cysts appear in formed stools and are 7–10 μm in length; they contain a single nucleus and vestiges of a cytostome. In fresh preparations they have to be differentiated from yeasts.

Infections with this parasite are very persistent, but there is no evidence of pathogenicity.

C. mesnili has been cultured on artificial media.

Trichomycin was obtained from a *Streptomyces* in soil in 1952. It is active against *Trichomonas* and is lethal in concentration of 2 μg/5 ml.

FAMILY: TRICHOMONADIDAE

GENUS: *Trichomonas*

Trichomonas hominis (Davaine, 1860) (Fig. 299)

This is the most common intestinal flagellate of man, inhabiting the caecum and large intestine, often in enormous numbers.

The body is pear-shaped, 10–15 μm in length by 7–10 μm in breadth. The spherical *nucleus* is at the anterior extremity and immediately in front of it are placed *blepharoplasts* from which 3 long flagella are directed forwards, while a fourth and stouter passes backwards to form the border of the undulating membrane, beyond which it is continued as a free flagellum. The cytostome is represented by a small aperture near the anterior end. A *stiffening rod*, arising from the blepharoplast, supports the undulating membrane. Running down the middle of the body is a second skeletal rod, or *axostyle*. The cytoplasm contains vacuoles with bacteria and food granules.

According to the number of flagella (3, 4 or 5), 3 varieties are recognized, although the triflagellate is the most common. Dobell thought that these varieties were merely strains of the same species. This flagellate progresses by lashing movements from the 3 anterior flagella, and the undulating membrane causes it to revolve on a longitudinal axis. The parasite is also capable of amoeboid movement, especially evident in degenerate individuals. Reproduction is by longitudinal fission, by duplication of the various parts. No *cysts* are known.

The abundance of *T. hominis* in diarrhoeic stools in the tropics has induced some observers to consider it pathogenic, and in one instance Wenyon found definite evidence of invasion of the intestinal mucosa by these organisms. Moreover, the closely allied *T. caviae* often causes ulceration of the large intestine in guinea-pigs.

On the whole, the pathogenicity of *T. hominis* in the intestinal tract of man is doubtful, and its presence in diarrhoeic stools may be due to liquid faeces which constitute a congenial medium for this flagellate.

T. hominis can be artificially cultured on blood agar with Locke's fluid for many generations, but subinoculations are necessary every few days, but now bacteria-free cultures can be obtained with antibiotics on egg-slants overlaid with bouillon serum and yeast extract.

A somewhat similar species, *T. elongata*, is found in the mouth cavity, as well as on the tonsillar surface. A third form, *T. vaginalis*, is present in the vaginal cavity of 10% of women. *T. vaginalis* can be grown easily in bacteria-free culture and its requirements are less exacting than those of *T. hominis*.

Most gynaecologists now regard *T. vaginalis* as a definite clinical pathogen, responsible for vaginitis, and the human analogue of *T. foetus*, which causes inflammation of the genitalia of cattle. The two species are physiologically different. On serological grounds it has now been shown that *T. hominis* and *T. vaginalis* are distinct species. *T. vaginalis* is sometimes found in the male urethra and can invade the epithelium and prostate. The male is the most important transmitter of this infection. It flourishes mainly during the reproductive period, but not, as a rule, in young girls, or after the climacteric. It appears to multiply when the vaginal state is favourable, at pH 4, and a symbiotic association with a non-haemolytic streptococcus is suggested. The parasite disappears when the urine becomes alkaline. *T. vaginalis* is said to be considerably larger than *T. hominis*, reaching 27 × 18 μm. Four anterior flagella are of equal length, a fifth flagellum on the margin of the relatively short undulating membrane protruding a considerable distance beyond the posterior tip of the organism. *T tenax* (*Tetratrichomonas buccalis*) Dobell, 1939, is probably a cosmopolitan parasite of man and has 4 anterior free flagella of equal length, a relatively short undulating membrane, a slender *axostyle* and a subspherical nucleus. On the average it is smaller than *T. hominis*. It inhabits the mouth, especially in diseased gums. It has been found in sputum from the lung and in pulmonary gangrene. It occurs in about 18% of individuals.

FAMILY: HEXAMITIDAE
GENUS: *Giardia*

Giardia intestinalis (Lambl, 1859)

Synonyms: *Giardia lamblia, Lamblia intestinalis* (Fig. 299)
This remarkable parasite lives in the upper part of the small intestine, particularly the duodenum. In shape it resembles a half-pear, split longitudinally. It measures 12–18 μm in length. The ventral surface is furnished with a concave sucking disc with a raised ridge at the anterior end, and the posterior extremity tapers into a fine tail and terminates in 2 flagella. There are altogether 4 pairs of flagella on the body, arising from as many blepharoplasts; the posterior 3 arise from the margins of the *axostyles*. There are 2 of these stiff supporting structures which pass down the centre of the body. Two oval *nuclei* are situated within the sucking discs at the anterior end. The cytoplasm also contains a characteristically curved parabasal body in the lower half of the body. This flagellate swims rapidly, like a flat fish, swaying from side to side. *Giardia* reproduces itself by a complicated process of binary fission.

The *cysts*, which may occur in the faeces in enormous numbers, are characteristic structures. They are oval, measuring about 10·5 × 7·4 μm. The body of the flagellate becomes rounded, while the various inner structures (flagella, axostyle, etc.) become detached and cannot always be identified, except for the crescentic parabasal body. There are at first 2 nuclei, which divide, giving rise to 4 in the mature cyst. When examined in iodine solution, the cysts stain faint yellowish-brown and the cytoplasmic contents shrink back from the thick wall.

A method of cultivation of *Giardia* together with a yeast, *Candida guillermondi*, has been described. For initial isolation the medium is composed of 25% inactivated serum, plus 5% chick embryo, plus 10% chick amniotic fluid and 60% Hanks solution. For maintenance, a mixture of 20% human serum with 5% chick embryo extract and 25% Hottinger's digest (tryptic meat digest) and 50% Earle's solution. Penicillin and streptomycin are added to prevent growth of extraneous bacteria. 0·2–0·5 ml of washed and centrifuged *Giardia* from duodenal drainage is placed into insulin bottles containing the medium previously seeded with fibroblasts. The bottles are plugged with rubber corks and incubated at 37°C. The growth of *Giardia* in bottles can be observed under low magnifications of the microscope.

For pathology and treatment see page 186.

SUBPHYLUM: CILIOPHORA
CLASS: CILIATA
GENUS: *Balantidium*

Balantidium coli (Malmsten, 1857)

This is a large protozoon belonging to the class Ciliata. Oval in shape and of variable size, it is 30–200 μm in length by 40–60 μm in breadth. The average is 50–70 μm. Various races are recognized by the size. The body is clothed with a thick covering of cilia arranged in longitudinal rows (Fig. 300).

The *nucleus* is represented by a large kidney-shaped *macronucleus* with a small *micronucleus* closely approximated. The protoplasm contains 2 *contractile* and a number of *food vacuoles*. At the anterior end there is a *peristome*, leading into a mouth, or *cytostome*; posteriorly there is an anus, or *cytopyge*. Nutrition is effected by ingestion of solid particles, leucocytes and red blood corpuscles.

Bal. coli reproduces asexually by transverse fission. Conjugation takes place by exchange of certain nuclear elements and, when once this has been effected, the conjugants once more separate.

The *cysts* (Fig. 300) are ovoid, 45–60 μm in length, and are passed in the faeces. They contain the parasite which may be seen moving actively. The enclosed balantidium then loses its cilia, and sometimes 2 individuals are found in the same cyst. Transmission of infection takes place by means of cysts.

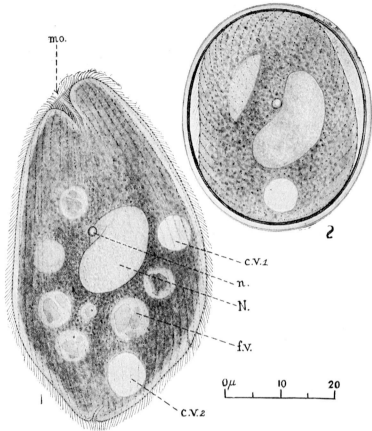

Fig. 300.—*Balantidium coli.* ×1200. (*After Dobell. By permission of the Medical Research Council*)

1, Living individual. N., Meganucleus; n., Micronucleus; c.v.1, Anterior contractile vacuole; c.v.2, Posterior contractile vacuole. f.v., Food vacuole; mo., Mouth. 2, Encysted form, showing nuclei, posterior contractile vacuole and remains of cilia.

Bal. coli has been cultured in human serum diluted with saline. The presence of symbiotic bacteria is necessary, at 30–37°C, but frequent subinoculations have to be made.

For pathology and treatment see page 188.

REFERENCES

ADLER, S., FONER, A. & MONTIGLIO, B. (1966) *Trans. R. Soc. trop. Med. Hyg.*, **60,** 380.
ALVARADO, C. A. & BRUCE-CHWATT, L. J. (1962) *Sci. Am.*, **206,** 86.
AREAN, V. M. (1971) in *Pathology of Protozoal and Helminthic Diseases.* (ed. RAUL A. MARCIA-ROJAS), p. 292. Baltimore: Williams & Wilkins.
BAND, R. N. (1959) *J. gen Microbiol.*, **21,** 80.
BRAY, R. S. (1965) *Am. J. trop. Med. Hyg.*, **9,** 455.
BURROWS, R. B. & SWERDLOW, M. A. (1956) *Am. J. trop. Med. Hyg.*, **5,** 258.
CARTER, R. F. (1968) *J. Path. Bact.*, **96,** 1.
CHIN, W., CONTACOS, P. G., COATNEY, G. R. & KIMBALL, H. R. (1965) *Science, N.Y.*, **149,** 865.

COATNEY, G. R., CHIN, W., CONTACOS, P. G. & KING, H. K. (1966) *J. Parasit.*, **52,** 660.

CUNNINGHAM, M. P., LUMSDEN, W. H. R. & WEBBER, W. A. F. (1963) *Exp. Parasit.*, **14,** 280.

DERRICK, E. H. (1948) *Trans. R. Soc. trop. Med. Hyg.*, **42,** 191.

FRENKEL, J. K. (1971) in *Pathology of Protozoal and Helminthic Diseases.* (ed. RAUL A. MARCIAL-ROJAS), p. 255. Baltimore: Williams & Wilkins.

FULTON, J. D. & VOLLER, A. (1964) *Br. med. J.*, **ii,** 1173.

GARNHAM, P. C. C. (1966) *Malaria Parasites and Other Haemosporidia.* Oxford: Blackwell.

HAWKING, F., WORMS, M. J. & GAMMAGE, K. (1968) *Trans. R. Soc. trop. Med. Hyg.*, **62,** 731.

HOARE, C. A. (1957) *Trans. R. Soc. trop. Med. Hyg.*, **51,** 304.

———— (1961) *Bull. Soc. Path. exot.*, **54,** 429.

KERNOHAN, J. W., MAGATH, T. B. & SCHLOSS, G. T. (1960) *Archs Path.*, **70,** 576.

LANHAM, S. M. (1968) *Nature, Lond.*, **218,** 1273.

MANDOUR, A. M. (1965) *Trans. R. Soc. trop. Med. Hyg.*, **59,** 423.

ORMEROD, W. E. & VENKATESAN, S. (1971) *Trans. R. Soc. trop. Med. Hyg.*, **65,** 722.

PHILLIPS, N. R. (1960) *Ann. trop. Med. Parasit.*, **54,** 397.

RIECKMANN, K. H., MCNAMARA, V. J., FRISCHER, H., STOCKERT, T. A., CARSON, P. E. & POWELL, R. D. (1968) *Am. J. trop. Med. Hyg.*, **17,** 661.

SHUTE, P. G. (1966) *Trans. R. Soc. trop. Med. Hyg.*, **60,** 412.

———— & MARYON, M. (1966) *Laboratory Technique for the Study of Malaria.* London: Churchill.

STAUBER, L. A. (1958) *Rice Inst. Pamph.*, **45,** 80.

UMLAS, J. & FALLON, J. N. (1971) *Am. J. trop. Med. Hyg.*, **20,** 527.

UPTON, A. J. (1969) *Trans. R. Soc. trop. Med. Hyg.*, **65,** 542.

WORLD HEALTH ORGANIZATION (1963) *Terminology of Malaria and of Malaria Eradication.* Geneva.

APPENDIX II

MEDICAL HELMINTHOLOGY

PHYLUM: PLATYHELMINTHES
CLASS: TREMATODA OR FLUKES
SUPERFAMILY: FASCIOLOIDEA

GENUS: *Fasciola*

Fasciola hepatica (Linn., 1758) is a parasite of sheep, causing 'liver rot'. Also found in 'Jack' and 'cotton-tail' rabbits in the U.S.A. and rats in the Old World.

Distribution

World wide.

Characters

Pale grey with dark borders, it measures 2·3 cm × 8–13 mm; large specimens in cattle (7·5 cm) are known as *F. gigantica*. The anterior extremity is narrow, containing the oral sucker; the ventral sucker is larger than the anterior and situated 3 mm from the anterior extremity. Branched intestinal caeca with diverticula are present. The ovary is racemose, placed anterior to the testes in the posterior end of the body. The uterus is short and anterior to the ovary. An exsertile cirrus is present, and the genital pore is median.

The *egg* is operculated, 130–140 × 63–90 μm, ovoid, brown and bile-stained, and contains the ovum and yolk cells. A cilated, eye-spotted miracidium develops in about 3 weeks, and enters fresh-water snails: *Lymnaea* (*Galba*) *truncatula* (Europe), *L. pervia*

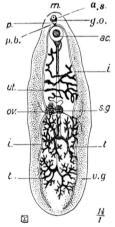

Fig. 301.—*Fasciolopsis buski.* (*After Odhner*)

The following is a key to the terminology of the anatomy of trematodes, as used in this and subsequent illustrations. *as*, anterior sucker. *m*, mouth. *p*, pharynx. *pb*, pharyngeal bulb. *ac*, acetabulum or ventral sucker. *go*, genital opening. *ut*, uterus. *vg*, vitelline glands. *ov*, ovary. *sg*, shell gland. *va*, vagina. *oo*, oötype. *ovd*, oviduct. *vs*, vesicula seminalis. *rs*, receptaculum seminis. *t*, testis. *vd*, vas deferens. *oes*, oesophagus. *i*, intestine. *ic*, branch intestine. *exp*, excretory pore. *nc*, nerve cord. *lc*, Laurer's canal.

(Japan), *L. vicetrix* (Cuba), *L. bulimoides* and *L. auricularia* (U.S.A.). Other snails are *Succinea, Fossaria, Praticolella* (a land snail in Cuba), *Bulinus* and *Ampullaria*. In these it becomes a sporocyst, daughter sporocysts, rediae (named after the Italian zoologist Redi) and cercariae. Development takes two months. The cercaria is blunt-tailed and settles in grass or on bark, where it secretes mucus to form a cyst with 2 prominent suckers (metacercariae). Then it is eaten by the mammalian host. Metacercariae excyst in the duodenum and migrate through the intestinal wall into the body cavity, then to the capsule of the liver to the biliary passages, where they grow to maturity.

For clinical features and pathology see page 320.

GENUS: *Fasciolopsis*

Fasciolopsis buski (Lankester, 1857) (Odhner, 1902) (Fig. 301)

A parasite of the pig which constitutes a reservoir for man.

Characters

F. buski inhabits the small intestine, rarely the stomach; only a small number of those infected show symptoms. This is the largest human trematode, measuring 3 cm × 12 mm, and 2 mm thick. It is flesh-coloured, elongated and oval, with transverse rows of spines, especially numerous near the ventral sucker. The oral sucker is sub-terminal, but ventral in position, and is only quarter the size of the ventral which is placed close to the oral, and prolonged into the cavity dorsally and backwards, a

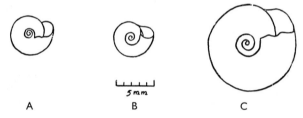

5 mm

A   B   C

Fig. 302.—Molluscan hosts of *Fasciolopsis buski*. A, *Segmentina hemisphaerula*. B, *Gyraulus convexiusculus*. C, *Hippeutis cantori*. (*C. J. Hackett*)

feature peculiar to this species. (For details of the anatomy see Fig. 301.) The intestinal caeca are simple, with two characteristic curves towards the midline. The genital pore is median, placed anterior to the ventral sucker. Branched testes are found in the posterior half of the body; there is a branched ovary and a fine, tortuous, Laurer's canal.

Development in the fresh-water snail resembles that of *F. hepatica* (Nagakawa, 1920). The egg (Plate XIII) is operculated and yellow, measuring 130–140 × 80–85 μm. Eggs are found in large numbers in the faeces, the egg capacity of each fluke being about 25 000/day. In water, after 3–7 weeks, they hatch a ciliated miracidium which develops in fresh-water snails—*Segmentina hemisphaerula* (China, Formosa, Japan), *Segmentina trochoideus* (Assam), *Hippeutis cantori* (China) and *Gyraulus convexiusculus* (*saigonensis*) (Formosa, Japan, Indo-China, Philippines, Indonesia, India). A sporocyst is formed in 3 days, followed by the rediae and daughter rediae, which eventually produce cerceriae (the whole cycle takes 2 months) (Fig. 302).

The cercariae, resembling those of *F. hepatica*, are oval, short-lived, lophocercous and measure 0·7 mm; they have a well developed digestive tract with a muscular bladder and collecting tubules. They encyst, as *metacercariae*, on fresh-water plants especially the outer cuticle of the water-calthrop (ling), *Trapa* (*Salvinia*) *natans* in China, *T. bicornis* in India, *T. bispinosa* in Formosa. As many as 20 encysted metacercariae may be found on a single leaf. In S. China the most important is the water-chestnut, *Eliocharis tuberosa*, also in *Zigania aquatica*, the water bamboo (Chekiang and Canton), *Eichornia crassipes*, the water hyacinth (Formosa). The outer layers of the plants are torn off by the teeth. All the plants are grown in ponds in China, and fertilized by human faeces, thus affording an opportunity for infection; *F. buski* is therefore limited in distribution to that of these plants. The cysts, when taken into the mouth, pass through the stomach, excyst in the duodenum, become attached to the intestinal wall.

For clinical features and pathology see page 322.

SUPERFAMILY: OPISTHORCHIOIDEA

GENUS: *Clonorchis*

Clonorchis sinensis (Cobbold, 1875) (Looss, 1907) (Fig. 303)

Synonym: *Opisthorchis sinensis*

Distribution

Far East, especially China (Kwangtung Province in S. China, Indo-China and Okayama, Japan).

Characters

This is a common parasite of man and also of the biliary passages of the dog, cat, pig, rat, mouse, camel and badger. It is found rarely in the gall-bladder of man, but often in the bile ducts, pancreas, pancreatic ducts and duodenum. It is spatulate, tapering anteriorly, reddish, semi-transparent and measures 10–25 × 2–5 mm. The cuticle is smooth; the oral sucker is larger than the ventral; the intestinal caeca are simple.

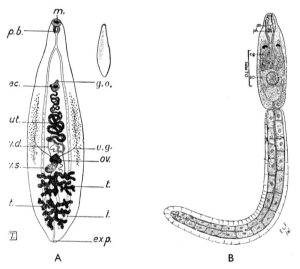

A   B

Fig. 303.—A, *Clonorchis sinensis*, magnified and natural size. (*After Loos*) B, Cercaria of *Clonorchis sinensis*. (*After Faust & Khaw; by permission of The American Journal of Hygiene*)

os, Oral sucker. *ph*, pharynx. *cg*, cephalic secretory gland. *vs*, ventral sucker.

The genital pore is median and placed anterior to the ventral sucker. The testes are branched, and situated posteriorly one behind the other. The ovary is trilobate, with coils anterior to the genital glands. Vitelline glands are moderately developed in the mid-third of the body. Cross-fertilization occurs; the spermatozoa develop before the ova; the sperms enter the female genital pore, pass into the immature uterus and thence to the *spermatheca* (Fig. 303), where they are stored, the ova are fertilized in the spermatheca and then pass on.

The egg measures 20–30 × 15–17 µm (Plate XIII); it is operculated, yellow-brown, and one of smallest trematode eggs found in man; it is fully embryonated when discharged. It resembles an electric light bulb, with the knob at the bottom. It withstands desiccation but not decomposition. It can remain viable in water for 5 weeks, and is ingested by the snail before the escape of the miracidium, which has a life-span of 20 minutes. Development continues in *Bulimus (Parafossarulus) striatula* (Japan, Korea and Formosa), *B. fuschianus, Alocinma longicornis* (China) (Fig. 304) and in *Melania cancellata*. The miracidium pierces the oesophagus of the mollusc, casts its cilia and soon becomes a sporocyst; later, the elongated rediae grow within the sporocysts and burst into the peri-oesophageal sinus and move tailwards into the liver, the whole process taking 3–4 weeks.

The cercariae (Fig. 303), 450–550 × 100–120 µm, escape from the rediae from the birthpore; they have 2 pigmented eyespots, a lophocercous blunt-ending tail, and burst through the space between the upper body surface and the shell, emerging into water. Within 24–48 hours they encyst, as metacercariae, in the muscles and underscales of fresh-water fish of families Cyprinidae and Anabantidae (of which 34 species

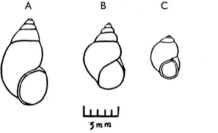

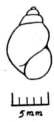

Fig. 304.—Molluscan hosts of *Clonorchis sinensis*. A, *Parafossarulus manchouricus*. B, *Bulimus fuschianus*. C, *Alocinma longicornis*. (*C. J. Hackett*)

Fig. 305.—*Bithynia leachi*, the molluscan host of *Opisthorchis felineus*. (*C. J. Hackett*)

are susceptible). Cercarial glands excrete a histolytic substance which dissolves the skin of the fish, thus admitting percolating water. The *metacercariae* secrete a viscous fluid which forms an inner true cyst, which in turn is encapsuled by a fibrous layer formed by the tissues of the fish. These are eaten half-raw, or pickled in *soy* sauce, by the Chinese. The adolescercaria, the fully developed cyst, possesses a capsule protective against the gastric juice. In some species of fish—*Carassius auratus* and *Eleotris swinhornis*—the parasite is found under the scales; in others it is in the flesh, so that domestic animals which eat the offal may become heavily infected while man escapes. The cysts withstand a temperature of 50–70°C for 15 minutes. The cyst wall is digested by the succus entericus in the duodenum near the papilla of Vater, and the adolescercariae escape and attach themselves to the mucosa. The young distomes at first have spines but these are soon lost. They attain maturity in 26 days. Attracted by positive chemotaxis, a small proportion of them reach the bile-ducts, but 95% are digested and destroyed. The size of the resulting fluke is determined by the calibre of the bile-duct. Egg production is very large; in the cat 2400 eggs are produced daily; but fewer in dogs. As many as 21 000 adults are found at autopsy. Life-span is 12 years. Adult men are more infected than women.

The following is a list of the molluscs and fishes which may be intermediaries.

Mollusca

Fossarulus stachei, F. loczy, F. sinensis, Parafossarulus subangulatus, P. manchouricus (striatulus), P. woodi, Pseudovivipara hypocrites, Hydrobiodes dautzenbergi, H. nassa,

Bulimus (Bithynia) striatulus, B. longicornis (Alocinma longicornis), B. chaperi, B. morelelania, B. poeteli, B. misella, B. umbilicaris, B. morleti, B. goniomphalos, B. thatkeana, B. robusta, B. minor, B. truncata, B. dautzenbergiana, B. siamensis, B. funiculata, B. fuchsianus, B. delavayana, B. toucheana, B. loevis, Melania hainanensis, M. cancellata, M. hongkongiensis, M. tuberculata, M. variabilis, Vivipara polyzonata, V. quadrata and *Hua (Namrutua) ningpoensis.*

The most important snail hosts are:

P. manchouricus	China, Formosa, Indo-China, Korea, Japan
B. fuchsianus	S. China
Alocinma longicornis	China
Hua ningpoensis	China

Pisces

Hemiculter kneri, H. clupeoides, Acanthorhodeus atranalis, A. gracilis, Carassius auratus, Pseudogobio rivularis, P. sinensis, Pseudorasbora parva, P. fowleri, Eleotris swinhornis, E. potamophila, Paracheilognathus rhombea, Rhodeus sinensis, R. notatus, Culter aburnus, Sacrocheilichthys nigripinnis, S. sinensis, S. morii, S. variegatus, Macropodus opercularis, Biwia zezera, Xenocyprus davidi, Pseudiperilampus typus, Abbotina psegma, Leucogobio guentheri, L. striatus, L. coreanus, L. mayedae, L. herzensteini, Ctenopharyngodon idellus, Acheilognathus lanceolata, A. limbata, A. cyanostigma, Labeo jordani, Hypothalmichthys nobilis, Mylopharyngodon aethiops.

The most important cyprinoid fish are *Mylopharyngodon aethiops, Ctenopharyngodon idellus* (Canton) and *Culter aburnus* (Peking).

For clinical features and pathology see page 325.

GENUS: *Opisthorchis*

Opisthorchis felineus (Rivolta, 1884) Blanchard, 1895 (Fig. 305)

The cat liver fluke (Europe, Near East, U.S.S.R.).

Characters

It inhabits the liver, pancreas, bile-ducts and lungs (in Russia). It is lanceolate, and measures 8–11 × 1·5–2 mm. The cuticle is smooth, the suckers equal in size and separated by 2 mm (Fig. 306). The egg measures 30 × 12 μm (Plate XIII) and is yellowish-brown with an operculum. At the posterior end there is a minute tubercular thickening.

Development

The snail intermediary host is usually *Bithynia leachi* (Fig. 305). The miracidium is fully formed in the egg and hatches in the snail, forming a sporocyst in the intestine measuring 1·2–1·85 mm. Rediae are formed in one month, and then cercariae which mature in four months.

Cercariae, 430–670 × 40–50 μm, leave the snail by daylight. They are shaped like a tobacco-pipe, with tail membrane; they are phototactic, and stimulated by agitation. The secondary intermediary hosts are fish—the tench (*Tinca tinca*), the chub (*Idus melanotus, Barbus barbus* and *Leuciscus rutilis*). The cercariae penetrate in 15 minutes, and grow to 3 or 4 times their original size, forming metacercariae, 220 × 160 μm. When ingested by man, they pass through the stomach, are freed by the succus entericus, attracted by the bile and travel up the bile duct in 5 hours. Infection is therefore contracted by eating raw fish. The entire life cycle requires a minimum of 4 months. This fluke is not specially pathogenic, although 200 or more have been found in the body at autopsies. Another variant (?) of this fluke (Rodriguez *et al.* 1949) has been described as a parasite of man in Ecuador; 32% of 214 persons in a village and 3% of dogs were found infected.

Other species of importance are *O. noverca* and *O. viverrini* (India and Siam), of which the normal hosts are the dog and civet cat respectively.

For clinical features and treatment see page 323.

GENUS: *Heterophyes*
Heterophyes heterophyes (Siebold, 1852)
(Fig. 307)

Distribution

Egypt, China, Japan (cases also reported from Missolonghi in Greece).

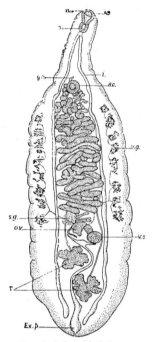

Fig. 306.—*Opisthorchis felineus*. ×9.
(*After Barker*)

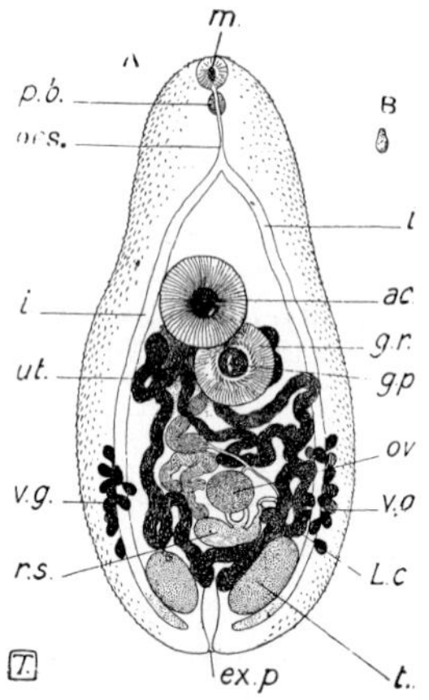

Fig. 307.—*Heterophyes heterophyes*.
A, Greatly magnified. B, Natural size.

Characters

It inhabits the small intestine of man in large numbers and also that of the rat, fox, dog, wolf, jackal and cat; also in the black kite (*Milvus migrans aegyptius*) and a bat (*Rhinolophus divosus acrotis*) in the Yemen. It imparts a coffee-grounds appearance to the intestinal wall. It is pyriform, grey and very small, measuring 1–1·7 × 0·3–0·7 mm. The uterus forms a brown patch in the centre. The oral sucker is subterminal and the ventral sucker is 3 times the size of the oral. The cuticle is thickly set with quadrate scales measuring 5 × 4 μm. There is a short prepharynx and long oesophagus. The intestinal caeca extend to the posterior extremity, converging close to the excretory vesicle. The vitelline glands are posterior, situated in 2 clumps; the genital pore is posterolateral, in the vicinity of the ventral sucker, and consists of a muscular ring armed with 70 chitinous cuticular teeth. The testes are oval and posterior, the ovary globular and median. There is a *receptaculum seminis* as large as the ovary; uterine coils are not numerous. Seminal vesicle and Laurer's canal are present.

The egg measures 20–30 × 15–17 μm (Plate XIII), being the same size as that of *C. sinensis*. Its greatest breadth is across the centre. There is no special ring to the operculum, which is light-brown and contains a ciliated miracidium when deposited. It hatches after ingestion by the appropriate snail.

Life history

H. heterophyes develops in brackish-water snails: *Melania tuberculata, Cleopatra bulimoides;* and in Lake Manzala (Egypt), in a conical snail, *Pirinella conica* (Fig. 308A). The cercaria, resembling that of *M. yokogawai*, is oculate and lophocercous (membranous-tailed); it was formerly known as *C. pleurolophocerca*. The second intermediary is a fish—the mullet (*Mugil cephalus*) and minnow (*Gambusia affinis*); in Japan a species of *Acanthogobius*. There is also a brackish fresh-water snail, *Tymphonotomus micropterus* (also known as *Cerithidea cingulata microptera*) which is the molluscan host.

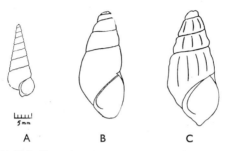

Fig. 308.—A, *Pirinella conica,* the molluscan host of *Heterophyes heterophyes*. B, *Semisulcospira libertina,* the snail host of *Metagonimus yokogawai*. C, *Hua amurensis,* the snail host of *Paragonimus westermani*. (C. J. Hackett)

Pathogenesis and treatment

The fluke occurs in enormous numbers, attached to the mucosa of the small intestine; it may give rise to diarrhoea. In Manila, heterophyes eggs are found in the walls of the intestines and in the myocardium and are said to produce symptoms resembling cardiac beri-beri. Africa has recognized two other human species—*H. brevicaeca* and *H. taihokui*. In Japan, in the vicinity of Kobe, *H. katsuradai*, a closely related stouter species, which has a relatively enormous acetabulum, is found. The eggs are smaller, measuring 25–26 × 14–15 μm. The flukes are removed by tetrachloroethylene, oleoresin of aspidium, and piperazine adipate and citrate, 0·9–4·5 grammes. Yomesan (Bayer) has also been used.

GENUS: *Metagonimus*

Metagonimus yokogawai (Katsurada, 1912) (Fig. 309)

Distribution

Korea, Formosa, Japan and Balkan States, very common in Far East.

Characters

This is found in the small intestine of man, higher up than *H. heterophyes*, and also in the cat, dog, pig and pelican. It is the smallest fluke parasitic in man, measuring 1·1 × 0·42–0·7 mm. The cuticle is covered with small spines; the ventral sucker is deflected to the right with its long axis in the diagonal plane. There is a genital pore in front; the ovoid testes are posterior; the ovary and *receptaculum seminis* are situated medially in front of the testes. The yolk glands are found in clumps in the posterior third. The uterus lies between the testes and the ventral sucker, and the seminal vesicle in front of the ovary (Fig. 309).

Egg. This measures 27 × 16 μm and resembles that of *C. sinensis*, but is more regularly ovoid (Plate XIII).

The first intermediaries are molluscs—*Melania* (*Semisulcospira*) *libertina* (Fig. 308B), *M. ebenina* and *M. obliquegranulosa* (50% of which are infected). Sporocysts, rediae and cercariae are formed; the last has an anterior end provided with armament. The tail is long and lophocercous, with lateral flutings, and is discarded on entering the fish—*Plecoglossus altivelis*, Japan and U.S.S.R. The metacercariae, 150 × 100 μm, encyst under the scales; the infected fish is eaten raw by the Japanese.

Pathogenesis

M. yokogawai causes a catarrhal condition of the intestinal tract and slight diarrhoea, but is easily removed by tetrachloroethylene.

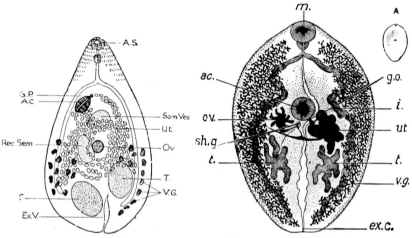

Fig. 309.—*Metagonimus yokogawai.* × 45. (*After Leiper*)

Sem. ves., seminal vesicle. *rec. sem.,* receptaculum seminis. *g.p.,* genital pore. Other lettering as previously.

Fig. 310.—*Paragonimus westermani* (*ringeri*), natural size and magnified. (*After Looss*)

SUPERFAMILY: PLAGIORCHIOIDEA

GENUS: *Paragonimus*

Paragonimus westermani (Kerbert, 1878) (synonym: *P. ringeri* Cobbold, 1880). Allied species have also been discovered: *P. kellicotti* (America), *P. compactus* (India) *P. africanus* (West Africa), *P. schechuanensis* (Skrjabini) and *P. tuanshanensis* (*heteroteirus*) (China).

Distribution

Far East from Japan to India, Indonesia, Pacific Islands, West Africa and South America.

Characters

P. westermani measures 8–20 × 5–9 mm and is oval (almost round in section), reddish-brown and translucent. The anterior extremity is rounded. The oral sucker is subterminal; the ventral sucker larger and placed anterior to the centre of the body. The pharynx and oesophagus are short, and the bifurcation of the intestine is anterior to the ventral sucker (Fig. 310). The intestinal caeca run a zigzag course; the common genital pore lies close to the posterior margin of the ventral sucker. The body is bisected by a large excretory vesicle. The testes are tubular and racemose; the branched ovary may be either to the right or the left of the midline and posterior to the ventral sucker. The uterus is short, sac-like and lies opposite the ovary. The vitellaria are well developed, extending through the whole body. Laurer's canal and shell-gland are present.

The cuticle is studded with wedge-shaped spines, which have been thought to differentiate the closely allied forms (see above), but these differences are not constant enough to justify this. In *P. westermani* the spines are arranged singly and in *P. compactus* they tend to be in clumps and are fewer and pointed.

The egg is brown and operculated, measuring 90 × 55 μm. It shows a thickening at the pole opposite the operculum (Plate XIII). The egg of *P. compactus* is smaller, 75 × 48 μm.

Life history

This is complicated (Fig. 311). The lung fluke can remain viable in the human body for 20 years. The eggs are first voided into cystic pockets in the lungs and then escape

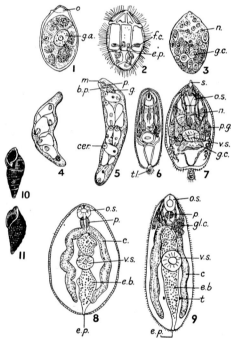

Fig. 311.—Life history of *Paragonimus westermani*. 1–9, × 15; 10–11, half natural size. (*After Belding & Chen*)

1, Egg showing yolk cells and germinal area. 2, Miracidium with excretory system and flame cells. 3, Miracidium with ganglionic mass and germ cells. 4, Mature sporocyst in snail containing well developed first generation rediae. 5, Mature second generation rediae. 6, 7, Stages of microcercous cercariae after emergence from the snail. 8, Metacercariae from the crab; the cyst wall is not shown. 9, Mature encysted metacercaria. 10, *Melania libertina.* 11, *Melania obliquegranulosa.*
b.p., birth pore. *c*, caeca. *cer*, cercaria. *e.b*, excretory bladder. *e.p*, excretory pore. *f.c*, flame cell. *g*, gut. *g.a*, germinal area. *g.c*, genital cells. *m*, mouth. *n*, nervous system. *o*, operculum. *o.s*, oral sucker. *p*, pharynx. *p.g*, periacetabular glands. *s*, stylet. *t*, testes. *tl*, tail. *v.s.* ventral sucker.

into water in the sputum and also in faeces from swallowed sputum. A ciliated miracidium hatches in 16 days to 7 weeks and has distinctive characters. There is a ciliated covering in 4 rows at the anterior cone. The excretory pore forms a rosette. It enters snails of the genus *Melania* (or *Thiara, Semisulcospira, Brolia*). *M. tuberculata* (Japan, China), *M. libertina* (Japan, China), *M. ebenina* (Korea), *M. obliquegranulosa* (Formosa), a synonym for this species in America is *Thiara (Tarelia) granifera*, and *M. paucicincta, Hua amurensis* (Fig. 308C), also known as *Brolia gottschei, M. nodiperda* (Korea), all these are common species living in fast flowing streams in S.E. Asia, Indonesia, Formosa, and W. Pacific Islands. In China, sometimes it develops in *Syncera lutea*; and in N. America in *Pomatiopsis lapidaria*. It develops in about 60 days into sporocyst and rediae, each containing 20 cercariae; the latter, ellipsoid and microcercous, have a short knob-like tail and measure $200 \times 70-80$ μm with an anterior stylet and body covered with spines. The cercariae bore into fresh-water crabs and become meta-cercariae in *Potamon obtusipes, P. rathbuni, P. dehaani* (Fig. 312), *Sesarma dehaani, S. sinensis, Eriocheir japonicus* (Fig. 313). Other hosts are the crayfish *Astacus japonicus*, in Korea the crab *Eriocheir sinensis* and crayfish *A. similis*, in Venezuela *Pseudothelphusa*

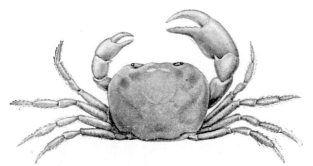

Fig. 312.—*Potamon dehaani*, half natural size.

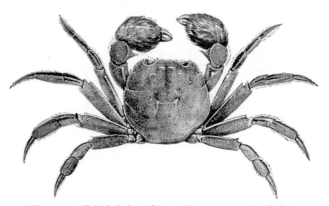

Fig. 313.—*Eriocheir japonicus*, male, quarter natural size.

iturbei and in the Philippines *P. mistis. P. africanus* has also been found in the West Cameroons, where the melaniid snail *Potadoma freethii* and the crabs *Sudanautes africanus* and *S. pelii* are the intermediate hosts.

In the crustacean (the second intermediary) the metacercariae encyst in the liver, muscles and gills. In Japan, crabs are eaten raw, but in Korea and Formosa they are not eaten; the supposition is that the crustacean phase is not always a biological necessity. In Venezuela the appropriate snails and crustacea are present and 30% of dogs are infected, but man is not. When the metacercariae enter the stomach of man, their cyst wall is digested and the adolescercariae emerge, pass through the jejunum, traverse the abdominal cavity, penetrate the diaphragm, pleura and lungs, reach the bronchioles forming cystic cavities. (For pathogenesis and treatment see pages 327–334.)

GENUS: *Dicrocoelium*

Dicrocoelium dendriticum (*D. lanceatum*), of which the normal host is the sheep, is rarely found in man, in biliary tract in Germany, Czechoslovakia, Italy, France, Egypt, China. The eggs passed in faeces are fully embryonated, resist desiccation and do not hatch in water. They are ingested by land-snails—*Zebrina detrita*, *Hellicella candidula*, *H. itala*, *Torquilla frumentum*, *Cochlicella acita*, *Clonella lubrica* and others.

The cercariae leave the snail in rains after a dry summer by migrating to the respiratory chamber and then agglomerating in hundreds in slime balls, cemented by mucus, which are dropped as the snail crawls along. A second intermediary is necessary in the brown ant (*Formica fusca*) and these are swallowed by man.

GENUS: *Plagiorchis*

Sandground (1939) found *Plagiorchis javanensis* in small intestine of Javanese, together with *E. iliocanum*. It is a small trematode belonging to group normally infecting birds, fish, amphibia and bats. Development takes place in a snail—*Stagnicola emarginata angulata*. Another species is *P. philippinensis*, recovered at autopsy in Manila from the small intestine of a patient who had eaten grubs of certain insects.

FAMILY: ACHILLURBANIIDAE

GENUS: *Poikilorchis*

Poikilorchis congolensis (Fain & Vandepitte, 1957) is a fluke which has been found in postaural subcutaneous cysts or abscesses in the Congo. The ova resemble those of *Paragonimus westermani*, but are smaller (60-68 × 38-41 μm).

SUPERFAMILY: ECHINOSTOMATOIDEA

GENUS: *Echinostoma*

A trematode of minor importance is *Echinostoma lindoensis*. Of this, a few cases from Celebes are reported, with flukes, sometimes in large numbers, in the jejunum. The reservoir host is the field rat. It causes diarrhoea, abdominal pains and eosinophilia. Development is as follows: first intermediary: planorbid snails (*Anisus sarasinorum* and *A. convexiusculus*); second intermediary (metacercariae), in snails (*Vivipara javanica rudipellis*) and two species of mussel (*Corbicula lindoensis* and *C. subplanata*). All snails in Lake Lindoe, near a heavily infected village, were found to harbour large numbers of echinostome cercariae, which have simple tails and a body resembling in miniature that of the adult worm. The eggs are straw-coloured, operculate and measure 83–116 × 58–69 μm. Immature when passed in the faeces, they mature in 6–15 days. Filix mas and tetrachloroethylene treatments are specific.

E. iliocanum and the closely allied *E. malayanum* (larger) are found in Singapore and Malaysia. The natural host is the pig. The snail host is *Gyraulus prashadi*. Also *E. jassyens* in Romania, *E. recurvatum* in Java and *Paryphostomum sufrartyfex* in Assam and Madras—all removed by filix mas.

PHYLUM: PLATYHELMINTHES

CLASS: TREMATODA Rudolphi, 1808

SUBCLASS: DIGENEA Carus, 1863

SUPERFAMILY: SCHISTOSOMATOIDEA Stiles and Hassall, 1926

FAMILY: SCHISTOSOMATIDAE Looss, 1899

GENUS: *Schistosoma* Weinland, 1858

The schistosomes commonly infecting man are:

Schistosoma haematobium (Bilharz, 1852) Weinland, 1858
Schistosoma mansoni Sambon, 1907

Table. 45 Differentiation of

Character	S. haematobium	S. mansoni
Habitat of adult	Vesical veins; occasionally veins of rectum and portal system	Inferior mesenteric and portal venous system
Adult male	10–15 × 0·75–1·0 mm	6–13 × 1·0 mm
Cuticle	Fine tubercles	Conspicuous tubercles and microscopic tufts of hair
Oesophagus	Single bulb	Single bulb
Caeca	Unite in anterior half; posterior caecum short, one-third of body length	Unite in anterior half; posterior caecum long, two-thirds of body length
Testes	4 or 5	2–14
Adult female	20–26 × 0·25 mm Darker than male, more blood pigment in gut	7–17 × 0·25 mm Darker than male, more blood pigment in gut
Cuticle	Transverse striations. Small tubercles at extremity	Transverse striations. Small tubercles at extremity
Ovary	In posterior third	In anterior half
Uterus	Anterior, long. Holds 10–100 eggs at one time. Produces 20–290 daily	Anterior, short. Holds 1–2 eggs only at one time. Produces 100–300 daily
Eggs	83–187 × 60 μm Terminal spine Pass through bladder wall Discharged in urine	112–175 × 45–70 μm Lateral spine Pass through bowel wall Discharged in faeces
Shell	Non-acid-fast with Ziehl-Neelsen stain in tissues	Acid-fast with Ziehl-Neelsen stain in tissues
Animal hosts	Occasionally baboons, monkeys, rats, pigs	(Occasional) baboons, rats

Schistosoma japonicum Katsurada, 1904
Schistosoma intercalatum Fisher, 1934

Three male and one female *Schistosoma intercalatum*, whose eggs are similar to those of *S. haematobium*, having a terminal spine, were recovered in 1922 by Dr C. C. Chesterman in the Congo, and were then regarded by Leiper as *S. haematobium*. Later investigation showed that *S. intercalatum* is a true species (Wright *et al.*, 1972). For a short account of this discovery see Chesterman (1969).

Infections of man have also been reported with:

Schistosoma mattheei Veglia and Le Roux, 1929
Schistosoma bovis (Sonsino, 1876) Blanchard, 1895

Many of the reports of *S. bovis* infection of man are of doubtful authenticity, but true infection has been recorded.

For notes on these two species see page 286, and for notes on the cercariae of swimmer's itch see page 319.

various species of *Schistosoma*

S. japonicum	S. intercalatum
Superior and inferior mesenteric, and portal venous system	Mesenteric and portal venous system
12–20 × 0·5–0·55 mm No tubercles; small acuminate spines	11–14 × 0·3–0·4 mm Tubercles and fine spines
Double bulb Unite in posterior half; posterior caecum medium, one-half of body length 6–8	Single bulb Unite in posterior half; posterior caecum one-fifth to one-quarter of body length 4–6
12–28 × 0·3 mm Darker than male, more blood pigment in gut Transverse striations. Minute spines	10–14 × 0·15–0·18 mm Darker than male, more blood pigment in gut Transverse striations, smooth
Central Anterior, long. Holds 50 or more eggs at one time. Produces 1500–3500 daily	In posterior half Anterior, long. Holds 5–50 eggs at one time
70–100 × 50–65 μm Rudimentary lateral spine Pass through bowel wall Discharged in faeces Acid-fast with Ziehl-Neelsen stain in tissues	140–240 × 50–85 μm Long terminal spine Pass through bowel wall Discharged in faeces Acid-fast with Ziehl-Neelsen stain in tissues
Rodents, dogs, cats, cattle, water buffalo, pigs, horses, sheep, goats	? Sheep, goats

The digenea are equipped with organs of attachment (suckers), one of which surrounds the oral cavity; they undergo an alternation of generations and of hosts, the hosts harbouring the intermediate stages being molluscs.

The schistosomes are digenetic trematodes, their life histories consisting of alternating generations, each with its own range of hosts. The adult worms inhabit vertebrates, the larval stages inhabit snails, which in the case of schistosomes pathogenic for man, are fresh-water snails.

The schistosomes are dioecious organisms, that is, the sexes are separate.

Adult schistosomes live in the veins of vertebrates; there is an oral cavity but no muscular pharynx; the eggs have no operculum; there is no encysted or metacercarial stage; the cercariae enter the definitive hosts through the skin (and possibly through mucous membranes).

Anatomy and physiology of schistosomes

Like other digenetic trematodes, the schistosomes are equipped with suckers. The *oral sucker* surrounds the mouth and is prehensile; the *ventral sucker* (*acetabulum*) is more posterior, on the ventral surface. With these suckers the worms can attach themselves to the walls of the vessels in which they live. The *mouth* itself is usually near the anterior extremity. The alimentary system consists of an *oral cavity* leading to the *oesophagus* and thence to the *gut* which soon divides into 2 *caeca* which reunite more posteriorly to form the *single posterior caecum* which ends blindly; there is no anus.

Food consists of the liquid material in which the worms live; unused material is rejected through the mouth. Schistosomes obtain oxygen from the blood in which they live.

The excretory system consists of 2 longitudinal canals opening posteriorly and fed by collecting tubules. There are flame cells whose function is to fan fluid wastes into the tubules by means of the vibratile cilia with which they are equipped.

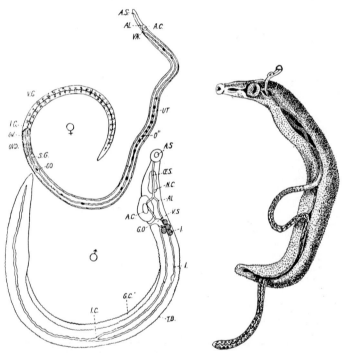

Fig. 314.—*Schistosoma haematobium.* × 10. (*Partly after Looss*)

A.C, ventral sucker. AL, bifurcation of the alimentary canal. A.S, anterior sucker. G.C, gynaecophoric canal. G.O, genital opening. I, intestine. I.C, union of intestinal caeca. N.C., nerve cord. O″, terminal spined ovum. OES, oesophagus. OO, oötype. OV, ovary. OVD., oviduct. S.G., shell gland. T., testes. T.B., tuberculations. UT., uterus. VA, vagina. V.G., vitelline glands. V.S., vesicula seminalis.

There is a rudimentary *nervous system* with an oesophageal ganglion and commissure encircling the oesophagus, and 2 longitudinal nerve cords running to the posterior end, and intercommunicating by lateral branches.

The *male reproductive organs* consist of testes dorsal to and posterior to the ventral sucker. Each testis discharges via a *vas efferens*; these unite to form the *vesicula seminalis* at the *genital pore* situated in the midline posterior to the ventral sucker.

The male worm is flat and leaf-like, but is folded to form the *gynaecophoric canal*, enfolding the very slender female for almost its entire length.

The *female reproductive organs* consist of an elongated *ovary* in the posterior half, from which the *oviduct* passes forward, to be joined by the *vitelline duct* from the *vitellaria* (*yolk glands*); the *shell gland* opens into the oviduct, which passes forward to a straight *uterus*. This contains eggs, and opens at the genital pore on the median surface posterior to the ventral sucker. The genital openings of both male and female face each other.

S. mansoni has been cultivated *in vitro*.

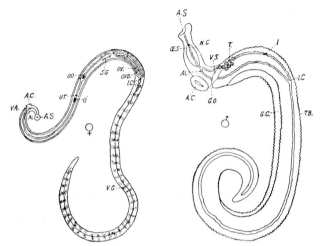

Fig. 315.—*Schistosoma mansoni.* × 10.

Key as to Fig. 314; *o'*, lateral spined egg.

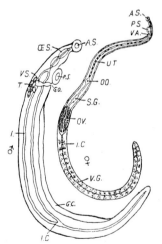

Fig. 316.—Male and female *Schistosoma japonicum.* × 10.

Key as to Fig. 314.

Life history

The eggs of the schistosomes are passed by the definitive hosts (vertebrates) in urine (*S. haematobium*) or faeces (*S. mansoni, S. japonicum, S. intercalatum*), but this is not an absolute rule, since eggs of *S. haematobium* may occasionally be found in faeces and in biopsy specimens of rectal mucosa. *S. mattheei*, a parasite of sheep and cattle which affects man in South Africa, is also found in both urine and faeces.

Eggs of *S. mansoni* and *S. japonicum* (but not *S. haematobium* or *S. mattheei*) are acid-fast when stained by the Ziehl-Neelsen method. Eggs of *S. intercalatum* in tissues stained in this way are also acid-fast, provided that the tissues are fixed initially in Bouin's fluid.

When an egg reaches fresh water it hatches within a few minutes, partly as a result of osmosis, partly owing to movements of the enclosed larva, to set free the *miracidium*, a highly motile larva which moves in the water for about 24 hours by means of the cilia which cover its integument. Miracidia tend to move to the upper layers of water where many of their snail hosts live, but in some circumstances they can infect snails inhabiting the bottoms of canals or lakes (e.g. Lake Victoria). These snails, however,

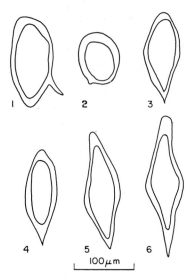

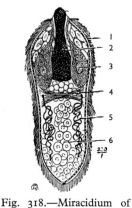

Fig. 318.—Miracidium of *Schistosoma haematobium*. (*After Looss*)

Fig. 317.—Eggs of *Schistosoma mansoni* (1), *A. japonicum* (2), *S. haematobium* (3), *S. intercalatum* (4), *S. mattheei* (5) and *S. bovis* (6). (*After Jordan & Webbe*)

1, Cilia. 2, Papillary beak and primitive intestine. 3, Cephalic salivary gland. 4, Nerve centre. 5, Excretory tubules. 6, Primitive genital cells.

frequently move up and down from the depths to the surface of such waters, and miracidia have the opportunity of infecting them in the upper reaches.

The miracidium has an apical papilla and a pair of cephalic penetration glands which enable it to make its way into the tissues of a snail into whose vicinity it swims. It does not discriminate between snails, entering species in which it cannot develop as well as species which are suitable hosts, in which it proceeds to change and develop to the next stage of its life history. Once inside the soft tissues of a favourable snail host, the miracidium develops within 96 hours into a mother sporocyst, an elongated sac almost filled with germinal cells. At 8 days it has become a non-motile convoluted tube from which daughter sporocysts develop, migrating to other parts of the snail. From these the final larva (*cercaria*) is formed, and from a single miracidium thousands of larvae are produced, all of the same sex. The cycle from penetration by the miracidium to the production of mature cercariae takes about 4–5 weeks for *S. mansoni*, 5–6 weeks for *S. haematobium*, and 7 weeks or more for *S. japonicum* (Jordan & Webbe 1969). The snails are damaged in the process, and their life span is shortened to about 1–2 months.

The mature cercaria escapes from the daughter sporocyst and enters the water, swimming vigorously by means of its bifurcated tail, usually tail first. Its body is less than 1 mm in length, with one oral and one ventral sucker, a mouth, oesophagus and a pair of short caeca, and an excretory system of tubules and flame cells. It has 6 pairs of cephalic glands, 2 pairs of which are in front of the ventral sucker (which probably secrete lytic enzymes whose function is to help to penetrate the skin of vertebrates), and 4 pairs behind the ventral sucker (which probably help the cercaria to attach itself to the skin).

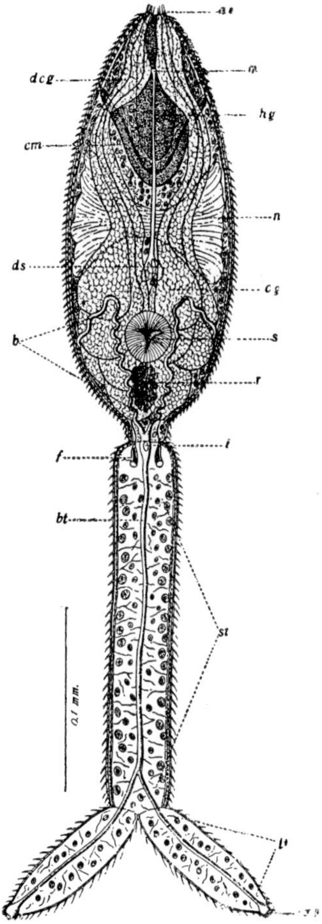

Fig. 319.—Cercaria of *Schistosoma japonicum*, ventral view. ×240. (*After Cort*)

as, anterior spines. *b*, excretory bladder. *cg*, cephalic glands. *cm*, circular muscles. *dcg*, ducts of cephalic glands. *ds*, digestive system. *exp*, excretory pore. *f*, flame cell. *hg*, head gland. *i*, island in excretory bladder. *lt*, lobe of tail. *m*, mouth. *n*, nervous system. *st*, stem of *r*, rudimentary genital cells. *s*, ventral sucker.

A snail may shed 500–3000 cercariae of *S. haematobium* or *S. mansoni* daily when in full production, but the figure for *S. japonicum* is much less (15–160), the snails being much smaller than those infected by the other species.

Cercariae tend to swim up to the surface of water, sinking from time to time and returning. They do not feed, and their life span is short, up to 48 hours. They are quickly killed at 50°C, and strong sunlight and lack of oxygen are rapidly lethal.

A cercaria can penetrate the skin of a definitive host within a few minutes. In doing so it sheds its tail, and in the tissues it becomes a *schistosomulum*, which within 24 hours enters the lymphatic or venous system, to be transported to the right heart and lungs.

Some schistosomules pass into the mesenteric vessels and thence to the vessels of the liver. Some may pass directly through the diaphragm to the liver and the portal vessels. Growth takes place in the liver, and paired worms may be found after about 26 days. Most worms leave the liver when they are sexually mature and have mated, and migrate to the veins of the vesical plexus (*S. haematobium*) or the mesenteric veins (*S. mansoni, S. japonicum* and *S. intercalatum*), where they begin to lay eggs. The period between penetration by the cercariae and egg laying may be 30–40 days or more.

The mated worms move as far as possible towards the fine terminal vessels, and the female then leaves the male, progressing to the finest vessels, where she deposits her eggs, retracting after having done so. The eggs escape from the venules into the tissues, those of *S. haematobium* largely into the wall of the bladder but occasionally into the wall of the lower bowel, those of *S. mansoni, S. japonicum* and *S. intercalatum* largely into the wall of the lower bowel. Many pass through the mucosa to be excreted in urine or faeces, but some remain trapped in the tissues, where they give rise to tissue

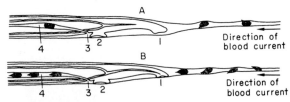

Fig. 320.—The deposition of eggs by *S. mansoni* (A) and *S. haematobium* (B) in the blood vessels and their passage to the exterior.

1, Anterior sucker. 2, Posterior sucker. 3, Vaginal orifice. 4, Uterus with contained eggs.

reactions. Some eggs of all species are usually also found in the genital tract, liver, lungs, central nervous system and other organs. Eggs are responsible for most of the pathological effects of the infection.

Intermediate hosts (snails). Strains of the species of schistosomes which infect man vary in their ability to infect snail hosts. Some schistosomes easily infect snails of one geographical area but either fail to infect, or infect only with difficulty, the same snails from a different area. The subject is complicated.

The following lists of proved and potential snail hosts have been constructed mainly from Jordan and Webbe (1969), and Wright (1962 and personal communication).

Snail hosts of S. haematobium. S. haematobium is now regarded as a composite species of 2 morphologically similar forms which at one time were regarded as different species, namely *S. haematobium* and *S. capense*. Strains from different areas are not always capable of infecting the same species of snails.

The intermediate snail hosts of *S. haematobium* are members of the genus *Bulinus*, with 2 exceptions: the strain found in Portugal is carried by *Planorbarius metidjensis*, and the strain found in India by *Ferrissia tenuis*.

Snail hosts of *S. haematobium* (*sensu stricto*)

Snail host	Locality
Truncatus group	
Bulinus (Bulinus) truncatus truncatus	Near East, Iraq, Arabia, N. Africa, E. Africa, W. Africa
B. (B.) truncatus rohlfsi	W. Africa
B. (B.) coulboisi	E. Africa, Congo (potential)
B. (B.) guernei	W. Africa
Tropicus group	
Bulinus (Bulinus) obtusispira	Malagasy Republic

Snail host	Locality
Forskali group	
Bulinus (Bulinus) forskali	Africa, Madagascar, Mauritius, Aden
B. (B.) reticulatus	E. Africa, Aden
B. (B) beccarii	Aden
B. (B.) cernicus	Mauritius
B. (B.) senegalensis	Senegal, Gambia
B. (B.) bavayi (potential)	Malagasy Republic

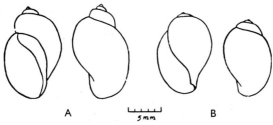

Fig. 321.—Molluscan hosts of *S. haematobium*. A, *Bulinus truncatus*. B, *B. africanus*. (*C. J. Hackett*)

S. haematobium (*S. capense* form)

Snail host	Locality
Africanus group	
Bulinus (Physopsis) africanus africanus	S. Africa, E. Africa
B. (P.) africanus ovoideus	S. Africa, E. Africa
B. (P.) globosus	Africa south of the Sahara
B. (P.) nasutus	E. Africa
B. (P.) nasutus productus	E. Africa
B. (P.) abyssinicus	Ethiopia, Somalia
B (P.) jousseaumei (= globosus)	W. Africa, Congo

Snail host of *S. intercalatum*

Snail host	Locality
Bulinus (Physopsis) africanus africanus	Congo, Gabon
B. (Bulinus) forskali	Cameroun, Gabon
B. wrighti (Reticulatus group)	Guinea, Congo

Snail hosts of *S. mansoni*. These snails are all members of the genus *Biomphalaria*; all the African species are susceptible.

Snail host	Locality
Pfeifferi group	
Biomphalaria pfeifferi (synonym B. ruepelli)	Aden, Yemen, S. Arabia, Africa, Malagasy Republic
Choanomphala group	
B. choanomphala choanomphala	
B. choanomphala elegans	
B. smithi	Round the great lakes of E. Africa
B. stanleyi	
Alexandrina group	
B. alexandrina alexandrina (synonym boissyi)	Egypt, Sudan
B. alexandrina wansoni	Congo
B. angulosa	E. Africa

Snail host	Locality
Sudanica group	
B. sudanica sudanica	E. and W. Africa
B. sudanica rugosa	Zambia
B. sudanica tanganyicensis	E. and W. Africa
B. camerunensis camerunensis	E. and W. Africa
B. camerunensis manzadica	E. and W. Africa
Australorbis group	
B. glabrata	Caribbean, S. America
Tropicorbis group	
B. centimetralis	Caribbean, S. America

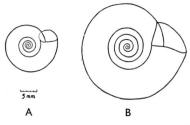

A   B

Fig. 322.—Molluscan hosts of *S. mansoni*. A, *Biomphalaria alexandrina*. B, *B. glabrata*. (*C. J. Hackett*)

Snail hosts of *S. japonicum*

Snail host	Locality
Oncomelania hupensis	China
O. nosophora	S.W. China, Japan
O. nosophora slateri	China
O. formosana*	Taiwan (Formosa)
O. quadrasi	Philippines

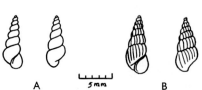

A   5 mm   B

Fig. 323.—Molluscan hosts of *S. japonicum*. A, *Oncomelania nosophora*. B, *O. hupensis*. (*C. J. Hackett*)

The snail host of *S. japonicum* in South East Asia is not known. Barbier and Brumpt (1969) report that species of *Oncomelania* have not been found there, and that attempts to infect *O. hupensis* with the local strain of *S. japonicum* have failed.

Interspecific antagonism between trematodes in snails

Kian Joe Lie *et al.* (1968) reported that if albino *B. glabrata* is infected with *S. mansoni* and also with *Paryphostomum segregatum* (an echinostome from Brazil), the rediae of *P. segregatum* will attack and breach the thin wall of the early mother sporocyst of *S. mansoni*, and ingest and destroy the daughter sporocysts within it. They fail,

* The Formosan strain of *S. japonicum* is not pathogenic for man.

however, to destroy mature daughter sporocysts, but they can cause degeneration of the schistosome sporocysts by other means. They can ingest whole cercariae. This biological antagonism between a dominant species and a subordinate species within a snail is also found with other trematodes, and could conceivably be the basis of some form of biological control, but however that may be, it is an observation of great biological interest.

SUPERFAMILY: PARAMPHISTOMATOIDEA
(AMPHISTOME TREMATODES)

GENUS: *Gastrodiscoides*

Gastrodiscoides hominis (Lewis and MacConnell, 1876); Leiper, 1913

Distribution

Malaysia, Assam, India, Burma, S. Viet Nam, British Guiana. In Kamrup District, Assam, 41% of the population are infected; in Burma 5%. The normal host is the pig or the mouse-deer.

Characters

The fluke is reddish from haemoglobin pigment. When alive, it is very expansile and can elongate to 1 cm. Preserved specimens measure 5–7 × 3–4 mm at the widest point. The anterior end is conical, the posterior discoidal flattened ventrally to form a concave disc. Prominent genital papillae are seen, and the common genital pore is 2·5 mm from the oral sucker. The ventral sucker (acetabulum) is ventrally situated in the caudal portion and measures 2 mm in diameter. The cuticle is smooth. The alimentary canal consists of a pharynx with 2 pear-shaped pharyngeal pouches. The oesophagus is 1 mm in length, and ends in a muscular bulb where the bifurcation of the intestine takes place and caeca run back to the edge of the acetabulum. There are 2 lobulated testes placed diagonally between the intestinal caeca. A seminal vesicle is present, but no cirrus. The ovary lies in the midline, posterior to the testes. An ovoid shell gland is placed near the ovary with a *receptaculum seminis* anterior to it. The uterus is short. Laurer's canal is present. The vitellaria lie in the mid-third. The ovoid egg measures 152 × 60 μm and has an operculum. Development outside the body takes place in a snail, probably a snail of the Family Thiaridae. The cercariae probably encyst on vegetation.

This fluke lives in the caecum in large numbers and usually produces no symptoms. Thymol, carbon tetrachloride and tetrachloroethylene are effective in treatment.

GENUS: *Watsonius*

Watsonius watsoni has been found in large numbers in an African in South West Africa. Its normal hosts are monkeys of the genera *Cercopithecus* and *Papio* (baboon).

CLASS: CESTOIDEA (kestos = a girdle) or TAPEWORMS

The head of these worms develops from the embryo after ingestion by the host, and shows independent co-ordinated movement. The *strobila*, or segments, have their own musculature, which relieves the strain on the head. The worms can live for several years. They absorb nutriment through the cuticle. They are hermaphroditic, the male segments fertilizing the adjacent female. Male organs develop before the female.

Human cestodes are divided into two orders:

1. *Pseudophyllidea*, with slit-like suckers, oval head, two long grooves with muscular walls, no hooks, and the genital orifice on the flat surface.
2. *Cyclophyllidea*, cup-like, or round suckers; genital orifice marginal.

ORDER: PSEUDOPHYLLIDEA
GENUS: *Diphyllobothrium*

Diphyllobothrium latum (Linn., 1758)

Synonym: *Dibothriocephalus latus*, broad tapeworm

Characters

It is greyish and more translucent and less fleshy than *Taenia* and may attain a length of 3–10 m, lying coiled up in the small intestine. Multiple infections are common. The scolex (3 mm) has no rostellum or hooklets, but 2 slit-like suckers with longitudinal grooves (bothria). The neck is thin; the proglottides number 3000–4000. The number of worms corresponds to the individual plerocercoids swallowed. Mature segments are broader than they are long. A single worm may discharge as many as from 36 000 to a million eggs per diem. The worm may be discharged from the bowel naturally, without treatment. (For details of anatomy of male and female elements, see Fig. 324).

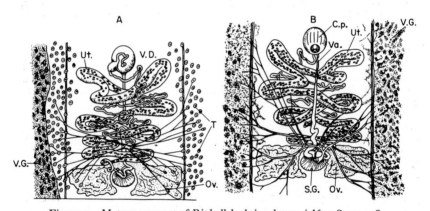

Fig. 324.—Mature segment of *Diphyllobothrium latum*. (*After Sommer & Landois*) A, Dorsal or male aspect. B, Ventral or female aspect.

T, testes. V.D, vas deferens. V.G, vitelline glands. C.p., cirrus pouch. Ov., ovary. S.G., shell gland. UT, uterus. Va, vagina.

The egg is operculated, with a brown shell, measuring 70 × 45 μm (Plate XIII). No segments are passed in faeces (unlike *Taenia*). The eggs, discharged by the uterus to the exterior, are found in vast numbers in the faeces, occupying one third of their bulk. The yolk-cells are tightly packed, crowded with steel-grey granules (thus differing from trematode eggs).

Life history (Fig. 325)

If the egg is passed in water the operculum is lifted, the ciliated 6-hooked *coracidium* emerges; resembling a ball (22–30 μm), it swims by means of its cilia, but dies in 24 hours. Normally it is swallowed by fresh-water crustacea, the first inter-mediary—*Cyclops strenuus, Diaptomus gracilis; D. graciloides* or *D. oregonensis, Cyclops brevispinosus*, and *C. prasenus* in U.S.A. The outer layer is then digested. The hooks tear a hole in the gut wall; it passes into the body cavity and may kill the cyclops. Lying outside the gut wall it becomes the *procercoid larva* (Fig. 325), which is ovoid, 50–60 μm long, with a terminal spherical appendix and 6 hooklets in the terminal appendage or *cercomer*. At most 2 of these are found in 1 *Cyclops*, which is then swallowed by fresh-water fishes of many species, the second intermediaries—pike, perch, salmon, trout, grayling; in Africa the barbel; in U.S.A. the pike, wall-eye and burbot. Reaching the stomach of the fish, the procercoid penetrates to the body cavity, and, after 3 to 4 days there, encysts as a plerocercoid or *sparganum* (6 mm) in the muscular and connective tissues. Sucking, cephalic grooves, nervous and excretory systems are developed. It is then ingested by man with raw roe (caviar) or insufficiently cooked fish and the *plerocercoid* develops in 5-6 weeks into an adult *Diphyllobothrium*. Fresh-water fishes harbour other spargana which cannot be differentiated in this stage.

The process of 'kippering' does not kill the plerocercoids, and ordinary smoking is ineffectual, but brine saturation is effective. This tapeworm can live as long as 29 years.

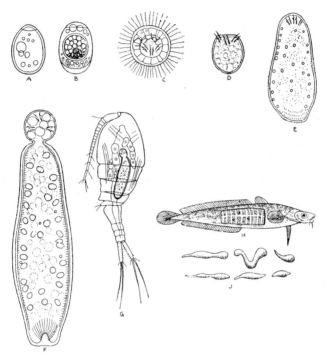

Fig. 325.—Evolutionary cycle of *Diphyllobothrium latum*. Various scales. (*After Brumpt*)

A, Egg of *D. latum*. B, Hexacanth embryo. C, Ciliated onchosphere or coracidium. D, E, F, Development of larva or procercoid in *Cyclops*. G, Procercoid in the body cavity of *Cyclops*. H, Development of plerocercoids in fishes. J, Plerocercoids of different shapes ingested by man, dog or cat.

Diphyllobothrium minus is a small variety which the Russians claim as a separate species. It has been found in Lake Baikal and has a similar life history to that of *D. latum*. Its second intermediary hosts are various species of salmon and grayling which are eaten salted or frozen by Mongolian peoples.

D. alascense is a species found in the Eskimos and is differentiated by the form of the scolex. The plerocercoids probably occur in two species of fish—*Pungitius* and *Dallia*.

For clinical features see page 349.

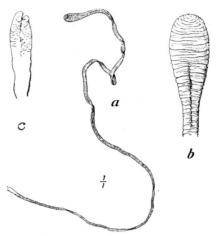

Fig. 326.—*Diphyllobothrium mansoni* plerocercoid, extracted from an abscess in a Masai. *a*, Natural size. *b*, Anterior extremity. *c*, Posterior extremity. (*After Sambon*)

Diphyllobothrium (Spirometra) mansoni (Cobbold, 1882)
Synonym: *Dibothriocephalus mansoni*

Characters

It resembles *D. latum*, is 6–10 m long and has a more delicate structure with a narrower and more ellipsoid egg than *D. latum*.

Life history

The adult stage occurs in the dog and other animals, the plerocercoid (sparganum) under natural conditions in the frog (*Rana nigromaculata*), or snake (*Elaphe climacophora*). The procercoid in *Cyclops leuckarti* shows the same stages as in *D. latum*.

Man is infected by accidentally swallowing a procercoid while drinking, thus becoming a second intermediary. The Chinese custom of applying raw split frogs to sores on the hands or to inflamed eyes may afford entry. The sparganum in man measures 8–36 cm × 0·1–12 mm × 0·5–1·75 mm thick (Fig. 327). Its body is flat and trans-

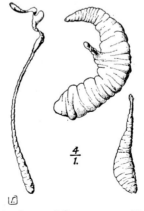

Fig. 327.—Different forms of *Sparganum proliferum*. (*After Ijima*)

versely wrinkled, with a longitudinal median groove. It is found in many parts of the body: kidneys and iliac fossae, pleural cavities, urethra and subcutaneous tissues.

D. *mansonoides* was formerly thought to be the parent form of *Sparganum proliferum* (Fig. 327). D. *mansonoides* is found in the intestine of the cat in the Southern United States, and is separable from D. *latum* and D. *cordatum* by the scolex, uterine characteristics and smaller size. Specimens vary from 20 to 60 cm in length, but may attain 1 m × 8 mm. Immature proglottides number 200–300.

The egg is pointed, 65 × 37 μm, with a conical operculum. The life history is as in D. *latum*.

The plerocercoids (*sparganum*) measure 3–12 × 2·5 mm (Fig. 327) and are contained in cysts, which are found in man in Japan and Florida. The body contains calcareous corpuscles. The cysts may be disseminated throughout the body in the subcutaneous tissues, intramuscular fasciae, walls of the alimentary canal, mesentery, kidney, lung, heart and brain. The prognosis in man is grave. Similar plerocercoids have been reproduced in macaque monkeys.

Sparganosis has been found in Korea and spargana, 23–50 cm in length, removed from the muscles of the abdomen and chest. All patients had eaten raw snakes—*Dinodon rufozonatum*. It has also been found in abscess of the leg. The adult form is *Dibothriorhynchus decipiens*. A new species, D. *sp.* type *grossum*, has been reported by Heinz from S. Africa.

Spargana are found near the Central African lakes (generally in swellings in the chest) and also in Ruanda-Urundi. The adults are probably D. *theileri* or D. *pretoriensis*.

For clinical features and treatment see page 329.

ORDER: CYCLOPHYLLIDEA
GENUS: *Taenia*

Taenia solium Linn., 1758, Pork tapeworm (Fig. 329)

Characters

It lives in the upper third of the small intestine. The name *solium* is derived from the resemblance of the rostellum to the conventional figure of the sun. It attains a length of 2–3 m (exceptionally 8 m), having 800–1000 segments. The head is globular, quadrangular, 1 mm in diameter, and the rostellum short and pigmented, with a double row of 20–50 hooklets (Fig. 328). The 4 suckers project slightly and are circular, measuring 0·5 mm in diameter. The anterior proglottides are small, broader than they are long, the more mature ones measuring 12 × 6 mm. Each proglottis has a marginal genital pore with thick lips; its situation alternates irregularly between the right and left margins. The uterus is median with 7–10 stout diverticula (Fig. 329). The testes consist of 150–200 follicles, distributed throughout the dorsal plane. Proglottides number less than 1000. Terminal ripe segments pass out in the faeces and have an independent movement which enables them to migrate outside the anus. Each gravid segment contains from 30 000 to 50 000 eggs.

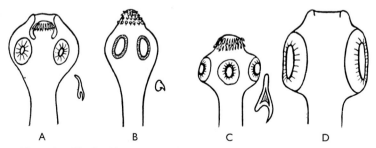

Fig. 328.—Heads of human cestodes, showing suckers and, when present, the arrangement of the hooklets. A, *Hymenolepis nana*. B, *Dipylidium caninum*. C, *Taenia solium*. D, *Taenia saginata*.

The egg measures 31–56 μm in diameter, and is round with no operculum. It has two radially-striated shells, the inner formed by the embryo (thus differing from pseudophyllidea), and a vitelline membrane when it is in the segment which is lost in the faeces. Small numbers of eggs are found in the faeces when the segments break. They contain the 6-hooked onchosphere (Plate XIII).

Life history

Mature segments are detached and pass out with the faeces; they disintegrate and the eggs are set free and eaten by the intermediary host (the pig). Man is occasionally infected by cysticerci (see Cysticercosis, page 337), so are other primates (macaque monkeys), occasionally sheep or dogs. The onchosphere penetrates the gut wall and enters the blood stream, settling in the muscles, especially the heart, where it loses its hooks, and becomes a *cysticercus* (5–20 mm). Known as *Cysticercus cellulosae*, it has a small, invaginated scolex and a neck, resembling a miniature adult taenia. Infected pork

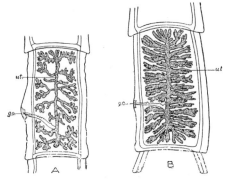

Fig. 329.—Segments of tapeworms, showing the characteristic branching of the uterus as seen in the mature segments. A, *Taenia solium*. B, *Taenia saginata*. (*After Blanchard*)

ut, Uterus. *g.o.*, genital opening.

is popularly known as 'measly pork'. In prevention thorough cooking of pork is essential. At 0°C the cysticerci can persist for 70 days.

In the alimentary canal of man or other definitive host the bladder of the cysticercus is absorbed by the gastric juices; the scolex and head are evaginated and then pass to the small intestine, where the scolex fixes itself to the gut wall and forms proglottides.

Taenia saginata Goeze, 1782, beef tapeworm (Figs 328, 329)

Characters

T. saginata is whitish and semitransparent, measuring 4–10 m; when fully adult it may contain 2000 segments. The scolex is pear-shaped, cubical and 1–2 mm in diameter with 4 lateral suckers but no rostellum or hooks. The suckers and sucker-like organ (Fig. 328) at the apex are frequently pigmented. The neck is long and half the width of the scolex. The older proglottides are elongated; gravid individuals are three to four times longer than they are broad. The genital pore is single, marginally placed at the hinder end of the proglottis, alternating regularly between the right and left margins. There are 20–35 lateral branches on each side of the uterus which may ramify (Fig. 329). The genital organs in the mature proglottid differ from those of *T. solium* in having about twice the number of testes (300–400) and in lacking the accessory ovarian lobe. Each gravid segment contains about 97 000 eggs and there may be 1000–2000 segments. The total output per year is reckoned at 594 million.

T. saginata, like *Enterobius vermicularis*, oviposits on the perianal skin. The ova are expelled when the proglottid has detached itself from the strobila. The gravid uterus carries lateral branches terminating in blind club-shaped sacs. There they form a separate organ resembling a tassel (*thysanus*), which when it distintegrates leaves behind a mass of ova. The thysanus then becomes an aperture for oviposition (*protocostoma*). The stimulus is provided by thousands of eggs compressed within the uterus. The yolk mass which envelops the embryophores of the ova causes them to adhere to the perianal skin.

The egg is globular, 30–40 × 20–30 μm, with a double-shelled striated embryophore, which contains the onchosphere (Plate XIII). It is indistinguishable from that of *T. solium*.

Life history

Gravid proglottides emerge in faeces or pass to the exterior independently; they then creep into grass or herbage, where they disintegrate. When the eggs are eaten by the ox, the onchospheres are set free and pass into the small intestine, where they bore through the wall, and are carried to the muscles, especially the pterygoids and the fatty tissues round heart, diaphragm and tongue. Then cysticerci (*Cysticercus bovis*) are formed, measuring 7·5–9 × 5·5 mm. They live for 8 months in the ox and develop further in man, who constitutes the normal definitive host. The bladder is digested, and the liberated scolex, passing to the small intestine, affixes itself by suckers to the gut-wall. The cysts die at 48°C. Infected meat is known to inspectors as 'measly beef'. In Egypt and Morocco the camel is the most important intermediary host. (Several varieties are described: *T. africana*, *T. hominis*, *T. philippina*, *T. bremneri* and *T. confusa*, have been attributed to new species, but are probably aberrant forms of *T. saginata*. Abnormal forms are common, such as *T. lophosoma*.)

For the pathogenesis and treatment, see page 337.

GENUS: *Echinococcus*

Echinoccus granulosus (Batsch, 1786) and *E. multilocularis* (Leuckart, 1863) Vogel, 1955

Synonym: *Taenia echinococcus* or hydatid.

Characters

E. granulosus is very small, 3–8·5 mm long, with a pyriform scolex, 0·3 mm in diameter, provided at the apex with a projecting rostellum, 4 suckers and 2 circular rows of hooks, varying in size and number. (Fig. 330). The neck is short and thick; the proglottides usually 4 in number. The last one is the longest (2–3 mm); only one is sexually mature and this contains up to 5000 eggs. The genital apertures are marginal, one to each proglottis, in an alternating arrangement. The testes are spherical and numerous. The cirrus pouch is large and pear-shaped. The uterus is tubular and median, with short unbranched lateral diverticula. The adult is difficult to remove from the small intestine of the dog without breaking its head. Eggs appear in the dog's faeces. Sometimes the fourth segment also comes away. Man is probably not a suitable intermediary, but is, of course, quite susceptible to hydatid infection.

The egg is spherical, 32–38 × 21–30 μm, and is double-shelled, the inner shell being thick. The egg is so similar to those of other tapeworms that it cannot be distinguished from them or from *Multiceps*. The onchosphere contains three pairs of embryonal hooklets. When swallowed, the shell is digested and the onchosphere escapes. After 8 hours embryos can be found in the portal vein and liver, whence they are filtered out. The next filter is the lung, where a smaller number lodge. In 3 weeks the larval worm becomes vesicular and visible to the naked eye; in 3 months it attains a diameter of 5 cm and 5 weeks later has doubled that size. The hydatid cyst wall is composed of a fibrous laminated layer formed by the host, a thick median striated layer secreted by the cyst, and an inner 'germinal' layer from which the brood capsules and daughter cysts arise. There are 2 types of proliferation: endogenous and exogenous. In the former, proliferation is inwards towards the cyst cavity; in the latter it is outwards. The varieties of hydatid are so striking that alveolar hydatid (*E. multilocularis*) has now been recognized as a distinct entity which has a limited geographical distribution.

The brood capsules are formed from small nuclear masses of the parenchymatous germinal layer; later, they become vacuolated to form vesicles. Larval scolices arise from a local thickening of the wall of the brood capsule; the wall evaginates to form a protective cup for the growing scolex. Near the head end the cuticle thickens and a circle of hooklets develops. The contractile part of the body of the scolex is capable of invaginating the head, so that in the typical resting position the scolex has the hooklets inside. Free brood capsules and free scolices in the hydatid cyst cavity are known as 'hydatid sand'. In other cysts the brood capsules never produce scolices and are known as acephalocysts.

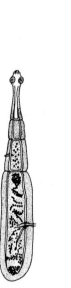
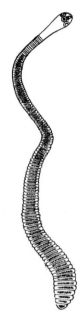

Fig. 330.—*Echinococcus granulosus.*   Fig. 331.—*Hymenolepis*
× 15. (*After Leuckart*)   *nana.* Magnified.

Daughter cysts may be produced by injury or by mechanical interference with the mother cyst, inside which they arise from the detached germinal layer, and also from the brood-capsule cells; rarely by vesicular changes from the detached scoleces. In the liver the daughter cysts are bile-stained. Intramuscular injection of scolices causes formation of new cysts (Dévé and Dew) and this accounts for the dissemination of hydatid cysts throughout the body which sometimes occurs after operation.

Exogenous daughter cysts in the omentum and bones are secondary, caused by herniation or rupture of both germinal and laminated layers through weakened parts of the adventitia from intracystic pressure. By final exclusion of these herniations new cysts form.

For clinical features see page 342.

ALVEOLAR HYDATID (*Echinococcus multilocularis*)

In the adult worm the differences are: the position of the genital pore in front of the middle of the proglottis. The number of testes is 21–29 (as against 45–65). These lie behind the posterior end of the proglottis in the region of the cirrus sac. The uterus

has no lateral branches. The length of the mature worm is 1·4–3·4 mm (as against 5–8 mm).
For clinical features see page 347.

GENUS: *Multiceps*

Multiceps multiceps

The adult worm is 40–60 cm in length and has a pyriform scolex about 1 mm in diameter with 4 scolices and a rostellum armed with a double rank of 22–32 large and small hooks.

Multiceps brauni

The adult worm has a scolex armed with 30 rostellar hooklets. The coenurus differs from that of *M. multiceps* in its larger hooks with bilobed glands.
For clinical features see page 348.

GENUS: *Hymenolepis*

Hymenolepis nana (Siebold, 1852) (Fig. 331)

Synonyms: *Taenia nana*, *H. murina*, dwarf tapeworm

Distribution

It is found in warm countries, Egypt, Sudan, Siam, India, Japan, South America (Brazil, Argentine, and especially Cuba), South Europe (Portugal, Spain and Sicily, where it affects 10% of the children). It lives in the small intestine (Grassi believed it to be identical with *H. fraterna* of the rat) and parasitizes the Syrian hamster (*Cricetus auratus*) (Fig. 331).

Characters

H. nana is 25–45 mm long by 0·5–0·9 mm and has 100–200 proglottides. The scolex measures 139–480 μm, is sub-globular with a well developed rostellum, a single crown with 20–30 hooklets (14–18 μm), and 4 globular suckers (80–150 μm) (Fig. 328). The neck is long, the proglottides short anteriorly, but the posterior ones increase in size and are broader than they are long. The genital pores are marginal and placed near the anterior border. There are 3 testes. The vas deferens widens into the seminal vesicle, and the gravid uterus occupies an entire segment.

The egg is oval and globular, and there are 8–180 in each segment. It has 2 membranes, outer (vitelline), 40–60 μm, and inner, 20–30 μm (Plate XIII). There is a conspicuous mammillate projection at each pole, enclosing an onchosphere with 3 pairs of hooklets.

The segments, when freed, are partially digested and the eggs, set free in the faeces, are easily detected.

Life history

This worm forms an exception to other members of the group, in that it has no intermediate host; the larva enters the villus of the intestine to become a cercocyst In 40–70 hours after infestation the scolex appears; in 80–90 hours the rostellum has hooklets and then passes into the lumen of the intestine attached to the epithelium of the villus by a short neck. The rapidity of development varies greatly. Strobilization is rapid; the proglottides mature in 10–12 days, and after 30 days eggs appear in the faeces. *H. fraterna* of the rat is morphologically identical, but its intermediary hosts are beetles and fleas (*Nosopsyllus fasciatus* and *Xenopsylla*).

Pathogenesis and treatment

H. nana appears in large numbers—hundreds or thousands. It may produce no symptoms, but occasionally there is abdominal pain and diarrhoea, rarely epileptiform convulsions, headache or strabismus. Nervous phenomena are due to the toxic products of the parasite. On account of its minute size, this worm is often overlooked. Diagnosis is made by finding the eggs in the faeces; care is needed because they are so transparent that they may be missed.

H. nana is not easy to dislodge by filix mas or oil of chenopodium; tetrachloroethylene (page 919) is said to be more effective. Chloroquine (page 901) has been recommended, and more recently Yomesan (page 916). The stools should then be examined by the flotation method. An infected patient should not sleep in the same bed with another person.

Hymenolepis diminuta (Rudolphi, 1819)

Distribution

This is a parasite of rats (*Rattus norvegicus (decumanus)*, *R. alexandrinus*) and mice (*Mus musculus* and *M. sylvaticus*); it is found in man in Italy, South America, the Congo and West Indies.

Characters

It measures 20–60 cm × 3·5 mm. The head is small and cuboidal with a small infundibulum. At the apex is a rudimentary rostellum with 4 small, unarmed suckers. The neck is shorter than the head. The proglottides increase in size as the tail is approached, and are broader than they are long.

The egg is circular or ovoid, measuring 60–80 μm. Its outer shell is yellowish and thickened, with indistinct radiations, and contains a hexacanth onchosphere.

Life history

The cysticercus stages occur in the body cavity of insects and fleas during their larval stages: *Nosopsyllus (Ceratophyllus) fasciatus*, *Xenopsylla cheopis*, *Leptopsylla segnis* (mouse flea); *Pulex irritans*; in coleoptera and lepidoptera such as *Asopia farinalis*, *Anisolabis annulipes*, *Tinea pellionella*, *Akis spinosa* and *Scaurus striatus*; also in South America, in *Dermestes vulpinus*, *D. peruvianus*, *Ulosonia parvicornis* and *Embia argentina*.

The rat becomes parasitized by eating infected fleas or other insects. The cysticercoids, when ingested by the definitive host, become adult in 17 days.

Treatment

Male fern is the drug of choice (page 899).

GENUS : *Dipylidium*

Dipylidium caninum (Linn., 1758)

Distribution

This is a common parasite of the dog, cat and jackal. There are 100 records of its occurrence in man, especially in children in European countries.

Characters

It lives in the small intestine, measuring 15–40 cm × 2–3 mm. The scolex is small and globular, 0·55 mm in diameter. The rostellum is retracted into the infundibulum and has 3–4 circles consisting of 28–30 hooklets (14–18 μm) of 'rose-thorn' shape and 4 elliptical suckers (Fig. 331). The proglottides are narrow and there are 200 or more of them. The segments measure 6–7 × 2–3 mm. Two sets of genital apparatus are found in each segment; the genital pores are placed symmetrically at the lateral margins. The uterine cavities contain egg-nests, each consisting of 8–15 eggs. Mature proglottides leave the intestine. The egg is round, 35–40 μm across.

Life history

The cysticercoid stage is passed through in the dog-louse (*Trichodectes canis*), dog-flea (*Ctenocephalides canis*), cat-flea (*C. felis*) and human flea (*Pulex irritans*). Eggs are eaten by the larval flea, and the hexacanth embryo develops in the adipose tissue and muscles, first appearing as a procercoid and later as a cysticercoid larva. Infection of man is accidental, due to swallowing infected fleas.

Pathogenesis and treatment

Usually there are no symptoms. Treatment is by filix mas, as for other forms of *Taenia*.

GENUS: *Railhetinu*

R. celebensis, *R. madagascariensis* (formerly *Taenia madagascariensis*), *R. quitensis*

These worms are found in Celebes, Thailand, British Guiana, Mauritius and Formosa, and the last has been reported by León in Ecuador and also by Baer and Sanders in Australia and from *Rattus assimilis*, a race of *R. rattus*. Two cases were reported by Chandler from Thailand as *R. siviragi*. They are characterized by numerous hooklets of 'coal-hammer' shape on the suckers and rostellum, and by unilateral genital pores on the proglottides. Ripe segments contain egg capsules. The ovoid eggs possess conspicuously large hooklets. Usually they are parasites of birds, more rarely of rats. Their intermediary hosts are probably flies.

GENUS: *Bertiella*

Bertiella studeri has often been found in man, and D'Alessandro *et al.* (1963) report a case of infection with *Bertiella mucronata*, a tapeworm of monkeys, in a woman in Paraguay; 3 others have previously been reported.

GENUS: *Inermicapsifer*

This genus closely resembles the foregoing and cannot be distinguished from it by the ripe proglottides, but the head and the suckers are unarmed. *I. arvicanthidis*, a parasite normally of the field-rat, was found by the late Editor in a European child from Kenya; since then others have been reported by Fain in Ruanda-Urundi and Baer in Arusha, Tanzania. It is suggested that it is commoner than has been supposed. No fewer than 12 species of *Inermicapsifer* are parasites of hyraxes and rodents in Africa. *I. cubensis* appears to be common in Cuba where 76 cases in man have been described by Kouri. It is identical with the foregoing; *I. madagascariensis* is also identical.

PHYLUM: NEMATHELMINTHES
CLASS: NEMATODA OR ROUNDWORMS

The sexes of these worms are separate. They are cylindrical, non-segmented and taper at both ends. They are white or yellow, sometimes semi-transparent and their eggs are characteristic (Plate XIII).

SUPERFAMILY: ASCARIDOIDEA
GENUS: *Ascaris*
Ascaris lumbricoides Linn., 1758, round worm

Characters

A. suum of the pig is indistinguishable from *A. lumbricoides* and allied species are found in the cat, dog and horse. The worm inhabits the small intestine. The female measures 20–35 cm × 3–6 mm; the male 15–31 cm × 2–4 mm. Both are pale yellow or brown, with whitish longitudinal lines, round, tapering at both ends. The mouth is at the anterior end, guarded by thin lips with finely denticulated margins (Fig. 332). The anus is subterminal. In the female there are paired genital tubes, containing the uterus, receptaculum seminis, oviduct and ovary. Tubules and ducts attain a length of 12 cm. The total capacity of the genital tubules at one time has been estimated at 27 million eggs; the average day output is 200 000. The male has the tail curved into a semicircle and has 2 rows of tactile papillae and two chitinous spicules. The life span is about 10–12 months.

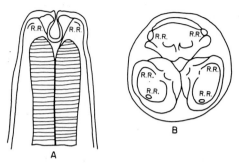

Fig. 332.—Head of *Ascaris lumbricoides*. A, Ventral view. B, Anterior view, showing the oral labia. (*After Faust*)

The egg (Plate XIII) measures 50–70 × 40–50 μm and is elliptical, encased in a rough albuminous coat giving it a mamillated appearance. It is usually stained by faecal pigments.

Life history

When the eggs are passed in the faeces, there is no segmentation or differentiated embryo. In water, or in moist earth, at 36–40°C within 2–4 months the embryo is seen coiled up and moving inside the egg-shell. The larva undergoes a moult before hatching and must be transformed into a second stage larva of the 'rhabditoid' type before it is infective. The embryo does not emerge from the egg until it is swallowed. The egg-shell is then softened by the gastric juice and hatches in the small intestine. The rhabditiform

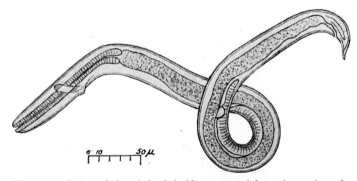

Fig. 333.—Larva of *Ascaris lumbricoides* recovered from the trachea of a rat 8 days after ingestion of the eggs. (*After Brumpt*)

larva penetrates the mucous membrane, enters the blood via the heart and lungs, and reaches the alveolar capillaries where it has a 'blood bath'. As the larvae cannot pass through they burrow through the wall of the alveolus and enter the respiratory tree, finally being carried up the trachea by ciliary action. Eventually, on reaching the vocal cords, the majority of the larvae are swallowed for the second time and reach the small intestine. The second invasion is often accompanied by severe allergic reactions, urticarial reactions and fall in blood pressure. The whole process occupies 10–14 days. During this time the larva moults twice (once after 5–6 days and the second time after the tenth day). The larvae measure 1·3–2 mm on the tenth day (Fig. 333) and 1·75–2·37 mm on the fifteenth. Larvae may reach the intestine as early as the fifth day. The fourth ecdysis takes place in the intestine between the twenty-fifth and twenty-ninth days. In man the incubation period (to time of first oviposition) occupies a period of 60–75 days. The diameter of the migrating larvae from the pulmonary capillaries to the terminal air spaces is considerably larger than that of the capillaries.

Hundreds of these larvae have been removed from a swelling in the neck and ramifying loculi.

For clinical features see page 248.

GENUS: *Toxocara*

Toxocara canis (Werner 1782; Johnston 1916)

Toxocara canis (the dog ascarid) is a cosmopolitan infection of dogs.

Morphology

The morphology is similar to that of *Ascaris*. The male worms are 4–6 cm long and the females 6·5–10 cm. In addition to the 3 characteristic lips of ascarids there are distinct cervical alae or wings, which are much longer than they are broad and extend some distance from the anterior extremity along the lateral margins. The perianal papillae of the male worms are characteristic. The ova are pitted superficially and measure 85 × 75 μm. They are dark or greyish brown and unembryonated when passed.

Life cycle

The life cycle is similar to that of *Ascaris lumbricoides* with 4 larval stages. In endemic areas young pups are born infected and may die during the first few weeks of life, after which they acquire some immunity.

Toxocara cati (Shrank 1788; Brumpt 1927)

This worm is the common ascarid of the domestic cat and some of its wild relatives.

Morphology

The male worms are 4–6 cm long and the females 4–12 cm. The anterior end has the characteristic ascarid lips and is provided with a pair of broad lateral cervical alae or wings, which give a pyriform outline to the anterior end of the body. The eggs are similar to those of *T. canis*, as is the life cycle.

For clinical features see page 253.

GENUS: *Lagochilascaris*

Lagochilascaris minor (Leiper, 1909)

Lagochilascaris minor resembles a small *Ascaris* and is normally found in the intestine of the clouded leopard. It is found in Surinam and in the Caribbean. It causes subcutaneous, tonsillar and mastoid abscesses. A case of this infection is reported from Tobago, it was thought to have been acquired through eating raw meat of the Manakou opossum.

The adult worm is recognized by a longitudinal furrow with indentations. The hare-lip-like parts of the mouth have given the worm its name. The eggs which occur in profusion resemble small ascaris ova. The male is 9 × 0·4 mm: the female 15 × 0·5 mm. Both have a triangular keel-like cuticular ledge along the entire extent of the lateral line.

Treatment with diethylcarbamazine has been successful.

SUPERFAMILY: SPIRUROIDEA

GENUS: *Gnathostoma*

Gnathostoma spinigerum (Owen, 1838)

Morphology

The adult worms (Fig. 334) in the feline host vary in length from 11 to 25 mm for males and 25 to 54 mm for females. They are stout, reddish-coloured, slightly transparent nematodes with a subglobose cephalic swelling separated from the remainder of the worm by a cervical constriction. One or more individuals are found in each tumour. The anterior half of the nematode is covered with leaf-like spines which are broader and tridented just behind the cervix and narrower and singly pointed more equatorially. These spines are species characteristic.

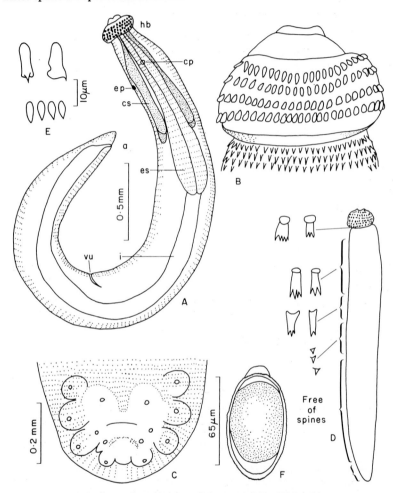

Fig. 334.—*Gnathostoma spinigerum*. (*After Miyazaki*)

A, Lateral view of third stage larva. B, Head bulb of third stage larva with 4 rows of hooklets. C, Posterior end of male, ventral view, with minute cuticular spines omitted. D, Diagram of the types of spines at different levels of the body. E, Detail of the spines on the head bulb. F, Fertilized egg.
a, anus. *cp*, cervical papilla. *cs*, cervical sac (gland ?). *ep*, excretory pore. *oes*, oesophagus. *hb*, head bulb. *i*, intestine. *vu*, vulva.

The cephalic portion of the body is covered with 4–8 transverse rows of sharp recurved hooks. Four conspicuous cervical glands, arranged symmetrically around the oesophagus, fuse in pairs and open through 2 ducts which perforate the lips. The male has a pseudobursa which is provided with 4 pairs of perianal papillae. The copulatory spicules are chitinoid rods measuring 1·1 mm and 0·4 mm respectively. The vulva of the female is slightly postequatorial in position. The vagina is long and is anteriorly directed. The other genital tubes are paired.

The eggs (Fig. 334) are ovoid and 65–70 × 38–40 μm in size. They are transparent, superficially pitted, have a mucoid plug at one end and are unembryonated when laid.

A motile first stage larva, measuring 223–275 × 13·4–17·4 μm and having a rounded anterior end provided with spines, emerges from the shell and actively enters a species of *Cyclops*, bores its way into the haemocoele and metamorphoses in 10–14 days into a second stage larva (350–450 × 60–65 μm), which is provided with a head bulb armed with 4 rings of spines and 2 pairs of cervical glands. A second intermediate host is required, which can be a snake (rock python, cobra in India), fresh-water fish (Philippines) or a frog (Thailand). In Japan third stage larvae are found in crayfish, crabs, amphibia, reptiles and mammals which had eaten infected fish flesh. Complete maturation to the adult stage in the stomach occurs only in the stomach of dogs, cats and other felines.

Life cycle in nature

The adult lives in tumours in the stomach wall of felines and dogs. Eggs are extruded from lesions and evacuated via the faeces into water where they embryonate and hatch. Larvae are ingested by *Cyclops*, which are then eaten by fish, frogs or snakes and the larvae develop into the third stage in the flesh of these animals. A dog or cat then eats the infected fish, frog or snake and the infection develops into maturity in the stomach wall in about 6½ months.

For clinical features see page 281.

GENUS: *Physaloptera*

Physaloptera causasica (Linstow, 1902)

Synonym: *P. mordens* (Leiper, 1907)

Distribution

Normal hosts are monkeys. In man it has been found in Central Africa, Mozambique, Uganda and Malawi. It lives in the oesophagus, stomach, small intestine and occasionally the liver.

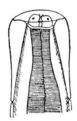

Fig. 335.—The head of *Physaloptera caucasica*. (*After Leiper*)

Characters

The female (2·4–10 cm × 1·14–2·8 mm) has a posterior end tapering to a sharp point, 2 ovaries, a single uterine tube, and a vulva in the anterior part of the body. The male (1·4–5 cm × 0·7–1 mm) has 2 lateral alae on the tail, formed by expansion of the cuticle, 4 pairs of pedunculated papillae—6 pairs sessile—1 unpaired postanal papilla, and 2 spicules of unequal length. In both sexes the mouth is guarded by 2 large lips, armed with 2 papillae and rows of teeth, which serve to grip the mucous membrane (Fig. 335).

The egg (45 × 35 μm) has a double contour, smooth, thick, colourless shell.

Life history

The life cycle is unknown; insects possibly act as intermediaries. The clinical symptoms are indeterminate. The worms live with heads embedded in the digestive tract from the oesophagus to the ileum.

GENUS: *Anisakis*

Anisakis (Eustoma) (Van Thiel, 1962)

This is an ascarid parasite of herrings and marine animals. Its larval stages have caused symptoms in man.

The adult form inhabits the intestines of sea mammals (whales, dolphins and porpoises) and the larval stages are found in a variety of fish (haddock, mackerel, cod, pike, herring, bonita, squid, salmon and Alaskan pollack).

The infective larva, as seen in the infective stage, is slender and threadlike, measuring 1·5–2·6 cm long and 0·1 cm in diameter. Its outer surface is somewhat striated and there is a ventriculus between the oesophagus and the intestine, with the latter two structures meeting on an oblique plane. There is an excretion pore in the anterior part of the head, ventral to a small larval tooth, and there are 3 anal glands near the rectum. Transverse sections show the lateral cords arranged in a Y-shaped structure along the upper intestine or oesophagus or intestine. The cuticle consists of three layers and shows no alae.

For clinical features see page 280.

GENUS: *Gonglyonema*

Gonglyonema pulchrum (Molin, 1857)

This is a spirurate nematode of a genus in which there are 6 species. It is a rare infection in man and pig, but all ruminants are optimum hosts.

The worm lives most commonly in the upper portion of the digestive tract, where it forms sinuous galleries in the mucosa and submucosa of the oesophagus, buccal cavity and tongue. The male is 62 × 0·15–0·3 mm and the female much larger, 145 × 0·2–0·5 mm. The anterior extremity is covered with a variable number of bosses or scutes arranged in 8 longitudinal series.

The transparent thick-shelled oval eggs are embryonated when laid and are 50–70 μm in length by 25–37 μm. Development takes place in dung beetles of genera *Apodius* and *Onthophagus*, as well as in a small cockroach. About 10 human cases are recorded in tongue, mouth and oesophagus, mostly in southern U.S.A. One was recorded from the lower lip of a man in Georgia (Dismuke & Routh 1963). Treatment is to remove the worm from its tunnel; antiseptic mouthwashes or novacaine applied locally help to extrude it.

SUPERFAMILY: STRONGYLOIDEA

GENUS: *Ancylostoma*

Ancylostoma duodenale Dubini, 1843, Old World hookworm, miner's worm

Characters

Both sexes are cylindrical, white, grey, or reddish brown (from ingested blood). The female (1–1·3 cm × 0·6 mm) (Fig. 336), is cylindrical and slightly expanded posteriorly. The vagina is in the posterior third. The body cavity is occupied by the ovary and coiled uterine tubes packed with eggs. The maximum egg-output occurs 15 to 18 months after infection. The male (0·8–1·1 cm × 0·4–0·5 mm) has a copulatory bursa consisting of an umbrella-like expansion of the cuticle; the dorsal ray is divided towards the distal end into smaller rays, which again divide into 3 unequal portions (Fig. 337). There are 2 long delicate spicules. The genital papillae are tactile, finger-like projections near the ano-genital opening. Owing to the situation of the genital openings in both sexes the worms in copulation assume a Y-shaped figure.

Two well marked cephalic glands occupy the anterior third in both sexes and secrete an anticoagulating ferment. The mouth end is bent dorsally. The excretory pore is ventral, placed at the level of the oesophagus. The buccal capsule is lined with chitin, and contains 2 pairs of sharp teeth on its ventral aspect (Fig. 338). The worm lives mostly in the jejunum, and to a lesser extent in the duodenum, but not in the ileum.

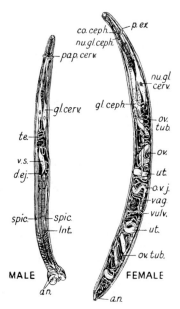

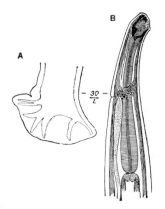

Fig. 336.—Male and female *Ancylostoma duodenale.* × 14. For actual size see Fig. 96. (*After Looss*)

An, anus. *co. ceph,* cephalic nerve commissure. *d. ej,.* ejaculatory duct. *gl. cerv,* cervical gland. *int,* intestine. *nu. gl. cerv.,* nucleus of cervical gland. *ov,* ovary. *ov. tub,* ovarian tubules. *ovj,* oveiector. *p. ex,* excretory pore. *pap. cerv.,* cervical papilla. *spic.,* spicules. *te,* testes. *ut,* uterus, *vag,* vagina. *v.s.,* vesicula seminalis. *vulv,* vaginal opening.

Fig. 337.—Bursa (A) and head (B) of male *Ancylostoma duodenale.* (*After Looss*)

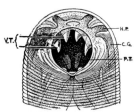

Fig. 338.—Head of *Ancylostoma duodenale,* showing the hook-like ventral teeth. × 50. (*After Looss*)

C.G., cephalic gland. H.P., head papillae. P.T., pharyngeal teeth. V.T., ventral teeth.

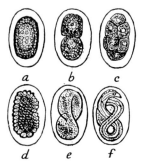

Fig. 339.—Development stages of *Ancylostoma duodenale* of the larva in eggs. *a, b* and *c* are seen in fresh stools, and *d, e,* and *f* when the stools are stale. × 300. (*After Looss*)

At autopsy 500–1000 or more worms may be found. They have a life-span of 4–7 years. The interval between active infection and the final disappearance of eggs from the faeces may be 76 months. The female produces 25 000–35 000 eggs each day, and some 18–54 million eggs during its lifetime.

For the pathogenesis and treatment see page 256.

Ancylostoma braziliense De Faria, 1910

Distribution

It is found in dogs and cats in Brazil. In Ceylon it was described as *A. ceylanicum* from the civet cat.

Characters

It is rarely found in the small intestine, and then is part of a mixed hookworm infection in man in India, Malaysia, and Thailand. It is smaller than *A. duodenale* and the internal pair of ventral teeth are smaller than the corresponding teeth of that species. The female is 1 cm long and the male 8·5 mm. The rays in the copulatory bursa differ (Fig. 340) from those of *A. duodenale*, and are distinctive.

The egg is indistinguishable from that of *A. duodenale*.

Life history

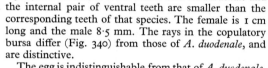

Fig. 340.—Dorsal ray of *Ancylostoma braziliense.* (*After Leiper*)

This is the same as *A. duodenale*. Man is apparently an unsuitable host. The larva does not penetrate into the blood stream easily, but wanders under the skin, causing irritation (larva migrans, page 263).

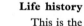

Table 46. Differentiation of third stage larva of
Necator and *Ancylostoma*

	Necator	Ancylostoma
Oral capsule	Sharply defined; visible dorsally and ventrally	Hardly visible; more marked dorsally than ventrally
Tail	Rather blunt	Pointed
Zone of closing cells	Leaves only small space between oesophagus and intestine	Leaves considerable space

GENUS: *Necator*

Necator americanus (Stiles, 1902), New World hookworm

Characters

It is found in the small intestine of man, and also of the gorilla, patas monkey, rhinoceros, pangolin and a rodent (*Caendu villosus*) and develops also in puppies. On the whole, *N. americanus* is a shorter and more slender worm than *A. duodenale*. The female (0·9–1·1 cm × 0·4 mm) has the vulva placed slightly in front of the middle of the body, so that it copulates at a Y-shaped angle, as in *A. duodenale*. The male (7–9 × 0·3 mm) has the copulatory bursa closed and blunt, and a short dorso-median lobe which appears as if divided (Fig. 341). The dorsal ray branches at the base into divergent arms with bipartite tips (tridigitate in *A. duodenale*). The base of the dorsal and dorsolateral rays is short (Fig. 342). Two separate spicules unite to form a single terminal 'fish-hook' barb. The living worms are greyish-yellow, at times reddish.

The sudden dorsal bend of the head, especially in the female, is distinctive. The buccal capsule is smaller than in *A. duodenale*, with an irregular border. In place of 4 hook-like teeth there is a ventral pair of cutting plates (Fig. 343). The first pair of dorsal teeth are represented by chitinous plates. The outlet of the dorsal gland constitutes a 'dorsal rib' or tooth which projects into the oral cavity. Deeply placed in the capsule are 1 pair of dorsal and 1 pair of sub-median lancets.

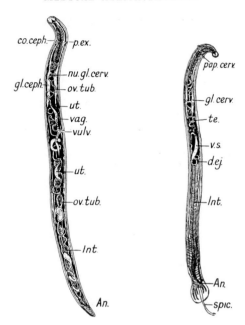

Fig. 341.—*Necator americanus.* × 12.
Key as for Fig. 336.

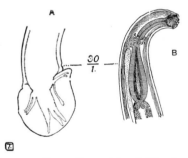
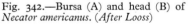

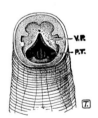

Fig. 342.—Bursa (A) and head (B) of *Necator americanus.* (*After Looss*)

Fig. 343.—The head of *Necator americanus*, showing the pharyngeal teeth (P.T.) and the ventral plates (V.P.) × 50.

The egg is slightly larger than that of *A. duodenale* (64–75 × 36–40 μm), but otherwise similar. The infective larva can be differentiated from that of *S. stercoralis* by the larger buccal vestibule and the intervening space between the oesophagus and midgut. Forty-four eggs/gramme of faeces are reckoned to represent one female worm. The female lays from 6000 to 20 000 eggs/day. The estimated duration of life is about 5 years.

Life history

This is identical with that of *A. duodenale*, except that it infects via the skin only.

SUMMARY OF LIFE HISTORY OF HOOKWORMS

The eggs are deposited in the lumen of the intestine with 2, 4, or 8 blastomeres. They develop and hatch, after expulsion in the faeces, if they are deposited in damp, shaded soil.

1. The embryo moves about inside the shell and alters its shape, then escapes and gives rise to

2. The rhabditiform larva which burrows into the faeces and feeds especially on bacteria. At first it has a double-bulbous oesophagus (Fig. 344). Feeding voraciously, it stores oil globules in its intestinal wall. It moults on the third day; on the fifth the

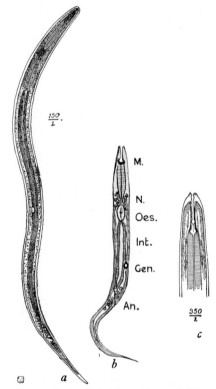

$\frac{150}{1}$.

M.

N.

Oes.

Int.

Gen.

An.

$\frac{350}{1}$

c

b

a

Fig. 344.—*Ancylostoma duodenale. a,* Mature larvae. *b,* Rhabditiform larva. × 120. *c,* Head of larva. (*After Looss*)

oesophageal bulb disappears, and the larva becomes elongated and fully developed at 20–30°C; the larva on the third day is 400 μm, and on the fifth it is 500–700 μm long. It then moves away from the faeces into the earth, moults again and becomes

3. The infective filariform, or third stage larva, with a well developed mouth capsule, a simple muscular oesophagus and protective sheath, the walls of which are seen as two bright lines in the living specimen. It moves towards the oxygen supply, but cannot swim in water. The larvae are most numerous in the upper 2·5 cm of the soil. They can ascend from deeper layers, but lateral movements are limited. Attracted by warmth, it is quiescent in the cold; it moves along a thin film of water as well as in the earth. Enabled by the sheath to withstand a certain degree of desiccation, it can live in warm damp soil under optimum conditions for 2 years. This is the

infective stage (Fig. 344). Direct sunlight, drying, flooding or salt water are fatal. On penetrating the skin of the host, the sheath is left behind, and the larva then enters the lymphatics, gains the blood stream, and reaches the lungs on the third day. If pyogenic bacteria enter the skin with the larvae an open lesion may develop, producing 'ground itch'. *A. duodenale* can infect via the mucous membrane of the mouth, as well as the skin, whereas *N. americanus* infects via the skin. Breaking through the alveoli of the lungs, it enters the bronchioles, and travels via trachea and oesophagus to the stomach. During this migration the third moult takes place and the buccal capsule is formed. On arrival in the intestine on the seventh day it undergoes its fourth moult; the terminal buccal capsule is changed into the 'provisional buccal capsule' with the mouth opening directed dorsally, as in the adult, but without teeth. On the fifteenth day the 'provisional buccal capsule' is cast off, and it then assumes the adult form with adult buccal capsule and bursa in the male. In 3–5 weeks it becomes sexually mature, copulates and then produces fertile eggs. Females of *A. duodenale* lay about 2½ times as many eggs as do females of *Necator americanus*.

Cultivation of hookworm larvae

A small portion of faeces is rubbed over a Petri dish with warm water, making a uniform layer like pea-soup. Inside the cover is placed a circle of wet blotting paper. This is kept moist and incubated at 23·9°C under a shade. If there is too much water the eggs will not develop. The larvae climb up the sides of the dish on to the blotting paper where they can be studied.

The striation of the sheath is indistinct in *A. duodenale*, but very distinct in *A. braziliense*. Rhabditiform ancylostome larvae are similar to those of *S. stercoralis*, but are slightly more attenuated posteriorly and possess a much longer buccal vestibule. Infective (third stage) *duodenale* larvae are differentiated from *Necator* by the oesophageal shears which are unequal in thickness in *Ancylostoma* but equal in *Necator*.

For clinical features and treatment see page 258.

GENUS: *Oesophagostomum*

Oesophagostomum apiostomum (Willach, 1891)

Distribution

This worm has been found in 4% of prisoners in the jails of North Nigeria. It is a common parasite of the caecum and colon of Old World monkeys in Africa, the Philippines and China.

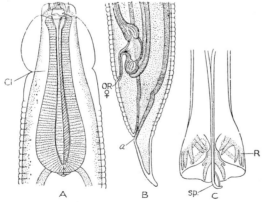

Fig. 345.—*Oesophagostomum apiostomum* (*brumpti*). A, Head, showing cuticular expansion and the oral vestibule. B, Tail of the female. C, Tail of the male, showing copulatory bursa. (*After Railliet & Henry*)

a, anus. *Cl,* ventral cleft. *OR,* vaginal orifice. *R,* characteristic rays of bursa. *Sp,* spicule.

Characters

When free or encysted under the mucous membrane of the large intestine it produces a condition like polyposis.

The female (1 cm × 0·325 mm) terminates posteriorly in a sharp point and has a vulva in its anterior half. The male (0·8–1 cm × 0·35 mm) has a copulatory bursa with a dorsal ray bifurcating into branches and forming a horse-shoe-shaped structure, each limb giving off a short lateral horn near its base (Fig. 345).

The egg (60 × 40 μm) closely resembles that of *Ancylostoma*, but is passed in an advanced stage of development.

Life history

The larvae hatch from the eggs in the soil. When mature, they are unsheathed. The rhabditiform stage is swallowed, and passes through the stomach and intestine. Then it invades the wall of the caecum where it forms nodules and, on occasions, it may penetrate the bowel and form intraperitoneal abscesses. The immature worms break out into the lumen, attach themselves to mucosa and become adult.

Treatment with intestinal anthelmintics is indicated.

Oesophagostomum stephanostomum var. *thomasi* (Railliet & Henry, 1909)

Distribution

This is a common parasite of monkeys (*Cercopithecus callitrichus*) and gorillas. The first case reported in man was in Brazil; the patient died of dysenteric symptoms and peritonitis. It has also been reported in French Guiana and in Northern Nigeria.

Characters

The morphology resembles that of *O. apiostomum*, but both sexes are larger and is distinguished by a corona radiata with 38 leaf-like spines.

The eggs in the faeces resemble those of *Ancylostoma*.

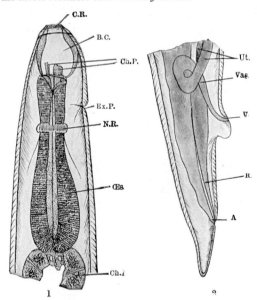

Fig. 346.—Female *Ternidens deminutus*. 1, Anterior extremity. 2, Posterior extremity. (*After Leiper*)

A, anus. B.C., buccal cavity. Ch. I., chyle intestine. C.R., corona radiata. Ch.P. chitinous plates. N.R., nerve ring. Oes, oesophagus. R, rectum. Ut, uterus. Vag, vagina. V, vaginal opening.

Life history

This is probably similar to that of *O. apiostomum*.

GENUS: *Ternidens*

Ternidens deminutus Railliet & Henry, 1905

Distribution

This strongylid nematode is relatively common in monkeys and baboons in Africa and Asia—*Macaca sinicus*, *M. cynomolgus*, *Cercopithecus pygerythrus* and *Papio porcarius*. In the small intestine of man it is not uncommonly found in Malawi, Mozambique, the Transvaal and Southern Rhodesia. It is not pathogenic, unless present in large numbers.

Characters

The female (14–16 × 0·73 mm) has a genital orifice posterior and subterminal, and a short vagina opening into two uterine tubes. The male (9·5 × 0·56 mm) has the dorsal ray of the copulatory bursa dividing into two distal extremities, and each branch bifurcates again (Fig. 347).

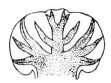

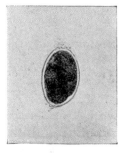

Fig. 347.—Bursa of male *Ternidens deminutus*. (*After Brumpt*)

Fig. 348.—Egg of *Ternidens deminutus*. (*After Blackie*)

The worm resembles a female ancylostome; its anterior extremity is not bent, and the mouth capsule is terminal, with a corona of setae. At the base of the cup-like buccal capsule 3 serrated teeth guard the entrance to the oesophagus; this is characteristic of the genus *Ternidens* (Fig. 346).

The egg (84 × 40 μm) is delicate, transparent, and in an advanced stage of segmentation resembles that of an ancylostome (Fig. 348).

Life history

The rhabditiform larva (0·3 mm), with flagellar tail, hatches from the egg in soil, becomes sheathed, and the infective filariform larva (0·6–0·7 mm) is formed. These can survive desiccation, reviving in water; thus they withstand drought. The larvae fail to penetrate human skin. Carbon tetrachloride and tetrachloroethylene are effective in treatment.

SUPERFAMILY: METASTRONGYLIDAE

GENUS: *Angiostrongylus*

Angiostrongylus cantonensis (Chen, 1935)

The male is 15·5–22·0 mm in length by 0·25–0·35 mm in breadth. It is transparent and smooth with faint transverse striae. The head is smoothly rounded and the mouth is without lips. There are 4 pairs of minute, submedian papillae which are sometimes visible *en face*, and 2 clearly defined minute triangular teeth present at the base of the oral cavity. There may possibly be a third which is difficult to define. The oesophagus is 0·29–0·33 mm long by 0·05 mm at maximum breadth at the posterior end. The intestine is a wide thin-walled tube. The excretory pore opens just posterior to the oesophageal–intestinal junction. The spicules are unequal, flexible and striated rods 1·2 mm in length. The bursa is well developed, but the gubernaculum is absent and there is one pair of large adanal papillae.

The female is 18·5–33 mm long by 0·28–0·5 mm in maximum breadth. Cuticle, head, papillae, oesophagus and intestines are as in the male. In life, the spirally wound, milky white uterine tubules and the blood-filled intestine can be seen through the transparent cuticle and form a striking 'barber's pole' pattern. The uterine tubules unite about 2 mm from the posterior end to form the thin-walled vagina. The vulva is a transverse slit. The tail is obliquely truncated. The anus is 0·06 mm and the vulva 0·25–0·28 mm from the tip of the tail which bears a minute terminal projection. The male: female ratio is usually 2:3.

Life history

The adult *A. cantonensis* lives in the pulmonary arteries of rats. Unsegmented ova are discharged into the blood stream and lodge as emboli in the smaller vessels. The first stage larvae which hatch from these eggs break through the respiratory tract, migrate up the trachea and eventually pass out of the body in the faeces. In Hawaii, the land snail, *Achatina fulica*, and the slug, *Veronicella leydigi*, and the land planarian, *Geoplana septemlineata*, have been found naturally infected.

Slugs (*Agriolimax laevis*) act as intermediary hosts. Two moults occur in the slug about the seventeenth day. The slugs are then eaten by rats (*R. rattus*) and the larvae remain in their cast skins until freed in the stomach of the rat by digestion. They then pass quickly along the gut as far as the ileum where they enter the blood stream and congregate in the central nervous system some 17 hours after ingestion. The anterior part of the cerebrum is the favourite site and there the third moult takes place on the sixth or seventh days and the final one on the eleventh to thirteenth. Young adults emerge on the surface of the brain from the twelfth to fourteenth days and spread during the next 2 weeks on the arachnoid surface. From the twenty-eighth to thirty-first days they migrate to the lungs via the venous system, passing through the right side of the heart to their definite site in the pulmonary arteries. The prepatent period in the rat usually lies between the forty-second and forty-fifth days.

For the pathogenesis and treatment, see page 277.

SUPERFAMILY: TRICHOSTRONGYLOIDEA

GENUS: *Trichostrongylus*

Trichostrongylus colubriformis (Giles, 1892) and allied species

Distribution

Normally, this is a parasite of the upper small intestine of the sheep and goat; it is not infrequently found in the duodenum and upper jejunum of man in agricultural districts of India, Central Africa, Egypt, Java, Australia, Japan, Korea and especially in Abadan (Iran), where 70% of inhabitants are infected (Stewart). It has been found by Bonne in Java in scrapings from the duodenum, where the adults live with head embedded in the mucosa. By flotation technique the eggs of this species can be found in the faeces, together with ancylostomes, fairly frequently in India and Assam. Though rare in Europeans it has been found in a doctor and his wife from Kenya. The worms suck blood and may cause anaemia.

Characters

The females (4–6·5 mm) usually outnumber the males. They are very slender and pink, with an attenuated anterior extremity, and the vulva in the posterior quarter. The males (4–5 × 0·07 mm) have a bilobed copulatory bursa and 2 spicules. These parasites are found, a third to a half buried in mucus. When scraped on to a slide they appear as delicate red streaks. When the slide is shaken in saline in a Petri dish they can be seen against a dark background. The adult worms are never found in faeces. The mouth is unarmed.

The egg (63 × 41 μm) is relatively large, oval, thin-shelled and contains a morula when deposited (Plate XIII). It is apt to be mistaken for that of *Ancylostoma duodenale*, but is translucent and smaller.

Life history

The eggs hatch outside the body; the rhabditiform larvae metamorphose into infective filariform in 6 days at 22–25°C and can be distinguished from similar stages in *Strongyloides* and *Ancylostoma* by the bead-like swelling at the tip of the tail. The semi-filariform third stage larvae are very resistant to desiccation. These enter the body via the skin or mouth, undergoing 2 ecdyses, and follow the same course as ancylostomes.

Bephenium is effective in treatment.

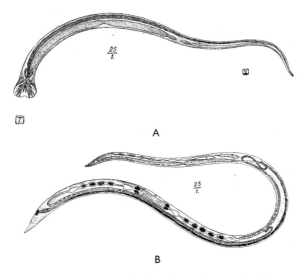

Fig. 349.—*Trichostrongylus colubriformis*. A, Female. B, Male. ×25.

An Eastern form has been separated in Japan (*T. orientalis*). *T. probolurus* (Railliet, 1896) is rarely seen in man; it is a natural infection of the gazelle and camel. *T. orientalis* is common in people who look after donkeys and goats.

SUPERFAMILY: RHABDITOIDEA
GENUS: *Strongyloides*
Strongyloides stercoralis (Bavay, 1876)

Characters

Formerly it was thought that embryos were produced by a parasitic, partheno-genetic female, in the absence of a male, but it is now known that a parasitic male exists, shorter and broader than the female. The oesophagus is characteristic, with a club-shaped anterior part, a post-central constriction and a posterior bulb (Fig. 350). Later, 2 copulatory spicules and a gubernaculum are said to become apparent and, when developed, the adult male resembles the free-living form (Fig. 351). Parasitic males are found in experimentally infected dogs, but not in human infections, owing to the fact that they do not invade the intestinal wall and so are eliminated from the bowel soon after the females begin to oviposit. Although adolescent parasitic females may be inseminated, probably the majority are parthenogenetics. This is a process of *reversive metamorphosis*, in which it loses the ability of penetrating tissues and remains a lumen parasite.

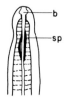

Fig. 350.—*Strongyloides stercoralis.* Anterior end of the parasitic male. (*After Faust*)

b, buccal chamber. sp, buccal spears.

The female (2·5 × 0·034 mm) (Fig. 351) tapers anteriorly and ends in a conical tail, The mouth has three small lips and leads to an oesophagus occupying a quarter of the length of the body. The vulva lies in the posterior third. There is a prominent uterus containing 50 eggs (50–58 × 30–34 μm) which are laid in the lumen of the bowel in an advanced stage of development and may occasionally be found in the faeces. They hatch immediately to embryos (0·2–0·3 × 0·013 mm), which have a double-bulb oesophagus,

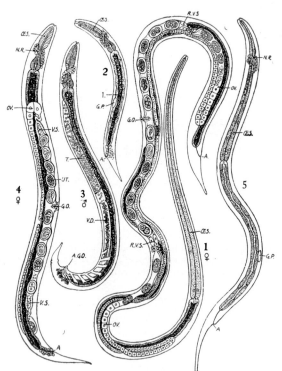

Fig. 351.—The life history of *Strongyloides stercoralis.* 1, Parasitic female. 2, Rhabditoid embryo. 3, Fully grown male. 4, Fully grown female. 5, Fully developed filariform larva. × 30. (*After Looss*)

A, anus. A.G.O., combined anus and genital pore. G.O., genital opening. G.P., primitive genital organs. I, intestine. N.R., nerve ring. OES., oesophagus. OV., ovary. R.V.S., rudimentary vesicula seminalis. T., testes. UT., uterus. V.D., vas deferens. V.S., vesicula seminalis.

apt to be confused with the rhabditiform stage of *Ancylostoma* and *Necator* (Figs 351, 352). They are passed active in faeces, and in 3–5 days are converted into free-living male and female forms, both of which have a rhabditiform, double-bulb muscular oesophagus. The male is a free-living form (0·7 × 0·035 mm) (Fig. 351), with the tail curved ventrally, 2 spicules and an accessory piece. The free-living form of the

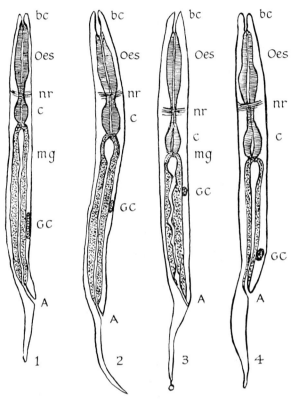

Fig. 352.—Distinguishing features of nematode larva in the faeces. 1, *Strongyloides stercoralis*. 2, *Ancylostoma duodenale*. 3, *Trichostrongylus colubriformis*. 4, *Rhabditis hominis*.

A, anus. b.c., buccal cavity. Oes, oesophagus. C, cardiac oesophageal bulb. mg, midgut. GC, genital cells. nr, nerve ring.

Characters	Strongyloides	Ancylostoma	Trichostrongylus	Rhabditis
Average size	225 × 16 μm	275 × 17 μm	275 × 16 μm	240 × 12 μm
Posterior tip	Blunt	Sharp	Sharp with bead-like swelling	Sharp
Buccal chamber	Shorter than width at tip of head	Longer than width at tip of head	Longer than width at tip of head	Longer than width at tip of head
Genital primordia	Fairly large	Small	Very small	Very small

female measures 1 × 0·05 mm. The vulva lies behind the middle of the body. The uterus contains thin-shelled eggs, measuring 70 × 40 μm (Fig. 351).

Copulation between the sexes takes place in faeces. The rhabditoid larvae produced are indistinguishable from those derived from the parasitic female. After 3–4 days they develop into host-feeding, mature filariform larvae, which are the infective stage, and re-enter the definitive host *via* the skin or buccal mucosa, as in *Ancylostoma* or *Necator*, but may remain alive in the soil for many weeks. The distinguishing feature is that the oesophagus in filariform larvae is half the length of the body (Fig. 351, 5); in *Ancylostoma* and *Necator* it occupies about a quarter. Filariform larvae find their way into the small intestine and develop into female parasitic forms. Under unsuitable climatic conditions, the sexual phase in the faeces may be omitted, and rhabditiform embryos produced by the parasitic female may develop directly into filariform larvae capable of infecting the definitive host. (Fig. 351, 5). The larvae of *S. stercoralis* may be confused with those of *Rhabditis hominis*, a free-living worm which may gain entry by accident to the digestive tract of man. These larvae measure 240–360 μm in length by 12 μm in diameter and resemble the parent worm in shape and structure of the oesophagus (Fig. 352, 4).

Life history

There are 2 stages: parasitic and free-living in soil (Fig. 99, page 270).

The parasitic stage

1. *Filariform* (infective) larvae from infective soil penetrate exposed skin or the mouth.

2. They may travel to the lungs via the intestine, and copulate as male and female.

Filariform larvae enter man by penetrating the skin or through the mouth, and migrate through the lungs to the oesophagus; on arrival in the pulmonary capillaries the larvae produce haemorrhages which form the avenue of escape into the alveoli; followed by cellular infiltration into the respiratory passages with output of eosinophil cells. The changes result in strongyloides pneumonitis. These develop in 2 weeks.

3. Females, with or without males, enter the mucosa (especially of the duodenum) and lay eggs.

4. Eggs hatch and larvae escape into the intestine. They may either

    a. Pass down and be evacuated, or

    b. Become filariform larvae (infective) and re-enter the mucosa or perianal skin (autoinfection) and pass to the organs (e.g. lungs).

Free-living stage

Larvae from faeces in soil are either rhabditoid or filariform (infective). Rhabditoid larvae can either become filariform and invade exposed skin or become male and female and produce rhabditoid larvae which continue the cycle indefinitely.

For the pathogenesis and treatment, see page 269.

Strongyloides fülleborni, a parasite of the monkey, chimpanzee and African baboon and recovered by Wallace and colleagues from an American soldier in the S.W. Pacific, is identified by prominent vulvar lips and narrowing behind the vulva in the free-living females. The prominent oesophagus in the free-living stages is also characteristic.

SUPERFAMILY: OXYUROIDEA
GENUS: *Enterobius*
Enterobius vermicularis (Linn., 1758), threadworm or pinworm

Synonym: *Oxyuris vermicularis*.

Characters

This is the only nematode of man with a double-bulb oesophagus in the adult. It is small and white, its mouth surrounded by a cuticular expansion, and its skin transversely striated. The male is seldom seen, and does not migrate like the female. Much smaller than the female (2·5 mm), its posterior third is curved spirally, and its caudal extremity blunt, with 6 sensory papillae and a single spicule, 70 μm (Fig. 353). The female (9–12 mm) has a long pointed tail, the anus 2 mm from the posterior extremity, and a transverse, slit-like vulva in the anterior fourth of the body (Fig. 353). The gravid female lays eggs in a stream of 10 000–15 000 in a few minutes and dies when egg-laying is completed.

The egg (50–54 × 20–27 μm) has a characteristic shape, flattened on one side, and is almost colourless, with a bean-shaped double-contour shell, which contains a more or less fully-formed embryo (Plate XIII).

Life history

There is no multiplication of worms inside the body. The egg-shell is weakened by the intestinal juices and the larva breaks out of the shell. Soon afterwards it invades the glandular crypts and penetrates into the glands and stroma, where it coils up, causing some liquefaction of the tissues, but no cellular reaction.

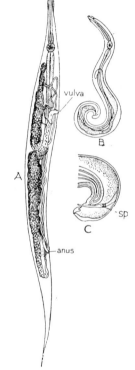

Fig. 353.—*Enterobius vermicularis*. A, Female. B, Male. C, Caudal extremity of male. × 12. (*After Leuckart*)

According to Schüffner the length of life of *E. vermicularis* ranges from 37–93 days. As soon as the ovary becomes packed with eggs the female worm looses her hold on the intestinal wall and lies passive in the faecal stream. The fertilized female migrates out of the anus to deposit her eggs in the perianal skin and perineum. The crawling of the gravid females produces intense pruritus. After few hours the embryo develops rapidly and attains a length of 140–150 μm. The egg is ingested, generally as a result of deposits of faeces under the finger nails, conveyed to the mouth, and hatches in the digestive juices. Liberated larvae after 2 moults pass from the small into the large intestine, where they become mature. The whole cycle takes 2–4 weeks. Eggs can be inhaled through the nose from infected garments at some distance (Lentze), and embryonated eggs have been found in dust. Damp conditions with minimal ventilation are necessary for survival. The eggs require a 6-hour exposure to air before they can hatch.

SUPERFAMILY: TRICHINELLOIDEA
GENUS: *Trichuris*
Trichuris trichiura (Linn., 1771)

Synonym: *Trichocephalus dispar*, whipworm.

Characters

The male (30–45 mm) has an anterior attenuated portion, containing the cellular oesophagus, which is half as long again as the thicker posterior portion. The caudal extremity is curved ventrally through 360 degrees and there is a single spicule in the sheath, studded with spines (Fig. 354).

The female (30–50 mm) has an anterior attenuated portion, twice as long as the posterior half, which is occupied by a stout uterus, tightly packed with eggs. A sacculate tubular ovary runs forward from the posterior end for over half the thick part of the body. Females preponderate over males in a proportion of over 400 to 1.

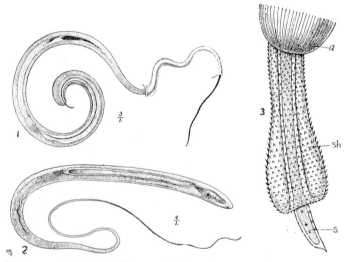

Fig. 354.—*Trichuris trichiura*. 1, Male partly embedded in the mucous membrane of the intestine. 2, Female. 3, Copulatory apparatus, greatly magnified. × 3. (*After Brumpt*)

a, posterior extremity of body. *s*, spicule. *sh*, sheath.

The egg (50 × 22 μm; Plate XIII) is brown and has a characteristic barrel shape, and a single shell with a plug at each end. It contains an unsegmented embryo.

The worm is greyish-white or slightly pink and lives in the caecum, where it maintains its position by transfixing a superficial fold of mucous membrane with its slender neck, and lying embedded in mucus between the intestinal villi.

Life history

Infection is spread chiefly by stale faeces. The egg is unsegmented; embryonation takes at least 21 days. It can withstand a low temperature owing to its thick shell. Moisture is necessary and it cannot withstand desiccation. Development is direct. The embryo hatches only when the egg is swallowed: the egg-shell is digested by the intestinal juices, the larva emerges in the small intestine, penetrates the villi where it develops for a week, re-entering the lumen. It then passes to the caecum or large intestine, where it attaches itself to the mucosa and becomes adult.

Trichuris suis of the pig, whose eggs are indistinguishable from those of *T. trichiura*, has been transmitted to man in an experiment in which 1000 infective eggs were swallowed. The volunteer had no symptoms, but eggs appeared in the faeces in about 60 days, and continued to be excreted for at least 10 weeks after maturation. *T. suis* may therefore be a cause of trichuriasis in man, especially if in contact with pigs (Beer 1971).

For clinical features and treatment, see page 272.

GENUS: *Capillaria*

Capillaria hepatica (Bancroft, 1893)

Synonyms: *Trichocephalus hepaticus; Hepaticola hepatica*

The adult worms are very similar to *Trichuris* but are much smaller and more delicate. It is normally a parasite of the liver of the rat where the eggs are deposited in masses. The eggs resemble those of *T. trichiura* but have an outer shell distinctly pitted and measuring 51–67·5 × 30–35 μm. It has a direct life cycle like that of *Trichuris*. For clinical features and treatment, see page 275.

Capillaria philippinensis

The adult worms resemble *C. hepatica*. The male worms measure 2·1–3·7 mm in length and the female 2·6–4·9 mm. The eggs measure 45·5 × 21 μm and are of 2 types: 'typical', with thick walls, and 'atypical', with thin-walled embryonated eggs resembling *Strongyloides* ova.

For clinical features and treatment, see page 275.

GENUS: *Trichinella*

Trichinella spiralis (Owen, 1835)

Morphology

Trichinella spiralis (Fig. 355) is a white worm just visible to the naked eye which inhabits the small intestine. The male (1·6 × 0·04 mm) has a cloaca situated posteriorly between two caudal appendages and 2 pairs of papillae. The female (3–4 × 0·06 mm) has a vulva in the anterior fifth, an ovary in the posterior half and an anterior portion occupied by a coiled uterine tube. The anus is terminal. Normally the female lives for 30 days and produces 1500 or more larvae which measure 100 × 6 μm.

The egg (20 μm in diameter) lies in the upper uterus but the embryo soon breaks out from the shell and lives free in the uterine cavity.

The larvae are shed mainly into the lymphatics and blood stream, reaching all parts of the body and encysting.

The cyst is formed by a larva encapsulated by the host tissues. The capsule is an adventitious ellipsoidal sheath with blunt ends which results from round cell and eosinophilic infiltration round the tightly coiled larva (Fig. 356). The long axis parallels that of the muscle fibres. Host amino acids can be transferred into the cyst and converted into larval protein so that an encysted larva remains viable for many years.

Life history

When consumed by a carnivorous host the cysts are digested in the stomach and, after excysting, the larvae invade the duodenal and jejunal mucosa and develop through 4 ecdyses into adult males and females, which then enter the lumen of the bowel. Later they re-enter the mucosa and penetrate the villi, even reaching the mesenteric glands. Larviposition takes place over a period of from 4 to 16 weeks or more. The larvae are carried through the right heart and lungs to the arterial circulation which they reach between the ninth and thirteenth day finally reaching the striated muscles where they encyst.

For clinical features and treatment see page 264.

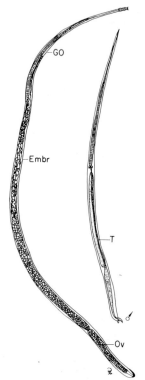

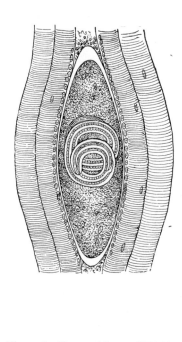

Fig. 355.—Female and male *Trichinella spiralis.* × 45. (*After Brumpt*)
Embr., embryos. *G.O.*, genital opening. *Ov.*,
ovary. *T.*, testes.

Fig. 356.—Encysted larva of *Trichinella spiralis,* 15 days after entering
muscle. × 300. (*After Claus*)

FILARIOIDEA

SUPERFAMILY: FILARIOIDEA

This group includes spirurate filiform nematodes adapted to inhabit the deeper
tissues, such as the circulatory, lymphatic and connective tissue layers. Some insect
intermediary is necessary to complete their development.

GENUS: *Wuchereria*

Wuchereria bancrofti (Cobbold, 1877) Seurat, 1921

Synonym: *Filaria bancrofti* (Cobbold, 1877)

Characters

It is a thread-like white worm found in lymphatic vessels and glands. The sexes are
coiled together, and can be separated with difficulty (Fig. 357). Buckley has shown
that the cuticle is adorned with small cuticular bosses.

The male (4 cm × 0·1 mm) is coiled, with a corkscrew-like tail and 2 spicules,
the larger of which measures 500 μm. The smaller (300 μm) is grooved on its ventral
aspect. There is a short, thick proximal and a whip-like distal portion ending in a hook,
and 15 pairs of minute sensory caudal papillae. A saddle-shaped thickening of the

cuticle on the posterior wall of the cloaca forms a shield, and there is an accessory piece peculiar to *W. bancrofti* (Fig. 357). There are 12 pairs of circumanal papillae, of which 8 are preanal and 4 postanal in position. There are also 2 pairs of large sessile papillae, and at the tail a solitary pair of minute size. The female (6·5–10 cm × 0·2–0·28 mm) has a tapering anterior end with a rounded swelling. There are sessile papillae on the head and an oral aperture leading to a cylindrical oesophagus. The mid-intestinal tube is one-third to one-fifth of the total diameter and opens into the rectum posteriorly. The caudal extremity is narrow and abruptly rounded (Fig. 357). The vulva is 0·8 mm behind the anterior extremity. A swollen vagina (0·25 mm in length) leads into the uterus, which divides into 2 tubuli, which are much coiled, occupying the greater portion of the body with a diameter three times that of the mid-intestine (Fig. 358). Two ovaries and ducts extend to within 1 mm of the tail.

The eggs lie in the upper uterus enclosed in a chorionic membrane which becomes a sheath to the living embryos (microfilariae) (Fig. 359). They are emitted by the viviparous female and travel via the lymphatics into the blood stream, whence they are abstracted by various species of mosquito. Their size in the distal part of the uterus is 38 × 25 µm, but as they are pushed to the vagina they become more elongated. The microfilaria develops from an oval egg and measures at first 216 µm. The embryo often lies curled up in its shell which becomes lobed, resembling a Dutch twist or pretzel.

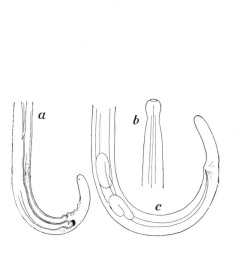

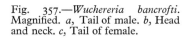

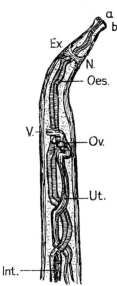

Fig. 357.—*Wuchereria bancrofti.* Magnified. *a,* Tail of male. *b,* Head and neck. *c,* Tail of female.

Fig. 358. Diagram of the head of *Wuchereria bancrofti,* female. × 50.

a, mouth. b, circomoral papillae. Ex, excretory pore. Int, intestine. N, nerve ring. Oes, oesophagus. Ov, oviduct. Ut, uterus. V, vulva.

Examined in the living state with a low power the embryo (microfilaria), 280 × 7 µm, appears structureless. With higher magnifications the entire embryo is seen to be enclosed in a sheath (structureless sac), which is longer than the enclosed embryo, so that this can move backwards and forwards, and the collapsed portion trails after the head or tail. The sheath has been the subject of controversy. It is generally held to be the outstretched vitelline membrane, but in the microfilariae of *Litomosoides carinii* of the cotton rat it has been found that a true larval sheath is developed during its sojourn in the blood. In the middle third is some granular material, or primitive gut (*Innenkörper*). There is transverse striation of the muscular layer throughout. At one-seventh of the length from the head there is a break which denotes the nerve ring (n.r.) and one-fifth of the length there is a triangular V-shaped patch, demonstrated by light staining with dilute haematoxylin, known as 'anterior V-spot', or the excretory pore and excretory cell (e.p. and e.c.). A short distance from the tail a second pore represents the anus, cloaca or terminal part of the primitive alimentary canal, and is known as the 'posterior V-spot'. Deeply staining cells are known as genital cells (g.c.). When stained, the body of the embryo is seen to be composed of closely packed cells, and by focusing, when the movements of the living microfilaria have subsided, the head appears to be covered by a delicate prepuce. A short fang is from time to time shot out from the uncovered cephalic end and suddenly retracted (Fig. 362, page 1042).

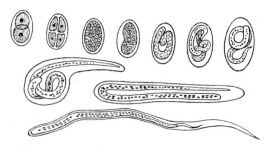

Fig. 359.—Evolution of sheathed microfilaria from ovum in the uterus of the parent worm. The later stages may occasionally take place after emission from the vagina. (*After Penel*)

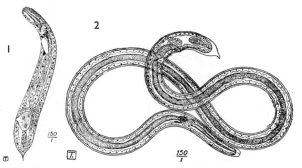

Fig. 360.—Stages of the larval forms of *Wuchereria bancrofti* from the thoracic muscles of *Culex fatigans*. × 150. (*After Looss*)

Microfilariae pass with difficulty through the peripheral capillaries and they are less active in day than in night blood. They are capable of movement and of transit from place to place.

Microfilaria vauceli. The microfilaria of *W. bancrofti* var. *vauceli* is described by Galliard from the west coast of Madagascar. It differs in its smaller length 250 μm, in the larger excretory pore and cells, in the disposition and size of the genital cells, which are larger, and in the larger anal pore. The 'inner body' is granular. The attitude lacks the graceful curves of *W. bancrofti*. In certain respects it is intermediate between it and *Brugia malayi*, but differs in the absence of the 2 terminal nuclei in the tail and in the shorter cephalic space. It exhibits nocturnal periodicity.

Timor microfilaria (David & Edeson, 1965). This microfilaria was discovered in Timor. It is close to *Brugia* species, which it resembles in general morphology, but is distinguished by a sheath which does not stain bright pink with Giemsa as does that of

B. malayi. In periodicity and symptomatology it resembles *Wuchereria bancrofti.* There is no animal reservoir and the vector is unknown.

Periodicity

Microfilariae of *W. bancrofti* exhibit a nocturnal periodicity in certain parts of the world, in West Indies, South America, North, West and East Africa, China, Indonesia, New Guinea and Melanesia, i.e. they are present in peripheral blood in larger numbers during the night than during the day. The maximum concentration is from 10 p.m. to 2 a.m. It appeared to Manson that this nocturnal periodicity was an adaptation to the habits of night-biting mosquitoes—*Culex fatigans, C. pipiens* and certain Anophelines— but the mechanism has never been satisfactorily explained. The numbers of the microfilariae are influenced by sleeping, and respond to waking and bodily activity. By reversing the hours of sleeping and waking the periodicity is disturbed for 3

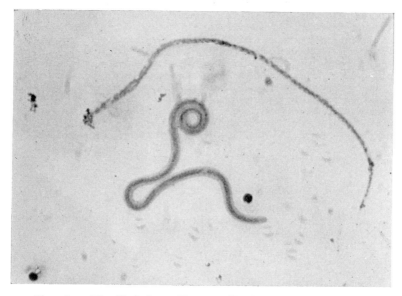

Fig. 361.—*Microfilaria bancrofti* var. *pacifica* in hydrocoele fluid. The embryo on the right has escaped from its sheath.

days and then reversed to diurnal periodicity. Observations on microfilariae of animals (*Dirofilaria repens* of dog, filaria of American crow and that of Malayan monkey, *Macaca speciosa*) show that they also maintain nocturnal periodicity and reversal is easily established. Periodicity is probably a quality inherent in the microfilaria itself and persists unchanged in transfused blood. This was demonstrated in a patient injected with blood containing microfilariae, and in whom a nocturnal periodicity was maintained for 14 days.

Many years ago Manson had an opportunity of ascertaining that, during their diurnal absence from the peripheral circulation, the microfilariae retire principally to the larger arteries and to the lungs where, during the day-time, they may be found in enormous numbers.

Considerable light has been shed upon the mechanism of periodicity in general by the discovery of Hawking and Thurston of a non-sheathed microfilaria in a monkey (*Macaca speciosa*). In the animal, as in man, the curve of microfilarial density in the venous blood follows closely that of the capillary blood. They have shown that an increase of microfilariae in the blood at night is due to the periodic liberation from accumulations in the small blood vessels of the lungs.

McFadzean and Hawking (1956) proved that the microfilariae of *W. bancrofti* are affected by the oxygen concentration in inspired air and by muscular exercise. The periodicity of *W. bancrofti* and *B. malayi* may depend on changes in the difference of oxygen tension between venous and arterial blood by day and night. During the day-time the microfilariae accumulate in the lungs where the oxygen tension is high. They manage to hold themselves in the pulmonary capillaries by some force which is increased by the rise in the oxygen tension and decreased by its fall. This force seems to be switched on and off every 12 hours by some unknown mysterious mechanism inside the microfilariae (Hawking 1954). A curious agglutinative phenomenon has been described by the injection of anticoagulant (heparin) to the drawn blood. Intravenous injection of this substance during day-time releases microfilariae of *W. bancrofti* into the peripheral blood for a short period. It is presumed that microfilariae gather together in the capillaries and other vessels of the lung during their absence from the peripheral blood by the power of agglutination and thigmotaxis.

A general anaesthetic does not affect the periodicity of *W. bancrofti* but markedly reduces the numbers of *L. loa* microfilariae in the peripheral blood (Hawking 1956).

Formerly it was thought that nocturnal periodicity was uniformly observed by the microfilariae of *W. bancrofti* the world over, but in 1896 Surgeon-Commander Thorpe remarked that in Tonga and Fiji the microfilariae were abundant in the blood both by day and by night; those in the W. Pacific, the Solomon Islands, New Guinea and Bismarck Archipelago are nocturnally periodic, but in New Caledonia the microfilariae are non-periodic. As shown by Buxton, the demarcating line between the two lies in longitude 170°E and this also coincides with the distribution of malaria. On the west of this line there are *Anopheles* and malaria, on the east there is neither. It was originally

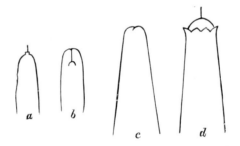

Fig. 362.—Structure of the head end of *Microfilaria perstans* (*a*, *b*) and of *Microfilaria bancrofti* (*c*, *d*).

demonstrated that in Indian and Solomon Island immigrants in Fiji these microfilariae maintain their nocturnal periodicity amongst the non-periodic Fijians, but, if they and the Europeans also, contract the infection in Fiji, the microfilariae are non-periodic. An attempt was made to explain this anomaly by the day-biting habits of the mosquito intermediaries, *Aedes s. pseudoscutellaris* and *Ae. s. polynesiensis* which have a regional distribution in the Pacific corresponding to that of the non-periodic filariae. As the microfilariae remain true to type after transfusion it was suggested that they are the progeny of a parent distinct from *W. bancrofti*; this has been named *W. bancrofti* var. *pacifica*. The microfilariae of both varieties are morphologically indistinguishable. The non-periodic Pacific type in Fiji differs from that of periodic African *W. bancrofti* in that increased oxygen content of the blood brings about a *slight rise* of the microfilarial counts.

Periodicity is a biological rhythm inherent in the microfilariae but influenced by the rhythm of the host, which itself is influenced by the changes in body temperature which occur every 24 hours.

The two forms of *B. malayi* from Malaysia exhibit different periodicities which correspond with the biting habits of their chief vectors. Therefore attempts have been made to see whether it is possible to change periodicity by feeding mosquitoes by day on a nocturnal periodic infection and transmitting the few filarial larvae which develop in them to experimental animals. Thus when a human infection was transmitted to a cat it was found that the nocturnally periodic microfilariae became semi-periodic.

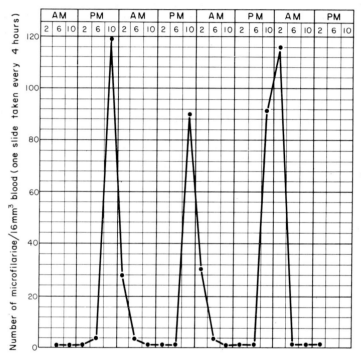

Fig. 363.—Filariasis (*Wuchereria bancrofti*, *Microfilaria nocturna*). Showing the nocturnal periodicity.

Life history

The life history was first worked out by Manson in *Culex fatigans* in China in 1878. Within one hour of entering the mosquito's stomach, the microfilariae cast the sheaths and bore through the stomach wall. At the end of an infective feed the embryos collect at the anterior end of the stomach and then enter the anterior cylindrical portion of the midgut. Forward transportation is effected by reversed peristalsis until they are distributed over the whole of this cylinder. At the end of 16 hours they form a writhing mass behind the valve which prevents their progress into the foregut. The proboscis of the mosquito exerts positive chemotaxis upon microfilariae. Therefore *Culex fatigans* or *C. pipiens* can abstract more embryos than would be present in a similar quantity of circulating blood. The mosquito abstracts 1 mm³ of blood at each feed and, in so doing, concentrates the embryos ten-fold. They next enter the thorax, where they lie between the muscular fibres (Fig. 365). Within 2 days they increase in girth, the 'posterior V-spot' (or anal pore) enlarges, and the excretory vesicle becomes more prominent. By rapid nuclear proliferation the larval filaria now assumes a squat 'sausage' form (Fig. 360, 1), the tail shrinks and is then absorbed. Mouth and oesophagus are apparent from the fifth day onwards. According to Iyengar the Gc.2 and Gc.3

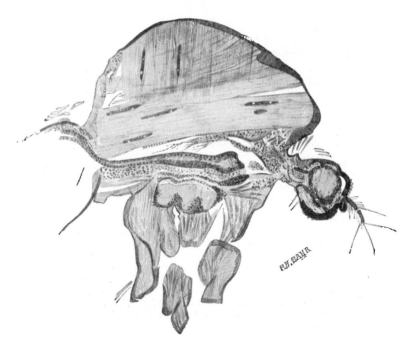

cells (Fig. 370) divide several times and give rise to a column of cells which form the mid-intestine (large gut). The posterior intestine (rectum) is formed from 4 cells derived from] the Gc.4 cell. The genital primordium is formed from the Gc.1 cell.

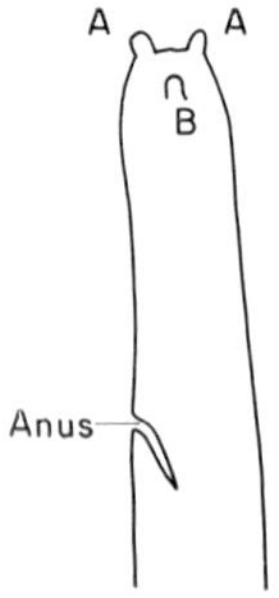

When the larva is 0·5 mm in length, a bulbar oesophagus appears at the first and second fourths of the alimentary canal. Now, elongated and worm-like, the larva moves sluggishly about. Three caudal papillae develop which function in progression and facilitate penetration of human skin (Fig. 364). About the tenth day (in favourable circumstances) the larval filaria, 1·4 mm long, travels forward into the head of the mosquito,

Fig. 364.—Larval filaria from the proboscis sheath of *Aedes scutellaris pseudoscutellaris.*

A, terminal. B, postanal papillae. Length 1·4 × 0·018 mm.

where it coils up and enters the proboscis sheath, but occasionally it may penetrate into the abdominal cavity and legs. Two or more ecdyses take place. At high temperatures and in moisture the complete cycle occupies 10 to 14 days, but it is retarded to 6 weeks by cold. Sometimes the larvae die in the thoracic muscles and are enclosed in chitin, producing a curious mummy-like structure (Fig. 369, page 1046). When an infected mosquito bites man, the larvae, attracted by warmth, break through the terminal portion of the proboscis sheath at the ligula at the central point of 'Dutton's membrane', wriggle out on to the skin, which they penetrate near the seat of

Fig. 365.—Section of the thoracic muscles of *Aedes scutellaris pseudoscutellaris,* the second day after feeding on the filariated patient.

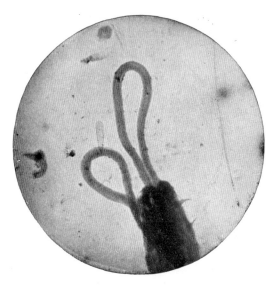

Fig. 366.—Larval *Wuchereria bancrofti* var. *pacifica* emerging from the proboscis of *Aedes s. pseudoscutellaris.*

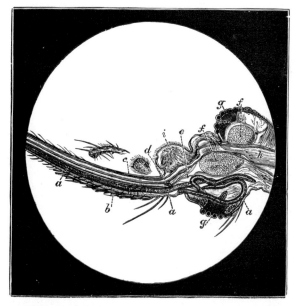

Fig. 367.—*Wuchereria bancrofti* in the head and proboscis of the mosquito. (*G. C. Low*)

a, filariae. *b,* labium. *c,* labrum. *d,* base of hypopharynx. *e,* duct of venenosalivary gland. *f,* cephalic ganglia. *g,* eye. *i,* pharyngeal muscle.

the puncture caused by the stylets of the mosquito (Fig. 366). Complete development of *W. bancrofti* has been observed in the species of mosquitoes listed on page 197.

Some 22 species are known in which partial development may occur.

In the human host the infective larvae pass through the peripheral blood vessels to the lymphatics where they become mature in an estimated period of 3 months to 1 year. Man is the only known definitive host.

In view of the fact that considerable confusion has been caused in recent years by the discovery of larval filariae in wild-caught mosquitoes, in the course of surveys upon the natural infection rate, it has become necessary to differentiate between the larval

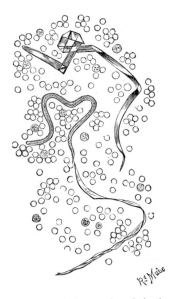

Fig. 368.—Microfilariae casting their sheaths.

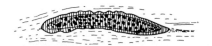

Fig. 369.—Chitinized larval filaria in the thorax of a mosquito.

characters of human and allied species of animal origin. It has to be realized that the filariae of some animals, fruit bats and birds develop in those species of mosquitoes which normally transmit human filariasis.

The infective larva of *B. malayi* is 1–2 mm in length and has 3 poorly defined caudal papillae; that of *B. patei* is about the same length and has a marked dorsal protuberance resembling a dog's head, in lateral position. The larva of *Dirofilaria corynodes* of monkeys (*Cercopithecus* and *Colobus*) from *Aedes pembaensis* has the typical cigar-shaped tail but less pronounced narrowing between the anus and the extremity, with three small papillae. The larva of *D. repens* of the dog and cat resembles the foregoing, but with only one terminal papilla: it develops in *Aedes aegypti*, *Ae. pembaensis* and *Mansonia africanus*; that of *D. immitis* of the dog, from *Ae. aegypti* and *Culex fatigans*, cannot be distinguished from that of *D. repens*. The larva of *Setaria equina* of the horse, mule and donkey in *Ae. aegypti*, *Ae. pembaensis* and *Culex fatigans* is about the same length, but can easily be distinguished by one large terminal papilla and two subterminal ones, looking like little ears. Distinguishing features are illustrated in a key by Nelson (1959).

Wuchereria bancrofti var. *pacifica* (Manson-Bahr, 1941)

It has been suggested that the filaria found in Central and Southern Pacific might be a separate species. As far as can be ascertained, embryos (microfilariae) are morphologically identical with those of *W. bancrofti*. Certain small differences have been noted in the morphology. The average length is smaller—females 58 mm, males 27 mm. The tail of the female lacks the bulbous swelling which characterizes those from British Guiana. The anterior end of the Fijian specimens is oval in outline.

Microfilariae in Polynesians (Fiji, Samoa, Tonga, Cook Islands, New Caledonia) are non-periodic. In these islands as well as in Tokelau, Wallis, Ellice, Gilberts, Marquesas and those beyond 'Buxton's line' (longitude 170° E) they do not exhibit nocturnal periodicity, but occur in equal numbers in the blood by day and night. Development of this filaria is confined to mosquitoes indigenous to the S. Pacific Islands, *Ae. scutellaris pseudoscutellaris* and *Ae. s. polynesiensis*, in both of which maximum development occurs. A third species, *Ae. fijiensis*, has also been incriminated. The non-periodic microfilaria does not develop readily in *C. fatigans*, which is the optimum host for the nocturnal periodic *W. bancrofti*. *Ae. s. pseudoscutellaris* and *Ae. s. polynesiensis* are adapted to the coconut palm and have peculiar habitats; they bite by day. In New Caledonia the vector of the non-periodic form is *Ae. vigilax*, a species which is also found in N. Australia and Queensland.

GENUS: *Brugia* (Buckley, 1959)

The genus *Brugia* contains 8 representatives: *B. malayi*, *B. pahangi*, *B. patei*, *B. beaveri*, *B. buckleyi*, *B. ceylonensis*, *B. guyanensis* and *B. tupiaz* (Fig. 371).

Brugia malayi (Brug, 1927; Rao & Maplestone, 1940)

Distribution

This is the common form in Malaysia, Indonesia, Timor, Central India, Ceylon, South China, Korea, Indo-China and Koshima Island (Japan). It has not been found in Africa, America, Australia or the Pacific Islands.

Characters

The adults are practically identical with *W. bancrofti* in nearly all characters; the females are indistinguishable. The female measures 55 mm in length by 160 μm. The vulva is situated 0·92 mm from the anterior extremity. The caudal end is bluntly rounded. The male is 22–23 mm in length by 88 μm in diameter. The posterior extremity has about 3 turns and the anus is 0·1–0·14 mm from the tip of the tail. One pair of large papillae are just in front of the cloaca and 1 behind. There are also 2 smaller pairs. There is a small naviculate gubernaculum and 2 spicules which are unlike in size and structure. The longer is 0·34–0·36 mm: the shorter 0·11–0·12 mm in length. There are morphological differences in the microfilariae and the mosquito intermediary is distinct—*Mansonia annulifera*. Poynton proved that it is identical with the microfilaria of the 'kra' monkey (*Macaca irus*) which is transmitted by the same mosquitoes. It is common in domestic dogs and cats in Malaysia and has been found also in the slow loris (*Nycticebus coucang*), the banded leaf monkey (*Presbytis melalophos*) as well as in the pangolin (*Manis javanica*).

The microfilaria of *B. malayi* was first discovered by Lichtenstein in Celebes, and was studied further by Brug in 1927. Brug and de Rook found natural infection in the mosquitoes, *Mansonia longipalpis* (also known as *dives*) and *M. annulata*.

The animal representative of *B. malayi* is widespread. It has been found in cats in the island of Pate in N. Kenya, but not in humans, who are infected with *W. bancrofti*. Although the human form of *B. malayi* is common in dogs and cats in Malaysia, yet there is a species, *B. pahangi*, which is confined to these animals and which has distinctive morphological characters (Fig. 371).

The human form of *malayi* can be transmitted to cats by the bite of *Mansonia longipalpis*. The period of full development of the adult filaria in this animal varies from 81 to 96 days before microfilariae appear in the blood. The adult forms recovered from the cat correspond to the descriptions of *B. malayi* in man. *Malayi*-like microfilariae have been found in cats in Orissa, India, and dogs and genet cats in Pate Island,

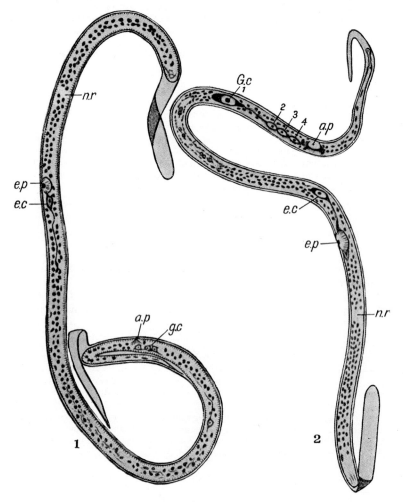

Fig. 370.—1, *Microfilaria bancrofti*, 2, *Microfilaria malayi*. (*After Feng*)

n.r., nerve ring. e.p., excretory pore. e.c., excretory cell. G.c. 1–4, genital cells. a.p., anal pore.

Kenya. The nocturnal periodic form in Malaysia does not develop well in cats and is transmitted by species of *Anopheles* and *Mansonia*. A semi-periodic form occurs in man and commonly in cats, in fresh-water swamps and forest. It is transmitted by *Mansonia annulata* and *uniformis*.

Microfilaria *malayi* has a nocturnal periodicity like that of *W. bancrofti*, or it may

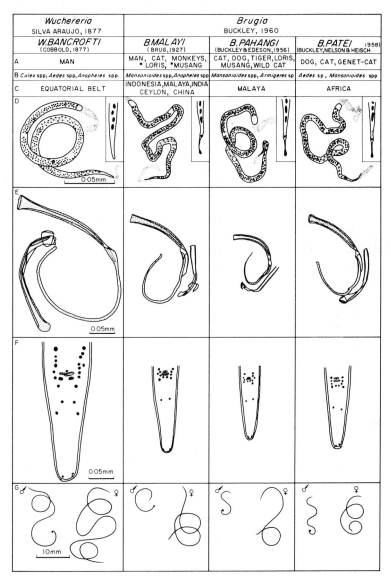

Wuchereria	Brugia		
SILVA ARAUJO, 1877	BUCKLEY, 1960		
W.BANCROFTI (COBBOLD, 1877)	**B.MALAYI** (BRUG,1927)	**B.PAHANGI** (BUCKLEY & EDESON,1956)	**B.PATEI** 1958) (BUCKLEY,NELSON & HEISCH)
A MAN	MAN, CAT, MONKEYS, * LORIS, *MUSANG	CAT, DOG, TIGER,LORIS, MUSANG, WILD CAT	DOG, CAT, GENET-CAT
B *Culex* spp,*Aedes* spp,*Anopheles* spp.	*Mansonioides* spp,*Anopheles* spp	*Mansonioides* spp, *Armigeres* sp	*Aedes* sp , *Mansonioides* spp
C EQUATORIAL BELT	INDONESIA,MALAYA,INDIA CEYLON, CHINA	MALAYA	AFRICA

Fig. 371.—The morphological distinctions between the genera *Wuchereria* and *Brugia*. (*After Buckley; by permission of Annals of Tropical Medicine and Parasitology*)

A, Definitive hosts. B, Intermediate hosts. C, Geographical distribution. D, Microfilariae and (inset) tail nuclei of microfilariae. E, Spicules of male, lateral view. F, Tails of males, ventral view. G, Adult worms, actual size. * indicates an experimental infection only.

be semi-periodic. It is nocturnal on the west coast of the Malaysia peninsula but non-periodic in the Huantan district on the east coast. It measures 200–250 × 5–6 μm. Its chief points of distinction are the elongated nucleus at the tip of the tail and the absence of nuclei in the cephalic space. (Fig. 370, 2).

Table 47 summarizes the main points of distinction between microfilaria *malayi* and microfilaria *bancrofti*.

Table 47. Differentiation between *Microfilaria malayi* and *Microfilaria bancrofti*

Microfilaria malayi	*Microfilaria bancrofti*
It is often found closely folded with head close to tail, and is irregularly disposed for, besides major curves, minor angulations are typical	Usually seen lying with head and tail well separated, and commonly shows 3 or 4 major curves of graceful appearance
The nuclei are blurred and inter-mingled so that they cannot be easily counted	The nuclei are well defined and spaced and can be easily counted
The tail tapers to a fine point, continued as a fine thread. There is *typically* 1 nucleus at the extremity of the tapered portion and 2 in the terminal thread	The tail tapers to a point and the terminal portion contains no nuclei
The cephalic space is twice as long as broad	The cephalic space is as long as it is broad
The excretory pore and cell are separated	The excretory pore and cell are close together and a thread of proto-plasm runs posteriorly from the latter
The anal pore is clear space about 40 μm from the tail end	

Life history

The most favoured mosquito intermediaries belong to the genus *Mansonia* which are crepuscular or nocturnal feeders. Development in the mosquito is similar to that of *W. bancrofti*, but more rapid, in 6–8½ days. Difficulties have been encountered in Malaysia in distinguishing larval forms of ornithofilariae of birds from those of human *W. malayi* in the routine dissection of mosquitoes.

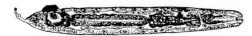

Fig. 372.—Development stage of *Brugia malayi*, showing the terminal nucleus in the tail. (*After Feng*)

The larval forms of *B. malayi* in *Mansonia* undergo 2 ecdyses. The buccal cavity is formed from the cephalic space; the oesophagus from the nuclei of the anterior part of the nuclear column; the rectum and anus from the 4 G cells of Rodenwaldt and the anal pore. The premature genital pore mass is derived from the nuclei of the *Innenkörper*, and the muscles of the body wall from the so-called 'subcuticular cells' of Rodenwaldt. The tail of the microfilaria, with its two nuclei, is shed with the first moult. As in the case of *W. bancrofti*, the larva, when in the thoracic muscles, feeds by absorbing food through the cuticle. It does not feed at the expense of these muscles as has been stated.

GENUS: *Dirofilaria*

Dirofilaria (Nochtiella) magalhaesi (Blanchard, 1896)

This filaria was discovered in Rio de Janeiro in 1887 in the left ventricle of the heart of a child. For a long time its classification and significance remained obscure. Then Faust and his colleagues reported a similar discovery in a Negress in New Orleans. The specimen was a solitary male closely allied to, if not identical with, the dog heart worm, *Dirofilaria immitis*, which is transmitted by *Culex fatigans*, *C. annulirostris*, *Aedes aegypti* and *Ae. polynesiensis* in the Pacific. This filaria may therefore sometimes occur as an accidental infection in man. The female is 155 mm; the male 83 mm in length. For clinical features see page 237.

GENUS: *Mansonella*

Mansonella ozzardi (Manson, 1897) Faust, 1929

Synonyms: *Filaria ozzardi; F. demarquayi*

Distribution

West Indies, South America, Peru, northern provinces of Argentina (20–30% infected). Common in St Vincent (West Indies) in aboriginal Indians (Caribs) of British Guiana, often together with *Dipetalonema perstans*. It was originally discovered by Manson in the blood of Carib Indians, and is now considered identical with *F. demarquayi*. The parental forms were discovered by Daniels in Demerara Indians and by Galgey in St Lucia.

Characters

The male, 3·2 cm, has a coiled tail and 1 spicule. The female (6·5–8·1 cm × 0·21–0·25 mm) has a vulva 0·76 mm from the anterior extremity, and an anus 0·23 mm from the tail. The caudal extremity has 2 prominent papillae with a terminal thickened cuticle. The worms live in body cavities, embedded in adipose tissues. The microfilaria (173–240 × 4–5 μm) is unsheathed and closely resembles that of *D. perstans*, but has a sharp tail (Fig. 61, page 194). Transfusion experiments, using 100 ml of blood containing 120 000 microfilariae, have determined that they can live in the blood of the recipient for more than 2 years.

Life history

This was worked out by Buckley in St Vincent, British West Indies (37·7% of the inhabitants infected). The intermediary insect is a midge, *Culicoides furens* (page 1103), a common pest; 27·5% experimentally infected contained larval forms of this filaria. The ingested microfilariae migrate within twenty-four hours to the thorax; developmental stages are similar to those of *D. perstans*. Two ecdyses occur; the largest (third stage) larvae in the head measure 0·7 mm. Emergence from proboscis takes place within 8 days. *C. paraensis* is possibly a vector in St Vincent: *C. furens* in Antigua. Development occurs in *Simulium amazonicum*, which may be a vector in Brazil. For clinical features see page 238.

GENUS: *Loa*

Loa loa (Guyot, 1778), eye worm

Characters

The body is filiform, cylindrical, whitish and semi-transparent, with numerous round, smooth, translucent protuberances of the cuticle, 12–16 μm in diameter, and

9–11 μm above the surface. These chitinous bosses are more numerous in females. Their distribution is irregular. In the male they are absent at the extremities; in the female they extend on the tail and also the cephalic end. The mouth is unarmed and destitute of papillae; there is no distinct neck, but a shoulder 0·15 mm from the mouth where there are 2 papillae, one dorsal, the other ventral. The alimentary canal commences at a funnel-shaped mouth as a slender straight oesophagus, going on to an intestine 65 μm wide, and a short attenuated rectum. The male (3–3·4 cm × 0·35–0·43 mm) has its maximum breadth anteriorly (Fig. 373); posteriorly it tapers to a tail, which is curved ventrally, with 2 lateral expansions of the cuticle (0·7 × 0·029 mm) (Fig. 375). In the middle, 0·08 mm from the tail-tip, is the opening of the anogenital orifice with 2 unequal spicules (123–176 μm and 88–113 μm) surrounded by thick labia. There are 4 large globular, pedunculated papillae, decreasing in size anteroposteriorly, and a fifth pair of small postanal papillae. The female (5–7 cm × 0·5 mm) has a straight, attenuated, broadly rounded posterior extremity and a vulva 2·5 mm from the anterior extremity placed on a small eminence. The vagina, 9 mm long, branches off into 2 long

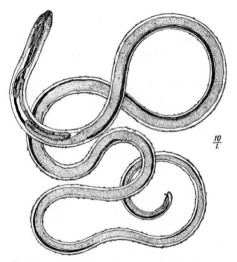

Fig. 373.—Male *Loa loa*. × 10. (*After Looss*)

uterine tubes extending through the length of the body. At the narrow end are the ovaries, with eggs in all stages (Figs 374, 375). Reproduction is ovoviviparous; the embryos develop within the egg envelope and uncoil themselves on expulsion from the vagina. When dead the adult worm often becomes cretified.

The embryo is known as microfilaria loa, or diurna, and is similar in size (298 × 7·5 μm) and structure to microfilaria bancrofti. In fresh blood it may be impossible to distinguish them. In dried stained films (1) it assumes a stiff angular attitude, (2) the tail end is disposed in a series of sharp flexures, giving it a corkscrew appearance, with the extreme tip flexed, (3) the nuclei of the central column of cells of microfilaria loa are larger and less deeply stained. (4) The cephalic end of the column is more abruptly terminated (Fig. 61, page 194). By special staining methods a large genital cell at the beginning of the posterior third constitutes a marked feature. Microfilaria loa takes up methylene blue (1 in 5000) in 10 minutes. In microfilaria bancrofti, absorption is much slower, but it shows up the excretory pore. Microfilaria loa may not be found in the peripheral blood until 6 or even 7 years have elapsed from the primary infection. It is strictly diurnal, from 8 a.m. to 8 p.m.—the reverse of microfilaria bancrofti. Inversion of periodicity takes place very gradually, as, for instance, when daily observations are made on a voyage round the world (Külz).

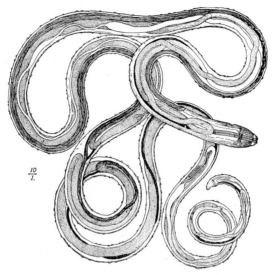

Fig. 374.—Female *Loa loa.* × 10. (*After Looss*)

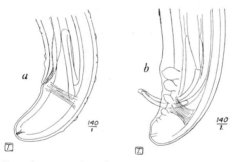

Fig. 375.—Posterior extremity of *Loa loa. a*, Female. *b*, Male. (*After Looss*)

Life history (Fig. 376)

This proceeds in much the same manner as in *W. bancrofti*, but in the thoracic muscles, connective tissue and fat-body (Stevenson) of the bloodsucking 'mangrove flies', *Chrysops silacea*, *C. dimidiata*. The simian *Loa*, which is indistinguishable from the human form, undergoes similar development in *C. langi* and *C. centurionis*. On entering the stomach the embryo casts its sheath in 3 hours, and, piercing the stomach wall, enters the thoracic muscles and fat-body of the thorax, but principally that of the abdomen. Development is complete in 10 days. In 3 days it becomes broad and torpedo-shaped; on the fourth and fifth days the squat form is lengthened to 0·8–1 mm; on the sixth, the corkscrew-like appearance is replaced by gentle curves. Then occurs the first ecdysis, and the sharp tail is replaced by a rounded trilobed extremity. By the tenth day it measures 2 × 0·025 mm and 3 ecdyses have occurred. Larvae congregate in the head in large numbers, the majority at the root of the proboscis, and make their way on to the skin of the human host by piercing the proboscis sheath when the fly feeds (Fig. 377). It is capable of carrying infection for

5 days. In Calabar 3·5% of wild-caught chrysops are found naturally infected with *Loa loa*. When an infected fly feeds, large numbers of infective larvae emerge and are deposited on the surface of the skin, from which they disappear rapidly, by burrowing in. Escape of the larva is usually made by stripping the membrane joining the hypopharynx at the base of the labium. In the mammalian host the worms migrate along the

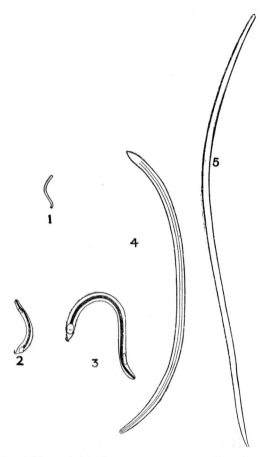

Fig. 376.—Development of *Loa loa* in *Chrysops*. × 30. (*After A. & S. L. M. Connal, from Transactions of the Royal Society for Tropical Medicine Hygiene*)

1, Larva, 24 hours old. 2, Fourth day, length 390 μm. 3, Fifth day. 4, Seventh day. 5, Tenth day, length 2 mm, breadth 0·025 mm.

inter-fascial planes. Lavoipierre has shown that the worms, on the way to the head proceed along the haemocele spaces and avoid air sacs. Infective forms rarely penetrate the brain.

Chrysops, the intermediary, feeds to repletion once every 14 days (the gestation period is 12 days). It is a 'pool feeder', straining the blood from the subcutaneous haemorrhages caused by its bite.

For the clinical features and treatment, see page 218.

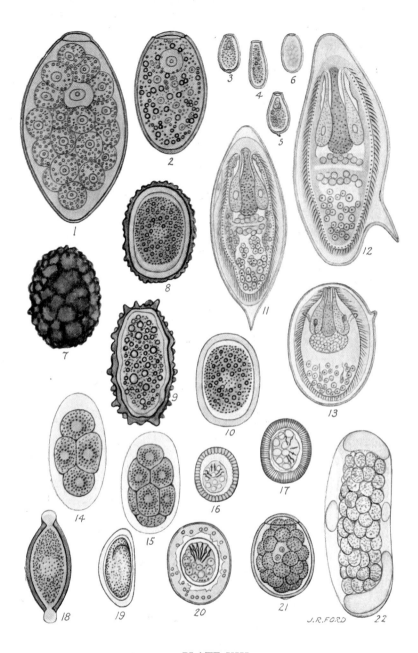

PLATE XIII

Eggs of the commoner helminths found in man. × 400

1, *Fasciolipsis buski.* 2, *Paragonimus ringeri.* 3, *Heterophyes heterophyes.* 4, *Opisthorchis felineus.* 5, *Clonorchis sinensis.* 6, *Metagonimus yokogawai.* 7, 8, *Ascaris lumbricoides,* external aspect. 9, *Ascaris lumbricoides,* unfertilized egg. 10, *Ascaris lumbricoides,* decorticated egg. 11, *Schistosoma haematobium.* 12, *Schistosoma mansoni.* 13, *Schistosoma japonicum.* 14, *Ancylostoma duodenale.* 15, *Trichostrongylus colubriformis.* 16, *Taenia solium.* 17, *Taenia saginata.* 18, *Trichuris trichiura.* 19, *Enterobius vermicularis.* 20, *Hymenolepis nana.* 21, *Diphyllobothrium latum.* 22, *Heterodera radicicola,* non-parasitic, ingested with vegetables.

[*To face p. 1054.*

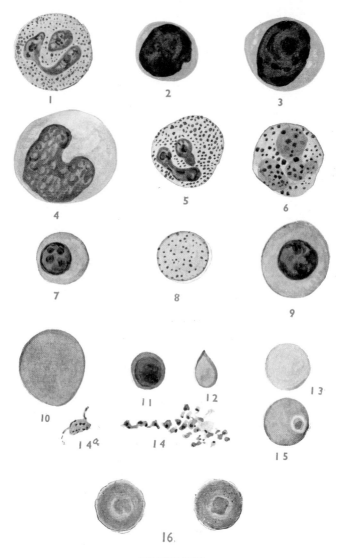

PLATE XIV

Normal and abnormal blood cells.

1, *Neutrophil polymorphonuclear leucocyte.* 2, Small *lymphocyte.* 3, Large *lymphocyte.* 4, *Monocyte.* 5, *Eosinophil leucocyte.* 6, *Basophil leucocyte* (mast cell). 7, *Normoblast* (nucleated red cell). 8, *Basophilic* dots in red cell. 9, *Megaloblast.* 10, *Megalocyte.* 11, *Microblast.* 12, *Microcyte* showing *poikilocytosis.* 13, *Polychromatophilic* degeneration of the red cell. 14, 14a, Various appearances of blood platelets. 15, Blood platelets superimposed on a red cell. 16, Target cell (Mexican hat red cell) found in sickle cell anaemia and thalassaemia.

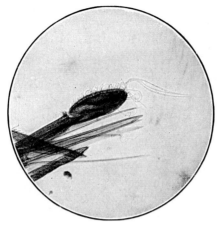

Fig. 377.—Development of *Loa loa* in *Chrysops silacea*, showing several mature larvae at the tip of the labella. (*After A. & S. L. M. Connal, from Transactions of the Royal Society for Tropical Medicine and Hygiene*)

GENUS: *Dipetalonema*

Dipetalonema perstans (Manson, 1891) Railliet, Henry and Langeron, 1912

Synonyms: *Filaria perstans; Acanthocheilonema perstans; Tetrapetalonema perstans*

Characters

It has a long cylindrical, smooth body, and a simple, unarmed mouth. The tail in both sexes is characteristic: incurvated, with a chitinous covering at the extreme tip split into 2 minute appendages, giving a mitred appearance (Fig. 378). The female possesses 4 cuticular appendages at the posterior extremity, not 2 as hitherto believed. The male (4·5 cm × 0·06 mm) is smaller than the female. The head is 0·04 mm in diameter, and the cloaca has 4 pairs of pre-anal and 1 pair of postanal papillae, and 2 unequal spicules (Fig. 378). The female (7–8 cm × 0·12 mm) has a club-shaped head

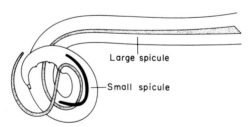

Large spicule

Small spicule

Fig. 378.—The tail of *Dipetalonema perstans*, showing 2 unequal spicules and papillae. (*After Leiper*)

0·07 mm in diameter, and a vulva situated 1·2 mm from the head. The anus opens at the apex of a papilla in the concavity of the curve formed by the tail; its diameter is 0·02 mm.

The microfilaria (200 × 4·5 μm) is unsheathed (Fig. 61, page 194). It possesses in a remarkable degree the power of elongation and contraction. Therefore the measurements vary considerably. Long and short forms (90–110 × 4 μm) have been described. It is smaller than microfilaria bancrofti or loa and its caudal end is truncated and abruptly rounded. The tapering tail extends two-thirds of the entire length. The anterior 'V-spot' is 30 μm from the anterior extremity. There is no marked tail spot, no central granular mass, and no cephalic prepuce. It moves freely in the blood. The microfilariae are found mostly in the heart, lungs, aorta and large vessels and spleen, rarely in the pancreas.

The embryos occur in equal numbers both by day and night; according to the self-inflicted experiment of Gönnert this embryo can persist in the recipient 3 years after blood transfusion.

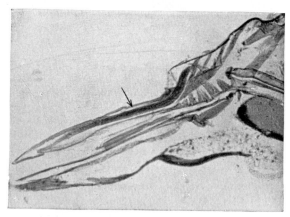

Fig. 379.—The larva of *Dipetalonema perstans* in the proboscis of *Culicoides austeni*. (*Dyce Sharp*)

Life history

Development has been described in midges, *Culicoides austeni* (Fig. 379) and also to a lesser degree in *C. grahami*. It proceeds in the thoracic muscles, and, within 6–9 days, the larval filariae (0·7 mm) are ripe for emergence from the proboscis. Before they emerge they cause a globular expansion of the labrum of *Culicoides* which then collapses and gives exit to larval filariae; 7% of wild-caught midges are infected in Cameroon.

For clinical features see page 236.

Dipetalonema streptocerca (Macfie & Corson, 1922)

Synonym: *Agamofilaria streptocerca* (Macfie & Corson, 1922) Stiles and Hassall, 1926; *Acanthocheilonema streptocerca*.

This sheathless microfilaria is found commonly in the corium of the skin, but not in the blood of people in Ghana (22 out of 50 in Accra). It probably has a wide distribution, especially in Cameroon. The microfilaria (Fig. 380) is distinguished by the 'walking-stick handle' of the tail extremity. It is 215 μm in length. The arrangement of nuclei in the head and the 4 prominent ones in the tail constitute an index of differentiation from the microfilaria of *O. volvulus* and *D. perstans*. Development takes place in *Culicoides grahami* and is similar to that described for *D. perstans* (Henrard & Peel 1949).

Microfilariae were found in the skin of 6 out of 11 chimpanzees (*Pan paniscus* and *P. satyrus*) in the Congo. Two adult female worms found in the connective tissue were closely similar to *D. perstans*. The microfilariae of this species, *D. vanhoofi*, closely resemble those of the latter. The incubation period of *D. streptocerca* is 3–4 months.

For clinical features see page 237.

Tetrapetalonema berghei (Chardome & Peel, 1951)

This is found in the Congo together with *D. streptocerca*. It is a white nematode, 60·9 × 0·271 mm, with almost imperceptible striations. The head is hemispherical and a relatively large genital opening is situated anteriorly. The uterus divides into 2 branches. Microfilariae in all stages are visible in the uterus. There are several enlargements of the body at intervals. The caudal extremity narrows rapidly showing 4 excrescences. The tail is recurved. The microfilaria which is found in the skin resembles that of a small microfilaria perstans and measures 179 × 3·55 μm. The adult form may turn out to be similar to *D. perstans.*

GENUS: *Onchocerca*

Onchocerca volvulus (Leuckart, 1893) Railliet and Henry, 1910

Characters

The body is white and filiform, tapering at both ends. The head is rounded. The cuticle is marked by transverse ridges, and raised, with prominent angular and oblique thickenings, more distinct posteriorly. It is usually found in nodules, but can reproduce outside them. The male (2–4 cm × 0·2 mm) has a straight alimentary canal ending in a subterminal anus. The tail ends in a slight spiral, and is bulbous at the tip. There are 2 pairs of pre-anal, 2 post-anal, an intermediate large papilla, and 2 unequal spicules (82 μm, 77 μm) protruding from the cloaca (Fig. 381); the former has a fluted

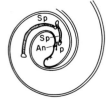

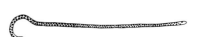

Fig. 380.—Embryo of *Dipetalonema streptocerca,* showing the characteristic curvature of the tail. × 200. (*Dyce Sharp*)

Fig. 381.—The caudal extremity of a male *Onchocerca volvulus.* (*After Brumpt*)
Sp, spicules. *An,* anus. *p,* papillae.

end and the latter a narrow neck and knob. The female normally measures 60–70 cm × 0·4 mm, but is often smaller, 35–40 cm. The head is round and truncated (0·04 mm), the vulva 0·85 mm from the anterior extremity and the tail curved. Cuticular striations are not so marked as in the male. It is ovoviviparous and the egg has a striated shell with a pointed process at each pole (like an orange wrapped in tissue paper) measuring 30–50 μm in diameter. Usually males outnumber females by 2 to 1 (4 males and 2 females in each tumour). (Brumpt separated a South American form as *O. caecutiens,* which is said to differ in the size and shape of the papillae in the male and in the size of the spicules, but this is doubtful.)

The microfilariae (300 × 8 μm) are sheathless and are found in the fluid of the cyst cavity and in the surrounding skin: they are of two types, large and small. The body tapers from the last fifth and ends in a sharply-pointed, recurved tail (Fig. 61, page 194). In the anterior fifth is a marked anterior V-spot. The cephalic cone is thickened at the commencement of the nuclear column. This microfilaria is non-periodic; it is found in skin, in the femoral, inguinal and cervical lymph-glands and in the expressed juice of tumours, but rarely in blood (2%), and has also been described in urine. It is also present in the skin of widely separated portions of the body in apparently healthy people, without producing any nodules or tumours. Microfilariae are easily demonstrated in the skin by biopsy. They are often associated with eye symptoms, in the absence of tumours, and, by aid of the slit-lamp may be seen in the cornea.

Life history

This was worked out in Sierra Leone, where 45% of the inhabitants were infected. Development takes place in the 'buffalo gnat', *Simulium damnosum* (Fig. 427, page 1103) and in *S. neavei* in Kenya. The fly abstracts microfilariae from the deeper layers of the skin near the nodule; they then enter the stomach, pierce its walls, and pass to the thoracic muscles where they undergo further development. During growth one or more ecdyses take place. At the seventh day the larva measures 0·65 mm. Development has been traced to the tenth day when the larva escapes from the proboscis; *Simulium* is a day-biting fly (6 a.m.–6 p.m.) and 2·6% may be naturally infected. They probably attract and then abstract microfilariae by scraping the skin with their prestomal teeth.

In the South American form development is similar to that of the Central African, but occurs in *Simulium metallicum* (*avidum*), *S. ochraceum* and *S. callidum* (*mooseri*), which are common in endemic areas in Guatemala. Developing larvae are frequently found in the abdomen and Malpighian tubules of these flies. Two caudal papillae are seen in fully developed larvae, which measure 0·45–1·14 mm. In Guatemala 11% of *Simulium* are naturally infected. Non-human filariae can occur in *Simulium*, and a key to their identification and distinction from human *Onchocerca* is given by Nelson and Pester (1962).

For eye symptoms, see page 860 and for clinical features page 230.

SUPERFAMILY: DRACUNCULOIDEA

GENUS: *Dracunculus*

Dracunculus medinensis (Linn., 1758), guinea worm

Characters

The female is the thickness of a knitting needle and usually 60 cm in length (60 cm × 1·5–1·7 mm; 90 cm is probably exceptional, but 120 cm has been recorded). It lives in connective tissues, and does not harm its host until about to produce its young, when it exhibits 'geotropism', i.e., it is drawn towards earth, towards the limbs—to the fingers, if in the arms; to the scrotum or penis, if in the abdomen; to the breasts in the female, though 90% migrate to the legs and feet, especially behind the outer malleolus.

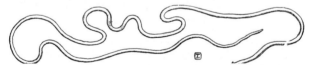

Fig. 382.—Female *Dracunculus medinensis*. One-third natural size.

The body is cylindrical, white and smooth (Fig. 382). The tip of the tail is pointed forming a blunt hook which was formerly thought to be used for holding firm in tissues, but this is not correct. The head is rounded, terminating in a thickened cuticle cap or 'cephalic shield'. The mouth is triangular, small and surrounded by 6 papillae and an outer circle of 4 double papillae. A lateral pair of cervical papillae is situated behind the nerve ring (Fig. 383). There is a single-bulb oesophagus. The secretion from the head glands is very irritating, and blisters the skin of the host. The alimentary canal is small and is thrust to one side by the branched uterus. There is no definite anus. The vulva is difficult to see and has been only recently discovered as a very small tube in the centre of the worm. The whole worm is occupied by the double uterus packed with embryos (Fig. 384). The coiled uteri, distended by 3 million larvae, fill the body. There is a double ovary and double oviducts at the posterior extremity. When douched with water, waves of contraction force the uterine contents forward, and then the thickened cuticle gives way and the 'cap' is blown off. The uterus is extruded up to a length of 1·25 cm; this also bursts and the contained embryos are shed into the water. The worm dies when its nervous system is destroyed. The sinus containing the dead worm easily becomes septic, but it may coil itself round tendons and, if pulled upon, may break. It often becomes cretified and can then be demonstrated by X-rays.

The male is known from a single specimen in man 40 mm in length, but was discovered by Moorthy (1937) in experimental dogs. It measures 1·2–2·9 cm × 0·4 mm, has sub-equal spicules (490–730 μm), and a gubernaculum (200 μm). The posterior end is coiled on itself one or more times. There are 10 pairs of caudal papillae of which 4 are preanal and 6 postanal. The copulatory spicules are subequal, 490–730 μm in length. After copulation it dies and is absorbed. It lives in between the muscles of the groin. Copulation probably takes place in the deeper tissues.

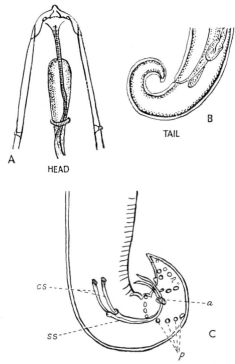

Fig. 383.—A, Anterior end of *Dracunculus medinensis*, female. B, Tail of *D. medinensis*, female. C, Posterior end of *D. medinensis*, male. Ventro-lateral aspects. × 10. (*After Faust*)

a, anus. *cs*, copulatory spicules. *p*, pre-anal and postanal papillae. *ss*, spicular sheath.

The embryo (Fig. 385) measures 500–750 × 17 μm and shows transverse striations of the cuticle. It is flattened, not cylindrical, with a long, slender tail, and a rounded head. The alimentary canal has a rudimentary anus and a bulbous oesophagus. There are 2 glands at the root of the tail. In water the embryos cannot swim, but sink and coil up and release again, moving by side-to-side lashing of the tail and tadpole-like movement of the body. Abnormal embryos, with prominences on the dorsal and ventral caudal surfaces, are not uncommon, but do not survive long.

Life history

In water they live for 6 days; in muddy water or moist earth 2–3 weeks. If slowly desiccated, they can be revived by water. They are swallowed by *Cyclops* when coiled up in rounded masses (*Cyclops* has a very small mouth). The efficient intermediaries are *Cyclops quadricornis*, or allied species (*C. strenuus, C. viridis, C. coronatus, C. bicuspidatus, Mesocyclops leuckarti* and *M. hyalinus*), but in the true tropics *Tropocyclops multicolor* and other species; in S. Nigeria it is *Thermocyclops nigerianus*. Jerky movements of the embryo attract *Cyclops* as a trout is attracted by a fly. As many as 20 may be found in 1 crustacean, but usually they die out when there are more than 4. The pointed tail

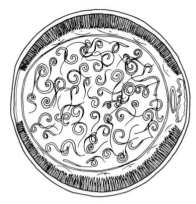

Fig. 384.—Transverse section of *Dracunculus medinensis*, showing the contained embryos. (*After Leuckart*)

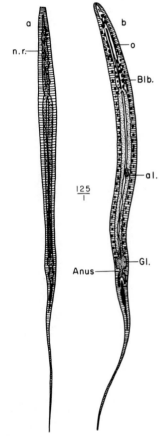

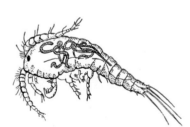

Fig. 386.—Larvae of *Dracunculus medinensis* in the body cavity of *Cyclops*. (*After R. P. Strong*)

Fig. 385.—Embryo of *Dracunculus medinensis. a*, Side view. *b*, Front view. (*After Looss*)

o, oesophagus. *Blb*, bulb. *al*, alimentary canal. *Gl*, glands. *n.r.*, nerve ring.

penetrates the gut wall; they then migrate into the body cavity and feed on the ovary or testes of the cyclops. There is no growth in size, but 2 to 3 ecdyses take place. The tail is absorbed and they become cylindrical and the posterior extremity trilobed. Development takes 4–6 weeks, but the larva may survive for 4 months. When 1 mm in length they acquire a simple muscular oesophagus (Fig. 385) and the tail is truncated. This distinguishes the infective stage.

Cyclops is swallowed by man; in the gastric juice the body of the cyclops is dissolved and the larvae become active and burst out. Onabamiro (1956) has to some extent cleared up the migration of the early stages in the mammalian host. It takes 3–4 months for the full development of both sexes. Immature stages were recovered 43–48 days while undergoing the fourth ecdysis. The route of the larvae from the alimentary canal to the subcutaneous tissues of the mammalian host takes place via the lymphatic system. The worms reach the subcutaneous tissues by the forty-third day. In this situation the sexes live in equal numbers and sexual differentiation is distinct, though the males have not developed spicules. The final ecdysis takes place in the subcutaneous tissues. The adult worm takes 1 year to develop.

REFERENCES

BARBIER, M. & BRUMPT, V. (1969) *Trans. R. Soc. trop. Med. Hyg.*, **63**, Suppl. S–66.
BEER, R. J. S. (1971) *Br. med. J.*, **ii**, 44.
CHESTERMAN, C. C. (1969) *Trans. R. Soc. trop. Med. Hyg.*, **63**, Suppl. S–92.
D'ALESSANDRO, B. A., BEAVER, P. C. & PALLARES, R. M. (1963) *Am. J. trop. Med. Hyg.*, **12**, 193.
DAVID, L. & EDESON, J. F. B. (1965) *Ann. trop. Med. Parasit.*, **59**, 193.
DISMUKE, J. C. jun. & ROUTH, C. F. (1963) *Am. J. trop. Med. Hyg.*, **12**, 73.
HAWKING, F. (1956) *Trans. R. Soc. trop. Med. Hyg.*, **50**, 397.
—— (1964) *Trans. R. Soc. trop. Med. Hyg.*, **58**, 212.
HENRARD, R. D. C. & PEEL, E. (1949) *Ann. Soc. belge Med. trop.*, **29**, 127.
JORDAN, P. & WEBBER, G. (1969) *Human Schistosomiasis*. London: Heinemann.
KIAN JOE LIE, BASCH, P. W., HEYNEMAN, D., BECK, A. J. & AUDY, J. R. (1968) *Trans. R. Soc. trop. Med. Hyg.*, **62**, 299.
MCFADZEAN, J. S. & HAWKING, F. (1956) *Trans. R. Soc. trop. Med. Hyg.*, **50**, 543.
MOORTHY, U. N. (1937) *J. Parasit.*, **23**, 220.
NELSON, G. S. (1959) *J. Helminth.*, **33**, 233.
—— & PESTER, F. N. R. (1962) *Bull. Wld. Hlth. Org.*, **27**, 473.
ONABAMIRO, S. D. (1956) *Ann. trop. Med. Parasit.*, **50**, 157.
RODRIGUEZ, M. J. D., GOMEZ, L. L. & MONTALUAN, C. J. A. (1949) *Revta ecuat. Hig. Med. trop.*, **6**, 11.
SANDGROUND, J. H. (1939) *Geneesk. Tijdschr. Ned.-Indie*, **79**, 1722.
WRIGHT, C. A. (1962) *Ciba Foundation Symposium on Bilharziasis*, p. 103. London: Churchill.
—— SOUTHGATE, V. R. & KNOWLES, R. J. (1972) *Trans. R. Soc. trop. Med. Hyg.*, in the press.

APPENDIX III

MEDICAL ENTOMOLOGY

PHYLUM: ARTHROPODA
CLASS: ARACHNIDA
ORDER: ACARINA (Ticks and Mites)
GENUS: *Sarcoptes*
Sarcoptes scabiei (Linn., 1758), itch mite, scabies mite

Morphologically similar species are found on domestic animals, foxes, wolves, and llama.

Scabies

Scabies is widespread in the tropics, especially in North Africa.
The female (0·3–0·4 mm) of *S. scabiei* is bigger than the male (0·2 mm). The sexes may be further distinguished by the epimera of the second pair of hind legs which unite near the sexual orifice in the male; in the female they are free. There are suckers (ambulacra) on the much reduced legs of the female, and on the first, second and fourth legs of the male. The greater part of the surface of the female is covered with fine transverse folds. The upper surface bears a number of specialized spines and conical scales. The gravid female lays eggs in a burrow in the skin.

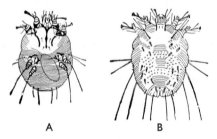

A   B

Fig. 387.—*Sarcoptes scabiei*. A, Ventral aspect with egg. × 35. (*After Canestrini*). B, Dorsal view. × 40. (*After Brumpt*)

The oval eggs measure 150 × 100 μm; in 3–5 days they give rise to larvae and nymphs which live like adults, and pass through 4 stages in 3 weeks. Finally the nymphs moult, become sexually mature and pair off on the surface of the skin. The average life of the adult is 4 to 5 weeks.

Sarcoptic mange (animal scabies). This is sometimes contracted by contact with dogs, cats and cattle infested with their own biological races of *Sarcoptes*. They may be distinguished from human scabies by the distribution of papules and vesicles on the arms, shoulders, trunks and thighs, and by the absence of burrows on the hands. Sarcoptic mange is much more amenable than scabies to treatment with sulphur compounds.

Treatment and prevention of scabies. Scabies is unlikely to be spread by blankets, but may be passed on in underclothes. Lack of washing facilities aids in its dissemination. 'Norwegian scabies' is a severe type accompanied by profuse crusting and pustulation, and is often encountered in leprosy patients. The objection to sulphur ointments, which formerly were extensively used in treatment, is liability to sulphur dermatitis.

Application of 25% emulsion of benzyl benzoate is effective, though sometimes causing dermatitis. The treatment is completed in 45 minutes and is inexpensive. The whole body is anointed with soft soap and the patient soaks in a warm bath (37·8°C) for 10 minutes. Using a brush of pigs' bristles, the body is brushed with 40 ml of the

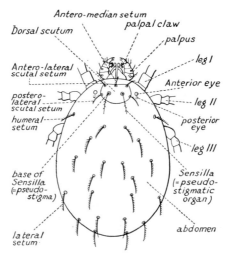

Fig. 388.—Anatomical features of a trombid larva. (*After Finnegan*)

application. A second course is taken next day. The introduction of this method was an important advance, particularly for large numbers; it is rapid and simple. Or *Tetraethylthiuram monosulphide* (ICI) in 5% solution is rubbed over the body, with the exception of the face and head, twice daily and does not cause dermititis. It is cheap, clean and effective. Another method of treatment consists of 0·5% gammexane (BHC) in vanishing cream. One application is said to suffice.

FAMILY: DEMODECIDAE

GENUS: *Demodex*

Demodex folliculorum (Simon, 1842) (Fig. 389)

This mite is found in sebaceous glands and hair follicles, and is universally distributed. Usually it produces no symptoms, but it may give rise to dermatitis, and some species in animals to mange. A minute degenerate acarid, 0·3–0·4 mm in length, it is not found in infants. Its structure is primitive. The head is provided with elongated rostrum. The female lays heart-shaped eggs (60–80 × 40–50 μm), from which hexapod larvae develop. All the stages of development are passed within the follicles. The mature parasites migrate over the skin. To demonstrate them, sebum, expressed from the mouth of the sebaceous glands, or comedones, is examined with a drop of xylol. This parasite may give rise to a chronic dry erythema with follicular scaling. Gammexane 0·5% in vanishing cream is effective.

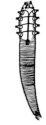

Fig. 389.—*Demodex folliculorum*. × 100. (*After Brumpt*)

Pediculoides and mites

Pediculoides ventricosus, found in cotton and cereals, usually feeds on caterpillars. In dock labourers and others handling cotton and crops it gives rise to dermatitis. The abdomen of the pregnant female is swollen with eggs like that of a miniature chigger; in it the eggs hatch and the young complete their development. Treatment by carbolic lotion or gammexane ointment or cream may be used.

Tyroglyphus mites are found in cheese, flour and sugar, and cause copra itch or grocer's itch. The dermatitis may also be partially due to food sensitization. Gammexane cream is effective.

SUB-ORDER: TROMBIDIFORMES
FAMILY: TROMBICULIDAE
GENUS: *Leptotrombidium* (*Trombicula*)

These are small, orange-red, 'velvet mites', predaceous on their own kind, and on other insects and on plants. The larvae resemble minute larval ticks, but bear bristles on their backs. The harvest-mite, the larva of *Trombicula autumnalis*, is small (0·5 mm), just visible to the naked eye; it hatches out from eggs laid on the ground. These mites are normally parasitic on moles and hares; they live a few days on man, causing intense itching points with purpuric blotches. Inunction with dimethyl phthalate or treatment of clothing with dibutyl phthalate can protect against infestation.

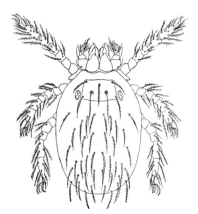

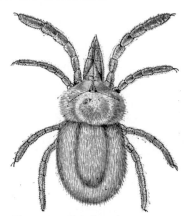

Fig. 390.—Larva of *Leptotrombidium akamushi*. × 80. (*After Hirst*)

Fig. 391.—Fully grown imago of *Leptotrombidium akamushi*. × 35. (*After Mizajima & Okumura*)

Trombiculid larvae live on various plants and parasitize many animals and man. They abound in late spring, summer and autumn. The legs above the shoe tops are commonly attacked, less frequently the belt line.

The bite is inflicted in a curious manner, assisted by the secretion of a salivary substance which liquefies the skin in a tubular structure called a histosiphon or stylostome, extending through the skin of the host. The cutaneous reaction takes the form of an erythematous macule which becomes a papule in a few hours, surrounded by an erythmatous halo.

The sudden appearance of severe pruritic bites in a person who has walked through grass suggests the presence of these mites.

Eutrombicula batatas (*Trombidium irritans*), the 'chigger mite' of America, is widely distributed, from Long Island and California to Mexico. In Florida the species is *E. alfreddugesi*. The larvae attach themselves to the skin, but do not burrow in;

secondary infection is produced by scratching. Local application of kerosene or 95%
alcohol is curative. Dusting the clothes with flowers of sulphur is preventive. In
Mexico *Neoschöngastia nunezi* produces an irritating impetiginous rash. Similar mites
occur all over the world; the adult stages, known as 'money spiders', are non-parasitic.
Schöngastia indica is the commonest mite parasite of rats of Java and it is believed to
transmit rickettsiae to them. Of medical interest are *Leptotrombidium akamushi*,
L. schüffneri, *L. deliensis*, *L. pallida*, *L. intermedia*, *L. scutellaris* and *L. hirsti*, 'Kedani
mites', the larval stages (*microtrombidium*) of which carry rickettsiae of 'scrub typhus'
(Figs 388, 390, 391). The hexapod larvae live on the ears of the field vole (*Microtus*)
and the house-rat of Formosa (*R. rattus rufescens*), whilst other rodents may act as
reservoirs.

The adult form (*Leptotrombidium*) (Fig. 391) is characterized by having spicular
openings of the tracheate system at the side of the beak (*capitulum*). It lives in soil and
measures 0·9 × 0·5 mm. It is pale grey or red, with rudimentary eyes, 4 pairs of legs,
the anterior pair stout, situated on the anterior part of the cephalothorax parallel to the
pedipalps. On the ventral surface are suckers, close to the genital orifice and anus
(2 pairs in the nymphs and 3 pairs in the adult). The mites feed on insect eggs. They
deposit their own eggs in late spring or early autumn in loose top soil under leaves in
damp places. The hexapod larvae, ochre-coloured to orange-red, become active in the
presence of a potential host, swarm on to any warm-blooded animal and feed in crowded
colonies on the ears of rats and the rump of insectivores. They hang on by palpal claws
and by inserting their fangs or chelicers. They remain attached to their mammalian
host, feeding for 3–4 days. The engorged larvae then leave the host, absorb water
and become pupa-like *nymphophanes* from which 8-legged nymphs emerge which are
carnivorous and feed on the eggs of certain mosquitoes. After a week these pass into a
second pupa-like stage (*teleophane*) from which the adults emerge, resembling the
nymphs in appearance, but larger and sexually mature. The adults lay eggs in 3–4
weeks, producing 30–50 viable eggs daily and living 15 months.

The males deposit their sperm in stalked capsules when the females lower their
genitalia. Audy has described *Laurentella*, a new subgenus of 22 species in Oriental and
Australian regions, of which one, *L.* (or *Euschöngastia*) *indica*, is a widespread species
and common as a commensal on rats in urban areas. *L. audyi* is dominant and parasitic
on mammals of Malaysia and Borneo. *Tetranychus molestissimus* is a mite which may
cause larva migrans (see page 262). This belongs to a group known as 'red spiders',
which invest vegetation and are well known as the 'Bicho Colorado' of South America.
Persons employed in picking hops often complain of the itching produced by it.

For critical review of acari as transmitting agents, see Finnegan (1946).

SUPERFAMILY: IXODOIDEA (Ticks)

Ticks are cosmopolitan, and important carriers of disease. These large, blood-sucking
Acarina are larger editions of mites. With the exception of *Argas* and *Ornithodorus*,
they rarely attack man voluntarily in their adult stage. The females are invariably
larger than the males. The shell is often highly ornamented, and has 4 pairs of segmented legs and a single spiracle on each side between the third and fourth legs. There
is a special series of tooth-like lumps on the protarsus of the first pair of legs. When
ticks are gorged the posterior end expands, but the males never gorge themselves on
blood to the same extent as the females.

Ticks are divided into Argasidae (soft) and Ixodidae (hard). In the former there is no
shield. The mouth-parts are not visible from above and there are no festoons. The
genital pore is situated in the midline on the ventral surface, not far behind the
capitellum. All ticks lay shiny spherical eggs in enormous numbers—up to 5000. The
excretory organs, or Malpighian glands, open into the rectum, and the coxal glands
open between the first and second coxae. Eggs hatch into hexapod larvae, which
become octopod nymphs, three series of which usually develop before the adult
stage is reached. All are endowed with a phenomenal capacity for fasting—some for
4–5 years.

Argasidae live apart from their host, in burrows or crevices, and have the habits of a bug. All stages of Ixodidae attach themselves to the host, and drop off when gorged; and after fertilization the male dies. In some species—*Margaropus*—the metamorphosis from larva to nymph, and from nymph to adult takes place on the same host; in others —*Haemaphysalis*—the tick drops off before each moult, to find a new host three times in its life.

FAMILY: ARGASIDAE (Soft Ticks)

GENUS: *Ornithodorus* (contains 20–30 species)

Ornithodorus moubata (Murray, 1877)

This tick is widely distributed in East, Central and South Africa. The body is rounded and mammillated and the legs tuberculated. The integument is greenish-brown, hard and leathery, marked above and below with symmetrically-arranged grooves, and numerous hard, shiny trabeculations. The carapace contains no 'eyes'. The females (12–14 mm) are larger than the males (8 × 7 mm). The habits resemble those of the bed-bug, and they live in mud huts, thatched roofs and cracks in floors and walls, emerging at night to suck the blood of man and beast, and in doing so may inject an anticoagulant and analgesic. *O. moubata* is found in burrows excavated by ant-eaters and porcupines, associated with wart-hogs, far from human habitations in Kenya and there they breed in large numbers. The presence of these ticks is not consistently associated with relapsing fever. Three forms are now recognized which feed on man, chicken and wart-hog respectively. In Kenya, in the Digo district, where ticks are very numerous, but relapsing fever is infrequent, the ticks have micro-environmental conditions of hot and moist (relative humidity of 77%). Man-feeders are more characteristic of cooler, wet climates. The tick feeds slowly and cannot abstract much blood, except from a sleeping host. It is important as a vector of relapsing fever (*Borrelia duttoni*). Spirochaetes pass through the gut wall, and small infective forms arise in the body cavity and settle in various tissues, especially the ovaries and salivary glands. Transmission is frequently effected by the bite. Spirochaetal infection is transmitted in a hereditary manner, and the organisms have been found in the eggs. Eggs are laid in batches of 50–100 and the fertility of the female is favoured by liberal feeding. They hatch within 20 days and the larval stage is practically absent. On the thirteenth day the egg-shell splits, and about the same time the skin of the contained larva splits also, and an 8-legged nymph emerges, throwing off simultaneously both egg shell and larval skin. There are several nymph stages, the largest of which may equal the adult in size.

O. moubata is common on travel routes. Rest-houses are always most infested, and ticks may be carried long distances in mats and bedding. In parts of Africa, the people try to protect themselves by plastering their huts with mud and cow-dung and by frequently smoking them. Pyrethrum powder is a valuable preventive. This tick is comparatively resistant to DDT, but can be killed easily by BHC at 20 mg/900 cm² in dusting the floors of houses, etc. The tick is difficult to dislodge and burning may not completely eradicate it. Old camping sites and mud houses are to be avoided, and travellers must never sleep on the floor.

Precipitin tests show that in cool, wet habitats of the Kenya Highlands and N.W. Tanganyika, 94% of *O. moubata* feed on man and 2% on chickens, but in hot, moist habitats these percentages are reversed. Walton (1962) has named biological races: *O. compactus* from tortoises in S. Africa, *O. apertus* from porcupines and wart-hogs, *O. porcinus porcinus* in animal burrows and baobab trees. *O. p. domesticus* is widely distributed in African dwellings—it is the most persistent form and the best vector, but has cycles of low and high seasonal incidence.

In certain parts of Africa, Ethiopia and Somalia, *O. moubata* is overlapped by *O. savignyi* (Audouin, 1827), which prefers market-places and cattle byres in the vicinity of wells. It is distinguished by having eyes, larger processes on its legs and more minutely pitted dorsal surface. It can transmit *B. duttoni* (in the laboratory) but its exact role under natural conditions is doubtful, though suspected in Somaliland.

It has been reported from Northern Nigeria, Egypt, the Sudan, East Africa, India and Arabia.

O. lahorensis (Newman, 1908), resembles *O. moubata* and has an anterior projecting hood. The adult lives in cracks of houses and walls in Iran and North India. The nymphal stages are passed on sheep. It is suspected of carrying relapsing fever (see page 586).

O. tholozani (Lab. and Mégn., 1895), syn. *O. papillipes* (Birula), the 'Persian bug', is widely distributed in Israel, Jordan, Iran, India and Turkmenistan. In nature it is found in porcupine and jerboa burrows. The male is 4–6 mm in length, the female 8–9 mm. It transmits *Borrelia persica* (see page 584) and on biting injects an analgesic substance. Other species in Asia are *O. asperus* and *O. tartakovskii*.

O. talajé (Guerin-Menéville, 1849) resembles *O. venezuelensis*, and is found from Mexico to Paraguay. The female measures 5–6 × 3–4 mm. It transmits *B. venezueleniss* (see page 584). *O. turicata* is also a vector with similar habits from the same region.

O. venezuelensis, syn. *O. rudis* (Brumpt, 1921), is related to the foregoing, and found in Venezuela and Colombia at the higher altitudes (900–1500 m). The female is larger than the male (5–6 × 3–4 mm). It lives in the walls of huts in company with bed-bugs and is very voracious. Eggs are laid in batches of 50–100. Hexapod larvae, on emerging, feed actively within a few hours on mammalian blood. The nymphs feed without undergoing ecdysis, as in *O. talajé*, but thereafter they moult after each feed, becoming adult at the fourth. This tick conveys relapsing fever in the districts in which it occurs.

O. hermsi (Wheeler, Herms and Meyer, 1935) is a small ovoid species, sandy-coloured when not engorged. The female (5 × 3·1 mm) resembles the male (3·8 × 2·4 mm). It differs from *O. talajé* in minor details and in the smaller size of the male. It is found in the burrows of many rodents and in chipmunks' nests, at an elevation of 1200–2100 m near Big Bear Lake, San Bernardino County, California. It transmits *B. turicatae* in California and Nevada, though tick-transmitted relapsing fever has now been reported from Colorado, California, Texas, Arizona, Nevada, Kansas, New Mexico, Washington and Montana.

O. turicata (Dugès) is closely allied to the foregoing and is found in Mexico, Texas, Arizona, and possibly Kansas. Normally it lives on goats, sheep, foxes and rabbits.

O. erraticus (Lucas, 1849), like. *O. marocanus* (Velu, 1919), under natural conditions, lives in burrows far from human habitations. In Morocco it inhabits piggeries. In Senegal and Dakar it transmits *Borrelia duttoni* (syn. *B. crocidurae*), and in Spain and Morocco *B. hispanica*, in the hexapod larval stage (see page 584).

O. normandi (Larousse) is found in Tunisia where it transmits *Spirochaeta normandi*, a parasite of gerbils (*Meriones shawi*).

Argas persicus (Fisher, 1824) is common in northern and eastern Iran, Syria, Turkestan, Russia, China, Algeria, South Africa, North and South America, West Indies, Western Australia and Queensland, attacking poultry and man. It lives in old houses, in cracks of the walls and floors. Normally it transmits *S. gallinarum* of fowls and ducks.

FAMILY: IXODIDAE (Hard Ticks)

GENERA: *Rhipicephalus, Dermacentor, Haemaphysalis, Amblyomma*, etc.

There are 12 genera, all parasitic on mammals, except *Aponomora*, which is parasitic on reptiles. All species of ixodid ticks pass through 4 stages—egg, larva, nymph and adult. They may have one or multiple hosts. The eggs are deposited on the ground where they hatch and give rise to hexapod larvae which soon seek a blood meal. In the case of multiple host ticks the engorged larvae drop from the host after several days of feeding and seek a cool place where they remain till moulting takes place. The resulting octopod nymphs then feed on a second host, again drop to the ground and await moulting. The ticks emerge from the second moult as adult males and females. An interval of 10 days is required for engorgement of the female, during which time mating takes place. The life-cycle normally extends from a few weeks up to 10 or more years. After egg-laying is complete, the female dies. Eggs are laid in enormous num-

bers, and the larvae wait in herbage for their hosts. Some feed and drop off: others have
different hosts (cattle, rabbit, etc.); others, again, have different hosts at different
stages. Debility is produced by multiple bites and secondary infections. Tick paralysis
(page 813) is a toxic manifestation from the saliva when the tick has been attached for
several days in the region of the head and neck. Coma, respiratory paralysis and death
may ensue. In other cases the hypostome, plunged into the skin, may break the
capitulum which, being left behind, gives rise to a septic focus.

Rhipicephalus sanguineus (Latreille, 1804) is a brown cosmopolitan species in many
countries, present throughout all months of the year. It attaches itself to the dog, in
association with which the whole cycle is completed. Each individual normally has
3 hosts, 1 for each of the larval, nymphal and adult stages. The female engorges
with blood and then immediately separates from the dog and lays 1000–3000 brown
eggs which hatch at 25°C; the larvae attach themselves to a new host. At 15–20°C they
can live 3–4 months. This species transmits the *Rickettsia* of tick typhus in Texas,
South America and South Africa, *fièvre boutonneuse* of Marseilles, and also conveys
canine piroplasmosis.

R. appendiculatus closely resembles the foregoing. The larval forms transmit the
Rickettsia of tick typhus in South Africa.

Haemaphysalis leachi (Audouin, 1827) does not readily attack man. Its larval and
nymphal stages are spent on carnivora, quitting the host at each stage. It is the active
carrier of canine piroplasmosis in South Africa and has been incriminated there as a
vector of tick typhus also.

H. humerosa, an Australian species, has been found by Derrick to transmit the
Coxiella of Q fever (*C. burneti*) to man and parasitizes the bandicoot (*Isoodon torosus*).

H. spinigera is the vector of Kyasanur Forest disease of man. Ticks infest small
mammals, birds, monkeys and man in the forests.

Amblyomma americanum (Linn., 1758), known as the 'lone star' tick, from the bright
spot on the carapace of the female, is important as the vector of Rocky Mountain fever
in Texas, where it is abundant. Recently the pocket-gopher (a small rodent) which is
parasitized by this tick has been found to constitute the reservoir of *Rickettsia rickettsii*.
Found throughout North America and Brazil, it infests dogs, cattle and fowls. The
larvae frequently attack man and live in scrub and high grass.

A. hebraeum (Koch), an African species, is widely distributed on lizards and birds,
and occasionally attacks man. It has 3 hosts of the same species. The female may
lay as many as 20 000 eggs and transmit the *Rickettsia* of 'tick-bite' fever in South
Africa.

A. cajennense (Koch, 1844) is a large tick found in America from Texas to Argentina.
The males are adorned with a carapace of silvery design. The natural host is the cavy,
it transmits the *Rickettsia* of tick typhus in São Paulo and of Rocky Mountain spotted
fever in Mexico, Panama and Colombia.

A. paulopunctatum, a parasite of the giant forest hog in W. Uganda, produces
immature nymphs which are apt to infect the nostrils of man and cause considerable
irritation.

Dermacentor andersoni (Stiles, 1908), syn. *D. venustus* (Banks, 1897), is an important
carrier of Rocky Mountain fever in the western United States, where it is known as the
wood-tick. Primarily a rodent infection this is probably normally maintained by
Haemaphysalis, but rodents are also attacked by *Dermacentor*, so the infection 'over-
flows' to man as in parallel cases of murine typhus. Tularaemia (page 493) is also
occasionally transmitted. Abundant in the Rocky Mountains, the adults appear during
the summer, parasitic on horses, big game and other wild animals, and frequently on
man (Figs 392, 393). Larvae and nymphs occur on small rodents and ground-squirrels.
The female, when engorged, deposits 5000–7000 eggs 4–6 days after quitting the host.
Hexapod larvae appear on the sixteenth day and in 2–8 days engorge. After the larva has
fallen to the ground and moulted, the nymph produced can survive for 300 days and,
after itself feeding, falls to the ground and moults. Fully developed males and females
can fast 2 years. After attaching themselves to a mammalian host they copulate in
4 days. The males remain attached, the females fall to the ground and deposit their
eggs. Under natural conditions the cycle takes 2 years.

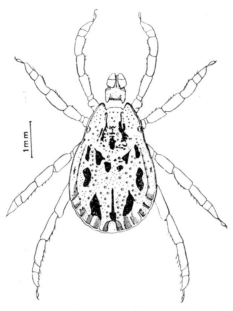

Fig. 392.—Female *Dermacentor andersoni*. (*After Nuttall*)

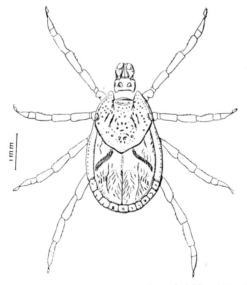

Fig. 393.—Male *Dermacentor andersoni*. (*After Nuttall*)

D. variabilis (Say, 1821), the dog-tick, is widely distributed in North America, most abundantly on the Atlantic coast. In its immature stages it feeds on small rodents, especially mice; the adults attack dogs and other large animals. It resembles the foregoing. It is the principal vector of spotted fever in central and eastern United States (see page 622) and may cause paralysis in dogs. Arsenical dipping of sheep and goats acts as a control, and the rodents should be killed off.

Hyalomma spp. and *Dermacentor* spp. are vectors of viral haemorrhagic fevers.

Ixodes persulcatus and *I. ricinus* are vectors of Russian spring–summer encephalitis in the far east of the U.S.S.R. and in Central Europe.

Ixodophagus is a small wasp parasite of ticks found in Europe and introduced into America to combat *Dermacentor*.

CLASS: PENTOSOMIDA
FAMILY: LINGUATULIDAE

The lingulatids, pentastomes or 'tongue worms' are neither protozoa nor helminths, but occupy an intermediate position between the annelids and the arthropods. Two species may infect man as a dead-end infection: *Linguatula serrata* and *Armillifer armillatus*.

GENUS: *Linguatula*
Linguatula serrata (Frohlich, 1789)

This is found in southern Germany, Switzerland, the Middle East and Brazil.

Life history

The adult *Linguatula* lives in the lungs of snakes and the nasopharynx of mammals, usually dogs, foxes and wolves, but occasionally sheep and goats. These are the definitive hosts. Eggs are passed in the faeces or saliva, and hatch in the gut of an intermediate host, a reptile or mammal, including man. A first stage larva emerges, penetrates the gut wall and migrates to the tissues, where it undergoes several moults, eventually forming a third stage larva, which is the infective stage and which forms a cyst. The third stage larvae are eaten by the definitive hosts, and there develop into nymphs, which migrate to the lungs and nasopharynx, where they become adults.

Man can be infected by the ingestion of eggs, in which case the third stage larvae encyst in various tissues of the body, or by the ingestion of third stage larvae, which migrate as nymphs from the stomach to the nasopharynx and cause halzoun.

Morphology

The body of the adult *Linguatula* (Fig. 394) is somewhat pear-shaped, flattened and transversly striated with about 90 rings; the mouth is roughly quadrangular and surrounded by hooks. The intestine is simple. The male is white, 18–20 mm long and 3 mm broad anteriorly and 0.5 mm posteriorly. The female, 8–10 mm in length, is grey, but may be brown when packed with eggs; she measures 8–10 mm broad anteriorly and 2 mm posteriorly.

The eggs are ovoid and 90 μm in length by 70 μm in breadth. They contain ripe embryos which hatch into first stage larvae; these are stumpy, and have 4 'legs' which each bear a bifurcate claw. The posterior end is drawn into a rounded or 'forked' tail. The third stage larvae (Fig. 394) are worm-like and 5–6 mm in length; they have distinctive spines arranged in transverse rows at the posterior margin of each annulus. These are sufficient to distinguish *Linguatula* spp. in any section.

Infection in man

Cysts. Encysted larvae are well tolerated and are met with frequently in the mesenteric glands of domestic animals, as well as in rabbits and hares, and they have been found in 4·6% of human livers, where they appear to cause no symptoms. Occasionally single cysts in certain locations may obstruct bile-ducts or bronchi or cause cerebral compression. When they occur in the anterior chamber of the eye glaucoma may result (see Chapter 44).

Halzoun (parasitic pharyngitis, Marrara syndrome (Sudan)) (Schacher *et al.* 1969; Hopps *et al.* 1971). Halzoun was formerly thought to be caused by the immature fluke of *Fasciola hepatica* being ingested in uncooked liver. It is now known that this syndrome is caused by the cysts of *Linguatula* being ingested in the raw liver or lymph glands of sheep or goats into the stomach, where they develop into nymphs. They then migrate to the throat and nasopharynx and attach themselves. This syndrome occurs mainly among the Lebanese. As early as several hours after eating infected tissues there is pain and itching in the throat, paroxysmal coughing and sneezing and lacrimal and nasal discharge. Often there is hoarseness, dyspnoea, dysphagia and vomiting, less frequently haemoptysis and temporary loss of hearing. There may be enlargement of the submaxillary and cervical lymph glands. The disease is self-limiting, with spontaneous recovery within a week or 10 days. Very occasionally death has been recorded by asphyxiation, possibly caused by a sensitivity reaction. Cases of recurrent epistaxis have occurred as a result of an adult *Linguatula* in the nose.

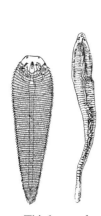
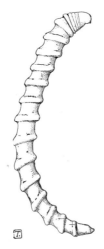

Fig. 394.—Third stage larval form (× 6) and mature form (natural size) of *Linguatula serrata*. (*After Brumpt*)

Fig. 395.—*Armillifer armillatus*, natural size. (*After Sambon*)

Diagnosis

In tissue sections the pentastomid presents as a well defined body cavity which contains an intestinal tract and distinctive reproductive organs. The muscle fibres are striated and the spines on the cuticle distinctive. These characteristics will serve to distinguish them from *Sparganum*.

GENUS: *Armillifer*

Armillifer (Porocephalus) armillatus (Wyman, 1848)

A. armillatus occasionally infects humans, especially in Negroes in Central Africa. In oriental regions *A. moniliformis* is the usual cause and human infection has been recorded from Malaysia, Java, Manila, Sumatra and China.

Characters

The adult parasite is found in pythons and other snakes; the nymphal form in the lion, mandrill, giraffe and African hedgehog. The arachnid is vermiform, yellowish and translucent. The anterior part is cylindrical, the posterior tapering into a blunt-pointed cone. In the male there are 17 and in the female 18–22 prominent opaque rings (each 1–2 mm). The male is 3–5 cm long, the female 9–12 cm. There is no clear separation between the cephalothorax and the abdomen. The mouth opening is capped by two prominent papillae on the ventral surface, lipped by a chitinous ring. On each side are 2 protractile chitinous rings; the anus is terminal. The genital orifice of the male lies at the anterior end of the abdomen; that of the female opens in the middle of the ventral surface of the caudal cone. *A. moniliformis* is more slender and has more rings than *A. armillatus*. The female is oviparous. The eggs are broadly elliptical, double-shelled, and measure 108 × 80 µm.

The nymph lies coiled within the cyst, with its ventral surface corresponding to the convexity of the curve. In shape and structure it resembles the adult. Calcification may take place in the liver and other organs.

The life-history of *A. armillatus* is similar to that of *L. serrata*. The ingested eggs hatch in the intestine and the larvae bore through the wall to lodge in any viscus, where they undergo 9 moults in 6 months to a year to form infective nymphs. Man acquires the infection by drinking pond water contaminated by snakes or by eating snake meat.

In man the infection comes to a dead end and the larvae or nymphs encyst on the surface of the liver, in the intestinal mucosa, peritoneal cavity or lungs. Infection of man has been found in 33 of 133 post mortems in the Congo and in 45% of Malaysian aborigines. A large number of parasites were found within the lumen of the small intestine and encysted in the lungs. Pathological changes occur around the dead parasites and vary from very little reaction around live parasites to the formation of a necrotic granulomatous reaction followed by fibrosis and calcification round the dead parasites. The dead parasites may be seen on X-ray pictures as characteristic horse-shoe or crescent-shaped bodies 4–7 mm in size.

Rarely the parasite has caused intestinal obstruction, pneumonitis, meningitis, pericarditis, nephritis and obstructive jaundice. A blood eosinophilia occurs especially after death of the larva. Two cases of infection with *P. crotali* of the rattlesnake have been reported in U.S.A.

CLASS: INSECTA

ORDER: DIPTERA

FAMILY: PSYCHODIDAE

SUB-FAMILY: PHLEBOTOMINAE

IMPORTANT GENERA: *Phlebotomus**, *Sergentomyia* (Old World)

*Lutzomyia**, *Brumptomyia* (New World)

PHLEBOTOMINE SANDFLIES

BY D. M. MINTER, PH.D., B.SC.

The phlebotomine sandflies, of which there are more than 500 known species, are small (1·5–2·5 mm), hairy flies with long slender legs. The lanceolate wings, also very hairy, are held in a vertical V over the back of the resting fly (Fig. 396). The antennae are filamentous and similar in both sexes.

The female sandfly feeds on blood: one or more meals are needed to complete the maturation of each batch of eggs. Male flies probably feed on the juices or secretions of plants but do not suck blood. The biting mouth-parts are, however, similar in both sexes and consist of a pair each of toothed mandibles and maxillae, with a median labium and hypopharynx. The labrum is short and forms part of the head. The mouth-parts are flanked on each side by hairy labial palps.

Phlebotomine sandflies are the vectors of visceral leishmaniasis (kala-azar; see page 119), the various forms of cutaneous leishmaniasis (oriental sore, espundia etc.; pages 133, 139), bartonellosis (oroya fever, Carrión's disease; page 633) and sandfly fever (papataci fever, 3-day fever etc.; pages 359, 368).

The distribution of the group is mainly tropical and subtropical but extends into

* These genera include all species of known medical importance.

north temperate latitudes to the Channel Isles and southern Canada. Southern limits are less well known but sandflies occur in southern parts of Australia and in South America to about 40°S. The vertical distribution of sandflies extends to 2800 metres or more (Peru, Ethiopia) in warm parts of the world.

Sandflies are mainly crepuscular and most species are inactive in daylight hours and seek shelter in dark, moist places. Typical daytime resting places include dark corners and crevices of houses and out-buildings, in pit latrines, crevices in stone walls, tree-holes, soil and rock crevices, caves, animal burrows and, where suitable termitaria are found, the ventilation shafts of termite hills (e.g. East, West and South-west Africa; Philippines; Australia).

The normal flight of a sandfly is more like a slow and leisurely hop, usually of less than a metre. Nonetheless, sandflies can cover long distances, sometimes more than a kilometre overnight. Movements of up to 100 metres during the night are not un-common. Perhaps such long-range travel is mainly the result of passive carriage by air movements rather than of sustained flight, although most species cease activity in the

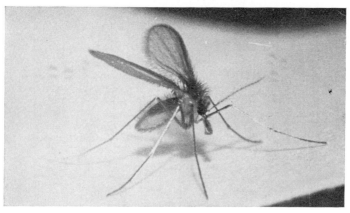

Fig. 396.—Adult female *Phlebotomus longipes*. Note the presence of partly digested blood (dark) and developing ovaries (light) in the abdomen. (*Photograph by Mr Teferi Gemetchu*)

lightest perceptible breeze. Most individual sandflies probably live and die within a few tens of metres from the place of their birth.

Female sandflies of different species feed on the blood of a wide variety of warm- and cold-blooded hosts: these include man, domestic pets such as cats and dogs, rodents and other small mammals, cattle, wild carnivores (jackals, foxes etc.), bats, birds, lizards, tortoises, snakes, frogs and toads. Each species probably has a more or less limited range of preferred hosts: members of the genus *Sergentomyia* frequently favour birds and reptiles etc., while members of the genus *Phlebotomus* more frequently favour mammals and, sometimes, man. A few species, such as *P. papatasi* of the Near and Middle East, readily become domestic in habits and man becomes a preferred host.

Life history

Breeding sites are always dark, damp places which are rich in organic matter, humus, leaf debris, animal faeces, insect remains and so forth. Suitable places include tree-holes, leaf litter in tropical rain-forest, rubble and loose earth, caves and rock holes, etc.

Female sandflies are ready to oviposit 3–10 days after taking a blood meal as a rule, although some autogenous species are known to produce eggs, at least occasionally, without the necessity for a previous blood meal (e.g. *P. papatasi* and some South American sandflies).

The eggs are small (generally less than 0·5 mm), elliptical and brown or black in colour with a sculptured or reticulated surface and are laid in batches of 15–80. Flies are very weak after oviposition and many die. Hatching occurs in 1–2 weeks and the young larvae emerge from the egg with the aid of an egg-tooth on top of the head capsule. The first instar larvae which hatch from the eggs are very small (0·5–1·0 mm) and have a white, caterpillar-like body with a black head capsule. From the darkened posterior end arise a pair of dark, stout caudal bristles that are at least as long as the body. Within a few days the larvae moult to the second instar in which, as in later instars, the caudal bristles are increased to two pairs (except in the South American genus *Brumptomyia*, which retain only a single pair throughout larval life). These long caudal hairs are characteristic of sandfly larvae and enable them to be recognized with ease. With each successive moult up to the fourth and final instar there is a progressive increase in size; up to 3 mm in the case of large species, with caudal hairs as long again. The larvae have 12 body segments, 9 of which bear false legs that are locomotory in

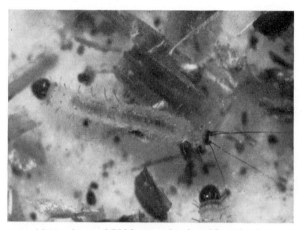

Fig. 397.—Mature larva of *Phlebotomus longipes*. Note the dark head and terminal abdominal segment, the latter bearing 2 pairs of long, stout, caudal bristles. The body bears a small number of characteristic stout, branched hairs. (*Photograph by Mr Teferi Gemetchu*)

function. Each of the similar body segments bears a small number of characteristic club-shaped branched hairs (Fig. 397).

The larvae are sensitive to desiccation, especially the younger instars, and therefore require a high humidity. However, the presence of free water is also deleterious and young stages may actually drown in a film of water. The larvae feed on particulate organic matter of various kinds. The period of larval life is very variable between species and is also dependent upon ambient temperatures. Under favourable conditions some species can complete larval development in less than 3 weeks; other species, living under colder conditions, may take as many months (e.g. *P. longipes* in cold highland areas of Ethiopia). Some species are able to enter a period of larval diapause in the fourth instar and thus survive, in an inactive state, conditions which would be unfavourable for the adult flies. Some species, such as *P. papatasi*, overwinter in larval diapause in temperate climates; some tropical species living in arid areas probably survive the long dry season, wholly or partly, in larval diapause.

When about to pupate, the mature larvae seek drier conditions and climb out of the larval food medium. The larvae attach themselves by the posterior end and cast the skin of the last instar; the cast skin remains attached, complete with caudal hairs, to the tail of the pupa. No coccoon is formed. The naked pupa completes development to the eclosion of the mature adult fly within 1-2 weeks as a rule, during which time it remains immobile and does not feed. Shortly before eclosion, eye pigment is laid down inside the pupal skin and is visible through the integument (Fig. 398).

The adult insects emerge during the hours of darkness, often just before dawn: male insects usually emerge first and are then ready to fertilize the females when they

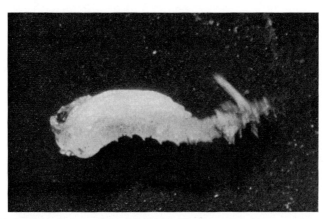

Fig. 398.—Mature pupa of *Phlebotomus longipes*. Note the eye pigment and developing wings and legs visible through the integument. The cast skin of the last larval instar is still attached to the larval end of the pupa. (*Photograph by Mr Teferi Gemetchu*)

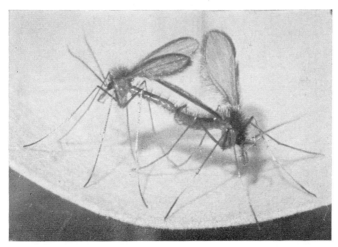

Fig. 399.—Male and female *Phlebotomus longipes in copula*. (*Photographs by Mr Teferi Gemetchu*)

emerge an hour or so later (Fig. 399). Female flies store sufficient sperm in their spermathecae to fertilize the eggs laid at intervals throughout their life. The adult flies emerge to feed on warm still evenings; even a slight breeze is sufficient to discourage activity of most species. The life cycle, from egg to adult, may occupy a period that varies from less than 1 month to more than 3 months, depending upon the species and

Table 48. Phlebotomine sandflies and human disease

Disease and aetiological agent	Sandfly species implicated	Animal reservoir	Area	Remarks
Visceral leishmaniasis (kala-azar)	Lutzomyia longipalpis	Dogs, foxes	Central America; north and central South America	
Leishmania donovani	Phlebotomus perniciosus, P. ariasi, P. major, P. longicuspis	Dogs, foxes	Mediterranean basin	Infantile kala-azar
	P. chinensis, ? P. caucasicus, ? P. mongolensis	Dogs, jackals, foxes	Central Asia	
	P. chinensis, ? P. mongolensis	Dogs	China	
	P. argentipes	None	India	
	P. orientalis	Wild rodents and carnivores	Sudan	Transmission confined to areas of Acacia 'forest' 'Termite-hill kala-azar'
	P. martini, ? P. vansomerenae ? P. celiae	Unknown	Kenya	
Old World cutaneous leishmaniasis (Oriental sore), Leishmania tropica	P. sergenti, P. papatasi, P. perfiliewi, ? P. caucasicus, ? P. mongolensis	Various, wild rodents (L. tropica tropica) and dogs (L. tropica major)	Mediterranean basin to Central Asia and India	Only in Central Asia is the disease clearly differentiated into two distinct nosological forms; rural and urban
	? P. dubosqi, ? P. bergeroti P. longipes	? Dogs, ? rodents ? Hyrax	W. Africa (Senegal) E. African highland areas above 2000 m: Ethiopia and Mt Elgon (Kenya)	Cases of diffuse cutaneous leishmaniasis also occur: thought to be due to failure of normal immune response to L. tropica
New World cutaneous leishmaniasis I. Chiclero's ulcer Leishmania mexicana	Lutzomyia olmeca, ? other Lutzomyia spp. (e.g. Lu. ylephiletrix, Lu. geniculata, Lu. paraensis, Lu. pessoana Lu. cruciata)	Various forest rodents	Mexico and Central America	A forest zoonosis: infection of man is an occupational hazard

Disease and aetiological agent	Sandfly species implicated	Animal reservoir	Area	Remarks
II. South American mucocutaneous leishmaniasis (Espundia etc.) *Leishmania braziliensis* and related forms	Many *Lutzomyia species* probably concerned in the zoonotic cycle: some undoubtedly transmit infection to man. The following species, and probably others, may act as vectors: *Lutzomyia flaviscutellata, Lu. panamensis, Lu. trapidoi, Lu. whitmani, Lu. intermedia, Lu. anduzei, Lu. cruciata, Lu. migonei, Lu. gomezi, Lu. fischeri, Lu. pessoai, Lu. ylephiletrix*	Various rodents and other forest animals	Central and South America	Infection in man is due to contact with a complex of zoonotic leishmanial diseases in forest areas or areas bordering forest. Infection is frequently an occupational hazard
III. *Uta* *Leishmania peruana*	*Lutzomyia peruensis* *Lutzomyia verrucarum*	Dogs	Highland areas of South America, especially Peru	Transmission mainly associated with caves and rock fissures of a barren upland landscape up to 2800 m
Bartonellosis (Oroya fever; Carrion's disease etc.) *Bartonella bacilliformis*	*Lutzomyia verrucarum*, possibly also related species	?. ?.	Highlands of Peru, Ecuador and Colombia	The only bacterial disease associated with sandflies
Sandfly fever (papataci fever, 3-day fever)	*Phlebotomus papatasi*	?.	Mediterranean basin to W. Pakistan	The only human viral infection in which sandflies have been incriminated with certainty

prevailing conditions of temperature. The life cycle of the adult insect in nature is probably rarely more than a few weeks and often much less. Female flies may acquire infection of pathogenic organisms with the first blood meal and can then transmit infection to new hosts at intervals throughout the remainder of their lives.

The transmission of disease organisms by sandflies (Table 48)

Leishmania species. Sandflies are the vectors of several leishmanial diseases to man and animals; the parasites undergo cyclical development in the gut of the female before reaching the infective stage. Some species of *Leishmania* (mainly those of lower vertebrates) multiply as promastigotes (leptomonads) in the lumen of the midgut and later migrate to the hind-gut or rectum to reach the infective stage: this is the so-called 'posterior station', in which infection of a new host is by contamination. Infection takes place when flies are crushed on the skin while feeding or are eaten—by lizards or other insectivorous vertebrates.

Most leishmanial parasites of man and the higher vertebrates are, however, transmitted by the bite of infected sandflies. In these cases development of the flagellates in the gut of the fly follows a different pattern. Firstly, promastigotes (leptomonads) multiply in the midgut as described but then they migrate forward into the anterior part of the midgut—frequently referred to as the cardia—where they may form a dense mass, often attached by the flagella to the wall of the cardia; this is the so-called 'anterior station' characteristic of parasites whose transmission is inoculative. From the cardia, flagellates may actively move forward to contaminate the mouthparts, or be regurgitated into the bite wound when feeding commences.

The cycle of *Leishmania* spp. in sandflies is always as an active flagellate, usually as a promastigote (leptomonad) but sometimes with an epimastigote (crithidial) intermediate stage. Amastigote (leishmanial) stages do not occur in the insect host. Development of the parasites to the infective stage is normally synchronous with the gonotrophic cycle of the host (variously, 5–10 days) so that infections acquired with one blood meal are transmissible when the infected insect is ready to feed again, usually after oviposition has taken place.

Infection rates in wild sandflies are generally very low (mostly below 1%) and it is likely that repeated attempts to probe and feed are made by infected flies so that multiple infections are possible from one insect attempting to feed on several hosts in order to obtain the blood meal necessary to mature the next batch of eggs.

Because newly emerged flies have not yet had a blood meal they cannot be infected with *Leishmania* and are therefore not of epidemiological importance. It is useful if such young (i.e. nulliparous) flies can be distinguished from older (i.e. parous) flies that have fed at least once, have laid eggs and are thus capable of harbouring infections. This can be done, as with mosquitoes and other insects, by examination of the condition of the ovarioles, but because of their small size this is seldom practicable for sandflies. Microscopic examination of the accessory glands, lying close to the rectum within the posterior part of the abdomen of female sandflies, is a useful guide to separate nulliparous (uninfected) females from parous (and hence potentially infected) older females. The presence of granules or secretion in the glands of flies with empty guts indicates that they are parous and dissection for the presence of parasites is warranted. The absence of secretion in the accessory glands indicates a nulliparous fly which cannot be infected. This method is useful for many species of sandflies in the Old World, with a margin of error that may be neglected for most practical purposes, but breaks down with some sandflies, especially many South American species, where autogeny occurs or in which the accessory glands of nullipars may contain secretion for some other (unknown) reason. Females which contain blood, or the residues of a blood meal, cannot be separated into nulliparous and parous groups by this method since the glands fill with secretion very quickly after the initial feed. Lewis, Lainson and Shaw (1970) discuss the subject of the determination of parous rates in sandflies, with particular reference to New World species.

Fig. 400 shows the anatomy of the alimentary canal of sandflies insofar as this relates to the site of development of various *Leishmania* species and also indicates the location

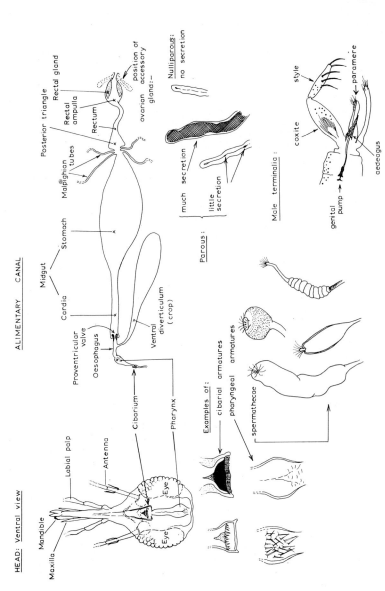

Fig. 400.—The anatomy of the alimentary canal of sandflies.

and appearance of the accessory glands of, respectively, nulliparous and parous unfed female sandflies.

Transmission of pathogens other than *Leishmania* by sandflies

Bacteria. The causative organism of Carrión's disease (Oroya fever; verruga peruana) is *Bartonella bacilliformis* and the disease occurs in Peru, Colombia and Ecuador. The only established vector is *Lutzomyia verrucarum* in Peru and a species close to, if not identical with it, in Colombia. Infections in these sandflies are confined to the proboscis and transmission, it would seem, is essentially mechanical, but the problem deserves further study. The epidemiology of the disease is not adequately known and future study may implicate other sandflies as potential or actual vectors.

Viruses. Sandfly fever (papataci fever; 3-day fever) is a viral disease of man commonly occurring during the summer months in many countries of the Mediterranean basin and the near East, including West Pakistan and part of India. The only established vector is *P. papatasi*. Epidemiological evidence strongly suggests that transovarial transmission of the virus occurs.

It is quite possible that sandflies are vectors of other viral diseases clinically similar to sandfly fever. The virus of vesicular stomatitis, a disease of livestock, has been recovered from sandflies in Panama.

Reaction to sandfly bites: harara. Persons newly exposed to the bites of *P. papatasi* and other species in parts of the Middle East often experience a severe urticarial reaction to sandfly bites after a variable time. This period of sensitization may later be followed by desensitization. Such sensitization phenomena as a result of sandfly bites are occasionally met with in a proportion of individuals exposed to sandflies in other parts of the world.

Classification and identification

Classification. Several systems of classification have been used from time to time. This results from differences of opinion concerning the status of groups of related species and whether these should be given generic or sub-generic rank or be regarded, more loosely, as 'species groups'.

The system adopted here of 4 main genera (each containing sundry subgenera and/or species groups)—2 (*Phlebotomus* and *Sergentomyia*) in the Old World and two (*Lutzomyia* and *Brumptomyia*) in the New World—is most widely used in the recent literature. Most earlier systems used a single genus (*Phlebotomus*) divided into various subgenera.

Identification. More than 500 species are recognized: most are very similar in size and outward appearance and cannot be identified with certainty until they have been suitably prepared and mounted on microscope slides. Although there are various regional keys for the identification of sandflies in different parts of the world it is always advisable to submit representative material to a specialist in the group for confirmation.

The most important taxonomic characters are found within the head capsule: these are the cibarium (buccal cavity of the early literature) and the pharynx, which vary in their morphology and armature and are similar in both sexes, although less strongly developed in the male as a rule. Other characters of major importance are the spermathecae in the female and the external genitalia of males. The genitalia of male sandflies are complex structures made up, mainly, of paired structures. Usually only one half the pair is shown in diagrammatic illustrations accompanying keys or descriptions of species. Fig. 400 gives a few examples of the characters mentioned.

Preparation and preservation of specimens. It is preferable to clear out the soft internal tissues (by soaking in potassium hydroxide solution, phenol or chloral hydrate solutions) as soon as possible after specimens are collected. Cleared specimens can be mounted on slides for examination immediately after or may be preserved in 70% alcohol indefinitely. Gum chloral mounting media are the simplest to use and in most cases are the most satisfactory. For mounting, the sandfly is placed in a drop of medium on a slide, the head is removed wholly or partly and arranged so that its ventral side is uppermost. The body, legs and wings are extended as fully as possible and a coverslip carefully lowered in place with the help of a needle, care being taken not to roll the head over.

In the absence of proper equipment and facilities, sandflies can be preserved quite satisfactorily in a dry condition, in wisps of toilet tissue loosely packed in small tubes. Specimens stored dry are, naturally, rather brittle and easily damaged.

Collection

Sandflies can be collected from their daytime resting places with simple aspirators: a torch is a useful adjunct and tobacco smoke will disturb the flies if they are not easy to see. Aspirators, or merely glass or plastic tubes of suitable size, can be used to collect sandflies attracted to human or animal baits. A few species are attracted by lights. Plastic or paper sheets *thinly* smeared with castor oil or sesame oil and put out overnight in likely places are a simple and often very effective method of catching flies. These are picked off with the tip of a brush moistened with spirit, and dipped quickly into alcohol to remove the oil. The cleaned specimens are then treated in the usual way.

Control

In areas where biting sandflies are numerous and troublesome the use of repellants, such as dimethyl phthalate and others, is warranted. The use of fine-mesh sleeping nets will also keep sandflies—and other insects—at a comfortable distance. Sandflies, moreover, are very susceptible to modern insecticides of all types and, where the cost is not prohibitive, these can be widely but selectively applied to known resting or breeding places. With domestic pests or vectors, effective control is often a fortunate by-product of antimalarial spraying of habitations (e.g. *P. papatasi* in the Middle East and *P. argentipes* in India). In areas where sandfly vectors are exophilic, house-spraying is ineffective (e.g. *P. orientalis* in the Sudan, *P. martini* and related species in Kenya).

FAMILY: CULICIDAE (Mosquitoes)

Mosquitoes (see Fig. 401) are not confined to tropical regions; many genera (including *Anopheles*) are found even within the Arctic Circle. The adult insects feed on vegetable juices; the males almost exclusively. The females of most species suck the blood of mammals and birds. Many act as carriers of disease. They lay eggs singly on the surface of water, in groups, or in raft-like masses. Hatching out depends upon temperature. In some species the eggs remain dormant throughout the winter, or in drought. In ordinary circumstances the larvae hatch out in 2 or 3 days, then feed upon organic matter suspended in water. They breathe in air through the respiratory siphon situated near their tails. The larval stage lasts from 6 days to several weeks, usually 10 days. They moult 4 times before pupating.

The pupa is free and active for 2–4 days. It does not feed, but rests on the surface. Eventually the pupal case splits and the mosquito works its way out. The abdomen is contracted, and blood is forced into the wings, which then expand. The mosquito rests $\frac{1}{4}$–$\frac{1}{2}$ hour on its pupal case until its wings and body have hardened.

In Europe the whole process from egg to imago occupies about 1 month, but in the tropics 7 to 10 days. During colder weather development of the larva is temporarily suspended and the surviving adults, especially females, hibernate in dark and sheltered places. In this manner the species is carried over the winter. In some varieties there is evidence that hibernation is carried out in the egg and larval stages. The life of an adult mosquito is variable, but some species, if supplied with suitable food, can live for several months.

Although most mosquitoes are singularly local, yet migrations are occasionally observed, and the insects are often transported great distances in ships, railway carriages or airplanes, and widely diffused. A few species in most genera are domestic. The majority feed at night, though some *Aedes* spp. do so by day.

For classification various structures need to be identified as follows. There are 3 recognizable divisions: head, thorax and abdomen (Fig. 401). The head is rounded and attached to the thorax by a slender neck. It is provided with large eyes, antennae and mouth-parts. The antennae (Figs 401–3) are composed of 15 segments. Each bears a whorl of hairs in the female, but in the male the hairs are profuse, giving a bristly appearance. The mouth-parts consist of a proboscis in the female fitted for piercing and sucking. Externally, a chitinized labium (Fig. 404) encloses the other mouth-parts,

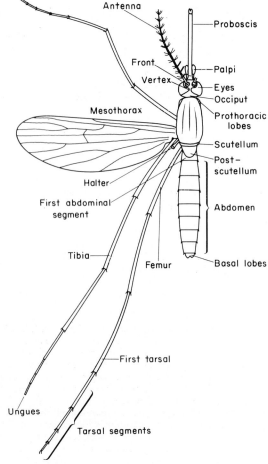

Fig. 401.—The anatomy of the female culicine mosquito. Note the short palps: those of anophelines are much longer.

except the maxillary palpi, and ends distally in 2 pointed labellae clothed with scales and hairs. The labrum is a hollow cylindrical tube with a narrow opening on the ventral surface. In the act of biting, the labellae part and are applied to the surface of the skin, forming a sheath for the delicate piercing organs, and do not enter the wound made for obtaining blood. Within is the labrum epipharynx, composed of 2 thin chitinous lamellae imposed on each other, forming a V-shaped channel which is open on the ventral surface. This extends along the whole length of the labium and ends in a sharp point. Lying directly beneath the labrum-epipharynx, closing the ventral slit, is the hypopharynx, consisting of a thin, chitinous lamella, fitting closely to the ventral surface of the labrum epipharynx, thus forming a tube through which blood is sucked. In the longitudinal chitinous thickening runs a very fine channel extending from base to tip of the hypopharynx; through this the salivary secretion is poured into the wound (Fig. 405). The mandibles are delicate chitinous structures at the side of the hypopharynx. The labium buckles in the act of biting, and the mouth-parts emerge. Each of these tapers slightly towards the tip, ending in a sharp point. The maxillae are more

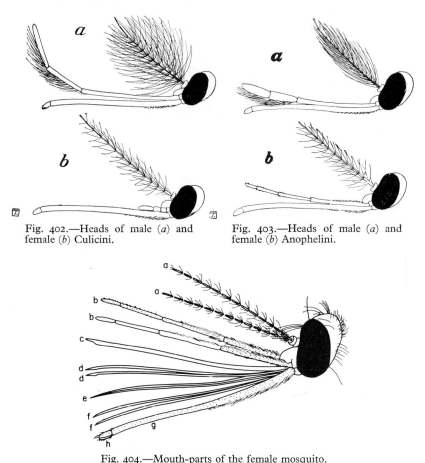

Fig. 402.—Heads of male (a) and female (b) Culicini.

Fig. 403.—Heads of male (a) and female (b) Anophelini.

Fig. 404.—Mouth-parts of the female mosquito.

a, antennae. b, palpi. c, labrum-epipharynx. d, mandibles. e, hypopharynx. f, maxillae. g, labium. h, labella.

robustly constructed, but have the same general form, the tip is generally provided with a row of backward projecting teeth. The maxillary palpi consist of 3–5 segments. In the male the mouth-parts are greatly modified and not adapted for piercing. The maxillary palpi are elongated, extending beyond the top of the proboscis, but the mandibles and maxillae are greatly reduced and may be lacking altogether.

In the female anophelines the palpi are as long as the proboscis and usually closely applied, but in female culicines the palpi are short. In both male anopheline and culicine mosquitoes the palpi are as long as the proboscis. The palpi of the male culicines are bushy, and the 2 terminal joints tend to turn upwards; those of the male anophelines are rather club-shaped.

The thorax is wedged-shaped: the sides form the pleura, whilst the apex bears the legs and spiracles which are prominent black-rimmed apertures. The various sclerites composing the side of the thorax bear stiff setae or hairs, arranged in definite groups. The scutellum is separated by a transverse suture from the mesonotum. In all genera, except *Anopheles*, it is trilobate, and each lobe bears a group of stiff setae. In anophelines

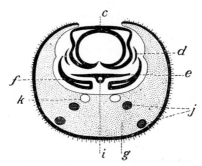

Fig. 405.—Section of the mosquito's proboscis. (*After Nuttall & Shipley*)

c, labrum-epipharynx. *d*, mandible. *e*, hypopharynx. *f*, maxillae. *g*, labium. *i*, salivary duct. *j*, muscles. *k*, trachea.

the scutellum is arcuate. The region behind the scutellum is known as postnotum and is generally nude. The wings are long and narrow with venation (Fig. 406); the scales are characteristic. Situated immediately posterior to the base of the wings is a pair of halteres or balancers, which are sense organs connected with flight (Fig. 401).

The legs are long and slender, composed of coxa, trochanter, femur and tibia, and a tarsus of 5 joints, the last of which is long and slender, especially in the hind legs. The last tarsal joint bears a pair of claws (ungues), which vary greatly in size and shape, but

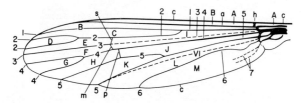

Fig. 406.—Wing of a male *Culex*, illustrating the male terminology.

a, auxiliary vein. *c*, costa. 1–6, first to sixth longitudinal veins and branches. 7, seventh or false (unscaled) longitudinal vein. *h*, humeral transverse vein. *p*, posterior transverse vein. *s*, supernumerary transverse vein. *A*, costal cells. *B*, subcostal cells. *C*, marginal cells. *D*, anterior fork cell of first submarginal cell. *E*, second submarginal cell. *F*, First posterior cell. *G*, Hinder fork or second posterior cell. *I*, first basal cell. *J*. second basal cell. *K*, anal cell. *L*, axillary cell. *M*, spurious cell. *VI*, unscaled vein between fifth and sixth longitudinal veins.

those of the hind legs are generally smaller than those of others. The abdomen is nearly cylindrical, narrow and elongated, consisting of 10 segments. The first 8 are quite similar, but the terminal segments are modified for sexual purposes. The terminal segment in the female is pointed. The ninth is reduced, and in the intersegmental area between it and the eighth lies the opening of the reproductive organs. The tenth segment is greatly reduced and bears the basal lobes (cerci) and anal opening. The abdomen of the male is frequently longer than that of the female. The terminal segments are greatly modified and bear clasping organs. In the male the seventh and eighth segments undergo torsion through an arc of 180° after emergence from the pupa, with the result that the eighth tergite and those distal to it become ventrally situated, and the sternite dorsal.

The foregut and midgut are ectodermal, lined with chitin, continuous with the cuticle. Columnar epithelium lines the midgut. The entrance of the 5 Malpighian tubes marks the junction of hind and midguts. There are 3 salivary glands on each side. In the

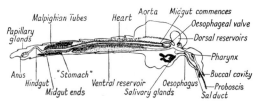

Fig. 407.—Longitudinal section of a female mosquito to show the anatomy.

genus *Anopheles* the middle lobe of the trilobal salivary gland is always shorter than the lateral lobes, whereas in culicines the three lobes are of approximately equal length. In the female anopheline only one spermatheca is present, whereas in culicines there are 2 or 3. Various diverticula branch off from the gut.

Dissection of mosquito

After chloroforming, the insect is placed on a slide in a drop of saline; the wings and legs are cut off. For dissection of the salivary glands one needle is applied behind the head and a second held horizontally on the thorax. The head is pulled forward, dragging out the salivary glands: this movement should be done in stages, with frequent jerks. Next the head is removed from the glands and the preparation covered with a coverslip. Examined under 4 mm objective, refractile sporozoites can be seen in a malaria-infected *Anopheles*. For dissection of the gut, the rectum is pressed up and down with pointed needle and then the body is cut through near the termination of the rectum. Gentle traction draws out the rectum and gut in a series of jerks. These are covered with a coverslip and examined. The tracery of fine black lines over the stomach denotes the tracheae, and this feature can be used for focusing down with 4 mm objective in order to demonstrate malarial oöcysts.

SUBFAMILIES: ANOPHELINAE; CULICINAE

TRIBE: ANOPHELINI

GENUS: *Anopheles*

The palpi in both sexes are as long, or nearly as long, as the proboscis. The scutellum is rounded, without lobes, and the eggs are laid singly.

The subfamily Anophelinae was divided by Edwards into 3 genera: *Chagasia* (scutellum slightly trilobed), *Bironella* (scutellum evenly rounded, wing with stem of median fork wavy) and *Anopheles* (scutellum evenly rounded, wing with stem of median fork straight). The genus includes over 160 species. The commoner kinds, whilst resting, hold the proboscis, head and abdomen nearly in a straight line, and give the appearance of a splinter lifted at an angle from a surface; exceptionally, as in *A. culicifacies*, the resting position adopted is more culex-like (see Fig. 417). Usually the hum produced by these mosquitoes is low-pitched, almost inaudible unless close to the ear. Most of them are not strong fliers, and seek cover, even in a moderate breeze, yet dispersal flights may carry individuals 10 or more miles from their breeding places. The flight range is usually 3–4·5 km.

Fertilization of the female takes place directly upon emergence from the pupa. The males emerge first, and swarm over the breeding places awaiting the females; when the

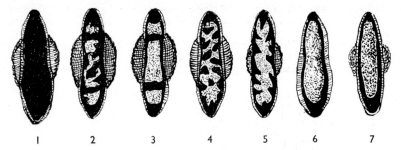

1	2	3	4	5	6	7

Fig. 408.—Eggs of the *Anopheles maculipennis* complex. 1, *Melanoon*. 2, *Messeae*, 3, *Typicus*. 4, *Atroparvus*. 5, *Labranchiae*. 6, *Sacharovi* (summer). 7, *Sacharovi* (spring and autumn). The main difference between 2 and 3 is that 2 has 2 chevrons. 6 has no floats, 5 very small, and 4 medium; 1, 2 and 3 have large floats. 1 has about 20 ribs in the float without striations; 2 and 3 about 20 ribs with coarse striations; 5 has 10–12 ribs with striations. (*After Shute*)

insects dart into a dancing mass, mating occurs. Most species require wide spaces for mating, rendering it difficult to propagate them in captivity. Over-wintering females are fertilized by the last brood of the males during autumn; the eggs are deposited soon after the spring dispersal flight. The boat-shaped eggs (Fig. 408), with rare exceptions, have an investing membrane inflated laterally to form a pair of floats. These represent an air-filled space between the exochorion and the endochorion of the egg shell to resist submersion. The anopheline eggs are 1 mm in length. They are white

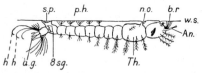

Fig. 409.—Larva of *Anopheles maculipennis*, showing the feeding position. (*After Marshall*)

An, antennae. *a.g.*, anal gills. *b.r.*, mouth brush. *h*, hooked (grapnel) hairs. *n.o.*, notched organ. *p.h.*, palmate (float) hairs. *s.p.*, spiracles. *Th.*, thorax. *w.s.*, water surface. 8 *sg.*, eighth abdominal segment.

when freshly laid, but change to dull brown or black within a few hours. They arrange themselves in a distinct pattern on the surface of the water. They are laid singly on the surface of the water and hatch in 2–3 days. The larva during growth undergoes 4 moults The cuticle is laid down by a single layer of epidermal cells, which form a new and folded cuticle, the larva inflating itself by swallowing water before the new cuticle hardens. The larva feeds on small floating particles swept into its mouth by two feeding brushes which can be folded under its head. When *Anopheles* larvae lie on the surface,

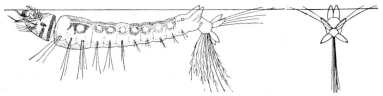

Fig. 410.—Larva of *Anopheles maculipennis* Meigen, showing the breathing position at the surface of the water. (*After Howard*)

the dorsal aspect of the thorax and abdomen faces upwards, but the head is rotated 180° so that its ventral surface lies upwards (Fig. 409). Food consists of living organisms, bacteria and protozoa obtained beneath the surface. The head of the larva is complex: the central portion is known as the clypeus, the anterior plaque as the preclypeus. It has a pair of short antennae, eyes, a pair of feeding brushes, and preclypeal and clypeal hairs. The respiratory opening is composed of two dorsally placed spiracles on the eighth abdominal segment. There is no respiratory syphon (Fig. 410).

The larva maintains itself on the surface in a horizontal position by a row of dorsoabdominal plaques, palmate hairs and a series of scales in rosette form on its back. The terminal segment is provided with four anal papillae (gills), dorsal and ventral,

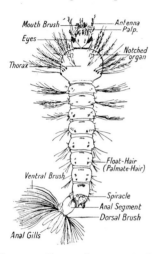

Fig. 411.—Larva of an anopheline (*A. maculipennis*) from above. The anal segment is twisted round to display the dorsal and ventral brushes. (*After Marshall*)

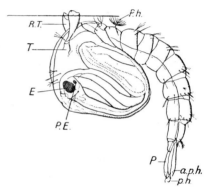

Fig. 412.—Pupa of *Anopheles maculipennis*. (*After Marshall*)

E, eye. P, paddle. P.E., pupal eye. P.h., paddle hair. A.p.h., accessory paddle hair. R.T., respiratory trumpet. T, trachea leading to anterior thoracic spiracle.

and swimming brushes (Fig. 411). The gills have no respiratory function, but take up chlorides from the water. The eighth segment is adorned with a chitinous plate lying between the two openings of the spiracles, and just below it there is a row of teeth arising from a chitinized base and the structure is known as the *pecten*. Trachae run the length of the body with branches extending to all regions. Small glands secrete a waxy substance near the spiracles, which therefore cannot be wetted. (It is important to note this fact in oiling water to kill larvae.) Respiration also takes place through the cuticle, but the oxygen intake from the water is not sufficient to maintain life, except when the temperature is low and metabolism is reduced. The pupae are distinguished by the shape of the respiratory trumpets and by the presence of a paddle hair (Fig. 412).

The stages of metamorphosis are egg, larva, pupa and imago. The casting of successive larval skins is termed *ecdysis*. In each stage the head remains unchanged. The fourth ecdysis determines the final larval stage (fourth stage larva) and results in *pupation*, followed by emergence of the imago. The deposition of eggs is *oviposition*.

Gonotrophic cycle

Fertilization is evidenced by packing the spermatheca with spermatozoa and as blood is digested so the ovaries enlarge. The complete cycle from feeding to oviposition completes the gonotrophic cycle and extends over a period of 2–3 or more days.

The blood meal may be obtained from man, cattle or other animals or birds. *Anthro-*

pophilic, Zoophilic and *Neutrophilic* are terms which indicate preferences for feeding upon man, cattle or both indiscriminately. Animals, especially cattle, can be used to lure some species from feeding on man.

Only the adult females are able to suck blood, but they do also feed on fruit juices in late summer when the grapes are ripe. The males feed on flower and fruit juices. The females can survive, but cannot lay eggs, on a diet of vegetable juices; this function needs a rich protein meal. They usually suck blood at night, but times vary with the species, and in dark rooms they may feed during the daytime.

The capabilities of any particular species of anopheles to transmit malaria are regulated by a number of factors, such as the numbers present, whether the parasites of malaria can complete their development in the mosquito, anthropophilism (readiness to feed in nature on human blood), and whether the insects feed in the open or readily enter houses. The term 'zoophilism' is employed when the insect is deviated by animals, i.e. cattle, as habitually happens with races of *A. maculipennis*.

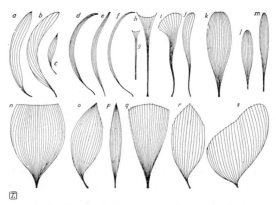

Fig. 413.—Graphic key to distinctions based on scale characters. *a, b, c,* Narrow curved scales. *d, e, f,* Hair-like curved scales. *g, h,* Upright forked scales. *i, j,* Long twisted scales. *k,* Large lanceolate scale. *l, m,* Small narrow lanceolate scales. *n,* Large expanded scale. *o, p,* Spindle-shaped scales. *q,* Broad flat scale. *r, s,* Broad irregular scales.

The terms 'exophily' and 'endophily' are applied to those mosquitoes which feed and rest outside and inside dwellings, respectively. Exophilic species do not come into contact with insecticides sprayed inside dwellings, and are therefore difficult to kill.

A species proved to be a natural carrier in one situation does not necessarily play an important part somewhere else.

There is a striking correlation between the incidence of malaria and of *Anopheles* as seen in the case of *A. punctulatus* complex, which occurs on some islands in the South Pacific, but not on others. Where these species occur there is malaria; where they do not, there is none.

Nomenclature is a vexed question. A great many species have been renamed in recent years. In case of doubt recourse should be made to the *Index Insectorum* and the monumental publications of the British Museum by Edwards, and the *Synoptic Catalog of the Mosquitoes of the World*.

In making a malaria survey an attempt should be made to identify female ano-phelines; they should be collected and dissected to find out which species is infected. It is necessary to dissect several hundred insects and to examine the gut and salivary glands. An infection rate of 5% is usually heavy, though higher rates are recorded in Africa. Adults and larvae should be identified to determine dangerous carriers. The locality should be studied for at least a complete year. Seasonal transmission is important; one species may be responsible in spring and another during the autumn.

Identification of the many diverse species of *Anopheles* is specialized work. The following points are of specific importance: size, general coloration, colour of frontal tuft on the head (yellow or white), and character of the scales (Fig. 413). The distal half of the proboscis may be pale, the palpi may be smooth or shaggy, depending on the scales. The markings (banding) on palpi may be entirely dark or there may be pale bands. The general coloration of the thorax and scales on the mesonotum is helpful. The scales on the wings may be entirely dark, or may have 4 pale areas. The third vein may be entirely dark or pale. Pale spots may be present on the fringe opposite the various veins. Speckling, or banding, of the legs is an important point, and the presence or absence of lateral tufts or buttons of the large scales on the abdomen. In scientific entomology, besides morphological characters of adult females, those of fourth instar larvae and of eggs are important in identification. These features are too intricate to be detailed here, and identification depends upon detailed characters listed in the published keys.

The distribution and importance of some species of *Anopheles* have been changed in recent years as a result of control or eradication programmes in which residual insecticides have been used. Some strains and species have shown resistance to insecticides,

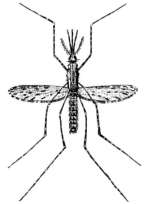

Fig. 414.—*Anopheles gambiae*. One of a series of drawings made by the late Sir Philip Manson-Bahr, showing the wing markings characteristic of *Anopheles*. × 6.

and some species are less susceptible than others to insecticides sprayed indoors because either they tend to leave buildings after feeding, without resting on treated walls, or they tend to bite and rest in the open and therefore do not come into contact with insecticides.

Much success has been achieved in eradication programmes in subtropical areas, and in some parts of the tropics, but even where eradication has been almost complete, there have been renewed outbreaks of malaria, as in Ceylon. Such outbreaks can occur if surveillance is insufficient, and mosquitoes are allowed to breed, even in small numbers, to multiply enormously if conditions change so as to stimulate breeding.

In most parts of tropical Africa malaria transmission has hardly changed, though where intensive insecticide spraying has been carried out, *A. funestus* has been eliminated, though it could re-enter the area from the periphery when spraying is discontinued. The main vectors, members of the *A. gambiae* complex (*A. gambiae* A and B, *A. melas*) breed so prolifically in so many collections of water, and bite man so voraciously indoors and in the open, that control by insecticides is extremely difficult. *A. gambiae* C and *A. merus* (which breeds in crab holes in East Africa) are not important carriers.

In addition to malaria, *Anopheles* species transmit *Wuchereria bancrofti*; most of the malaria-carrying species being implicated (see page 197). *Anopheles* also transmit several arboviruses, for instance EEE, WEE, VEE, o'nyong-nyong.

Table 49.* Geographical distribution of the main malaria-carrying species of *Anopheles* (Subgenera: *Anopheles* (*A.*), *Cellia* (*C.*), *Kerteszia* (*K.*) and *Nyssorhynchus* (*N.*)

Palearctic region	North Europe	East Europe	North U.S.S.R.	Mediterranean	Balkans	North Africa	Near East	South U.S.S.R.	Iran, Iraq	Pakistan, Afghanistan
(A.) claviger (Meigen)	+			+		+	+	+	+	+
(C.) hispaniola (Theobald)				+		+				
(A.) labranchiae Falleroni				+		+				
(A.) l. atroparvus van Thiel	+	+	+	+						
(A.) maculipennis Meigen	+	+					+		+	+
(A.) m. messeae Falleroni	+	+	+	+				+		
(C.) multicolor Cambouliu				+		+	+	+	+	+
(A.) sacharovi Favre	+			+		+	+		+	+
(C.) sergenti (Theobald)						+	+			+
(C.) superpictus Grassi				+	+	+		+	+	+

Nearctic region	Canada	U.S.A.	South U.S.A., Mexico
(A.) freeborni Aitken	+	+	+
(A.) quadrimaculatus Say	+	+	+

Neotropical region	South U.S.A., Mexico	Central America	Caribbean	South America
(N.) albimanus Wiedemann	+	+	+	+
(N.) albitarsis Lynch Arribálzaga			+	+
(N.) aquasalis Curry			+	+
(K.) bellator Dyar & Knab			+	+
(K.) cruzi Dyar & Knab				+
(N.) darlingi Root	+	+		+
(N.) nuñez-tovari Gabaldón				+
(A.) pseudopunctipennis Theobald	+	+	+	+
(A.) punctimacula Dyar & Knab	+	+		+

* Tables 49, 50 and 51 are constructed on the basis of Faust and Russell (1964) with modifications from other sources.

Table 49.—continued.

Oriental region	Persian Gulf	Indian subcontinent	Malaya, Indochina	Indonesia	Philippines	Borneo	South China	North China
(C.) *aconitus* Dönitz		+	+	+		+		
(C.) *annularis* van der Wulp		+	+	+	+	+	+	
(C.) *balabacensis* Baisas		+	+	+	+	+		
(A.) *barbirostris* van der Wulp			+	+	+		+	
(C.) *culicifacies* Giles	+	+	+				+	
(C.) *fluviatilis* James	+	+	+				+	
(C.) *jeyporiensis* James		+	+				+	
(C.) *jeyporiensis candidiensis* Koizumi		+	+				+	
(A.) *letifer* Sandosham			+	+		+		
(C.) *leucosphyrus* Dönitz		+	+	+		+		
(C.) *maculatus* Theobald		+	+	+	+		+	
(C.) *mangyanus* (Banks)					+			
(C.) *minimus* Theobald		+	+				+	
(C.) *minimus flavirostris* (Ludlow)				+	+	+		
(A.) *nigerrimus* Giles		+	+				+	
(C.) *pattoni* Christophers								+
(C.) *philippinensis* Ludlow		+	+	+	+	+	+	
(A.) *sinensis* Wiedemann		+	+				+	+
(C.) *stephensi* Liston	+						+	
(C.) *sundaicus* (Rodenwaldt)		+	+	+		+	+	
(A.) *umbrosus* (Theobald)		+	+	+	+			
(C.) *varuna* Iyengar		+						

Ethiopian region	West Africa	East Africa	Central Africa	Sudan, Arabia	Near East
(C.) *funestus* Giles	+	+	+	+	
(C.) *gambiae A & B* Giles	+	+	+	+	
(C.) *melas* (Theobald)	+				
(C.) *moucheti* Evans	+	+		+	
(C.) *nili* (Theobald)	+	+	+	+	
(C.) *pharoensis* Theobald	+	+		+	+

Australasian region	Australia	New Guinea	Pacific Islands
(C.) *farauti* Laveran	+	+	+
(C.) *koliensis* Owen		+	+
(C.) *punctulatus* Dönitz		+	+

Table 50. Feeding and resting habits of the main malaria-carrying species of *Anopheles* (Subgenera: *Anopheles* (*A.*), *Cellia* (*C.*), *Kerteszia* (*K.*) and *Nyssorhynchus* (*N.*))

	Usually feed on man indoors	Usually feed on animals	Feed on either man or animals	Usually feed on man outdoors	Usually rest indoors in day-time	Usually rest outdoors in day-time	Rest either indoors or outdoors
Palearctic region							
(*A.*) *claviger* (Meigen)			+				+
(*C.*) *hispaniola* (Theobald)			+				+
(*A.*) *labranchiae* Falleroni	+				+		
(*A.*) *l. atroparvus* van Thiel	+				+		
(*A.*) *maculipennis* Meigen			+		+		
(*A.*) *m. messeae* Falleroni		+					+
(*C.*) *multicolor* Cambouliu	+						+
(*A.*) *sacharovi* Favre	+				+		
(*C.*) *sergenti* (Theobald)	+				+		
(*C.*) *superpictus* Grassi	+				+		
Ethiopian region							
(*C.*) *funestus* Giles	+				+		
(*C.*) *gambiae A & B* Giles	+				+		
(*C.*) *melas* (Theobald)	+				+		
(*C.*) *moucheti* Evans	+				+		
(*C.*) *nili* (Theobald)			+				+
(*C.*) *pharoensis* Theobald			+	+			+
Oriental region							
(*C.*) *aconitus* Dönitz			+		+		
(*C.*) *annularis* van der Wulp			+				+
(*C.*) *balabacensis* Baisas	+			+			+
(*A.*) *barbirostris* van der Wulp			+			+	
(*C.*) *culicifacies* Giles			+		+		
(*C.*) *fluviatilis* James	+					+	
(*C.*) *jeyporiensis* James	+					+	
(*C.*) *jeyporiensis candidiensis* Koizumi	+					+	
(*A.*) *letifer* Sandosham	+					+	
(*C.*) *leucosphyrus* Dönitz	+				+		
(*C.*) *maculatus* Theobald			+			+	
(*C.*) *mangyanus* (Banks)			+			+	
(*C.*) *minimus* Theobald	+				+		
(*C.*) *minimus flavirostris* (Ludlow)			+			+	
(*A.*) *nigerrimus* Giles		+				+	
(*C.*) *pattoni* Christophers			+				
(*C.*) *philippinensis* Ludlow			+				+
(*A.*) *sinensis* Wiedemann		+				+	
(*C.*) *stephensi* Liston	+				+		
(*C.*) *sundaicus* (Rodenwaldt)			+	+			+
(*A.*) *umbrosus* (Theobald)	+					+	
(*C.*) *varuna* Iyengar			+		+		

Table 50.—continued.

	Usually feed on man indoors	Usually feed on animals	Feed on either man or animals	Usually feed on man outdoors	Usually rest indoors in daytime	Usually rest outdoors in daytime	Rest either indoors or outdoors
Australasian region							
(C.) *farauti* Laveran	+					+	
(C.) *koliensis* Owen	+				+		
(C.) *punctulatus* Dönitz			+			+	
Nearctic region							
(A.) *freeborni* Aitken	+				+		
(A.) *quadrimaculatus* Say	+				+		
Neotropical region							
(N.) *albimanus* Wiedemann			+			+	
(N.) *albitarsis* Lynch Arribálzaga			+			+	
(N.) *aquasalis* Curry			+		+		
(K.) *bellator* Dyar & Knab	+			+		+	
(K.) *cruzii* Dyar & Knab			+			+	
(N.) *darlingi* Root	+				+		
(N.) *nuñez-tovari* Gabaldón	+			+			+
(A.) *pseudopunctipennis* Theobald			+		+		
(A.) *punctimacula* Dyar & Knab			+		+		

Table 51. Common breeding waters of the main malaria-carrying species of *Anopheles* (Subgenera: *Anopheles* (*A.*), *Cellia* (*C.*), *Kerteszia* (*K.*) and *Nyssorhynchus* (*N.*))

	Household utensils	Puddles	Pools, ponds, lakes	Seepages, springs	Wells, cisterns	Rice fields	Running streams, canals	Brackish swamps, marshes	Shade	Sunlight	Shade or sunlight	Bromeliads
Palearctic region												
(*A.*) *claviger* (Meigen)		+	+	+								
(*C.*) *hispaniola* (Theobald)		+			+					+		
(*A.*) *labranchiae* Falleroni		+	+	+	+	+	+			+		
(*A.*) *l. atroparvus* van Thiel					+			+		+		
(*A.*) *maculipennis* Meigen					+	+				+		
(*A.*) *m. messeae* Falleroni		+								+		
(*C.*) *multicolor* Cambouliu		+		+				+			+	
(*A.*) *sacharovi* Favre		+	+					+			+	
(*C.*) *sergenti* (Theobald)		+	+			+	+	+		+		
(*C.*) *superpictus* Grassi		+				+	+			+		
Ethiopian region												
(*C.*) *funestus* Giles			+	+			+					
(*C.*) *gambiae A & B* Giles	+	+	+				+	+			+	
(*C.*) *melas* (Theobald)								+				
(*C.*) *moucheti* Evans				+			+					
(*C.*) *nili* (Theobald)							+			+		
(*C.*) *pharoensis* Theobald			+		+	+	+			+		
Oriental region												
(*C.*) *aconitus* Dönitz			+				+	+				
(*C.*) *annularis* van der Wulp			+				+	+				
(*C.*) *balabacensis* Baisas			+	+					+			
(*A.*) *barbirostris* van der Wulp			+	+	+	+	+	+	+			
(*C.*) *culicifacies* Giles			+	+	+	+	+	+				
(*C.*) *fluviatilis* James			+	+			+					
(*C.*) *jeyporiensis* James			+	+			+	+				
(*C.*) *jeyporiensis candidiensis* Koizumi			+	+	+		+					
(*A.*) *letifer* Sandosham	+	+								+		
(*C.*) *leucosphyrus* Dönitz	+	+		+						+		
(*C.*) *maculatus* Theobald			+	+		+	+				+	
(*C.*) *mangyanus* (Banks)				+			+					
(*C.*) *minimus* Theobald			+	+		+	+				+	
(*C.*) *minimus flavirostris* (Ludlow)				+			+					+
(*A.*) *nigerrimus* Giles			+				+					
(*C.*) *pattoni* Christophers			+				+					
(*C.*) *philippinensis* Ludlow			+		+	+						
(*A.*) *sinensis* Wiedemann			+		+	+						
(*C.*) *stephensi* Liston	+				+							
(*C.*) *sundaicus* (Rodenwaldt)								+				
(*A.*) *umbrosus* (Theobald)			+					+	+	+		
(*C.*) *varuna* Iyengar			+		+	+						

Table 51.—continued.

	Household utensils	Puddles	Pools, ponds, lakes	Seepages, springs	Wells, cisterns	Rice fields	Running streams, canals	Brackish swamps, marshes	Shade	Sunlight	Shade or sunlight	Bromeliads
Australasian region												
(C.) *farauti* Laveran		+	+	+			+				+	
(C.) *koliensis* Owen		+								+		
(C.) *punctulatus* Dönitz		+	+				+				+	+
Nearctic region												
(A.) *freeborni* Aitken		+	+	+		+	+		+			
(A.) *quadrimaculatus* Say		+					+				+	+
Neotropical region												
(N.) *albimanus* Wiedemann			+	+	+	+		+		+		
(N.) *albitarsis* Lynch Arribálzaga	+		+				+			+		
(N.) *aquasalis* Curry							+	+	+			
(K.) *bellator* Dyar & Knab												+
(K.) *cruzii* Dyar & Knab												+
(N.) *darlingi* Root			+						+			
(N.) *nuñez-tovari* Gabaldón			+									
(A.) *pseudopunctipennis* Theobald			+	+					+			
(A.) *punctimacula* Dyar & Knab			+					+	+			

TRIBE: CULICINI

This large tribe contains over 500 species and some 20 genera. The scutellum is trilobed, each lobe bearing bristles. The abdomen is blunt and completely clothed with broad flat scales. The eighth segment of the larva is drawn out into a respiratory siphon with a well developed pecten and 4 gills provided with tufts of hairs situated on a projection anterior to the respiratory siphon. Culicines living in water with little chloride have large anal gills. There are no rosettes or palmate hairs as in *Anopheles*. The pupae are similar to those of *Anopheles*, but the respiratory trumpets are longer.

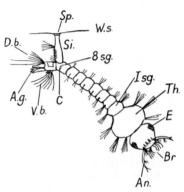

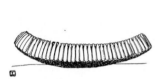

Fig. 415.—Egg raft of *Culex fatigans*. (*After Sambon*)

Fig. 416.—Larvae of *Culex fatigans*. (*After Marshall*)

A.g., anal gills. *An.*, antennae. *Br*, mouth brush. *C*, comb on eighth abdominal segment. *D.b.*, dorsal brush. *E*, eye. 1 *sg*, first abdominal segment. 8 *sg*, eighth abdominal segment. *Si.*, siphon. *Sp.*, spiracle. *Th.*, thorax. *W.s.*, water surface. *V.b.*, ventral brush.

The following are the main characteristics of culicines in contradistinction to those of anophelines:

1. The eggs are not provided with air floats, and are either laid separately or stacked in rafts (Fig. 415).

2. The larva breathes through a pair of spiracles, situated at the tip of a tail-like tube or siphon, projecting dorsally from the eighth abdominal segment. It hangs head downwards from the water surface, supported by the capillary action of five hinged valves surrounding the tip of the siphon. It sweeps for floating, as well as suspended,

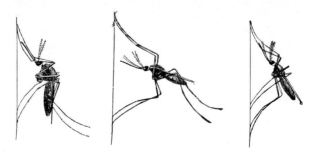

Fig. 417.—The resting positions of *Culex fatigans*, *Anopheles hyrcanus* and *Anopheles maculipennis*.

particles of food with mouth brushes below surface level, or else dives to the bottom (Fig. 416).

3. The pupa has cylindrical respiratory trumpets and usually a branched hair at each 'apical' corner of 3–7 abdominal segments. It has no accessory hair on the ventral surface of the paddle.

4. The adult has an abdomen densely covered with scales. The female has short and slender palps, from one-fifth to one-half as long as the proboscis. The male has, as a rule, long hairy palps which have a 'plume-like' appearance. These mosquitoes usually rest with proboscis and abdomen forming an obtuse angle, the abdomen being more or less parallel with the supporting surface (Fig. 417).

GENUS: *Culex* (Linnaeus)

Species of *Culex* are important because they transmit *Wuchereria bancrofti* from man to man (see page 197), and some arboviruses from birds, horses and other animals to man. The fact that some species of *Culex* have been found to be infected with arboviruses in nature does not necessarily mean that they transmit them, but transmission experiments have been conducted on a number of species, with positive results.

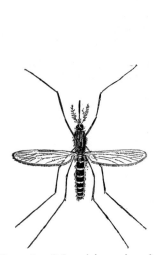
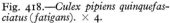
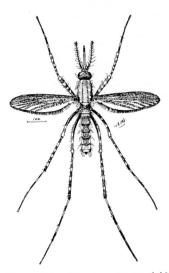

Fig. 418.—*Culex pipiens quinquefasciatus* (*fatigans*). × 4.

Fig. 419.—Female *Mansonioides annulifera* (Theo.). (*After McKay*)

The following species have been found infected with arboviruses in nature (they are all of the subgenus *Culex*):

C. (C.) *annulirostris*
C. (C.) *gelidus*
C. (C.) *tarsalis*
C. (C.) *thalassius*
C. (C.) *tritaeniorhynchus*
C. (C.) *univittatus*

Many of these harboured more than one type of arbovirus. C. (C.) *pipiens pipiens* and C. (C.) *pipiens quinquefasciatus* (*fatigans*) have also been found infected, but rarely.

In mosquitoes susceptible to filariae the parasite penetrates the gut wall and develops normally in the cells of the thoracic muscles. In refractory mosquitoes it reaches the thoracic muscles and develops no further. The gene controlling susceptibility (f^m) is sex-linked and susceptibility is recessive. Heterozygotes for the gene (f^m/F) are refractory (MacDonald 1962).

Since the arthropod hosts of filariae can be damaged by the larval stages their mortality depends upon the relative susceptibility of the strain of mosquito.

Species of *Culex* also transmit malaria parasites of several species in birds.

Some species of *Culex* breed in water which would not attract anophelines. For instance the characteristic habitat of *C. quinquefasciatus* (*fatigans*) is fresh water polluted by decaying organic matter, in which there is a complete absence of all living organisms other than bacteria. In Rangoon it breeds in underground drains (it can breed in the dark), culverts, septic tanks, grit chambers, soakage pits, latrine pits, wells, tanks and pools. It also breeds in water tubs and other domestic sources. A disturbance of a road drainage system or of a sewerage system (for instance by failure of upkeep) can cause enormous increase in a *Culex* population, and could lead to an increase in the diseases these mosquitoes carry.

Females are avid of human blood, and less so of animal blood; they also feed on fruit, as do males. They are nocturnal in habit.

Adult *Culex* are resistant to many insecticides, but fenthion 50% emulsifiable concentrate, diluted in water and sprayed at 0·38% dosage to make a concentration of 1 ppm has been successful as a larvicide in Rangoon.

GENUS: *Mansonia* (*Taeniorhynchus*) (Edwards)
SUBGENUS: *Mansonioides* (Theobald) (Fig. 419)

This genus occurs in tropical and Central America, tropical Africa, and in Asia especially Malaysia, but is less important in temperate North America, Europe, and

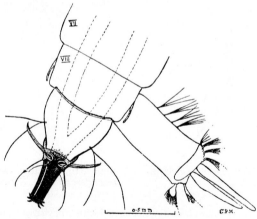

Fig. 420.—Respiratory syphon and terminal segments of larva of *Mansonioides* (dorsal view). (*After Poynton & Hodgkin*)

Australia. These mosquitoes are recognizable by the very broad asymmetrical wing scales, which are of two colours, white and grey, like salt and pepper, but which do not make conspicuous pale and dark areas. The palpi of the male are longer than the proboscis; the penultimate segment is turned upwards, while the last segment is minute, and is turned downwards. The end of the abdomen of the female curves upwards, so that only 6½ segments are visible dorsally. The eighth segment is entirely retracted, is of a peculiar form, and carries a row of strongly chitinized teeth on the tergite. The arrangement of these teeth and the shape of the lobes of the sternite are of value in identification. There are 5 species of importance which are concerned with the transmission of *Brugia malayi*: *M. annulata* Leic., *M. annulifera* Theo., *M. indiana* Edwards, *M. dives* (Schiner) and *M. uniformis* Theo. The members of this subgenus are of little or no importance as vectors of *W. bancrofti*.

The larvae of *Mansonioides* are readily recognizable by the peculiar form of the respiratory siphon, which is adapted for piercing plant tissues (Fig. 420). This structure is short, and has a conical base and a distinctive black tip made up of several parts, one of which has a saw edge and ends in a ring of retractable hooks. The known larvae closely resemble one another. The pupae are also distinguishable by the form of the respiratory horns which, like the siphon of the larvae, are modified for piercing plant tissues (Fig. 421). Each horn is long and terminates in a narrow, strongly chitinized portion, which bears a pair of feather-like structures and ends in a sharp point. All species of *Mansonia* are man-hunters and fierce biters, and attack either in or out of doors. Primarily night-biters, in the jungle they feed at any time. The eggs are laid in small batches, containing 100 or more, on the underside of leaves of water plants

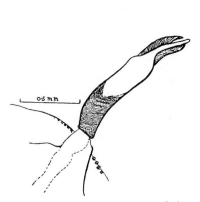

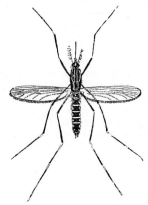

0·5 mm

Fig. 421.—Respiratory horn of the pupa of *Mansonioides*.

Fig. 422.—Female *Aedes aegypti*. × 4.
A magnifying glass is necessary for identification from this drawing.

just above the surface of the water. The most characteristic peculiarity, and the one which defines the distribution of the genus, is the habit of the pupae and larvae of obtaining air from the submerged portions of water plants.

The larva of *Mansonioides* inserts its respiratory siphon into the air-containing tissues, and remains there until forcibly removed. The pupae do likewise. The roots appear to be the part of the plant most favoured. Different species have a preference for certain water plants, and the type of water in which they prefer to grow. *M. annulifera*, *M. indiana* and *M. uniformis* are most easily found among the roots of water plants floating and growing in exposed situations, especially *Pistia stratiotes*, a plant which floats with hanging roots in still water. *M. uniformis* has a preference for the water hyacinth (*Eichornia crassipes*) and swamp grass (*Isachne australis*). The food of the larvae includes fine particles of organic matter which are freed from coconut husks in the process of coil and rope-making.

Mansonia (*mansonia*) *titillans* (Walker) is a vector of virus encephalitis in South America.

GENUS: *Aedes* (Meigen, 1818)

Abbreviations for classification of the *Aedes* group:

A. = *Aedimorphus*   F. = *Finlaya*
H. = *Howardina*   O. = *Ochlorotatus*
S. = *Stegomyia*

This genus is widely distributed. These are mostly black and white insects with white, silvery yellow bands or spots on the thorax and legs, for which reason they are generally known as 'tiger mosquitoes'. Certain species (*Ae. aegypti* and *Ae. albopictus*) are frequently found in ships.

Aedes (*S.*) *aegypti* (Fig. 422). Syn *Ae. argenteus, Stegomyia fasciata*

The reader is referred to the authoritative work on *Ae. aegypti* by Sir S. R. Christophers (1960).

This occurs all over the tropics and subtropics, 40° North and South of Equator, and in Europe at the level of Gibraltar. It is a domestic species rarely breeding more than 90 m from houses, and can be recognized by the peculiar lyre-shaped design— 2 dull-yellow parallel lines in the middle and curved silvery line on each side of the thorax. The proboscis is not banded, but the abdomen is banded basally. The last hind tarsal joint is all white and some of the other tarsal joints are marked basally by light bands. It bites avidly, mostly by night. The eggs are laid in small dark receptacles, e.g. water in tree-rot holes, tins, pots, coconut shells, cut bamboo, sagging eaves, plants, tops of pineapples, sisal leaves, vases in cemeteries, bilges of ships, old beer bottles and car tyres. When deposited they are white, but darken in a few hours. If kept moist, the larvae develop in 12–24 hours; the eggs can resist drying for as long as 6 months. The larvae then emerge when they are moistened.

Ae. aegypti transmits the virus of yellow fever and dengue (page 374).

Ae. (*F.*) *leucocelaenus* Dyar and Shannon represents a complex species, which extends from Costa Rica along the east coast of America to Argentina. It divides into 2 subspecies at the extremity of its range, one of which, *Ae. leucocelaenus clarki* Galindo, is found in Panama and Costa Rica.

Ae. (*S.*) *vittatus* (Bigot), with 6 white spots on the thorax, has a wide range throughout tropical Africa, but extends to Pakistan, India, Ceylon, Burma, Indo-China and Malaysia. It is a species which readily becomes domesticated and it may act as a vector of yellow fever in W. Africa.

Other species also transmit yellow fever (see page 375).

Ae. (*S.*) *albopictus* (Skuse) (Fig. 424) is commonly distributed in Australasia, Mariana Islands, Hawaii, Japan, Somalia, and Malagasy. It usually breeds in bamboos in the vicinity of dwellings. It resembles *Ae. aegypti* in general habits, but can be distinguished by the single broad median stripe on the scutellum. It transmits dengue virus in Japan.

Ae. (*O.*) *vigilax* (Skuse) has a wide range in the coasts of Australia, New Guinea, New Hebrides, New Caledonia, Indonesia, Siam, Indo-China, Formosa, Seychelle Islands and Fiji. It is the main vector of the non-periodic filaria in New Caledonia, but has proved to be a poor vector in Fiji. It breeds in the saline and brackish water of coastal mangrove swamps.

Members of the *Aedes scutellaris* complex are found throughout Indonesia and the Pacific Islands. A subspecies with minor differences is to be found in almost every island group.

Ae. (*S.*) *pseudoscutellaris* is found solely in the Fiji group (Fig. 423). A second closely allied species is *Ae.* (*S.*) *polynesiensis* Marks, which has an extensive range in the Pacific, in Fiji, Ellice Islands, Samoa, Cook Island, Tokelau, Marquesas, Society Islands, Tuamotus, Austral and Hoorn Island; it breeds commonly in holes made by the land crab (*Cardisona carnifex*), but also in coconut shells and tree holes, as does *Ae. pseudoscutellaris*. It closely resembles *pseudoscutellaris*. There are some small differences in the scales on the scutellum, but the main distinction is found in the genitalia of the male where the basal lobe of the coxite is simple with setae extending nearly to the base dorsally but without specialized setae. There are also minor distinctions in the papillae of the tail of the larvae.

A third species, *Ae.* (*F.*) *fijiensis* Marks, which breeds in the axils of *Pandanus* (*P. thurstoni, P. tectorius,* and *P. joskei*) and in those of the Taro (*Colocasia antiquorum*), has been found to be a host of the Pacific filaria in Fiji. Some 18 members of the *Ae. scutellaris* group are recognized, such as *tongae, hebrideus, marshallensis,* etc.

Ae. horrescens is found in Fiji, and possibly also Tahiti. The larvae are clothed in hairs. *Ae.* (*S.*) *upolensis* Marks is a species from W. Samoa which is distinguished by absence of a distinct patch of white scales on the lateral thorax; there are also differences in the structure of the basal lobe of the male coxite.

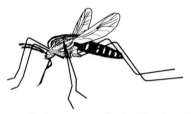

Fig. 423.—*Aedes scutellaris pseudoscutellaris*, side view, showing buckling of the proboscis sheath in the act of biting. × 4.

A magnifying glass is necessary for identification from this drawing.

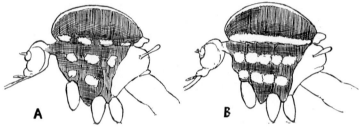

Fig. 424.—The markings on the thorax of *Aedes albopictus* (A) and *Ae. scutellaris pseudoscutellaris* (B), lateral view.

Members of the *Ae. scutellaris* group are the main vectors of the Pacific filaria—*Wuchereria bancrofti* var. *pacifica*—and are also vectors of the dengue virus. They are diurnal in habit, bite man, but also feed on birds, pigs, horses, fowls, and dogs. Their chief biting activity is in the afternoon (3–6 p.m.) with a low peak in the morning (6–8 a.m.). They do not rest in houses but in the bush. Their dispersal is limited, not exceeding 90 m in 2–3 weeks. The distinguishing marks are 3 parallel white strips on the mesothorax, and the incomplete white abdominal crossbands (Fig. 423). The larvae resemble those of *Ae. aegypti*, but are distinguished by the lateral bands of the comb scales which are distinctly smaller and more delicate. Though readily entering houses, they are not domestic mosquitoes. They breed, mostly in small collections of

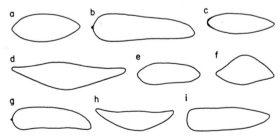

Fig. 425.—Various forms of mosquito eggs. *a*, *Grabhamia dorsalis*. *b*, *Culex pipiens*. *c*, *Culex scapularis*. *d*, *Mansonia titillans*. *e*, *Aedes aegypti*. *f*, *Taeniorhynchus fulvus*. *g*, *Culex fatigans*. *h*, *Janthinosoma lutzi*, *i*, *Taeniorhynchus fasciolatus*.

fresh water containing decaying vegetable matter, in the shells of coconuts, in crevices and holes in trees, in the artificial reservoirs in coconut trees used by Polynesians, in holes in coco-pods gnawed out by Pacific rats, in crab holes, in bottles and tins lying about in the bush. The eggs and pupae can withstand considerable desiccation. These species are intolerant of sun and wind. Their main haunts are in still, shady, bush around villages. Much has been done in the Gilbert and Ellice Islands to control them by the removal of undergrowth, creating a through draught to the trade winds. Somewhat similar measures are now undertaken on a large scale in Fiji.

In campaigns against these mosquitoes, the introduction of predatory Megarhine larvae has been attended in the Pacific by some success. It has been found that unless rotten wood from tree holes is completely excavated, filling in holes with a mixture of sand and tar is unsatisfactory.

GENUS: *Haemagogus*

This genus of mosquitoes is closely related to *Aedes*. It occurs in S. America; the adults are metallic blue and green due to their covering of scales on thorax and abdomen. Several species are vectors of sylvan (jungle) yellow fever: *Haemagogus equinus*, *H. mesodentatus*, *H. spegazzinii falco* and *H. capricorni*. They are separable only on the characters of the male genitalia and not at all as larvae and pupae. The larvae of the group are 'hairy' and are thus distinguishable from other species of *Haemagogus* which are not vectors. They have been reared from captured females.

GENUS: *Sabethes*
SUBGENUS: *Sabethoides*

These are jungle mosquitoes, suspected of transmitting jungle yellow fever in Brazil. In all 3 stages of their existence they are so characteristic that they have been distinguished as a separate tribe. The adults have a metallic lustre. The scales of all parts of the body are flat. There is a pair of very large procumbent bristles projecting from the crown of the head, and a tuft of hair on the mesonotum. The antennae are similar in both sexes; the palpi short in the female and usually also in the male. The larvae are generally predaceous and live in the water which collects in the axils and bracts of leaves, in tree holes, or is secreted by pitchers or other modified parts of plants. They are usually rather hairy and have smooth or stumpy antennae. A siphon is present and there is a single row of scales on the sides of the eighth abdominal segment. The pupae are characterized by the conspicuous fan of bristles at the postero-lateral angles of the eighth and ninth abdominal segments and by the small tail-fins. *Sabethes (Sabethoides) chloropterus* transmits yellow fever.

LARVICIDAL FUNGI

The discovery of fungus *Coelomomyces stegomyiae* Keilin, a parasite of mosquito larvae, may be of some importance, as indicated by the work of Marshall Laird. It was introduced from Singapore into atolls of the Tokelau Islands for the destruction of *Aedes polynesiensis*, and later it was applied to *Anopheles gambiae* in Zambia. Adults and pupae do not harbour these parasites as frequently as do larvae, which suffer a heavy mortality through massive destruction of their organs, including the fat body.

FAMILY: CERATOPOGONIDAE (midges, gnats)

These are very small (1–3 mm in length), slender, bloodsucking gnats, generally known as midges. In biting habits they resemble Simuliidae and are frequently mistaken for them. The antennae are plumose in the male, pilose in the female. Among 20 or more genera comprising the family, the most important from the medical aspect are *Culicoides* (Fig. 426), *Ceratopogon* and *Leptoconops*. All bite man viciously, mostly at dusk or night.

GENUS: *Culicoides*

The genus *Culicoides* measure 1·4–1·8 mm in length. The eyes are large. The antennae are long and thread-like; the wings contain pigment in the membrane, not scales like mosquitoes.

The species of *Culicoides* which transmit *D. perstans*, like other midges, lay their eggs on plants or vegetable matter on the shallow water containing decaying substances round the margins of ponds, in puddles and smaller collections of water and in a variety of habitats such as organic matter. Thus the rotting tissues of banana stumps are a favourable breeding site in some localities. The larvae wriggle around feeding on decaying organic matter. The adults swarm during the day near ponds, swamps and other collections of water and do not fly more than 1 km from their breeding places. The females attack man aggressively, particularly through the night from twilight to early morning and in shady places near water during the day. *C. grahami* is primarily a day biter. *Culicoides austeni* and *C. grahami*, which breed in stumps of banana plants, have been proved intermediary hosts of *Dipetalonema streptocerca*. *C. furens* transmits *Mansonella ozzardi* in Guyana and *C. paraensis* does so in Antigua. The malaria-like parasite, *Hepatocystis kochi*, is transmitted by *Culicoides adersi* (Garnham).

FAMILY: CHIRONOMIDAE

These are midges which look like mosquitoes, but do not bite man. When resting they raise the front pair of legs. The proboscis is vestigial, and there are no scales on the wings. They occur near lakes and rivers in large swarms.

FAMILY: SIMULIIDAE
GENUS: *Simulium*
(Black flies, buffalo gnats, turkey gnats)

The Simuliidae are small flies (1–5 mm long); the females suck blood and have blade-like piercing mouth-parts; in the males these are more or less rudimentary. The flies have a characteristic prominent hump caused by strong development of the scutum

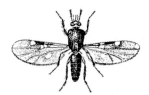

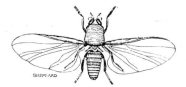

Fig. 426.—Female *Culicoides grahami*.
× 50. (*After Byam & Archibald*)

Fig. 427.—*Simulium damnosum.* × 10.

and reduction in the size of the prescutum. They occur in enormous numbers in favourable localities during late spring and early summer in northern countries, and are abundant in the north temperate and subarctic zones, and also in the tropics. They can be a severe nuisance on account of their bites, irrespective of their role as transmitters of serious disease to man and cattle. The females attack viciously in the open, and some species (*S. damnosum* and *S. ochraceum*) are exclusively anthropophilic, but do not enter houses. They shun bright sunlight, however, and bite principally in the early morning and towards evening, but will attack at any time of the day in shade or when the sky is cloudy, being more aggressive before storm or after rain.

The females lay their triangular eggs in running (and therefore oxygenated) water, in masses of 300–500, which are attached to rocks, grass and other objects by a gelatinous fluid. The eggs hatch in 4–12 hours and the emerging larvae attach themselves to stones (*S. damnosum*), crabs (*S. neavei* complex), prawns or mayfly nymphs. The larvae feed by means of fan-shaped brushes near their mouth parts. There are 5 larval instars, ending in 13 days or more. The pupal period is 2–10 days, and the complete life cycle 2–3 weeks. The *Simulium damnosum* and *Simulium neavei* complexes have been separated into a number of different genotypes by chromosome studies. These genotypes differ in their behaviour and in feeding preferences for different hosts, which affect their importance as vectors of human onchocerciasis.

The following species are actual or potential vectors of *Onchocerca volvulus* in man:

Africa. The *Simulium damnosum* (Jinja fly) complex which contains more than one biological variety, including 'Guinea zone' and a 'savanna zone' forms in West Africa, which are vectors of the *Onchocerca* only of their own zones. The *S. neavei* complex, which includes *S. woodi*, common in East Africa and South-west Ethiopia.

The *S. damnosum* complex breeds in large rivers and the outflows of dams, the larvae attaching to stones in the river beds. Females are capable of very long flights; Waddy (1968) refers to flights of 100 miles along a river. The *S. neavei* complex is confined to small streams in thick forest, which it never leaves; its flight range is very short. The larvae attach to crabs.

Central and South America. *S. ochraceum* is the main vector in the 2 foci in Mexico (States of Oaxaca and Chiapas) and the 3 in Guatemala. It breeds in minute trickles of water, often under leaves, and in innumerable streams in rugged country with heavy vegetation cover; these breeding places are therefore difficult to reach. It also breeds close to villages in the coffee plantation zone, in very limited conditions between 500 and 1200 metres above sea level. It bites man avidly and is a very efficient vector.

S. metallicum breeds in small streams but travels some distance to feed. In Central America it is a secondary vector, but in Venezuela it is the main vector, though relatively inefficient.

S. callidum is a secondary vector in Central America.

S. exiguum is possibly a minor vector in Central America, but in Colombia it is the only anthropophilic species so far caught in the endemic focus on the western slopes of the Andes.

African species tend to bite below the waist, but Guatemalan *S. ochraceum* tends to bite above the waist, possibly by natural inclination, or possibly because people mostly work with their legs covered by clothing. *S. metallicum* and *S. callidum*, however, tend to bite below the waist (De Leon & Duke 1966).

BLOOD-SUCKING FLIES
FAMILY: TABANIDAE

Horseflies, gadflies and deer flies are large insects with well developed bodies (10–25 mm). They are strong fliers, notorious pests of cattle and deer, and readily attack man, especially *Chrysops*. The males feed on vegetable juices, and do not bite warm-blooded animals. The eyes are very large and widely separated in the female, contiguous in the male. The antennae consist of 3 dissimilar segments; the third is usually elongated. The venation of the wings is complex; the second longitudinal vein

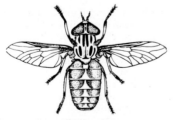

Fig. 428.—Male *Tabanus ustus*, natural size. (*After Austen; by permission of the Trustees of the British Museum*)

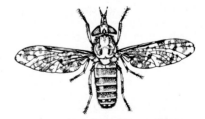

Fig. 429.—Female *Haematopota*. × 2½. (*After Austen; by permission of the Trustees of the British Museum*)

is not forked. The family *Tabanidae* includes gadflies, *Tabanus* (Fig. 428), *Haematopota* (Fig. 429), *Pangonia* and *Chrysops* (Fig. 430). They are most frequent near water, being semi-aquatic in their breeding habits, some breeding in moist earth, or leaf would. Eggs are laid near water in layers, and are narrow and cylindrical (1·0–2·5 mm), vary from 100–700 and are covered with a secretion binding them tightly together. The larvae are slender and cylindrical, have 11 segments, a head, and taper at both ends. The pupae resemble those of lepidoptera. Adult flies emerge from the pupal case through a slit along the dorsum of the thorax.

GENUS: *Chrysops*

The deer or mango flies of the genus *Chrysops* which transmit *L. loa* are generally found in shady woodlands, especially forest swampland. The females attack man throughout the day, but most actively in the early morning and the late afternoon. Males do not suck blood. Dark-skinned persons are more readily bitten than whites. The eggs are laid on vegetable matter or rocks in or overhanging water and the larvae drop into the water or mud below on hatching. The larvae are found especially in densely shaded streams when the course is impeded by vegetation, the flow is slow and the bottom is covered by decaying leaves over soft mud, overlaid by fine sand. The complete life cycle requires 4 months or more. *C. silacea* is the most important species

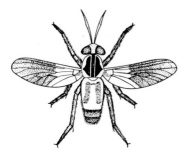

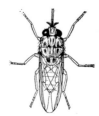

Fig. 430.—Female *Chrysops dimidiata* (v.d. Wulp). × 2½.

Fig. 431.—Tsetse fly at rest. × approx. 1½.

transmitting *Loa loa* to man. It is a day biter attracted to wood smoke, and therefore to human dwellings and clothes, and it is more numerous and widespread than *C. dimidiata*.

C. zahrai may transmit *L. loa* to man in Cameroon.

Chrysops discalis is grey or yellowish grey; in the female black spots are seen on the abdomen. The male (8–10 mm) is predominantly black, with yellowish grey spots on the abdomen. This fly is a transmitter of tularaemia in Central and North America, where it is a common species.

C. dimidiata (v.d. Wulp) (Fig. 430), a West African species, is particularly abundant during certain times of the year in Nigeria and Cameroon, and acts as an intermediary of *L. loa* (page 217). In Cameroon 7·2% of wild-caught flies harbour this worm. The face and palpi are yellow, the scutum black with yellow stripes and the abdomen yellow with a dusky brown tip. The legs are yellow, with dark tibia and tarsi. The distal half of the wing is smoky.

C. silacea (Austen) is a common species in West Africa, also an intermediary for *L. loa*, and is found infected with this filaria in Cameroon. It differs from the former species in having a red or bright orange abdomen and legs with dark brown tarsi. *C. distinctipennis* may also transmit *L. loa* in the Sudan.

C. silacea is responsible for the transmission of infection from man to man and possibly between man and monkey. *C. longicornis* and *C. langi*, which bite at night, feed on monkeys and transmit simian loiasis. Adult females of *C. silacea* and *C. dimidiata* are normally canopy dwellers and are day feeders. *C. zahrai*, a newly discovered species, is crepuscular.

FAMILY: MUSCIDAE
SUB-FAMILY: GLOSSININAE
GENUS: *Glossina* Wiedemann 1830
TSETSE FLIES

By D. M. Minter, Ph.D., B.Sc.

The unique viviparous genus *Glossina* contains some 30 species and subspecies nowadays confined to tropical Africa between latitudes 15°N and 30°S. Until the early years of the twentieth century an isolated population (of *G. tachinoides*) still existed in the south-western part of the Arabian peninsula, but seems likely to have died out since then. Fossil tsetse flies occur in Oligocene deposits in North America (Colorado), suggesting that the distribution of the genus was once considerably wider.

Nonetheless, tsetse flies still occupy a very large area in Africa; about 10.4×10^6 km² are infested, roughly half of the surface of the continent.

The tsetse flies are large, brown to greyish, narrow-bodied flies, 6–15 mm long, with a stout proboscis projecting forward well in front of the head (Fig. 432). The proboscis is adjoined laterally, except during the act of biting, by the paired labial palps. The mouth-parts consist of a horny labrum, a slender hypopharynx (through which an

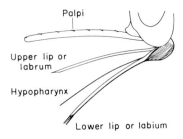

Fig. 432.—Mouth-parts of *Glossina*.

anticoagulant saliva is injected into the bite wound) and a stout ventral labium (Fig. 432). These 3 parts enclose a space, the food canal, through which blood is sucked by muscular action into the alimentary canal of the fly. During feeding the mouth-parts, but not the palps, are lowered some 90° from the line of the body axis. Male and female tsetse feed exclusively on the blood of vertebrates.

Characteristic features which distinguish *Glossina* species from other large biting flies, such as *Stomoxys, Haematobia, Lyperosia, Haematopota, Tabanus* and *Chrysops*, include the long straight proboscis with a basal bulb, the presence of branched hairs on the arista (the prominent bristle on the largest, distal, segment of the antenna) and the length of the labial palps (as long as the proboscis in *Glossina*). The manner in which the wings are folded, scissors-like, over the back of the resting fly is also a very characteristic feature (Fig. 431). The presence of the 'hatchet' or 'cleaver' cell, enclosed between the fourth and fifth longitudinal wing veins, is diagnostic of *Glossina*. This cell is clearly seen in the central area of the wings (Figs 433–6) and contrasts with the triangular shape of the corresponding cell of related flies (e.g. *Stomoxys*, Fig. 437).

The genus *Glossina* is usually divided by modern taxonomists into 3 species-groups (sometimes given subgeneric status) as follows:

a. The *fusca* group (subgenus *Austenina*).
b. The *palpalis* group (subgenus *Nemorhina*).
c. The *morsitans* group (subgenus *Glossina*).

This taxonomic separation is, in a general way, reflected in the ecological requirements and distribution of the species included in each group: characteristically, flies of the *fusca* group are associated with dense humid tropical forest or forest edges; members of the *palpalis* group are basically dependent on more or less dense riverine or lacustrine vegetation but their distribution extends into savanna zones well away from forested, or formerly forested, areas. Species of the *morsitans* group are the least hygrophilic and occupy vast areas of bushland and thicket vegetation often far from lakes and rivers. Strangely, however, one of the least hygrophilic species, occupying arid and semi-desert areas, is *G. longipennis*, a member of the *fusca* group. *G. brevipalpis*, also a *fusca* group species, has a distribution which also extends into dry savanna zones. Though flies of the *fusca* group include important vectors of trypanosomes pathogenic to livestock, especially species of the *Trypanosoma vivax* group (subgenus *Duttonella*) and *T. congolense* group (subgenus *Nannomonas*), they have never been associated with the transmission of trypanosomiasis to man and will not be considered further in this section. Fig. 438 indicates the distribution of the species of main medical importance.

The pictorial key (Table 52) to the principal species reproduced on pages 1108–1109 includes some species of the *fusca* group and indeed divides the group into two sections that are no longer accorded taxonomic recognition. Potts (Mulligan 1970) and Ford (1971) summarize modern views on the taxonomy and distribution of species and subspecies included in the *fusca*, *palpalis* and *morsitans* groups and Potts gives a detailed key for the identification of all members of the genus.

Life history

Tsetse flies, in common with a very few other Diptera, have a method of viviparous reproduction uncommon among the higher insects, by which a single larva is produced at a time and is retained and nourished within the body of the female fly. Associated with the production of single offspring is a reduction in the number of ovarioles in the 2 ovaries to a single pair in each: 4 ovarioles in all, from which fertilized eggs pass into the uterus in a regular rotation. Female flies are normally fertilized only once, shortly after emergence, and store sufficient viable sperm from this single mating to last throughout life, during which, under favourable conditions, they may produce, at intervals of about 11 days, some 20 individual larvae.

Each successive fertilized egg (1·5 mm long) passes from the oviduct into the uterus where it hatches into a small, white, grub-like larva. The young larva obtains nutriment solely from the secretion of the uterine (or 'milk') glands of the mother, in which it is bathed. The larva grows, and twice moults, during the 8–12 days of intra-uterine development. The mature larva, by now in the third instar, is finally extruded by the mother (by breech delivery) while she is perched on the ground, or on vegetation a few centimetres above it, in a site selected for its shady situation and suitable soil texture. The newly deposited larva, creamy white in colour with shiny, black posterior polyneustic lobes through which it breathes, actively burrows below the surface soil to a depth of a few millimetres, using vigorous peristaltic movements. Having reached a point below the surface where conditions are suitable, it becomes immobile and begins to pupate, still within the third larval skin, that darkens and hardens. During emergence from the puparium, and in reaching the soil surface, the young fly is aided by an eversible bladder extruded from the front of the head and known as the *ptilinum*. During the first few days of life, this bladder can still be everted, while the body is still soft and 'soapy' in texture, if the young fly is carefully pressed between the fingers. Flies in this stage, so far unfed, are referred to as *teneral* flies: older flies as *non-teneral*, in which the head and body are hardened and horny and the ptilinum can no longer be everted.

After the quiescent period, the young teneral flies seek their first blood meal. Flies of each sex normally feed at intervals of 3–4 days, sometimes less, and die of starvation if deprived of a blood meal for 10–12 days. The average life span of female *Glossina* is 2–3 months: exceptionally, up to 6 or 7 months. Male flies have a much shorter life-span.

Male flies exhibit a progressive fraying of the trailing edge of the wings; this can be used to estimate the average age of *groups* of males from the same population. The wings of females also fray with age, usually less rapidly than those of males. With females, however, careful examination of the 4 ovarioles enables an estimation of the

Table 52. Synopsis of the genus *Glossina*

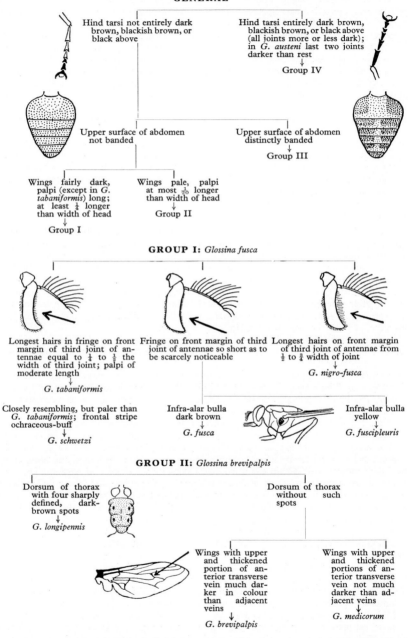

NOTE.—Two new species are: *G. vanhoofi* Henrard, 1952, *G. nashi* Potts, 1955, both members of the *fusca* group. *G. severini*, of which only two specimens (from Congo) are at present known, is not included in the above table, since its precise affinities are as yet uncertain; although in some respects resembling *G. fuscipleuris*,

GROUP III: *Glossina morsitans* (subgroup *Glossina*)

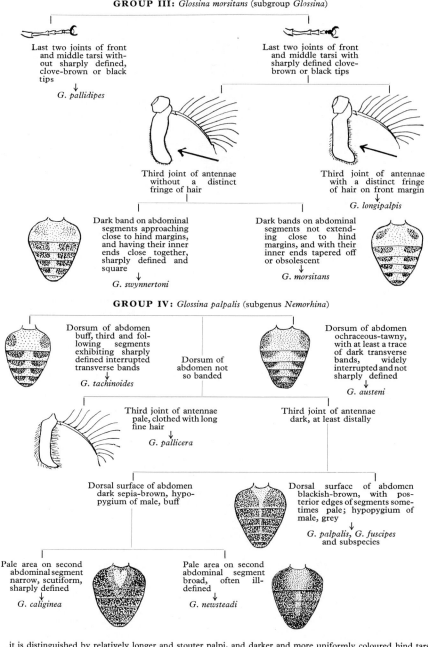

Last two joints of front
and middle tarsi with-
out sharply defined,
clove-brown or black
tips
↓
G. pallidipes

Last two joints of front
and middle tarsi with
sharply defined clove-
brown or black tips

Third joint of antennae
without a distinct
fringe of hair

Third joint of antennae
with a distinct fringe
of hair on front margin
↓
G. longipalpis

Dark band on abdominal
segments approaching
close to hind margins,
and having their inner
ends close together,
sharply defined and
square
↓
G. swynnertoni

Dark bands on abdominal
segments not extend-
ing close to hind
margins, and with their
inner ends tapered off
or obsolescent
↓
G. morsitans

GROUP IV: *Glossina palpalis* (subgenus *Nemorhina*)

Dorsum of abdomen
buff, third and fol-
lowing segments
exhibiting sharply
defined interrupted
transverse bands
↓
G. tachinoides

Dorsum of
abdomen not
so banded

Dorsum of abdomen
ochraceous-tawny,
with at least a trace
of dark transverse
bands, widely
interrupted and not
sharply defined
↓
G. austeni

Third joint of antennae
pale, clothed with long
fine hair
↓
G. pallicera

Third joint of antennae
dark, at least distally

Dorsal surface of abdomen
dark sepia-brown, hypo-
pygium of male, buff

Dorsal surface of abdomen
blackish-brown, with pos-
terior edges of segments sometimes pale; hypopygium of
male, grey
↓
G. palpalis, G. fuscipes
and subspecies

Pale area on second
abdominal segment
narrow, scutiform,
sharply defined
↓
G. caliginea

Pale area on second
abdominal segment
broad, often ill-
defined
↓
G. newsteadi

it is distinguished by relatively longer and stouter palpi, and darker and more uniformly coloured hind tarsi.
G. haningtoni, of Cameroon, very few specimens of which have yet been captured, is closely allied to *G. fusca*,
but is distinguishable externally from that species by its relatively much shorter palpi and slightly more robust
appearance. *G. martinii* described in 1935, is a subspecies of *G. fuscipes*, with which, in all external characters,
it is identical. *G. fuscipes fuscipes* comes from forests of the Congo and gallery forests to the north. *G. fuscipes
quanzensis* from the basin of Kasai, affluents of the lower Congo on the south bank.

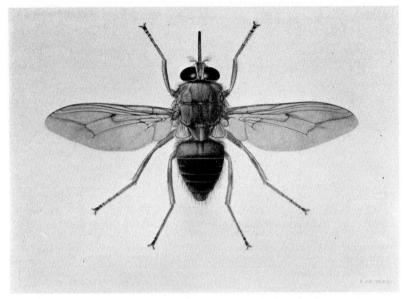

Fig. 433.—Female *Glossina brevipalpis* Newstead. × 4½. (*Figs 433–436 from Austen; reproduced by permission of the Trustees of the British Museum*)

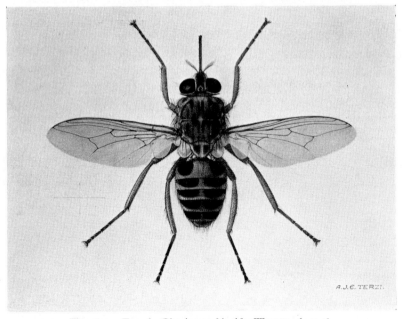

Fig. 434.—Female *Glossina tachinoides* Westwood. × 6.

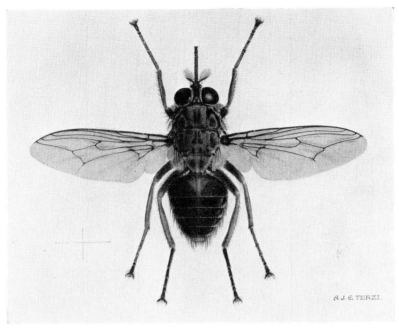

Fig. 435.—Female *Glossina palpalis* Robineau-Desvoidy. × 6.

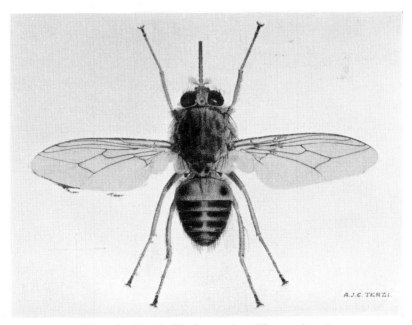

Fig. 436.—Female *Glossina morsitans* Westwood. × 6.

Table 53. Biotype, distribution and medical importance of *Glossina*

Species group/subgenus	Habitat type	Distribution	Species of medical importance
fusca group (*Austenina*)	Mainly rain forest areas	Chiefly forest areas of W. and Central Africa. Relict species in dry areas of E. Africa	None. But several vectors of livestock trypanosomiasis
palpalis group (*Nemorhina*)	Mainly linear: shores of lakes and rivers in forested or formerly forested areas	15°N to 12°S, approx. 17°W to 15°E, approx.	*G. palpalis*, vector of *T. brucei gambiense* in W. Africa
		10°N to 12°S, approx. 10°E to 40°E, approx.	*G. fuscipes* (and subspecies), vectors of *T. brucei gambiense* (W. Africa, Central Africa) and *T. brucei rhodesiense* (E. Africa)
		12°N to 4°N, approx. 12°W to 40°E, approx.	*G. tachinoides*, vector of *T. b. gambiense* in W. Africa and of *T. b. rhodesiense* in S.W. Ethiopia
morsitans group (*Glossina*)	'Game' tsetse of the savanna zones: open woodland ('miombo'), bushland and thicket	15°N to 20°S, approx. 17°W to 45°E, approx.	*G. morsitans* (and subspecies), vectors of *T. b. rhodesiense* in E. and S.E. Africa
		8°N to 20°S, approx. 25°E to 48°E approx.	*G. pallidipes*, vector of *T. b. rhodesiense* in E. Africa
		Limited area S.E. of Lake Victoria; mainly in Tanzania	*G. swynnertoni*, vector of *T. b. rhodesiense*

age of *individual* females to be made on a physiological basis. This method of 'ovarian ageing' is accurate to within a few days up to an age of about 40 days; with older flies there is a greater margin of possible error. For a fuller discussion of ageing methods, the reader is referred to Mulligan (1970).

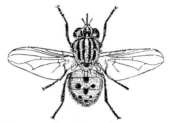

Fig. 437.—*Stomoxys calcitrans.* × 3.

Female *G. fuscipes* in the field mate soon after emergence: female *G. pallidipes* are frequently fertilized near the host while seeking the first blood meal. Copulation may last from 2 to 24 hours and, at least in the laboratory, older males (about 14 days) are more potent than younger males.

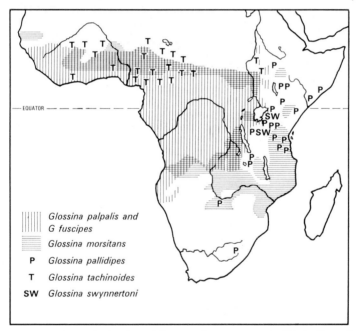

Fig. 438.—The distribution of the more important tsetse flies in Central Africa. (*After Buxton*)

The *palpalis* and *morsitans* groups: bionomics and ecology in relation to sleeping sickness

Species of these two groups are active only during daylight hours: flight and feeding activities decrease markedly even during dull and overcast weather; few species show evidence of purposive behaviour after dusk. Tsetse flies hunt their prey mainly by sight, although scent becomes increasingly important at close range; the flies are often aware of movements at a considerable distance and will fly to investigate any large moving object in their environment. Such objects can include cars, trains, canoes and lake steamers as well as animals and man.

When not actively seeking food, the flies normally rest on woody elements of the vegetation. Horizontal or inclined branches, 2–5 cm thick and 1–3 m from the ground, are favoured resting sites during the day for most species. Resting flies are most numerous where such perches provide a good field of view, as along the edge of thickets or the margins of lakes and streams. Flies in the course of digesting a meal and females seeking to deposit larvae are found in more sheltered places. By night, both sexes of those species so far investigated change from their daytime resting sites on the larger woody elements, to spend the hours of darkness on leaves and small twigs; the change-over takes place very rapidly, during the last few moments of twilight, and a reverse movement occurs at first light in the morning. The change of resting sites has, perhaps, the function of protecting the flies from the activities of nocturnal predators.

Sleeping sickness vectors

G. palpalis, G. fuscipes and *G. tachinoides*. Until the closing years of the 1950's it was generally considered, firstly, that flies of the *palpalis* group were limited to, and dependent upon, the woody vegetation along streams and lake shores, and that the flies could not maintain themselves elsewhere except during limited sorties at favourable times of the year. Secondly, flies of the *palpalis* group were considered to be solely responsible for the transmission of Gambian sleeping sickness; while flies of the *morsitans* group transmitted only the acute, Rhodesian, type of disease. These distinctions are no longer completely tenable, though they remain as useful generalizations that apply under most circumstances. However, not only have *G. fuscipes* and *G. tachinoides* been implicated in epidemic outbreaks of the Rhodesian type of disease (in Kenya and Ethiopia, respectively) but the same two species have been found (in Kenya and Nigeria) sometimes to live and breed in peri-domestic environments far from water. It is now realized that neither species is quite so dependent upon particular vegetational associations as was formerly thought. Many instances of tsetse behaviour once labelled as atypical are now known to be quite commonplace: present-day views of the factors which influence tsetse ecology and behaviour, especially in relation to different types of vegetation, are now less rigid than once was the case.

In natural circumstances, where there is no close contact with man and domestic animals, flies of the *palpalis* groups show a preference for feeding on large reptiles, such as monitor lizards and crocodiles. Reptiles form more than half of the feeds of wild flies in these conditions; bushbuck (*Tragelaphus scriptus*) account for about a quarter and other animals the remainder. Where man and domestic animals are available, they too are attacked readily by species of the *palpalis* group. In circumstances where man, domestic animals and flies of the *palpalis* group come into close proximity (such as at river-crossings, water-holes etc.) people and their livestock become a major source of food for the flies, and sharp outbreaks of sleeping sickness are likely to occur, especially in the dry seasons when man, cattle and small populations of flies are likely to depend upon the same limited water sources.

G. morsitans, G. pallidipes and *G. swynnertoni*—the '*game*' *tsetse*. Unlike flies of the *palpalis* group which commonly occupy waterside habitats of an essentially linear type, often intersected by patterns of human activity that may lead to close and personal contact, species of the *morsitans* group occupy vast areas of xerophytic woodland, dry bushland and thicket vegetation, particularly in the eastern parts of Africa. Under these conditions contact between man, his livestock and the wild fly populations is seldom close and intense. Species of the *morsitans* group obtain most of their blood meals from the wild game animals, especially Bovidae and Suidae, that roam the savannas and 'miombo' woodlands, and among which trypanosomes of the *T. brucei* subgroup are circulated and maintained as a zoonosis. Some of the zoonotic strains are infective to man and give rise to symptoms, characteristically, of the acute, Rhodesian type of disease. Human infections are, however, comparatively rare because of the infrequent and mainly accidental contact between the *morsitans* group and man. The number of cases of Rhodesian sleeping sickness contracted in eastern Africa is very small in comparison with the number of mainly Gambian cases in West Africa and the Congo basin, where man is the principal—if not the only—reservoir of infection.

Exposure to *T. rhodesiense* strains is largely occupational: hunters, honey-gatherers, pole-cutters and charcoal burners are among groups likely to enter fly-infested bush. In recent years the rapid growth of the tourist 'package' industry in East Africa has put another large group of itinerants at risk: the tourists themselves. Although species of the *morsitans* group are relatively little interested in man as a source of food if game animals are locally abundant, they often attack in sufficient numbers to be a considerable nuisance. Flies of the *morsitans* group are likely to acquire strains pathogenic to man from prior feeds on bushbuck (the only proved reservoir) or other ungulates. In this latter category should be included, perhaps, domestic cattle: strains causing acute disease in man were isolated from cattle during a localized outbreak in Kenya (Alego) some years ago. It is thus possible that cattle may act as temporary reservoirs, at any rate, under circumstances in which cattle survive in the presence of fly, or when cattle are moved through fly-infested areas. Cattle can seldom be kept long in the presence of heavy or moderate fly infestation, however, owing to the damaging incidence of infections with *T. vivax* and *T. congolense*.

Natural infection rates and methods of fly dissection

Infective metacyclic trypanosomes of the *T. brucei* subgroup (subgenus *Trypanozoon*) are found in the salivary glands of the tsetse fly. To reach their final station in the glands they undergo a complex migration in the fly that takes nearly 3 weeks to complete; hence it follows that only flies more than 3 weeks old can be infected with trypanosomes infective to man. Even among older flies, infection rates with the *T. brucei* subgroup are always low (commonly $0 \cdot 1\%$ or less: rarely more than 1%), especially when compared with infection rates with the *T. vivax* ($=Duttonella$) and *T. congolense* ($=Nannomonas$) groups in the same flies. The *T. vivax* group have a short and simple life cycle in the fly: infection rates may reach 75% or more. The *T. congolense* group have a longer and slightly more complex cycle in the fly: infection rates may reach 18–25%.

The full dissection of a tsetse involves the removal and microscopic examination of the elongate salivary glands, the midgut and the mouth-parts. There are several possible methods of dissection, but given some practice there is probably little to choose between them. The method preferred by the writer is as follows:

1. The fly is killed (with ether, chloroform or by judicious finger pressure against the sides of the thorax), wings and legs may be removed at this stage, or left.

2. The fly is placed on a slide in a *small* amount of physiological saline (or 5% glucose solution).

3. The tough, membranous connection between head and thorax is 'frayed' carefully with the point of a needle to weaken it.

4. The proboscis is held (under a needle or with forceps) by the basal bulb and drawn slowly away from the head. With practice, the proboscis comes away from the head still attached to the salivary glands; continued slow, careful traction enables these to be pulled gradually clear of the body. If the glands break at this stage they can be recovered later.

5. The labrum, hypopharynx and labium are preferably separated with needles and examined in saline under a coverslip. Or the intact semi-transparent proboscis can be examined without separating the parts.

6. If removed with the mouth-parts, the salivary glands are separated from the former and mounted in a small drop of saline under a coverslip.

7. If the salivary glands were broken during stage 4, the fly is now turned so that its abdomen lies flat on the slide, dorsal side uppermost. The thorax is pulled off and discarded and needles are inserted through the two anterolateral corners of the abdomen, at a point roughly half-way from the corners towards the long axis of the abdomen, with sufficient pressure to pierce well below the dorsal integument. Firm traction in

the direction of the forward corners of the abdomen, to tear them open, will usually result in the recovery of the glands at this stage: they may be recognized by their glass-like, refractile appearance. Continued needle traction will normally pull the glands clear of the abdomen, for examination in a separate drop of fresh saline under a cover-slip.

8. With a needle or scalpel the sides of the posterior tip of the abdomen are cut and the gut is extracted; the covering of fat-body is stripped off with a needle and the gut is placed in a drop of saline, teased open and examined under a coverslip for the presence of trypanosomes.

Trypanosome infections of tsetse are identified, in the organs dissected, by reference to their location and morphology. Infections of the mouth-parts only are likely to be *T. vivax* group; infections in the mouth-parts and gut only are likely to be *T. congolense* or a mixed infection of *T. vivax* and *T. congolense* groups. Infections involving the salivary glands, gut and mouth-parts certainly include the *T. brucei* subgroup but may also be complicated by the presence of *T. vivax*, *T. congolense*, or both. Gut and mouth-parts infections could also include immature infections with *T. brucei* subgroup.

Control of tsetse flies

The subject of tsetse control is a large one and its detailed treatment is beyond the scope of this section. The interested reader is referred to Mulligan (1970) for a full review. Control methods now available, or likely to have practical application in the near future, are either chemical or biological.

Chemical methods. The main chemical control method depends on the applica-tion of residual insecticides to the vegetation of tsetse habitats. Tsetse flies are suscep-tible to all the usual insecticides and resistance does not normally occur. Insecticides can be applied either from the ground or from the air; applications may be total or partial. Ground application is usually cheaper and has the advantage that it can be applied selectively to the vegetation known to be favoured as resting sites by different species. At least 2 applications of insecticide are normally required for adequate control, the second and subsequent applications are made at intervals sufficient to ensure the exposure of flies emerging from puparia after the first application. In very dense thickets, the prior use of defoliants might offer advantages in aerial applications but in most instances this is precluded on the grounds of the additional cost. A chemical method which may be practicable in future is the application of chemosterilants, either to vegetation used as resting sites, or in combination with an effective attractant yet to be developed.

Biological methods. Other than insecticide application, the control methods most widely in use depend on the destruction, or radical alteration, of vegetational associa-tions which provide suitable habitats for tsetse flies. Bush clearing may be total or partial (i.e. selective), or limited to barrier areas, usually about 3 km wide, to prevent re-invasion of areas cleared of fly by other means. Clearing may be effected by hand labour or machines: 'chain-dozing' is a rapid and effective method, in which a ship's anchor chain is linked to two heavy bulldozers that are driven slowly forward on parallel courses. The heavy chain between them tears down thick bush and trees. By whatever means bush clearing is undertaken it is vitally necessary that it is followed promptly by settlement and effective use of land, to prevent the rapid regeneration of bush which otherwise occurs. The vegetation cut or torn down is first gathered into windrows, allowed to dry and then fired; the cleared land is then available for agriculture.

The use of parasites and predators of tsetse flies as a form of biological control has a potential value but has yet to reach a point at which it can be applied widely in practice. A method of control which, although successful in Rhodesia, has now been replaced by less destructive measures, involved the deliberate elimination of the game animal populations which supported species of the *morsitans* group.

A method which has great theoretical and practical advantages in the field of tsetse control depends upon the release of sterilized male flies, able to compete adequately with wild males, in sufficient numbers to ensure that most females are inseminated with infertile sperm and thus fail to produce viable young. Sterile but fully competitive males can be produced by irradiation of puparia or by the topical application of chemo-sterilants. The practical limitation yet remaining to be overcome is that of rearing sufficient pupae simultaneously, in the vast numbers necessary for this form of control to be effective. Improved methods of rearing tsetse flies may eventually overcome this difficulty and place a new and potent tool in the hands of those concerned with the control of tsetse flies.

MUSCIDAE THAT DO NOT SUCK BLOOD
GENUS: *Musca*

The common housefly, *Musca domestica* (Fig. 439), is a domestic species. On account of its insanitary habits it acts as a vector of pathogenic micro-organisms, especially dysentery bacilli, cysts of *Entamoeba histolytica*, other intestinal protozoa and helminth eggs.

M. domestica (8 mm in length) is dark grey, with 4 parallel black stripes on the dorsum of the thorax. Eggs are laid in masses in manure and other refuse, hatching in 24 hours in hot weather. The larvae are legless maggots with large stigmal plates, bearing posterior spiracles on the abdomen. Pupation under favourable conditions occurs in 5 days. The puparium is an elongated barrel shape, and in the tropics the pupal stage

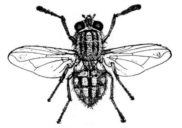

Fig. 439.—Female *Musca domestica*. × 4.

lasts 3 days. The adult fly lives about 1 month. Larvae are capable of traversing considerable thicknesses of soil in order to reach the surface. In the tropics houseflies are in evidence throughout the year; in dry deserts they may die off during the hot season. In temperate zones they are most numerous in the early autumn. Larvae survive the winter buried in decaying vegetable matter. The best method of storing manure is to ram it so tight that fermentation is intense enough to destroy maggots.

FAMILY: CHLOROPIDAE

These are Hippelates flies, members of the family Chloropidae (Oscinidae) and commonly known as 'frit flies'. Small members are known as 'eye flies' because of their liking for the lacrimal and sebaceous secretions, and also for blood and pus. They are extraordinarily persistent in their attentions.

Siphunculina funicola, the 'eye fly' of India, Ceylon and Java, is responsible for the spread of conjunctivitis. It has been shown that the seasonal prevalence of this fly in Assam closely coincides with that of epidemic conjunctivitis, and there is a similar belief for an allied species in southern United States. In parts of California these flies are a veritable pest.

Hippelates pallipes has been suspected of transmitting yaws mechanically in Jamaica (see page 567). They are small black flies with aristate antennae. The eggs are deposited on decaying organic matter and the larvae feed on the same material.

H. pusio, known as the 'eye gnat' or *mal de ojo*, is particularly abundant in Florida and causes great annoyance to men and animals.

FLIES PRODUCING MYIASIS

Myiasis is the condition produced when fly larvae invade living tissue, or when they are harboured in the intestine or bladder.

Dipterous flies causing myiasis are:

1. *Obligatory* myiasis producers, whose larvae develop only in living tissue.
2. *Facultative* myiasis producers, whose larvae usually develop on decaying tissue, but may also invade wounds.
3. *Accidental* myiasis producers, whose eggs or larvae are ingested and are not killed in the intestine, where they may even develop further.

OBLIGATORY MYIASIS PRODUCERS

Calliphoridae (including bluebottles, greenbottles) and Sarcophagidae flesh flies)

Auchmeromyia luteola (Fabr., 1805) (Fig. 440) is widely distributed throughout tropical Africa, from Northern Nigeria to Natal, and also in southern Sudan, in latitudes from 18°N to 26°S from sea level to 2250 m in dry or wet climates. Its general colour is orange-buff, but numerous small black hairs impart a smoky appearance. It measures 10–12 mm with a stoutly built body. The head is large, with the eyes

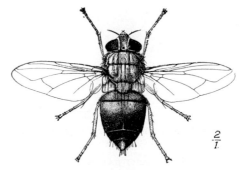

Fig. 440.—Female *Auchmeromyia luteola.*

well separated in both sexes. The thorax shows two indistinct, dark, longitudinal stripes. The abdomen differs in the sexes, the second segment in the female being twice the length of the same segment in the male. In the female the dark band on the second segment is so wide that it occupies almost the whole (Fig. 440). The third segment is almost black in both sexes. The wings are smoky-brown with conspicuous venation. Human and simian faeces constitute the most important source of food. First batch of eggs is laid 2–3 weeks after emergence. The larva (Fig. 441), known as the 'Congo floor-maggot', is dirty white, semi-transparent, 15 mm in length and composed of 11 segments. The central part of its ventral surface is flattened. At the posterior margin of each segment are 3 short limbs, transversely arranged, provided with backwardly directed spines which enable the maggot to move about like a caterpillar. The anterior segment is roughly conical and bears a mouth which is placed between 2 black hooks protruding from the apex and curving backwards towards the ventral surface. Paired groups of minute teeth are placed around 2 hooks, forming a sort of cupping apparatus. There is a remarkable dorsal diverticulum, corresponding to the food reservoir of the muscid larva which opens into the oesophagus near the anterior end.

After the larva has fed it forms a conspicuous red object filled with blood. After taking its meal it retreats into the cracks in the floor from which it emerged. It feeds by scraping with the mouth-hooks until it reaches a blood vessel. The first segment is then retracted and the sucker apparatus applied as in wet-cupping. The host must be

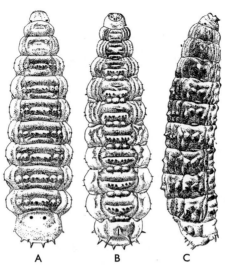

Fig. 441.—Larva of *Auchmeromyia luteola*. A, Dorsal view. B, Ventral view. C, Lateral view. × 5. (*After Brumpt*)

hairless and remain quiet, e.g. a man asleep. It also attacks the aardvark (anteater) and nestling birds. Larvae are frequently found under the mats on which people sleep and in the earth to a depth of 7·6 cm. They feed mainly at night, and drop off at once, if disturbed. They can be recognized by the characteristic shape of the stigmata or openings of the respiratory tubes.

When ready to pupate, the larva selects a suitable spot, and lies dormant. The puparium is a dark, reddish brown, oblong body, 9–10·5 × 4·5 mm. This stage lasts 2–3 weeks.

The adult fly (Fig. 440) is usually found sitting motionless among the thatch, beams and cobwebs of the walls and roofs of huts and, on account of its protective coloration, is difficult to detect. It deposits its eggs in the crevices of the floor, particularly mud floors, in spots where urine has been voided. To avoid being bitten, travellers should sleep on beds or in hammocks. Bites are painless.

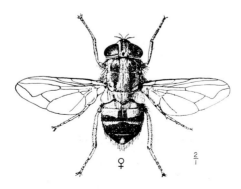

Fig. 442.—*Cordylobia anthropophaga*.

Cordylobia anthropophaga (Grünberg, 1903) (Fig. 442), the Tumbu Fly or Ver du Cayor, is widely spread in Central Africa. It measures 8·5–11·5 mm, and is yellowish grey, with black spots on the abdomen and brown wings, and resembles *Auchmeromyia luteola*. The male *Cordylobia* is distinguished from the male of *A. luteola* by its closely-set eyes. In the female *Cordylobia* the abdominal segments are of equal size, while the

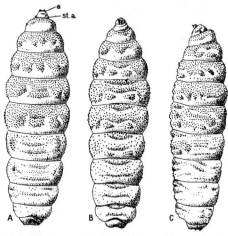

Fig. 443.—Adult larvae of *Cordylobia anthropophaga*. A, Dorsal view. B, Ventral view. C, Lateral view. × 5. (*After Brumpt*)

a, antennae. *t.a.*, anterior spiracle.

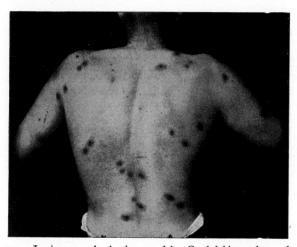

Fig. 444.—Lesions on the back caused by *Cordylobia anthropophaga*.

female *Auchmeromyia* has a triangular abdomen with the second segment long. They differ in life history and habits. *Cordylobia* is an obligatory myiasis producer and gives rise to lesions in man or animals. Usually, it is inactive; when disturbed, it flies away with great rapidity. The eggs, white and visible to the naked eye, are laid on the ground, or on clothing if it is contaminated by urine or sweat. Larvae are activated by the warm body of the host, and in the early stages are provided with structures, such as cuticular spines, to assist penetration of the skin. There are 3 moults or instars (Fig. 443). Development in subcutaneous tissues is completed in 12 days. The cavity containing the larvae breaks down to form a swelling, resembling a boil which bursts without much inflammation. The larvae emerge from the swellings (Fig. 444), which are situated on the forearm, scrotum, and other parts of the body; they fall to the ground and pupate in 36 hours. The pupa has a characteristic shape with a square truncated extremity. Pupal cases are commonly found in rat holes. The adult hatches in 10–20 days according to the temperature prevailing.

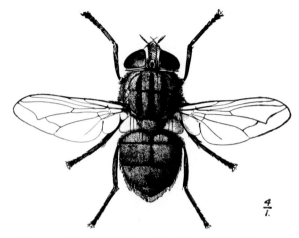

Fig. 445.—Female *Callitroga (Cochliomyia) hominivorax*.

Larvae can be extracted by pouring water over the hole in the skin, thus stopping their oxygen supply; they then extend their posterior spiracles, and can be squeezed out. They also die when covered by an adhesive dressing. All underclothes and towels should be ironed on both sides, and drip-dry clothing should be hung indoors with windows closed (Radcliffe 1972).

The tumbu fly provides a remarkable example of metazoan immunity. In guinea-pigs the degree of immunity produced by previous infection is not general, but local. No antibodies are present in the serum. Larvae penetrating into the immune area die in 40 hours, and immune skin grafted elsewhere retains and imparts its immunity.

Chrysomyia bezziana (Villeneuve, 1914) is metallic blue with a bright green thorax. The females lay numerous eggs in the nasal cavities, especially where there is chronic

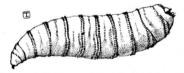

Fig. 446.—Larva of *Callitroga (Cochliomyia) hominivorax*. × 5.

nasal discharge, or in ulcers or skin wounds (for instance in leprosy), or even in the gums, conjunctivae, ears or vaginae. The larvae require living tissue in which to develop; they hatch in a few hours and burrow into the tissues, even to the bones of the nose, producing foul, infected, discharging and disfiguring lesions. These can be treated with a douche of 15% chloroform in light vegetable oil. A few drops of chloroform applied to an infested wound will cause the larvae to appear, and they can be removed with sinus forceps. This fly is common in India and tropical Africa.

Callitroga (formerly *Cochliomyia*) *hominivorax* (Coquillett, 1858) (syn. *C. americana*, screw worm) is found in the Western hemisphere. It lays its eggs in wounds, ears and nasal passages, and even in the vulva and vagina. The larvae hatch in a few hours and invade the skin, producing deep, discharging and disfiguring wounds, which may destroy cartilage and bone, even reaching the brain. A case mortality rate of 8% has been recorded. People in contact with infested cattle are particularly at risk. The fly has been eradicated from several areas in the Caribbean region by releasing millions of male flies, reared in captivity and sterilized by X-rays. Males mate several times, but females once, and the intrusion of enormous numbers of sterile males competing with the normal male population has been successful in eradicating the species.

In nasal myiasis the initial symptoms are tickling pain and nasal obstruction. Epistaxis is common, but the discharge soon becomes purulent and fetid. Inhalation of chloroform or packing with chloroform gauze, or the careful local use of weak carbolic acid and turpentine, have been advocated, but the nasal sinuses may need to be opened.

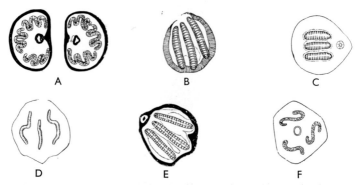

Fig. 447.—Stigmata of muscid larvae, a means of rapid identification. A, *Musca domestica*. B, *Wohlfahrtia magnifica*. C, *Auchmeromyia luteola*. D, *Stomoxys calcitrans*. E, *Calliphora vomitoria*. F, *Cordylobia anthropophaga*. Magnified.

Wohlfahrtia magnifica (Schiner, 1862) (Old World flesh fly, sheep maggot) is found in the Near East and the U.S.S.R. It deposits its larvae in skin lesions, nasal sinuses, ears, sore eyes and vagina, producing serious disfigurement. Like the larvae of *W. vigil* and *C. bezziana*, these larvae rely entirely on living vertebrates for their nutrition; they do not infest dead tissues or excreta.

Wohlfahrtia vigil Walker (the Nearctic flesh fly) deposits its larvae in lesions of the skin or mucous membranes, or even on the uninjured skin. It is attracted by foul odours from secretions of the eyes or nose, and possibly from the soiled diapers of infants; young children are particularly attractive to the flies, but they do not enter houses. Other species of *Wohlfahrtia* have also been incriminated.

Sarcophaga fuscicauda Böttcher, 1912 sometimes deposits its larvae on ulcerated areas, but it and other species normally do so on decaying flesh and excreta.

Gasterophilidae (horse bots, warble flies)

Gasterophilus species are common parasites of horses, and occasionally of man, especially in people in contact with horses. It is said that they can introduce their eggs directly under the skin, but more commonly the larvae are picked up, and these penetrate the skin, causing a swelling and a wandering tunnel in the lower epidermis, in which they may progress for long periods. These tunnels resemble the lesions caused by *Ancylostoma braziliense*, constituting one form of larva migrans (creeping eruption): they itch but do not discharge unless infected. If a small amount of clear mineral oil is smeared over the lesion, the larva can be seen and identified by the black transverse bands of spines on its body. It can be removed with a sharp needle.

Cuterebridae

Dermatobia hominis (*cyaniventris*) Linnaeus junior (Macquart, 1843) (Ver macaque, macaw worm, tropical warble fly) (Fig. 448) is widely distributed throughout South America. The larva occurs in the most diverse animals: cattle, pigs, dogs, agouti, jaguar, South American monkeys and birds; it is rare in the mule and never found in the horse. It can complete its development in man and is an example of obligatory myiasis. In man it is found in the head, arm, back, abdomen, thigh, axilla or orbit. It is a common cause of ocular myiasis in Colombia. When the larvae are hatched out they penetrate the skin and produce an inflamed swelling about the aperture of entrance, from which exudes a seropurulent fluid containing the dark faeces of the larvae. At an

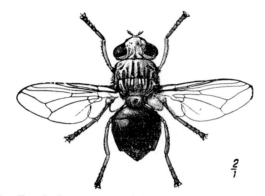

Fig. 448.—Female *Dermatobia hominis* (Lynn Jr.) syn. *cyaniventris*.

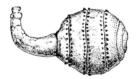

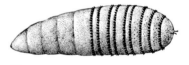

Fig. 449.—Early stage larva of *Dermatobia hominis*. (*After Blanchard*)

Fig. 450.—Later stage larva of *Dermatobia hominis*. (*After Brauer*)

early stage the larva has the curious appearance depicted (Fig. 449) and is known as ver macaque; and later, when larger (Fig. 450), it is called torcel or berne. This myiasis is acquired in a curious manner. On attaining maturity, *D. cyaniventris* lays eggs on wet leaves in damp places where mosquitoes feed, especially *Psorophora* (*Janthinosoma*) *lutzi* (Fig. 451). Other species can take on this function—mosquitoes: *Psorophora posticata, P. tovari* and *Goeldia longipes*; flies: *Sarcophaga terminalis, Musca domestica, Stomoxys calcitrans*; and a tick, *Amblyomma cajennense*. Packets of eggs are enclosed in a cement which, becoming softened by moisture, adheres to the arthropod's thorax, and the eggs are thus conveyed to man or other vertebrates when the mosquito next feeds. This process is known as phoresis or hitch-hiking. The eggs develop, and the larvae, attracted by warmth when the insect feeds, burrow into the the skin and develop like cordylobia. In Brazil this pest has been completely controlled by insecticides—DDT, BHC and toxaphene. In Curacao this fly has, in the space of 2 years, been exterminated by irradiating the males which, in turn, have sterilized the female flies.

The lesions caused by *D. hominis* are very painful and itchy. The larvae can be removed by stretching the exit aperture with forceps and applying some pressure; they then slip out. Otherwise surgical removal may be needed.

Oestridae (bot flies)

Oestrus ovis Linnaeus (sheep bot fly), which is found in the U.S.S.R. and the Mediterranean region, deposits its larvae on the conjunctivae (especially at the inner canthus), the outer nares, the lips or even the mouth. The larvae penetrate the mucous membranes, and may enter the eyelid or lacrimal duct, or even the eyeball itself. From the nares the larvae may reach the nasopharynx and the sinuses, causing secretion, pruritus and headache. Larvae about the eye can be removed with a needle or scalpel, and in the nares after treatment with chloretone or ephedrine drops. Gargles with strong salt solutions will probably help to expel the pharyngeal forms. The larvae spontaneously leave the tissues after a few days. Infestation of the eyeball is obviously serious and may require enucleation.

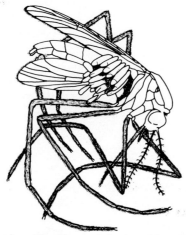

Fig. 451.—*Psorophora* (*Janthinosoma*) *lutzi* carrying eggs of *Dermatobia cyaniventris*. (*Reproduced by courtesy of the Tropical Diseases Bureau*)

Rhinoestrus purpureus (Brauer) (Russian gadfly) is found in southern and eastern Europe, the Near East and North Africa. It normally deposits its larvae in the nares of cattle and horses, but cases of ophthalmomyiasis in man have been reported.

The larvae of *Hypoderma bovis* (Linnaeus), *Hypoderma lineatum* (Villers) (cattle bots, warble flies) cause one form of creeping eruption, especially in persons closely associated with cattle. The eggs are deposited on the hairs of cattle, hatching within a week. In infested persons the larvae penetrate into the subcutaneous tissues, more deeply than *Gasterophilus*, producing an inflamed swelling resembling a boil, which is painful. They migrate, sometimes for considerable distances. The lesion can be treated by making a cruciform incision and removing the larva. Ophthalmomyiasis interna has been reported and is serious.

For ocular myiasis see Chapter 44.

FACULTATIVE MYIASIS PRODUCERS

Calliphoridae

Larvae of *Calliphora vomitoria* (Linnaeus), *C. vicina* (Robineau-Desvoidy) have been found in wounds, in which they feed on the necrotic tissues, but can also attack healthy tissues. They can even penetrate unbroken skin.

Larvae of other flies—*Lucilia, Phormia, Musca, Fannia* and others—have also been found in wounds. *Lucilia sericata* has been found in the nares.

At one time it was found useful to clean septic wounds or bones with osteomyelitis by introducing carefully cultivated larvae of *Lucilia* and *Phormia* into the septic area, to feed on diseased tissues and bacteria. The practice has now been abandoned.

Species of *Sarcophaga, Wohlfahrtia* and *Chrysomyia* are also facultative.

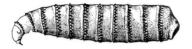

Fig. 452.—Larva of *Calliphora vomitoria*.

ACCIDENTAL MYIASIS PRODUCERS

Intestinal myiasis

Eggs, and sometimes larvae, of many species of flies are deposited on foodstuffs, and sometimes survive the journey down the intestinal tract. They may then develop in the folds of mucous membrane, even causing some irritation (pain, vomiting, diarrhoea) or even ulceration before being evacuated. If deposited round the anus, such larvae may crawl into the rectum to complete their feeding inside the body. This kind of infestation may persist for months, producing severe nervous symptoms as well as internal irritation. The larvae can be recognized in the faeces, sometimes in vomit.

The flies usually implicated include species of *Musca, Fannia, Chrysomyia, Calliphora* and others. Prevention entails the careful covering of food. Treatment with castor oil will probably expel these larvae.

Urinary myiasis

A mistaken diagnosis of urinary myiasis due to a larva from a contaminated vessel in which urine has been collected, or which has been introduced into the urine after it was passed, is not uncommon, but there have been a few true cases in which the larvae have been passed via the urethra from the bladder. If the vulva or vaginal area in women is infested, there are obvious opportunities for larvae to enter the bladder. The flies concerned are of the families Muscidae, Psychodidae, Piophilidae, Calliphoridae and Sarcophidae.

ORDER: ANOPLURA (Lice)
FAMILY: PEDICULIDAE
GENUS: *Pediculus*

Lice are obligatory parasites and spend the whole of their life on the body of some particular host. They cannot live, apart from their host, longer than 12 hours at 40°C or 10 days at 5°C. There is a great reduction in the size of the eyes and antennae. They have flattened bodies without wings, and an indistinctly segmented thorax. The integument is tough, to resist pressure. The number of abdominal segments ranges from 6 to 9, the last being bilobed. Spiracles stand out prominently on the sides of the abdominal segments. In the male the abdomen ends bluntly, bearing a spine-like penis. The legs are modified for holding on. The eggs or nits adhere to the body hairs of host, and the young which emerge are miniature editions of the adults. The sub-species of louse parasitic on man are 2 in number: *Pediculus humanus corporis*, the body-louse, and *P. humanus capitis*, the head-louse (Fig. 453). These interbreed and produce fertile offspring. The egg nits of *P. corporis* are laid on the body hair, but mostly on the inner surface of clothing. Those of *P. capitis* are laid on the head at the base of the hairs, which grow up with them. The female produces about 5 eggs a day and continues to do so for a month; the eggs hatch in 8 days at 32°C, but take longer at a lower temperature.

The immature louse, or nymph, moults 3 times, and becomes mature in 14 days. Like the adult, it feeds on blood twice a day. The life span of the adult is from 4 to 6 weeks. Lice cannot live for any length of time on discarded clothing. Under experimental conditions they can survive at the low temperature of 5°C.

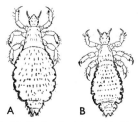

Fig. 453.—A, Female *Pediculus humanus*. B, Female *Pediculus humanus* var. *capitis*. × 5. (*After Cummings; by permission of the Trustees of the British Museum*)

Infection with lice occurs through close contact with verminous persons huddled together. Lice avoid light, and tend to leave patients with fever and sweating, so that this is a factor in the transmission of disease. They also leave a body which is undergoing hard physical exercise, and they leave a corpse.

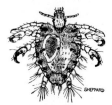

Fig. 454.—Female *Phthirus pubis*, showing the contained ovum. × 12.

Lice convey relapsing fever and the rickettsia of exanthematic typhus (*R. prowazeki*), and that of trench fever (*R. quintana*). They also play a part in the spread of taeniasis. *Dipylidium caninum* is occasionally found in children and has as its larval host *Trichodectes canis*, the dog louse, and it may also develop in *P. humanus*.

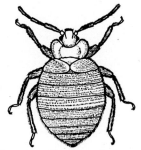

Fig. 455.—*Cimex lectularis*. × 7.

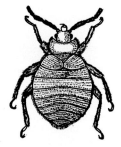

Fig. 456.—*Cimex hemipterus* (*rotundatus*). × 6.

Another species is *Phthirus pubis* (Fig. 454), the 'crab-louse', which lives chiefly in the genital and inguinal regions, and is acquired mostly during coitus. It is distinguished from other lice by its broad flat body and festooned abdomen of 6 segments. The second and third pairs of legs have massive talon-like claws. By these means the louse clings to 2 approximated hairs 2 mm apart. The life cycle is completed in 27 days. The lice of rats and pigs —*Haematopinus* and *Polyplax*—also belong to this order.

Prophylaxis

For destruction of lice and eggs in clothes on a large scale an efficient method is by dry or moist heat; a temperature of 50–55°C will kill in 40 minutes. The application of a hot iron to the seams is useful. For practical purposes, clothes should be exposed to 70°C for 30 minutes. Attention must be directed to folds and pleats.

For head lice the hair must be cut short, and a comb with square-edged teeth (*Sacker* patent), used with soft soap, is useful to remove nits. For destruction of adult lice all former methods have now been superseded by DDT or other insecticides.

ORDER: HEMIPTERA (Bugs)
FAMILY: CIMICIDAE
GENUS: *Cimex*

Bed-bugs (*Cimex*) have a world-wide distribution. The species parasitic on man are *Cimex lectularius* (Fig. 455), the bed-bug of Europe, and *C. hemipterus* (*rotundatus*), the bug of the tropics, which is distinguished by its elongated, narrow abdomen (Fig. 456). In West Africa a species of another genus—*Leptocimex boueti*—attacks man. The body of *C. lectularius* is broad and flat, the head short and broad, attached to the thorax, the antennae four-jointed, and the eyes present, but reduced in size. The mouth-parts (jointed proboscis) are normally folded back under the head. The maxillae are serrated at the tip. Lying in a groove between the head and the thorax are short pad-like hemi-elytra characteristic of the practically wingless condition. *Cimex* feeds only on blood, and can resist starvation well. The labium does not pierce the skin, but buckles up like that of a mosquito. The bodies of bugs give out a nasty, pungent odour. Bed-bugs are nocturnal in their feeding habits, hiding in crevices during the day-time. The eggs are shaped like a wine-bottle with a cap and stuck on to the surface of the crevices of woodwork in houses, beds, mattresses, behind pictures and nail holes. Nests can be located by finding the black faeces round holes.

The females deposit eggs in batches from 10 to 50, totalling 200–500: they are large, yellowish white and easily visible to the naked eye. The nymphs resemble adults and are white, with no elytra or rudimentary wings; they mature in about 6 weeks, if fed at each stage, but each can resist starvation for 2 months. Under less favourable conditions, development may be protracted to 6 months or more. Adults may live for many months. Bed-bugs are sensitive to high temperatures: even 37·8°C with a fairly high humidity will kill many. The most effective method is fumigation with sulphur. The dosage necessary varies from 0·34 to 0·74 kg/28 m³), with an exposure of at least 6 hours. Sulphur dioxide is cheap and, owing to its smell, free from hazard. It kills the active stages of the bug, but a few eggs may escape, and complete combustion must be ensured.

Hydrocyanic acid fumigation is very efficacious, but dangerous, and must be carried out only by skilled persons. For articles of furniture, which cannot be boiled in water, an emulsion of petroleum is used: 3 parts of soap to 15 of hot water, to which 70–100 parts of oil are added, should be forced into cracks and crevices with a brush.

Coal-tar naphtha is lethal to bugs and nymphs, but less so to eggs. The concentration which can be obtained at 15·6°C is 0·2% over a period of 24 hours. Bugs are also destroyed by some insecticides.

Though bed-bugs cause a great deal of irritation by their bites, they have not been actually proved to disseminate disease, with the doubtful exception of relapsing fever.

FAMILY: REDUVIIDAE

Reduviid bugs ('assassin or kissing bugs') include a number of species which feed on human blood, inflicting painful bites. They are classified into several genera—*Pan-*

strongylus, Eratyrus, Triatoma and *Rhodnius,* and are confined to America, from 41°N. to 41°S. One (*T. rubrofasciata*) has a cosmopolitan distribution.

These bugs live on wild animals in nests and burrows, but certain species become domesticated, living in crevices in the walls of mud houses. Larvae and nymphs are flightless, and can only bite human beings in their immediate vicinity, but the adults of both sexes can fly considerable distances. When engorged with blood after a feed they void from the cloaca a white or dark fluid which may contain *Trypanosoma cruzi.* The trypanosomes may thus gain entrance through the wound made by the bite. The bite itself is not infective. Eggs are laid singly.

The larvae, on emerging, engorge themselves with blood on 4 occasions, undergoing a moult after each; they then become nymphs, which, after several feeds, moult for a fifth and final time before becoming adult. The whole cycle of evolution takes 3 or 4 months to complete.

The life-span is on an average one of over 3 months, and when once infected with *T. cruzi* the insects remain so for the remainder of their life span.

GENERA: *Panstrongylus* (Burmeister, 1835) and *Triatoma* (Wolf, 1802)

The genera *Panstrongylus* and *Triatoma* were separated by Pinto on certain characteristics of the probosces and antennae.

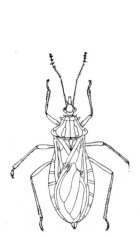

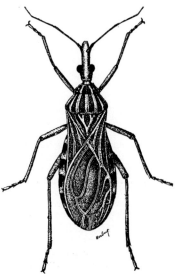

Fig. 457.—*Panstrongylus megistus,* natural size.

Fig. 458.—Adult male *Rhodnius prolixus.* × 2½. (*After Brumpt*)

GENUS: *Panstrongylus*

Synonym: *Conorhinus* (Laporte, 1832)

This genus is distinguished by its smooth body and elongated or conical head.

P. megistus (Burmeister, 1835) (Brazil) is a domestic species measuring 3 cm in length. The body is black, with red stripes (Fig. 457). The insect has feeble powers of flight. The life cycle takes a year to complete, and the adults can live about 6 months.

P. chagasi (Brumpt and F. Gomes, 1914) (Brazil) has a characteristic red band on the head, and lives in the burrows of *Kerodon rupestris* and those of armadillos. This species has been found infected with *Trypanosoma cruzi* at a considerable distance from human habitations.

P. dimidiatus (Erichson, 1848) (Brazil, Venezuela, British Guiana, and San Salvador) is also naturally infected with *T. cruzi* and possibly conveys the human disease in San Salvador.

P. geniculatus (Latreille, 1811) (Paraguay, Brazil, Peru, Venezuela and French Guyana) is a sombre-coloured species, living normally in armadillo burrows; it transmits *T. cruzi* to these animals.

GENUS: *Triatoma* (Laporte, 1833)

Triatoma infestans (Klug, 1834) (South America) is a domestic species and lives in cracks in the walls of houses or hen-roosts. It is found naturally infected with *T. cruzi* in Argentina.

T. protracta (Uhler, 1894) (the United States, from Utah to California) is known as the 'kissing bug', and lives in the burrows of rodents. Under natural conditions it harbours a trypanosome, *T. neotomae*.

T. rubrofasciata (de Geer, 1773), a cosmopolitan domestic species, can be infected experimentally with *T. cruzi*. It has been suspected, on rather imperfect evidence, of once transmitting kala-azar in India.

T. sanguisuga (Lecomte, 1855) (United States) is a common domestic species which associates with bed-bugs. Under experimental conditions it can be infected with *T. cruzi*.

T. sordida (Stal, 1859) (Brazil, Bolivia and Paraguay) is a small domestic species met with near the banks of the large rivers; it has been found naturally infected with *T. cruzi*.

T. vitticeps (Stal, 1859) (Brazil) is the largest known of these insects, and is a rare species.

GENUS: *Eratyrus* (Stal)

Eratyrus cuspidatus (Stal, 1859) (Venezuela) is rare, occurs at an altitude of 1380 m and is naturally infected with *T. cruzi*.

GENUS: *Rhodnius* (Stal, 1850)

This genus is characterized by a narrow attenuated head and by elongated antennae (Fig. 458).

Rhodnius prolixus (Stal, 1859) (Venezuela, Colombia, Guiana, Brazil and San Salvador) has nocturnal habits, and feeds voraciously on human blood. Normally it lives in the burrows of the armadillo and those of a rodent (*Coelogenys subniger*).

The adult is capable of flying considerable distances; the larvae and nymphs live in cracks in the walls and in the crevices of palm trees.

Under experimental conditions this species can transmit *T. cruzi*, and harbours *T. rangeli* (see page 963).

A list of the bugs infected with *T. cruzi* and *T. rangeli* in S. America is given by Dias.

Rhodnius prolixus is the chief vector and *Triatoma infestans* in Brazil; in São Paulo 25·19% infected; in Minas Geraes 18·54%; in Rio Grande do Sol 56·69%. In Paraiba *P. megistus* and *T. maculata* are chief vectors; Mexico *T. sanguisuga*, *R. prolixus*; Guatemala *T. dimidiata*; Panama *Eratyrus cuspidatus*, *R. pallescens*; Argentina *R. prolixus*, *Eutriatoma sordida*, *T. infestans*; Bolivia *Eutriatoma sordida*, *T. infestans*; Brazil *P. megistus*, *T. brasiliensis*, *Eutriatoma sordida*, *T. chagasi*, *T. vitticeps*; Chile *Mapraia spinolai*, *T. infestans*; Colombia *R. prolixus*, *R. pictipes*; Paraguay *E. sordida*; Uruquay *E. sordida*, *T. infestans*; Ecuador *Eratyrus cuspidatus*; Venezuela *Eratyrus cuspidatus*, *Eutriatoma nigromaculata*, *P. rubrotuberculatus*, *Psammolestes arthuri*, *P. geniculatus*, *R. prolixus*.

ORDER: SIPHONAPTERA
FAMILY: PULICIDAE
FLEAS

Fleas have laterally compressed bodies and are wingless, with mouth-parts adapted for piercing and sucking blood. They are active ectoparasites, almost exclusively of birds and mammals, and do not resist starvation. Many are moderately specific in their choice of host, but will migrate to another where necessary. The female is larger than the male, and in the former the curved *receptaculum seminis* forms a conspicuous feature. The eyes and antennae are reduced, the latter fitting into a pit on the side of the head. The maxillae are short and the mandibles function as cutting organs. Some have combs on the head and thorax. The body is contained in plates which represent a fusion of sternal, pleural and tergal portions. The ninth sternite is converted into a paired boomerang-shaped structure, and superficially looks like a clasper. White eggs are dropped by the female indiscriminately and hatch in summer time in 3 or 4 days. The larva lives in dust, feeds on debris, crumbs and faeces of adults, and is an active, footless maggot of a whitish colour, sparsely adorned with hairs (Fig. 459). When fully grown, it spins a cocoon and pupates; the duration of this stage depends on temperature. A resting larval stage occurs, in which it can remain dormant for months

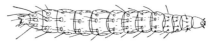

Fig. 459.—Larva of *Xenopsylla cheopis*. Magnified. (*After Bacot & Ridgway*)

The pupae are similar in shape to the adults, and encased in a cocoon. The adult may remain thus encased as a resting adult stage or hypopus. Inside the crop, or proventriculus, there is a patch of spines, about 800 in number, which help to crush up the red blood corpuscles of the host.

There are 2 main families: *Pulicidae* (ordinary fleas), 30 genera, and *Tungidae* (chiggers) a small group.

Of *Pulicidae* 5 genera are important, and the following points are used for identification:

1. Head and thorax without combs—*Pulex* or *Xenopsylla*.
2. Head, no comb; thorax with combs—*Nosopsyllus* (*Ceratophyllus*).
3. Head and thorax with comb—*Ctenocephalides* (*Ctenocephalus*).
4. Head pointed, without eyes—*Leptopsyllus*.
5. Distinction between *Pulex* and *Xenopsylla* is based on the mesopleural plate:

   Pulex has no vertical bar: *Xenopsylla* has vertical bar. Therefore, a flea without combs with vertical bar = *Xenopsylla*. But a flea without combs, with antennal groove forming a thickening extending to top of head = *Pulex*.

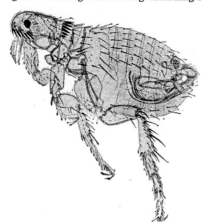

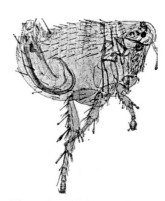

Fig. 460.—Male *Ctenocephalides canis*. × 16. (*After Bomford*)

Fig. 461.—Male *Xenopsylla cheopis*. × 16. (*After Bomford*)

Nosopsyllus fasciatus is the common rodent flea of temperate and tropical climates, and the dominant rat-flea of Europe. It will attack man in the absence of rats.

Ctenocephalides canis and *C. felis* are very similar and interchangeable between the dog and cat; they may also be found on rats. They attack man readily (Fig. 460).

Ctenopsyllus (Leptopsyllus) segnis is the mouse-flea and is also found on rats.

Hoplopsyllus anomalus infests ground squirrels and rats in the western U.S.A., has a pronotal comb, and plays a part in dissemination of rodent plague.

Pulex irritans, the common human flea, has decreased in Europe enormously during the last 30 years but has penetrated many parts of the tropics; it is occasionally found on rats and pigs (Fig. 462).

Xenopsylla contains 30–40 species which flourish in the tropics; they require a higher temperature to develop, and exist in heated buildings in England, America and Russia (Fig. 461).

In the male *X. astia* (Rothschild, 1911) the antepygidial bristle is similar to that of *X. cheopis*, but it is easily differentiated by the shape of the ninth sternite, which,

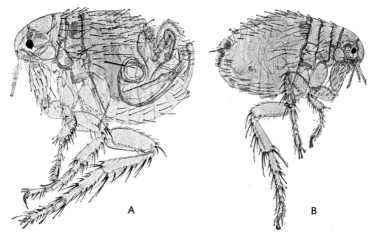

Fig. 462.—*Pulex irritans*. A, Male. × 25. B, Female. × 14. (*After T. L. Bomford*)

instead of being club-shaped, has the appearance of a ribbon, due to chitinization of its ventral margin. The outer flap of the organs of copulation is narrower than in *X. cheopis*, and bears fewer bristles. The 'tail' of the receptaculum is so strongly widened near the constriction that it is much wider than the head. The eighth segment has more than 30 bristles on the outer surface (Fig. 463).

In the male *Xenopsylla braziliensis* (Baker, 1904) the long dorsal bristle on the seventh abdominal segment in front of the pygidium is placed on a long pedestal. In the female the 'head' of the receptaculum seminis is very much wider than the 'tail' (Fig. 463).

In the male *X. cheopis* (Rothschild 1903) the antepygidial bristle is situated on a short pedestal. The outer flap of the copulatory organs is sole-shaped; its upper edge is more curved than the lower, and bears 9 or 10 bristles on its outer surface, all of them thinner than in *X. braziliensis*, and drawn out into a long, thin point. The ninth sternite has the appearance of a club, the upper side of which is flattened.

In the female the 'tail' of the receptaculum is much longer than in the preceding species and, near the constriction, is distinctly wider than the 'head' (Fig. 463).

X. cheopis must feed every 10 days, except in the adult resting stage and in temperate climates. It may hibernate as an adult and so may remain infected with plague throughout the winter, as occurs in the case of rodent-flea plague in Siberia.

X. cheopis is widely disseminated on rats—*R. rattus, R. norvegicus; X. braziliensis* on rats in Uganda, Kenya and Nigeria; *X. astia* on rats in India, Ceylon, Burma and Iraq; *X. nubica* on rats in tropical E. and W. Africa; *X. eridos* on wild rodents in S. Africa; *Pulex irritans,* universal in S. Africa on pigs and rodents; *Nosopsyllus fasciatus* on *R. norvegicus* in temperate zones; *Diamanus montanus* on ground squirrels in W. U.S.A.; *Rhopalopsyllus cavicola* in S. American cavies; *Ceratophyllus tesquorum* on ground squirrels on Russian steppes; *Oropsylla silantievi* on rodents in Manchuria.

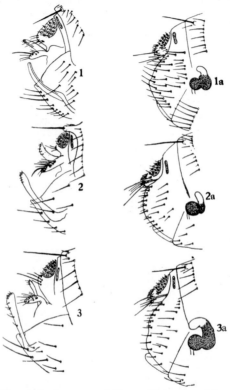

Fig. 463.—Diagnostic characters of *Xenopsylla* rat fleas. Magnified. (*After Cragg & Hirst*)

1, *X. astia*: pygidium of the male. 1a, *X. astia*: pygidium and spermatheca of the female. 2, *X. braziliensis*: pygidium of the male. 2a, *X. braziliensis*: pygidium and spermatheca of the female. 3, *X. cheopis*: pygidium of male. 3a, *X. cheopis*: pygidium and spermatheca of the female.

FAMILY: TUNGIDAE
GENUS: *Tunga*

Tunga penetrans (Jarocki, 1838), the 'chigger flea' (Fig. 464; Fig. 228, page 788), has a powerfully toothed mandible, a short thorax and slender legs. In the female the spiracles are massed at the hind end of the abdomen. In the early stages it behaves like other fleas, but when the female is impregnated, it attaches itself to the skin, especially of the feet, burrowing deeply with its mandibles until it becomes covered with skin with only the spiracles projecting. When filled with eggs the body swells enormously. When the eggs are discharged the female dies and sloughs away. The egg is oval, about 0·5 mm in length. A larva emerges in 3 days, resembling other flea larvae, but has a chitinous structure on its head, the 'egg breaker' with which it slits the egg shell. Then it feeds on organic matter in dust and passes through 2 larval stages. A pupa is formed in 14 days. In the second stage the larva spins a silken cocoon within which it casts its skin and becomes a pupa. The flea emerges in 1 week. *T. penetrans* originated in America, and has long been known in West and South Africa; but only comparatively recently in East Africa and West Coast of India.

Echidnophaga gallinacea, the stick-tight flea, is a dangerous pest of poultry, but also attacks man occasionally, dogs, rabbits, cats, rats and horses. The adults are very active, but during copulation the female flea attaches herself to the skin and then burrows into it, forming a swelling which may ulcerate. In the lesion so produced the female lays eggs that drop to the ground, where the larvae develop as do other fleas.

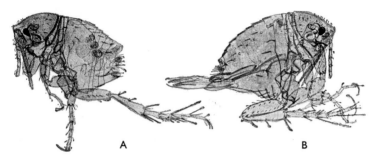

Fig. 464.—*Tunga penetrans* (*Dermatophyllus penetrans, Sarcopsylla penetrans*). A, Female. B, Male. × 38. (*After Bomford*)

Importance of fleas to man

Flea bites may cause severe irritation in some individuals. This is largely an anaphylactic response in persons who are sensitized; subsequent desensitization may take place. Tapeworm eggs are eaten by fleas and encyst in the larva, pupa and adult, e.g. *Hymenolepis diminuta* of rat and *Dipylidium caninum* of dog. Endemic murine typhus is normally spread by fleas in the following rhythm:

Rat—rat louse—rat—rat flea—man

Plague is essentially a disease of rodents spread by *X. cheopis* and other fleas by the method of 'blockage' (page 460), which is due to their peculiar type of proventriculus. *X. astia* can transmit the plague bacillus, but is not nearly so effective as *X. cheopis*.

Identification

Three species of *Xenopsylla*—*X. cheopis, X. astia* and *X. braziliensis*—are ectoparasites of the rat in India. It is not possible to make out the distinguishing features of the 3 species unless the specimens are suitably prepared. With the aid of a hand lens, the females can be recognized by the shape of the spermatheca after the soft parts have been dissolved by caustic potash, or rendered transparent by means of a clearing agent. For the certain identification of the males, a compound microscope is necessary, when it can be seen that the ninth sternite ends in a sharp point in *X. astia*, instead of a flattened projection, as in *X. cheopis*. The shape of the claspers differs in *X. astia*; they are more elongated. These differential characters can only be relied upon in fleas from the Indian area, because in that country only these 3 species exist.

After a short preliminary treatment with caustic potash, the fleas are treated with alcohol and xylol and placed overnight in a thin solution of balsam in xylol. Slides are prepared by coating the specimens with a thin layer of balsam and allowing them to dry overnight in the incubator. The fleas themselves are mounted and orientated on the slide; the insects can then be individually examined under the microscope in rows of 5.

Prophylaxis

To rid cats and dogs of these insects they should be washed with carbolic soap or a strong lather of 'vermijelli'. Cats that object to water may be powdered with DDT or other insecticides. The floors of the house should be washed with a solution of naphthalene in benzene. An emulsion of petroleum which will kill fleas when diluted with water, 1 in 20 or more, may be made from soft soap and ordinary petroleum, 3 parts of soap being dissolved by heat in 15 of water, and 70–100 parts of oil added while still hot, with much shaking and stirring. The final mixture should be white and creamy.

The irritation of flea-bites may be allayed by the application of 1 in 20 phenol. The good repellents for fleas are dimethyl phthalate, Rutgers 612 and indalone.

Rat flea survey

This consists of collecting information on an abundance of fleas and identifying the species at different seasons. Single rats should be caught alive and kept under observation. Fleas should be collected, counted and examined. Rats must be kept apart; if 2 are together they fight and interchange fleas. The rats are killed so as to preserve all their fleas. The trap should be put into a white bag in a chamber filled with cyanide gas, which kills rat and fleas together. The fleas should be mounted in pure phenol. Record should be kept of the species and sex of the rat, the species and numbers of fleas present.

The *flea index* is the number of fleas per rat and is used in making surveys of plague.

REFERENCES

BUXTON, P. A. (1955) 'The Natural History of Tsetse Flies', *Memoir Ser. Lond. Sch. Hyg. trop. Med.*, 10.

CHRISTOPHER, S. R. (1960) *Aedes aegypti (L), The Yellow Fever Mosquito: Its Life History, Bionomics and Structure*. London: Cambridge University Press.

DE LEON, J. R. & DURE, B. O. L. (1966) *Trans. R. Soc. trop. Med. Hyg.*, **60**, 735.

FAUST, E. C. & RUSSELL, P. F. (1964) *Craig & Faust's Clinical Parasitology*, 6th ed. London: Kimpton.

FINNEGAN, S. (1946) *British Museum (Natural History) Economic Series*, 16. London: British Museum.

FORD, J. (1971) *The Role of the Trypanosomiases in African Ecology: A Study of the Tsetse Fly Problem*. Oxford: Clarendon.

HOPPS, H. C., KEEGAN, H. L., PRICE, D. L. & SELF, J. T. (1971) *Pathology of Protozoal and Helminthic Diseases* (ed. Paul A. Marcial Rojas), p. 970. Baltimore: Williams & Wilkins.

LEWIS, D. J., LAINSON, R. & SHAW, J. J. (1970) *Bull. ent. Res.*, **60**, 209.

MACDONALD, W. W. (1962) *Ann. trop. Med. Parasit.*, **56**, 373.

MULLIGAN, H. W. (1970) *The African Trypanosomiases*. London: Allen & Unwin.

RADCLIFFE, W. (1972) *Br. med. J.*, **ii**, 164.

SCHACHER, J. F., SABB, S., GERMANOS, R. & BOUSTANY, N. (1969) *Trans. R. Soc. trop. Med. Hyg.*, **63**, 854.

Synoptic Catalog of Mosquitoes of the World (1959) Vol. VI. Washington: Entomological Society of America.

WADDY, B. B. (1968) *Trans. R. Soc. trop. Med. Hyg.*, **62**, 17.

WALTON, G. A. (1962) *Symp. Zool. Soc. Lond.*, **6**, 83.

APPENDIX IV

CLINICAL PATHOLOGY

VARIETIES OF BLOOD CELLS AND THEIR SIGNIFICANCE (PLATE XIV)

Leucocytes

THE mean total leucocyte count in adults is 7000 (5000–10 000), comprising:

Polymorphonuclear neutrophils	4500 (3000–7000)	66% (60–70%)
Eosinophils	100 (50–400)	1·5% (1–4%)
Basophils	25 (0–50)	0·5% (0–1%)
Lymphocytes	1800 (1000–3000)	26% (20–30%)
Monocytes	450 (100–600)	6% (2–6%)

At birth the total number is high (22 000 or more) but falls sharply within 3–4 days. In adult life a count above 10 000 indicates *leucocytosis*: a count below 5000 indicates *leucopenia*. Leucocytosis can occur as a response to infection, or when blood is concentrated (as in cholera), or in tropical eosinophilia and other conditions, for instance anaphylaxis.

Polymorphonuclear neutrophils (microphages). The name polymorphonuclear means cells which have nuclei of many shapes. The cells measure 10–12 μm in diameter, and each is equipped with a nucleus which is normally divided into 2–5 lobes joined by a thread of nuclear tissue. The younger the cell the fewer the lobes, and an excess of cells with only 1–2 lobes indicates rapid production and rapid extinction; it is therefore an indication of excess demand, such as occurs when those cells are called upon to combat bacterial infection by phagocytosis, as in acute pyogenic infections and many other conditions. The *Arneth index* is the mean number of lobes per polymorphonuclear cell, calculated by counting an adequate number of cells. An increase in the number having only 1–2 lobes per nucleus is called a shift to the left, and indicates an excess of young cells. Polymorphs are active phagocytes of foreign bodies or foreign antigens; in tissues their action can be detrimental in that they damage tissue cells. Polymorphonuclear leucocytosis occurs in response to many bacterial infections; leucopenia (agranulocytosis, meaning diminished numbers of granular cells) occurs in kala-azar and some other infections, and also as a result of the action of sulphonamides and other drugs.

The nuclei of polymorphonuclear neutrophils stain deeply with the Romanowsky stains, and their cytoplasm contains numerous reddish granules which, in spite of the name neutrophil, have taken up the eosin, acting as slightly acidophil bodies.

Eosinophils (12–14 μm) contain coarse granules staining bright red with Romanoswky stains. The nuclei are lobed, but not so much as the polymorphs. Eosinophils are increased in most helminthic infections, especially in filariasis of various kinds, schistosomiasis and trichinosis, when the proportion may reach 20–60% of the total leucocytes. Great increase is also a feature of tropical eosinophilia and Loeffler's syndrome, asthma and anaphylactic conditions. Eosinophils seem to be attracted to concentrations of histamine, which they detoxify; they also phagocytose antigen–antibody complexes.

Basophils (10–12 μm). The nuclei are kidney-shaped and may be lobulated. The cytoplasm contains large granules staining blue or purple with Romanowsky. Punctate basophilia is one feature of lead poisoning. The exact function of these cells is not clear.

Lymphocytes (small 5–8 μm; large 12–15 μm) are important cells, largely involved in the phenomena of immunity. The nucleus of each cell is large and single; the cytoplasm stains blue with Romanowsky. Lymphocytes arise from precursors in bone marrow, and take part both in cell-mediated immunity developed in response to antigens fixed in the tissues and in the production of humoral antibodies in response to soluble antigens. From the bone marrow lymphocytes the progeny may become sensitized by a foreign antigen (or even an auto-antigen), and proliferate in lymph nodes or the spleen, to produce immunologically active lymphocytes which can enter the blood to attack foreign antigens, provoking inflammatory response or, in the case of homografts, starting the process of rejection. This cell-mediated response is known to depend upon the integrity of the thymus during embryonic and early neonatal life. Macrophages appear to interact with lymphocytes in these processes (Turk 1969).

In the humoral antibody series the progeny of the bone marrow lymphocytes pass to intestinal lymph follicles and other lymph nodes and the spleen, where they may meet antigens from macrophages. They give rise to plasma cells which form the immuno-globulins which are the humoral antibodies. This whole process is not, however, clearly understood. The immunoglobulins in normal serum are:

$$\begin{array}{lll} \text{IgG} & 800\text{--}1680 \text{ mg/100 ml} & 78\% \\ \text{IgA} & 140\text{--}420 \text{ mg/100 ml} & 16\cdot6\% \\ \text{IgM} & 50\text{--}190 \text{ mg/100 ml} & 5\cdot0\% \\ \text{IgD} & 0\cdot3\text{--}40 \text{ mg/100 ml} & 0\cdot4\% \\ \text{IgE} & 0\cdot0001\text{--}0\cdot0007 \text{ mg/100 ml} \end{array}$$

(Turk 1969)

Monocytes (*macrophages, large hyalines*) (16–22 µm) are actively phagocytic. They are increased in protozoal diseases, and increase should lead to suspicion of these diseases. They may appear in urine and faeces; in faeces they are motile and their cytoplasm contains ingested material; they have often been mistaken for trophozoites of *Entamoeba histolytica*, with all the dangers of such a mistake.

Erythrocytes

Erythrocytes (7·2–7·5 µm) arise from precursor cells in bone marrow, and have a life span of 109–120 days, corresponding to a replacement rate of about 0·9% daily. Small forms (microcytes) are sometimes seen, and large forms (megalocytes) occur in anaemias of various kinds. Immature erythrocytes appear in the peripheral blood when the bone marrow is more than usually active, indicating the need to replace erythrocytes more than normally lost or destroyed, for instance in malaria and the anaemias. Immature forms stain pale violet or purplish blue (polychromasia), and basophilic stippling sometimes occurs. They lead to *reticulocytes*, which contain haemoglobin but have a basophilic reticulum shown on vital staining. In normal persons these average 6–9/1000 erythrocytes, more in infancy and in haemolytic anaemia or haemorrhage; a reticulocyte count is helpful in anaemic states. Some malaria parasites show partiality for reticulocytes.

Reticulocytes can be stained by mixing one drop of 0·2% brilliant cresyl blue (in 0·6% NaCl solution, and filtered) with one drop of blood on a slide, and covering. After 5 minutes the reticulum can be seen stained blue.

Normoblasts are also increased in anaemia.

Target cells are very thin erythrocytes; on staining they show a deeply stained centre and periphery, with a lighter zone in between.

Megaloblasts are large nucleated erythrocytes, with basophilic cytoplasm and a large pale nucleus; they do not contain haemoglobin.

Blood platelets (*thrombocytes*) (2–4 µm) stain blue or purple with Romanowsky; they also stain with cresyl blue. The normal count is 150 000–500 000/mm³. Purpura is usually present when the count is below 40 000; bleeding time is prolonged and clot retraction poor.

MICROSCOPICAL EXAMINATION OF THE FAECES FOR INTESTINAL PARASITES

Helminth eggs

The eggs of tapeworms, with the exception of *Diphyllobothrium latum*, and thread-worms (*Enterobius vermicularis*) (Plate XIII) are rarely found in the stools, as these parasites do not, as a rule, part with their eggs until the segments of the former, or the entire body of the latter, have left the alimentary canal. However, the eggs of hepatic and other parasites, such as *Schistosoma haematobium*, *S. mansoni*, *S. japonicum*, *Clonorchis sinensis*, *Fasciola hepatica*, *Fasciolopsis buski*, *Heterophyes heterophyes* and rarer helminths are encountered.

The microscopical examination of faeces for eggs is by no means difficult. Place on the slide a minute portion of the suspected faeces, the size of a hempseed, and apply the cover-glass, gently gliding it over the slide so as to spread out the mass in a thin, fairly uniform and transparent layer.

The points to be attended to in the identification of eggs are size, shape, colour, thickness, roughness, smoothness and markings on the surface of the shell; the presence or absence of yolk spheres, of a differentiated embryo or, in the cestodes, of the 3 pairs of embryonic hooklets; the existence of an operculum in certain trematodes and in the broad tapeworms (*Diphyllobothrium*). Eggs of the same species of parasite vary slightly, but are in every instance sufficiently stable and definite for correct diagnosis.

Of the three common nematodes—*Trichuris trichiura*, *Ascaris lumbricoides* and *Ancylostoma duodenale*—the eggs of the first are the most frequently met. Those of *T. trichiura* occur sometimes in enormous numbers, as many as 6 or 8 specimens being visible in one field of 2·5 cm objective. They form rather striking objects under the microscope. They are oval, measuring 51–54 × 22 μm, the ends of the long axis of the oval being slightly pointed, and tipped with a little shining projection or plug. Their general appearance suggests an elongated oval tray, the projections at the poles of the ovum representing the handles. They are dark brown, sharply defined, doubly outlined and contain no differentiated embryo.

Eggs of *Ascaris lumbricoides* are considerably larger (50–75 × 40–50 μm) than those of *Trichuris*. As a rule they are more spherical or, rather, more broadly oval; occasionally they are almost barrel-shaped. Like those of *Trichuris*, they are dark brown from bile staining, but they are much less sharply and smoothly defined, possessing a coarse thick shell, which is roughened by many warty excrescences. The yolk contents are not always easily made out, nor, when made out, can any indications of embryo or segmentation be discovered. In certain instances the eggs are smooth on the surface, the rough outer layer being almost or altogether absent. In this condition they are unfertilized.

A point of practical importance is that the rough outer layer of the shell of the egg of *Ascaris* is very easily detached, leaving it with a sharp, smooth outline suggesting some other species of parasite. To obviate this, in mounting faeces it is well to avoid too much gliding of the cover-glass over the slide.

Eggs of *Ancylostoma duodenale* contrast very markedly with both the foregoing, particularly in colour. *Trichuris* and *Ascaris* eggs are invariably dark and bile-stained; those of the *Ancylostoma* are beautifully clear and transparent, measure 55–60 × 32–40 μm and have a regular, somewhat elongated oval form, with a delicate, smooth, transparent shell, through which 2, 4, or 8 light grey yolk segments can be distinctly seen. Eggs should be looked for soon after the faeces have been passed; otherwise, owing to the rapidity with which, in favourable circumstances, development proceeds, the embryo may have quitted the shell and the egg be no longer visible. The eggs of *Necator americanus* cannot be differentiated from those of *A. duodenale* with certainty. The eggs of *Trichostrongylus colubriformis* also resemble those of *A. duodenale*, but they are relatively larger and contain a fully segmented morula.

The eggs of *Heterodera radicicola* (*H. marioni*) or *Meliodogne javanica*, which have a characteristic appearance, have been noted from time to time in the faeces of otherwise normal individuals since their discovery by Kofoid and White in 1919. *H. radicicola* is a common root-parasitic nematode living in a variety of plants, such as radishes, celery, carrots and turnips; it is therefore apt to be encountered in the excreta of individuals who have ingested these vegetables. Of conspicuous asymmetric appearance and size, 95 × 40 μm, it might well be regarded in human faeces as an indication of nematode infection of the intestinal canal. A feature of the egg is the presence of 2 highly refractile, flattened, bluish-green globules at the poles of the embryo. As a rule the eggs are kidney-shaped, and can pass uninjured through the alimentary canal.

The eggs of the cestodes may be distinguished from those of the nematodes and trematodes by their circular outline and, as a rule, by their smaller size.

The eggs of *T. saginata* and *T. solium*, which are indistinguishable from one another, are provided with a single brown striated outer membrane, which encloses a ciliated 6-hooked onchosphere. On the other hand, *Hymenolepis nana* eggs (40 μm) have 2 transparent membranes. Individual eggs of *T. saginata* are more ovoid than those of *T. solium*, and measure 31–43 μm in diameter. Eggs of *Diphyllobothrium latum* (70 × 45 μm) are translucent, oval and provided with an operculum.

Thick smear technique for rapid examination (Kato & Miura 1954). Place 100 mg faeces on a slide; cover with a Cellophane strip, 26 × 28 mm (not moisture-proof) which has been soaked in the following mixture for at least 24 hours (the strip can be stored indefinitely):

Distilled water	500 ml
Glycerin	500 ml
Malachite green 3% solution in water	5 ml

With a spatula press the Cellophane strip on to the faeces, and spread. Keep the slide at room temperature for ½–1 hour. The glycerin clears the specimen, and helminth eggs can be seen at magnification of 100.

Zinc sulphate centrifugal flotation for concentration of helminthic ova and protozoan cysts (Faust's method, modified by Watson). For this method, which is highly recommended, the following technique is employed. A sample of stool, the size of a pea, is placed in a glass centrifuge tube and broken up to form a fine suspension in distilled water. It is then centrifuged for 3 minutes at 1500 r.p.m., in an ordinary laboratory centrifuge with a radius of 14 cm. Supernatant fluid is then removed and the process repeated until it is clear. Zinc sulphate solution (33%; S. G. 1·18) is poured into the tube and the packed sediment is broken up into a uniform suspension. Then a chemically clean circular cover-slip, of slightly greater diameter than the glass tube, is smeared on one side with a thin film of Mayer's egg medium (white of egg 50 ml, glycerin 50 ml, sodium salicylate 1 gramme, shaken well together and filtered) and pressed firmly on top of centrifuge tube. The zinc sulphate solution must fill the tube to the brim so that the cover-slip is in contact with the solution. The suspension is again centrifuged for 3 minutes at 1500 r.p.m. The cover-slip is carefully lifted off the top of the tube and placed, prepared-surface downwards, on a drop of Weigert's iodine solution on a slide.

Simple flotation method (Hung). Two grammes of faeces are carefully rubbed up with a glass rod and saturated salt solution; the mixture is poured into a watch-glass or wide tube, which is filled to the brim. A slide or cover-glass is placed in contact with the fluid and allowed to remain for 10 minutes. When ancylostome eggs are present they will be found adhering to the under-surface of the slide or cover-glass.

Fülleborn's method for detection of schistosome eggs in the faeces. The diagnosis of intestinal schistosomiasis (*S. mansoni* and *S. japonicum*) by detection of the eggs in the faeces is not always easy. Faeces of the volume of a hazel-nut are placed in a conical glass, carefully rubbed up with a glass rod and a little 2½% salt solution, and put away to settle, in the dark, for 5 minutes. The solution is poured off from the sediment, and the process repeated 2 or 3 times. The schistosome eggs remain in the sediment, which is flooded with distilled water at 48·9°C and exposed to a bright light.

The miracidia now escape from eggs and can easily be detected with a hand lens, particularly against a dark background. On adding a few drops of perchloride of mercury solution, they are killed off and are found in the sediment.

Direct egg count. Direct faecal smears made by the same technician using the same size of cover-slip usually contain about the same amounts of formed faeces, and provide standards of comparison.

Stoll–Hausheer dilution egg count. A special flask is used, marked on the neck at 56 and 60 ml. It is filled to 56 ml with 0·1 N NaOH, and 4 ml (4 grammes) of faeces are added to reach the 60 ml mark. Glass beads are added and the stoppered flask is shaken vigorously to break up the faeces completely; it may be left for some hours and then reshaken if the faeces are hard. After a final shake 0·075 ml of this emulsion is with-drawn by pipette, placed on a clean slide and covered. The eggs are counted, and when the number is multiplied by 200 the result gives the number per gramme of faeces. Faeces vary in consistency, and to compensate for this the result should be multiplied as follows:

Mushy formed faeces	× 1·5
Mushy	× 2·0
Mushy diarrhoea	× 3·0
Flowing diarrhoea	× 4·0
Watery	× 5·0

Protozoa

Saline preparation. The specimen is emulsified in a drop of saline and covered with a cover slip. If the faeces are fluid the saline may not be needed. The preparation should be thin enough to see through. For trophozoites of amoebae the specimen must be absolutely fresh if good results are to be obtained with trophozoites of *Entamoeba histolytica*. Trophozoites and cysts can be seen under the 16 mm objective and × 10 ocular, but for identification higher magnification is necessary.

Iodine preparation. The specimen is emulsified in a drop of 1% iodine solution, covered and examined at once. Nuclei and glycogen are easily seen, but the organisms are killed and therefore do not show movement.

Eosin preparation. The specimen is emulsified in a drop of 0·5% aqueous solution of eosin, covered and examined after a few minutes. Live cysts remain as clear unstained bodies against a background of pink-stained detritus. Cysts which stain pink are thought to be dead.

Concentration techniques. *Sedimentation (for protozoa and helminth eggs).* 10 grammes of faeces are suspended in 250 ml water in a conical flask and allowed to settle for 10–15 minutes. The supernatant is diluted to 250 ml with water and again allowed to settle, and if the deposit is heavy this can be repeated. The final deposit is examined. If saline is used instead of water it is sometimes possible to concentrate living tropho-zoites of *Entamoeba histolytica*; eggs of schistosomes are prevented from hatching.

Flotation. The techniques described for helminth eggs apply.

One method makes use of a solution of cane sugar of specific gravity 1080. A mass of faeces is ground up with water in a small mortar and the emulsion is shaken with a large amount of water, poured into a glass cylinder and allowed to stand for 15 minutes. The supernatant is withdrawn and centrifuged, and the deposit from this is shaken with the sugar solution and again centrifuged. Cysts are left floating on the supernatant fluid, which is withdrawn, diluted with 4 times its volume of water, and centrifuged. The small deposit, containing many cysts, is then washed and centrifuged several times to wash away the sugar, and the final deposit is examined.

An efficient and practical method of concentration is that described by Ridley and Hawgood (1956). This concentrates the material 20–30 times. 1 gramme of faeces is emulsified in 7 ml of a 10% formol saline solution. The emulsion is passed through a filter of 16 mesh/cm wire gauze, into a centrifuge tube, and 3 ml ether are added; it is then shaken vigorously for 1 minute and centrifuged for 2 minutes at speeds increasing to 2000 r.p.m., and allowed to come to rest. After the debris is loosened with a swab stick, the supernatant is decanted, leaving 1–2 drops in the tube. The deposit is shaken and poured on to a slide for examination.

Various other elements

Blastocystis hominis (Fig. 465). Sometimes during examination of faeces, a yeast-like organism—*Blastocystis*—simulating an amoebic cyst, but less refractile, is encountered (Plate XII). Each cell contains a large central vacuole, while the cytoplasm is reduced to a thin layer in which are situated one or two small iodophilic nuclei at each pole. The cytoplasm contains refractile globules of *volutin* which should not be mis-taken for the nuclei. *Blastocystis* multiplies by gemmation and rapidly increases in culture media such as are suitable for *E. histolytica*, unless dextrose has been added. The organism varies a good deal in size and shape; single cysts measure from 5 to 20 μm in diameter. This organism has no pathogenic significance.

Muscle-fibres, derived from meat, practically always occur in the stools, and are recognized by their cross-striation. When present in large numbers they indicate defective intestinal digestion (Fig. 466).

Connective tissue, derived from meat, somewhat resembles mucus; it is distinguished by striation, which disappears on addition of acetic acid. When it is present in large masses, defective gastric digestion may be inferred. Elastic fibres have no significance.

Starch granules, derived from fruit and potatoes, are stained blue by iodine solution. They vary in size and shape, according to the food from which they are derived. Well preserved granules with concentric markings are seldom seen. They are often enclosed in a cellulose covering, and can readily be recognized, except those from peas and beans, which roughly resemble tapeworm eggs.

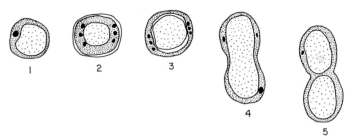

Fig. 465.—*Blastocytosis hominis.* 1–3, Resting forms. 4, 5, Dividing forms. × 1500.

Excess of starch is pathological, and such a stool is usually acid and shows signs of gas-bubbles, fermentation, and yeasts. The iodine test may be applied to ascertain the extent to which starch has been digested. A blue colour indicates unchanged granules; red, that digestion has begun.

Detritus derived from fruits and vegetables is easily recognized by spiral ducts, areolar tissue, vascular bundles and pigment cells.

Neutral fats, derived from fat, are recognized as colourless, highly refractile droplets, or sometimes as irregular bile-stained masses which are stained by Sudan III and are insoluble.

Fatty acids, derived from fat, occur as sheaves of colourless acicular crystals, which melt on being warmed and dissolve in ether (Fig. 466).

Soaps from the fat of food occur as greasy looking amorphous masses, or sometimes as needles, which are thicker and not so long as those of the fatty acids. They may be colourless, or stained with bile-pigments. Insoluble in ether, as are fatty acids, they do not melt on being warmed. If the film of faeces on a slide is treated with acetic acid and heated fatty acid crystals will separate out (Fig. 466).

Fats may be distinguished from mucus or from vegetable material by the following rough test; prepare a smear of the stool on a slide, put on a cover-slip, and press the latter down on to the smear; should the material be of fatty composition, the cover-slip will remain in place; if vegetable detritus or mucus, it will spring back when pressure is released (Fig. 466).

In a normal stool, fat is present almost entirely in the form of amorphous masses of soap, less often as crystals. Neutral fat is normally absent.

Mucus occurs as transparent shreds, sometimes bile-stained. It has always a pathological significance and, when it contains leucocytes and epithelial cells, indicates intestinal ulceration.

Intestinal sand. Sand grains in the faeces of persons who live in deserts are extremely frequent, but sand-like material is a pathological product sometimes present in diverticulitis.

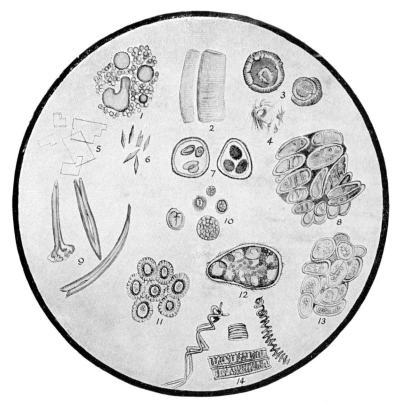

Fig. 466.—Microscopic appearance of common objects in the faeces. 1, Casein and fat droplets. 2, Muscle fibres. 3, Soap crystals. 4, Crystalline fatty needles. 5, Cholesterin crystals. 6, Charcot–Leyden crystals. 7, Truffle spores. 8, Portions of husks of cereals. 9, Hairs of wheat grain. 10, Spores of fungi. 11, Cells of pericarp of peas. 12, Parenchyma of beans. 13, Endosperm of rice. 14, Vegetable spirals. × 800.

Charcot–Leyden crystals are frequently found in stools containing *Entamoeba histolytica* (Fig. 466). These crystals have a chemical connection with eosinophil cells; they are therefore most evident in diseases with an eosinophilia. Originally seen in leukaemic blood, they are recorded in smear preparations from periarteritis nodosa, trichiniasis, intestinal infections, and in localized collections of eosinophils in nasal polypi and skin blebs.

Benzidine reaction for blood pigments

Benzidine and sodium perborate are required (tablets obtainable of 0·1 gramme each) and glacial acetic acid. Grind one of the tablets and dissolve in 5 ml of glacial acetic acid and 5ml of water. Filter and place 2 drops of filtrate on a clean slide. To one of the drops add a platinum loop of the material to be tested. If blood is present a green colour appears in less than one minute.

Occult blood. 1 ml blood gives a positive reaction with most methods in simple, infective or malignant ulceration anywhere in the bowel (including the pharynx) particularly hiatus hernia, peptic ulcer, duodenal ulcer, oesophageal varices, carcinoma of stomach, carcinoma of colon, piles, some worm infections—ancylostomiasis, schistosomiasis—amoebic dysentery, purpura and many bleeding and clotting diseases. False positives may be caused by ingestion of much green and vegetable matter, meat, or liver. Unless the test is strongly positive, positive results must be checked by repeating the test after a few days on 'occult blood diet'.

REFERENCES

KATA, K. & MIURA, M. (1954) *Jap. J. Parasit.*, **3**, 35.
RIDLEY, D. S. & HAWGOOD, B. C. (1956) *J. clin. Path.*, **9**, 74.
TURK, J. L. (1969) *Immunology in Clinical Medicine*. London: Heinemann.

INDEX

INDEX

£43·85.   ML

Books are to be returned on or before
the last date below.

DUE
- 1 JUN 2010

LIBREX-

996